PATHWAYS OF GROWTH

ESSENTIALS OF CHILD PSYCHIATRY

Volume 2
Psychopathology

WILEY SERIES IN CHILD AND ADOLESCENT MENTAL HEALTH

Joseph D. Noshpitz, Editor

PATHWAYS OF GROWTH

ESSENTIALS OF CHILD PSYCHIATRY

Volume 2
Psychopathology

ROBERT A. KING
Yale Child Study Center
Yale University School of Medicine

JOSEPH D. NOSHPITZ
Chesapeake Youth Centers

A Wiley-Interscience Publication
JOHN WILEY & SONS
New York   Toronto   Chichester   Brisbane   Singapore

Library of Congress Cataloging-in-Publication Data

Noshpitz, Joseph D.
    Pathways of growth : essentials of child psychiatry / Joseph D.
Noshpitz, Robert A. King.
        p.   cm. — (Wiley series in child and adolescent mental health)
    "A Wiley-Interscience publication."
    Includes bibliographical references.
    Contents: v. 1. Normal development — v. 2. Psychopathology.
    ISBN 0-471-09917-1 (v. 1). — ISBN 0471-53177-4 (v. 2). — ISBN
0-471-53178-2 (set)
    1. Child psychopathology.   2. Child development.   I. King,
Robert, A., 1943–   .   II. Title.   III. Series.
    [DNLM.   1. Child Development.   2. Child Psychiatry.   3. Mental
Disorders—in infancy & childhood.   WS 350 N897p]
RJ499.N68   1991
618.92'89—dc20
DNLM/DLC
for Library of Congress   90-12693

To our children, our spouses, and our parents

Series Preface

This series is intended to serve a number of functions. It includes works on child development; it presents material on child advocacy; it publishes contributions to child psychiatry; and it gives expression to cogent views on child rearing and child management. The mental health of parents and their interaction with their children is a major theme of the series, and emphasis is placed on the child as individual, as family member, and as a part of the larger social surround.

Child development is regarded as the basic science of child mental health, and within that framework research works are included in this series. The many ethical and legal dimensions of the way society relates to its children are the central theme of the child advocacy publications, as well as a primarily demographic approach that highlights the role and status of children within society. The child psychiatry publications span studies that concern the diagnosis, description, therapeutics, rehabilitation, and prevention of the emotional disorders of childhood. And the views of thoughtful and creative contributors to the handling of children under many different circumstances (retardation, acute and chronic illness, hospitalization, handicap, disturbed social conditions, etc.) find expression within the framework of child rearing and child management.

Family studies with a central child mental health perspective are included in the series, and explorations into the nature of parenthood and the parenting process are emphasized. This includes books about divorce, the single parent, the absent parent, parents with physical and emotional illnesses, and other conditions that significantly affect the parent–child relationship.

Finally, the series examines the impact of larger social forces, such as war, famine, migration, and economic failure, on the adaptation of children and families. In the largest sense, the series is devoted to books that illuminate the special needs, status, and history of children and their families, within all perspectives that bear on their collective mental health.

JOSEPH D. NOSHPITZ

Chesapeake Youth Centers
Cambridge, Maryland

Preface

The goal of this volume is to present what is currently known about the nature, course, and treatment of the major psychiatric disorders of childhood. We have tried to make this body of knowledge accessible to the interested nonspecialist, while still addressing the issues and controversies that occupy clinical researchers at the frontiers of the field. Our intended audience is all those who are concerned with children, whether as clinicians, researchers, educators, policy makers, or parents. We hope that graduate level students and postgraduate professionals alike will find this book interesting and helpful.

It is no easy task to summarize the current state of knowledge about childhood psychopathology. During the past 20 years, child psychiatry has been transformed by the development of new methodologies and approaches. Advances in neurobiology, behavioral genetics, clinical epidemiology, psychopharmacology, and developmental psychology have provided new insights and techniques and enlarged our theoretical frame of reference. Psychodynamic thinking about children has been enriched by the contributions of infant and family systems research, object relations theory, and self-psychology. Someday, it may be possible to give a fully integrated account of how genetic endowment, maturation, interpersonal experience, social context, and intrapsychic reality interact to produce the full spectrum of healthy development and adverse outcomes; as a corollary, we will then perhaps also know where and how to intervene to assure the child's optimal development. However, this visionary moment is not yet at hand. In the interim, our partial understandings and interventions all too often appear as competing or conflicting perspectives rather than as complementary ones. Thus, although new developments have enriched our traditional approaches to childhood psychopathology, those who work with children must struggle to make sense of the medley of theoretical and therapeutic paradigms.

A principal aim of this volume is to help those concerned with children to put these various paradigms into perspective. The causes of childhood disturbances range from the molecular through the cultural. We have tried to give each of these various frames of explanation due weight. However, the challenge of clinical work is to understand how these diverse processes interact in an individual child whose unique life unfolds in the context of a given family, community, and historical epoch. In this task, we have placed the inner life of the child at the center of our frame of reference. This phenomenological approach is not an assertion that all childhood psychopathology is "psychogenic." Instead, it reflects our conviction that the child's inner experience of the self and the world must be an abiding concern of those who care for the child. Furthermore, this sense of the self in relationship to the world serves as a "final common pathway," in which the contributions of a wide range of biological and experiential factors may be read.

Each major section of this volume addresses a particular broad realm of dysfunction. Most individual chapters deal with specific syndromes or diagnostic categories. However, several chapters are exceptions to this syndromic method of organization. For example, the chapter on the disorders of infancy deals with general principles of pathogenesis and treatment in the first two years of life; it discusses a variety of disorders of regulation, attachment, and parent–infant interaction. In exploring the topic of anxiety, an introductory chapter provides an overview of the problem of anxiety from diverse perspectives; the subsequent chapter deals in greater clinical detail with separation anxiety disorder, which in turn serves as an exemplar for the more general principles discussed in the introductory chapter. Similarly, an introductory chapter on psychosomatic disorders explores the means by which psychological factors might influence physical health. The chapter on asthma that follows illustrates the application of these principles to a specific illness.

Throughout this book we have used the traditional pronoun *he* in referring to the child. This stylistic convention is for ease of reading only; the information herein refers impartially to girls and boys unless the specific content states otherwise.

How best to classify the various psychopathological symptoms of childhood has been a recurrent question for the field that is echoed throughout this book. Although we have organized our discussion of childhood psychopathology by syndrome, alternative approaches to nosology exist. For example, children's abilities and behaviors can be organized by areas of functioning (e.g., social relations) or arranged along dimensions (such as verbal intelligence, impulsivity, aggression) that can be expressed quantitatively on a continuous scale, rather than as dichotomous variables that are either present or absent. Thus, an alternative classification scheme for psychopathology might be based on a dimensional rather than a categorical approach.

Throughout the text we have used the most recent version of the American Psychiatric Association's *Diagnostic and Statistical Manual of Mental Disorders, Third Edition, Revised* (DSM-III-R, 1987), which serves as the field's current standard. However, we have also tried to convey the limitations of this nomenclature as it applies to various areas of childhood psychopathology. One of our goals is to illustrate some of the difficulties that plague psychiatric nosology. These difficulties range from relatively pragmatic issues associated with current practice through deeper epistemological questions dating back at least to Plato.

Although these issues of classification may seem at first glance only of peripheral interest, they are important to understand if the reader is to be an "informed consumer" of the clinical and research literature. For example, because an official name and criteria set exist for a disorder, it might seem that the disorder must in some sense *exist* as a distinct entity. This understandable tendency toward reification is encouraged by the spurious air of precision with which the DSM-III-R lists diagnostic criteria. In reality, however, we do not yet know how to "carve Nature at the joints." With further advances in our understanding of underlying mechanisms, many currently accepted syndromes may come to seem as epiphenomenal as *fever* does today; at the very least, the outlines of many symptom constellations are likely to be drawn quite differently. Meanwhile, it is important to understand the limitations and practical implications of the definitions for any given syndrome. Wittgenstein once described philosophy as the struggle against the bewitchment of our intelligence by words; it is in this spirit that we have explored these nosological uncertainties surrounding each of the various current diagnostic categories.

The effective treatment of most childhood disorders is also a complex affair. There are few if any "magic bullets." We have tried to give the reader a picture of the range of therapeutic approaches available for each disorder, their relative strengths and weaknesses, and how they might be most effectively integrated. Whether the treatment modality is pharmacological, educational, behavioral, or psychodynamic, alone or in combination, the clinician must try to discern the impact of both the illness and the treatment on the diverse aspects of the child and family's developmental trajectory. For each disorder we describe the various areas of functioning that must be assessed to make an accurate diagnosis and to plan and monitor optimal treatment. These areas in turn become the foci for therapeutic intervention. We also address in detail the nature of the treatment alliance required over time with both parents and child.

Finally, we have tried to indicate the many unanswered questions in the field. Some arise directly from the exigencies of the clinical situation; others involve the elucidation of basic pathogenic mechanisms. Both in clinical work and basic research it is necessary to be clear about what we do not know. Only by formulating our uncertainties in ways that are susceptible to investigation is further progress possible.

ROBERT A. KING
JOSEPH D. NOSHPITZ

New Haven, Connecticut
Cambridge, Maryland
February 1991

Acknowledgments

Our intellectual endeavors condense the influence of many friends, colleagues, and teachers who, through the years, shape our way of thinking. As Socrates suggested long ago, teaching and learning involve more than intellectual passions; they are also affairs of the heart. For this reason, every author owes many debts. Some influences we can easily discern and name; others no longer can be distinguished from who we are.

My first and greatest debt is to my parents, Alfred and Clara King, whose curiosity and love of learning made the pursuit of knowledge seem at once the highest calling and greatest adventure in the world.

This volume would not have been possible without the support and encouragement of Dr. Dexter Bullard, Jr., the Medical Director of Chestnut Lodge Hospital and founder of its Adolescent and Child Division. Beyond the many tangible supports provided by my colleagues there, the special ethos of the Lodge was an important daily presence: the quest for intellectual rigor, a deep concern for the dignity of children and their families, and a long-term commitment to compassionate care.

I am also endebted to Dr. Donald Cohen for his many years of friendship and his vision of how our profession might best integrate the centrality of the inner life, the exigencies of neurobiological processes, the impact of the social environment, and the imperatives of compassionate care.

Of my many friends, colleagues, and teachers at the Washington Psychoanalytic Institute to whom I am grateful, William Granatir, Roger Shapiro, Robert Winer, Justin Frank, and Judith Viorst deserve special mention. Dr. Melvin Kohn, former chief of the Laboratory of Socio-Environmental Studies at the National Institute of Mental Health, and Dr. Albert J. Solnit, of the Yale Child Study Center, also provided encouragement at important junctures in my career.

Many colleagues provided thoughtful critiques and suggestions as this volume was under construction. Drs. Tom McGlashan, Wells Goodrich, Mark Riddle, Donald Cohen, Benson Foreman, Alex Adams, and Susan Bliss were particularly helpful.

Chestnut Lodge's librarian Karen Smith as well as Alisa Shreier, Susan Bliss, and Victor Fisher provided bibliographic assistance. The bulk of the manuscript was typed with diligence and skill by Ellen Rafferty, Bunny Thye, and Patricia Wershiner. Ellen Berman, Nestor Afable, Brian Yates, and David Bruce provided assistance with computerware, hard and soft.

I am especially grateful to my wife, Ruth, for her support and to my children, Benjamin, Claire, and Adam, for their love and affection during the long gestation of this book.

R.A.K.

Contents

PART II
MAJOR DISRUPTIONS OF DEVELOPMENTAL PROGRESS

PATHWAYS OF GROWTH

ESSENTIALS OF CHILD PSYCHIATRY

Volume 2
Psychopathology

PART I

Developmental Disturbances of Infancy

Chapter 1

Principles of Pathogenesis and Treatment in Infancy

INTRODUCTION

The basic tasks of infancy include achieving physiological homeostasis; learning to maintain a state and to make transitions between states; organizing basic rhythms such as wakefulness and feeding; dealing with novel stimuli; organizing experience into coherent patterns; learning to maintain a positive affective tone; learning to concentrate; establishing a specific relationship to a caretaker; developing channels of communication (including sending and receiving vocalizations, gestures, and facial cues); regulating the expression of emotion; forming initial schemata of causality, intention, and object permanence; and beginning to differentiate self from parents as well as parents from others (Greenspan, 1981). Development can go at a different pace in each area; it can go awry in any of these areas—or in all.

Infancy, more than any other age, illustrates the truism that the child cannot be diagnosed or treated apart from his parental environment (Cicchetti & Rizley, 1981; Sameroff, 1975). Winnicott (1964) emphasized this point in his typically aphoristic style: "There is no such thing as a baby!" Any evaluation of crises and problems in an infant's development must, to be sure, consider the child and the parent individually. Even more important, however, is the imperative to evaluate their interactions. To regard the mother–child dyad as a transactional unit is not to deny that each partner brings important and often enduring characteristics to their encounter. Parents bring to the task of child rearing a wide variety of personality styles, skills, and capacities. Each parent, from his or her own childhood experience, has developed explicit and implicit notions about what it means to be a parent or a child. Parental psychopathology, subtle or severe, may also be present.

Infants, too, possess specifiable constitutional differences in temperament that endure over time. Korner (1983), for example, showed early individual differences in how readily and by which means infants could be soothed. Thomas and Chess (1977) delineated nine stable dimensions of temperament that characterized the formal aspects of children's behavior during the first 5 years of life. These dimensions included approach–withdrawal, adaptability, threshold of responsiveness, intensity of reaction, quality (valence) of mood, distractibility, attention span, and persistence (see Volume 1). In addition to these temperamental differences, infants may have a wide range of frank physical handicaps and disabilities. Development will be determined by the interactions among these and other characteristics of the parents and infant.

Analyzing the interactive effects of infants and parents is a complex task. Even with infants who have a serious deficit such as blindness or deafness, the eventual emotional and cognitive outcome may depend on the parents' sensitivity and adaptability. The handicapped infant needs an environment that in large measure offers compensatory stimulation. Some method must be found to bypass or cope with the defect by opening up alternate pathways that foster the growth of human attachment and encourage exploration of the outside world. Much depends on how well the parents can meet these needs.

It is not only the parents, however, who influence the child. In recent years, interest has increased in the other dimension—the effect of the child on the caretaker. The child shapes his parents just as surely as they shape him (Anthony, 1984; Bell, 1974), and the baby's constitutional makeup strongly affects parental attitudes and caretaking style. In Thomas and Chess's (1977) study, for example, 10% of the sample were infants with a "difficult" constitutional temperamental configuration, that is, a low threshold for arousal, intense reactions, poor adaptability, and irregularity of biological functioning. Such difficult infants accounted for a disproportionate 25% of the children with later behavioral disturbances. For a given infant, however, temperament was not the sole predictor of outcome. Rather, a crucial factor was the parents' ability to adapt to their child's temperament. Differences in parental behavior were not predictable and apparently arose as a consequence of the parents' interaction with their child. As Sameroff (1975) observed:

> Knowing *only* the temperament of the child or knowing *only* the child-rearing attitudes and practices of the parent [does] not allow one to predict the developmental outcome for the child. It would appear, rather, that it is the character of the *specific transactions* that occur between a given child and his parents which determine the course of the subsequent development. (pp. 277–278)

Another example of the effect of interactional factors (modified from Sameroff, 1975) would be a premature child who is born to an alcoholic or drug-addicted, unwed teenage mother in a complicated delivery. The infant may be fussy, poorly modulated in his responses, difficult to soothe, and socially unresponsive. If so, he will further stress the already preoccupied mother, who is at best only marginally adequate. Such an infant fails to provide the gratification and positive feedback that might encourage and elicit whatever nurturing capacities the mother possesses. In turn, the mother's anxiety, inexperience, and preoccupation further frustrate the infant, who is already more than usually vulnerable and sensitive to unempathic care. The infant's increased distress and discomfort raise the mother's resentment to an even higher pitch, and their mutual anguish and reactivity spiral upward. Although the problematic outcome of such a case could be cited as proof of the determining effects of social factors, prenatal medication, infant temperament, or maternal personality, only interactional analysis does justice to the true complexity of the developmental process. An interactional perspective also implies that the strength and predominant direction of such mutual influences can vary with age, altering the pathogenic impact of a given deficit in the parent or child over time.

The mutual adaptation of mother and child begins to take place long before the infant has any stable image or concept of the mother as person. Indeed, the child constructs images of himself and his mother out of his developing expectancies of and responses to her (Stern, 1985). From the outset the infant is adapting to the specific feel, smell, look, and sound of his particular mother and her unique style and responsive rhythm; the mother meanwhile is adapting to her infant with his unique aspects and individual temperament. Careful developmental studies indicate that the process of mutual adaptation probably begins prenatally and certainly is underway from the first minutes of life.

Klaus and Kennell (1982) described the responses of young first-time mothers when given their babies to hold after birth. The mothers first explored and handled their babies with hesitant finger contact to the hands and feet and then caressed the newborn's trunk with increasing excitement. They attempted to make frequent eye contact with the baby by looking intensely *en face*.

Sander et al. (1976) studied infants cared for by their mothers during the first 10 days of life and compared them with infants receiving standard nursery care from various nursing staff. The authors demonstrated marked and enduring differences in the diurnal rhythmicity and other behaviors of these two groups.

Detailed frame-by-frame film analysis of face-to-face mother–infant play has greatly increased understanding of the intricate, reciprocal interplay of responses between mother and infant (Brazelton et al., 1974; Stern, 1977, 1985). Such analyses reveal a complex mutual give-and-take of gesture and vocalization, controlled alternately by the mother and the infant. During such play there is modeling back and forth of facial expression, vocal inflection, approach, and withdrawal. The mother varies the level of excitement, titrating her tempo and rhythm to the infant's reaction, at one moment producing an exciting and suspenseful discrepancy by stretching the interval of an anticipated beat, at another moment soothing the infant by slowing and regularizing the rhythm of her voice. With these and other building blocks of social exchange, the infant begins to construct the affective images and sensorimotor schemata of himself in interaction with others—the feel of what it is like to be with another person (Stern, 1985). By the end of the first month, the infant shows subtly differentiated responses to his father, mother, and strangers.

Fine-grain film analyses also demonstrate subtle "missteps in the dance"—specific repetitive miscarried interactions that may be the precursors of later pathology (Greenspan, 1981; Stern, 1977, 1985). Some mother–infant pairs seem poorly attuned. Film frames show that in some dyads, where the mother had trouble engaging the infant or reading his cues, the infant appeared understimulated. Other infants appeared over-stimulated by mothers who moved in too closely or did not modulate their behavior as the infants' excitement mounted to a high level. Sometimes the mother did not permit the infant to withdraw or break off an interchange but instead pursued the child intrusively with increased touching and vocalization, trying to elicit a response. Such recurring mistuned exchanges often left both mother and infant upset and frustrated.

In one experimental paradigm, the *still-face situation,* mothers are instructed deliberately to violate reciprocity by offering the infant a flat and expressionless face (Mayes & Carter, 1990). In response to this, infants as young as 7 weeks of age show a marked reaction. Many first attempt to make contact, then sober, and finally look away with a hopeless demeanor; some become frustrated, distressed, or disorganized. This experiment may capture a glimpse of the repeated experiences between an infant and a depressed mother (Tronick & Gianino, 1986). Nondepressed mothers often find it very difficult to comply with the experimenters' instructions to maintain an affectively neutral face in their baby's presence.

PRINCIPLES OF TREATMENT

The treatment approach to disorders of infancy varies with the nature of the disorder and the adaptive capacities of the parents. Often the clinician can formulate specific guidance or advice that is readily utilized by the parents. Sometimes, parents and therapist may recognize feelings that prevent the parents from interacting constructively with the child; sympathetic discussion of these feelings may help the parents to control their parenting more effectively and to act more adaptively. Even in interventions primarily focused on support and guidance, there must be careful attention to developing a working alliance with the parents. Resentment, suspicion, and guilt may become impediments to such an alliance and may, in turn, be exacerbated by sociocultural factors and family dynamics as well as by transference issues related to the parents' difficult childhood experiences. Such childhood memories, conscious and unconscious, are notorious for their capacity to interfere with the parent–infant relationship (Seligman & Pawl, 1984).

It is important not merely to give advice, but to cultivate the parents' perceptiveness and sense of competency. The therapist shores up parents' ability to read the infant's cues about his needs and reactions; improvement in this realm fosters the parents' sense of efficacy. While helping parents to understand the child's responses and to define suitable interventions, it is important to maintain the interactional focus by acknowledging the difficulties and challenges a given infant may present. Rather than "blaming the victim" or exonerating maladaptive parental behavior, using such an approach helps to stop the vicious "bad parent–bad baby" cycle of frustration. Effective intervention can produce a "virtuous circle" in which altered parental behavior produces a more positive infant response, which in turn reinforces the parents' self-esteem. Families who have infants with major developmental problems or handicaps may need help and guidance for an extended period, and the clinician must make clear his or her ongoing availability. The same long-term assistance is necessary for the vulnerable high-risk infants of schizophrenics and of affectively disturbed, abusive, or drug-abusing parents (Anthony & Cohler, 1987).

Unfortunately, in truly malignant cases of neglect or abuse, the parents may not only be unempathic and unresponsive to the infant, they may harbor deeply hostile and punitive feelings toward the child (often reflecting their unhappy treatment by their own parents). Selma Fraiberg (Fraiberg et al., 1975) labeled such destructive identifications with the aggressor as "ghosts in the nursery." Her striking article is a moving, insightful account of the vicissitudes encountered helping parents to exorcise these ghosts of their past and to redraw the family's protective "magic circle" about the child. Fraiberg emphasizes that such parents often reject formal office therapy or casework for themselves; indeed, the therapist tends to be seen as a critical intruder or a potential baby snatcher. Treatment entails observing the parents and child together, often during regular home visits (hence the term *kitchen therapy*); technically, it involves a demanding mixture of parent education and interpretive intervention.

Neglectful or abusive parents tend to perceive advice alone as being either critical or irrelevant. More effective interventions include underscoring positive interactions with comments such as "Did you see how the baby brightened when you did that?" or, speaking for the baby, "Isn't it good to have a mommy who knows what you need?" The goals of intervention are to promote greater empathy for the child and a greater sense of efficacy and nurturance in the parents. In terms of their own painful past, parents thus obtain some measure of reparation and relief through giving to their child what they themselves lacked as children.

The key questions that Fraiberg and her colleagues asked were, "Why can't this mother hear her infant cry?" and "Why does this mother avoid holding and touching her infant?" Although the mothers studied could frequently recall their painful childhoods, they could not remember the feelings they had experienced. Only as the parents recaptured these painful feelings, often tempestuously, were they able to develop empathy for their children as well as for the child they once had been.

Unfortunately, intensive clinical attention is available to only a few of the many children needing early intervention. The past two decades, however, have seen the development of an enormous range of preventive intervention programs, including infant stimulation programs, preschool programs, home-based counseling programs, and comprehensive clinical programs that address both the child and the family's physical, cognitive, and emotional needs. Although assessment of such programs continues, available evidence suggests that they have the potential for long-range improvement of family functioning (Provence, 1985).

To illustrate the normal vicissitudes of mutual adaptation, the following section describes the developmental crisis of *colic* in the context of providing and receiving comfort and helping the infant to achieve homeostasis. The next section examines the problems and obstacles in achieving a stable attachment between the parent and child. The reactions range from brief separation through the extremes of anaclitic depression and hospitalism. The final section in the chapter describes two psychosomatic disorders of infancy, *rumination* and *eczema,* to illustrate a powerful adaptive-defensive mode at this time of life. In the absence of an adequate nurturing or tension-modulating relationship with a caretaker, the infant may turn away from the world of people to the contents of his stomach and mouth or to sensations arising from his skin as substitute sources of comfort and gratification.

COLIC: A CRISIS OF INFANCY ARISING DURING NORMAL DEVELOPMENT

Definition.   The average 1- to 2-month-old cries about $2\frac{1}{4}$ hours a day, and much of this normal crying appears unrelated to identifiable needs. Fussy infants, however, may cry 4 or more hours a day (Brazelton, 1962b). Prolonged, unexplainable crying in the young infant is a common and sometimes a harrowing experience for parents. Fussiness or "colic" usually begins in the 1st month of life and wanes by the 3rd month, but it may persist throughout the first year. The colicky infant cries inconsolably, often screaming, arching his back, drawing up his arms and legs, and turning red with effort. Nursing, rocking, walking, singing to, and other attempts at comforting all seem ineffective, and the infant finally quiets down of his own accord, perhaps falling asleep from sheer exhaustion. The attacks may last for minutes or hours and tend to recur regularly at the same time of day, frequently in the evening. The colicky infant can induce feelings of desperation in his parents; new parents especially may feel overwhelmed by a sense of helplessness, inadequacy, and anger. A vicious cycle may arise in which the increasingly agitated parents become less and less able to cope with the increasingly agitated baby.

Prevalence.   Normative longitudinal studies show that significant periods of unexplained fussiness are virtually ubiquitous in early infancy.

About 25% of infants show extreme fussiness with crying and restlessness that may last an hour, a day, or more (Farran, 1983).

Etiology. The cause of colic is still a mystery (Farran, 1983). As Paradise (1966) observed, theories of colic have historically followed the periodic shifts in pediatric emphasis. Thus, feeding, allergies, the mother–child relationship, and constitutionally determined differences in physiologic regulation have all been invoked. The term *colic* is itself the remnant of an early theory that intestinal cramping or gas causes the upset; radiological studies have failed to bear out this theory. Secondarily, however, while crying or frantically feeding, the infant may swallow large amounts of air and exacerbate his distress. Some tense infants have trouble making a smooth transition from wakefulness to sleep; others appear to be overstimulated by their parents; still others seem to have too little stimulation during the day. Thus, in at least some instances, colic may arise when parents are out of tune with a particular infant's requirements for calming or for stimulation.

Some investigators view colic as a kind of attachment behavior, a normal phase of attempted homeostasis that facilitates bonding by promoting closeness to the caretaker at nonfeeding times.

Contagion of maternal anxiety is another common hypothesis. It is difficult, however, to distinguish between maternal anxiety as the cause of or the response to infant colic. Prospective studies that assessed mothers' personality style and anxiety levels during pregnancy found no correlation between maternal personality and the subsequent development of colic in their infants (Shaver, 1974). An ambivalent, anxious, or inexperienced mother, however, will be most severely tried by a colicky infant, who causes her to doubt her goodness and competency. The resulting maternal tension will probably serve further to upset the infant.

Treatment. The first step in dealing with colic is to rule out medical or surgical illness as a cause. The next approach is to find an optimal level of stimulation during the day. There have been innumerable studies proposing methods of treatment for colic, but these studies generally have been poorly controlled, and their outcomes are difficult to assess due to spontaneous remission of the condition. Among the measures that appear promising are smaller, more frequent meals; swaddling or rhythmic monotonous noise and motion (long car rides are a common remedy); use of a pacifier; a semiinclined posture for the infant during and after feedings; and decreased lactose and butterfat in formulas (Farran, 1983). Once these steps have been taken, the most important element in treatment is to help the parents to endure the crying with as little exacerbating rage or self-reproach as possible (Brazelton, 1962b, 1974). Explaining the adaptive meaning of the behavior is beneficial because once something makes sense, it is easier to endure even if it is unpleasant. Parents often suggest a soporific, remarking either humorously or bitterly that they might take it instead; experience indicates, however, that sedatives (like antispasmodics) are usually ineffective.

PROBLEMS OF ATTACHMENT AND SEPARATION

Primary Failure of Attachment—Hospitalism

In some situations the infant receives adequate physical care but cannot develop a stable attachment to a caretaker because none is available. Sander et al. (1976) demonstrated that even within the first 10 days of life, infants receiving nursery care from a rotating shift of nurses and infants cared for from birth by a consistent caretaker showed marked differences. The single-caretaker infants exhibited a clearer diurnal variation in sleep and wakefulness; even at 2 months of age their processing of visual stimuli and regulation of feeding differed from that of infants who had had no consistent caretaker for the first 10 days.

An all-too-frequent natural experiment of this sort occurs regularly in premature nurseries and neonatal intensive care units; in such a setting infants may remain isolated from their parents for several months while receiving care from a variety of nursing staff. These vulnerable infants and parents are delayed and handicapped in their ability to form a mutual attachment. Enlighted special care nurseries now encourage parents to visit daily and to participate as much as possible in the holding, feeding, and care of their infant.

Even when the physical care is adequate, where the infant remains deprived of a consistent attachment figure over many months, the effects on the child can be devastating. The study of this phenomenon, called *hospitalism,* was prompted by the observation in the early part of the century that despite good hygiene and nutrition, many foundling homes and orphanages had extremely high infant mortality rates as well as a high prevalence of retardation and psychiatric problems (Chapin, 1908, 1915).

In his classic study, Spitz (1945, 1965) compared a group of infants in the nursery of a penal institution for delinquent girls with a second group of infants reared in a foundling home. The girls in the penal institution looked after their own babies; rotating shifts of nurses in the foundling home provided care with no consistency of caretaker from day to day. Despite adequate food and medical care, the foundlings showed progressive deterioration from the age of 4 months on. Although initially, their developmental quotients were superior to the penal institution infants, as the first year of life advanced, the infants in the foundling home showed increasing retardation of motor and social development, increased susceptibility to illness, and poor physical growth. They showed no stranger anxiety and many developed bizarre mannerisms, including fecal play, rocking, pervasive anxiety, and shrieking. During the next 2 years, the foundling group suffered a striking 37% mortality; the survivors displayed poor physical growth and profound motor, social, and intellectual retardation. Spitz attributed the deterioration to the lack of stimulation and most important, to the lack of human contact with a mother or mother substitute.

In their landmark book, *Infants in Institutions*, Provence and Lipton (1963) recorded similar patterns of deficit. They noted institutionalized infants' diminished vocalizations, bareness of affective response, and failure to respond to holding. By 4 to 5 months of age the infants showed diminished interest in exploring inanimate objects, engaged in markedly decreased social play, and had a "spooky," highly vigilant, radarlike gaze, but poor and delayed visual discriminatory ability. Self-stimulation such as rocking was prominent. Provence and Lipton noted that similar symptoms could occur in certain children cared for at home, a topic discussed later in this chapter in the section "Nonorganic Failure to Thrive." These children received good physical care but little emotional involvement from their preoccupied and depressed mothers.

Separations—Brief and Prolonged

Once the infant has formed an attachment to his mother, his reaction to separation from her varies with his age and the length and context of the separation. Schaffer studied the response to hospitalization of a group of 76 children under 1 year of age, many of them healthy infants admitted for elective surgery (Schaffer, 1958; Schaffer & Callender, 1959). In addition to being without their mothers, the infants had little social interaction with nurses. Infants over 28 weeks (approximately 7 months) of age showed dramatic protest, with piteous fretting, crying, struggle, and restlessness. They also appeared negative and frightened and showed little friendly responsiveness to observers or to the nurses who cared for them. When the mother visited, the infant clung to her desperately and then cried long, loud, and frantically on her departure. On return home such an infant clung to his mother almost continuously and showed increased fear and crying when she left or when in the presence of strangers. Sometimes even formerly familiar figures such as the father or siblings were regarded with suspicion.

In contrast, infants under 28 weeks accepted the separation with little active protest or fretting but showed an uncharacteristic, bewildered silence. When the mother visited, these younger infants showed a friendly response to the nurses and the observers as well as to the mother. The mother's departure was also accepted without prolonged protest. On return home, however, these younger infants appeared "strange," with little of the active clinging of the older children. They were preoccupied with scanning the environment, usually without expression, but sometimes they showed a bewildered or frightened expression. They were quiet and less active than usual (save for the scanning) and seemed in many cases to ignore parental attempts to engage them. Both over and under 28 weeks of age the infants showed increased disturbance of sleep and night-crying.

Yarrow (1963) noted that children between 7 and 12 months of age who were moved from a temporary residence to a permanent adoptive home became disturbed, with the severity and pervasiveness of the disturbance increasing with age.

The results of these various studies seem in keeping with the development of stranger anxiety at about 7 months and parallel the infant's growing concept of his mother as a persisting, separate entity at about the same age. The young infant, however, accommodates to his caretaker (and vice versa) well before he has any concept of her as a person, and separation, even at a few days of age, can cause distress.

Working with children in the second year of life, the Robertsons (1971) demonstrated that if the child became familiar with an able and empathic full-time caretaker (and vice versa) prior to experiencing maternal separation, then the impact of subsequent separation was mitigated dramatically (albeit not completely). Thus, the optimal management for a young infant whose mother must be absent is to keep the child in familiar surroundings, along with his familiar possessions, and to have a consistent person, preferably one known to the child, provide his care.

In actual practice, the effect of separation from the mother is rarely seen in pure culture. During infancy, such separations usually occur in the context of illness or family stress, often in a family with ongoing disruptions. The impact of such disastrous events on the child may be further complicated by the effects of strange surroundings and new caretakers who are at best unfamiliar and at worst inadequate. The summed effects of these complicating pathogenic factors are difficult to disentangle.

Spitz and Wolf (1946) described a serious, life-threatening response to prolonged separation, termed *anaclitic depression,* in institutionalized infants between 6 and 8 months of age who had been separated from their mothers for more than 3 months. These infants showed weepiness, withdrawal, sleep disturbance, loss of appetite, poor growth, and retarded development. Spitz and Wolf observed that some infants who suffered similar separations from their mothers did not develop anaclitic depression because the institution had provided a substitute love object who was consistent and caring. When reunited with the mothers, the infants showed a dramatic and remarkable recovery of positive affect and interest in the outside world together with a striking advance in their developmental level. In the absence of the follow-up data, however, Spitz and Wolf cautioned that the long-term sequelae of separation were unclear. Where the mother was not reunited with the infant, deterioration continued to produce a "frozen, affect-impoverished expression," bizarre posturing, and "stupor." Spitz (1965) quoted a Spanish bishop of the 18th century who had observed: "In the foundling home the child becomes sad, and many of them die of sorrow."

Nonorganic Failure to Thrive

Introduction and Definition. *Failure to thrive* (FTT) is a common pediatric diagnostic problem. The term is used for children whose weight is below the third percentile on standard growth charts. Retarded growth may be due to a wide variety of organic conditions including malabsorption syndrome, cardiac or renal disease, central nervous system defects or tumors, and primary endocrine and metabolic disorders. Despite exhaustive workups, in many patients no organic etiology can be found (Sills, 1978). Such cases are referred to as *nonorganic failure to thrive.*

Growth failure associated with emotional deprivation was first noted in institutionalized children. In 1915, Henry Chapin observed that the "cachexia of hospitalization" produced a mortality rate of 42% in children under 2 years; he also demonstrated that a program of careful foster care could dramatically reduce this high mortality. Especially following the seminal work of Spitz (1945), nonorganic FTT came increasingly to be seen as a psychosomatic disorder, rooted in a failure of the mother–child bond formation. In recent years, however, there has been a growing realization that the etiology is more complex. Adequate diet and a nurturant environment lead to rapid weight gain only in about half of nonorganic FTT cases. Thus, the simple equation of nonorganic FTT with environmental or maternal deprivation is unwarranted (Kotelchuck, 1980).

Although many cases of FTT are indeed the product of gross neglect, others result from more subtle derangements of maternal attunement to the infant's needs. Furthermore, not all cases represent maternal malfeasance. Infant factors, such as poor sucking, developmental delays, temperamental difficulties, and general sickliness may represent not only the effects of FTT, but also contributing causes. The syndrome is most common in infancy, where it may represent but one facet of a failure of homeostasis, a primary attachment disorder, or a disorder of separation (Chatoor & Egan, 1987a). However, the condition also occurs in older childhood where it is most frequently referred to as *deprivation* or *psychosocial dwarfism* (W. H. Green, 1986). Other terms for the condition are *maternal deprivation syndrome* or *environmental failure to thrive*, titles that reflect specific causal hypotheses.

Diagnostic Criteria. In the *Diagnostic and Statistical Manual of Mental Disorders* (DSM-III-R) (APA, 1987), nonorganic FTT is referred to as *Reactive Attachment Disorder of Infancy or Early Childhood.* The DSM-III-R diagnostic criteria are:

A. *Markedly disturbed social relatedness in most contexts, beginning before the age of five, as evidence by either (1) or (2):*
    (1) *persistent failure to initiate or respond to most social interactions (e.g., in infants, absence of visual tracking and reciprocal play, lack of vocal imitation or playfulness, apathy, little or no spontaneity; at later ages, lack of or little curiosity and social interest)*
    (2) *indiscriminate sociability, e.g., excessive familiarity with relative strangers by making requests and displaying affection*
B. *The disturbance in A is not a symptom of either Mental Retardation or a Pervasive Developmental Disorder, such as Autistic Disorder.*
C. *Grossly pathogenic care, as evidenced by at least one of the following:*
    (1) *persistent disregard of the child's basic emotional needs for comfort, stimulation, and affection. Examples: overly harsh punishment by caregiver; consistent neglect by caregiver.*
    (2) *persistent disregard of the child's basic physical needs, including nutrition, adequate housing, and protection from physical danger and assault (including sexual abuse)*
    (3) *repeated change of primary caregiver so that stable attachments are not possible, e.g., frequent changes in foster parents*
D. *There is a presumption that the care described in C is responsible for the disturbed behavior in A: this presumption is warranted if the disturbance in A began following the pathogenic care in C. (p. 93)*

Prevalence. At many large urban pediatric centers FTT cases constitute about 1% to 5% of all inpatient admissions; in 33% to 50% of these hospitalized cases no organic etiology can be found (English, 1978; Glaser et al., 1968; Hannaway, 1970; Kempe et al., 1980).

Clinical Features and Course. Nonorganic FTT usually has its onset in the first few months of life, with hospitalization often occurring by 6 to 12 months. The distinguishing features of the condition are frequent feeding problems and failure to grow and gain weight. During these early critical months when growth is normally rapid, the child may actually lose weight to the point of emaciation, which frequently precipitates admission. As the disorder progresses, developmental delays as well as weakness, fatigue, and irritability become manifest. Socially the child may appear apathetic, fearful, or withdrawn (Bullard et al., 1967). Although these children are relatively inactive and display little exploratory behavior, they often appear hypervigilant, with what has been described as "radar gaze." They smile little, vocalize less, and lack cuddliness (Leonard et al., 1966). Additional physical findings include poor muscle tone, retarded bone age, and, frequently, protuberant abdomen.

A significant number of these infants show physical signs of frank neglect or abuse, such as fractures or burns. In such cases, the child is often poorly clothed and dirty with severe diaper rash; the back of the head may be bald from long periods of lying without stimulation.

In the absence of specific indications from the history or physical examination, extensive laboratory tests are rarely informative (Sills, 1978). A frequent and striking diagnostic clue to the nonorganic etiology of the child's state emerges when the hospitalization alone leads to prompt weight gain, often up to 80 grams a day. Hence, before embarking on an extensive array of intrusive tests, it is now common practice simply to observe the child's response to consistent good nursing care. Failure-to-thrive infants without detectable organic illness often respond with voracious appetite and rapid weight gain. Although this response suggests an environmental cause, only about half the infants make dramatic weight gains (Kotelchuck, 1980); whether the remainder suffer from undetected organic pathology or other less reversible factors remains to be seen. Such observations have prompted the suggestion that the dichotomy between organic and environmental FTT is too simple; in many intermediate cases organic factors, child-related factors (such as temperament), and psychosocial factors may interact (Kotelchuck, 1980).

Chatoor and colleagues (1984, 1987a, 1987b) have proposed a developmental classification of nonorganic FTT. They suggest that infantile feeding difficulties can result from disorders in homeostasis, disorders of attachment, or disorders of separation-individuation. The discussion that follows uses their conceptual framework.

● *Disorders of Homeostasis.* Feeding difficulties in the first 3 months of life often reflect the infant's temperamental or organic difficulties in sucking. The severity of the infant's impairment or the mother's trouble in reading and responding to his cues may make it difficult for her to help the infant compensate for these difficulties. The hunger and satiety cues of such infants may be hard to interpret; in addition, inexperience, preoccupation, or ambivalence may impair the mother's sensitivity and efficacy in responding to the infant's needs. As a result, a well-regulated "nursing couple" fails to develop.

These problems are particularly common in infants who are premature or who suffer from perinatal or congenital difficulties. The premature infant is often a poor feeder and can tax the resources of an inexperienced mother. Such infants may carry an especially high risk, particularly in light of prematurity's association with maternal youth, poverty, and poor prenatal care.

CASE EXAMPLE

Deniko was discharged from the preemie nursery at the age of 6 weeks when she had attained a weight of 5 pounds. At 3 months she was admitted on an emergency basis because of her failure to gain weight beyond that mark. On readmission she was lethargic and had poor skin and muscle tone; she was clad only in a dirty T-shirt and a diaper that appeared not to have been changed for a day. In addition to a severe diaper rash, the infant had a partially healed but infected cigarette burn that the mother attributed to a careless babysitter. Deniko could not hold her head up, sucked feebly, and did not smile.

The mother, 15 years old and unwed, was accompanied by her own 30-year-old mother, who complained that she had to care for her grandchild because her daughter was rarely home. Both stated that the baby was fussy and a poor eater.

On the ward Deniko did indeed choke easily and required careful, patient feeding with a preemie nipple. Close observation of Deniko and her mother revealed that she was both uncertain and abrupt in her ministrations. The mother responded to her daughter's choking with anger and withdrawal; her infant's difficulties made her feel rebuffed and inadequate. With attentive feeding, however, Deniko soon began to gain weight at a very rapid rate and became more responsive and alert. Involvement of Protective Services resulted in placement in a foster home.

- *Disorders of Attachment.* Feeding difficulties stemming from disordered attachment become prominent between 2 and 9 months if a specific, reciprocal affectionate bond has failed to develop between mother and infant. These are the infants described by the DSM-III-R (1987) criteria for Reactive Attachment Disorder of Infancy.

Careful direct evaluation of the mother–child interaction usually reveals serious pathology, especially in the mother's attunement to the child's needs and rhythms. Some infants suffer from global neglect, with lack of medical attention and inadequate physical care; overt abuse may be present. Other children may be well cared for physically, but their mothers are emotionally unavailable and unresponsive to their infant's more subtle cues. Compared to well controls, mothers of FTT children show less warmth and positive reinforcement, have less verbal and physical contact with their infants, and are more prone to use physical punishment (Kotelchuck, 1980; Pollitt et al., 1975).

In one unreplicated study, interactions with their mothers and strangers differentiated infants with nonorganic FTT from children with organic growth retardation (Rosenn et al., 1980). The children with organic illnesses responded positively to holding and touch, whereas the nonorganic FTT infants preferred play with inanimate objects and distant social encounters rather than intimate contact. Using Ainsworth's attachment classification system, more nonorganic FTT infants than controls were insecurely attached.

Findings conflict as to whether the mothers of nonorganic FTT infants have an increased incidence of diagnosable psychiatric illness or psychopathology. Several studies (Kotelchuck, 1980; Newberger et al., 1977; Pollitt et al., 1975) did not substantiate any such increase. Nevertheless, many such mothers suffer from a variety of psychological problems, sociological stresses, and poor mothering skills (often as a result of their own lack of adequate mothering during childhood) (Mrazek & Mrazek, 1985). A prospective study of low-income pregnant mothers found several characteristics correlated with the development of nonorganic FTT including marital strife, mothers' recall of feeling unhappy and unloved during childhood, short gestation, complications of pregnancy, and residual minor medical problems at discharge from the newborn nursery (Altemeier et al., 1985). To account for the data, the authors hypothesized that these factors interfered with the normal development of the mother–child relationship. This conclusion was also suggested by the finding that mothers whose infants subsequently failed to thrive spent less time looking at them during the first 2 days of life and were quicker to terminate interaction with their infants than mothers of controls (Vietze et al., 1980).

Evans and co-workers (1972) identified at least 3 subgroups of mothers and children with nonorganic FTT. The mothers in the first group saw the child's illness as just one more of the many crises and long-standing problems with which they had to deal. Living conditions were deprived, the often numerous older siblings were poorly cared for, and standard prenatal and well-baby care had never been obtained. These mothers seemed severely and chronically depressed; often suffered from persistent medical problems; and appeared, in some instances, to be of limited intelligence. They gave the impression of being helpless and overwhelmed, handled their children with great hesitancy, and had histories of deprivation and poor mothering. At follow-up, improvement was noted only where there had been a dramatic change in living arrangements (such as the departure of an abusive husband or the provision of a substitute caretaker).

The second group of children and mothers described by Evans et al. revealed more subtle defects in maternal care. In contrast to the first group, these children were generally well cared for physically and, despite frequent poverty, had adequate housing and medical care. Home life appeared less chronically chaotic. The most striking finding among the mothers in the second group was extreme depression, generally of recent origin, with a history of severe loss within a few months prior to the hospitalization. They were anxious about their children, but their efforts to feed or cuddle the babies were strained, constricted, and unsure. These mothers were usually eager for help and permitted the staff to be supportive. At follow-up the children had generally done well.

The mothers in the third group showed open hostility toward both the staff and their children. They were often antagonistic and belittling toward the hospital staff, handled their children abruptly and angrily, and tended to view the babies as "bad" rather than ill. The hospital course was stormy.

At follow-up, made more difficult because of the mothers' suspiciousness and reluctance to be involved with helping agencies, only those children who were no longer at home\showed adequate growth.

As Whitten (1981) summarized the matter, "Some mothers do not want to mother their infants and know it, some do not want to and are not aware of it, and some want to but are unable to mobilize the energy that is necessary to fulfill their desire" (p. 204).

Failure to thrive is also seen occasionally in the infants of mothers who hold strong faddist or cultist views concerning nutrition. Although it might be argued that the child's malnutrition is the result of maternal ideology rather than psychopathology, these mothers show a pathological lack of empathic concern for their child's serious debilitation, which appears to be less important to them than preserving their belief system.

CASE EXAMPLE

Sean, a 10-month-old boy, was admitted because of poor weight gain and slow development. Examination revealed moderate anemia and X-ray findings of early rickets. Mother and father were both ardent disciples of a local macrobiotic practitioner. The mother had breast-fed Sean through age 4 months; thereafter, in keeping with the group's dietary beliefs, the baby's diet had been extremely restricted. The parents had refused all immunizations for the child as a matter of principle and had stopped taking the child for well-baby visits because they felt hassled by their pediatrician, who had expressed his extreme concern.

Sociocultural factors also play a role in the genesis of nonorganic FTT. The families of these infants are more likely to consist of a single mother, to be poorer and more socially isolated, and to lack an adequate social support system (Newberger et al., 1977; 1986). When present, these factors burden the parents and further impair their functioning.

• *Disorders of Separation and Individuation.* Chatoor and Egan (1983, 1987a, 1987b) have described a form of nonorganic FTT in the second 6 months of life characterized by food refusal. This refusal is part of an oppositional struggle centered on eating.

From 6 to 12 months of age the infant normally starts taking a more active role in his meals. He begins to feed himself "finger foods" and develops stronger preferences and aversions for tastes and textures. For the now increasingly active infant, mealtimes are also the occasions for banging, smearing, grabbing the spoon, dropping food and utensils overboard, and generally squirming about. "The battle of the spoons [Levy, 1955]. . . becomes a battle of wills" (Chatoor & Egan, 1987a, p. 276), however, when mothers are unwilling to cede a measure of autonomy to the infant, instead forcing food on him in disregard of his tempo or satiety. The infant may respond by spitting food out or refusing to open his mouth. These maladaptive interactions may become entrenched when mothers have an intense need for control or are excessively concerned with the child's eating.

Such overconcern may stem from earlier problems with the infant's health or nutrition or may reflect the mother's difficulty regulating her own hunger and satiety. Chatoor (personal communication, 1987) suggests that eating disorders may be common among these mothers. Concerns with weight and diet may pervade their feeding relationship with their infants; such mothers worry groundlessly that their babies are overweight, attempt inappropriately to slim them down, and are excessively controlling with their infants' diet (Lacey & Smith, 1987). The term "infantile anorexia nervosa" is suggested by the parallel between this infantile oppositional syndrome and the adolescent anorexic's use of food refusal as a desperate weapon in the struggle for autonomy. In older children, growth retardation and delayed puberty have also been described secondary to food refusal prompted by such oppositional dynamics (Chatoor & Egan, 1983) or the fear of obesity (Pugliese et al., 1983). Like classic anorexia nervosa, this condition is reportedly more common in middle- and upper-middle-class families. Longitudinal studies suggest that early problematic eating behaviors often persist into adolescence and may be risk factors for the development of adolescent eating disorders (Marchi & Cohen, 1990).

● *Child Factors.* A perplexity associated with nonorganic FTT is that of several children in a family only one may be affected. Why a particular child should fail to thrive is a complex question. As noted earlier, prematurity and its complications may render some children vulnerable to feeding difficulties. Sometimes, a full-term infant's temperament may prove generally difficult or radically at odds with his mother's. Infants also may differ with age in their susceptibility to various defects in mothering. Kotelchuck (1980) and Newberger et al. (1977) found that child-related factors, especially developmental status and health prior to hospitalization, were the strongest discriminators for nonorganic FTT, whereas maternal factors were *not* discriminating.

● *Neuroendocrine Factors.* Spitz (1945) speculated that the growth retardation associated with maternal deprivation was due to secondary metabolic or endocrine abnormalities that interfered with the child's utilization of his food. Along with emotionally induced growth retardation, many older children with "psychosocial dwarfism" show deficiencies in growth hormone secretion that may simulate hypopituitarism (W. H. Green, 1986; Powell et al., 1967a, 1967b). Much debate has focused on whether the hormonal abnormalities and growth retardation of children with FTT or psychosocial dwarfism are caused simply by diminished nutritional intake or by other factors interfering with the utilization of nutrients.

Careful studies by Whitten (1981) indicate that FTT children *do* have a low food intake secondary either to not being offered adequate food or to not accepting it. However, recent studies suggest that although diminished food intake plays a role, maternal deprivation has growth-stunting effects independent of nutrition (Barnes, 1988; W. H. Green, 1986). In an ingenious series of experiments, Schanberg and his colleagues (1984) demonstrated that maternal touching promotes protein synthesis and weight gain in infant rat pups. Absence of such touching produced profound metabolic changes including a drop in crucial anabolic enzymes and a selective depression of growth hormone levels and tissue sensitivity to growth hormone; this drop occurred within a half hour of loss of tactile stimulation. Although such metabolic suppression could be produced by separating rat pups from their mother, it also occurred even when nutrition was maintained, as in the case of rat pups nursing from a motionless anesthetized mother. In contrast, maintaining tactile stimulation prevented this pattern of metabolic suppression, even in the face of diminished nutritional intake, as was demonstrated in rat pups whose mothers' nipples had been ligated. Although providing no milk, these mothers provided vigorous touching of their infants. The metabolic effects of maternal deprivation could also be blocked by stroking the pups' backs with a wet paint brush, simulating mother's licking.

Drawing on these observations, Schanberg and Fields (cited in Barnes, 1988) found that frequent stroking of premature human infants caused them to thrive better. Compared to controls, babies whose backs were massaged and limbs moved over a 12-day period showed a 50% better weight gain and enhanced neurological development. The touched babies continued to fare better, even at 8 months. These effects of touching appeared to be mediated via the β-endorphin opiate receptors.

These powerful effects of tactile contact shed new light on Harlow's (1961) classic experiments showing that contact was more important than food in fostering attachment behavior. The findings are also intriguing in view of emerging data that suggest the opiate receptor system plays a role in regulating attachment behavior (Sahley & Panksepp, 1987).

Treatment. Optimal treatment of nonorganic FTT must go beyond the infant's nutritional rehabilitation; dysfunctional mother–child interactions related to feeding and other aspects of development must be identified and addressed. In addition, families in "ecological crisis or adversity" (Newberger et al., 1986) may require support and assistance with a host of practical difficulties. Unless the mother is helped to feel more efficacious with her child, the hospital staff's ability to nourish the child where she has failed only reinforces her sense of inadequacy (Oates, 1986).

A careful diagnostic assessment is essential to effective treatment because different interventions are indicated for the different forms of nonorganic

FTT (Chatoor & Egan, 1987b; Drotar et al., 1981; Haynes et al., 1983, 1984). A multidisciplinary team can best carry out assessment and treatment. Direct observation of the mother and child together, feeding, at play, and in other care situations is essential to accurate identification of the problem.

The goals of intervention are to assist the mother in developing a warm, positive relationship with her infant and to increase her confidence in her efficacy as a mother (Ayoub et al., 1979). The mother should be involved in the care of her child from the time of admission (Oates, 1986). Mothers of young infants with feeding difficulties may need to learn effective feeding techniques that address specific problems; in addition, they may need assistance in reading and responding effectively to the infant's cues and signals of hunger or satiety (Chatoor & Egan, 1987b). When the problem lies in more general aspects of mother–infant attachment, basic help in other areas of child care may be necessary. To develop the mother's sense of adequacy, it is important to use a warm, encouraging, nonjudgmental approach that praises her efforts, helps her identify and respond more sensitively to the child's needs, and gives her credit for the child's advances (Leonard et al., 1966; Oates, 1986). Help in encouraging play and in fostering language and cognitive development stimulates the child's cognitive growth and increases the mother and infant's pleasure in each other.

The mother's lack of adequate mothering skills often reflects her own inadequate care as a child. Many of these mothers not only lack adequate role models and skills, they are haunted, in the words of Fraiberg et al. (1975) by persistent "ghosts in the nursery." These inner unconscious presences may dominate a mother's attitudes and reflect either her unexorcised identifications with the perceived harsh and uncaring aspects of her own parents or her identification of the infant with the perceived bad and defective aspects of herself. Practical advice alone is rarely effective. Treatment requires long-term committed work, combining support, education, psychotherapy, and active case work with the community and other agencies (Fraiberg, 1980, 1983). Some of the special technical problems in this kind of treatment are reviewed in the introduction to this section (see pp. 7–9).

When FTT is related to oppositionality and disorders of separation, the overanxious mothers need assistance in disengaging from struggles with the infant and in helping him learn to respond to his own signals of hunger or fullness (Chatoor & Egan, 1987b).

Intensive aftercare and active follow-up are essential. Without it two-thirds of families fail to keep return appointments, and as many as 25% of the infants are readmitted for recurrent FTT; even with intensive follow-up approximately 14% of the cases are readmitted (Ayoub et al., 1979). In intractable cases, foster placement may prove necessary. Although foster care may be most effective in maintaining weight gain and preventing rehospitalization, all too often it fails to provide the child with a long-term stable family setting (Holman, 1983).

Outcome. Different outcome studies suggest a wide range of prognoses. Oates's (1986) 6 to 12 year follow-up of FTT children treated at the Children's Hospital in Sydney, Australia, found an increased risk of emotional and academic difficulties (compared to controls), with half the FTT children rated by their teachers as having personality abnormalities. These infants were also at high risk for later physical abuse (Hufton & Oates, 1977; Oates & Hufton, 1977). Although less pessimistic findings were reported in the study by Mitchell et al. (1980) and the intensive intervention program of Malone and Drotar (1983), other follow-up studies report persistent growth deficits in 20% to 53% of the children, and intellectual and personality abnormalities in 15% to 65% of the children (Ayoub et al., 1979; Elmer et al., 1969; Glaser et al. 1968).

PSYCHOSOMATIC DISORDERS OF INFANCY

Rumination

Introduction and Definition. Rumination is a serious condition that occurs primarily in the first year of life but may infrequently appear in children as old as 7 years of age (Chatoor et al., 1984). Ruminators voluntarily regurgitate previously swallowed food, rechew this material, and partially reswallow it. In the first year of life rumination is an important variant of nonorganic FTT. If it persists, rumination can lead to cachexia, dehydration, hypochloremic alkalosis, and death.

As with nonorganic FTT, rumination appears to be rooted in a troubled mother–child relationship. However, the infant destined to ruminate may previously have had a bout of organically determined vomiting. It may develop directly into the ruminative pattern, or a period of weeks or months may intervene before the syndrome of deliberate regurgitation appears.

DSM-III-R Diagnostic Criteria for Rumination Disorder of Infancy
A. *Repeated regurgitation, without nausea or associated gastrointestinal illness, for at least one month following a period of normal functioning.*
B. *Weight loss or failure to make expected weight gain.* (APA, 1987, p. 70)

Incidence. Rumination is now rarer than it was 50 years ago, when it was relatively common and mortality ran as high as 20%. However, cases are still seen regularly at most pediatric centers.

DSM-III-R notes that the typical age of onset is 3 to 12 months. However, self-stimulating rumination may also be found in mentally retarded individuals of any age (Mayes et al., 1988).

Clinical Features.   In 1925, Cameron gave the following classical description of the ruminating infant:

> After taking the meal quite in the ordinary way, the baby, as a rule, lies quiet for a time. Then begin certain purposive movements, by which the abdominal muscles are thrown into a series of violent contractions—the head is held back, the mouth is opened, while the tongue projects a little and is curved from side to side so as to form a spoon-shaped concavity on its dorsal surface. After a varying time of persistent effort, sometimes punctuated by grunting or whimpering sounds, expressive of irritation at the failure to achieve the expected result, with each contraction of the abdominal muscles, milk appears momentarily in the pharynx at the back of the mouth. . . . Finally, a successful contraction ejects a great quantity of milk forwards into the mouth. The infant lies with an expression of supreme satisfaction upon its face, sensing the regurgitated milk and subjecting it to innumerable sucking and chewing movements. . . . It is very evident that achievement of his purpose produces a sense of beatitude, while failure results in nervous unrest and irritation. . . . The power to ruminate is not suddenly acquired. In the earliest stages, before dexterity has been achieved, the act differs relatively little from that of vomiting. . . . In its earlier development, therefore, rumination is very apt to be mistaken for habitual vomiting due to other causes, and it may require careful observation to make the distinction evident. Nor are such babies easy to observe. It is characteristic of the ruminating child that it sins its sin only in secret. To watch it openly is to put a stop to the whole procedure. . . . Only when the child is alone and in a drowsy, vacant state, while nothing distracts attention or excites curiosity, does the act take place. (Cameron, 1925, quoted in Richmond, Eddy, & Green, 1958, pp. 49–50)

The *voluntary and pleasurable quality* of regurgitation and the apparent self-absorption of the infant are key features of psychologically determined rumination. The rumination occurs primarily in two circumstances. First, it may happen in the absence of, and as an apparent substitute for, human interaction. Ruminating infants often show other self-stimulating behavior, such as head rolling, rocking, hair pulling, genital play, or head banging, suggesting an increased capacity or need for substitute gratification. Second, rumination may occur as a self-soothing, tension-reducing response to overstimulation. Some ruminators are described as having an alert, wide-eyed appearance with a radarlike, searching gaze.

The mothers of many ruminators appear to have difficulty developing a close and comfortable relationship with their babies. Such mothers tend to be immature and may show a variety of psychopathology; they are often locked in marital conflict with and do not receive emotional support from the infant's father. Richmond and co-workers (1958) suggested that "any factors which deprive the infant of intimate, stimulating relationships may predispose to the disorder" (p. 54). These infants are not completely deprived; indeed, feeding appears to have been their greatest source of gratification, though apparently an incomplete one. Richmond et al. (1958) speculated that "the lack of comfort and gratification which ordinarily comes from without (outside) causes [the baby] to seek and re-create such gratification from within" (p. 53). A small minority of infants appear tense and overstimulated, and their mothers seem unable to provide adequate comfort because of maternal or infant factors (or both) (Chatoor et al., 1984). For example, the mother may be unable to respond soothingly to the infant's cues because of her own psychopathology or stress. On the other hand, even a very competent mother may have difficulty comforting an infant with temperamentally poor regulation.

Given the high prevalence of emotional deprivation sufficient to cause FTT, a still unanswered question is what specific additional factors produce the rarer outcome of rumination. As noted, some infants have a history of organically caused vomiting (e.g., viral gastroenteritis) prior to the onset of rumination. There may be an underlying "somatic compliance" in the form of incompetency of the esophageal sphincter (such as a hiatal hernia) or a functional gastrointestinal motility disorder (including pylorospasm, delayed gastric emptying, and diarrhea) (Chatoor et al., 1984). On the other hand, many infants studied with barium swallow show no esophageal or diaphragmatic defect. However it initially occurs, the regurgitation of the habitual ruminator is clearly voluntary, pleasurable, and preceded by forceful, preparatory movements. The infant sometimes appears deliberately to gag himself with his hand. Like the adolescent bulimic, the infant ruminator becomes addicted to regurgitation as a form of tension release and self-soothing.

Treatment. Many treatments have been proposed for rumination ranging across thickened formula, the strapping of the infant upright in a chair, gavage or gastrostomy, splinting of the arms, aversive electric shocks, and antispasmodics. Like FTT infants, the ruminator is often exhaustively worked up with "an instrument in every orifice," a process that may exacerbate the child's condition. The prudent approach would be to attempt "emotional replacement therapy" first, reserving a more aggressive organic workup for cases that fail to respond. Barium swallow, however, is indicated to rule out surgically correctable hiatus hernia or other esophageal defects.

Lourie (1955) outlined the principles of psychological treatment for both rumination and cyclical vomiting in infancy:

(1) The primary goal was to help these children to trust those around them and reinvest their libido in the substitute mothers available. . . . (2) The second

step was to observe the patients for any pattern in their symptoms. . . . When such patterns were known, an effort was made to be sure that holding, carrying or other physical contact would overlap with those periods when the symptoms would be expected to occur. In other words, if substitute satisfaction, particularly relationship satisfactions, could be made available to the infants at the time when the symptoms seem to be needed, it was hoped that the symptoms would be foregone for the moment. . . . (3) The next step was to provide other forms of satisfaction and stimulation when these children were willing. Standard equipment on the wards began to include highchairs next to the nurses' desks, strollers, playpens and baby carriages. Toys that trial and error showed would interest individual infants were supplied for them. Their own motility patterns were used and encouraged as most of them emerged or reemerged into more purposeful and consistent standing and crawling. . . Once [these] stages were accomplished there was an improvement in the physical symptoms of almost all cases. (pp. 143–145)

Aversive negative conditioning, such as electric shock, lemon juice, or hot pepper sauce, has been used in attempts to extinguish ruminative behavior. The success of such methods is equivocal, and nursing staff and parents may resist such measures (Chatoor et al., 1984). As part of an integrated approach, Chatoor et al. designed a treatment plan that provided much attention (but not to the point of overstimulation); rumination, however, was met with a sharp "no" and turning away or leaving for a 2-minute period.

Careful evaluation of the parents and of their interaction with the child offers the key to treatment and to posthospital improvement. The nursing staff should help parents to utilize the principles outlined above in feeding and caring for their child. Ongoing casework or therapy is indicated to identify and remediate the deficits in parenting. It is important not to permit the successful aspects such as weight gain and resolution of the feeding problem to obscure serious ongoing pathological interactions between the child and parents. These require continuing intervention.

Infantile Eczema

Introduction and Definition. Infantile eczema, also known as atopic or neurodermatitis, is a complex psychophysiological skin disease, often arising in early infancy. The term *atopic* refers to its occurrence in individuals who have increased levels of IgE, a form of immunoglobulin serum protein predisposing those who have it to hay fever and asthma (see Chapter 16). Allergic mechanisms involving IgE-mediated hypersensitivity play a central role in the predisposition to infantile eczema and its pathogenesis (Kaplan et al., 1987). However, emotional factors also play an important role in the waxing and waning of its symptoms. Like pica and rumination, infantile eczema appears to be in part a disorder of tension regulation. Thus, its exacerbation often reflects a disturbance in the parent–child interaction, resulting in the infant's turning away from the interpersonal world to his own skin as a means of soothing and reducing discomfort.

Most children with infantile eczema suffer only a mild, fluctuating rash during the first few years of life. However, the seriously affected child suffers for years with a tormenting cycle of itching and scratching. Presently his red and oozing skin assumes a thickened, crusty appearance that may disgust both parent and child. The role of specific environmental and food allergens in the disease process remains unclear (Kaplan et al., 1987). The condition illustrates the intricate interplay of psychological and physiological factors in the genesis of physical disease and provides an object lesson in the way such diseases affect psychosocial functioning. Severe infantile eczema is critically affected by and, in turn, exacerbates anxiety, stress, and rage (Cohen & Nadelson, 1971). It partially arises from and contributes to failure in parental comforting. The infant becomes a social isolate, turning away from the external world to focus exclusively on his own skin and scratching (Cohen, 1975).

Epidemiology, Incidence, and Prevalence. The overall prevalence of atopic dermatitis in the general pediatric population is 1% to 3% (Kaplan et al., 1987). About 4% of all infants will develop the disease sometime before their 7th birthday. The disease usually appears in the first 6 months of life; in two-thirds of the patients it is present by the first birthday and there is a family or individual history of hay fever, asthma, or eczema. In more than half the cases, infantile eczema persists into early adulthood.

Clinical Features and Course. The condition begins with reddened, itchy, and papular skin lesions that the inevitable scratching soon exacerbates into oozing and crusting. The child experiences his scratching as relieving and pleasurable, but this practice leads to further itching and pain and the tormented, unhappy child may claw at his skin until it bleeds. This in turn provokes the parents into frantic efforts to restrain the infant. They feel helpless to comfort or soothe their irritable child. They want to help, but at the same time the oozing crusted skin appears repulsive. In the presence of such distress, the best-intentioned adult is torn between the impulse to reach out, hold, and comfort the child and an involuntary tendency to recoil. The infant in turn finds the parent's touch uncomfortable rather than soothing and soon can read the recoil in others' eyes (Cohen, 1975). The skin is the surface with which we greet the world; when it is diseased, it stirs powerful and archaic feelings about contamination and sinfulness: Witness the scourge of Job's boils, the plague that afflicted the biblical Egyptians, and the ancient stigmatization of the leper.

The child quickly learns that rather than reaching out to his parents, he can find his best comfort from his own body. Scratching thus becomes an established, preferred channel for relief from tension and may eventually replace more adaptive methods. Stress or upset further increases the itching and scratching, and a viciously exacerbated scratch–rash cycle becomes the final common path for expressing anxiety or anger. This pattern is associated with attendant serious defects in the child's ability to accept comfort or to comfort himself.

For eczematous children the skin is not a channel for pleasurable comforting and soothing interaction with the parents. (Think how much time a mother spends in patting, stroking, tickling, or ministering to her infant's skin with powder, lotion, and bath rituals.) Instead, as Cohen (1975) has poignantly described, the infant with eczema comes to mistrust both his body and the external world as reliable sources of pleasure. His attention becomes increasingly fixed on his own body; he turns away from the world of people and external objects and increasingly views it in terms of fantasies of attacking and being attacked. Both child and parents come to see the child's skin as a hated "thing" or foreign object. This estrangement between the child and his parents and between the child and his own body, coupled with the constant discomfort and a turning away from the outside world, results in a preoccupied, inhibited child.

CASE EXAMPLE

Mary was a 16-month-old girl who had been hospitalized twice, each time for several weeks, for exacerbations of her atopic, near-total-body eczema. Her red, thickened, exudative rash was worst over her hands, neck, face, and joint surfaces with areas of secondary pustular infection. Mary's interactions with her mother were largely irritable interchanges culminating in Mary's scratching at herself. Exasperated, the mother would try unsuccessfully to stop her and finally would turn away in disgust. Although Mary had walked at an early age, when alone she showed little interest in exploring. She often preferred instead to sit and rock or scratch. Nursing staff initially found her hard to hold and soothe; within seconds, frustration or limit setting led to crying and clawing at her skin.

Etiological and Pathophysiologic Factors. Eczema has often been cited as an example of multifactorial determination of disease (Cohen & Nadelson, 1971). Conflicting and controversial evidence suggests that at least some patients present a diffuse instability of the autonomic nervous system along with altered peripheral neurotransmitter responses. These factors may cause heightened itch sensation and vasculitis. There is also evidence of altered immunoglobulin, mast cell, and delayed hypersensitivity responses, although cause and effect are difficult to disentangle (Kaplan et al., 1987). The child's ability to modulate anxiety and stress (and his parents' capacity to help him do so) may also be a determining factor. An eczemateous child, who is often temperamentally difficult, sorely taxes any parent. When the parents are anxious, intolerant, or ambivalent, the coping ability of the parent–child unit is even further impaired.

The final clinical outcome is the result of three vectors: (1) biological predisposition to cutaneous itching and vasculitis, (2) psychobiological endowment (especially in the modulation of anxiety, stimulation, and stress), and (3) the quality of parent–child interaction (Cohen, 1975).

Treatment. Infantile eczema is difficult to treat and requires a coordinated approach to the child's skin as well as to the psychological functioning of the child and his parents. Topical treatment of the rash alone rarely succeeds. Even in the presence of positive skin test findings, substitution or exclusion of various foods or the maintenance of a dust-free environment is often not curative. The principles of an integrated treatment approach outlined by Cohen (1975) are as follows: The skin must be soothed (using steroid cream, hypoallergenic lotions, and cool baths); pleasant relations with the parents are encouraged and strengthened around soothing baths and other positive, shared activities; attempts are made to reduce the child's anxiety and redirect attention to the outside world; nonsoporific, antipruritic antihistamines, often in large doses, are given to reduce itching; and bedtime sedation for the child may help him and his parents to sleep comfortably through the night. Treatment of the parents is geared to helping them understand the child's dilemma rather than to see him as naughty, and to reestablishing their sense of efficacy and self-esteem in dealing with their difficult child. As with all chronic diseases, the treatment requires an empathic and active physician's ongoing involvement.

CASE EXAMPLE (*continued*)

Mary began a regimen of twice daily soothing colloidal oatmeal baths, which were made as pleasurable and as playful as possible. In addition, she received topical steroid creams, large doses of brompheniramine as an antipruritic, and bedtime chloral hydrate as a sedative. Although hesitant at first, the mother was encouraged by the nurses to join in the play while Mary was bathed on the ward. After a while, she was able to smile at Mary's splashing and to interest Mary in the bath toys that they passed back and forth, the first positive interaction noted by the staff. The mother applied the steroid cream with a grim and punitive air; nursing staff tried to demonstrate to her how this could be made into a game with Mary.

In casework, the mother spoke of Mary as "mean and ornery just like her father," who had abandoned the family at Mary's birth. The mother had liked Mary as a cuddly infant but could not tolerate her increasing autonomy as a toddler or her sporadic dependent clinging. The mother's view of Mary's scratching as willful defiance yielded only slowly. After discharge, many months of work were necessary before the mother was able to comfort Mary without resentment and to enjoy spending time with her. Casework with the social worker and outpatient visits to her pediatrician continued on a weekly basis after discharge. This treatment included time with Mary's former primary ward nurse and a review with the mother of the progress of Mary's treatment program. Mary's eczema improved to the point that further inpatient hospitalizations were unnecessary. She continued, however, to suffer exacerbations at crisis points in her relationship with her mother.

PART II

Major Disruptions of
Developmental Progress

Chapter 2

Mental Retardation

INTRODUCTION

Historically, interest in retardation has had two sources: the *medical* tradition, which has sought to delineate the underlying neurological defects and physical causes of retardation, and the *pedagogic* tradition, which has been concerned with identifying and teaching children with intellectual deficits. In recent years, there has been increased recognition that retardation may arise from multiple causes and that, in most cases, outcome and course are determined not only by the type of neuropathological lesion (if any) but by the family environment, cultural shaping forces, and the child's adaptive skills. Retardation is simultaneously a clinical, educational, and social phenomenon that must be viewed and treated in the broadest perspective.

DEFINITION

Currently mental retardation denotes the presence of *both* subaverage intellectual functioning and impaired social adaptation.

DSM-III-R Diagnostic Criteria for Mental Retardation

A. *Significantly subaverage general intellectual functioning: an IQ of 70 or below on an individually administered IQ test (for infants, a clinical judgment of significantly subaverage intellectual functioning, since available intelligence tests do not yield numerical IQ values).*

B. *Concurrent deficits or impairments in adaptive functioning, i.e., the person's effectiveness in meeting the standards expected for his or her age by his or her cultural group in areas such as social skills and responsibility, communication, daily living skills, personal independence, and self-sufficiency.*

C. *Onset before the age of 18.* (APA, 1987, pp. 31–32)

DSM-III also suggests that the clinician should note biological conditions causing or accompanying the retardation, along with additional psychiatric disorders or behavioral concomitants such as aggression, anxiety, or self-mutilation.

Therefore, the two key criteria in diagnosing mental retardation are IQ level and social adaptation. A curve showing the frequency of occurrence of different IQs in the general population is, for the most part, bell shaped and normal with a peak frequency at an IQ of 100. A second, smaller hump at the lower end of the curve represents a statistical excess of people with very low IQs because there are more people with very low IQs than with very high ones. The cutoff point for diagnosing retardation is usually an IQ two standard deviations below normal. One standard deviation equals 15 points on the WISC-R test and 16 points on the Stanford-Binet (Achenbach, 1982).

DSM-III-R (1987) uses the term *Borderline Intellectual Functioning* for deficits in adaptive behavior associated with borderline (low) intellectual functioning, that is, IQs between 71 and 84. DSM-III-R regards this condition as a potential "focus for attention or treatment" rather than as a mental disorder. By definition, 14% of the general population fall into this IQ range, because it represents all individuals with IQs lying more than one, but less than two, standard deviations below normal.

DSM-III-R distinguishes the following subtypes of mental retardation on the basis of IQ levels:

Subtypes of Mental Retardation	*IQ Levels*
Mild	50–55 to 70 (approx.)
Moderate	35–40 to 50–55
Severe	20–25 to 35–40
Profound	Below 20 or 25

To make the DSM-III-R diagnosis of retardation, impairment in *adaptation* must be present as well as low IQ. There is no ready quantitative measure of adaptive functioning comparable to standardized IQ tests. However, reliable tests, such as the Vineland Adaptive Behavior Scales (Sparrow et al., 1984), include competency on such practical behavioral items as dressing, bathing, and toileting ability. More important, although IQ may serve as a predictor of eventual academic attainment, there is no simple correlation between IQ scores and adaptive functioning, especially for the mildly and moderately retarded. Overall social competency involves more elusive factors such as personality, motivation, special talents, and, in the case of minority group children, degree of adaptation to their own subculture as well as to the mainstream.

The DSM-III-R approach, which follows that of the American Association on Mental Deficiency, is by no means universally accepted (Zigler and Hodapp, 1986). For example, Zigler and colleagues (1984) argued that use of low IQ alone as a criterion would provide a more circumscribed and reliable diagnosis. "Labeling theorists," on the other hand, have emphasized the social impact of the diagnosis. Mercer (1975) and others argued that the diagnosis of retardation is often made on the basis of factors extraneous to intellectual ability and constitutes assignment of a social role that in turn shapes the putatively retarded child's behavior and destiny (see p. 40).

EPIDEMIOLOGY

The diagnosis of mental retardation is age-dependent. The annual incidence of newly diagnosed mental retardation during the infancy and preschool period is 10 new cases per 100,000, rising to a peak of 37 per 100,000 during the middle school years, and declining to 7 per 100,000 by adolescence (Tarjan et al., 1973). There are several reasons for this age-related pattern of prevalence. First, because of the difficulty of accurately ascertaining levels of intellectual functioning in infancy, usually only the severest forms of retardation (generally associated with conspicuous physical signs and symptoms) are diagnosed in this period. Second, because retardation is defined in terms of adaptive as well as intellectual deficits, the impairments of many mildly or moderately retarded children do not become clear until they begin school. With its relatively rigorous social, behavioral, and academic demands, school acts as a proving ground for adaptive competence. Further, to the extent that mild retardation often appears to be the cumulative result of long-term environmental deprivation and trauma, it may not become manifest until middle childhood. All of these factors account for the marked peak in the number of newly diagnosed cases during the school years. Finally, after adolescence, the ability to attend, behave, and learn in school ceases to be a societal expectation. At any rate, the adult's intellectual and behavioral performance is not scrutinized as carefully as the child's. Thus, about 75% of individuals diagnosed as retarded are adolescents or school-age children. Subsequently, in late adolescence or early adulthood, two-thirds of those so diagnosed become reabsorbed into the general population, with their retardation no longer suspected or diagnosed (Tarjan et al., 1973). This phenomenon also highlights the degree to which the adaptive criteria for retardation are influenced by societal norms.

In the less educationally demanding agrarian society of the United States before the 20th century, many individuals with low IQs were never considered retarded. Not only was academic scrutiny less universal, more societal niches existed in which such persons could function without noticeable deficit. Improved health, education, and welfare programs in the past several decades have probably caused a slow decline in the number of persons of low IQ. It is ironic, however, that at the same time, our increasingly technological society, with its greater educational and vocational demands, has magnified the relative adaptive and occupational handicaps of persons with low IQ.

Because of the high frequency of their associated physical disorders, the more severely retarded have a markedly higher death rate than the general population. Thus, the proportion of severely retarded individuals in the population decreases gradually with age.

The overall distribution of the four subtypes of the retarded population is:

Mild	80%
Moderate	12%
Severe	7%
Profound	1%

Males outnumber females at every level of retardation (Vandenberg et al., 1986). The distribution of the different degrees of retardation by social class varies in striking ways (Birch et al., 1970; Tarjan et al., 1973). Because the most severe and profound cases of retardation are usually organic in origin, they occur at about the same rate in all social classes. Although some known physical factors associated with retardation, such as prematurity and the complications of poor prenatal care, are more common with low socioeconomic status (SES), many other organic factors appear to be relatively independent of it. (Low SES also exacerbates the maladaptive impact of perinatal vulnerabilities.) In contrast, mild to moderate retardation is an estimated 15 times more frequent in the children of the lowest socioeconomic class, compared with children of middle-class suburbia (Stein & Susser, 1963).

The majority of the mentally retarded population in large public residential institutions are persons with very low IQs, physical disabilities, and behavioral problems (Scheerenberger, 1983). With the growth of day classes for the educably retarded and the establishment of group foster homes, sheltered workshops, and other day facilities, the number of institutionalized mentally retarded patients has steadily decreased, as has the proportion of mildly retarded persons in institutions.

CLINICAL FEATURES

The development, education, and ultimate social and vocational status for the four levels of retardation are summarized in Table 2.1.

Two Categories of Retardation: Organic and Cultural-Familial

The mentally retarded compose an extremely heterogeneous group, and generalization from one individual to another is hazardous. Nonetheless, two broad categories of retardation can be delineated: (1) the *biological* or *organic* variety, with an organic basis; and (2) the *cultural-familial* or *psychosocially disadvantaged* type, with no identifiable physical cause and with apparent environmental and familial factors.

Table 2–1. Four Levels of Retardation.

Level	Maturation and Development (Preschool: age 0–5)	Training and Education (School age: 6–21)	Social and Vocational Adequacy (Adult: 21 and over)
Profound	Gross retardation: minimal capacity for functioning in sensori-motor areas; needs nursing care	Obvious delays in all areas of development; shows basic emotional responses; may respond to skillful training in use of legs, hands, and jaws; needs close supervision	May walk, need nursing care, have primitive speech; usually benefits from regular physical activity; incapable of self-maintenance
Severe	Marked delay in motor development; little or no communication skill; may respond to training in elementary self-help, e.g., self-feeding	Usually walks barring specific disability; has some understanding of speech and some response; can profit from systematic habit training	Can conform to daily routines and repetitive activities; needs continuing direction and supervision in protective environment
Moderate	Noticeable delays in motor development, especially in speech; responds to training in various self-help activities	Can learn simple communication, elementary health and safety habits, and simple manual skills; does not progress in functional reading or arithmetic	Can perform simple tasks under sheltered conditions; participates in simple recreation; travels alone in familiar places; usually incapable of self-maintenance
Mild	Often not noticed as retarded by casual observer but is slower to walk, feed self, and talk than most children	Can acquire practical skills and useful reading and arithmetic to a 3rd to 6th grade level with special education; can be guided toward social conformity	Can usually achieve social and vocational skills adequate to self-maintenance; may need occasional guidance and support when under unusual social or economic stress

Source: From *Chart Book: Mental Retardation, a National Plan for a National Problem,* the President's Panel on Mental Retardation, Washington, D.C., U.S. Department of Health, Education, and Welfare, 1963.

Organic Retardation. More than 200 physical disorders are associated with retardation (Grossman, 1983; Mackay, 1982). The major categories include genetic and chromosomal abnormalities, prenatal and perinatal difficulties, and acquired childhood diseases (see Appendix 2–1).

The physically determined forms of retardation are of great scientific and therapeutic interest. Prompt treatment of some conditions, such as phenylketonuria, hydrocephalus, cretinism, or malnutrition, can dramatically minimize or even prevent the development of subsequent mental retardation. Furthermore, the identification of heritable disorders is important for genetic counseling and prenatal diagnosis.

Organic causes can be found, however, in only about 25% to 50% of the retarded (Zigler & Hodapp, 1986). Although the majority of children in this group have severe to profound retardation, most Down syndrome children function in the mildly to moderately retarded range (Pueschel, 1983). Down syndrome is probably the commonest known organic factor. Phenylketonuria was once quite common; widespread mandatory neonatal screening and early dietary treatment have made it a much less frequent cause of retardation. The estimated contribution of different types of defects in a university hospital developmental evaluation clinic (Crocker & Nelson, 1983) was:

Defect	*Percentage of Total Group*
Single gene and polygenetic abnormalities	5%
Chromosomal abnormalities	10
Prenatal damage (e.g., intrauterine infections, drugs)	22
Perinatal difficulties	11
Acquired childhood diseases (including infection, accidents, toxins)	4
Environmental difficulties (e.g., deprivation and parental mental illness)	9
Childhood behavior problems (an ill-defined category including neurosis and childhood psychosis)	8
Unknown or multiple causes	31

The mix of conditions associated with retardation varies with the observational setting. Thus, a specialized academic medical setting, such as the one cited, draws more complex cases with mixed biological and social vulnerabilities. In school systems, on the other hand, milder cases of apparent environmental origin are more common. In third-world countries, and even in parts of this country, malnutrition and infections in pregnant women and children constitute a major, remediable cause of retardation.

Because of their severe retardation and frequently striking physical symptoms, most children in the organic group are diagnosed in infancy. Many of these children look abnormal, with a host of physical anomalies, including short stature, micro- or macrocephaly, wide-set eyes, abnormalities of dentition, palmar creases, epicanthal folds, and high-arched palate. Neurological findings are more common in the organic group. There is also a higher incidence of seizures, which may further compromise the child's development. Finally, other medical problems often accompany the many forms of retardation caused by chromosomal abnormalities or inborn errors of metabolism. For example, frequent concomitants of Down syndrome include congenital heart and gastrointestinal malformations and, in later life, leukemia, hypothyroidism, hearing loss, and instability of the cervical spine (Pueschel, 1983). As previously noted, the prevalence of organically diagnosable retardation is about the same in all socioeconomic classes, although environmental factors strongly influence the treatment and course of the disorder.

Cultural-Familial Retardation.   The cultural-familial group comprises about 50% to 75% of the population of retarded individuals (Zigler & Hodapp, 1986). These cases have no identifiable physical cause, and most are mildly to moderately retarded. Because of their milder disability and normal physical appearance, these children are often not diagnosed until the school years when their intellectual and adaptive impairments first become apparent in the school setting.

Adaptive abilities vary widely in this group. A host of behavioral, personality, and cultural factors may cause one child to be diagnosed as retarded and another not although they have the same tested IQ. Thus, in one Southern California community with a mixed English-speaking and Hispanic population, Mercer (1975) found that the children identified as retarded by the school were those with poorer academic and social adjustment to school and poor English competence. Some classmates with the same low IQ score on testing but who spoke better English, were better behaved in class, and were better liked by their peers were not labeled as retarded.

Because this form of retardation is most noticeable during the school day, Work (1979) and others have called it "six-hour retardation." In contrast, at home the same child's parents and peers may not regard him as deviant. Such retardation is commonest in the lowest socioeconomic group; indeed, about three-quarters of mildly to moderately retarded children come from poor, multiproblem families (Cytryn & Lourie, 1980). Thus, the diagnosis of mental retardation often is not simply a clinical matter but is also a social and administrative decision.

Patterns of Deficit

The pattern and the degree of intellectual deficit in mental retardation vary from child to child. Some retarded children are severely handicapped by attentional deficits; others show uneven cognitive functioning with particular weakness in verbal, visual-motor, or spatial organizational skills. Not only do many retarded children learn more slowly, they tend to generalize poorly, and show limited flexibility in moving from one context to another. In some youngsters, preservation and "stickiness" of focus can also be serious impediments. Further work is needed to elucidate the extent to which these various cognitive defects are intrinsic to low IQ or are secondary to social and sensory deprivation, such as occurs with many institutionalized retarded children (Balla & Zigler, 1979).

Whether the retarded child's intelligence is qualitatively as well as quantitatively different from the normal child's is a matter of considerable debate and has been termed the "developmental versus difference (or defect) controversy" (Zigler & Balla, 1982; Zigler & Hodapp, 1986). At stake is the question: To what extent does a retarded child cognitively resemble a normal child of the same mental age? For example, how much cognitive similarity is there between a normal 4-year-old and a retarded 10-year-old with an IQ of 40? The developmental position holds that the intellectual development of retardates is qualitatively similar to that of the normal child but merely progresses more slowly through the same sequence of stages and becomes arrested at an early stage. From a Piagetian perspective, the severely retarded are, for the most part, arrested at the sensorimotor stage; the moderately retarded, at the stage of intuitive thought; and the mildly retarded, at the stage of concrete operations. In contrast, difference theorists see major qualitative abnormalities in the cognition of retardates. Luria (1963) contends that the retarded show a general underdevelopment of the verbal system, which remains disassociated from their motor and action schemata. In this view, the retarded fail to use verbal mediators as a significant element in their thinking. Short-term memory span and the ability to incorporate recently learned material into long-term storage are impaired.

Over and above these cognitive issues, personality factors strongly influence the retarded individual's competency (Zigler & Balla, 1977b). For example, Balla and Zigler (1979) emphasized that given a long history of repeated failure, discouragement, and low self-esteem, retarded children approach their learning tasks with impaired motivation and set.

Research is just beginning in the correlation of patterns of cognitive deficit with specific causes of retardation.

Associated Features

Although attempts have been made to delineate a "typical mentally retarded personality pattern," few generalizations are in fact possible (Chess & Korn, 1970). Retarded individuals seem to show a wide range of personality traits complexly determined by the type of underlying organic pathology, family child-rearing practices, and unknown factors. Some retarded children show a tendency toward rigid and obsessional behavior. To what extent this represents the perseveration often associated with organic brain damage as against a combination of cognitive inflexibility and deliberate conscientiousness is not clear. Many retarded children show a related intolerance for change and an exaggerated degree of wariness, negativism, and oppositionality. The motivational difficulties of retarded persons may not be intrinsic to their cognitive deficits, but rather the maladaptive responses to social deprivation, negative reinforcement, or frustration; as such, they may also be ameliorated by altering their social milieu and pattern of reinforcers (Zigler & Hodapp, 1986).

Rocking, head-banging, compulsive masturbation, and other stereotypies may occur in severe retardation. Irritability, poor impulse control, and attention deficits with or without hyperkinesis may be variably present. In the more severely retarded, temper tantrums and aggressive behavior directed both toward the self and others are sometimes serious problems. In some instances, such as temporal lobe epilepsy or frontal lobe disinhibition syndromes, such behavior can arise from altered neurological functioning. Harsh or overindulgent parental behavior as well as inadequate alternative coping strategies may also contribute to intemperate and aggressive behavior.

Little is known about possible correlations between type of retardation and personality. Although Down syndrome children are frequently described as gregarious, friendly, and likable, there is no stereotypic temperamental profile (Gunn et al., 1981). Down syndrome children do appear to be better related and to display less withdrawal, impulsivity, and irritability than matched IQ classmates suffering from other forms of retardation (Cytryn & Lourie, 1980). The data are equivocal as to whether Down syndrome children differ from their retarded classmates on such variables as hyperactivity and aggression (Corbett, 1985; Cytryn & Lourie, 1980).

Retarded children have a generally higher incidence of psychiatric disorder than the population at large (Eaton & Menolascino, 1982). In various studies, the incidence of diagnosable psychiatric disorders in retarded children ranged from about 25% to 65%, with the frequency and severity of the psychiatric disturbance increasing with the severity of the retardation (Gillberg et al., 1986a; Reid, 1980). On the basis of their comprehensive epidemiological study of all 9- to 11-year-olds on the Isle of Wight, Rutter and colleagues (1970/1981) found that a general inverse correlation existed between the frequency of deviant behavior and intelligence and that this held true across the entire range of intelligence and not merely over the retarded spectrum.

The patterns of disturbance in the mildly retarded population approximate those among the nonretarded. However, within the ranks of the severely retarded, psychosis, stereotyped movements (e.g., head-banging, rocking), and attentional deficit with hyperactivity are especially common. The incidence of behavior disturbance is especially high in retarded persons in institutions, in part because severity of disturbance is often the reason for institutionalization, and in part because poor institutional conditions exacerbate disturbed behavior.

The mechanisms involved in the high incidence of psychiatric problems among the retarded are many and complex (Corbett, 1985). Organic damage that can produce retardation also predisposes to certain psychiatric disorders. At the same time, the poor socioeconomic conditions often associated with retardation frequently beget psychiatric problems. Even children of normal intelligence with the same difficult temperamental features of some retarded children develop a high incidence of psychiatric problems, especially if there is a poor parent–child fit. Retarded children are especially vulnerable and require more than the usual amounts of firm, loving, and consistent parental care and stimulation. Most mildly retarded children are aware of their deficits and have correspondingly poor self-esteem; they tend to regard themselves as bad, inadequate, or, most commonly, stupid. Their rejection by normal peers often exacerbates these feelings; the retarded child's behavioral deviations may be both a source of and a response to this rejection or scapegoating. All too often the result is a progressively intensifying feedback loop. The parents of retarded children may be rejecting, ambivalent, or overprotective, any of which are likely to deleteriously affect the growing child's developing self-image and object relations.

Certain childhood psychiatric syndromes appear to have a specific association with intellectual retardation. Infantile autism, for example, is typically accompanied by early-appearing symptoms of pervasive social unresponsiveness, gross language deficits, and bizarre behavior. Autism frequently occurs with retardation due to specific neurological syndromes such as phenylketonuria (Valente, 1971), congenital rubella syndrome (Chess, Korn, & Fernandez, 1971), and infantile spasms; it may also accompany retardation of unknown origin. High rates of autism have been reported with fragile-X syndrome. However, recent studies suggest that despite atypical speech and language and stereotyped behavior, most individuals with fragile-X have affectionate social relations and do not meet criteria for infantile autism (Bregman et al., 1987, 1988). (The relationship of autism to retardation is considered further in Chapter 4.)

Many retardates display pervasive hyperactivity, impulsivity, and attention deficit disorder (Reid, 1980). Psychosis, with symptoms of frank thought disorder such as delusions, hallucinations, and loosening of associations, also occurs with increased frequency. Kraepelin noted this association and coined the term "Pfropfhebephrenia" to describe "the psychotic states observed in a colony of mental defectives" (cited in May, 1979).

Although most common, stereotyped self-injurious behavior seen in retardation is nonspecific, it may occasionally represent a cardinal symptom of Lesch–Nyhan syndrome. Characteristic self-mutilation by biting is found in this disease, which is a form of retardation due to a sex-linked inherited defect in purine metabolism (Nyhan, 1978).

ETIOLOGY

The main categories of organic pathology that result in retardation account for only about 25% to 50% of mental retardation cases. Before turning to the possible causes of the more common category of cultural-familial retardation, a brief discursion into the hereditary and environmental determinants of intelligence is necessary.

Environmental and Nonpathological Genetic Effects on IQ

Intelligence is a complex phenomenon determined by the interplay of organic and environmental factors. Intelligence is often conceptualized as an underlying unitary competency; an alternative view is that it is a set of skills that are independent of each other. Studying the determinants of intelligence is further complicated, because both performance variables (such as set and motivation) and measurement factors (including cultural experience and English competency) affect its measurement.

Controversy still rages over the old question of the relative roles of heredity and environment in determining human intelligence (Achenbach, 1982; Gould, 1981; Scarr & Kidd, 1983; Zigler & Hodapp, 1986). Methodological complexities and passionate ideological polemics cloud the issue.

At one pole the extreme *environmentalists* hold that the variations in human intelligence stem from environmental differences such as physical factors (nutrition and medical care) and cultural, family, or child-rearing factors (intellectual stimulation, educational opportunities, and parental socioeconomic status). This hypothesis is obviously attractive to persons with politically egalitarian views and a commitment to ameliorating social ills.

At the other pole the extreme *hereditarians* hold that genetic endowment determines attained adult intelligence. Although the hereditarian view carries no necessary political implications, both its defenders and attackers have often regarded it as offering "scientific" legitimacy to social inequities and justifying a laissez-faire social policy. In one of the most controversial versions of the hereditarian hypothesis, Arthur Jensen (1980) proposed that racial differences in measured intelligence have their origin primarily in genetic rather than cultural or environmental factors. (For a proposed refutation of Jensen's hypothesis, see Scarr & Kidd, 1983.)

In between the extreme hereditarian and environmentalist hypotheses a variety of interactionist formulations attempt to account for the contribution of both environment and heredity. Most such theories assume (1) a polygenetic influence on intelligence (i.e., genes at several loci augment or diminish aspects of intellectual functioning) and (2) an environmentally influenced reaction range for each genotype (*reaction range* refers to the range of phenotypes that can develop from a given genotype under different environmental conditions). Thus, an interactionist hypothesis would suggest that children with a given set of genes might attain different adult IQs depending on their developmental environment. Conversely, if reaction ranges for different genotypes overlapped, a given IQ might be the product of several different genetic endowments unfolding under different environmental conditions.

It is easy to cite examples of obvious genetic and environmental influences on intelligence. Even dedicated hereditarians would acknowledge that severe malnutrition or extreme sensory deprivation might stunt a child's intellectual development. Similarly, the chromosomal aberrations and genetically determined metabolic disorders discussed earlier can disrupt the normal maturation of the nervous system and thus affect intellectual functioning. These extreme examples, however, shed little light on how genetic differences affect intelligence under "average expectable conditions." Another way of posing the question is: Within a given population, what are the sources of variation in intelligence (Scarr & Kidd, 1983)?

Although the data and methodological issues are complex, many behavioral geneticists have concluded that genetic differences account for about half the variance in measured IQ of the US and European white population (Plomin & DeFries, 1980; Rimland & Musinger, 1977; Scarr & Kidd, 1983). Evidence supporting this conclusion comes from studies of intelligence in adopted children and in twins and their families.

The correlation of IQ between monozygotic (identical) twins is high (about .85 for twins reared together and about .74 for twins reared apart). In contrast, the correlation of IQs between dizygotic (fraternal) twins is only about .53, the same as the correlation for singleton (nontwin) siblings reared in the same family (Rimland & Munsinger, 1977; Rowe & Plomin, 1978). It had been suggested that the higher correlation between monozygotic twins as compared to dizygotic twins was the result of more similar rearing environments for the monozygotic twins; considerable evidence, however, now indicates that this is not the case (Scarr & Kidd, 1983).

Comparison studies of parents and their biological offspring living together show a modest correlation in IQ, on the order of .3 to .5 (Rimland & Munsinger, 1977). Under such conditions, genetic and shared environmental factors cannot be disentangled. However by comparing the intelligence of children adopted shortly after birth with that of their biological parents and sibs as against their adoptive parents and sibs, it is possible to tease these two sets of influences apart. For example, the Texas Adoption Project found that the IQ of adopted children correlated more highly with that of the biological mother than that of the adoptive parents (Horn et al., 1979). Indeed the magnitude of the correlation between the biological mother and her adopted-away child was as high as that between the adoptive parents and their biological offspring. A study of French adoptees found that adoptees with biological parents of high-SES status attained mean IQs 15 points higher than did adoptees with low-SES biological parents (Capron and Duyme, 1989).

At the same time, environment does have its effects. Children of families with low SES who were adopted early in life by higher SES families showed generally higher IQs than their biological siblings who remained in the families of origin (Brand, 1987; Schiff & Lewontin, 1986). Similarly, the average IQ of French adoptees reared by high-SES adoptive families was 12 points higher than those reared by low-SES families (Capron & Duyme, 1989). In their classic study of 100 infants adopted from an Iowa orphanage, Skodak and Skeels (1949) compared the children's IQs through adolescence with both the IQs and education of the biological parents and the education of the adoptive parents (a proxy measure correlating with IQ). Although the biological mothers' mean IQ was 86, the adopted children's mean IQ (measured at age 14) was 106.

Are there limits to the apparently ameliorative effects of the child-rearing conditions in the adoptive environment? Some studies support the notion that individuals of different genetic backgrounds respond differently to adoption into an above-average intellectual environment (this notion is consistent with the concept of genotypes with different reaction ranges). For example, the Texas Adoption Project compared the outcomes for children of high-IQ (120 or above) biological mothers with the outcome for children of low IQ (95 or below) biological mothers (Willerman, 1979). Both sets of children were adopted by families with above-average parental IQs. Attesting to the influence of their adoptive environment, the children of the low-IQ biological mothers attained IQ scores in the average range, with a mean 13 points higher than that of their biological mothers. However, the scores of these children still fell far below those of the adopted children of the high-IQ biological mothers. Among the children with low-IQ mothers, none achieved a score of 120 or over and 15% fell below 95. In contrast, 44% of the adoptees born to high-IQ mothers attained scores of 120 or better, and none fell below 95. On the other hand, the French adoption study cited above failed to find evidence of inherited sensitivity to environmental differences (McGue, 1989). Regardless of biological background, the mean IQ of adoptees reared in high-SES homes was 12 points higher than those reared in low-SES homes (Capron & Duyme, 1989).

In summary, adoption studies support the notion of environmental effects on actual IQ levels, especially for children from disadvantaged backgrounds. However, within a normal child-rearing environment, genotypic differences have a dominant influence on the rank ordering of IQs and equal or outweigh parental socioeconomic indicators in determining phenotypic IQ differences (Achenbach, 1982).

Cultural-Familial Retardation

As noted earlier, in about 50% to 75% of the persons living in this country who are diagnosed as retarded, no organic cause can be identified. Most of these individuals have IQs above 50. This form of retardation has been variably labeled *cultural-familial* or *sociocultural* depending on the investigator's etiological perspective.

Whether the family and the subcultural clustering found in this condition are due to hereditary or environmental factors, the term *cultural-familial* is descriptively apt. Children with milder forms of retardation are *more* likely than severely retarded children to have siblings and parents who are also retarded (Scarr & Kidd, 1983). In contrast to retardation that is clearly of organic orgin, mild, apparently nonorganic retardation varies with social and cultural factors (Zigler & Hodapp, 1986). Severe organic retardation is equally prevalent across social class and occurs with the same frequency in both the United States and Sweden. With lower class status, however, the incidence of mild retardation increases 15 to 20 times (Birch et al., 1970; Stein & Susser, 1963) and is 8 to 10 times more frequent in the United States than in Sweden (Sameroff, 1986). In several countries, the incidence of retardation is higher in rural than in urban populations (Akesson, 1986).

One hypothesis proposes that cultural-familial retardation simply represents the lower end of the normal population distribution curve for IQ (excluding the excess of low IQs caused by organic abnormalities). From this perspective, cultural-familial retardation results from the same interplay of hereditary and environmental factors that accounts for the variation of IQ throughout the biologically normal population (Achenbach, 1982; Akesson, 1986).

In light of the genetic and environmental contributions to intelligence, both polygenic hereditary factors and environmental influences are likely to have an effect. From a genetic viewpoint, the clustering of mild retardation within families is consistent with the inherited nature of this handicap (representing, in part, the expression of genotypes for low IQ). On the other hand, if reared under adverse conditions, even an individual with a presumed genotype for high IQ might attain only a low phenotypic IQ. The complex interactions between genetic endowment and environment seldom are simply additive, nor does heredity merely set the upper limit on intellectual potential while environment determines the fulfillment of this potential. Much of the current research in behavioral genetics is devoted to developing transactional multifactorial models that more adequately define this interplay (Sameroff, 1986; Sameroff & Chandler, 1975; Scarr & Kidd, 1983).

Some polemicists have seen the high incidence of borderline intellectual functioning and mild-to-moderate retardation in the lowest socioeconomic class as evidence for a downward-drift hypothesis. They postulate that across the generations, genetically determined low intelligence has led the affected individuals to fall to an ever lower socioeconomic position. Environmentalists, however, have argued convincingly that low SES, particularly when it involves poor health care, nutrition, housing, and a chaotic pattern of family life, has a powerful detrimental effect on intellectual development.

Social status may be regarded as a summary variable with associated risk and protective factors that exert both independent and interactive influences on outcome (Sameroff, 1986). These risk factors include family characteristics, psychological characteristics of the parents, child-rearing practices, and stressful life events (Sameroff & Seifer, 1983). For example, high-SES status may not only protect against financial privation, it also may be associated with access to quality education and health care, intellectual stimulation, encouragement for academic achievement, and other positive child-rearing factors (Kohn, 1969; McGue, 1989). In contrast, the adverse conditions associated with low SES confront the developing child with cumulative emotional, intellectual, and physical hazards. Along with poor prenatal care and maternal malnutrition, premature delivery is more frequent among impoverished mothers, many of whom are unwed teenagers. Ongoing pediatric care is often absent, and deleterious organic factors such as prenatal alcohol exposure, poor nutrition, and lead poisoning are widespread.

From infancy onward, low-SES children frequently lack informal cognitive stimulation in their homes. Formal academic achievement is often little encouraged; indeed, school may be viewed as an alien, even a hostile, environment. Further, the presence of multiple, often inadequate, early caretakers and chaotic living conditions may be so damaging that the child does not develop the basic ego functions necessary for learning. In practice the picture of early FTT and early mental retardation may be clinically indistinguishable. Lack of concern for the child's emotional and intellectual development may result in delayed identification of problem areas. More than that, even when the difficulties are discovered, inadequate remediation is all too likely.

Although children's vulnerability to the hazards of poverty may vary with age, many studies indicate that the effect on IQ is progressive (Stein & Susser, 1971). Groups of middle-class and economically disadvantaged children who were compared during early infancy showed no significant differences in developmental quotients. By the age of 3, however, the disadvantaged group had five times as many children with IQs below 80. Other studies have shown that when children from the poorest social circumstances were compared to children from a less disadvantaged background, as the years advanced, the poorer children's IQ and their educational attainment both declined. These studies have at times been challenged as reflecting the influence of cultural biases and specific school experiences on IQ test performance. Because intervention programs and change of social environment can lead to marked improvement in IQ levels, scores are not immutable. Nonetheless, although children may retain the potential for improvement, in the absence of intervention, serious cumulative damage to their intellectual capacities does result.

Even when children have frank organic vulnerabilities, socioeconomic factors profoundly influence the eventual outcome, often in a decisive fashion. The Kauai study (Werner et al., 1968, 1971) longitudinally surveyed the medical and developmental progress from infancy onward of all children born in one year on that Hawaiian island. The study demonstrated the striking extent to which social and family factors exacerbate or ameliorate the influence of organic factors. One group of infants had suffered severe perinatal stress. At 20 months of age, those youngsters had lower IQ scores than the nonstressed group. However, when stressed infants with stable families, high SES, or mothers with high IQ were compared to children with normal birth histories, the test difference was only 5 to 7 points. In contrast, when the environmental conditions included unstable families, low SES, or mothers with low IQ, then the infants with perinatal complications scored 19 to 37 points *below* those with normal birth histories. The entire cohort was studied again at 10 years of age; at that point, the presence of intellectual, physical, or behavior problems correlated far more strongly with poor early environment than it did with the presence of perinatal complications. Thus, as childhood progresses, the importance of perinatal risk factors seems to diminish or even to disappear because more potent familial and socioeconomic factors exert an ameliorating or exacerbating influence.

Congenital cytomegalovirus infection provides another striking demonstration of the extent to which environmental factors modulate the impact of organic pathology (Sameroff, 1986). Occurring most frequently in the infants of teenage mothers with low SES, this prenatal infection occurs in about 1% of U.S. infants. Compared with noninfected controls, the infected infants as a group show lower IQ scores and a higher incidence of later neurological deficits. However, if the infected and control groups are broken down by SES, only the low-SES infected children appear vulnerable to reduced IQ relative to their uninfected peers. When infected and noninfected middle-class children were compared, no IQ differences appeared.

Other studies have demonstrated that poverty amplifies the intellectual deficits of vulnerable infants (Stein & Susser, 1971). Poor children who had scored low on infant IQ tests at 8 months continued to do so at 4 years. High-SES children, however, showed little correlation between these 8-month and 4-year scores. Further, by 4 years of age, the high-SES children who had been in the *lowest* IQ quartile at 8 months were doing better than the low-SES children who had been in the *highest* IQ quartile at 8 months.

PREVENTION AND TREATMENT

Primary Prevention

Recent advances in prenatal diagnosis and increased understanding of inherited metabolic disorders have improved primary prevention of many types of genetically determined mental retardation. It is now possible to identify asymptomatic carriers of recessive genes for Tay-Sachs disease, phenylketonuria, and a host of other inherited metabolic disorders, as well as carriers of mosaic trisomies. The increased risk of Down syndrome with advanced maternal age is now widely appreciated. Fetuses with inherited metabolic diseases and chromosomal abnormalities can frequently be identified prenatally by amniocentesis, and abortion is now a clinical option for individuals who find it ethically acceptable.

Good maternal nutrition, abstinence from drugs and alcohol, and adequate prenatal and obstetrical care are important in preventing prenatal and perinatal causes of retardation, as is immunization against rubella or confirmation of immune status prior to conception. The early identification and treatment of infantile jaundice can prevent significant retardation and cerebral palsy due to kernicterus. The prevention of pica, removal of lead-based paint from homes, and lead screening for children at risk (examining lead levels in hair and blood) are necessary to eliminate lead poisoning as a cause of retardation. Many retarded children have pica; ongoing vigilance against lead poisoning is needed with such children to prevent further neurological damage.

The primary prevention of sociocultural retardation lies beyond the scope of the medical profession alone. Adequate food, housing, medical care, and schooling are all necessary. Increased parental interest and involvement in the informal and formal aspects of children's learning are important. Developmentally sound day care and Head Start preschool programs are effective intervention methods that can produce short-term gains in young children's IQs and first-grade academic progress. However, the rapidity with which these cognitive gains wash out, in many cases within a year or two following the end of the program, gives testimony to the difficulty of effective long-term intervention in the face of pervasive environmental deprivation (Holden, 1990). Long-term intervention projects that identify at-risk children at an early age seem the most promising. For example, the Milwaukee Project (Garber & Heber, 1977) provided structured cognitive and language stimulation beginning at age 3 months for deprived children who had mothers with IQs below 80. This intervention produced striking and persistent improvements in the children's IQs. Similarly, in his classic studies, Skeels (1966) demonstrated that removing young children from the deprived conditions of certain orphanages to more nurturant and stimulating placements produced improvements in IQ and social adjustment that persisted into adulthood. During the same time frame, the IQ scores of unremoved controls deteriorated.

Secondary Prevention

Early detection of retardation through regular pediatric care and careful developmental surveillance is essential for optimal intervention. In many instances, prompt early treatment of medically and surgically correctable causes of retardation can minimize or prevent long-term pathology. Early detection and appropriate care are also important for the seizure disorders, motor handicaps, and visual and hearing defects that complicate many cases of retardation.

Early intervention programs such as special day care have beneficially affected the behavioral and cognitive progress of retarded children, particularly when combined with the training of parents in cognitive stimulation techniques. Such training helps increase parental involvement, while offsetting feelings of guilt. Similarly, behavioral modification techniques can shape language and self-help skills for more severely retarded children and reduce aggressive and stereotypic behavior. There have been promising results from training parents in the use of such methods.

Parents require long-term help concerning not only the specific medical, emotional, and educational needs of their retarded child, but also the familywide stresses created by such a child. Parental feelings of guilt and ambivalence are common, as are the tendencies toward overprotection or rejection. Normal siblings soon surpass the retarded child developmentally, and presently these more competent youngsters will come to resent or protect their retarded sibling. In either event, their inevitably complex feelings toward him must be taken into account. The ongoing availability of an informed and supportive clinician for advice or counseling around these issues is invaluable.

The retarded child's personality and behavioral style may play a greater role than his intellectual impairment in determining his ultimate level of social, educational, or vocational attainment. Consequently, the psychiatric care of the retarded is especially important (Szymanski, 1977). Paradoxically, many mental health facilities refuse to provide them with adequate services. Family, group, and individual psychotherapy are all feasible with the less severely retarded child, if due note is taken of the affected youngster's limited verbal and abstract capacities.

Stimulant medication may be useful for attention deficits and hyperactivity, whereas brief use of the phenothiazines is often helpful in treating psychotic, aggressive, or self-injurious behavior. (The dangers of oversedation and possible increased risk of tardive dyskinesias in brain-damaged individuals should be noted.) A few uncontrolled studies have also found lithium or the opiate antagonist naltrexone helpful for self-injurious behavior.

The decision to institutionalize a retarded child who is used to his own home is difficult and painful for both parents and clinician. For most retarded children, separation from home, parents, siblings and familiar surroundings is as stressful and traumatic as it is for the normal child. Most mildly and moderately retarded children probably make better cognitive progress in a supportive at-home environment than in the hospital.

Despite the present public policy emphasis on deinstitutionalization, the effect of an institution on children is not always deleterious; much depends on the specific home and hospital environment (Zigler & Balla, 1977a). Permanent institutionalization can often be avoided with an adequate spectrum of community-based supportive services, including short-term treatment facilities and short-term foster or respite care. Although some families may scapegoat or seek to extrude their retarded children, many more families have great difficulty in letting go. The decision to institutionalize often is forced on the family by some combination of profound retardation, parental age and illness, or severe behavior problems that do not respond to treatment or exceed the tolerance of the family and neighbors. In the face of the crisis of institutionalization, ongoing casework with families helps to minimize the trauma for both family and child. When placing a child in an institution is unavoidable, it may be difficult to select the best setting. In general, small well-staffed units that are run along family lines provide optimal care. Unfortunately, many public institutions for the retarded continue to have poor physical facilities and insufficient staff, who tend to be undertrained, inadequately motivated, and poorly compensated.

During the past 25 years, the emphasis on deinstitutionalization has led to a marked decline in the proportion of retarded persons in large institutions. In the period from 1970 to 1982, the institutionalized retarded population decreased from 190,000 to 120,000 (Zigler & Hodapp, 1986). A community-oriented philosophy of care has emphasized alternative placements such as group homes, halfway houses, sheltered workshops with dormitory living, and foster family care. However, such alternatives can succeed only with adequate community and family support (Schalock, Harper, & Genung, 1981); without such support deinstitutionalization may prove a bitterly empty promise. The Federal Education for All Handicapped Children Act (P.L. 94-142, 1975) has gone far in affirming the right of retarded children to an appropriate education in a least restrictive setting at public expense. However, the appropriateness of various types of institutional placements for different retarded persons remains an issue requiring empirical study (Zigler & Hodapp (1986)).

One of the clinician's most valuable roles is serving as an advocate for the child and family in their dealings with the school system concerning educational placement. The clinician can also help parents choose a suitable educational facility. What mix of special and mainstream instruction is optimal must be decided on an individual basis. Careful clinical assessment identifies the child's emotional and intellectual strengths and weaknesses, permitting the selection of a classroom situation that will neither overtax nor understimulate the child. The assessment can go far toward helping parents establish realistic educational and vocational expectations for their child.

Vocational planning and assistance in the areas of self-maintenance and the daily routines of living require a life-span perspective. Although many mildly retarded persons disappear from the statistics of the handicapped after leaving the demands of the school setting, at least 50% continue to have adjustment problems as adults (Zigler & Hodapp, 1986). Moderately and severely retarded young people face lifelong difficulties in self-maintenance. Many retarded young adults will outlive their parents, yet still will need a sheltered and protected environment.

Organized advocacy and consumer groups (such as the local and national Association for Retarded Citizens and the National Down's Syndrome Congress) provide invaluable support and are important sources of information concerning programs and resources.

APPENDIX 2-1
ORGANIC ABNORMALITIES ASSOCIATED WITH
RETARDATION*

Genetic Disorders

- *Inborn Errors of Metabolism.* A defect at a single gene locus causes disruption of a crucial metabolic pathway. Nearly a hundred such disorders have been identified, involving errors in the metabolism of various amino and organic acids, carbohydrates, and essential structural compounds (oligosaccharides, glycoproteins, and mucopolysaccharides) (Leroy, 1983). Many of these disorders, such as phenylketonuria, cogenital hypothyroidism, Tay-Sachs disease, and Lesch-Nyhan disease, cause progressive neurological disease or mental deficiency. Aminocentesis and special tissue culture techniques have made possible the prenatal diagnosis of a growing number of these conditions.
- *Other Single Gene Abnormalities.* These include muscular dystrophy and tuberous sclerosis.

Chromosomal Anomalies

In these aberrations part or all of a given chromosome is missing, duplicated, transposed to another chromosome, or otherwise abnormal in structure. Many conditions can cause such anomalies, including radiation, drugs and toxins, viruses, and advanced parental age (Gerald & Meryash, 1983). Chromosomal anomalies are responsible for about 10% of institutionalized persons with mental retardation.

- *Autosomal Trisomies.* The commonest chromosomal aberration, Down syndrome, is caused by an extra copy (or trisomy) of chromosome 21.
- *Autosomal Chromosomal Deletion Syndromes.* An example is deletion of the short arms of chromosome 5 (the *cri du chat* syndrome), characterized by retardation, facial anomalies, and the high-pitched infant cry from which it draws its name.
- *Multiple Sex Chromosome Syndromes.* An example is Klinefelter's syndrome (XXY), which is characterized by mild retardation and eunuchoid features at puberty.
- *Fragile X Syndrome.* The second commonest known genetic cause of retardation, fragile X syndrome is caused by a structural abnormality on the long arm of the X-chromosome.

---

*After Crocker & Nelson, 1985; Grossman, 1983.

Prenatal and Perinatal Difficulties

- *Prenatal Infections.* Cytomegalic inclusion disease, rubella, syphilis, and toxoplasmosis are the commonest infections related to retardation. In the future, congenital human immunodeficiency virus (HIV) infection will no doubt join this list.
- *Fetal Malnutrition.* Maternal malnutrition or placental insufficiency are the usual causes.
- *Toxins.* Examples are maternal medication, drug abuse, or alcohol abuse.
- *Perinatal Difficulties.* These include prematurity, hypoxia, intracranial hemorrhage, neonatal jaundice. Cerebral palsy or hydrocephalus may be a concomitant.

Acquired Childhood Disease

- *Infections.* Examples are viral encephalitis, bacterial meningitis.
- *Accidents.* Examples are cranial trauma, drowning.
- *Toxins.* Examples are lead, mercury, carbon monoxide.

Chapter 3

Schizophrenia in Childhood and Adolescence, with an Overview of Childhood Psychosis

INTRODUCTION AND DIAGNOSTIC CONSIDERATIONS

Among the most striking and tragic children seen by the child psychiatrist are those labeled as suffering from *childhood psychosis* or *childhood schizophrenia*. This heterogeneous group of severely and pervasively disturbed children shows serious developmental deviations in the cognitive, perceptual, emotional, and interpersonal spheres.

The classification of such children continues to cause confusion and controversy. Under the rubric of *childhood psychosis,* different authors have included notably disparate groups of children. In the past, for example, the term might have referred to both a mute, retarded autistic child with no meaningful social interaction and an intelligent, verbal child with bizarre preoccupations, delusions, and intense, ambivalently chaotic social attachments. Even in adult psychiatry the term *psychosis* is poorly defined; when applied to children, it has traditionally implied severe and pervasive disturbance, especially in the sphere of relatedness to people. With children, however, the term historically has not necessarily carried the connotation of impaired reality testing or formal thought disorder that it does with adults.

Before examination of these diagnostic controversies, it is useful to consider the diverse symptoms that such children may present. A working group of British child psychiatrists under the leadership of Creak (1961) compiled one of the most influential and broadly inclusive summaries about 30 years ago. This group attempted to define the then-current usage of the term *child psychosis* by detailing the various features of children to whom the label had been applied. Their list included:

1. *Gross and Sustained Impairment of Emotional Relationships.* Behavior is characterized by aloofness, empty clinging, and abnormal behavior toward other people as persons.

2. *Apparent Unawareness of Their Personal Identity.* Abnormal behaviors toward self, such as posturing and scrutinizing parts of the body, are common. The presence of repeated self-directed aggression, even to the point of injury, and confusion of personal pronouns may also represent an unintegrated sense of personal identity.

3. *Pathological Preoccupation with Particular Objects Without Regard to Their Conventional Use.*

4. *Sustained Resistance to Change in the Environment.* The child strives to maintain sameness, using repetitive behaviors that may produce a state of perceptual monotony.

A portion of Chapter 3 is adapted from "Disturbances in Early Adolescent Development," by J. D. Noshpitz, in S. I. Greenspan and G. H. Pollock (Eds.), *The Course of Life: Psychoanalytic Contributions Toward Understanding Personality Development,* Vol. II, 1980, pp. 309–356. Washington, D.C.: NIMH (U.S. Government Printing Office).

5. *Abnormal Perceptual Experience.* The child demonstrates excessive, diminished, or unpredictable responses to sensory stimuli.

6. *Acute, Excessive, and Seemingly Illogical Anxiety.* It may be precipitated by change in routine, material environment, or temporary interruption of symbiotic attachments to persons or things. Apparently commonplace objects may become invested with terrifying qualities, whereas an appropriate sense of fear in the face of real dangers may be lacking.

7. *Distortions in Motility Patterns.* Common manifestations are immobility, bizarre posturing, or ritualistic mannerisms, such as the child's rocking and spinning himself or objects.

Three additional symptom areas were less uniform and controversy continues regarding the appropriate diagnostic categorization of these children.

8. *Language Disorder.* The British group specified that such children show "speech that has been lost or never acquired or that failed to develop beyond a level appropriate to an earlier stage. There may be confusion of personal pronouns, echolalia, or other mannerisms of use and diction. Although words or phrases may be uttered, they may convey no sense of ordinary communication" (Creak, 1961, p. 890). As discussed below, however, there are also children who are quite fluent and whose peculiarities of speech do not lie predominantly in the area of syntax or communicative intent. Instead, their speech, much like that of the adult schizophrenic, is striking in its looseness of associations and bizarre content.

9. *Level of Overall Intellectual Functioning.* The British group was impressed that most psychotic children showed "a background of serious retardation in which islets of normal, near-normal, or exceptional intellectual function may appear" (Creak, 1961). Although this description is true for many such children, others have apparently normal intelligence (although their disturbed relatedness may pose serious obstacles to adequate testing).

10. *Symptoms Similar to Those of Adult Schizophrenia.* A final controversial area (not included in the British group's discussion) is the presence or absence of *defective reality testing* with *hallucinations* or *delusions* and a *formal thought disorder* characterized by incoherence or marked loosening of associations (tangential thinking). Ascertaining whether a child has such symptoms is possible only if the child has reached a sufficiently mature chronological and mental age to allow adequate evaluation and has enough intelligible speech to permit the necessary communication.

DEFINITION

Different authors have proposed a bewildering array of classificatory schemes for these seriously disturbed children (Cantor et al., 1982; Fish & Ritvo, 1979; Kolvin, 1971; Kolvin et al., 1971; Tanguay & Asarnow, 1986). The nosology of these disorders continues to be highly controversial. Several crucial issues are at stake in the seemingly contradictory assertions made by various authorities.

A major axis of dissension concerns the relationship of the various forms of childhood psychosis both to adult schizophrenia and to each other. The two major camps might be termed the "lumpers" and the "splitters." In the opinion of the lumpers, who include such writers as Bender (1947), Fish (1977), and Goldfarb (1970), the clinical presentations of childhood psychosis represent the variable phenotypic manifestations of a single basic underlying disease process similar to or identical to the fundamental defect in adult schizophrenia. From this viewpoint, a similar pathogenic process is presumed at work in both the autistic child who, from infancy on, has shown a profound aloofness and little social language, and the more classically schizophrenic child who develops hallucinations in the school years, after a long period of deviant emotional and cognitive development. Implicit in such a perspective is a rather broad definition of schizophrenia. Thus, as early as 1906, De Sanctis (1906/1971) applied the term *dementia praecoccissima* to children with a mixed picture of developmental lags, intellectual deficits, inappropriate affect, social isolation, bizarre behavior, and language abnormalities (such as echolalia). Similarly, Bender (1971) saw schizophrenia in children as "the same process as schizophrenia in adulthood" (p. 651). She defined it broadly as:

> A clinical entity, occurring in childhood before the age of eleven years, which reveals pathology in behavior at every level and in every area of integration and patterning within the functioning of the central nervous system, be it vegetative, motor, perceptual, intellectual, emotional, or social. (p. 40)

In contrast to the lumpers, the splitters, such as Rutter (1972) and Kolvin (1971), believe that criteria such as age of onset and the presence or absence of hallucinations, delusions or thought disorder can phenomenologically define discrete groups of psychotic children. Beginning in 1943, Kanner described a group of dramatically disturbed children characterized by what he termed "an inborn autistic disturbance of affective contact." Although the children showed a variety of linguistic and motor peculiarities, Kanner believed their cardinal symptoms stemmed from "a powerful desire for aloneness" (p. 249) and "an anxiously obsessive desire for the maintenance of sameness" (p. 245). Kanner came to regard this condition as distinct from both retardation and childhood schizophrenia. After studying several series of psychotic children categorized by age of onset of psychosis, Rutter and Lockyer (1967) and Kolvin (1971) concluded that children with very early onset were quite different clinically from those with later onset. The early-onset group symptomatically resembled Kanner's autistic children. Furthermore, they rarely developed hallucinations, delusions, or thought disorder and had a low frequency of schizophrenia among family members. Compared to the later-onset group, children with early-onset had an increased prevalence of mental retardation, perinatal risk factors, EEG abnormalities, and seizures. In contrast, the late-onset group had hallucinations, delusions, and thought disorder similar to adult schizophrenics as well as a higher prevalence of schizophrenia among family members. On this basis, the splitters concluded that the early-onset psychoses are not related to adult schizophrenia and should be regarded as a separate category (Lotter, 1978; Rutter, 1978). These authors proposed that children who had been labeled psychotic actually fell into three distinct categories:

1. Early-onset infantile autism.
2. Late-onset "pervasive developmental disturbances" without hallucinations, delusions, or thought disorder.
3. Schizophrenia with hallucinations, delusions, or thought disorder, occurring in childhood.

In their view, each condition represented a clinically and presumably etiologically distinct diagnostic entity with its own genetics, epidemiology, and clinical course.

The "splitting" camp strongly influenced the DSM-III (APA, 1980) diagnostic schema that was adopted after much debate and revision; this schema eliminated a unitary notion of childhood psychosis altogether. In its place, the DSM-III nosology recognized three entities:

1. *Infantile Autism.* Characterized by early onset (before 30 months); pervasive lack of social responsiveness; gross deficits in the social use of language; and bizarre responses to the environment (cases with delusions, hallucinations, or thought disorders excluded).
2. *Childhood-Onset Pervasive Development Disorder.* Characterized by late onset (after 30 months); impaired social relationships; primitive anxiety; inappropriate affect; cognitive rigidity; and motor, sensory, and linguistic abnormalities (cases with delusions, hallucinations, or thought disorders excluded).
3. *Schizophrenia (initially appearing in childhood).* Defined by the standard DSM-III adult criteria, including delusions, hallucinations, or formal thought disorder.

The classification of these disorders has recently been revised again in DSM-III-R (APA, 1987), a change that many professionals feel is premature. The criteria for Schizophrenia (initially appearing in childhood) remain essentially those of the adult disorders. For several reasons, however, Infantile Autism and Childhood-Onset Pervasive Developmental Disorder have been folded into a single, broader condition called *Autistic Disorder.* First, age of reported onset proved to be a poor criterion. The age when symptoms are first noted (or recalled to have first occurred) appears to depend as much on the degree of parental sophistication or denial as on the intrinsic nature or severity of the disease process (Volkmar et al., 1985b). With careful retrospective study, early deviations in development are almost always found (D.J.Cohen et al., 1986a). Second, the difference between the two disorders appeared to be more a matter of severity than of kind (Dahl et al., 1986); in practice, cases often could not easily be assigned to one or the other (Waterhouse et al., 1983).

The two current DSM-III-R categories are thus:

1. Schizophrenia (initially appearing in childhood).
2. Autistic Disorder.

DSM-III-R Diagnostic Criteria for Schizophrenia (Abridged)

A. *Presence of characteristic psychotic symptoms in the active phase: either (1), (2), or (3) for at least one week (unless the symptoms are successfully treated):*
   (1) *two of the following*
      (a) *delusions*
      (b) *prominent hallucinations (throughout the day for several days or several times a week for several weeks, each hallucinatory experience not being limited to a few brief moments)*
      (c) *incoherence or marked loosening of associations*
      (d) *catatonic behavior*
      (e) *flat or grossly inappropriate affect*
   (2) *bizarre delusions (i.e., involving a phenomenon that the person's culture would regard as totally implausible, e.g., thought broadcasting, being controlled by a dead person)*
   (3) *prominent hallucinations [as defined in (1)(b) above] of a voice with content having no apparent relation to depression or elation, or a voice keeping up a running commentary on the person's behavior or thoughts, or two or more voices conversing with each other*

B. *During the course of the disturbance, functioning in such areas as work, social relations, and self-care is markedly below the highest level achieved before onset of the disturbance (or, when the onset is in childhood or adolescence, failure to achieve expected level of social development).*

C. *Schizoaffective Disorder and Mood Disorder with Psychotic Features have been ruled out.*

D. *Continuous signs of the disturbance for at least six months.*

E. It cannot be established that an organic factor initiated and maintained the disturbance.

F. If there is a history of Autistic Disorder, the additional diagnosis of Schizophrenia is made only if prominent delusions or hallucinations are also present. (APA, 1987, pp. 194–195)

DSM-III-R Diagnostic Criteria for Autistic Disorder

These include qualitative impairment in reciprocal social interaction; impairment in verbal and nonverbal communication and imaginative activity; and marked restriction and peculiarities of activities and interests; with onset during infancy or childhood. (For detailed DSM-III-R criteria for autistic disorder, see Chapter 4, "Infantile Autism.")

Whether the DSM-III's diagnostic approach is valid is a question for ongoing study (D. J. Cohen et al., 1986; Dahl et al., 1986; Waterhouse et al., 1983). The clarity with which the DSM-III treats this area is, however, spurious (Cantor et al., 1982; Tanguay, 1982). In clinical practice it may be difficult to tell when bizarre ideas, preoccupations, phobias, or obsessions become extreme enough to warrant being labeled delusions (Volkmar et al., 1986; Rumsey et al., 1985).

The presence or absence of hallucinations may also be difficult to determine, especially in a nonverbal child (Wing & Attwood, 1987). The illogical, tangential thought and incoherent speech of verbal autistic children may resemble the formal thought disorder of schizophrenia.

In addition, many intermediate, difficult-to-classify cases exist (Howells & Guirguis, 1984). Some of these patients resemble the children described by earlier workers as suffering from "atypical personality development" (Rank, 1949, 1955), Asperger's syndrome (Volkmar et al., 1985a; Wing, 1981b), symbiotic psychosis (Mahler, 1952), schizoid (Wolff & Barlow, 1979), and borderline children (Robson, 1983) (see Chapters 4 and 5).

In addition, the DSM-III-R category of Schizotypal Personality Disorder may apply to many of the children, at least at some point during their development. Such children are characterized by oddities of speech, poorly modulated anxiety, and inappropriate or constricted affect that interferes with normal social relationships. They also show peculiarities of thought, such as bizarre preoccupations, beliefs, or fantasies that are not sufficiently severe to be called delusions or hallucinations. This diagnostic category may also apply to some patients who later go on to develop full-blown schizophrenic symptoms (McGlashan, 1986a). On the other hand, it may also represent a condition that is stable and does not further decompensate. The notion of a "schizophrenic spectrum" of disorders has evolved to include conditions like *schizotypal personality disorder,* which shares several diagnostic criteria of schizophrenia (especially the prodromal ones (Baron et al., 1985;

Kendler, 1985). This concept implies that such a disorder represents either a milder (*forme fruste*) phenotypic expression of a presumed schizophrenic genotype or else an attenuated genetic loading for the disorder. Congruent with this notion, schizotypal personality disorder has a higher prevalence in families of schizophrenics than of controls (Kendler, 1986; Kendler & Tsuang, 1988). The genetic relationship of the other atypical cases to schizophrenia proper is still unknown.

DSM-III-R Diagnostic Criteria for Schizotypal Personality Disorder

A. *A pervasive pattern of deficits in interpersonal relatedness and peculiarities of ideation, appearance, and behavior, beginning by early adulthood and present in a variety of contexts, as indicated by at least* five *of the following:*

   (1) ideas of reference (excluding delusions of reference)

   (2) excessive social anxiety, e.g., extreme discomfort in social situations involving unfamiliar people

   (3) odd beliefs or magical thinking, influencing behavior and inconsistent with subcultural norms, e.g., superstitiousness, belief in clairvoyance, telepathy, or "sixth sense," "others can feel my feelings" (in children and adolescents, bizarre fantasies or preoccupations)

   (4) unusual perceptual experiences, e.g., illusions, sensing the presence of a force of person not actually present (e.g., "I felt as if my dead mother were in the room with me")

   (5) odd or eccentric behavior or appearance, e.g., unkempt, unusual mannerisms, talks to self

   (6) no close friends or confidants (or only one) other than first-degree relatives

   (7) odd speech (without loosening of associations or incoherence), e.g., speech that is impoverished, digressive, vague, or inappropriately abstract

   (8) inappropriate or constricted affect, e.g., silly, aloof, rarely reciprocates gestures or facial expressions, such as smiles or nods

   (9) suspiciousness or paranoid ideation

B. *Occurrence not exclusively during the course of Schizophrenia or a Pervasive Developmental Disorder.* (APA, 1987, pp. 341–342)

Although there are reservations about the DSM-III treatment of childhood psychosis, for expository purposes this volume follows the DSM-III-R (APA, 1987) in splitting off autistic disorder as a separate descriptive entity (see Chapter 4 "Infantile Autism"). The balance of this chapter deals with schizophrenia first appearing in childhood. The term *childhood schizophrenia* in this volume refers to the DSM-III-R's restricted notion of *schizophrenia with childhood onset*. Because the bulk of the clinical literature that predates the DSM-III often fails to define precisely the criteria used in diagnosing childhood psychoses, much of the discussion that follows may also apply to the atypical categories discussed above. Schizotypal personality disorder is discussed further in Chapter 5, "Borderline Children."

EPIDEMIOLOGY

Prepubertal schizophrenia is rare. Although pre-DSM-III studies suggested a prevalence rate among 2- to 12-year-olds of 1.4–4.5 cases per 10,000, a more recent study using DSM-III criteria found a low prevalence of only 0.19 cases per 10,000 (Burd & Kerbeshian, 1987). About 72% of children with onset of schizophrenia under age 15 years are male; males also appear to have an earlier onset (Kallman & Roth, 1956).

With puberty, schizophrenia becomes much more common. In England, age-specific hospital admission rates for schizophrenia rise from about 0.1 per 10,000 under 15 years of age to about 2.5 per 10,000 between the ages of 15 and 20 (Holzman & Grinker, 1977).

The differential diagnosis of adolescent psychosis is often difficult (Aarkroog & Mortensen, 1985; Feinstein & Miller, 1979; Steinberg, 1985); schizophrenia is but one of several possible diagnoses. Psychotic disorders comprise about 1% to 5% of adolescent psychiatric cases (Steinberg, 1985). In one of the few general population surveys, 0.54% of all teenagers in one Swedish town were hospitalized for a psychotic disorder sometime during the 13- to 19-year-old age period; criteria included one or more of the following symptoms: hallucinations; delusions; formal thought disorder; confusion with loss of sense of time, place, or person; mania; or major depression with mood-congruent psychotic features (as defined in DSM-III) (Gillberg et al., 1986). The prevalence rate rose from a low of 0.9 cases per 10,000 among the 13-year-olds to a peak of 17.6 per 10,000 among the 18-year-olds. The breakdown by diagnostic category was schizophrenia, 41.0%; major affective disorder, 27.9% (approximately half being psychotic depressions and half bipolar disorders); substance-induced disorder, 21.3%; and atypical psychosis, 9.8%.

Most childhood schizophrenics do not have schizophrenic parents. Nonetheless, the relatively high prevalence of adult schizophrenics implies that their offspring constitute a very large group of children at risk for schizophreniclike disorders, even though many schizophrenics do not have children. By their adult years, about 10% of the offspring of schizophrenics develop schizophrenia, and an additional number develop other "schizophrenia spectrum disorders" such as schizotypal personality disorder. In general, although the most vulnerable 10% to 30% of offspring of schizophrenics manifest pathology from middle childhood, it is rare for frank schizophrenic symptomatology to appear before adolescence.

CLINICAL FEATURES

The Early Development of Schizophrenic Individuals

Current knowledge of the early development of individuals who later become schizophrenic comes from three types of studies. The first approach is to gather data retrospectively about patients who have developed schizophrenia in adolescence or adulthood. Such retrospective data has serious limitations. Patient and parents' recollections obtained after the onset of illness may be subject to distortion. *Follow-back* data, which consist of retrospectively reviewed school and clinical records, home movies, and similar data, are undistorted by the vagaries of memory but are often incomplete and unstandardized. The second approach involves studying offspring of schizophrenic parents. This *high-risk* strategy makes it possible to study prospectively the development of vulnerable individuals at increased risk for developing schizophrenia. The third approach to shedding light on the early developmental course of the disorder is to study individuals with onset of schizophrenia during childhood.

All three types of study suggest that many, but not all, individuals who develop the pathognomonic symptoms of schizophrenia in childhood or adolescence will have displayed earlier signs of disturbed development, often from infancy on (Cantor, 1988; Eggers, 1989; Russell et al., 1989; Watkins et al., 1988). Common early difficulties include soft neurological signs and disturbances in cognition, language, socialization and the regulation of affect, anxiety, and autonomic functioning (J. Asarnow, 1988; Erlenmeyer-Kimling & Cornblatt, 1987a; Fish, 1986, 1987; Kron & Kestenbaum, 1988; Nuechterlein, 1986). However, it remains unclear how specific these early problems are for subsequent schizophrenia (as opposed to later psychopathology in general).

High-Risk Studies: Offspring of Schizophrenic Parents.
About 10% to 12% of the offspring of schizophrenics subsequently also develop schizophrenia, generally in adolescence or adulthood. Studying these offspring to identify predictors of subsequent schizophrenic decompensation has proven to be a promising research strategy. Several samples of vulnerable offspring have been followed into the period of greatest risk for developing schizophrenia (J. Asarnow, 1988; Marcus et al., 1985a, 1985b, 1987; Watt et al., 1984); Fish (1977, 1986, 1987) has followed some of her subjects for up to 35 years. Fish's cohort was unusual in that two offspring were diagnosed as schizophrenic as early as 10 years of age.

A variety of early neuromaturational abnormalities have been inconsistently associated with later schizophrenia (J. Asarnow, 1988). Fish (1977, 1986, 1987) described an irregular maturational pattern, which she termed *pandevelopmental* retardation. From the first few months of life on, the most vulnerable children showed a strikingly disorganized pattern in the timing and integration of neurological maturation, with fluctuations in the rate of physical and perceptual motor development. These shifting rates resulted in marked upward and downward swings in the infants' developmental quotients over a few months' time. Other studies have found preschizophrenic infants to be abnormally quiet, underactive, flaccid with abnormal "doughy" muscle tone, and impaired sensory motor coordination. Some children may show extreme sensitivity to certain sensory modalities (Bergman & Escalona, 1949). As infants, children who later develop schizophrenia may have more difficult temperaments and show abnormal patterns of interactions with their mothers. Nonspecific factors, such as maternal psychopathology and socioeconomic status, also influence patterns of mother–child interaction, however.

By early and middle childhood, many children of schizophrenics already show disturbed behavior and impaired social functioning, as well as persistent neurointegrative problems. These children may form few friendships and are regarded negatively by teachers and peers because of passive, irritable, immature, negativistic, or labile behavior. As adolescents, these vulnerable children often show poor affective control and ongoing social isolation.

Preschizophrenic children manifest cognitive and attentional anomalies. Their verbal IQ is often lower than their performance IQ (Green & Deutsch, 1990; Kron & Kestenbaum, 1988; Nuechterlein, 1986). The most specific predictors of later schizophrenic difficulties in the offspring of schizophrenics appear to be impaired attention and information processing, as measured on complex tests of sustained focused attention with high processing demands (Cornblatt & Erlenmeyer-Kimling, 1985; Erlenmeyer-Kimling & Cornblatt, 1987a, 1987b; Erlenmeyer-Kimling et al., 1984).

Because the nonspecific effects of a parent with severe parental psychopathology may be difficult to disentangle from the genetic and environmental impact of schizophrenia, it is necessary to interpret data from high-risk studies of the offspring of schizophrenics with caution. In addition, it may not be possible to generalize across the different subject groups. About 90% of schizophrenics do *not* have a schizophrenic parent. It is thus not clear to what extent conclusions drawn from the study of high-risk individuals are applicable to the larger group of preschizophrenic individuals who do not have schizophrenic parents. Similarly, only a very small number of offspring of schizophrenics develop schizophrenia prior to adolescence. Hence, the applicability of the findings from high-risk studies to childhood-onset schizophrenia is also unclear.

The Early Development of Childhood-Onset Schizophrenics. The onset of childhood schizophrenia is generally insidious, although a few children display apparently normal development until an illness or psychological trauma seems to trigger acute symptoms. In most cases, serious developmental difficulties have been present from infancy onward (Cantor, 1988; Eggers, 1978; Kydd and Werry, 1982; Russell et al., 1989; Volkmar et al., 1988; Watkins et al., 1988).

Motor development may be abnormal with delays, incoordination, poor motor tone, and unusual mannerisms. Sensory preoccupations, such as perseverative smelling, may exist alongside sensory hypersensitivities, such as hyperacusis.

Attention and circadian rhythms may be disturbed. Infants and toddlers who later develop schizophrenia in childhood may spend long periods staring at or perseveratively manipulating various objects on which they fix their attention. On the other hand, at the toddler stage, they may wander aimlessly about, flitting from one activity to another.

The abnormality of these children's interactions with parents and peers often becomes increasingly apparent in the preschool years. Their affect may be labile, constricted, or inappropriate, with moments of inexplicable laughing or smiling. These children form few friendships and are avoided (or in later grades teased) by schoolmates. They have difficulty with cooperative play and possess few social skills; these deficits stem in part from a lack of empathy and a striking failure to appreciate that others have feelings, opinions, and preferences of their own.

Premorbidly and prodromally, schizophrenic children may suffer from excessive social anxiety and suspiciousness (Watkins et al., 1988). Thus, chaotic, fragmented behavior may fluctuate between clinging and hostility. Poorly modulated anxiety also manifests itself in unusual fears, severe panic attacks, or seemingly unprovoked tantrums. Bender (1947) believed that persistent, pervasive, and disorganizing anxiety in childhood was virtually pathognomonic of childhood schizophrenia.

The early language of most schizophrenic children is either delayed or disturbed (Cantor, 1988; Watkins et al., 1988). Language processing and usage are deviant in several ways. Language may be delayed, sparse, and limited to short utterances, or it may be fluent but overelaborative with excessive, poorly related details. Associations may be loose and difficult to follow, as when words are linked by rhyming or assonance ("clang associations"). Abnormalities in word usage may reflect not only word-finding difficulties but also deviant categorization or idiosyncratic concept formation. Neologisms are frequent, syntax may be disordered, and the use of personal pronouns is often abnormal. Illogical thinking may also be apparent in contradictory assertions and hard-to-follow jumps in reasoning (Caplan et al., 1989).

Beyond these formal defects, the social use of language by such children is usually also deviant. Language may be noncommunicative because it is muttered or echolalic. Context may be disturbed or incomprehensible to anyone who does not know the child intimately. Prosody, pitch, and intonation may all be unusual and poorly modulated.

Cognitive abnormalities are often apparent in the form of magical thinking, perseveration, ritualistic behavior, and unusual preoccupations. As the child grows older, these preoccupations may become increasingly bizarre and morbid; they often concern the child's bodily functions or involve machines, ghosts, or monsters. Such children may show a precocious intellectual grasp in the area of their usual preoccupations; behind their concerns, an anxious involvement with aggression, fragmentation, death, and devitalization is usually readily apparent. Pervasive rituals, obsessions, and compulsions may serve to fend off primitive anxiety and aggressive concerns. As preschoolers, their tantrums, bizarre rituals, and preoccupations are far more extreme than those of the normal preschooler. Such children may strenuously resist or react catastrophically to changes in diet, schedule, or physical setting. Cantor (1988), for example, described a preschizophrenic toddler who screamed for hours when his mother attempted to replace the calculator that he regularly took to bed with a teddy bear.

Given their premorbid impairments in a wide range of adaptive realms, it is not surprising that schizophrenic children show a generally poor overall premorbid adjustment, even when compared with other psychiatrically impaired children, such as those with a depressive disorder (Asarnow & Ben-Meir, 1988).

Pathognomonic Symptoms of Schizophrenia

Despite the presence of nonspecific difficulties and vulnerabilities from the earliest years of life, the pathognomonic signs of schizophrenia—delusions, hallucinations, and formal thought disorder—are rarely apparent before the age of 5 or 6 years. However, the onset of such symptoms as early as 3 years of age has been noted in a few cases (Russell et al., 1989).

Mahler (1968) described a group of children who, during the 2nd to 4th years of life, showed a sharp deterioration of behavior, which she termed *symbiotic psychosis*. It is not clear from her clinical description to what extent these children met the DSM-III criteria for schizophrenia. Although Mahler postulated constitutional vulnerabilities in these children, she saw their psychotic decompensation, which included panic attacks, desperate clinging behavior, bizarre preoccupations, and in some cases hallucinations, as a response to the stresses of the separation–individuation process in vulnerable toddlers who failed to differentiate from their mothers. Mahler regarded the symptoms, including hallucination, as attempts to reinstate and maintain a delusional omnipotent fusion with the mother.

Although the onset of hallucinations, delusions, and thought disorder may be acute, in most childhood schizophrenics it is insidious. It is frequently difficult to identify the exact moment at which fantastic or hypochondriacal preoccupations become bizarre or somatic delusions, or when extreme suspiciousness and sensitivity to slights cross the line and become persecutory delusions.

Auditory hallucinations are the commonest, followed by mixed visual and auditory types (Cantor et al., 1982; Kemph, 1987; Kolvin, 1971; Russell et al., 1989; Volkmar et al., 1988). Auditory hallucinations are usually of voices, often that of a relative, and contain upsetting tone or content such as insults or orders to "do bad things," including hurting or killing themselves or others. Visual hallucinations also often have ominous content, for example, ghosts, monsters, the devil. When hallucinating, children may look about in a distracted manner. Developmental and cognitive factors influence the form of these failures of reality testing. Fixed elaborated delusional systems are rare in latency children, although striking cases have been reported, such as Bettelheim's (1959) Joey, "the mechanical boy." Childhood themes of animals or monsters are more common than sexual concerns (Russell et al., 1989). With the approach of adolescence, delusional themes may be more abstract (Eggers, 1978). Adolescent schizophrenic patients often show more hallucinations, perplexity, preoccupation with internal stimuli, paranoia, and ambivalence than do prepubertal schizophrenics (Cantor et al., 1982).

CASE EXAMPLE

Sam, age 12, first came to psychiatric attention when he was brought to the emergency room by his schizophrenic mother for treatment of a cough. Although his mother did not report any concerns about his mental status, the emergency room staff noted that he was floridly hallucinating. He heard alternately the voices of Muhammed Ali and the Fonz, each of whom, he felt, had taken over half his body and were fighting for possession of him. He stared blankly or looked distractedly about the room where he hallucinated unfamiliar, malevolent faces glaring at him. He retained his urine and voiced fears that his voiding would poison the city. Speech was mumbled almost inaudibly and fragmented in content.

History was scanty, but teachers had noted that he was extremely shy, withdrawn, and "fell between the cracks" in class; they had not previously observed him hallucinating overtly or showing delusional behavior. Sam's family was riddled with severe chronic schizophrenia; father, mother, older brother, and three grandparents had all been hospitalized for schizophrenia and two relatives had spent their entire adult lives in mental hospitals. Despite several years of subsequent hospitalization, special education, and antipsychotic medication, Sam remained floridly psychotic and seemed unfortunately destined for a similar course.

The psychotic child's inner world—his fantasy life and emotionally colored images of himself and others—is chaotic, fragmented, and frightening

(Kernberg, 1979). Affects, such as guilt, anxiety, anger, or frustration are poorly modulated and frequently experienced as overwhelming, catastrophic, and even annihilatory. The results are often panic attacks or rageful tantrums that are really terror tantrums.

CASE EXAMPLE

David, age 11, would shriek or pummel himself whenever he made a mistake in a school problem. Frustrated by his poor dexterity, he would often pound to pieces his art projects or model kits that thwarted him. Given an after-school detention, he would immediately fly into a tantrum and "trash" his work area. After he had accidentally caused some minor damage to another child's toy, David rushed off in a panic and precipitiously smashed his own.

Images of the self and of others and the fantasied interactions between them are contradictory, primitive, and terrifying. Such children feel in danger of falling apart, fragmenting, exploding, or disappearing. Minor bodily injuries or even states of bodily tension seem to them cataclysmic.

CASE EXAMPLE

Mary, an 8-year-old schizophrenic girl, picked relentlessly at her scabs; when they bled, she would panic and shriek "I'll die!" or "My arm's falling off!"

At the same time, the child may feel himself to be dangerous and often tries to protect others from what he fears is his murderous rage.

CASE EXAMPLE

David (described above) accidentally kicked two teachers whom he liked while being restrained during a tantrum. He became even more panicky, wanting to know if he had killed them. Later that day he announced solemnly and contritely to his therapist, "I nearly caused the death of two innocent people today."

Concomitantly, the child often experiences other people as dangerous or persecutory because of his tremendous sense of vulnerability and the projective attribution of his own rage onto others. Such children do not experience castration anxiety only in reference to their genitals, but rather fear multiple mutilation or total body disintegration (Kernberg, 1979).

CASE EXAMPLE

Peter, a precociously bright 10-year-old special education student, hurt his finger in a ball game. He was panicky and told his teacher that he had been "assassinated, just like Indira Ghandi." When his parents attempted to trim his hair or nails, he would become terrified and fly into a tantrum. On one occasion he did not want to go on a field trip to an unfamiliar part of town for fear of "being assassinated."

The psychotic child may fear merging with others, especially those to whom he is close; on the other hand, he may experience minor disappointments by others (such as temporary unavailability or lapses in empathy) as overwhelming abandonment. He may fear endlessly falling (Winnicott, 1975) or disappearing. One articulate schizophrenic girl late in her therapy explained, "I feel like a piece of dust on a shelf, which someone is about to blow away."

CASE EXAMPLE

An 18-year-old schizophrenic boy explained that he could not permit himself to ejaculate while having intercourse with his girlfriend. "I'm a pistol that will go off and explode—we'll both disappear."

Separation anxiety may be experienced as fragmentation of the self.

CASE EXAMPLE

An 8-year-old schizophrenic boy became upset over his therapist's impending vacation. The boy wrapped himself, the therapist, and his favorite playroom toy together with a ball of twine so as to stay connected and not fall apart. Under similar circumstances, a schizophrenic 6-year-old announced that he was Jaws and would eat the therapist up (both to punish him for leaving and to keep him safe forever inside).

Similar to the normal attitudes of much younger children, psychotic children may regard their bodily products, such as feces, as being alive. They may become distraught at what they experience as the loss of part of themselves, or they may endow their saliva, urine, feces, or blood with magical properties.

CASE EXAMPLE

Mary (see Case Example on preceding page) would panic when constipated or suffering from diarrhea. At other times, she would smear her mucus or saliva on favorite staff members and murmur "You're mine."

In summary, schizophrenic children experience intense, primitive, and unmodulated anxieties (Ekstein, 1966). Among such primitive agonies, Winnicott (1965, 1975) included fears of fragmentation, complete isolation, annihilation, paralysis, and "having no relation to the body." As Stern (1985) observed, these psychotic states represent disruptions of the basic experiences of self-coherence, agency, self-continuity, and affectivity that constitute the sense of a core-self.

Schizophrenia in Adolescence

Prepubertal schizophrenia is rare; adolescence is the characteristic age of onset. Adolescents are prone to a host of other psychoses that may be initially difficult to distinguish from schizophrenia. They include affective psychoses associated with bipolar and depressive disorders; drug-induced psychoses; transient psychotic decompensations in borderline personality disorders; organic psychoses, including temporal lobe epilepsy; and acute confusional and schizophreniform reactions. Only about 25% of the cases of schizophrenia are correctly diagnosed at time of onset (Masterson, 1967).

Schizophrenia in adolescence may present in at least three patterns (Masterson, 1967): (1) a childhood schizophrenic condition exacerbated by puberty; (2) an insidiously developing disturbance in a child with significant vulnerability; and (3) an acute decompensation without previous significant psychopathology, often following a major stress or separation, such as going away to college.

Many adolescent schizophrenics have histories of emotional difficulties prior to the onset of psychosis, such as excessive worries, fearfulness, and shyness (Hellgren et al., 1987). In grade school, the girls are often moody, introverted, and passive, whereas in high school preschizophrenic boys are often increasingly unpleasant, aggressive, and self-centered (Watt, 1978). Such children are also more likely to have a history of attentional and motor-perceptual difficulties, neuromuscular problems, and other neuro-developmental problems. Stressors such as loss of a parent prior to adolescence may also be more common (Hellgren et al., 1987).

The onset of schizophrenic symptoms apparently represents the response of an inherently predisposed ego to the developmental and maturational stresses inherent in adolescence (Kestenbaum, 1985). (The neurobiological determinants of overt psychotic symptoms are discussed further below.) The developmental stresses of adolescence include the psychobiological changes associated with pubertal sexual development as well as the increased adaptational demands posed by high school graduation, vocational pressures, or departure from home for college. Developmental factors may combine with external demands so that the vulnerable ego begins to fail to cope, leading to behavioral maladjustment that begets negative social responses and hence more stress. A downward spiral ends with the appearance of psychosis.

Of the varying modes of onset, the most common is the acute outbreak of symptoms. There can also be a gradual onset with a slow progressive slipping away from reality into a more and more withdrawn lifestyle. Not infrequently, the onset appears as a turning toward aggressive acting-out, and the patient is considered to be, and all too often is managed as, a delinquent. In any case, there is a loss of boundaries, a cloudiness about the body outlines, a loosening of the ego's perimeter, and a sense of withdrawal from people and external reality. Things slide and slip; thoughts and daydreams become as real or more real than external perceptual elements. The patient loses the distinction between the two and responds to his mind's creations and to the distortions he has introduced into his perceptual world. He experiences the fragile boundaries of his ego as open and vulnerable; sights, sounds, meanings intrude with enormous force; sounds reverberate strangely with hints of inner dread; visual images are too sharp; the boundaries are less a defensive perimeter than a ravaged no-man's-land.

Initially, the youngster has some awareness that the real world is slipping away and seeks to cope by sharpening his sensibilities; he hears more clearly, sees more brightly, feels all keyed up. His affects come in gusts with intense rushes of emotion; sexual fantasies dance before his eyes; he feels curiously alive. At the same time, he is less able to sleep; a sense of dread or imminence hovers over him; something is about to happen. Then his thoughts gain ever greater autonomy; they march alone and in unusual forms. He begins to note strange phenomena (ideas of reference). People are signaling, laughing about him, or trying to influence him. He becomes frightened because he is being menaced, insulted, threatened, hounded and makes all sorts of restitutive attempts to overcome his losses. One kind of youth flails out at the environment and becomes a delinquent; another child may take a mystical, philosophical, or religious turn and have a sense of moving into another plane. Great forces are at work in the world, and the child begins to seek and find evidence for them.

As the youngster senses that the ego's basic structure is crumbling, losing its boundaries, he attempts to construct a logical explanation for what is happening based on delusional formations. Now it all makes sense; he understands. The pseudologic of magical thinking permits him to regain some coherence and reduce his overwhelming anxiety. In effect, he has regrouped at an infantile level of ego development and object relations where self and others flow into one another, and he loses, in large measure, the distinction between what is inside and outside the self. Distancing devices come into play, and he feels far from his own affective life. As the ego loses its integrity, islands of function, isolated identifications, voices from the superego, memories, and fantasies may become tangible; they speak to him or appear visually. It is hard to put thoughts together because ideas are blocked or running too fast and without control.

In the face of this enormous threat the youngster falls silent or becomes incoherent. More intellectual youths, with less ego fragmentation, feel a constant pressure to reorganize a sense of self and self-in-the-world. The adolescent may turn to vast generalizations about religion, philosophy, science, or political ideology and seek to make sense out of what is happening by addressing the forces implicit in the particular system. He is one with God; he is possessed by the devil; he is persecuted by communists or is losing himself in the great proletariat movement; he is partner to the third world mystique, involved in mystical union with unearthly forces, solving the Unified Field Theory, or lost in some other high-order abstraction. The combinations and permutations are endless, but the loss of a coherent distinction between inner and outer experience and between magical and rational thinking is universal.

The duration of the condition is highly variable. The acute state may resolve rapidly. In a few cases, however, generally those with poor premorbid histories and more pathological family background, the psychotic symptoms may be unremitting, requiring long-term hospitalization (McGlashan, 1986b). After the initial surge of symptoms, there is usually a gradual reintegration so that the florid psychotic manifestations presently disappear. Feinstein and Miller (1979) noted a postpsychotic phase characterized by progressive lessening of the vestiges of the illness, heightened vulnerability to stress, and particular fragility in the face of separation. In addition, apathy and postpsychotic depression may persist for some time (McGlashan, 1982). These residual disabilities may make it difficult for the youngster to work in school. Thus, after the overt psychosis clears, the slow process of reconsolidation may take as long as a year. It is a time for continued active treatment, often for continuing hospitalization, and it needs the most careful attention to allow for adequate emergence from the previous pathological state.

The prognosis may be best when onset is acute and the symptoms resolve rapidly, especially for inpatients with good premorbid social functioning; absence of blunted affect; and confusion, disorientation, or perplexity at the height of the psychotic episode (APA, 1987; Coryell & Tsuang, 1986). This acute stormy syndrome generally comes on abruptly with frightening behaviors that resemble major psychosis. The youngster is terrified, confused, depersonalized, and feels totally lost. He may transiently fail to recognize familiar people, assert that he no longer knows who he is, break up furniture, and act drunk without being drunk. Moments of perfect lucidity alternate with this wild, confused behavior. Often, however, no real thought disorder, true delusions, or hallucinations are present, and the reaction may clear up as abruptly as it appeared. Albeit frightening, such a reaction does not ordinarily lead to prolonged illness.

This *acute confusional syndrome* seems to come on as a consequence of massive developmental stresses; in effect, it represents a transient overwhelming of the defenses by the tide of impulse that comes with puberty. The existing ego structures simply cannot support the load, and for a while the whole apparatus is shaken. But the ego does not fragment, it recoups and reestablishes control, and, as a rule, the youngster seems to recover; he is frightened, but not otherwise damaged. The panicky agitation that accompanies the syndrome represents the fear of loss of control over the forbidden impulses as well as the response to the threat to the ego's basic integrity.

Under DSM-III-R, when reality testing is impaired or a thought disorder is present, the acute condition is diagnosed as a *Schizophreniform Disorder* or, where the precipitant is an identifiable major stressor and the duration of the disturbance is less than a month, a *Brief Reactive Psychosis*.

The relationship of this acute condition to classic schizophrenia remains unclear (Pao, 1979). Feinstein and Miller (1979) consider this more transient *acute confusional state of adolescence* to be a separate entity, an acute psychotic reaction of adolescence, and not properly a schizophrenic syndrome. Others consider the condition to be closely related to schizophrenia proper. Family and genetic studies are contradictory concerning whether this condition shows vulnerability factors in common with schizophrenia (APA, 1987).

Although major tranquilizers are widely used in acute psychotic states, their influence on the course of this syndrome is unclear (Carpenter et al., 1977). In general, the syndrome responds well to various supportive measures.

Differential Diagnosis

A child who manifests psychotic symptoms requires a thorough diagnostic evaluation. Clinicians must search for organic causes with great care, especially when there is any suggestion of progressive deterioration. Toxic and febrile deliria and viral encephalopathies should be considered, and, if possible, excluded. An adequate EEG study including nasopharyngeal leads and sleep record can identify seizure disorders (especially temporal lobe or *petit mal* status epilepticus). A careful neurological examination, including electroencephalogram and computed X-ray tomographic scan or magnetic resonance imaging scan is important to rule out brain tumor, vascular malformation, or intracranial hemorrhage. Early authors described a *disintegrative psychosis* of childhood with apparently normal development up to age 3 or 4 years, followed by profound behavioral regression, including loss of language and social skills (Evans-Jones & Rosenbloom, 1978; Volkmar & Cohen, 1989). In retrospect, some of these cases may have been organic degenerative diseases, such as the leucodystrophies or lipid storage diseases. Other cases appear to involve viral encephalitides or postencephalitic processes (Nunn et al., 1986). Metabolic screening should be done to rule out these biochemical disorders, but also other inborn errors of metabolism, such as Wilson's disease, porphyria, and various organic acidurias. Psychotic symptomatology may be the first manifestation of these diseases (Propping, 1983).

In adolescents, *organic psychoses secondary to illicit drug use* (especially of cocaine, stimulants, and hallucinogens) are an important part of the differential diagnosis. The task is difficult because in the prodromal phase of schizophrenia many prepsychotic adolescents abuse drugs heavily, perhaps in an attempt at self-medication. Rarely, transient psychotic symptoms (such as delusions, hallucinations, or disorientation) can occur premenstrually in adolescent girls and resolve with the menses, only to reappear during the next menstrual cycle (Berlin et al., 1982). With such a history, the syndrome of *periodic psychosis of puberty* should be considered. In ways still not understood, the dramatic symptoms in this condition appear linked to hormonal changes of the luteal phase.

As diagnostic sophistication develops, clinicians will likely be able to identify more cases of specific organic etiology.

Bipolar Affective Illness. The early symptoms of children who later develop manic-depressive illness usually do not include hallucinations and delusions (see Chapter 6, "Affective Disorders"). However, when full-blown manic symptoms do make their first appearance in adolescence (as they do in 20%–35% of manic-depressives), these early episodes may show many schizophrenic features including bizarre delusions, hallucinations, and ideas of reference or other paranoid ideation (Ballenger et al., 1982). At the time, the condition may be difficult to differentiate from a schizophrenic break, especially in the absence of a positive family history (McGlashan, 1988). Associated features such as hyperactivity, pressured speech, decreased sleep, grandiosity, and euphoria may be the only indicators of the underlying pathology's affective nature. As such patients move into adulthood, their subsequent attacks of psychosis show fewer schizophrenic-like symptoms and assume more typical manic features.

Attention Deficit Hyperactivity Disorders (ADHD) and Language Disorders. In certain children with severe attentional deficits or language processing difficulties, it may be difficult to rule out a mild thought disorder that takes the form of loose associations or tangential thinking. A few ADHD children, when anxious or when in an unstructured situation, jump so quickly from topic to topic that their thoughts are virtually impossible to follow. Not surprisingly, many children with pervasive developmental disorders or childhood schizophrenia also have severe attentional and language deficits.

Borderline and Schizotypal Personality. Many borderline children and adolescents experience transient hallucinations and near-delusional thinking, often of a paranoid cast.

"Benign" Hallucinations in Younger Children. Hallucinations may occur transiently in nonpsychotic children, especially when young and under stress (Kotsopolous et al., 1987; Ravenscroft, 1980; Rothstein, 1981). Although such symptoms in older children may indicate a borderline personality organization, in young children it need not be diagnostically ominous. Transient hallucinations in an otherwise healthy preschooler are usually of acute onset and involve tactile and visual hallucinations of insects and animals. The child may experience panic, phobia, and delusions concerning these creatures, which he often imagines as crawling on his skin or in his clothing or bed. The symptoms occur when the child is anxious about aggressive and oedipal concerns and usually pass within minutes to days, although apprehension may linger for a much longer interval. Dynamically, the hallucinations and accompanying phobia seem to represent "a more intense regressive variant of an acute anxiety attack of childhood" (Ravenscroft, 1980). The similarity of these symptoms to the animal phobias of childhood led Ravenscroft to characterize this syndrome as "acute phobic hallucinosis."

Generally, the preschool child has a poorly developed reality sense and imaginary fears (as well as imaginary companions and imaginative games) loom large in his life. In the face of severe anxiety or under the burden of physiologic impairment, the child's reality testing may transiently break down. Febrile delirium in the form of hallucinations is common with high fever whereas the children with phobic hallucinations are usually physically well. In many cases, however, the hallucinations originate in a twilight sleep state, that is, as hypnogogic or hypnopompic hallucinations that persist abnormally long after awakening.

Rothstein (1981) suggested examining the following features to assess the diagnostic implications of a childhood hallucination: (1) the age and general level of adaptive and defensive development, (2) the state of the child's object relationships (e.g., to what degree the hallucinated object occurs in the absence of significant relationships); (3) whether the hallucination occurred when the child was drowsy or asleep; (4) the readiness with which the child becomes aware that the hallucination is not real; (5) how readily the hallucination disappears with reassurance and parental presence. More systematic follow-up studies are required to clarify the long-term prognostic significance of childhood hallucinations (Del Beccarro et al., 1988).

ETIOLOGY

The etiology of schizophrenia remains an enduring enigma of psychiatry. Most of the many theories advanced and debated through the years can be categorized as psychodynamic, familial-interactional, neurobiological, or genetic. Although researchers have advanced each category as a contender for "*the* cause," from a broader biopsychosocial perspective, the categories might be viewed as different levels of discourse about a related group of phenomena (Carpenter, 1987). Thus, genetic factors may determine certain vulnerabilities in the neurobiological constitution of both child and parent. In turn, these constitutional vulnerabilities influence (and are influenced by) the interaction among the child, his parents, and the environment, which includes not only physical factors, but also community and sociocultural influences. Psychodynamic factors represent a psychological description of the child's personality from an intrapsychic perspective.

Application of this perspective to schizophrenia research has important consequences (Carpenter, 1987). First, the clinician must study the nature of the schizophrenic's disordered functioning at multiple levels. Second, it is necessary to consider how interactions between these levels influence the manifestations of the disease. For example, do family and child-rearing factors exert an exacerbating or ameliorating influence on children with a presumed genetic susceptibility to the illness? How are such influences psychologically and biologically mediated? Third, dysfunction occurring simultaneously on several levels does not itself establish the level that is primary or "causal."

Ignorance about the etiology of childhood schizophrenia is even more extensive than ignorance about adult schizophrenia. Many children with the syndrome become schizophrenic adolescents or adults. However, most persons who develop schizophrenia in adolescence or adulthood do not appear schizophrenic in childhood, although they may manifest developmental disturbances (Hellgren et al., 1987; Nuechterlein, 1986; Watt, 1978). Even if the causes of childhood schizophrenia prove similar to those of the adult form, researchers do not yet understand what determines the age at which pathognomonic symptoms first appear (King, 1988; Weinberger, 1987). Nor do they know whether the relationship of childhood schizophrenia to adult schizophrenia is that of a distinct disorder, a genotypic variant, or a phenotype with especially severe and early presentation.

The research into the causes of schizophrenia is vast and rapidly evolving (Barnes, 1987; Pardes et al., 1987). A complete review of the field is beyond the scope of this book, but several excellent reviews offer detailed information (e.g., Special Report: Schizophrenia, 1987; Strauss & Carpenter, 1981). The difficulty in defining and identifying the condition precisely is a major impediment to progress (Andreasen, 1987); research results are powerfully determined by whichever of the many competing and overlapping definitions of schizophrenia defines the study population. Additional complexity occurs because schizophrenia is clinically or phenotypically heterogeneous (i.e., it has a varied clinical presentation and course); the extent to which it is also etiologically heterogeneous remains unclear. As early as 1911, Bleuler (1911/1950) emphasized this pluralism in the title of his classic work, *Dementia Praecox or The Group of Schizophrenias.*

The search for the cause of schizophrenia is complicated because "apparently similar symptoms may be caused by radically different etiologies, and a single biological factor can produce very different overt symptoms" (Buchsbaum & Haier, 1978, p. 474).

Thus, as noted in the section on differential diagnosis, genetically determined neurological and metabolic diseases can produce schizophreniclike symptoms and may thus be thought of as "genocopies" of schizophrenia proper (if such an entity exists) (Gottesman et al., 1987; Propping, 1983). "Phenocopies" of schizophrenia also exist, such as schizophreniform psychoses caused by drugs (e.g., cocaine or amphetamine) or nongenetic organic neurological disorders (Davison & Bagley, 1969; Gottesman et al., 1987). The extent to which any study population includes such cases will strongly influence the findings, for example, by altering or diluting patterns of family transmission. As pointed out in the discussion of other syndromes, the inability to define homogeneous groups of patients for study is a powerful impediment to research. To the extent that a sample is descriptively or etiologically diverse, abnormalities may not be apparent or may cancel each other out.

Models of Explanation in Schizophrenia

The multitudinous biological theories of schizophrenia tend to cluster around several basic models or paradigms (Strauss & Carpenter, 1981). For example, theories of a *static* model postulate that an abnormal substance or a derangement of some specific mechanism purportedly produces the symptoms of schizophrenia.

In contrast, *dynamic* models look beyond single variables and examine altered interactions between physiological systems. Thus, a neurotransmitter dysfunction not only may alter amounts of transmitter at the synapses, it may also alter receptor sensitivity, complex feedback mechanisms, and the reciprocal balance with other hormonal and neurotransmitter systems. Although a dynamic model is complex, it can account for many interacting variables. The *adaptational* model is a special dynamic model that attends not only to disruptions in homeostasis but to the organism's response to the disruption (Strauss & Carpenter, 1981). Such a broad model requires taking into account neurobiological adaptation over time to external psychological pressures (e.g., separation, stress, overstimulation), as well as to changes in the internal milieu (e.g., altered enzyme activity, medication, etc.). The *vulnerability-stress,* or *diathesis-stress model* is a currently popular adaptational model for integrating constitutional, developmental, and environmental factors in the genesis of schizophrenia (Goldstein, 1987a, 1987b; Zubin & Spring, 1977). The model proposes that certain children are vulnerable to schizophrenia because of presumed early or congenital defects. Whether the child actually develops schizophrenic symptoms will depend on the stressors that he experiences and the presence or absence of protective or exacerbating influences in the environment.

Commonly presumed vulnerabilities include neuroregulatory defects such as dysfunction of the dopaminergic system (Weinberger, 1987); impaired attention and information processing (Erlenmeyer-Kimling et al., 1984); and autonomic or affective instability (Kestenbaum, 1986; Nuechterlein, 1986). Various biological origins for these neurointegrative defects have been proposed: genetic predisposition (Kendler, 1986), viral infections (perhaps perinatal) (Mednick et al., 1988; Torrey, 1986), perinatal trauma, immunological factors (DeLisi, 1986), and so on. Proposed environmental stressors potentiating the development of schizophrenia range from the nonspecific, such as stressful life events, through specific familial factors, such as communication deviance or negative affective family climate (termed "high expressed emotion" or "high EE") (Goldstein, 1987a, 1987b; Leff & Vaughn, 1985; Wynne et al., 1977).

Biological Theories

With only a few exceptions, the vast literature on the biological aspects of schizophrenia is derived from work with adult-onset schizophrenics (Green & Deutsch, 1990; Tanguay & Cantor, 1986). The applicability of this research to childhood-onset schizophrenia will remain equivocal as long as the relationship of the two conditions is uncertain. Nonetheless, because adult-derived work remains the basis for the present understanding of the disease, it compels attention. The following material will note where research has dealt explicitly with childhood-onset schizophrenia.

Dopaminergic Factors. During the past two decades the predominant area of interest for biological researchers has been the neurotransmitter systems, especially those mediated by dopamine (McKenna, 1987; Weinberger, 1987). The dopamine hypothesis postulates that schizophrenia is related to excessive activity in the dopaminergic system (Meltzer, 1987).

The original evidence for the dopamine hypothesis came from pharmacological observations. First, it has long been known that indirect dopamine agonists such as amphetamine and phencyclidine (PCP) can induce an acute paranoid psychosis that resembles acute paranoid schizophrenia. Also, amphetamine and other dopamine agonists exacerbate the psychotic symptoms of schizophrenics. Second, most known antipsychotic drugs (i.e., the neuroleptics) block dopaminergic transmission by blocking the postsynaptic dopamine receptors sites in the central nervous system. Further, the antipsychotic potency of each drug correlates closely with its potency in binding to dopamine receptors in the basal ganglia (Synder, 1980).

Researchers have made direct attempts to demonstrate deranged dopaminergic functioning in schizophrenia. For example, postmortem assays of schizophrenics' brains have found increased dopamine receptor levels in the limbic system (Weinberger & Kleinman, 1986). As yet unconfirmed in vivo positron-emission tomographic studies of drug-naive schizophrenics have also shown increased dopamine receptor activity in the striatal region (Wong et al., 1986).

The variegated symptomatology of schizophrenia and its fluctuating clinical course have prompted the suggestion that different symptoms may have different pathogenic mechanisms. Thus, Crow (1985) speculated that the *positive* symptoms of schizophrenia, such as hallucinations and delusions, might be linked to altered dopaminergic activity; patients showing many of these symptoms, he believed, were more responsive to neuroleptic medication and less likely to show structural abnormalities of the ventricular. Crow speculated that the *negative* symptoms of chronic schizophrenia, namely affective flattening, apathy, and social withdrawal, might have other causes; for example, these symptoms may be linked to brain cell loss and structural brain changes, such as enlarged ventricles, and hence less reversible or responsive to medication.

Can Schizophrenia Be Localized in the Brain? Through the years, many researchers have speculated that the symptoms of schizophrenia relate to specific abnormalities in brain function and structure (Andreasen, 1986, 1987). The typical schizophrenic defects in affective responsiveness, social judgment, volition, planning of future actions, attention, language, and abstract thought all involve functions believed to reside in the frontal lobes. Because these are the functions most compromised in negative schizophrenic symptoms, frontal lobe abnormalities may be responsible for such symptomatology (Pardes et al., 1987; Weinberger, 1987). Positive symptoms, including hallucinations, delusions, and thought disorder, are harder to localize but may functionally represent dysfunction in the temporal cortex or limbic system structures such as the amygdala or hippocampus (Andreasen, 1987; Weinberger, 1987). As the psychopathology associated with temporal lobe epilepsy indicates, abnormal discharges involving these structures can cause perceptual distortions, hallucinations, strange experiences (e.g., *déjà vu*), and anxiety (Gloor et al., 1982). Recent postmortem studies of brain cell architecture in schizophrenics show variable, nonspecific abnormalities of cell density or patterning, especially in the prefrontal cortex and periventricular limbic and diencephalic areas (Kirch & Weinberger, 1986; Weinberger, 1987).

Defects in dopaminergic transmission are widely suspected to provide the neurochemical basis for such dysfunctions (MacKay, 1980). Although dopaminergic neurons compose only about 1% of the brain's total, they link many of the key structures that may play a role in schizophrenia. The dopaminergic system, for example, includes the mesolimbic and mesocortical pathways that connect the midbrain ventral tegmental areas to the limbic system and the prefrontal cortex respectively (Weinberger, 1987).

Sophisticated computerized brain imaging has provided tantalizing clues about possible structural and functional neurological abnormalities in living schizophrenics (see reviews by Buchsbaum and Haier, 1987; Meltzer, 1987; Shelton & Weinberger, 1986). The following paragraphs describe some of these new methods.

- *Computed X-ray Tomography (CT Scan)*. CT scan studies have identified a subgroup of schizophrenics who show ventricular enlargement and cortical atrophy, especially in the prefrontal area. In some studies, but not others, these nonspecific changes correlate with poor premorbid adjustment, a preponderance of negative symptoms, unresponsiveness to neuroleptics, and a more chronic course. The neuropathological mechanisms that underlie such hypoplasia or atrophy of brain tissue remain obscure. To what extent different abnormalities reflect the impact of genetic factors, acquired conditions (such as perinatal complications, viral infections, immune reaction, or toxins) or an interaction between genetic and acquired factors remains unclear (Cannon et al., 1989; Meltzer, 1987; Shelton & Weinberger, 1986).

- *Positron-Emission Tomography (PET)*. This method, by applying the mathematical techniques of CT scanning to the emissions of radio-isotope-tagged chemicals in the brain, generates "brain-slice" images of those chemicals' distribution and concentration. Because radio-labeling techniques can be applied to diverse substances such as glucose, neurotransmitter precursors, and psychoactive drugs, PET can provide in vivo "snapshots" of various metabolic and neurochemical processes.

PET studies of schizophrenics have shown relative metabolic underactivity of the frontal lobes (Buchsbaum & Haier, 1987). Similar *hypofrontality* in schizophrenics is found in cerebral blood flow imaging studies of the cortical surface. The specific frontal region with the greatest patient versus control differences in PET and cerebral blood flow is also the very region that shows greatest activation in normals during tests of attentional ability. In addition, several studies point to the importance of dopamine and the basal ganglia. PET studies of the basal ganglia of schizophrenics show decreased metabolic activity, which can be reversed with neuroleptic medication. Some, but not all PET studies also show greater dopamine D_2-receptor densities in the caudate nuclei of drug-naive schizophrenics compared with normal controls (Wong et al., 1986).

• *Magnetic resonance imaging (MRI).* MRI techniques distinguish grey and white matter in the brain with great sensitivity. Using analytic techniques similar to PET and CT, MRI constructs images from the signals of hydrogen atoms in the brain that have been oriented by a high-strength magnetic field; the signals are emitted as the atoms resonate to precisely timed radio frequency pulses. Unlike PET and CT techniques, MRI reduces or eliminates the hazards of radiation exposure. MRI studies of schizophrenics show reduction in anterior frontal and temporal white matter and suggest that schizophrenics have generally smaller frontal lobes and cerebrums than controls (Andreasen et al., 1986; Smith et al., 1987).

These new technologies, together with others, such as computer electroencephalographic topography, promise exciting new insights into the defects in cerebral structure and function that may underlie the symptoms of schizophrenia (Andreasen, 1986).

A variety of psychophysiological and electrophysiological measures have been employed with adult-onset schizophrenics, childhood-onset schizophrenics, and offspring of schizophrenics (Asarnow et al., 1986; Erlenmeyer-Kimling & Cornblatt, 1987; Holzman, 1986; Patterson, 1986). These studies suggest that vulnerability to schizophrenia is associated with attentional deficits and abnormalities in sensory information processing (as evidenced by altered sensory-evoked potentials). In schizophrenia, both the spatial distribution of the electrophysiological abnormalities and the nature of the attentional deficits suggest dysfunctioning of the tertiary associative areas of the cortex, especially the prefrontal areas (Asarnow et al., 1986). How these abnormalities in attentional and informational processing functions might cause the pathognomonic schizophrenic symptoms of hallucination, delusion, and thought disorder has been the subject of much speculation (Asarnow et al., 1986; Holzman, 1986; Matthysse, 1987; Meehl, 1989).

Neuromaturational Factors. Weinberger (1987) attempted an ambitious synthesis of the existing neurobiological data that describes the development of the pathogenesis of schizophrenia. His theory tries to account for the diverse neuroanatomical findings in schizophrenics, the role of the dopaminergic system, the dichotomy between positive and negative symptoms, and the tendency for overt schizophrenic symptoms first to become manifest in late adolescence.

Weinberger proposes that the underlying lesion(s) in schizophrenia may have diverse origins: genetic, viral, perinatal insult, and so on. Although present early in the life of the future schizophrenic, the lesion remains silent throughout childhood except, presumably, for the subtle signs and deficits seen in at-risk infants and children (Erlenmeyer-Kimling & Cornblatt, 1987). According to Weinberger's hypotheses, these silent lesions in some way compromise the dopamine-mediated pathways to the prefrontal cortex, which subserves important cognitive, motivational, and social functions. Because this brain area does not mature and become fully active until myelination is complete in the late teens or early 20s, lesions affecting it are not functionally apparent earlier in life. Thus, animal experiments confirm that prefrontal cortical functioning is not "rate limiting" for many behaviors until adulthood, when these cortical structures normally come "on-line." During late adolescence, however, deficits in prefrontal cortical functioning may become dramatically obvious as social and cognitive demands increase and the functional ascendency of this cortical area fails to develop.

Such deficits in prefrontal cortical capacity could account for many negative symptoms of schizophrenia: cognitive impairment, motivational and planning difficulties, poor insight, and poor social judgment (Berman et al., 1988; Goldberg et al., 1987). Furthermore, Weinberger (1987) proposes, the lack of age-appropriate activation of the prefrontal cortex has other far-reaching consequences, such as the disruption of the inhibitory feedback regulation that the prefrontal cortex normally exerts to prevent limbic system overactivity. This limbic system overactivity in turn might produce the more florid psychotic positive symptoms of schizophrenia, such as hallucinations and delusions.

The specifics of Weinberger's hypothesis are speculative. The theory, however, has heuristic value because, by taking normal neuromaturation into account, it suggests how early lesions might, after a long silent period, become symptomatically manifest at a later developmental epoch. Data suggest, for example, that prenatal exposure to viral infection during the second trimester may predispose individuals to develop schizophrenia as adults (Mednick et al., 1988).

A major limitation of Weinberger's model is its difficulty in explaining childhood-onset schizophrenia (King, 1988). Neurophysiological and neuropsychological studies in these prepubertal children do suggest dysfunction of the prefrontal cortex (Asarnow et al., 1986); the functional and neuromaturational "coming of age" of these brain structures with puberty, however, was clearly not a prerequisite for developing full-blown schizophrenic symptomatology.

Genetic Factors

Genetic investigations of schizophrenia have been hampered by the difficulty in specifying the appropriate phenotype to study, as well as by the unknown degree of etiological heterogeneity (Gottesman et al., 1987; Meehl, 1989). Nonetheless, genetic factors exercise a strong influence in many cases of schizophrenia. After reviewing the entire genetic literature,

McGuffin and colleagues (1987) concluded that "genes probably account for about two-thirds of the variation in liability to the disorder" (p. 582). Studies of adult cases have shown that schizophrenia in a parent greatly increases the risk of schizophrenia in the offspring. Children with one schizophrenic parent have a markedly increased risk (about 12%) of manifesting the condition by middle adulthood, compared with the general population (about 1%); with two affected parents, the morbid risk rises to about 39% (Erlenmeyer-Kimling & Cornblatt, 1984). It had long been debated whether such an increased incidence was due primarily to the pathogenic effects of being reared by a seriously disturbed parent or to a shared genetic vulnerability. Unfortunately, when children are reared by a disturbed biological parent, the relative contributions of heredity and environment are difficult to disentangle.

Adoption studies have proven to be a powerful method for teasing apart genetic and environmental factors. Although debate over their design and interpretation continues (Clerget-Darpoux et al., 1987), these studies have provided evidence that hereditary factors play a major role in shaping the development of schizophrenics' offspring. Rosenthal and co-workers (Rosenthal et al., 1971) studied a population of children whose biological parents were schizophrenic. These youngsters were reared from infancy by nonschizophrenic adoptive parents. When followed into adulthood, the offspring showed a much higher rate of schizophrenia than was found in the adopted-away offspring of nonschizophrenic biological parents (Lowing et al., 1983). Indeed, the prevalence of schizophrenia in adopted-away offspring of schizophrenics did not differ significantly from that of offspring reared by the schizophrenic biological parents (Higgins, 1976). Further, it did not matter *which* biological parent was schizophrenic; schizophrenia in the father increased the child's risk for schizophrenia as much as schizophrenia in the mother (Wender et al., 1974). Conversely, children who had nonschizophrenic biological parents but were adopted by a parent who subsequently became psychotic tended *not* to develop schizophrenia (Wender et al., 1974). Thus, who the child's biological parents were, rather than who reared the child, appeared to be the major determinant of risk for schizophrenia.

Does the rearing environment have any modulating effect? Rosenthal and co-workers (1975) attempted to answer this question with a crude, retrospective assessment of the quality of the adoptive parent–child relationship in each of the different child-rearing groups. They then correlated this measure with the degree of illness in the child. They estimated that for adopted-away offspring, environmental rearing factors on the average accounted for only about 9% of variance in outcome with respect to schizophrenia. However, the adoptive parent–child relationship correlated more highly with schizophrenic outcome for the children of nonschizophrenic parents (0.37) than for the children of schizophrenics (0.23); the quality of this relationship accounted for 5% and 13% of the variance respectively. Rosenthal and colleagues concluded, "These findings suggest that rearing patterns have only a modest effect on individuals who harbor a genetic background for schizophrenia, but an appreciable effect on persons without such a background" (p. 474).

Preliminary results from a different adoption study, still underway, indicate an interaction of psychosocial and genetic factors (Tienari et al., 1985, 1987a, 1987b). Although many of the offspring have not reached the age of maximum risk for schizophrenia, this study so far agrees with earlier studies in finding an increased incidence of schizophrenia spectrum disorders (7 out of 112) in the adopted-away offspring of schizophrenic mothers, compared with those of control mothers (2 out of 135). However, the quality of relationships in the adoptive families was also an important variable; the adoptive families of the seven index offspring who developed a schizophrenic-spectrum disorder were all rated as seriously disturbed.

Another strategy to separate genetic from rearing factors was employed in Israel with high-risk children of schizophrenic parents (Mirsky et al., 1985; Marcus et al., 1987). Half the children were reared by their own ill parents, whereas the other half lived on kibbutzim, where communal child-rearing practices greatly reduced their exposure to their ill parents. Preliminary results suggest that decreased exposure to an ill parent did little to reduce the development of schizophrenia-spectrum disorders.

Twin studies also demonstrate the powerful effects of heredity. When one dizygotic (fraternal) twin is an adult schizophrenic, by mid-adulthood, in about 6.5% to 12% of the cases, so is his cotwin. This is about the same concordance rate as for nontwin siblings. When the twins are monozygotic (identical), the concordance rate rises to about 31% to 48% (Gottesman et al., 1987; Kendler & Robinette, 1983). The increased prevalence exists even when the twins have been separated from their biological parents and reared apart from each other. Why the genotype for schizophrenia might be expressed in one monozygotic twin, but not in the other is unclear. However, the offspring of the nonschizophrenic twin have as high a risk for schizophrenia spectrum disorders as do those of the schizophrenic twin, suggesting the genotype can remain unexpressed in one generation only to manifest itself in the next (Gottesman & Bertelsen, 1989).

Childhood schizophrenia also shows a strong genetic influence (Hanson & Gottesman, 1976). In various studies, the prevalence of schizophrenia in the parents of childhood schizophrenics (8.8%–12%) is markedly greater than in the general population (Fish & Ritvo, 1979). This increased prevalence rate equals or exceeds that found in the parents of adult schizophrenics. Twin studies of childhood schizophrenics show both a strong genetic influence and an even higher penetrance than in adult schizophrenics. Thus, the concordance rate in monozygotic twins for schizophrenia appearing before age 15 years is 70.6% in contrast with 17.1% for dizygotic twins. Including cotwins who become schizophrenic in adulthood causes the concordance rate to rise to 88% versus 23% (Kallman & Roth, 1956). Whether this high rate simply reflects the severity of disturbance in childhood schizophrenia is unclear. Gottesman and Shields (1972) showed that in adult twins, severity of schizophrenia (as measured by time spent in the hospital) corresponded with a higher concordance rate. In the Kallman and Roth (1956) study although most of the schizophrenics among the siblings of childhood schizophrenics resembled the index cases in having a prepubertal onset, adult-onset schizophrenia also tended to cluster in the family of childhood schizophrenics. Rosenthal (1970) concluded that there is a strong case for the biological unity of preadolescent and adult schizophrenia, with pre-adolescent schizophrenia representing "a more virulent form which has virtually complete penetrance" (p. 146).

The exact mode of the genetic transmission of schizophrenia is unknown (Faraone & Tsuang, 1985). Many behavior geneticists favor a multifactorial, polygenic model, suggesting that schizophrenia is caused by combinations of genes at several loci, in combination with environmental factors, presumably both biological and psychological (Gottesman et al., 1987).

Recent advances in pedigree analysis and linkage techniques utilizing DNA markers may soon shed more light on these questions. Linkage studies of a small number of Icelandic families with a high density of schizophrenia spectrum disorders suggest that in these families vulnerability to these disorders is linked to an unknown dominant gene somewhere on chromosome 5 (Sherrington et al., 1988). However, the conclusions that can be drawn from this study have important limitations (Lander, 1988). First, the results do not apply to all families with schizophrenia. Kennedy et al. (1988) showed that the vulnerability to schizophrenia in a large Swedish pedigree was *not* linked to chromosome 5. Second, it is not clear how best to define the underlying vulnerability that is apparently linked to the putative chromosome 5 locus. The strongest linkage to the putative gene was not for schizophrenia but rather for a broad range of disorders that also included schizotypal personality disorder and miscellaneous psychopathology such as anxiety disorders and depression. The current definitions of various mental disorders may not reflect the underlying patterns of inheritance. Like many family studies of psychiatric illness, linkage studies of schizophrenia are complicated by the difficulty of specifying the phenotype whose putative genetic roots are being sought. As Lander (1988) has cautioned, "Good genetics requires good phenotypes" (p. 106).

Thus it is not yet clear *what* is inherited from a schizophrenic parent. Even those adopted-away children of schizophrenic biological parents who did not develop schizophrenia were at high risk for other significant psychiatric disorders. In some studies, those offspring who did not develop classic schizophrenia showed an increased prevalence of both schizophrenic spectrum disorders, such as borderline schizophrenia and schizotypal personality disorders, and psychopathic and neurotic personality disorders.

It is likely that what is inherited is not schizophrenia itself, but rather a vulnerability to certain types of deviant development. Many researchers have speculated about the nature of this postulated "core" vulnerability (Kestenbaum, 1986; Meehl, 1989). A recurrent hypothesis is that a subtle neurointegrative deficit renders the affected offspring vulnerable to developing a range of psychopathology, including schizophrenia. Since only about 10% to 15% of the offspring of schizophrenics develop schizophrenia much research has focused on identifying the distinguishing features of this vulnerable subgroup. Various high-risk longitudinal studies confirm that a significant subgroup of children of schizophrenics, perhaps 10% to 30%, show early neurodevelopmental deviance (Erlenmeyer-Kimling et al., 1987; Fish, 1987; Marcus et al., 1985b, 1987). The symptoms include soft neurological signs, uneven maturation, and poor performance on various cognitive, perceptual, motor, and attentional tests. The offspring most at risk for later developing significant psychopathology have attentional, information-processing, and motor abnormalities (Nuechterlein, 1986; Watt et al., 1984). Laboratory studies with these high-risk children also show abnormalities in such neuropsychological measures as cognitive event-related evoked potentials (Erlenmeyer-Kimling & Cornblatt, 1984). Even when not clinically psychotic, children of psychotic parents show conspicuously high levels of thought disorder, as evidenced by fluid associations, confabulation, autistic logic, incoherence, and neologisms (Arboleda & Holzman, 1985).

Genetics, however, do not tell the whole story. Despite the increased incidences of parental and sibling schizophrenia, most childhood schizophrenics do *not* have schizophrenic parents, just as 80% of adult-onset schizophrenics do not have any schizophrenic first-degree relatives (Gottesman et al., 1987). Whether such apparently sporadic cases should be considered nongenetic is open to debate. For example, apparently nonfamilial cases may reflect chance isolates, complex polygenic or non-Mendelian modes of transmission, incomplete penetrance, as well as truly nongenetic causal factors (McGuffin et al., 1987). Furthermore, researchers have not yet established whether the clinical and developmental features of familial and apparently nonfamilial cases differ in significant ways. Because most longitudinal and adoptive data come from the offspring of schizophrenic parents, far less is known about the course or genetics of the apparently nonfamilial cases. For example, prior to developing psychotic symptoms, do the nonfamilial cases show the same neurointegrative defects as familial cases?

A major unanswered question is whether a genetic vulnerability is a necessary precondition for developing schizophrenia or whether there are other biological or environmental pathways to this outcome. Conversely, it is unclear whether possessing the presumed genotype is sufficient or whether particular environmental stressors are necessary to develop the illness (Kron & Kestenbaum, 1988).

Corollary questions concern the factors that exert a protective or exacerbating effect in children who have an inherited vulnerability to schizophrenia (Anthony & Cohler, 1987). Some risk and protective variables relate to environmental factors (Sameroff et al., 1987). For example, severity and chronicity of parental disturbance are variables that may be as important as the parent's specific diagnoses. Socioeconomic and family variables are among the most important protective factors; they include socioeconomic status, race, family size and degree of support, and stressful family life events.

Why some children appear relatively invulnerable to parental schizophrenia, whereas others are not, has been the subject of much study (Anthony & Cohler, 1987; Garmezy, 1987).

Anthony (1987) found that a small proportion of children with psychotic parents (about 15%) remained relatively well adjusted and asymptomatic; a smaller group, about 10%, not only remained asymptomatic, but thrived, showing excellent coping skills and many creative and constructive capacities (Anthony, 1987). These resilient or invulnerable children appeared to be those who resisted becoming engulfed in their parents' psychopathology; they maintained a "compassionate yet detached" attitude toward the sick parent and were able to see that parent in objective terms as disturbed. Perhaps most important, these children could reach out to adults, especially the well parent, and receive emotional support. Intelligence, creativity, and personal and physical attractiveness were assets in engaging relatives, teachers, and other supportive adults (Anthony, 1976; Cohler, 1987). How these assets relate to other family and genetic variables remains to be explored. The availability of a well parent, able and willing to reach out to the child, is a key variable; the length and timing of the sick parent's hospitalization or the child's out-of-home placement may also be important. Prospective studies using DNA marker techniques may someday tell researchers whether these resilient children carry less genetic vulnerability to schizophrenia.

Family Factors

Clinical and research studies of the families of young adult schizophrenics have found frequent aberrant patterns of communication and relating (Goldstein, 1987a, 1987b; Liem, 1980). Early theoretical and clinical speculation emphasized how these aberrant patterns of relating and communicating might *cause* schizophrenia in offspring. Whether the stress was on the schism or skew of family roles or on the pseudomutuality or double-bind communication in the family, most causal theories were heavily "parento-genic."

For example, in the families of schizophrenics, roles often were found to be poorly differentiated and generational boundaries were blurred. Parents failed to preserve appropriate boundaries of age and sex within the family, often treating the child as a spouse or parent. Other studies of schizophrenics' families (Summers & Walsh, 1977) suggested that an abnormal degree of symbiotic fusion characterized relationships between family members with difficulties in separation, self–other differentiation, and intrusiveness.

Studies of deviant communication in schizophrenics' families demonstrated familywide difficulties in establishing and maintaining a shared focus of attention (Wynne et al., 1977, 1987). In such families, communications were often amorphous, loose, and indefinite to the point of unintelligibility. Utterances tended to be fragmented, easily disrupted, or lacking in closure. These disturbances were apparent in the thought and speech of individual family members as well as in the family's attempts to work together on tasks or to elaborate a consensually shared view of reality. Individuals in such families often failed to acknowledge each other's communications, thereby rendering discourse less instrumental and depriving members of a sense of efficacy or validity.

Family theorists thus spoke of "the transmission of irrationality" (Lidz et al., 1958). Wynne et al. (1977) and Singer et al. (1978) hypothesized that the schizophrenic's fragmentation of experience, identity diffusion, anxiety, and disturbed thinking derived, by processes of internalization, from pathological aspects of the family organization.

Such etiological conclusions concerning the direction of effects must be viewed with caution (Goldstein, 1987a, 1987b; Reiss, 1976). Cause and effect are notoriously difficult to distinguish in a family system, and a disturbed offspring has a severe impact on his parents and siblings. Finally, when both parent and child are disturbed, difficulties in their relationship may represent shared genetic (or other risk) factors, rather than child-rearing effects per se. If family factors are at work in childhood schizophrenia, where deviant development is apparent so early, it seems plausible that family variables must work synergistically with an already present vulnerability in the child. Parents of children with schizophrenia and schizotypal personality disorder have higher rates of communication deviance than do parents of children with depressive disorders (J. Asarnow et al., 1988). Schizophrenic and schizotypal children from families with high communication deviance were the most severely impaired and had the poorest attention. These complex interactions will require well-designed prospective longitudinal studies for further clarification.

Family style can have an important exacerbating or ameliorating influence on the difficulties of the growing child; once schizophrenic symptoms are manifest, family factors strongly influence both the symptomatic course of the illness and how treatment is used (Leff & Vaughn, 1985).

Mother-Infant Factors

The area of early mother–child interaction has also seen heated debate concerning the nature versus nurture issue. Much research has focused on the infantile experience of the schizophrenic child because of his apparent failure to master the developmental tasks of earliest childhood. These tasks include the development of a cohesive self, with stable body images and self-images that are adequately differentiated from the mother. Here, too, early theories tended to be parentogenic. Frieda Fromm-Reichmann (1948) spoke of a "schizophrenogenic" mother who subjected her child to "severe early warp and rejection" early in his life. (See also the debate regarding the role of parents in the etiology of autism in Chapter 4.)

Mahler (1968) took a more cautious view. She saw the core problem of infantile psychosis as the child's inability to relate to the mothering partner. In her view, the child could not communicate with his mother in a way that allowed him to acquire a sense of her as a reliable, comforting object external to himself. Thus, the infant did not develop a pleasurable, need-satisfying relationship with mother and was subsequently unable to internalize her as a facilitator of homeostasis. Consequently, he could neither fully relate to her nor let her go. Mahler postulated that such infants and mothers lacked adequate mutual cuing. Because of this lack, both being held close and being apart could be distressing to the uncomforted infant. In later life, this discomfort might be reflected in the profound "ambitendency" or "need–fear" dilemma of the schizophrenic (Burnham et al., 1969). Like the porcupines of Freud's parable, who attempted so unsuccessfully to huddle together for warmth, the schizophrenic wants to relate to others, but is afraid to do so because closeness becomes either painful or terrifying (Fromm-Reichmann, 1950; Pao, 1979).

In Mahler's view, the crucial failure of adequate mother–infant relatedness might originate in either the mother or the infant or in the match between them. Thus, for a "constitutionally greatly predisposed oversensitive or vulnerable infant," normal mothering may not adequately buffer or counteract the infant's difficulties. Likewise, even a constitutionally sturdy infant could subsequently become psychotic if he were to receive severe cumulative trauma during the phases of infancy that are critical for the formation of sustaining and stabilizing relationships.

Propensity to overwhelming panic, abnormal development of affective experience and expression, and a disturbed sense of self may accompany a disturbed early mother–child relationship (though whether as a cause or effect is unclear). The child may come to experience the external world and internal states as predominantly bad and painful, rather than as good and pleasurable. As a result, attachment to others becomes problematic, and aggressive tendencies may be exacerbated.

Further work is necessary to define whether specific pathogenic interactions are predictive of psychotic outcome. The observation that child abuse, sensory impairment, parental absence, and inadequate caretaking in infancy often lead to serious psychopathology, but not necessarily to psychosis, is difficult to reconcile with any simple "parentogenic" theory. How child-rearing variables interact with and relate to the constitutional vulnerabilities and strengths of both mother and child remains an important area of investigation (Anthony & Cohler, 1987; Goldstein, 1987a, 1987b; Sameroff et al., 1987).

Some direct studies of mother–infant interaction indicate that the infants of schizophrenic mothers appear less competent in a variety of ways than the infants of control mothers; furthermore, the high-risk infants' degree of competency shows less correlation with measures of their mothers' skill in handling them than does that of normal infants (R. Clark, personal communication, 1983). This finding is reminiscent of Rosenthal and colleagues' (1975) conclusion (on the basis of less adequate retrospective data) that rearing variables may have less influence in children with a greater genetic loading for schizophrenia. Longitudinal prospective studies, especially in high-risk populations, may soon shed greater light on these questions (Garmezy, 1987; Sameroff et al., 1987).

TREATMENT

As with adult-onset schizophrenia, the treatment of childhood schizophrenia remains uncertain and controversial. In light of the developmental issues facing the schizophrenic child, it is unclear how far treatment methods used with adult-onset schizophrenics can be usefully adapted to such children (Tanguay & Cantor, 1986). In recent years psychodynamic psychotherapy has been deemphasized, partly because of increased skepticism about the role of psychological factors in schizophrenia's primary etiology. Paralleling this shift has been an increased use of behavioral and psychopharmacologic treatment approaches.

Although a purely psychogenic theory of etiology appears untenable, the schizophrenic child manifests multiple areas of impaired psychological and social functioning. These defects include extensive developmental deficits and deviations in the ability to communicate and relate to others, in the sense of self, in the perception of reality (particularly its interpersonal aspects), and in the regulation of affect (especially an intolerance of unpleasant affects and a tendency to overwhelming "organismic" panic). Medication may reduce or eliminate hallucinations, delusions, hyperactivity, social withdrawal, and aggressive outbursts, but it leaves many core impairments untouched. Thus, even the optimal medication response does not alleviate the need for psychotherapy, special education, and rehabilitation to permit previously stunted or deviant development to proceed in a healthy direction.

Psychotherapy

A large, rich, but unsystematic, literature distills several authors' thoughtful and heroic psychotherapeutic work with deeply disturbed children (Cantor, 1982; Cantor & Kestenbaum, 1986; Des Lauriers, 1967; Ekstein, 1966; Goldfarb, 1970, 1974; Sechahaye, 1951). Many of the controversies about theory, efficacy, and technique resemble the unresolved issues in the treatment of adult schizophrenics (McGlashan, 1983c, 1986c). Despite the diverse theoretical orientations and etiological assumptions, several common themes emerge.

First, establishing contact or a "bridgehead" of relatedness is a difficult but central task (Kestenbaum, 1978). Schizophrenic children are difficult to engage because of the massive deficits in their interpersonal capacities and their ready resort to primitive defenses such as passive or active withdrawal, regression, projection, or attack in the face of the anxieties stirred by human contact. Whether from their social deficits or active defenses against painful engagement, such children are profoundly ambivalent about human attachment. With a nod to Freud's adage that neurotics have "preconditions for loving," Ekstein (1966) observed that psychotic children have stringent "conditions for contact." The therapist, while maintaining expectations for higher levels of function, may have to establish contact at the child's present functional level, however archaic it may be (Sechahaye, 1956). This effort may entail engaging the psychotic child with limited language around any available islands of pleasurable activity or need-satisfying communication. Paraverbal techniques, such as rhythm, music, and body movements, not only provide an avenue for positive engagement, but also help the child define his body image and sense of self (Cantor & Kestenbaum, 1986; Heimlich, 1972). Cantor's (1988) multimodal treatment team approach utilizes intensive gross motor therapy to foster the emergence of the schizophrenic preschooler's still inchoate body–self concept. Play therapy provides an entrée only to the less autistic children because many of the more disturbed youngsters are unable to use toys in any imaginative or projectively expressive way. Even in better functioning children, play may be repetitive, impoverished, and unelaborated (Cantor & Kestenbaum, 1986). For those youngsters who can play imaginatively, Ekstein (1966) proposes "interpretation within the metaphor" as a means of establishing empathic contact, while avoiding further ego regression.

The therapeutic goals with schizophrenic children are to strengthen the ego, supply cognitive structure, clarify areas of conflict, encourage the development of a sense of autonomous identity, and foster more adaptive defenses. Goldfarb (1970, 1974) emphasized the mutative power of "corrective socialization" to fill in the gaps in the development of the child's ego capacity for self-regulation and self-direction.

The technical means for accomplishing these goals are diverse; selection among them should be based on systematic assessment of the individual child's strength and deficits, including cognitive and linguistic development, motivation, interpersonal modes of relating, and defensive style.

One dilemma concerning technique is whether to foster expression or suppression (Escalona, 1964; Federn, 1952). Federn noted that whereas the usual analytic technique encouraged *de*-repression, the schizophrenic is all too readily aware of and overwhelmed by primitive affects, thoughts, and fantasies; the goal in schizophrenia, as he saw it, was to foster *re*-repression. Escalona (1964) saw the task as "discouraging the expression and acting out of fantasies, and providing as much gratification as possible in more realistic pursuits, and. . . strengthening reality testing by all possible means" (p. 54). The dichotomous hazards of the two approaches are that they may either exacerbate ego weakness or fail to help the patient confront and cope with his primitive concerns (Ekstein, 1966). This may be a false dilemma. Although the therapist's activity with such children is sometimes referred to as giving "interpretations," his or her crucial activity is not interpretive in the usual sense of making the unconscious conscious or linking current reactions with their genetic roots. The therapist's interventions are more on the level of confrontation and clarification (Khantzian et al., 1968). Although the troublesome affects and conflicts that disturb the psychotic child are not unconscious, he may avoid, deny, or feel overwhelmed by them. The therapist's job is to help label and put these feelings into perspective, which renders them more bearable and strengthens the child's mastery of them. In the child's relationship with the therapist, he or she offers the child not simply an object of transference, but a real person—a helper, a teacher, a comforter, and a model for identification. From this perspective, the therapist should resort to interpretation of the transference primarily to deal with resistances that interfere with the unfolding and deepening of the therapist–patient relationship.

The goals and techniques of various therapeutic approaches to childhood schizophrenia are predicated on their implicit view of the disorder's underlying pathogenesis (McGlashan, 1986c). Deficit theories dictate remedial measures to encourage compensatory strengthening of remaining areas of competency and potential growth. Such measures might include social skills training and special education (including speech therapy and gross and fine motor training), in addition to the ego-strengthening, psychotherapeutic approach. Conflict psychodynamic models emphasize utilizing the therapeutic relationship to explore, contain, and resolve the schizophrenic child's intense ambivalence toward human relationships. Vulnerability-stress models mandate a wide range of interventions to strengthen coping skills, minimize stress, or reduce underlying vulnerability factors. Such interventions might include all of the above-mentioned measures as well as family therapy (to reduce family-induced stresses) and the judicious use of medication.

A specialized milieu such as a therapeutic day school (or day hospital) program designed for schizophrenic children usually best integrates these therapeutic modalities. Severe cases may require either long-term residential treatment or intermittent hospitalization at times of symptom exacerbation. The treatment setting should be appropriate for the child's age and level of cognitive, linguistic, and social functioning. Involvement of parents in the various therapeutic modalities and parental support and self-help groups help maintain the child's functioning at home. Cantor (1988) described the functioning of a well-integrated treatment program for multiply impaired schizophrenic children. In the older literature, Ekstein (1966), Szurek and Berlin (1973), and Bettelheim (1974) gave accounts of several decades of heroic efforts, often unsuccessful, in their psychodynamically oriented treatment programs. Unfortunately, with only a few exceptions, such as Goldfarb (1974), there is little systematic treatment outcome data from this work that might more precisely define the indications for psychotherapy.

Drug Therapy

The neuroleptics (major tranquilizers), which form the mainstay of psychopharmacological treatment of adult schizophrenia, have a more limited usefulness in childhood-onset schizophrenia (Campbell, 1985; Campbell et al., 1985; Green et al., 1984; Green & Deutsch, 1990). In various patient samples drugs from each of the major classes of neuroleptics, including haloperidol, loxapine, thiothixene, thioridazine, and pimozide, have produced positive effects. The number of systematic studies is extremely small, and few deal primarily with prepubertal children. Hallucinations, delusions, thought disorder, social withdrawal, hyperactivity, assaultiveness, and excitability were among the symptoms showing improvement. In some studies, only about 50% to 60% of the children showed improvement (Campbell, 1985; Green & Deutsch). Not only do younger schizophrenics appear less responsive to these medications than adults, they are also more likely to respond with anergy, apathy, and withdrawal. In addition, the medications, especially the more sedative drugs such as chlorpromazine, may cause some cognitive dulling. Whether higher potency neuroleptics such as haloperidol produce less deleterious effects on learning ability remains under investigation.

In addition to oversedation, side effects may include dysphoria; increased separation anxiety (Mikkelsen et al., 1981); and extrapyramidal side effects, such as acute dystonic reactions, parkinsonian rigidity, and akasthisia (restless legs). Tardive and withdrawal dyskinesias can occur in children after as few as 3 months on these medications (Campbell, 1985; Gualtieri et al., 1984). These involuntary abnormal movements, most often of the face, tongue, and mouth, may be disfiguring and irreversible. For all of these reasons, neuroleptics should be used in as low doses and for as short a time as possible.

PROGNOSIS OF CHILDHOOD-ONSET SCHIZOPHRENIA

Most children with childhood-onset schizophrenia do poorly and many go on to become schizophrenic adults. Reliable data on the long-term outcome of the condition are difficult to come by as most older studies are flawed by overly inclusive standards for diagnosing schizophrenia in childhood and by failure to exclude cases of early-onset bipolar disorder, which may initially resemble schizophrenia, but may run a less intractable long-term course. Eggers (1978) conducted a 20-year follow-up of children with onset of schizophrenia between the ages of 7 and 14 years. The children with onset before 10 years had a uniformly chronic course; poor premorbid functioning and low IQ were associated with poorer outcome. The prognostic importance of schizoaffective features was revealed in a subsequent reanalysis of the same cohort. Eggers (1989) divided the children into two groups: the 28% who met criteria for schizoaffective disorder and the remaining 72%, who were classified as simply schizophrenic. Compared with the schizophrenic children, the schizoaffective group had better premorbid adjustment, acuter onset, and family histories with more affective psychoses and suicide and less schizophrenia. These schizoaffective children also had a significantly better prognosis; at follow-up 31% were found to be in "complete remission," 44% had "slight" residual defects, and only 25% had "severe deficits." In contrast, only 27% of the schizophrenic patients were in complete remission at follow-up, 24% had "slight defects," and 49% had severe residual defects.

Kydd and Werry (1982) found an even bleaker picture in their 1–10-year follow-up of children diagnosed with schizophrenia prior to age 16 years. Insidious onset, disorganization, and poor premorbid functioning were associated with poor outcome; children with affective features or a paranoid presentation did better. At follow-up, 60% of the children still had active or residual psychotic symptoms and were on antipsychotic medication. Even among the remaining 40% who were less impaired and classified as "in remission," all save one were still in treatment and on antipsychotic medication.

Chapter 4

Infantile Autism

INTRODUCTION

During the second year of life the child's initial imaginative use of toys and imitative role-playing reveal the beginnings of a rich inner fantasy life. The normally developing toddler manifests an increasingly complex sense of himself and others as interacting beings, each with emotions, motives, and an identity of his or her own. Concurrently, the child's language grows in vocabulary, sentence length, and syntax. More than that, he puts language to new uses in games, metaphors, and a panoply of social exchanges and communications. Firmly rooted in a mutual attachment with his parents, the toddler reaches out to explore the world of social roles with other adults, siblings, peers, and pets even more intensely than he explores the world of inanimate objects.

These crucial developmental steps form an initiation into the human community; tragically, however, some children fail to make such advances. Although they have adequate sensorimotor intelligence, evidenced by skill at mechanical tasks, these children show little interest in the social world and their language is usually rudimentary. Occasionally they show prodigious verbal imitative capacities, echoing long passages verbatim. Even here, however, such children do not utilize language flexibly and adaptively for social intercourse; instead, they use whatever language they possess in inappropriate or self-stimulatory ways. Communication at best remains limited to indicating basic wants. Because these children fail to develop normal play and language, they most often come to professional attention as toddlers, but careful history taking usually reveals defects in relatedness from the earliest months of life.

Leo Kanner, in 1943, first described this group of children systematically. He coined the term *infantile autism* to depict their "extreme aloneness" or "self-isolation," which, together with an "anxiously obsessive desire for sameness" (p. 245) he saw as the cardinal feature of the condition. Although Kanner (1943) originally used the term *autistic* as an adjective (the title of his classic paper was "Autistic Disturbances of Affective Contact"), the noun form *autism* is now used to refer to the syndrome he delineated. Kanner (1943) took the concept of autism from Bleuler, who had used the term in 1911 to describe a particular kind of relationship with reality that he postulated as one of the primary pathognomonic defects in adult schizophrenia. Bleuler wrote:

> The most severe cases of schizophrenia, who no longer have any contact at all with others, live in a world by themselves; they have retreated into cocoons with their wishes. . . , and they set themselves off as much as possible from any contact with the external world. This cutting themselves off from reality, together with the relative and absolute predominance of their inner lives, we call autism. (Bleuler, 1911/1950, p. 63, modified translation)

Kanner's borrowing of the term from Bleuler raised two questions that have plagued the history of infantile autism: (1) What is the relationship of infantile autism to schizophrenia? (2) Is the autistic child's aloofness the result of a *withdrawal*, perhaps defensive, from a position of potentially better relatedness; or is it, instead, the outcome of an *inability* to develop social attachments that is present from the start? Chapter 2 touched on these topics, and this chapter will return to them in the section on the etiology of autism.

DEFINITION

DSM-III-R Diagnostic Criteria for Autistic Disorder

At least eight of the following sixteen items are present, these to include at least two items from A, one from B, and one from C. Note: *Consider a criterion to be met* only *if the behavior is abnormal for the person's developmental level.*

A. *Qualitative impairment in reciprocal social interaction as manifested by the following:*
   (The examples within parentheses are arranged so that those first mentioned are more likely to apply to younger or more handicapped, and the later ones, to older or less handicapped, persons with this disorder.)
   (1) marked lack of awareness of the existence or feelings of others (e.g., treats a person as if he or she were a piece of furniture; does not notice another person's distress; apparently has no concept of the need of others for privacy)
   (2) no or abnormal seeking of comfort at times of distress (e.g., does not come for comfort even when ill, hurt, or tired; seeks comfort in a stereotyped way, e.g., says "cheese, cheese, cheese" whenever hurt)
   (3) no or impaired imitation (e.g., does not wave bye-bye; does not copy mother's domestic activities; mechanical imitation of others' actions out of context)
   (4) no or abnormal social play (e.g., does not actively participate in simple games; prefers solitary play activities; involves other children in play only as "mechanical aids")
   (5) gross impairment in ability to make peer friendships (e.g., no interest in making peer friendships; despite interest in making friends, demonstrates lack of understanding of conventions of social interaction, for example, reads phone book to uninterested peer)
B. *Qualitative impairment in verbal and nonverbal communication, and in imaginative activity, as manifested by the following: (The numbered items are arranged so that those first listed are more likely to apply to younger or more handicapped, and the later ones, to older or less handicapped, persons with this disorder.)*
   (1) no mode of communication, such as communicative babbling, facial expression, gesture, mime, or spoken language
   (2) markedly abnormal nonverbal communication, as in the use of eye-to-eye gaze, facial expression, body posture, or gestures to initiate or modulate social interaction (e.g., does not anticipate being held, stiffens when held, does not

> *look at the person or smile when making a social approach, does not greet parents or visitors, has a fixed stare in social situations)*
>
> *(3) absence of imaginative activity, such as playacting of adult roles, fantasy characters, or animals; lack of interest in stories about imaginary events*
>
> *(4) marked abnormalities in the production of speech, including volume, pitch, stress, rate, rhythm, and intonation (e.g., monotonous tone, questionlike melody, or high pitch)*
>
> *(5) marked abnormalities in the form or content of speech, including stereotyped and repetitive use of speech (e.g., immediate echolalia or mechanical repetition of television commercial); use of "you" when "I" is meant (e.g., using "You want cookie?" to mean "I want a cookie"); idiosyncratic use of words or phrases (e.g., "Go on green riding" to mean "I want to go on the swing"); or frequent irrelevant remarks (e.g., starts talking about train schedules during a conversation about sports)*
>
> *(6) marked impairment in the ability to initiate or sustain a conversation with others, despite adequate speech (e.g., indulging in lengthy monologues on one subject regardless of interjections from others)*
>
> C. *Markedly restricted repertoire of activities and interests, as manifested by the following:*
>
> *(1) stereotyped body movements, e.g., hand-flicking or -twisting, spinning, head-banging, complex whole-body movements*
>
> *(2) persistent preoccupation with parts of objects (e.g., sniffing or smelling objects, repetitive feeling of texture of materials, spinning wheels of toy cars) or attachment to unusual objects (e.g., insists on carrying around a piece of string)*
>
> *(3) marked distress over changes in trivial aspects of environment, e.g., when a vase is moved from usual position*
>
> *(4) unreasonable insistence on following routines in precise detail, e.g., insisting that exactly the same route always be followed when shopping*
>
> *(5) markedly restricted range of interests and a preoccupation with one narrow interest, e.g., interested only in lining up objects, in amassing facts about meteorology, or in pretending to be a fantasy character*
>
> D. *Onset during infancy or childhood. (APA, 1987, pp. 38–39)*

The current DSM-III-R diagnostic criteria for infantile autism borrow heavily from Kanner's (1943) original description, but specifically exclude children who show signs of a classic schizophrenic thought disorder.

DSM-III-R both broadens and gives greater specificity to the criteria for the disorder, which was termed *Infantile Autism* in the DSM-III (APA, 1980). That edition had defined *Infantile Autism* as a pervasive developmental disorder characterized by (1) onset before 30 months of age; (2) pervasive lack of responsiveness to other people (autism); (3) gross deficits in language development; (4) peculiar speech patterns such as immediate and delayed echolalia, metaphorical language [unclear idiosyncratic usages], and pronomial reversal; (5) bizarre responses to various aspects of the environment, e.g., resistance to change, peculiar interest in or attachments to animate or inanimate objects; and (6) absence of delusions, hallucinations, loosening of associations, and incoherence as in Schizophrenia (pp. 89–90).

In DSM-III-R the rubric *Autistic Disorder* combines the DSM-III categories of Infantile Autism and Childhood-Onset Pervasive Developmental Disorder. Criticism of the dichotomous DSM-III scheme had included the unreliability of age of onset as a criterion and overlap between the behavioral descriptors for the two categories. The DSM-III-R revision of these criteria also has been under attack for being premature, confounding legislation and service-delivery regulations that embody DSM-III criteria, and widening the diagnostic category so broadly that it includes children without the "core" disorder (for a further discussion of diagnostic issues, see Cohen et al., 1986a, 1986b; Dahl et al., 1986; Denckla, 1986; Volkmar et al., 1986; Volkmar & Cohen, 1988).

The National Society for Autistic Children has officially adopted a complementary definition of the syndrome of autism. With minor modifications the key features of this definition may be summarized as follows (Ritvo & Freeman, 1978):

Autism is a behaviorally defined syndrome. The essential features are typically manifested prior to 30 months of age and include:

1. Disturbances of developmental rates and sequences. Normal coordination of the three developmental pathways (motor, social-adaptive, cognitive) is disrupted. Delays, arrests, and/or regressions occur within one or more of the pathways.
2. Disturbances of responses to sensory stimuli.
3. Disturbances of speech, language-cognition, and nonverbal communication.
4. Disturbances of the capacity to relate appropriately to people, events, and objects, manifested by failure to develop appropriate responsivity to people and assignment of appropriate symbolic meaning to objects.

EPIDEMIOLOGY

In various surveys, the general-population prevalence of infantile autism is about 2 to 5 cases per 10,000; the rate varies with the strictness of the diagnostic criteria (Zahner & Pauls, 1987). The condition is found throughout the world and in all social classes. Some of the many feral or "wild" children reported through the years (e.g., Itard's *Le Sauvage d'Avignon*) may well have been autistic children abandoned by their families. There is a marked excess of boys over girls, with the ratio ranging from two-to-one to four-to-one in different studies (Tsai et al., 1981; Wing, 1981a). The section on etiology discusses familial and social class distribution patterns.

CLINICAL COURSE

Early Development

The development of most autistic children goes awry from earliest infancy (Kanner, 1943; Rutter, 1985a, 1985b; Wing, 1985). Mothers often report that even in the first weeks of life the affected infant was somehow "different" from his normal siblings. Some are flaccid and lethargic "good" babies, whereas others are irritable. Some may show unusual sensitivities and overreact to sound, light, or touch (Bergman & Escalona, 1949). Such infants are often not cuddly; when they are held, they fail to mold to the mother and instead remain either limp or rigid. Eye-to-eye gaze is attenuated or aberrant. Babbling develops abnormally and is impaired in both its inflection and playful social use. Later, unlike normal infants, they do not reach up with their arms to anticipate being picked up. Social imitation, such as waving bye-bye, does not develop, and the autistic infant has no interest in interactive games such as pat-a-cake or peekaboo.

Thus, by the time the infant is 6 to 9 months of age, the clinician often can suspect the diagnosis of autism. The child cannot meet all the criteria, however, until the second year of life when the full extent of the language disorder, bizarre behavior, and social aloofness becomes clear. At the toddler stage, and beyond, autistic children fail to develop make-believe play and do not imitate their parents' everyday activities such as telephoning, sweeping, or brushing their hair. They do not follow their parents about or seek physical affection and attention. To the extent that the autistic toddler's motor coordination permits, peculiar mannerisms and repeated stereotyped behaviors such as hand-flapping, rocking, or spinning may appear. Language is absent or delayed; if and when it appears, it is characterized by echolalia, reversal of pronouns, and a striking lack of reciprocal, to-and-fro chatter.

Some autistic children (perhaps as many as 20%) are reported to have developed normally up to 2 or 3 years of age; at that point disturbances of language, alertness, and social responsiveness were first noted (Rutter, 1985a, 1985b; Volkmar & Cohen, 1989). It is unclear whether these children had milder early symptoms, less observant parents, or a different pathogenic process that does not manifest itself until later in infancy. In this connection Folstein and Rutter (1978) studied one monozygotic twin pair who were both autistic, but with markedly different ages of onset.

In addition to the stated difficulties, many autistic children are mentally retarded (see below). Unlike the nonautistic retarded individual, the autistic retarded individual's social relatedness is far more impaired than would be expected from his overall cognitive abilities or mental age.

Autism may also coexist with other serious handicaps such as congenital rubella syndrome (with frequent concomitant blindness or deafness) (Chess, 1977), retrolental fibroplasia, chromosomal disorders (such as fragile X syndrome), and metabolic disorders (such as phenylketonuria) (Golden, 1987; Young et al., 1990). In cases of *secondary* autism, the severe sensory defects or global retardation may obscure the autistic deficits until the child reaches a sufficient mental age that his bizarreness, language defects, and social aloofness become apparent.

Areas of Disturbance

The symptoms of autism can be considered under five headings (modified from Ritvo & Freeman, 1978): social relatedness, language and cognition, perception, motility, and developmental rate.

Disturbances of Social Relatedness.   The disturbed interpersonal relatedness of autistic children is apparent in their lack of sociability and sparse social communications, their impaired capacity for empathy and constricted affective range, and their failure to develop a normal pattern of attachment to familiar figures (Cohen et al., 1986a).

The autistic child's lack of social bonding and specific attachment behavior toward his caretakers are cardinal features of his illness (Fein et al., 1986; Shapiro et al., 1987b; Volkmar, 1987). He treats adults as if they are relatively interchangeable. Unlike the child who may be indiscriminately but superficially affectionate because of being reared by multiple caretakers, the autistic child is indiscriminately indifferent. When hurt, these children usually do not turn to their parents either for affection or for comfort. Autistic children may suffer from sudden panic attacks or outbursts of aggression directed at themselves or others. At such times they appear unable to use their parents for calming or consolation. The presence of strangers or the absence of parents can lead to extreme agitation; however, a new refrigerator or a moved table might evoke a similar response because the panicked child seems to be reacting more to change than to fearing or missing a *person*. To the extent that the autistic child attaches to others at all, he often relates to people as part-objects. An autistic child, for example, might use his mother's hand to open the refrigerator door, but he does not address her or ask her to get him something to eat.

Autistic children appear aloof, preferring self-stimulatory activity or solitary manipulation of physical objects to the company of either peers or adults. They tend to "look through" people, as if others were not present or of no special interest (Fein et al., 1986). Although their eye contact may not be quantitatively diminished, their gaze bears little relationship to the interpersonal context and is not used to modulate social interactions (Rutter, 1985b). Such a child pays little attention to and has little understanding of others' emotions or feelings. He has severely impaired ability to read the nonverbal gestures and cues, such as facial expression, body posture, and verbal intonation, that convey emotions and subtle interpersonal signals (Hobson, 1986a, 1986b, 1989); and he, himself, makes little or no expressive use of facial expression, symbolic gesture, or vocal inflection.

The most striking deficit is thus the autistic child's inability to see himself or others as persons, that is, as stable, sentient loci of feelings, wishes, and initiative. His world is populated primarily with things, rather than with people.

In adolescence, some high-functioning autistic children develop language and perhaps a desire for friendship; even they, however, remain socially inept, lacking empathy for others' feelings or perspectives (Kanner et al., 1972; Volkmar & Cohen, 1985). To the extent that they can describe their inner lives, these youths seem curiously impoverished and empty of feelings, warmth, or imagination. This emotional void led Bettelheim (1967) to call the autistic condition "the empty fortress."

This lack of human responsiveness is perhaps most heartbreakingly painful to the parents of such a child, who may devote their lives to his care. Cohen and colleagues (1978, p. 72) reported the poignant feelings of one such mother, who, after having spent every day with her son for 17 years, finally placed him in a residential treatment center. "I knew that as soon as I brought him there he would be as happy as he was at home. He didn't seem to miss me for a moment."

Disturbances of Language and Cognition. Approximately 50% of autistic children never develop useful speech. Those children who do learn to speak usually do so only after serious delays and with striking characteristic abnormalities of style, syntax, and social usage (Paul, 1987). Their speech is often poorly inflected and modulated and may be accompanied by echolalia and syntactic peculiarities.

Echolalia is the immediate or delayed repetition of heard words and phrases. In its rigid persistence, lack of playfulness, and other formal characteristics, autistic echoing differs markedly from the normal phase-appropriate imitation of the toddler who is learning to speak. Although the determinants of this parroting are complex, from one perspective it is an extension into the linguistic sphere of the autistic child's perseverative tendencies and insistence on sameness (Paul, 1987).

Echolalia may also represent the child's recognition that his interlocutor has requested some sort of response; as such, it may be the best he can do (Caparulo & Cohen, 1977; Shapiro, 1977). One morning, for example, 6-year-old Billy and his teacher were greeted by a classmate. The teacher prompted Billy to respond by suggesting, "Say 'Good morning,' Billy." Billy replied, "Say good morning Billy."

Some autistic children have remarkable verbal recall. One 7- year-old girl, who had no useful communicative language, would frequently repeat verbatim minute-long TV ads after she heard them only once or twice.

Other conspicuous and common peculiarities of autistic speech include the absence of the usual "I–you" pronoun reversal in conversation and the frequent failure of the child to refer to himself in the first person. These difficulties may represent the lack of a developing sense of self, a tendency for echolalia and perseveration, and difficulty in grasping the grammatical concept of shifting reference (Paul, 1987). Thus, when the mother of an autistic 5-year-old asked, "Do you want your chocolate pudding now?" the child replied, "Want your pudding now." Such a child may say of himself, "He go to the store." In contrast, the normal 2-year-old may walk about the house, intoning with both pride and assertiveness, "*My* teddy, *my* dolly, *my* table, *my* mommy."

The most strikingly abnormal aspect of austistic children's language, however, lies in its aberrant social usage rather than in its deviant syntax or lexical features (Cohen, et al., 1986a; Paul, 1987; Prizant & Wetherby, 1987; Shapiro et al., 1987a). Such children do not understand the situational, communicative, or social use of language, that is, the features that linguists term the *pragmatics* of speech. An autistic child's speech has little or no give-and-take. This deficit may be apparent in the first year of life, for normally even the babbling preverbal infant shows marked attention to and alternation with the vocalizations of his partner.

The autistic child pays little attention to how his utterances are being received or to what others are saying. On a more subtle level, even high-functioning autists have difficulty assessing what others are interested in discussing or whether people know or understand what they are saying. Metaphors and idioms, irony, and other nuances of expression may be lost on them. As Wing and Attwood (1987) have observed, what autistic children say often appears unrelated to what they have heard. They give the impression of talking *in the presence of* someone rather than *with* someone.

The autistic child's communicative deficits are not confined to verbal usage. Although capable of gestural requests, autistic children are deficient in many nonverbal areas of communication, such as pointing, that involve coordinating their own focus of attention with that of a social partner (Mundy et al., 1986).

The cognitive deficits of the autistic child also lie at a deeper level than the purely linguistic (Fein et al., 1986; Sigman et al., 1987). Although autistic children may show a prodigious ability to repeat long strings of words, draw complex pictures from memory, or remember the route to places visited only once, they have little appreciation of the *meaning* or *significance* of patterns, events, or relationships (Rutter, 1983). Unlike normal children, many autistic youngsters can recall strings of random words as readily as meaningful phrases of the same length. In perceiving and producing patterns, autistic children have difficulty appreciating abstract rules and general features. For example, Caparulo and Cohen (1977) cited a bright 10-year-old autistic boy who would repetitively draw accurate scale pictures of a local restaurant but could not arrange a set of geometric shapes according to size.

When confronted with a complex stimulus, autistic children frequently seize on only one aspect, ignoring all others, including elements that would seem most salient to the normal child. In both the perceptual and cognitive realms, autistic children's rules of salience differ greatly from those of nonautistic individuals. In the Embedded Figure Test, for example, many autists show outstanding skill locating hidden figures, as though not distracted by the surrounding welter of detail. Yet when putting together picture puzzles (at which many also excel), autistic children in one study ignored the picture and used the shape of the edges as a guide (Frith & Baron-Cohen, 1987).

Although autistic children may do well on discrimination tasks involving nonemotional cues, they do poorly on tasks involving affective or social stimuli (Fein et al., 1986; Hobson, 1986a, 1986b, 1989). For example, in matching photographs or videos, autistic subjects tend to ignore emotional facial expressions or gestures and instead rely on clothing, accessories, or other nonsocial cues; in general they do better on tasks involving inanimate objects rather than human stimuli (Jennings, 1973, and Hobson, 1982, cited in Fein et al., 1986).

Thus, in a variety of areas, autistic children use eccentric cognitive and perceptual strategies. Their idiosyncratic use of words often reflects this impaired conceptual ability. One of Kanner's patients, for example, was asked to solve a practical arithmetic problem to which the answer was 6 cents. He replied, "I'll draw a hexagon."

In later life, autistic children can show preemptive, fascinated preoccupation with telephone directories, airplane schedules, maps, or other abstract circumscribed areas of interest.

CASE EXAMPLE

Sam, a bright, 10-year-old, autistic boy, was preoccupied with maps, which he pored over for hours and drew with remarkable accuracy, most often from memory. On meeting his doctor for the first time, his opening gambit was to say, "We're right near Routes 28 and 270." He proceeded to draw from memory an accurate map of the school's surroundings, carefully indicating all of the local cemeteries (correctly including in one a tombstone that read "F. Scott Fitzgerald, 1896–1940"). As Sam got to know the school better, he drew maps of the school grounds but idiosyncratically focused on such features as the speed bumps. If asked how he had spent the weekend, he would describe the routes he had traversed, but it was difficult to impossible to ascertain with whom he had traveled, what he had done, or whether he had enjoyed the outing.

His preoccupations did little to engage his peers, and as a teenager, he complained that his classmates ignored him. In their therapeutic work, his therapist focused constantly on "how to have better talks with others." As a result, Sam gradually shifted his interests, first to sports and later to rock music. Here too, his prodigious but eccentric memory permitted him to recall quantities of facts and statistics that he would often relentlessly repeat to his peers, albeit with mixed results. Despite his difficulty with linguistic nuances, he would assiduously study compendiums of jokes, which, like Proust's Mme. Verdurin, he would carefully rehearse at home for later use.

Disturbances of Perception. The perceptual difficulties of autistic children lie in the processing of sensory inputs rather than in any gross sensory defects (Frith & Baron-Cohen, 1987). Autistic children show an apparently faulty modulation of both external and internal sensory input. The same child may underreact to some sensations and overreact to others with unusual sensory preferences and aversions. The taste, smell, and feel of objects may preoccupy autistic children. Some fail to react to sounds or voices to a degree that suggests deafness, whereas other children startle exaggeratedly or panic in response to sounds or bright light. Some appear unresponsive to painful injuries. Fine visual patterns, smells, and textures fascinate and capture the attention of many autistic children, who can spend hours staring intently, smelling a familiar object, or rubbing their faces or hands against a fabric. Many of these behaviors may be an attempt to induce a state of perceptual monotony, one aspect of what Kanner (1943) referred to as "an anxiously obsessive desire for the maintenance of sameness" (p. 245). A need to induce actively a monotonous rhythmic proprioceptive and vestibular or visual sensation may account for the repetitive rocking, whirling, and hand-flapping characteristic of this disorder (Ornitz, 1974; Ornitz & Ritvo, 1968). Repetitive and limited play patterns frequently involve aligning household objects or toys in the same pattern over and over, without regard for their usual function. These children may insist on the same food and the same clothes to an extent far beyond the demands of the normal preschooler. Such a child may compulsively carry some object like a piece of paper around with him, but without any of the affection that most children show a teddy bear or security blanket. The concern for sameness transcends the purely sensorimotor realm. Making even minor changes in the child's familiar environment, such as moving a vase or table, may produce panic, disorganization, or tantrums.

Disorders of Motility. Certain characteristic repetitive stereotyped behaviors and peculiar mannerisms give a strikingly bizarre appearance to the often attractive autistic child. Seemingly endless and virtually uninterruptible hand-flapping, rocking, or twirling at a monotonous rhythm is common (Freeman et al., 1981). Repetitive turning on and off of light switches or faucets for hours at a time may occur despite attempts at pleasant distraction. These stereotypies are more common in retarded autistic children and are exacerbated by barren, unstimulating environments (Rutter, 1985c); children may also use them to ward off excessive stimulation.

The autistic child may show unusual opisthotonic posturing (arching back and neck), toe-walking, and staccato darting movements. A spinning top can elicit twirling or posturing in the watching autistic child. Ornitz and Ritvo (1968), who studied this phenomenon as well as spontaneous repetitive twirling, were impressed by the abnormal nystagmus and disturbed vestibular functioning of these children.

Disturbance of Developmental Rate. The overall unevenness of the developmental process in autistic children is striking. Spurts and plateaus may alternate with delay and regression. Thus, certain motor skills, such as sitting up, may appear on schedule or early, whereas others, such as walking or fine motor manipulation, may be delayed. Striking disparities between lines of development may occur; social adaptive skills, for example, lag far behind the intelligent manipulation of objects. A few autistic children show precocious "splinter skills," such as prodigious mnemonic, computational, musical, or drawing skills (Cain, 1969; Rimland, 1978; Sacks, 1985; Selfe, 1977; Treffert, 1989). When children display these skills against a background of otherwise serious intellectual, social, and linguistic retardation, they are sometimes referred to as *idiots savants.* Some autistic children of otherwise quite limited verbal ability may show *hyperlexia*—the ability to read aloud complex written material—albeit with little or no comprehension (Burd et al., 1987).

Nonspecific Problems. In addition to these characteristic disturbances, autistic children may show various nonspecific problems that frequently cause serious management difficulties (Rutter, 1985c). These include hyperactivity, temper tantrums, aggressive outbursts, self-destructive behavior (such as head-banging), and idiosyncratic fears and phobias.

The Relationship of Retardation to Autism

The cognitive capacities of autistic children and the relationship of infantile autism to mental retardation have been the subjects of considerable research. Originally Kanner (1943) thought autistic children were of normal intelligence because of their alert facial expressions, absence of physical stigmata, skillful fine motor abilities, and relatively good performance on a form board test. Unlike the simply retarded child, whose social skills are often better than his cognitive ones, autistic children's aloofness and social isolation exceed their cognitive impairment (Fein et al., 1986).

Subsequent studies have failed to confirm Kanner's (1943) conclusion that most autistic children are of normal intelligence. Autistic children are notoriously difficult to motivate and engage in testing; in addition, their cognitive performance is highly variable across tasks and situations (Koegel & Mentis, 1985). Their apparent intellectual deficits, however, are not due solely to their poor relatedness or lack of motivation. With careful testing, only about 20% of autistic children have IQs of 70 or more; another 20% have IQs between 50 and 70; the remaining 60% have IQs below 50 (Ritvo & Freeman, 1978). Most autistic children thus function in the retarded range in both the verbal and nonverbal realms (Freeman et al., 1985).

Autism and mental retardation can and frequently do coexist. In a significant number of cases autistic behavior accompanies retardation from many organic causes, such as inborn metabolic disorders (i.e., phenylketonuria (PKU) and histidinemia), tuberous sclerosis, viral infections, congenital hypothyroidism, and chromosomal abnormalities (Golden, 1987; Yuwiler et al., 1985). Why and to what extent some forms of organic retardation may be more highly associated with autistic symptoms than others is unclear. For example, autism appears to be common with congenital rubella and rare with Down syndrome (Rutter & Schopler, 1987).

The degree to which researchers include severely retarded and grossly brain-damaged children in any clinical sample of autistic children markedly influences the conclusions they are likely to draw from such a sample. For example, a significant number of autistic children (as high as 25% to 33% in some samples) develop seizures by late adolescence (Rutter, 1985a; Volkmar & Nelson, 1990). Such seizures, however, occur most frequently in severely retarded children. Similarly, the prevalence of perinatal complications, abnormal EEGs and CAT scans, soft neurological signs, and other pathological findings depends on the population from which the sample is selected. In particular, findings vary according to the number of retarded children with frank neurological disease in the sample.

Referral patterns may strongly influence the type of autistic children seen in different settings. For example, Knobloch and Pasamanick (1975) studied young children referred from a general pediatric service for developmental evaluation. In their sample, half of the children who met their criteria for autism had frank neurological disease ranging from cerebral palsy through Down syndrome, obstructive hydrocephalus, brain tumors, encephalitis, meningitis, or metabolic disorders such as hypothyroidism. The authors estimated that children with such severe neurological damage make up as much as 5% of the retarded population. These children, however, are rarely referred to psychiatric services (such as those from which Kanner's original sample was drawn).

In practice, it may be extremely difficult to determine whether a severely retarded child is autistic. Rutter (1985a) has pointed out that because of the absence of social relations and speech, the label of "autism" might sometimes be applied to a 5-year-old child with an IQ of 20 and a mental age of 1 year; to do so, however, would totally ignore developmental considerations. To make the diagnosis, the child's language and social relatedness must be more impaired than that predicted from his mental age. Thus, unless a retarded child has a mental age of 2 years or more, it is difficult to know if his social development is out of line with his cognitive development. Differential diagnosis may also be complicated because many moderately or severely retarded children show some of, but not all of, the features of autism necessary to meet the full spectrum of DSM-III criteria. Finally, many of the bizarre mannerisms of autistic children such as rocking, perseveration, and hand-flapping are common in nonautistic retarded children.

Differential Diagnosis

Evaluation of the autistic child includes a current assessment of the child's social, emotional, and cognitive functioning. It also requires a careful history of the child and his family (including medical history and family pedigree). Thorough medical and neurological examination and evaluation are essential to identify any associated neurological disorders, especially potentially treatable ones. The evaluation should include an EEG, CT scan, visual and auditory testing, lead level, and screens for metabolic disorder and infectious agents such as toxoplasmosis, rubella, and cytomegalovirus. Cases with abnormal physical or laboratory findings or significant retardation may warrant further studies such as chromosomal analysis.

In addition to the numerous organic conditions associated with retardation, the clinician must rule out the conditions described below.

Disintegrative Psychosis. The term *disintegrative psychosis* has been used to describe those rare children, who after a period of clearly normal development, suddenly manifest a marked loss of previously acquired social and communicative skills (Evans-Jones & Rosenbloom, 1978; Volkmar and Cohen, 1989). Although this profound and mysterious developmental regression is sometimes associated with a stressful life-event or medical illness, the causal implications are unclear. Recovery is usually very limited. These children must be differentiated from children with progressive neurological disease (such as the so-called storage diseases) who may show autisticlike symptoms, often after an initial period of apparently normal development.

Language Disorders. Problems such as congenital or acquired childhood aphasia, which may be associated with neurological abnormalities, can pose a diagnostic dilemma (Caparulo & Cohen, 1977; Cohen et al., 1976).

Language-disordered children usually show normal social reciprocity and attachment, symbolic imaginative play, and an interest in nonverbal communication. Some aphasic children, however, especially those with acute acquired aphasia, which abruptly leaves the child communicatively isolated, may show social withdrawal and agitation.

Asperger's Syndrome and Related Conditions. Some children display unusual patterns of social relatedness in the presence of relatively normal intelligence and good language skills. The terms *Asperger's syndrome* (Szatmari et al., 1990; Volkmar et al., 1985a; Wing, 1981b) and *schizoid personality of childhood* (Wolff & Barlow, 1979) have been used to describe such youngsters. Similarly, many children who satisfy the criteria for the DSM-III category of *Schizotypal Personality Disorder* resemble high-functioning autistic individuals. Many questions remain concerning the relationship of these disorders to autism and whether these labels reflect valid diagnostic distinctions.

Subtypes

By definition, autistic children suffer from severe impairment of reciprocal social interaction and verbal communication and restricted or abnormal activities and interests. There have been various attempts to subclassify these children to highlight common etiological, clinical, or prognostic factors (Cohen et al., 1987; Siegel et al., 1986; Volkmar & Cohen, 1988; Wing & Attwood, 1987). For example, IQ or the absence of useful speech are important measures of overall severity, with important prognostic implications.

Wing and Gould (1979) have proposed the notion of an "autistic spectrum" to describe the wide range of social impairment in this disorder. Using this dimension, they divided autistic individuals into three types: *aloof, passive,* and *active-but-odd* (Volkmar et al., 1989; Wing & Attwood, 1987). The *aloof* group of children are the most socially isolated with no evidence of an inner imaginative life; they reject social contact, are largely mute, and remain preoccupied with repetitive, stereotyped activities. In contrast, the *passive* group of children do not reject social or physical contact. Less globally impaired than the aloof group, they have better developed speech, although it is repetitive and idiosyncratic. They have fewer stereotypies but may have repetitive routines and circumscribed eccentric interests. Finally, the *active-but-odd* group may seek out social contact with others but in a peculiar, awkward fashion that is poorly attuned to the other person's interests, feelings, or perspective. These individuals may resemble the children described above under the rubric *Asperger's syndrome* or *schizoid personality of childhood*.

Prognosis

Researchers have now followed several groups of autistic children into adulthood (Kanner, 1971; Lotter, 1978; Rumsey et al., 1985; and Rutter, 1978). Prognosis generally depends on IQ and attainment of useful language by age 5. Appropriate play with toys is also a positive prognostic sign. By the time they become adults, about 60% to 70% of autistic children will test in the mentally retarded range. As adults, almost all of these individuals are severely handicapped and remain totally dependent for care on their families or institutions. About 15% of autistic children grow up to lead independent existences, holding down a job and making a fair social adjustment. Even in the group of children with IQs above 70, who lack gross behavioral oddities and attain some measure of social independence, half are unable to hold a job and continue to need some supervision.

Despite showing slow improvement in interpersonal relationships, those autistic children with the most favorable outcome and social adjustment in adulthood usually remain shy, introverted, and aloof without close friendships or good social judgment. They do best in jobs that do not involve many social skills. Although they may excel at abstract technical work, they are often literal-minded and inflexible in their human interactions (Volkmar & Cohen, 1985a). Concrete thinking, stereotyped movements, generalized anxiety, flat affect, obsessive-compulsive phenomena, and language peculiarities frequently persist into adulthood (Rumsey et al., 1985).

As autistic children grow older, most do not develop a formal thought disorder with hallucinations or delusions (Kolvin, 1971; Kolvin et al., 1971). By the time they reach adolescence or adulthood, only a very small number of autistic children develop defects in reality testing of sufficient magnitude to merit the diagnosis of either schizophrenia or schizotypal personality disorder (Petty et al., 1984; Watkins et al., 1988). On this basis, it is likely that autism and schizophrenia constitute distinct disorders. Diagnostic confusion may arise because, as adults, autistic individuals may show many *negative* symptoms of schizophrenia, including flat affect and social isolation (Howells & Guirguis, 1984); however, the *positive* schizophrenic symptoms of hallucinations and delusions are usually absent. Occasionally, it may be difficult to distinguish between true delusions and the false beliefs, obsessions, or idiosyncratic thoughts of autistic individuals (Rutter & Lockyer, 1967; Wing & Attwood, 1987); in contrast to the usual schizophrenic delusions, the autistic phenomena appear to be relatively unelaborated (Rumsey et al., 1985). Of course, the presence of autism does not protect an individual from developing schizophrenia, although the pathognomonic signs of schizophrenia are not easily detectable when language is limited. Autistic individuals who do develop schizophrenia often resemble those individuals described in the literature as "simple schizophrenics."

ETIOLOGY

The cause of autism is not known. Whether it represents a single disease process or the final functional expression of several causes (as with fever or cerebral palsy) is unclear. There is an increased incidence of autism in various neurological disorders, including congenital and postnatal viral infections such as rubella (Chess, 1977), retrolental fibroplasia, genetic and chromosomal disorders (i.e., PKU), and other congenital and acquired neurological conditions. As diagnostic knowledge advances, many cases of autism previously considered idiopathic (of unknown etiology) can be re-classified as secondary to (or associated with) identifiable conditions. Such associations strongly suggest that autism can be, but is not always, the common symptomatic outcome of various central nervous system disorders. It is also likely that there is one or more primary or idiopathic forms of the disorder, perhaps genetic in origin and less often associated with severe neurological symptoms or retardation. The findings of the UCLA group (Mason-Brothers et al., 1987) provide support for this notion. They studied the prevalence of potentially pathogenic pre-, peri-, and postnatal factors in the histories of 181 autistic children both from families with a single autistic offspring and from multiple-incidence families. During the gestations of the autistic children, single-incidence families showed a higher incidence of maternal flulike symptoms, bleeding, and taking medication.

If there is more than one type of autism, the family and clinical correlates of each type may well differ (Pauls, 1987; Young et al., 1990). As a result, research on heterogenous groups of autistic children must be interpreted carefully. Thus, if a given sample includes a predominance of severely retarded, frankly brain-damaged children, their predominance might obscure the clinical features and correlates of a more genetically deter-mined form of autism that could be present in other children in the sample.

The relationship of both the primary and secondary forms of autism to the schizophrenic disorders remains unclear—and has been hotly debated. Researchers agree that autistic children suffer from a profound distur-bance of central integration. Some experts view autism as the earliest expression of the same (as yet unidentified) defect that is responsible for adult schizophrenia. The two disorders, however, have divergent clinical features: the family and class distribution of schizophrenia and autism differ, and in later life, most autistic children fail to develop the hallucina-tions, delusions, or formal thought disorder of schizophrenia. Because of these differences, most experts now see autism and schizophrenia as sepa-rate entities (Rutter, 1972). This debate will not be completely resolved until researchers discover the causes of schizophrenia and autism. (Chapter 3 discusses the relation of these two disorders in further detail.)

A related controversy concerns whether the autistic child's symptoms are direct expressions of a defect or deficit (presumably congenital) or represent a psychologically determined defensive withdrawal from disturbing affects or experiences (Fein et al., 1986). This debate will be considered further in the following sections, which examine some of the specific causes that have been proposed for autism.

Familial Factors

Psychogenic theories of infantile autism have been elaborated by Bettelheim (1967), Szurek and Berlin (1973), Mahler (1952), and others. Although these theorists acknowledge the importance of constitutional vulnerabilities, they see the autistic child's aloofness as the product of a defensive withdrawal from traumatic aspects of his family environment rather than as the result of an organically determined ego deficit. Thus, the child's early and global withdrawal is seen as a desperate attempt to avoid intolerable pain or anxiety caused by some pathogenic pattern of communication between the mother and infant. Kanner (1943) initially felt that the parents of autistic children were themselves aloof, emotionally cold, and "refrigerator"-like, but later rejected the suggestion that the children's condition was due to defective rearing (Schopler et al., 1981).

Bettelheim (1967) maintained that the home environment of the autistic child was psychologically akin to that of the concentration camp. The parental message to the child was "Don't be!" The autistic syndrome was the child's attempt to comply. In this view, parental ambivalence repeatedly confronts the child with impossible (double-bind) choices. In despair, the youngster withdraws.

In recent years, there has been a growing consensus that although familial factors may affect outcome and the ability to utilize rehabilitative therapy, infantile autism is not primarily *caused* by emotional or interpersonal factors (see review by Cantwell et al., 1978). Most studies of the parents of autistic children have failed to show convincing evidence of increased thought disorder, aberrant communication patterns, or pathogenic child-rearing styles. Further, the presence of an autistic child in the home represents a tremendous emotional strain on parents; hence, when family problems occur in later childhood, it is difficult to establish the direction of cause and effect. (The careful research analysis of home movies now offers some hope of ascertaining the early status of mother–child relations in certain cases.) Because so much about the condition is in fact unknown, to add to the guilty burden of an autistic child's parents by implying that they have caused the child's tragic condition is to be a miserable comforter indeed.

Kanner's (1943) original impression that autistic children spring from intelligent, middle-class families has also continued to be controversial.

Although some studies show a disproportionate middle class prevalence, others show that the class distribution for autism parallels that of the general population (Zahner & Pauls, 1987). In this respect, autism apparently does *not* show the same class distribution as schizophrenia, which has a markedly increased incidence in lower socioeconomic groups. To what extent referral and selection biases affect the apparent socioeconomic distribution of autism is unclear. Some studies suggest that the parents of autistic children tend to be more intelligent than the general population; these studies, however, may reflect similar biases (Cantwell et al., 1978).

Genetic Studies

Genetic influences are now believed to play a role in at least some cases of autism. What is inherited may not be autism itself, but rather a predisposition to developmental difficulties and language and cognitive impairment, of which autism represents the severest expression (Rutter, 1985a).

Evidence for genetic influence comes from twin and family studies (Pauls, 1987; Ritvo et al., 1985a, 1985b; Rutter & Schopler, 1987; Young et al., 1990). For example, a concordance study of fraternal and identical twins found a low rate of concordance for the full autistic syndrome among the identical twins in the sample (4 of 11 pairs of identical twins concordant), but this low figure nonetheless exceeded the concordance rate for the fraternal twins (no pairs of fraternal twins concordant) (Folstein & Rutter, 1978). When the sets of twins were examined for the simultaneous presence of cognitive abnormalities or language delay in both members of each twin pair, the concordance rate rose to 9 of 11 monozygotic pairs versus only 1 of the 10 fraternal pairs. Finally, the study showed that the autistic children who had a nonautistic twin tended to show evidence of organic brain damage. These findings suggest that autism might arise from either a genetic predisposition (as in the concordant sets of twins) or some more general, nongenetically determined form of neurological impairment (as in the disconcordant sets).

Despite methodological limitations, a more recent twin study also found evidence for a genetic factor in autism on the basis of a high concordance rate of 95.7% for monozygotic twins, compared with only 23.5% for dizygotic twins (Pauls, 1987; Ritvo et al., 1985a).

Studies of nontwin siblings of autistic children yield similar findings. August et al. (1981), for example, found that the siblings of autistic children had a higher rate of autism (2.8%) and a much higher rate of other forms of cognitive impairment (15.5%) than a control group of siblings of Down syndrome children. Among the control group, none were autistic and only 2.6% showed cognitive impairment.

Family studies also support the distinction between autism and childhood schizophrenia. Most recent studies have concluded that the parents of autistic children do *not* show an increased prevalence of schizophrenia. In this respect, autistic children differ markedly from both adult- and late-childhood-onset schizophrenics, whose families show a high prevalence of schizophrenia.

Although autism appears to be uncommon in some chromosomally determined forms of mental retardation such as Down syndrome (trisomy 21), much attention has focused on the possible association of autism and the fragile X syndrome. (See Chapter 2 and Volume I, Chapter 1, for a more detailed discussion of this condition.) This common chromosomal defect is quite variable in its phenotypic expression, often producing distinctive facial features, enlarged testicles, and a variety of cognitive, linguistic, and attentional difficulties. The strength of the association between autism and the fragile X syndrome varies widely in different studies (Bregman et al., 1987, 1988). The frequency of autism in male subjects with fragile X syndrome ranges from 7% to 46% in different samples; how this correlates with the presence or absence of mental retardation in these samples is unclear. Conversely, screening of different autistic male populations found frequencies of the fragile X condition ranging from 0% to 15.8%. One source of confusion arises from the diagnostic criteria used for autism (Payton et al., 1989). Although many fragile X patients have stereotyped behaviors, atypical speech and language, and socially anxious gaze avoidance, most are otherwise socially engaged, rather than aloof (Bregman et al., 1988). Whether the fragile X syndrome increases the risk of autism above that associated with mental retardation in general remains unclear (Payton et al., 1989). Because a few fragile X individuals show improvements of attention and expressive language ability following dietary folate supplementation, folate treatment of prepubertal autistic patients with fragile X warrants further research (Bregman et al., 1987).

Biological Studies

A vast number of metabolic, biochemical, and physiological parameters have been studied in autism without revealing significant characteristic abnormalities. These studies have been reviewed by Anderson and Hoshino (1987), Ornitz (1985, 1987), Young et al., (1990), and Yuwiler et al. (1985).

Imaging studies utilizing CT and PET scans have so far failed to reveal consistent structural abnormalities in autistic children (Rutter & Schopler, 1987). In about 25% of autistic children, CT scans reveal nonspecific abnormalities (such as enlarged ventricles or asymmetries in ventricular or hemispheric size (Ornitz, 1987). Such findings, however, do not appear to correlate with severity of symptoms (Caparulo et al., 1981). Magnetic resonance imaging (MRI) studies also suggest subtle cerebellar abnormalities, enlargement of the lateral ventricles (especially the anterior horn), and cerebral cortical malformations (Gaffney et al., 1989; Piven et al., 1990; Gaffney & Tsai, 1987; Courchesne et al., 1988).

No unique neuropathologic defects have been identified in association with autism. Researchers have reported decreased numbers of Purkinje cells in the cerebellar cortex in the majority of the small number of cases that have come to autopsy (Ritvo et al., 1986).

Neurotransmitters and neuromodulators, especially the serotonergic, dopaminergic and neuropeptide systems, continue to be areas of promising research. Some autistic children, especially the more retarded, show markedly elevated peripheral levels of serotonin, although such levels also may occur in some nonautistic retardates (Yuwiler et al., 1985). High serotonin levels may run in some families. Studies of cerebrospinal fluid tentatively suggest altered central nervous system levels of the breakdown products of dopamine and serotonin, either absolutely or in relation to each other (Cohen et al., 1978; Gillberg et al., 1983; Gillberg & Svennerholm, 1987). A possible role for the dopaminergic system in the pathogenesis of autism is suggested by the observation that some autistic symptoms improve with the use of dopamine-inhibiting drugs such as haloperidol, whereas drugs such as amphetamine (which stimulate the dopaminergic system) markedly exacerbate symptoms. Sahley and Panksepp (1987) have emphasized the possible role of the brain opioid system in disorders of attachment and social relatedness.

The presence of hyperserotoninemia in about one-third of autistic children led Ritvo et al. (1983) to employ fenfluramine, a drug that lowers brain and blood levels of serotonin, with initially promising results (see below). However, the equal efficacy of the drug in patients with normal, as well as elevated, serotonin levels raises the question whether the drug's therapeutic action is from reducing serotonin per se.

Because autistic children are often labile and uncooperative in test situations, it is difficult to perform neurophysiological studies of arousal and attention with them. Several studies, however, indicate persistently heightened autonomic arousal and abnormalities in processing sensory stimuli; as a result, the autistic child may have great difficulty "making sense out of sensation" (Ornitz, 1987).

Clinically, autistic children show profound and puzzling deficits in understanding the symbolic, affective, and human aspects of language and the world. A still unanswered question is the extent to which these deficits reflect the autistic child's serious disturbances in modulating anxiety, arousal, attention, and sensory input (Fein et al., 1986). On a neurological level, these deficits imply extensive malfunctioning of many areas of the neo- and paleocortex as well as the mid-brain, limbic system, and their interconnections (Ornitz, 1985, 1987). Although attempts at localization are speculative and premature, such widespread dysfunction could relate to defects in the various neurotransmitter pathways.

Models of Autism

The above discussion makes clear that the causes of autism have not been identified. Any satisfactory working model of autism must explain the autistic child's puzzling pattern of profound social, communicative, and attentional deficits that frequently occur side by side with relatively intact cognitive and intellectual skills.

The normal child's social and cognitive development are intricately inter-twined (Cohen et al., 1978). From the earliest days of life, the infant's most compelling and engrossing stimuli are other human beings. As Bowlby (1982) and Stern (1985) have postulated, the normal infant has an innately determined propensity to attend to and to interact with his human partner. These interactions in turn serve as the major organizers for his developing ego. Such social attachment and bonding require an available adult partner as well as relatively intact perceptual, attentional, and cognitive capacities in the infant. Experiments of nature, such as deafness, blindness, severe retardation, and failure to thrive (FTT) demonstrate the deformations of social attachment and ego development that can occur when maturational or environmental preconditions are not met. Nonetheless, the child's at-tachment to his caretaker is not simply the product of intellectual and maturational developments but is in itself a major shaper and organizer of the child's cognitive, perceptual, and affective development (Decarie, 1965; Fraiberg, 1969; Stern, 1985). Social interactions provide the context in which the developing infant forms and refines his ability to deploy atten-tion, to modulate anxiety and arousal, to appreciate the permanence of objects, and to conceive of himself, like others, as a participant in a social world with feelings, intentions, and perspectives of his own.

In autism, this complex interweaving of the strands of social and cogni-tive development becomes unraveled (Cohen et al., 1978; Fein et al., 1986). There are several possible causes for this mishap. The biological and maturational determinants of the innate attachment system may somehow go awry, whereas other cognitive capacities remain relatively intact. Some theorists have tried to explain autism as a derangement of central language capacities, but these language deficits seem to be grafted onto an even more profound deficit in the social uses of communication, verbal and nonverbal alike. Given the interdependence of social and cognitive development, children who fail to attach and attend to others may miss essential interac-tive opportunities which provide the context for learning critical linguistic and social communicative skills. At the same time, sensorimotor and visual-spatial development, which is more autonomous from social interaction, might proceed relatively unimpaired (Fein et al., 1986). Although autistic children do show subtle defects in processing sensory stimuli, their greatest difficulty is with stimuli that carry social or emotional meaning (Rutter, 1983a). Thus, one possibility is that autism reflects a primary deficit in social relatedness, rather than in linguistic, sensory, or information processing. As yet, researchers know little about which brain systems subserve attachment and social behavior, much less what abnormalities might produce specific dysfunctions in these areas. Most speculation has focused on limbic and brain stem structures (Fein et al., 1986; Ornitz, 1985, 1987).

Another possibility is that the autistic child's difficulty in modulating arousal, attention, and perceptual input makes the world in general, and the domain of human interaction in particular, seem frightening and chaotic, "swept with confused alarms." Unlike the normal child who finds interpersonal stimulation fascinating and seeks out interactions with his parents, the autistic child may prefer the world of inanimate things. By remaining locked in his rigid, repetitive behavioral patterns he can protect himself from the chaos that *human* interactions, with all their richness and variability, entail for him (Cohen et al., 1978). Just as the autistic child cannot categorize or extract salient conceptual features from his physical environment, so too his inability to process interactions with people coherently results in a failure to develop stable internal representations of himself or others. From this viewpoint, autism may represent both a deficit and a defense. The child defends himself against the trauma of human relatedness by withdrawing to the simpler and more dependable inanimate world. The pain, here, stems not so much from pathogenic or toxic styles of parenting as from the autistic child's constitutional inability to order his perceptual and social world.

TREATMENT

At one time or another, clinicians have tried almost every therapeutic modality known to psychiatry on autistic children. The list includes psychotropic medication, electroconvulsive therapy, intensive psychoanalytically oriented psychotherapy of the child and/or parents, behavior modification, social skills training, and special educational techniques.

Psychodynamically oriented psychotherapeutic approaches have traditionally focused on establishing a meaningful emotional relationship with the child as an initial bridge to the human world. Overcoming the autistic child's tremendous aloofness is no easy matter. The therapist is as sorely tried by the child's apparent indifference as by the periodic outbursts of panic, fury, or self-aggression. Bettleheim (1967) eloquently outlined the principles of treatment in a residential setting and provided an extraordinary statement about its taxing demands. Unfortunately, with few exceptions (Goldfarb, 1974), systematic outcome data are not available concerning this approach. Although a psychotherapeutic approach to such children need not be predicated on "parentogenic" theories of etiology (Riddle, 1987), the parent-blaming bias of some programs has had an unfortunate hurtful and guilt-inducing impact on autistic children's already traumatized families (Kysar, 1968).

In recent years, as enthusiasm has faded for psychogenic theories of autism, attention has turned increasingly to more direct methods that utilize special educational and operant conditioning techniques targeted at the child's social, linguistic, and cognitive deficits (Cohen & Donnellan, 1987; DeMyer, 1987; Rutter, 1985a, 1985c).

Rutter (1985a, 1985c) distinguished five goals of treatment with the autistic child: (1) fostering normal cognitive, social, and language development; (2) promoting learning; (3) reducing rigidity and stereotypy; (4) eliminating nonspecific maladaptive behaviors; and (5) alleviating family distress.

Several difficulties in the instruction of autistic children require specific attention (Rutter, 1985c). Not only do these children have major skill deficits, they also have limited comprehension of the teacher's communications to them. In addition, they are isolative, lack initiative, and give up easily, often retreating into stereotypic behavior when frustrated (Koegel & Mentis, 1985). Consequently, their learning situation should be structured and directive and provide planned periods of pleasurable interaction. Communications should be simple, and instruction should build on the child's areas of strength and interest.

Language instruction should teach and reinforce communication and the social use of language rather than the acquisition of words or syntax. Thus, it is important to determine the motivating social context for encouraging communication (Prizant & Schuler, 1987a, 1987b; Schuler & Prizant, 1987). Such approaches are most useful with children who already possess at least rudimentary communicative interests and skills. Instruction in sign language may prove helpful in selected cases (Kiernan, 1983).

Similar structure, directiveness, and attention to context promote the autistic child's social development. Rutter (1985c) emphasizes that personal interactions encourage attachment and social relationships when they are pleasurable and responsive to the child's needs and provide comfort at times of stress. Because the autistic child lacks spontaneous social overtures and responsiveness, deliberate measures are necessary to engage him and overcome his isolative tendencies. Rutter emphasizes the importance of (1) deliberate intrusion into the child's solitary activities to provide opportunities for pleasurable activities in a reciprocal, socially interactive context; (2) the prevention of an institutional upbringing with multiple caretakers, and (3) the direct teaching of social skills (Frankel et al., 1987).

In general, regardless of subject area, several factors complicate the instruction of autistic children: their short attention span and lack of self-motivation; their tendency to learn by rote rather than by meaning or concept; and their difficulty in generalizing what they have learned beyond the specific context (Rutter, 1985c). The teacher must present the material in manageable, "bite-sized" steps and emphasize its meaning and application across the diverse settings of home, school, and neighborhood. Behavioral techniques and the shaping of alternative responses can reduce stereotypies, disruptive behaviors, and fears (LaVigna, 1987; Lovaas, 1978).

The most effective programs begin with a careful, formal evaluation in which the teacher (or therapist) and parents work collaboratively to identify the most pressing cognitive and behavioral problems. The most promising approaches actively involve the child's parents, who learn how to provide an ongoing home-based treatment program that utilizes the techniques used at the school or treatment center (Lovaas, 1978). Institutional behavior modification programs that fail to involve the parents show disappointingly little generalization of benefits outside the treatment setting or persistence of the improvement following discharge. Parents receive training in special education techniques as well as in developmentally oriented behavior modification methods such as modeling and shaping procedures for language and social skills; extinction procedures for tantrums, self-stimulation, and self-injurious behavior; and gradual desensitization procedures for phobic anxiety. In recent years behavioral approaches have increasingly emphasized social cues and rewards, rather than material ones (Rutter, 1985c). Parents are taught how to interrupt self-stimulating and stereotypic behavior with attractive, individually identified pleasurable interactions. The family and school maintain consistency and continuity of approaches either by means of frequent parental involvement in the classroom or through home visits.

Outcome studies indicate that classes for autistic children should include a good deal of specific teaching in a well-ordered classroom environment and appropriate task orientation. Such classroom situations lead to more improvement in social interaction and scholastic achievement than do less structured programs. In evaluating and reviewing various treatment programs, Rutter (1985c) concluded that "total push" programs that utilized a home-based therapy approach were superior to other approaches over both the long and the short term. In outlining the benefits and limits of treatment programs, he noted that in general, over time, even optimal long-term treatment appeared to make little difference in the child's actual IQ (unless there had been serious environmental deprivation). In addition, only minimal improvement was noted in formal language competence. Good long-term treatment, however, *did* result in marked amelioration of social and behavioral problems and improvement in the social *usage* of language skills (as opposed to basic linguistic competency). In terms of eventual overall social adjustment, these areas are perhaps the most crucial.

Medication can be a useful adjunct in the treatment of autism by helping to make the child more amenable to education and other treatment modalities (Campbell, 1985; Campbell et al., 1987); beneficial effects on long-term outcome have yet to be demonstrated. Haloperidol and the less sedating phenothiazines (such as trifluoperazine) diminish symptoms such as withdrawal, uncooperativeness, aggression, self-destructive outbursts, stereotypies, or panic attacks (Perry et al., 1989). In carefully titrated doses, haloperidol may not only reduce maladaptive behaviors but may also beneficially affect attention and cognition (Anderson et al., 1984). Careful monitoring, however, is essential, as some autistic children respond to such drugs with lethargy, withdrawal, and cognitive blunting (Fish et al., 1966). Caution is also necessary concerning the many side effects of these drugs, especially the possibility of tardive dyskinesia with long-term administration (Gualtieri et al., 1984). Dopamine agonists, especially stimulant medication such as methylphenidate or dextroamphetamine, usually lead to marked distress and exacerbation of symptoms. The neurobiological implications of these drug responses have been the object of much speculation about possible underlying serotoninergic and dopaminergic mechanisms in autism (Campbell et al., 1987; Young et al., 1982) (see section on etiology).

The elevated blood serotonin levels of many autistic children has led to interest in fenfluramine, a drug that markedly lowers brain serotonin. This action may also produce the appetite-suppressing effect for which the drug was first developed. Following an initially promising pilot study (Ritvo et al., 1983), fenfluramine was evaluated in a large, collaborative multicenter study; results from this larger sample have been less promising (August et al., 1987; Campbell et al., 1986, 1988). Some individuals show clinically significant improvement in hyperactivity, irritability, aggressiveness, and motor stereotypies. Despite conflicting reports, there appears to be no significant improvement of cognitive and linguistic functioning. Indeed, Campbell et al. (1988) found that fenfluramine retarded discriminant learning and had no positive effect on behavior. Thus, the efficacy and safety of long-term fenfluramine administration remain an open question (Aman & Kern, 1989; Campbell et al., 1988).

Recent work suggesting that the endorphins play a mediating role in the development of attachment behavior as well as pain perception has led to the experimental use of opioid antagonists such as naltrexone. In preliminary studies with autistic patients naltrexone has decreased self-injurious behavior and stereotypies and caused occasional dramatic improvement in social responsiveness (Herman, personal communication, 1988; Herman et al., 1986; Sahley & Panksepp, 1987; Walters et al., 1990). More extensive clinical trials are underway.

There is no convincing evidence that nutritional approaches are helpful; isolated reports of improvement on various vitamins or minerals have been difficult to replicate (Raiten & Massaro, 1987; Rimland et al., 1978).

Specific and supportive work with parents is essential in treating this chronically disabling condition. Parents are often bewildered and anguished by their child's profound unresponsiveness to them. They need help in detecting whatever responses their child does show and assistance in finding regular, meaningful interactions that are mutually pleasurable and that foster more normal attachment. Practical help and casework concerning parental guilt and frustration, marital stress, reactions of the normal siblings to the patient, respite care, and long-term educational planning are essential. Many parents turn to unorthodox or cultist modes of treatment, not so much because of the limitations of established approaches, but because of the lack of ongoing sympathetic support for their herculean task of rearing an autistic child.

High-functioning, verbal autistic adolescents are often painfully aware of their social awkwardness and isolation and may be eager for help. Individual psychotherapy can be very useful, especially when coupled with explicit training social skills such as decoding social and conversational cues and formulating appropriate responses.

Chapter 5

Borderline Children

INTRODUCTION

Evolution of the Borderline Concept in Adults

When applied to adults, the diagnostic term *borderline* has at least two different meanings: First, it describes a broad range of behavioral disorders that are more severe and pervasive than commonly associated with the neurotic but are less bizarre and extreme than seen with the psychotic. These intermediate and symptomatically diverse disorders are postulated by some clinicians to share an underlying pathological character organization—the *borderline personality* (Kernberg, 1975, 1977).

The second use of borderline is exemplified by the term *borderline schizophrenia*. Referring to a "schizophrenic spectrum" of disorders (Kendler, 1985), this usage denotes a cluster of persisting "schizphrenialike" personality features such as poor rapport; constricted, inappropriate affect; referential ideation, deviant communication; and odd perceptual experiences that resemble the symptoms of schizophrenia but fail to meet the full criteria for the disorder.

The first concept, that of the borderline personality, is still evolving. Because it is a diagnostic grouping that probably contains many heterogeneous clinical subentities, researchers continue to debate its validity and proper definition in both the adult and child psychiatric literature (McGlashan, 1983a, 1983b, 1987; Petti and Vela, 1990; Shapiro, 1983, 1990; M. H. Stone, 1984). Its fuzzy outlines result not only from the limitations of our current knowledge, but also from the protean nature and chaotic shifts in behavior that characterize these patients. Indeed, lability of affect, rapidity of disorganization in the face of anxiety, and quick fluctuations in attachment to others are the very hallmark of the borderline patient, who has been aptly described as "stably unstable" (Schmideberg, 1959) or "predictably unpredictable" (Pine, 1974).

On the one hand, the borderline's perpetually chaotic life is characterized by impulsive, often self-destructive, action and manipulative, coercive conduct toward others. Such behavior wards off intense, disorganizing rage, anxiety, or emptiness (especially in response to separation). On the other hand, although adult borderlines may become extremely confused and may even appear transiently psychotic, their reality testing is generally intact. For the most part they remain intensely (albeit ambivalently) involved with the people around them, and they do not run the deteriorating course of the schizophrenic.

Many of the descriptions of this first group of patients originated with psychoanalytically oriented researchers, such as Otto Kernberg (1975, 1977); Knight (1953); and Gunderson and Singer (1975). These workers were impressed by these patients' primitive, intense, and labile object-relations with others and by the affectively stormy transference relationship that characteristically developed during psychotherapy.

In contrast, interest in borderline schizophrenia has long been present in various other guises. Thus, designations such as "pseudoneurotic schizophrenia" or "ambulatory schizophrenia" were described many years ago (Hoch & Cattell, 1959; Zilboorg, 1957). The more recent use of the term *borderline schizophrenia* sprang from family and adoptive studies of schizophrenia and descriptive studies of schizophrenia-like traits in nonpsychiatric populations (Gunderson & Siever, 1985; Kendler, 1985). These studies noted that the families of schizophrenics included an increased number of relatives with mild schizophrenialike symptoms and traits, including paranoid attitudes, constricted affect, social isolation, peculiar communication, eccentric behavior, and bizarre perceptual experiences. These observations led to an attempt to define the phenotypic variants of a postulated underlying schizophrenic genotype. For example, to describe the presumed genetic vulnerability in schizophrenics' families, Meehl (1962, 1989) introduced the notion of "schizotaxia," an inherited neurointegrative defect. He suggested that persons possessing this genetic trait ("schizotypes") suffered from mild thought disorder, interpersonal sensitivity, ambivalence, withdrawal, and anhedonia. Depending on the degree of genetic loading and environmental stress, this constitutional vulnerability might result in a clinical picture ranging from a "well-compensated schizotype" to a severe schizophrenic (Kendler, 1985).

Genetic factors thus seem to play a decisive role in "borderline schizophrenia," although the nature of the presumed common heritable trait remains in question (Torgersen, 1984, 1985). In contrast, although the affectively unstable type of borderline pathology may have genetic links to the affective disorders (Stone, 1980) or even genetic heritability in its own right, experiential factors also appear to be very important. For example, some researchers see its roots in the early miscarriage of the mother–child relationship, especially in the separation–individuation process (Shapiro, 1978a).

The Borderline Child

The notion of the *borderline child* evolved parallel to but separate from developments in adult psychiatry (Chethik, 1979; Petti & Vela, 1990; Shapiro, 1983; Vela et al., 1983). The nosology of severe, pervasive childhood developmental disturbance has long been a controversial issue (see Chapter 3). During the 1950s and 1960s, several authors described "borderline children," whose development was more pervasively disturbed than that of neurotic children (Ekstein & Wallerstein, 1954; Frijling-Schreuder, 1969; Geleerd, 1958; Rosenfeld & Sprince, 1963, 1965; Weil, 1953). Despite excessive magical thinking, suspiciousness, and withdrawal into fantasy (especially of an omnipotent nature), these children did not show sufficiently severe or persistent delusions or hallucinations to warrant a diagnosis of schizophrenia or "childhood psychosis." In addition to these weaknesses in reality sense, common elements in early descriptions of the borderline child included disturbed interpersonal relationships; excessive, intense anxiety; severe impulsive behavior; a plethora of "neurotic-like" symptoms (including phobias, obsessions, compulsions, and somatic concerns); and uneven motor, language, cognitive, or physiological development (Vela et al., 1983).

Whether the borderline concept will prove to be a valid diagnostic construct remains unclear (Anthony, 1983; M. H. Stone, 1984). Researchers have not determined whether diagnostic criteria can delineate a group of patients who share common genetic factors, etiology, clinical course, or response to treatment. These questions are especially important with borderline children, who form a very heterogeneous group (Kernberg, 1990; Petti & Vela, 1990; Shapiro, 1990). Some critics have argued that, at least in childhood, *borderline* does not denote a discrete disorder; instead, it is used to describe a disparate group of children with severe difficulties and multiple, overlapping diagnoses (Greenman et al., 1986; Gualtieri & Van Bourgondien, 1987; Shapiro, 1990). Many clinicians share Robson's (1983) suspicion that "ultimately most borderline children . . . will turn out to be at biogenetic risk for major mental illnesses and their variants." Certainly, follow-up studies (Kestenbaum, 1983) and longitudinal studies of high-risk children (Kron & Kestenbaum, 1988) suggest that many youngsters who appear initially to be borderline children in adolescence or early adulthood develop schizophrenia or major affective disorders. In the future, the discovery of "markers" for genetic vulnerability to such conditions may permit clearer delineation of their childhood precursors.

DEFINITION

Although common usage is often ambiguous as to which meaning of borderline is being employed, DSM-III (APA, 1980) and DSM-III-R (APA, 1987) attempt a formal division into two distinct entities: borderline personality disorder (i.e., stably-unstable) and schizotypal personality disorder (i.e., schizophrenialike).

DSM-III-R Diagnostic Criteria for Borderline Personality Disorder

A pervasive pattern of instability of mood, interpersonal relationships, and self-image, beginning by early adulthood and present in a variety of contexts, as indicated by at least five of the following:

(1) a pattern of unstable and intense interpersonal relationships characterized by alternating between extremes of overidealization and devaluation

(2) impulsiveness in at least two areas that are potentially self-damaging, e.g., spending, sex, substance use, shoplifting, reckless driving, binge eating (Do not include suicidal or self-mutilating behavior covered in [5].)

(3) affective instability: marked shifts from baseline mood to depression, irritability, or anxiety, usually lasting a few hours and only rarely more than a few days

(4) inappropriate, intense anger or lack of control of anger, e.g., frequent displays of temper, constant anger, recurrent physical fights

(5) recurrent suicidal threats, gestures, or behavior, or self-mutilating behavior

(6) marked and persistent identity disturbance manifested by uncertainty about at least two of the following: self-image, sexual orientation, long-term goals or career choice, type of friends desired, preferred values

(7) chronic feelings of emptiness or boredom

(8) frantic efforts to avoid real or imagined abandonment (Do not include suicidal or self-mutilating behavior covered in [5].) (APA, 1987, p. 347)

DSM-III-R Diagnostic Criteria for Schizotypal Personality Disorder

A. A pervasive pattern of deficits in interpersonal relatedness and peculiarities of ideation, appearance, and behavior, beginning by early adulthood and present in a variety of contexts, as indicated by at least five of the following:

(1) ideas of reference (excluding delusions of reference)

(2) excessive social anxiety, e.g., extreme discomfort in social situations involving unfamiliar people

(3) odd beliefs or magical thinking, influencing behavior and inconsistent with subcultural norms, e.g., superstitiousness, belief in clairvoyance, telepathy, or "sixth sense," "others can feel my feelings" (in children and adolescents, bizarre fantasies or preoccupations)

(4) unusual perceptual experiences, e.g., illusion, sensing the presence of a force or person not actually present (e.g., "I felt as if my dead mother were in the room with me")

(5) odd or eccentric behavior or appearance, e.g., unkempt, unusual mannerisms, talks to self

(6) no close friends or confidants (or only one) other than first-degree relatives

(7) odd speech (without loosening of associations or incoherence), e.g., speech that is impoverished, digressive, vague, or inappropriately abstract

(8) inappropriate or constricted affect, e.g., silly, aloof, rarely reciprocates gestures or facial expressions, such as smiles or nods

(9) suspiciousness or paranoid ideation

B. Occurrence not exclusively during the course of Schizophrenia or a Pervasive Developmental Disorder. (APA, 1987, pp. 341–342)

Prior to DSM-III (APA, 1980), these two borderline conditions were often lumped together under the same rubric or seen as diagnostic "near neighbors." Further refinement of the DSM-III distinction between schizotypal and borderline personality disorder has led to seeing these two entities as quite distinct and at best only "distant cousins." The clinical child psychiatric literature is only just beginning to reflect this diagnostic dichotomy (Petti & Vela, 1990).

Several lines of evidence support the validity of separating borderline adult patients into these two disorders (McGlashan, 1983a, 1983b, 1987). Descriptively, schizotypal personality disorder patients show aloofness and social isolation, affective detachment, suspicious/paranoid relationships, and odd communications; in contrast, the distinguishing core symptoms of borderline personality disorder are intense, unstable relationships, impulsivity, and self-damaging acts (McGlashan, 1987). The clinical course and family pedigrees of these disorders also differ. These findings suggest that schizotypal personality disorder is part of the schizophrenic spectrum and is probably genetically linked to schizophrenia proper. Schizotypal features occur with increased frequency in the relatives of schizophrenics (Torgersen, 1985); a significant proportion of inpatients diagnosed as having a schizotypal personality disorder develop frank schizophrenia in later life (McGlashan, 1986b). Schizotypal personality disorder represents one of the first attempts to define a diagnostic category along biogenetic lines (Gunderson & Siever, 1985). Further revisions of the criteria for this disorder have been proposed to improve its specificity for a presumed schizophrenic genotype (Frances, 1985; Kendler, 1985; Kety, 1985; Torgersen, 1985). In contrast, borderline personality disorder may represent a variant of affective disorder (Gunderson, 1984; Loranger et al., 1982; McGlashan, 1983b; M. H. Stone, 1980, 1984; for a critique of this view, see Torgersen, 1984).

In addition to these unresolved questions, a broader controversy exists about the optimal way to conceptualize, define, and subdivide personality disorders in general (Cloninger, 1987; Millon, 1986a, 1986b; Rutter, 1987; Widiger et al., 1987a, 1987b).

One area of controversy concerns the best way to classify maladaptive personality features—as discrete, specific categorical disorders (as in DSM-III-R) or as separate traits arranged along dimensions that can be expressed quantitatively on a continuous scale (as in some personality tests).

Another area of uncertainty concerns the relationship of the major mental disorders, which DSM-III-R places on Axis I, to the specific personality disorders, which are coded on Axis II. DSM-III-R treats the borderline conditions (borderline personality disorder and schizotypal personality disorder) as personality disorders, coded on Axis II. These diagnoses are thus compatible with various other Axis II personality disorders (such as histrionic or narcissistic personality), as well as with the clinical syndromes that code on Axis I. Indeed, borderline personality features may be found in many children with Axis I diagnoses (such as attention deficit–hyperactivity disorder, conduct disorder, anxiety disorders, eating disorders) and other Axis II diagnoses (such as the specific learning disorders). Axis II personality disorders are defined in DSM-III-R (1987) as enduring maladaptive "patterns of perceiving, relating to, and thinking about the environment and oneself. . . . [that are] not limited to discrete episodes of illness" (p. 335). In some patients, however, personality disorder is *not* independent of other illnesses. For example, some patients may meet the criteria for various personality disorders when depressed, but not when their depression is in remission (Korenblum et al., 1988).

The developmental aspects of personality disorder also require further study (Rutter, 1987). Adult borderline patients often report that their difficulties began in childhood (Kernberg, 1990). Although many children manifest distinctive, persistent, and even maladaptive personality traits from their toddler years on, it is unclear how early a child may be said to have an enduring personality *disorder* (Shapiro, 1990).

"Borderline" thus remains a controversial and evolving concept (M. H. Stone, 1980, 1984). It is particularly important for the child psychiatrist to note the lack of clarity in the relation of the adult borderline syndromes to the childhood borderline syndrome (Bemporad et al., 1987a, 1987b; Greenman et al., 1986; Vela et al., 1983; Shapiro, T., 1983). Because the adult and childhood concepts developed with relative independence (Bemporad et al., 1987a; Shapiro, 1983), controversy continues about the degree of descriptive overlap between the adult and childhood conditions and whether the childhood borderlines become adult ones. Several of the DSM-III-R criteria for borderline personality disorder are not developmentally appropriate for children. Consequently, Vela et al. (1983) and Bemporad et al. (1982, 1987a, 1987b) have proposed alternative criteria. Vela et al. suggest a "consensus definition" gleaned from several early descriptions of borderline children (see Table 5.1).

Many of the descriptions of the childhood borderline syndrome do not draw the DSM-III distinction between schizotypal personality disorder and borderline personality disorder; borderline children are usually described as showing features of both (Bemporad et al., 1982, 1987a; Vela et al., 1983). Unfortunately, except for a few studies, researchers have not systematically studied the validity of the schizotypal/borderline (proper) distinction in children (Petti and Vela, 1990). Because of the paucity of data using the DSM-III or DSM-III-R criteria with children, the discussion that follows will use the term *borderline* to refer to children from both the borderline personality disorder group (stably-unstable) and the schizotypal group, except where otherwise indicated.

EPIDEMIOLOGY

Although the borderline disorder(s) are apparently common, there are few or no systematic data on their prevalence in childhood and adolescence. The prevalence of borderline personality has been estimated at 2% to 4% of

Table 5–1. Consensus Symptoms for Borderline Conditions in Children

1. Disturbed interpersonal relationships characterized by the following:
    a. Behaving in a controlling, overdemanding, extremely possessive, clinging, overdependent way with adults in a relationship in which the child constantly demands to have his needs satisfied.
    b. Excessively outgoing social interactions without appropriate discrimination of the situation.
    c. Periods of being extremely withdrawn and aloof.
    d. Extreme outbursts of love and hate toward the same person or exaggerated but superficial love for one parent and outbursts of hate toward the other parent.
    e. Frequent exaggerated copying of another person's behavior, e.g., imitating every action, gesture, or movement the person makes.
    f. Isolation from peers and lack of friends.
2. Disturbances in the sense of reality manifested by the following:
    a. Fantasies of being all-powerful, including not only believing them, but behaving as if they were true, e.g., the child behaves as if he were a superhero, and engages in dangerous behavior.
    b. Withdrawal into fantasy more often than would be appropriate for a child of the same age. The fantasies are too idiosyncratic, too sustained, or appear at inappropriate moments.
    c. Excessive self-absorption in pretend play to the degree that the child has difficulty differentiating play from reality, e.g., playing with toy soldiers and reacting to the other person as if the person were actually an enemy.
    d. Paranoid ideation, but not delusions, involving the belief that the child is being harassed or unfairly treated, e.g., "The kids are always out to get me."
    e. Excessive use of magical thinking, with the fear that these thoughts will actually come true, e.g., fearing the mother will be hurt as a result of the child's thinking it.
3. Excessive, intense anxiety manifested by the following:
    a. Chronic, constant anxiety, often diffuse and free floating which interferes in most areas of the child's functioning and which may be manifested by driven restlessness, sleeplessness, and inability to concentrate.
    b. Panic states manifested by intense anxiety reaching panic proportions which the child may verbalize as fear of body disintegration, a major catastrophe, or fear of becoming another person. These states may also be demonstrated by the child's appearing frantic, disorganized, and severely agitated, with striking facial immobility, dead still or stiffened body, mechanical movements, and disturbed and unintelligible speech.
    c. Excessive anxiety to a wide variety of stimuli or new situations. Anxiety resulting from the child perceiving the world as a dangerous place to the point that it interferes with the child's functioning.
    d. Intense fear of separation from other persons, clinging to adults for protection, and getting very anxious when contact with them is temporarily broken.

(continued)

134

Table 5–1   (Continued)

4. Excessive and severe impulsive behavior, resulting from minimal provocation or frustration, occurring in a child past the age when this behavior would be normal and characterized by the following:
   a. Repetitive, unmitigated fits of rage.
   b. Loss of control, e.g., biting others, destroying objects indiscriminately.
   c. Total unmanageability due to aggressive behavior.
   d. Loss of contact with reality during these episodes.
   e. Tantrums lasting for an hour or more.
   f. Paranoid ideation during the tantrum, e.g., the child shouts, "Let go of me" when no one is touching him.
5. "Neurotic-like" symptoms, e.g., rituals, somatic concerns, obsessions, multiple phobias, or intense self-imposed restrictions and inhibitions which are fleeting and interchangeable.
6. Uneven or distorted development characterized by the following:
   a. Deviant or erratic physiologic patterning, e.g., hypertonic states, erratic feeding and sleeping patterns, hypo- or hypersensitivity to stimuli, or vomiting and diarrhea without demonstratable medical cause.
   b. Apathy, never crying to show their needs, poor sucking, lack of response to mother's face for months, poor molding into mother's arms, or lack of anticipatory gesture when picked up.
   c. Excessive rubbing, rolling, or head banging.
   d. Delay in motor or language areas.

Source: From "Borderline Syndromes in Childhood: A Critical Review" by R. Vela, H. Gottlieb, and E. Gottlieb, in *The Borderline Child: Approaches to Etiology, Diagnosis, and Treatment* by K. S. Robson (Ed.), 1983, pp. 40–43. New York: McGraw-Hill. Copyright 1983 by McGraw-Hill. Reprinted by permission.

the general population (Gunderson & Zanarini, 1987). Because it is unclear what proportion of adult borderlines (or for that matter adults with any other forms of psychopathology) show this pathology as children, few inferences can be drawn from this figure.

CLINICAL FEATURES

The borderline child shows marked and erratic fluctuations in his functioning along with a propensity for rapid decompensation and massive regression. His capacity to display more mature behaviors is highly dependent on external structure and on ready access to his need-gratifying attachment figures. Given such support, he can often appear remarkably intact, sometimes for fairly extended intervals. In the absence of support, however, the borderline child is exquisitely vulnerable to disorganizing panic or outbursts of rage. These reactions are all too readily provoked, sometimes by a mere hint of frustration or abandonment.

The characteristics of the borderline condition do not reside in the individual symptoms, many of which overlap other diagnostic categories. In fact, there are no pathognomonic findings. The essence of the disorder is rather in the matrix of deviant ego development, primitive defenses, and disturbed object relations in which the specific symptoms are embedded (O. F. Kernberg, 1975, 1977; P. F. Kernberg, 1983a). The borderline child may display neurotic-like symptoms such as phobias, obsessional thoughts, or psychosomatic problems; these symptoms, however, are multiple, poorly organized, and rapidly shifting. The patient may make transient use of high-level defenses such as isolation, intellectualization, and sublimation, but these defenses are fragile at best and give way readily to more primitive mechanisms such as denial, projection, and splitting. The borderline child often lacks a predominant libidinal style appropriate to his age and phase of development; rather, he seems to be a cauldron of seething, poorly integrated, oral, anal, phallic, and aggressive impulses that are constantly in danger of bubbling over.

In the realm of object relations, the borderline child experiences wide swings in his attitude toward himself and others; indeed, his sense of these relationships may move between polar opposites. Despite this, he has little trouble with any sense of contradiction or incongruity. Although he can differentiate between himself and others, he cannot integrate the good and bad aspects of either self or others (O. F. Kernberg, 1975; P. F. Kernberg, 1983a). In a desperate way the child attempts to ward off the threat of merger and loss of autonomy. Expressions of clinging dependency with panic at the prospect of separation may alternate abruptly with angry assertions of independence. Corresponding to this lack of internal integration are both a poor sense of personal identity ("identity diffusion") and an inability to perceive other people as whole persons in their own right. Instead, the child sees others merely as sources of gratification or frustration and hence as all-good or all-bad, depending on whether they give or deny. As a result, the borderline child's attachments, although intense, appear shallow and fickle; sometimes he seems to view other people as interchangeable so long as his needs are met.

Anxiety

The borderline child's anxiety is chronic, diffuse, and disorganizing. Normally, anxiety or guilt functions as a signal that calls into play appropriate coping or adaptive mechanisms. Rather than remaining circumscribed, however, and serving as an adaptive signal, the borderline child's anxiety readily overwhelms him (Pine, 1974, 1986). These children are often extremely sensitive to separation or criticism. Such children experience anxiety or guilt as threatening annihilation or as a dangerous attack from without. Their response is often a desperate panic or temper tantrum (really a "terror tantrum") marked by disorganization, paranoia, and transient loss of contact. Many clinicians see these "micropsychotic" episodes as pathognomonic of the borderline personality.

Because of the weakness of their coping and control mechanisms, borderline children are constantly anxious concerning abandonment or external attack as well as loss of control and the possible breakthrough of their own powerful impulses. The ego of such children is like "a delicate permeable membrane through which the primary process penetrates with relative ease from within and which external forces puncture easily from without" (Ekstein & Wallerstein, 1954, p. 349). Anthony (1981) observed that these children feel "peculiarly 'skinless' " (p. 5). Some schizotypal children may withdraw into an obligatory aloofness or fantasy world to protect themselves from the powerful anxieties they experience when around others.

Polysymptomatic Neuroses and Shifting Defenses

On superficial observation some borderline children may appear merely neurotic. At times, their disturbance takes the form of apparent oedipal level conflicts with associated neurotic symptoms and some high-level defenses. In the neurotic child, although much suffering may occur, conflict, symptom, and defense remain relatively well circumscribed in the context of a more-or-less healthy ego and object relations. In contrast, the borderline child's symptoms and defenses are more shifting and more poorly structured; they fail to contain his anxiety, regression, and disorganization. More important, his conflicts and defenses occur in the context of generally deviant ego functions and primitive object relations.

CASE EXAMPLE

Ray, age 12, complained of many fluctuating somatic problems, including headache, joint pains, dizziness, and hyperventilation. These symptoms at times appeared to accompany anxiety or guilt and to serve as direct physiological expressions of anxiety or tension. They may also have been pleas for attention. His myriad physical complaints were so variable that it was hard for nursing staff to keep up with them. None of the symptoms lasted long, but any failure on the part of the staff to provide prompt attention resulted in vituperative reproaches or tantrums. Periodically Ray would resolve to reform his chaotic and destructive ways and would compulsively rearrange his room, decorating it with charts recording his progress and posters filled with self-exhortations. He established an elaborately decorated barrier or "customs post" at the entrance to his room to prevent the staff or other patients from entering without permission or, worse still, inadvertently moving anything in the room. In between these spells of orderliness, within a few seconds of being frustrated or angered, Ray frequently reduced his room to rubble. In therapy,

Ray would intellectualize about himself and sometimes talk pseudomaturely about working on problems, complete with diagrams; however, he consistently repudiated any truly reflective stance and was unable to use play for sublimating aggressive and competitive feelings. He excelled at various competitive games, but the slightest setback led him to assault the other players or to rush sulkily out of the game.

Ray often had a macho swagger and would taunt female nursing staff with crude boasts of what he intended to do to them. His phallic strivings were pervaded with thinly disguised sadistic and destructive fantasies. There was, however, little true consolidation of either a latency or a phallic genital position. He was intermittently enuretic and encopretic, delighted in smearing and messing, and hoarded food avidly (sometimes gorging himself to the point of vomiting).

Impulsivity

The borderline child has little ability to contain and moderate strong affects or impulses. When he wants something, he grabs it; when angry, he hits; and when disappointed or frustrated with himself, he hurts himself or shrieks. Disappointments feel like the end of the world, and severe temper tantrums with attempts to injure himself or others are common. In adolescence, drug and alcohol abuse are frequently present. This behavior arises out of the inability to delay gratification and functions as an attempt at self-calming and self-medication.

Disordered Object Relations

Unlike the schizophrenic child, the borderline child can differentiate between himself and others. However, vulnerability in this area may persist as a fear of being taken over by or engulfed in intense relationships. At the same time, separation anxiety can be overwhelming and may require the actual presence of the significant other to allay it. Because of their intense needs and poor ability to delay gratification, borderline children are often manipulative and coercive in their relationships. Some children seek to avoid the pain of separateness by modeling themselves completely on another person or insisting that the other shares all of their ideas, feelings, and preferences.

Coexisting with this intense longing to fuse with a needed other is the borderline's terror at losing his fragile identity in intimate relations, which may provoke strenuous counterdependent flight or angry outbursts at the suddenly dangerous other.

Another closely related and striking aspect of the borderline child's disordered object relations is his inability to integrate the good and bad aspects of himself or of others, meanwhile remaining unaware of any contradiction in his shifting views. Thomas Sydenham observed of certain patients in the 17th century: "All is caprice; they love without measure those whom they will soon hate without reason" (cited in Groves, 1981, p. 259). In the heat of anger, the normal or neurotic child may yell at his parents or friends that he hates them. In a sober moment, however, he feels remorse and acknowledges that he both loves and is displeased with someone at the same time. ("*Odi et ami* . . . ," Catullus put it; "I hate and I love at the same time. You ask how can that be? I know not, but I feel the pain.") Not so the borderline patient. The borderline's previously expressed affection for another does not mitigate his rage when he is frustrated. Similarly, when feeling at one with his often (temporarily) idealized object, the borderline seems unaware that he ever had any negative feelings toward that person. These rapid oscillations between apparently unmitigated hate and unmitigated love led Schmideberg (1959) to coin the phrase "clinging antagonism." Such vacillations between longing for and angry rejection of a needed other resemble the toddler in the rapprochement phase, whose vigorous need to assert his fragile independence alternates with a frightened realization of his desperate dependency on his mother. The anger that tinges the borderline's counterdependency is also reminiscent of the angry detachment of young children who have been separated for too long or too often from their parents. "They feel like toddlers whose mothers are permanently out of the room" (Frijling-Schreuder, 1969, p. 322).

CASE EXAMPLE

Following a fight with her paranoid mother, B, a 10-year-old girl, deliberately shot herself in the abdomen. Despite their hostile and near-murderous (yet clinging) relationship, B, during her long and painful recuperation, would speak of mother and home only in glowing terms. On the other hand, the hospital staff could do nothing right. In B's view, they were uncaring, incompetent, and cruel. The mother also in describing her relationship with B, insisted that there had never been anything but harmony and love between them. During visits, the mother hovered over B, listened to her daughter's complaints about the nurses, and berated the hospital staff in front of B. Paradoxically, however, the visits usually ended with B and her mother yelling and shouting at each other hysterically. Following these episodes, B would cling frantically to her favorite nurse (whom, only minutes earlier she had been denouncing to her mother) and tell her how terrible mother was. Only after several months of inpatient psychotherapy could B tentatively admit that although her mother was often suffocatingly affectionate, she could also suddenly fly into paranoid rages, beating B and hurling racial epithets at her. B then began to realize that she both desperately loved and feared her mother.

Reality Testing

Although the borderline's reality testing is generally intact, his underlying ego weakness may result in feelings of depersonalization or unreality, paranoid trends, and vulnerability to transient psychosis under stress

(Gunderson & Zanarini, 1987). Because the borderline child or adolescent lacks a coherent sense of self, he often reports feeling unreal. Poorly integrated and conflicting identifications create an unstable sense of identity. The borderline patient may experience himself as forever playing a theatrical role; behind the mask of this "false self" he does not know who he is (Winnicott, 1965). Helene Deutsch (1942) labeled this clinical phenomenon the "as-if" personality.

Several authors see a disturbed sense of identity as a core feature of the borderline syndrome (O. F. Kernberg, 1975; P. F. Kernberg, 1983a; Rosenfeld & Sprince, 1963). Although adolescence is normally a time when the question "Who am I?" takes on a special urgency, the borderline adolescent characteristically shows a dramatic inability to elaborate a comfortable, coherent, livable identity. Trying on one role or persona after another, such adolescents flip dramatically, abruptly, and chaotically from one trial identity to another in a desperate attempt to resolve inner conflicts.

CASE EXAMPLES

A 17-year-old borderline youth alternately boasted of his plans to become a pornographic film star and piously recited his rosary in class while making plans to enter the seminary. Another teenager fluctuated between plans to join the Peace Corps and the goal of becoming a Green Beret. The borderline features of these adolescents did not lie in the age-appropriate conflicts between ideals on one hand and sexual and aggressive instincts on the other. Rather, it resided in their lack of integration and their inability to experience themselves as conflicted. When in his throes of piety, the first young man could not acknowledge that he was struggling against unsettling urges. Only a few days later, when trying to impress classmates with his sexual prowess, it was hard for him to admit that he felt any guilt about these impulses or had any doubts about how girls saw him.

Because of such patients' egocentric point of view, they experience the external world as unreal and evanescent. At times of stress or disappointment, the borderline patient may show paranoid tendencies, feeling that others are belittling or demeaning him. His neediness and ready recourse to projection and splitting impair his perception of other peoples' feelings and motives making it difficult for him to maintain stable friendships or family ties.

When stressed or under the influence of alcohol or drugs, some borderline patients experience transient psychotic episodes with ideas of reference, delusions, or hallucinations. (It is unclear whether those patients vulnerable to transient psychosis form a subgroup which is distinctive in other respects.) In contrast to the schizophrenic psychoses, these borderline psychotic episodes usually have clear-cut precipitants (most prominent of which are loss or rage toward someone important in the patient's life), and they are mercifully brief (usually lasting only a few minutes or hours). The borderline patient sees such psychotic episodes as ego-alien and distressing; usually they are readily reversible. The borderline's dissociative experiences and lapses in reality sense are highly sensitive to the degree of structure and external reality testing provided by the surrounding milieu (Gunderson & Zanarini, 1987). This sensitivity to structure has important implications not only for the therapeutic management of such patients, but also for their diagnostic assessment. Projective testing, especially the Rorschach, is extremely useful in assessing borderline features that may not be apparent on more structured instruments (Leichtman & Shapiro, 1983). Intense, albeit ambivalent, involvement with other people further distinguishes the patient with borderline personality disorder from the schizophrenic. In practice, however, the differentiation between childhood schizophrenia and a borderline condition may be difficult to make (Pine, 1974).

In childhood, immersion in fantasy and make-believe play are common and normal and serve simultaneously adaptive, defensive, and cathartic functions. The fantasies and make-believe of the borderline child, however, are different. In the movement between fantasy and reality, "There is more slippage in these children—the fantasy being too idiosyncratic, too sustained, coming at wrong moments, not easily enough given up" (Pine, 1974, p. 352). Such fantasies also tend to show a morbid preoccupation with death, monsters, body injury, torture, poisons, and other versions of the harmful and the harmed.

Pervasive Aggression

Borderline children often show pervasive aggression, either turned outward in impulsive, hostile action or inward as intense masochism or self-injury. Persistent underlying fears and fantasies of death, destruction, or mutilation usually dominate their inner lives. A common defense is to identify with the aggressor, and concern about attack and counterattack heavily color the child's relationships. In some children this preoccupation with aggression may represent an only partially distorted internalization of a harsh and chaotic environment; in other children, poorly understood constitutional defects of integration may result in a cruel and partially projected superego and an overconcern with aggression. Childhood and adolescent suicide attempters frequently have histories of impulsiveness and overt aggression toward others, often within a framework of borderline personality organization (Cohen-Sandler et al., 1982a).

Self-cutting is common in adolescent borderline patients, especially females (Doctors, 1981). Such patients are most often "delicate cutters," a term introduced by Pao (1969) to describe patients who made "superficial, delicate, carefully designed incisions" (p. 195). Delicate wrist-cutting is sometimes a dramatic effort to communicate desperation—"a cry for help."

Although these same patients may sometimes make deep life-threatening cuts (and other suicide attempts), delicate cutting in itself is not life-threatening and is often not intended as a suicide gesture. Indeed, delicate cutting may be done furtively and involve the breasts, genitals, or torso as well as visible parts of the body such as arms, legs, and face. Such cutting appears to release tension in reaction to real or threatened separation, rejection, or disappointment. Rather than experiencing hurt, anger, or sadness as such, the cutter more often feels an unspeakable isolation and tension, accompanied by depersonalization, numbness, emptiness, and a sense of unreality (Pao, 1969). At least initially, cutting evokes no pain and continues until blood flows. The patient finds the flow of blood and the return of pain satisfying because they relieve tension and restore a sense of being alive (Kafka, 1969). Only later do these feelings of satisfaction and even triumph give way to disgust, shame, or guilt. Often triggered by real or imagined disappointments in others, cutting may be accompanied by angry, vengeful fantasies.

Delicate cutters often have early histories of illness, injury, and physical distress; in addition, disturbed relations with their mothers have given them little sense of empathic understanding and comfort, with concomitant failure to develop the capacity for self-soothing (Doctors, 1981).

With treatment cutting usually diminishes as the patient comes to feel held and contained in the therapeutic relationship and becomes better able to verbalize feelings and to act constructively in the face of upsets (Nelson & Grunebaum, 1971). In the opening phases of treatment, however, cutting may occur in response to disappointment and anger at the therapist. One disturbed adolescent cut herself repeatedly in response to disappointments or fights with her mother or boyfriend. The behavior diminished dramatically following one episode that she described to her therapist: "I kept cutting, and it didn't hurt. I had the idea it was my mother's leg I was cutting, getting her back. Then I thought about what you said last time and it began to hurt, and I realized it really was *my* leg I was cutting."

Diagnostic Subgroups

Although there have been several attempts to divide the confusingly heterogeneous spectrum of borderline children into discrete diagnostic subgroups (Petti & Vela, 1990), none has met with universal acceptance.

As noted earlier, the DSM-III distinguishes two subgroups: (1) the *Borderline Personality Disorder* group of "stably unstable" personalities and (2) the *Schizotypal Personality Disorder* group, which is symptomatically (and perhaps genetically) more closely related to schizophrenia. These schemata are derived from adult psychiatry, and their applicability to child psychiatric patients is still uncertain.

In one study (Petti & Law, 1982), on the basis of the DSM-III (1980) criteria, the authors could satisfactorily divide a group of ten hospitalized children into schizotypal or borderline personality disorder. Many symptoms, however, such as ideas of reference, social isolation, recurrent illusions, and undue social anxiety were common to both subgroups. Magical thinking, bizarre fantasies and preoccupations, odd speech, and inadequate rapport best distinguished the schizotypal subgroup, whereas impulsivity, intense and unstable relationships, inappropriate anger, affective instability, and physical self-damage were the most distinctive features of the borderline personality disorder group. A substantial proportion of children in both diagnostic subgroups also met the DSM-III criteria for childhood-onset pervasive developmental disorder. This lack of diagnostic specificity resembles adult samples; for example, Spitzer and colleagues (1979) found that about 54% of an adult sample of patients fit the criteria for both borderline and schizotypal personality disorders. However, Russell et al. (1987) found that although 80% of the children in their study diagnosed as having a schizotypal personality disorder also met DSM-III criteria for other disorders, none met the criteria for borderline personality disorder.

Pine (1974, 1983) attempted to subdivide borderline children as follows:

1. Children with *chronic ego deviance,* with ongoing chronic anxiety and a tendency to panic, fluid object relations, and marginal reality testing.
2. Children with *shifting levels of organization,* who moved abruptly from a state of better compensation to a world of fantasy and disorganization; this helped them avoid anxiety, but at the price of poor adaptation to reality.
3. *Reactive* borderline children, who became massively disorganized in response to environmental chaos, but who could appear well-integrated within a stable therapeutic setting (despite persistence of subtle character pathology).
4. *"Identificatory"* borderlines whose psychotic trends represent partially internalized aspects of an actively psychotic parent.
5. *Inadequate* borderline patients, with dull, meager, or inadequate intellect, judgment, self-care, and sense of self, due either to early restrictions in ego development or to intense anxiety.
6. *Schizoid* borderlines, with a constricted affective life, impoverished relationships, and a preoccupation with their own fantasy life.

Differential Diagnosis

In adolescence, the differential diagnosis of borderline personality disorder may be difficult and often requires an extended evaluation. Although a significant minority of young people have a stormy adolescence marked by emotional lability, identity crises, and rebellious conflicts with family and authority (Offer et al., 1984), diagnostic conclusions cannot be based on these symptoms alone. Otto Kernberg (1977, 1984) utilizes a structural interview to assess the status of the adolescent's identity, object relations, reality testing, and current defense-impulse configuration. In assessing possible borderline features, Kernberg looks for evidence of (1) lack of integration in the teenager's concept of significant others as well as of the self (identity diffusion); (2) the predominance of primitive defenses, especially splitting; and (3) the maintenance of reality testing. In Kernberg's view, normal and neurotically disturbed adolescents, even when in turmoil, can be distinguished from borderline cases by their capacity for guilt and concern, their ability to establish enduring nonexploitative relationships with others, and their preservation of a realistic, balanced view of others. In addition, the nonborderline adolescent evidences superego integration in a consistent, expanding, and deepening set of values. Kernberg points out that a normal or neurotically rebellious adolescent may clash bitterly with his parents, but the capacity to appreciate other aspects of the parents usually mitigates the youngster's criticism and devaluation. In addition, the nonborderline adolescent can maintain relationships with others that are not pervaded by either extreme devaluation or unrealistic idealization.

An important subgroup of schizotypal or borderline children comprises those children who may be at later risk for developing a major mental illness, that is, a full-blown schizophrenic or manic depressive condition (Akiskal et al., 1985; Kestenbaum, 1983, 1986; Kron & Kestenbaum, 1988). Prior to developing pathognomonic symptoms of schizophrenia or a major affective disorder, such children may receive a variety of characterological and syndromic diagnoses, including borderline or schizotypal personality disorder. Drug or alcohol abuse may further complicate the picture. Harbingers of possible impending decompensation include evidence of depression or hypomania (especially when periodic or recurrent); progressive social withdrawal; intense, isolative preoccupation with idiosyncratic concerns; and signs of poor reality testing. Symptomatic children with a close relative suffering from schizophrenia or major affective disorder need especially careful evaluation (Kron & Kestenbaum, 1988). For further discussion of these high-risk children, see Chapter 3, "Schizophrenia in Childhood," and Chapter 6, "Affective Disorders." Although systematic data are unavailable, early vigorous psychotherapeutic intervention and the judicious use of appropriate medication sometimes may avert a catastrophic breakdown (Kestenbaum, 1983). These children, who bear the double burden of both genetic vulnerability and a disturbed upbringing, remain at risk and benefit most from the long-term availability of a therapist or caseworker who has known them and other family members through the years.

Course of Illness

The outcome and the natural course of childhood borderline personality disorders have not been adequately studied (Petti & Vela, 1990). Many borderline children undoubtedly go on to become borderline adults. Others may be at risk for the later development of schizophrenia or major affective illness (Kron & Kestenbaum, 1988).

ETIOLOGY

The causes of the borderline and schizotypal personality disorders are as yet imperfectly understood. Environmental, constitutional, and hereditary factors all appear to play a role. There are probably many paths to a final borderline outcome. Whether it is possible to link specific etiologies with specific borderline subgroups or with different treatment outcomes remains to be seen.

Genetic Factors

Genetic studies relevant to the borderline conditions include family studies of borderline index cases, twin studies of borderline and schizotypal patients, and studies of the biological and adoptive families of borderline or schizophrenic adoptees (Gunderson & Elliott, 1985; Torgersen, 1984, 1985). Although some samples include adolescent patients, systematic genetic or family data on borderline children are not available.

Family studies of patients with borderline personality disorders suggest an increased family incidence of personality disorders generally and borderline personality disorder in particular (Loranger et al., 1982; Pope et al., 1983; Soloff & Millward, 1983). However, a small study of monozygotic versus dizygotic cotwins of borderline patients failed to find evidence of genetic transmission (Torgersen, 1984).

Genetic factors are more evident in schizotypal personality disorder. Family, twin, and adoption studies indicate that biological relatives of schizotypal patients have an increased incidence of schizotypal personality disorder and suggest further that this familial clustering reflects genetic transmission (Torgersen, 1984, 1985). Although schizotypal biological relatives occur with increased frequency in the families of chronic schizophrenics, the genetic relationship of schizotypal personality disorder to schizophrenia remains unclear (Gunderson & Siever, 1985; Kendler, 1985; Torgersen, 1984, 1985). In any sample the specific criteria that define schizotypal personality disorder heavily influence the degree of association with schizophrenia.

Finally, borderline personality disorder may be more closely related to affective disorder than to schizophrenia. The symptoms of borderline personality disorder and affective disorder often overlap (Gunderson & Elliott, 1985). Many borderlines of the stably unstable type show marked affective instability as well as a chronic depressivelike emptiness or dysphoria; although usually lacking guilty self-reproach, this dysphoria may be severe enough to warrant a concurrent diagnosis of depression (Gunderson & Zanarini, 1987). In these patients, the affective symptoms are frequently more striking than any cognitive peculiarities. Researchers have advanced a variety of theories to account for this overlap (Gunderson & Elliott, 1985). Family studies suggest that relatives of borderlines may have an increased prevalence of affective illness; however, this finding is for the most part limited to index patients who themselves have a concurrent diagnosis of affective disorder (Loranger et al., 1982; Torgersen, 1984).

Additionally, hereditary factors other than those related to schizophrenia or affective illness might also predispose toward borderline conditions. Constitutional vulnerabilities, such as severe attention deficit disorders, can be important predisposing causes of borderline personality disorder. As discussed in Chapter 13, many cases of attention deficit disorder show evidence of hereditary factors.

Constitutional Factors

Signs of "organicity," such as nonspecific EEG abnormalities, poor fine and gross motor coordination, abnormal neuropsychological test findings, and a history of hyperactivity, are common in children with borderline or schizotypal personality disorder (Greenman et al., 1986; Petti & Vela, 1990).

Paulina Kernberg (1978) and Cohen et al. (1983) have detailed the ways in which attention–deficit hyperactivity disorder (ADHD) may predispose children to the development of a borderline personality disorder. Over and above the classic impulsivity and difficulty in focusing attention that children with ADHD typically display, they frequently show uneven synthetic ego functions. Such children tend to have cognitive defects that impair their ability to make adaptive sense of incoming stimuli. The same defects alter the way that these children "gate," level, or sharpen incoming stimuli; in particular, they have limited ability to inhibit their responses to irrelevant material. Memory for various modalities may also be impaired. These deficits not only affect the handling of external sensory data, they also impair the processing of internal and external affective stimuli and somatosensory input. Irrelevant external stimuli readily distract such a child, and he is also vulnerable to poorly modulated internal stimuli, which he experiences as peremptory and acts on readily. Because of these deficits, the ADHD child finds it difficult to develop and to integrate stable, coherent, and realistic internal representations of himself and others. Over and above these neurobiological difficulties, the ADHD child also induces considerable impatience and irritation in parents, peers, and teachers. These children are often difficult infants, unpopular playmates, and poor students. They have difficulty in self-organization and self-calming, straining the ability of parents and the community to provide containment for their impulses or a nurturant, growth-promoting "holding environment" (Winnicott, 1975). The negative responses provoked by the ADHD child create a vicious circle that leads him to experience lowered self-esteem, frustration, and guilt, which in turn cause even more disorganization and further maladaptive behavior. Without help, such children soon come to see themselves as "bad," damaged children surrounded by "bad," ungratifying, and punitive others.

ENVIRONMENTAL FACTORS

The proportion of borderline children who owe their symptoms to hereditary or constitutional factors as opposed to environmental influences is unclear. If a poorly integrated internal world and a propensity to primitive defenses, anxiety, intolerance, and low self-esteem can result from constitutional vulnerabilities, it is equally apparent that a sufficiently pathological or chaotic upbringing may overwhelm the integrative and adaptive capacities of even a biologically intact child. Stone (1984) suggests that most likely there is an etiological spectrum, with "purely psychogenic" cases at one end, and, at the other, cases with predominant constitutional or genetic factors. Presumably, the majority of cases would lie somewhere on the continuum between the extremes and represent an interaction of these factors.

During the first 2 to 3 years of life, the toddler gradually learns to separate from his mother; in the course of normal development he will learn to do this with a prevailing sense of confidence and basic trust. If the mother is able to titrate her absences and the inevitable frustrations she must visit on the infant in keeping with his growing ego capacities, the child will not feel overwhelmed by helplessness. He can then develop and maintain a conviction that the mother who may at times frustrate or leave him is the same mother whom he loves and who also sustains and gratifies him. This ability to integrate the "bad mother" (or "mother of separation") with the "good mother" (or "mother of symbiosis") enables the infant to maintain a stable and sustaining image of the mother even in her absence (Fraiberg, 1969; Mahler et al., 1975). Such an infant is able to be separate from mother; when she is away, he tends to experience sadness rather than rage or a feeling of being attacked. This development requires what Winncott (1965, 1975) termed a "good enough" mother, one who is able to sustain a maternal "holding environment."

A crucial aspect of this holding environment is the mother's ability to continue providing love and to tolerate the child's expressions of anger or growing independence without retaliatory abandonment or counterattack. The vital catalyst for such development is "an ordinary devoted mother" who empathizes with her infant's upsets rather than repudiating his feelings or retaliating against him. Over the course of many separations and reunions, blowups and reconciliations, the infant acquires a sustaining sense of his own lovability along with a sense of trust in the prevailing goodness and availability of others. Maternal constancy crucially strengthens the infant's confidence in the strength of the good self and the good object, and it mitigates his fear concerning his own and others' aggressive tendencies (Kernberg, 1975, 1976).

In contrast, the chaotic inner world of the borderline child is suffused with aggression and fear of attack; it is a world that lacks stable images of a calming, comforting other or of a self that can be calmed or comforted. Such a development may reflect the infant's experience of a mother who is excessively erratic, unempathic, severe, ungratifying, retaliatory, or abandoning. However, the child's failure to develop benign, sustaining internal images need not be due to poor parenting or emotional trauma. As discussed earlier, constitutional defects may interfere with the child's regulatory and integrative abilities. Early illness, especially when frequent pain and discomfort are present, may also leave the child with a sense of the world as persecutory or lacking in comfort. Furthermore, the child with a constitutional intolerance to anxiety or frustration or with an innate dysregulation of mood will in turn sorely tax the holding capacities of the average mother. Her attempts to cope with the ensuing state of chronic stress may cause the infant's experience of his mother to be excessively frustrating or ungratifying.

The effects of such difficulties on the developing child are far-reaching. Whether from constitutional integrative defects, failure of adequate mothering, or other unfortunate circumstances, the infant is unable to develop a sense of basic trust or to elaborate a stable inner image of his mother that is sustaining rather than terrifying. Such an infant experiences the anxiety of separation as attacking and overwhelming; throughout his later life he persists in angry clinging. The mechanism of splitting involves an unrealistic experiencing of the self or others as all-good or all-bad (Kernberg, 1975). It may originate passively when, faced with an excessively erratic or frustrating mother, the infant cannot integrate and internalize a single coherent caretaking image. Instead, he forms two separate and opposite images, in keeping with his experience, usually with the hostile and frightening image predominating. Kernberg (1975), however, suggests that children, in fact, actively resort to such splitting in later life in a defensive attempt to keep alive a fragile good image of the mother and the self (see the Case Example of B earlier in this chapter). As a rule, the child can maintain this state of affairs only by denying or projecting the bad aspects of the mother and self onto the external world, which accordingly becomes and remains frightening and destructive. The cost of building an inner world around such a split is the loss of a realistic sense of self and others; the youngster never achieves a perspective that includes both disappointing faults and mitigating virtues.

The effects of such maldevelopment extend beyond the realm of basic trust, adequate self-esteem, and libidinal constancy (Pine, 1986). Primitive organismic anxiety fails to develop into better modulated signal anxiety that can help the child to anticipate and cope adaptively. Correspondingly, more flexible, mature defenses fail to develop, or the child clings desperately and rigidly to primitive maladaptive ones. Relationships remain indiscriminate and exploitively focused on need gratification.

Unfortunately, many children reared in deprived, harsh, or neglectful homes have an inner sense of abandonment and attack that may only partially exaggerate their actual experience. Patterns of abuse, violence, and disorganization are common in the families of borderline children (Bemporad et al., 1987a; Bentivegna et al., 1985; Kernberg, 1983a).

In later life, physically abused children are prone to self-hurtful behavior, whereas sexually abused children may show various forms of dissociation including multiple personality disorder. (See Chapter 21, "Child Physical Abuse," and Chapter 22, "Child Sexual Abuse.") Thus, many borderline symptoms—impulsivity, aggression toward self and others, and impaired identity formation—may be the consequences of an abusive upbringing.

The families of borderline children, however, need not be overtly abusive or neglectful. Family studies and the increased use of family therapy in treating borderline children have permitted the delineation of more subtle kinds of pathological family behavior. Some clinicians postulate that a major cause of borderline pathology is a specific developmental failure in separation–individuation. They attribute this failure to a particular mode of mother–toddler interaction in the 2nd and 3rd years of life (Masterson, 1981; Rinsley, 1980, 1982). According to this view, adverse mother–child interactions during the separation–individuation phase of development may take various forms that, when combined with constitutional factors, may seriously deform the child's personality structure.

Because of difficulties of separation from her own mother, a mother may pathogenically project her experience onto her infant, seeing him alternately as completely helpless or ragefully assertive. As a result, she tends to reinforce the child's dependent clinging to her while failing to support his growing capacities for self-sufficiency. At the same time, in response to the child's normal, often angry, efforts to assert himself, she retaliates by threatening withdrawal or abandonment. Such a mother may have been close and nurturing during the first few months of life, when the infant made few demands for autonomy; to the struggling toddler, however, her implicit message is, "If you grow up, I will abandon you." The outcome is a child with a high level of separation anxiety manifested by angry clinging (Rinsley, 1980).

Some theorists emphasize that one characteristic of the families of borderlines is their heavy reliance on projection or splitting (Shapiro, 1975; Zinner & Shapiro, 1975), which parallels the patient's ready resort to such primitive defenses. In such families, "members split off disavowed or cherished aspects of themselves and project them into others within the family group" (Zinner & Shapiro, 1975, p. 107). These families parcel out good attributes and bad attributes so that each individual's *internal* conflicts (frequently concerning autonomy, separation, and aggression) are externalized. Instead of being personal problems, they assume instead the appearance of interpersonal conflicts between family members. Parents' projections of split-off aspects of themselves onto their children may be a replication within the current family of how things were within the parents' families of origin. In effect, these parents reexperience their own childhoods through their children. In their more virulent forms, such projections and splittings may exacerbate and magnify the vulnerable child's already defective integration.

Being seen and treated as someone other than who he is leads to a serious failure in the development of the child's personality. As a result of his mother's misperception and mishandling of him the child early develops a distorted self-image and later a disturbed self-identity based on his mother's projections, to which he responds accordingly (Rinsley, 1980). The outcome of what Rinsley terms "the child's pathological, pseudocomplementary responses" is a "false self" (Winnicott, 1965) or an "as-if personality" (Deutsch, 1942)—"a pseudo identity based upon and developing in relation to mother's own pseudo identity" (Rinsley, 1980, p. 151). This false self may take many forms. One child may opt to remain "mommy's good baby" at the expense of individuation and develops thereafter as an excessively compliant child. Another child may embrace as her own the repudiated needy, but defiant aspects of the mother's own personality that the mother has projected onto the child. In a similar fashion, certain delinquents, described by Johnson and Szurek (1952) as having "super-ego lacunae," appear to act out in their sexual and aggressive behavior the unconscious and disavowed impulses of their parents. Because the child's false self remains so intertwined with the parent's poorly integrated personality, the child never feels he is his own person. "Thus in significant measure unseparated and unindividuated, the child feels inadequate, impotent and empty; as the scapegoat, he paradoxically feels evil and powerful, yet rejected and abandoned" (Rinsley, 1980, p. 155).

One empirical study of families of hospitalized borderline adolescents (Gunderson et al., 1980) showed increased parental pathology and fewer effectual or dominant fathers in the borderline group than in the control groups. Such families were also more likely to see some siblings as especially good and other siblings as especially bad. Gunderson et al., noted that these families were intact but showed "a rigid tightness of the marital bond to the exclusion of the attention, support, or protection of the children" in contrast to the findings of those clinicians who were struck by the frequency of "an overinvolved, hostile-dependent, sado-masochistic, or even symbiotic bond between mothers and their borderline offspring" (p. 31).

TREATMENT

The borderline child's poor impulse control, capacity for regression, and intense rage and neediness make treatment difficult and demanding; the therapist must have a long-term commitment. The multiple developmental difficulties of the borderline child usually require the simultaneous use of several therapeutic modes. Without collateral work with the parents, psychotherapy for the child is rarely sufficient. Depending on the severity of the child's ego defects, vulnerability to psychotic regression, and degree of social impairment, special school placement and even residential treatment may be necessary. In some cases medication may also be a useful adjunct for the child's most disabling symptoms.

It is no easy task for a therapist to establish and maintain contact with the schizotypal child. Such a youngster can tolerate only a narrowly constricted range of relatedness and defends his fragile sense of self by maintaining "stringent conditions of contact" (Ekstein, 1966). The unstable borderline child's splitting and intense neediness and rage toward the therapist are also likely to result in a tenuous treatment alliance. With both types of borderline children, the therapist must work actively to contain the child's profound anxiety and precipitous regressions. Helping the child control impulsive destructive behavior is important, not only to protect the child, the therapist, and the environment, but to aid the child in bearing his tensions. Too passive a stance by the therapist leaves the child a frightened prey to his own impulses; the child may misinterpret the therapist's permissive neutrality as a dangerously seductive encouragement to express directly primitive feelings, which can lead to explosive regressions.

The tenuous relatedness and fragile defenses of the borderline child profoundly influence both the strategy and tactics of psychotherapy (Kernberg, 1983b; M.H. Stone, 1985). The first task of the therapist is to establish and maintain empathic contact. The touchstone for every intervention is its likely impact on the child's relatedness to the therapist. Interpretation of instinctual material must be approached with great caution, especially in the early phases of treatment. Borderline children often hear the content of the therapist's statements in highly idiosyncratic ways. Because the borderline child has difficulty distinguishing language from action, he may hear the therapist's recognition and reflection of his feelings as an enticement to action. (The therapist says, "You're feeling angry," and the child responds, "I'll show you what I do when I'm angry!" and proceeds to act up.) Or the child may feel accused rather than understood, as though the therapist were saying, "Aha, I've found you out!" The result is often an upsurge of anxiety or aggression. Although some therapists maintain that early interpretation of primitive material fosters increased integration, uncovering or making the unconscious conscious is never the primary goal of work with the borderline child. Indeed, the goal of therapy is ultimately to foster more appropriate and mature defenses, to facilitate repression and sublimation, and to help the child become aware that he can tolerate tensions. Although in some children strengthening of high-level defenses may entail fostering more obsessive-compulsive character traits, it is important not to force on the child an imitative facade, thereby reinforcing a pseudocompliant false self.

Dealing with the borderline's transference toward the therapist is a central, demanding task. Intense sensitivity to separations may lead to stormy behavior at the end of treatment hours or acting-out around vacations and holidays, and the narcissistic resistances of some borderline children may leave the therapist feeling relentlessly denigrated and devalued. Finally, the therapist must be prepared to tolerate intense, long-lasting dependence, often for years (Bemporad et al., 1987b).

Pauline Kernberg (1983b) has outlined several technical goals and considerations in the treatment of the borderline child. She emphasizes (1) fostering the child's reality testing and strengthening the therapeutic relationship through clarification of actual ongoing "here and now" interactions with the therapist; (2) advancing ego and superego integration through thorough discussion of splitting and contradictory behaviors, especially when they occur within the session; (3) helping better integration of the child's self-representation by containing and verbalizing contradictory self-images; (4) improving tolerance of anxiety through anticipating and verbalizing potentially disruptive experiences; (5) addressing lack of empathy for others and deficient social skills as manifested with the therapist; and (6) clarifying the source of real and perceived difficulties in the child's relationship with his mother and family.

Special aspects of work with borderline adolescents and their families have been discussed by Otto Kernberg (1984), Masterson (1972), Masterson and Costello (1980); Rinsley (1980); and Roger Shapiro's group at the National Institute of Mental Health (NIMH) (Shapiro, 1978b; Shapiro et al., 1975; Shapiro, Shapiro, Zinner, & Berkowitz, 1977; Zinner & Shapiro, 1975).

Otto Kernberg (1984) favors a dynamically oriented psychotherapeutic approach that explores the "internal consistency of the adolescent's picture of himself, his significant object relations, and the integration and adequacy of his view of the world" (p. 131). The therapist must carefully attend to the adolescent's use of splitting as manifested by primitive idealization and devaluation of the therapist, parents, and peers. During periods of regression and intense negative transference, the therapist is often hard-pressed to maintain a sufficient working alliance to contain the patient's primitive rage and propensity toward destructive acting-out. It is essential to explore the anxieties and conflicts that the youngster is attempting to express or to fend off. Often, however, interpretation of splitting and other primitive defenses within the transference is not enough to contain acting-out; firm administrative limit-setting and even hospitalization may be necessary.

Controversy exists over the usefulness and indications for adding family therapy to the individual therapy of the borderline adolescent. Some authors feel that having the same therapist serve both the individual and the family threatens the adolescent's exclusive relationship to his therapist and encourages splitting and dilution of the transference (Kernberg, 1984; Masterson, 1972); on the other hand, Shapiro and colleagues (1977) believe active participation of the individual therapist in concurrent conjoint family therapy facilitates both the working alliance and the resolution of pathological family interactions.

Outpatient treatment of the borderline adolescent is feasible when (1) the family setting provides sufficient structure and support for treatment and (2) acting-out in the form of antisocial behavior, promiscuity, substance abuse, and other self-destructive behavior does not threaten the safety of the adolescent or others. Often, however, disturbed adolescents require hospitalization to control dangerous behavior, to disengage the adolescent from escalating conflict at home, and to enable the teenager to "hold still" long enough to become involved in treatment. In addition, an inpatient setting permits a wide focus on the adolescent's pattern of interaction with peers, parents, teachers, and other adults. Exploration of how pathological internal object relations and defenses become activated and manifested in the hospital milieu provides a valuable avenue of treatment (O. Kernberg, 1975, 1976; Noshpitz, 1962). In addition, the hospital also provides a locus for special education, group work, and social skills training. With intensive long-term psychotherapy and hospitalization, many borderline adolescents show marked improvement (Masterson & Costello, 1980).

The role of medication in borderline children and adolescents remains controversial. Although adequately controlled studies of medication in adult borderline patients are beginning to be available (Cowdry, 1987; Cowdry and Gardner, 1988; Soloff, 1987), there is little systematic data with younger patients. Borderline children vary widely in their response to medication. Clinically, the impression is that many borderline children respond poorly or even adversely to medication; some show only transient nonspecific improvement, and a few show impressive and sustained benefit.

Nonetheless, within the context of an overall treatment plan and well-developed therapeutic relationship, a trial of medication may be a useful adjunct (Petti & Vela, 1990).

There are no precise indications for choosing among the various psychoactive medications in childhood borderline conditions. In the future, methods of identifying valid genotypic or phenotypic subgroups may make such choices easier.

Meanwhile, relative indications consist of specific target symptoms or comorbid conditions (Cowdry, 1987). Thus, affectively labile children with evidence of a bipolar diathesis (especially when a strong family history is present) may benefit from lithium, whereas those with strong depressive or dysphoric features may benefit from tricyclic or monoamine oxidase inhibitor (MAOI) antidepressants. Tricyclic antidepressants have far-reaching effects beyond alleviating depressive symptoms. Thus, Petti and Unis (1981) found that imipramine ameliorated borderline children's peer interactions, noncompliance, and bizarre behaviors. Inattentive, hyperactive children may also benefit from a trial of tricyclic antidepressants or stimulant medication. Children with an abnormal paroxysmal EEG and episodic dyscontrol may warrant a trial of carbamazepine, whereas low doses of neuroleptics may benefit both schizotypal children (whose symptoms include impaired reality testing or cognitive disorganization) and affectively labile patients with anger, hostility, suspiciousness, referential thinking, and behavioral dyscontrol (Soloff, 1987). Minor tranquilizers, such as the benzodiazepines, may be disinhibiting and actually cause increased rage reactions. As always, empirical trials of medication in children require careful monitoring for side effects such as cognitive blunting. Detailed ongoing observations from both parents and teachers are essential for adequate evaluation.

PART III

Dysregulations of Affect, Anxiety, and Movement

Chapter 6

Affective Disorders

INTRODUCTION AND DEFINITIONS

Affective illnesses are mood disorders characterized by a persisting inappropriate mood (i.e., depression or elation) coupled with changes in cognition, motivation, and sense of the self. The depression or elation is excessive relative to the environmental conditions and interferes with either the sufferer's functioning or enjoyment of life.

Depression

The term *depression* is used in at least three distinguishable senses: (1) as an *affect state or mood,* which may occur transiently and normally under appropriate circumstances; (2) as a persisting, pathological mood that constitutes a *symptom* and that may be a part of a variety of psychiatric conditions; (3) as a distinctive clinical *syndrome* or collection of related symptoms (Angold, 1988).

The *affect* of depression includes a feeling of unhappiness accompanied by a sense of the self as "poor and empty." In his classic paper "Mourning and Melancholia" Freud (1917/1957) distinguished depression from simple sadness or grief where the world—but not the self—appears "poor and empty." Adults experience depression as a *syndrome* (or symptom-complex) with several key features: (1) *affective components,* with persisting unhappiness, sadness, or loss of interest or pleasure (anhedonia); (2) *cognitive components,* with ideas that define the self as being helpless, unworthy, or defective; the world as presenting insuperable obstacles to satisfaction; and the future as offering hopeless, unremitting suffering (Beck, 1976); (3) *motivational components,* with strong convictions that it is useless to try, that no effort is worth making; and (4) *vegetative and psychomotor disturbances,* with altered libido, appetite, sleep, and temperature sense, decreased movement, and social withdrawal.

Controversy and research continue concerning the extent to which normal sadness, grief, or demoralization are part of the same continuum as severe depressive feelings. It is not clear under what conditions grief, mourning, or discouragement become a qualitatively (as well as quantitatively) distinct disease entity (Rutter, 1986a, 1986b).

Important developmental differences exist between children and adults. As a result another heated and complicated controversy during the past two decades has been whether a depressive syndrome in childhood exists at all, and, if it does, whether it is descriptively or etiologically similar to the adult syndrome (Carlson & Garber, 1986). To clarify these issues, the following paragraphs briefly review these developmental differences in the affective, cognitive, and social domains (Cytryn & McKnew, 1974, 1979; Emde et al., 1986).

The normal moods of children are labile and readily manifested; childhood has many joys and sorrows to which most youngsters give free expression. A treat can often dispel the young child's sobs in a moment and sudden tears at some perceived frustration can blight even the happiest activity. The child's sense of time and degree is different from the adult's; joys seem boundless, whereas disappointments feel unmitigated and endless. Although children have difficulty conceptualizing long periods of time, the promise of continued growth holds out the hope for a better future. The child's weak reality sense may exaggerate disappointments but may also permit him to deny, ignore, or shift the responsibility for his unhappiness. Because the child has immature judgment and egocentric orientation, he often cannot realistically sort out responsibility for untoward events. At best the child is not articulately self-reflective, and, when something bad happens, may deprecate the environment rather than himself. The tendency to perceive unhappiness as coming from without rather than within, combined with childhood's greater impulsivity, frequently leads an unhappy child to lash out angrily or greedily rather than to experience sadness. Under similar circumstances, however, another child may inappropriately blame himself.

Children readily express emotional pain and distress in somatic terms, complaining of aches and pains rather than of sadness. Cognitive and linguistic immaturities may limit the prepubertal child's ability to discriminate and articulate his moods and feelings. In addition, during the school years, a reluctance to appear vulnerable or dependent may encourage defenses against directly experiencing and acknowledging painful affects such as guilt, anxiety, and depression (Glasberg & Aboud, 1982).

Thus, the key developmental differences between adults and children are the latter's less articulated sense of self, instability of affect, and disinclination to experience guilt. Because of these factors, until recently many experts held that, although certain children were undoubtedly prone to sadness, childhood depression could not be a valid condition (Rochlin, 1959). In recent years, however, researchers have discarded these a priori objections in favor of empirical attempts to determine whether there are affective disorders in childhood that share features of the adult conditions. Consequently, they have tried to develop reliable descriptive criteria for a syndrome of childhood depression as a heuristic empirical guide to further research. These diagnostic schemes attempt to define a childhood syndrome similar to that of adult depression, while taking age-specific differences into account. Behind the debate about criteria, several conceptual questions are at stake (Carlson & Garber, 1986). In comparing the childhood syndrome of depression with adult depression, what sorts of comparability are important? The developmental differences between children and adults make it unlikely that depression would express itself in behaviorally isomorphic ways throughout the life-span (Cicchetti & Schneider-Rosen, 1986). The search for basic pathogenic processes common to children and adults necessitates moving beyond a focus on symptomatic identities and instead exploring how such processes might manifest themselves at different developmental epochs (Carlson & Garber, 1986). Thus, as Carlson and Garber suggest, a productive approach might be to (1) identify which symptoms of the adult depressive syndrome require developmental accomplishments that make their appearance unlikely in childhood and (2) determine if some symptoms are empirically associated with depressive symptoms in childhood but are not typically part of the adult depressive syndrome.

The most widely accepted and disseminated scheme for classifying affective disorders is in the DSM-III-R.

DSM-III-R Diagnostic Criteria for Major Depressive Episode

A. *At least five of the following symptoms have been present during the same two-week period and represent a change from previous functioning; at least one of the symptoms is either (1) depressed mood, or (2) loss of interest or pleasure. (Do not include symptoms that are clearly due to a physical condition, mood-incongruent delusions or hallucinations, incoherence, or marked loosening of associations.)*

   (1) *depressed mood (or can be irritable mood in children and adolescents) most of the day, nearly every day, as indicated either by subjective account or observation by others*

   (2) *markedly diminished interest or pleasure in all, or almost all, activities most of the day, nearly every day (as indicated either by subjective account or observation by others of apathy most of the time)*

   (3) *significant weight loss or weight gain when not dieting (e.g., more than 5% of body weight in a month), or decrease or increase in appetite nearly every day (in children, consider failure to make expected weight gains)*

   (4) *insomnia or hypersomnia nearly every day*

   (5) *psychomotor agitation or retardation nearly every day (observable by others, not merely subjective feelings of restlessness or being slowed down)*

   (6) *fatigue or loss of energy nearly every day*

   (7) *feelings of worthlessness or excessive or inappropriate guilt (which may be delusional) nearly every day (not merely self-reproach or guilt about being sick)*

   (8) *diminished ability to think or concentrate, or indecisiveness, nearly every day (either by subjective account or as observed by others)*

   (9) *recurrent thoughts of death (not just fear of dying), recurrent suicidal ideation without a specific plan, or a suicide attempt or a specific plan for committing suicide*

B. *(1)* *It cannot be established that an organic factor initiated and maintained the disturbance*

   (2) *The disturbance is not a normal reaction to the death of a loved one (Uncomplicated Bereavement)*

   Note: Morbid preoccupation with worthlessness, suicidal ideation, marked functional impairment or psychomotor retardation, or prolonged duration suggest bereavement complicated by Major Depression.

C. *At no time during the disturbance have there been delusions or hallucinations for as long as two weeks in the absence of prominent mood symptoms (i.e., before the mood symptoms developed or after they have remitted).*

D. *Not superimposed on Schizophrenia, Schizophreniform Disorder, Delusional Disorder, or Psychotic Disorder NOS.* (APA, 1987, pp. 222–223)

In addition to Major Depressive Disorder, DSM-III-R includes two other depressive disorders: *Dysthymia* (also called "Depressive Neurosis") and *Adjustment Disorder with Depressed Mood.*

DSM-III-R Diagnostic Criteria for Dysthymia

A. *Depressed mood (or can be irritable mood in children and adolescents) for most of the day, more days than not, as indicated either by subjective account or observation by others, for at least two years (one year for children and adolescents)*

B. *Presence, while depressed, of at least two of the following:*
    (1) poor appetite or overeating
    (2) insomnia or hypersomnia
    (3) low energy or fatigue
    (4) low self-esteem
    (5) poor concentration or difficulty making decisions
    (6) feelings of hopelessness

C. *During a two-year period (one year for children and adolescents) of the disturbance, never without the symptoms in A for more than two months at a time.*

D. *No evidence of an unequivocal Major Depressive Episode during the first two years (one year for children and adolescents) of the disturbance.*

    Note: There may have been a previous Major Depressive Episode, provided there was a full remission (no significant signs or symptoms for six months) before development of the Dysthymia. In addition, after these two years (one year in children or adolescents) of Dysthymia, there may be superimposed episodes of Major Depression, in which case both diagnoses are given.

E. *Has never had a Manic Episode or an unequivocal Hypomanic Episode.*

F. *Not superimposed on a chronic psychotic disorder, such as Schizophrenia or Delusional Disorder.*

G. *It cannot be established that an organic factor initiated and maintained the disturbance, e.g., prolonged administration of an antihypertensive medication.* (APA, pp. 232–233)

DSM-III-R Diagnostic Criteria for Adjustment Disorder with Depressed Mood

A. *A reaction to an identifiable psychosocial stressor (or multiple stressors) that occurs within three months of onset of the stressor(s).*

B. *The maladaptive nature of the reaction is indicated by either of the following:*
    (1) impairment in occupational (including school) functioning or in usual social activities or relationships with others

(2) symptoms that are in excess of a normal and expectable reaction to the stressors(s)

C. *The disturbance is not merely one instance of a pattern of overreaction to stress or an exacerbation of one of the mental disorders previously described.*

D. *The maladaptive reaction has persisted for no longer than six months.*

E. *The disturbance does not meet the criteria for any specific mental disorder and does not represent Uncomplicated Bereavement.*

[F.] *The predominant manifestation is symptoms such as depressed mood, tearfulness, and feelings of hopelessness.* (APA, 1987, pp. 330, 331)

Currently, the DSM-III-R criteria are gaining acceptance as a useful starting point for diagnosing childhood depression, although many professionals feel that additional modifications are needed to better reflect the developmental difference between children and adults (Carlson & Garber, 1986; Shaffer, 1985a). In recent years, clinical studies have increasingly employed the DSM-III-R (1987) or original DSM-III (1980) criteria, often operationalized in semistructured interviews such as the K-SADS (Chambers et al., 1985) and self-report scales such as the Childhood Depression Inventory (Kovacs, 1985a). Although many methodological questions remain concerning validity and reliability (Costello, 1986; Costello & Angold, 1988; Rutter, 1988), these structured interviews and questionnaires for depressive symptomatology have also proved helpful in identifying cases that would otherwise be missed. The National Institute of Mental Health (NIMH, 1985) has published an overview of these studies.

Several other proposed diagnostic schemes exist, such as those developed by the Group for the Advancement of Psychiatry (1966), Weinberg et al. (1973), Kovacs and Beck (1977), and Cytryn and McKnew (1972, 1979). They differ from one another and from the DSM-III in details such as their emphasis on the presence or absence of low self-esteem, on the classic adult vegetative signs of appetite and sleep disturbances, and on whether increased aggression, irritability, and somatic complaints are criteria that suggest depression. Some of these schemata are far broader than DSM-III and diagnose many more conduct-disordered children as depressed than do the DSM-III criteria (Cantwell, 1983). More empirical work is necessary to determine to what extent these different schemata define the same or different sets of children and to explore whether these groups of children are homogeneous with respect to etiology, clinical course, physiological characteristics, or response to treatment.

Mania and Manic-Depressive Illness (Bipolar Affective Disorder)

In adults, mania is a pathological condition with inappropriately elevated, expansive, or irritable mood accompanied by such symptoms as grandiosity, pressured speech, flight of ideas, hyperactivity, decreased need for sleep, distractibility, and poor judgment (APA, 1987). Grandiosity may be extreme to the point of being delusional. The manic may embark on vast schemes or unrealistic projects for which he has no preparation: to compose an opera, to organize a worldwide rally for universal peace, or to invent a cancer vaccine and win the Nobel Prize. These delusions may involve a fantasied special relationship with God or other celebrities. Such delusions may, at times, be difficult to distinguish from those of schizophrenia. A commonly drawn distinction is whether the content of a delusion is clearly consistent with the person's predominant mood or *mood-congruent.* For example, a young man with manic-depressive illness, in his manic state, felt certain that he had been selected to take John Lennon's place and organize an international reunion tour for the Beatles. When depressed, he felt certain that his body gave off a repulsive odor because his insides were rotting. Such delusional thoughts were present only when he was in a manic or depressed state. These delusions were mood-congruent. It is controversial whether the mood congruity or incongruity of delusions or hallucinations provides a reliable guideline for distinguishing the psychotic features of manic-depressive illness and schizophrenia.

Kraepelin was the first to define "manic-depressive insanity," in which periods of mania alternate with melancholia; in the DSM-III-R diagnostic schema, the condition is known as Bipolar Disorder. Kraepelin also noted milder forms of this disorder, so mild, in fact, that the more subtle cases "pass over without sharp boundary into the domain of personal predisposition" (cited in Loranger & Levine, 1978).

Over the past two decades, the childhood and adolescent manifestations of bipolar disorder have drawn increased attention. There is growing recognition that full-blown symptoms of bipolar disorder often appear in adolescence and, much more rarely, in young children. Interest in the early natural history of the illness has prompted study of the disorder's prodromal manifestations. Finally, as the children of bipolar parents in various prospective studies reach adolescence, a clearer picture is emerging of the various phenotypic forms that a genetic loading and environmental sensitization for this disorder can take during the early years of life.

DSM-III-R Diagnostic Criteria for a Manic Episode

Note: A "Manic Syndrome" is defined as including criteria A, B, and C below. A "Hypomanic Syndrome" is defined as including criteria A and B, but not C, i.e., no marked impairment.

A. *A distinct period of abnormally and persistently elevated, expansive, or irritable mood.*

B. *During the period of mood disturbance, at least three of the following symptoms have persisted (four if the mood is only irritable) and have been present to a significant degree:*

(1)   inflated self-esteem or grandiosity

(2)   decreased need for sleep, e.g., feels rested after only three hours of sleep

(3)   more talkative than usual or pressure to keep talking

(4)   flight of ideas or subjective experience that thoughts are racing

(5)   distractibility, i.e., attention too easily drawn to unimportant or irrelevant external stimuli

(6)   increase in goal-directed activity (either socially, at work or school, or sexually) or psychomotor agitation

(7)   excessive involvement in pleasurable activities which have a high potential for painful consequences, e.g., the person engages in unrestrained buying sprees, sexual indiscretions, or foolish business investments

C.   *Mood disturbance sufficiently severe to cause marked impairment in occupational functioning or in usual social activities or relationships with others, or to necessitate hospitalization to prevent harm to self or others*

D.   *At no time during the disturbance have there been delusions or hallucinations for as long as two weeks in the absence of prominent mood symptoms (i.e., before the mood symptoms developed or after they have remitted).*

E.   *Not superimposed on Schizophrenia, Schizophreniform Disorder, Delusional Disorder, or Psychotic Disorder NOS.*

F.   *It cannot be established that an organic factor initiated and maintained the disturbance. Note: Somatic antidepressant treatment (e.g., drugs ECT) that apparently precipitates a mood disturbance should not be considered an etiologic organic factor.* (APA, 1987, p. 217)

EPIDEMIOLOGY

Because of the methodological problems, there are few reliable prevalence studies of childhood depression (Fleming & Offord, 1990). Many studies fail to differentiate between sad or depressed feelings and depression as a clearly defined psychopathological syndrome (Angold, 1988).

Among preschoolers, depression is rare, occurring in only about 0.3% of the general population of preschoolers and in 0.9% of preschoolers seen in a child development unit (Kashani & Carlson, 1987; Kashani et al., 1984, 1986). It is unclear to what extent this low prevalence of diagnosable depression reflects the difficulty of diagnosing very young children, with limited ability to verbalize their feelings.

In school-age children, sad or depressed affect is relatively common although full-blown (major) depression, as defined by DSM-III-R or other diagnostic schemes, is rarer, occurring in less than 3% of prepubertal children (Fleming & Offord, 1990). For example, Kashani and Simonds (1979) interviewed 103 children and their parents; the youngsters were randomly selected from among the patients at a family practice clinic or infants born at a university hospital. The investigators reported sadness as an affect occurred in 17.4% of these 7- to 12-year-olds. The subgroup of children who appeared sad showed a higher incidence of low self-esteem, school refusal, overactivity and somatic complaints; however, only 1.9% of the total sample met the full DSM-III (1980) criteria for depressive disorder.

Similar findings resulted when a representative sample of 9-year-old New Zealand children were studied by means of parent and teacher questionnaires and the K-SADS interview (Kashani et al., 1983). Using the Research Diagnostic Criteria (Spitzer et al., 1978), the current prevalence of "major" and "minor" depression was estimated as 1.7% and 2.5% respectively. A more recent survey of New Zealand 11-year-olds found a prevalence of 1.8% for either major depressive disorder and/or dysthymic disorder. Of the children so diagnosed, 80% also met the criteria for other disorders such as attentional deficit, anxiety, and/or conduct disorder (Anderson et al., 1987).

As children approach puberty, feelings of depression and diagnosable depressive disorder appear to increase; estimated prevalence rates for major depressive disorder in adolescents range from 0.4% to 6.4% (Fleming & Offord, 1990). Albert and Beck (1975) studied 63 suburban 7th and 8th graders, ages 11 to 15 years, who attended a parochial school. They administered a modified form of the Beck Depression Inventory, a self-report questionnaire that assesses the presence and severity of the various component symptoms of depression. The scores of this population were surprisingly high. Over 50% of the students reported significant concerns about self-dislike and dissatisfaction. Between 29% and 49% reported thoughts of failure, guilt, social withdrawal, self-harm, pessimism, or sadness. About one-third of the children showed total scores that would indicate moderate to severe depression in an adult. The large proportion of students with such scores led the researchers to question whether they were measuring genuine depression or instead tapping into developmental concerns characteristic of this age group (Kovacs & Beck, 1977; Shaffer, 1985a).

Similarly, the general population study of 10- to 11-year-old children on the Isle of Wight found that 13% showed a depressed mood in the interview and 9% appeared preoccupied with depressive themes. Parent and teacher questionnaires reported 10% to 12% of the children as "very miserable" (Rutter et al., 1970/1981). When the same population was reassessed at ages 14 to 15 years, depressive feelings were even more common (Rutter, 1986a). Thus, in reassessment interviews, over 40% of these adolescents reported "substantial feelings of misery and depression"; 20% were self-deprecatory; and 7% to 8% reported suicidal feelings.

Despite the widespread prevalence of depressed feelings, a much smaller proportion of children were diagnosed as having an overt depressive disorder as defined by criteria that included both "abnormal psychological function" and "persisting social impairment or handicap" (Rutter, 1986a, p. 12). The same increase with age was also noted. Thus, at 10 years of age, among approximately 2000 children, only 3 cases of depressive disorders were found, whereas at ages 14 to 15 years, 9 cases of "pure" depressive disorder and 26 cases of mixed affective disorders were found in the same sample.

In agreement with the Isle of Wight data, other studies suggest that depression becomes more prevalent with age, especially with the onset of puberty. A community-based survey of adolescents, ages 14 to 16, in Missouri reported a prevalence rate for major depression of 4.7% (Kashani et al., 1987; Kashani & Carlson, 1987). It remains unclear to what extent this increase represents an ascertainment artifact, due in part to adolescents' greater ability to report their inner feelings. Although adolescence is a period of increased psychosocial stress, the direct impact of pubertal hormonal factors cannot be discounted. In the Isle of Wight study, the prevalence of depression in adolescence was not due simply to older chronological age. Within a 14- to 15-year-old cohort whose pubertal status was known, "scarcely any" of the prepubertal boys showed depressive feelings, whereas about one-third of postpubertal boys did; the figures for the boys in midpubescence were in between (Rutter, 1986a).

In adulthood, women are more prone to depression than men. Data on gender distribution in childhood are spotty. There is some evidence that prior to puberty, depressive disorders are more common in boys, whereas following puberty more girls than boys are affected (Fleming & Offord, 1990; Rutter, 1986a). In the mid-Missouri community study of adolescents ages 14 to 16 years, the prevalence of major depression in girls was 13.3%, almost five times the prevalence of 2.7% for boys (Kashani et al., 1987). It is unclear to what extent apparent gender differences in the prevalence of adolescent depression reflect a truly higher rate of depression in girls (perhaps due to cultural or neuroendocrine factors or a greater tendency for boys to deny depression or to express it in disordered conduct).

The prevalence of depression increases in populations at special risk. After reviewing a variety of studies, Kashani et al. (1981a, 1981b) estimated that approximately 7% of pediatric inpatients and 30% to 60% of child psychiatry patients meet the DSM-III (or comparable) criteria for depression. Separation and loss also predispose children to depression. For example, at time of admission to a private residential school for children who had experienced loss of one or more parents through death, divorce, or separation, 31% of entering students were identified as depressed (Handford et al., 1986).

Recent epidemiological studies suggest that with each successive generation in this century depression is more common and has an earlier onset (Klerman, 1988). Especially in those born after World War II, depression and related disorders such as suicide, alcoholism, and drug abuse are especially common. Speculative hypotheses to account for the increased rate of depressive disorders in more recent birth cohorts have included demographic pressures associated with the baby boom, increasing social anomie, rising divorce rate, and greater availability and abuse of depressogenic drugs.

CLINICAL FEATURES AND DEVELOPMENTAL CONSIDERATIONS

Depression as a Normal Affect

Depression as an affect occurs normally throughout the life cycle (Anthony & Benedek, 1975; Jacques, 1965). Admittedly, knowledge of the inner world and sense of self of the preverbal child is largely inferential. During the second year of life the infant's verbal expression of emotions becomes increasingly differentiated (Lewis & Michalson, 1983); somber periods are often visible even with optimal mothering, and frustration, separation, or the presence of strangers cause incipient tearfulness. Mahler and colleagues (1975) have poignantly described how the recognition dawns on the growing, previously exuberant toddler that the world is not his oyster, nor is he the world's center. Periods of "low-keyed" subdued affect appear that are easily transformed into angry or tearful squalls. Although to an adult, the immediate cause of the child's frustrations and disappointment may seem minor, the toddler is gradually losing faith in his parents' omnipotence and his ability to command them at will. Beyond the external disappointments, the child's sense of self undergoes a sobering shift. Mahler suggests that growth and individuation require further renunciation of the child's belief in the magic omnipotence of his parents and himself. If all goes well, the child buffers the greater sense of his and his parents' limitations with a more realistic "good enough" evaluation of his real skills, capacities, and ability to love and be loved. Even with optimal development, however, the growing child sometimes feels discouraged and hopeless, not only about external slights and disappointments but about his own worth, competence, and lovability. Capacity for self-reflection and guilt accelerates around the age of 5 or 6 and transforms previously global feelings of helplessness and discouragement into more clearly focused feelings of self-reproach and personal unworthiness.

In adolescence, self-doubt, depression, and *weltschmertz* ("world sadness") are normal as the teenager grows apart from his parents and struggles to consolidate a separate identity and set of values. The process that psychoanalysts describe as object removal is under way. The protective magic circle of the family wanes, the "silver cord" is loosed. With his wider experience, progressive deidealization of his parents, and growing capacity for abstract, formal thought, the adolescent sees that his family and his home with its customs comprise only one way of many. He is increasingly on his own in a larger world, and the loneliness can be both exhilarating and frightening.

The thoughts of youth are thus "long, long thoughts," and high spirits and dreams of glory may alternate with depressive brooding. The hormonal changes of puberty may also predispose the adolescent to depression, either as a direct effect of endocrine factors or as a result of the psychosexual stresses accompanying sexual maturation (Rutter, 1986a). Finally, the end of adolescence requires renouncing the omnipotence of youth. The young person must give up the sense of being able to choose to do anything, be anything, and love or be loved by anyone, accepting instead a specific identity, a delimited set of life interests and goals, and a given circle of friends. The person's ability to tolerate and cope with depressed feelings becomes a major determinant of the later form of his personality (Zetzel, 1970b).

When losses, frustration, or disappointment are too great, however, or when the blows to a youngster's self-esteem are too severe, then hopelessness, discouragement and self-reproach can become fixed aspects of the sense of self; with this, the full-blown syndrome of depression may ensue (see Etiology).

Depression as a Clinical Syndrome

Depression in Infancy. In their classic studies of hospitalization and institutionalized infants, Spitz (1946) and Bowlby (1980) first noted that features suggestive of adult depression could be seen in infants who had never had a stable attachment figure as well as in infants who had formed a bond to their mother and had then been separated from her (see also Chapter 1). Although these symptom patterns have been well substantiated, controversy continues as to (1) whether such reactions are homologous to adult depression and (2) to what extent disturbances of attachment in early childhood predispose to later depression and/or other psychopathology (Harmon et al., 1982; Rutter, 1986a).

In the first half year of life, frequent changes in caretaker or lack of adequate, attentive, affectionate caretaking by parents may prevent an infant from forming a specific emotional attachment. The resulting disorder has been variously described as reactive attachment disorder, primary attachment failure of early infancy, "hospitalism," or failure to thrive. Such infants are apathetic, move little, and show diminished or absent social responses (such as sucking, smiling, or engaging in vocal play). They do not visually track the parent's face and they exhibit such vegetative signs as poor appetite, sleep disturbance, deranged pituitary functioning, and retarded physical growth. Without intervention, further deterioration and sometimes even death may follow. From 6 months to about 3 years, the child who has formed an attachment to his caretaker responds to prolonged separation in characteristic fashion, first with *protest,* then *despair,* and finally, upon reunion with the caretaker, *detachment.* Bowlby (1980) and James and Joyce Robertson (1971) described these three stages, now regarded as classic, most clearly in situations where children were separated from parents and left in the care of strangers. During the *protest* phase, which may last from hours to days, the child cries vigorously, searches urgently for the missing parent, and is inconsolable. The second phase, *despair,* sets in as the likelihood of the parent's return fades. Active crying and searching cease. Apathy, withdrawal, and quiet misery prevail, punctuated occasionally by intermittent, listless weeping. Although the child becomes quiet, a muted longing for and persistent orientation to the lost parent remain.

Any reminder of the mother may renew active crying. Along with this low-grade dejected longing is often a general irritability and hostility. Finally, if and when the child is reunited with his parent, the child often shuns her or shows an apparent complete absence of attachment behavior. This *detachment,* which is usually more evident with the mother than the father, appears to be both a reproach to the mother and a defense against the child's own painful memories of grief and abandonment. If the child's previous attachment has been adequate, if the separations are not repeated, and if the child and parent are promptly reunited (or an adequate caring replacement for the parent is quickly found), these early loss reactions appear to be reversible.

If the love object is not restored (or a substitute provided), some young children may remain withdrawn, weepy, and show signs of developmental retardation, insomnia, and proneness to illness. Spitz (1946) was the first to describe this condition, which he termed "anaclitic depression" (from the term *anaclitic,* meaning "leaning up against"). Spitz noted that such children often progress to "stuporous deteriorated catatonia" or in other cases "agitated idiocy," with death in many cases.

Actual loss or separation are not the only causes of depressive symptoms in toddlers. Mahler (1966) noted that even in infancy affective reactions of helplessness, sadness, and grief may occur in response to disturbances in the mother–child relationship, especially if they impinge on the separation–individuation process. In some children, the usual periods of subdued affect associated with the rapprochement phase are exacerbated and persist as a "basic depressive mood." Mahler noted that such reactions may occur with infants whose mothers, although physically present, are emotionally unavailable or aloof. The depletion of "confident expectation" and "basic trust" (Erikson, 1950) and the collapse of the child's belief in his omnipotence and in his mother's goodness lead to diminished self-esteem and a profound sense of helplessness. Symptomatically, Mahler observed, such children are clingy, moody, demanding, and regard their primary objects with great ambivalence.

The despairing, grieving infant or toddler manifests many features of the depressed adult: withdrawal, listlessness, loss of pleasure, irritability, and disturbed sleep and eating. Adult features that are lacking in the younger child include a clearly articulated feeling of self-blame, worthlessness, and inadequacy. The section on etiology will consider to what extent early separations and loss may predispose to later depression and under what circumstances transient despair or detachment can crystallize into a depression that permanently alters the child's sense of self.

Depression in the Preschool Years. Although diagnosable depression is uncommon in the preschool years, there are very young children who meet the full DSM-III criteria for major depression (Kashani & Carlson, 1985, 1987). A larger number of preschool children exhibit enough depressive symptoms to concern their parents and teachers, even though they do not meet the full array of DSM-III criteria (Kashani et al., 1986). Expressed sadness or sad appearance, feelings of worthlessness, sleep disturbances, appetite changes, fatigue, and self-injurious behavior or wishes are the commonest core depressive symptoms. Irritability, apathy, and uncooperativeness appear to be more common in such children than in their nondepressed peers. Somatic complaints, such as medically ambiguous headaches and abdominal pain are also frequent. Moreover, the parents of depressed preschoolers reported a higher incidence of stressful life events than did the parents of nondepressed classmates, a finding of probable etiologic significance (Kashani et al., 1986). Many of these children suffered from parental abuse or neglect.

Depression in Middle Childhood. With advancing age, depressive symptoms are more frequent; as adolescence approaches they also become more adultlike (Carlson & Garber, 1986; Carlson & Kashani, 1988). Among 7- to 13-year-olds, depressive symptoms appear "more fully expressed and pronounced" with age (Ushakov & Girich, 1971, cited in Carlson & Garber, 1986). In addition, as children grow older, they become increasingly aware of their illness. Older children, with their expanding verbal and conceptual abilities, can directly express feelings of sadness, as well as symptoms of hopelessness and worthlessness (McConville et al., 1973).

In school-age children, the symptoms and course of depression may be quite variable. The depressed child appears sad, withdrawn, listless, hopeless, and passive. He takes little enjoyment in formerly pleasurable activities, and he may complain of boredom and of having nothing to do.

The depressed child may also verbalize feelings of being no good, "dumb," or unlovable. He may assume exaggerated responsibility for family events such as illnesses, divorce, or separations. Indeed, such events are common precipitants of depressive reactions (Wallerstein & Kelly, 1980). Nihilistic and somatic delusions resembling those of adult depressive psychoses are uncommon, but occasional cases of self-reproachful delusions have been reported at the approach of adolescence (Carlson & Garber,

1986; Chambers et al., 1982; McConville et al., 1973). Hallucinations in preschool children are not rare but may lack the diagnostic specificity of adult depressive psychoses (Carlson & Kashani, 1988).

Vegetative signs of psychomotor retardation and sleep disturbance are rarely as severe in children as in full-blown adult melancholia; they do occur but to a more limited extent. Loss of appetite or joyless overeating and obesity can be present. There may also be numerous somatic complaints such as aches, pains, dizziness, and fatigue, all of which defy physical diagnosis. However, somatic complaints, which are ubiquitous manifestations of depression in preschoolers, decrease with age. They are less common in adolescents than in preadolescents and still less common in adults (Carlson & Kashani, 1988).

The depressed child may voice the wish that he were dead, and there may be suicidal thoughts or attempts (see section on suicide below). In the absence of conscious self-injurious fantasies, accident proneness may take the form of frequent mishaps; these are in part due to the child's increased preoccupation and/or to masochistic tendencies. The depressed child has little energy for school or peers. Academic work frequently suffers, and teachers complain of his daydreaming, apathy, and inattention. Poor grades and their consequences may further erode the child's damaged self-esteem. Irritability often accompanies depression. Interpersonal relations with parents and peers deteriorate (Puig-Antich et al., 1985a, 1985b). Some depressed children, particularly if they have other psychopathology predisposing them to poor impulse control, show antisocial behavior such as minor thefts and increased aggression (Puig-Antich, 1982; Woolston et al., 1989).

Depression in Adolescence. With puberty, depression increasingly resembles the adult form and is more often complicated by alcohol and illicit drugs. Guilt, shame, and self-reproach appear more prominently in adolescent depression (as compared with younger children). Slights to the teenager's self-esteem or rejection by significant others are frequent precipitants. Compared with younger children, adolescent suicide attempts are more common and are of greater lethality. Vegetative symptoms, such as hypersomnia and weight changes are more common (Ryan et al., 1987a). Boredom, restlessness, and stimulation seeking may accompany or alternate with frank depression (Anthony, 1975c).

Diagnostic Considerations. Cytryn and McKnew (1979) divided childhood depression in the middle years into three categories: acute, chronic, and masked. Children with the acute and chronic varieties showed signs of *overt* depression with feelings of despair, helplessness, and hopelessness; *withdrawal,* with impairment of social and academic performance; and often *agitation, anxiety,* and *impairment in eating and sleeping.* The authors also noted persistent depressive themes in dreams, drawings, and other fantasy material (including projective testing), even when the child was able to defend against direct acknowledgment of unhappy feelings. Many children tend to avoid directly experiencing sadness or acknowledging it to themselves or others (Glasberg & Aboud, 1982). In Cytryn and McKnew's experience, the *acute* and *chronic* group were differentiated by: (1) duration; (2) in the acute syndrome, clear evidence of precipitating events (such as loss) immediately preceding the onset of illness; and (3) in the chronic cases, poorer premorbid adjustment and greater family psychopathology.

The authors' third category, *masked depression*, proved controversial, so much so that Cytryn and McKnew (1987) have now recommended dropping the category in favor of the DSM-III criteria. According to Cytryn and McKnew's (1980) description, in masked depression:

> The depression does not manifest itself in a clearly recognizable form; rather the child shows a variety of emotional disorders, including hyper-activity, aggressive behavior, psychosomatic illness, hypochondriasis, and delinquency. The underlying depression is *inferred* [italics added] from the presence of depressive fantasy material and periodic displays of overt depressive affects. (p. 2799)

Thus, the category of "masked depression" was intended to cover those children who seemed defended against the direct experiencing and verbal expression of depressive affect, but who expressed their presumed underlying depression in action, aggression, or other symptoms.

Although the general consensus is that depressed children often show concomitant aggressive, somatic, and anxiety symptoms, the concept of masked depression has proven difficult to operationalize; in recent years it has fallen out of favor (Kovacs & Beck, 1977; Gittleman-Klein, 1977). For example, there was no way to determine how much evidence of overt depressive affect was necessary to establish the diagnosis, and what the relationship must be between the episodes of overt depressive affect and the putative masked depressive equivalent.

Nonetheless, the frequent association of depression and conduct disorder poses a common diagnostic quandary and raises important theoretical questions (Carlson & Cantwell, 1980; Woolston et al., 1989). Puig-Antich (1982) found that more than one-third of prepubertal boys with major depressive disorders also met the DSM-III criteria for conduct disorder. For example, consider a deprived, disorganized, abused child from a chaotic and unsympathetic background who is suffering from attentional deficits and a hungry impulsivity. Such a child may show sad, joyless, and hopeless affect together with aggressive and antisocial behavior. A destructive cycle may exist: In order to vent his rage and to alleviate feelings of hopelessness and emptiness the child lashes out or steals. This action in turn begets either punishment or self-reproaches and thus leads to further deterioration in his self-esteem.

How should such a child be diagnosed? To the extent that problems of impulse control have predated the depressive symptoms and dominate the clinical picture, a diagnosis of conduct disorder with depressive features seems more appropriate than masked depression. If, on the other hand, the symptoms of depression seem to predominate or to have preceded the conduct problem, then a primary diagnosis of depression (or a double diagnosis of concomitant depressive disorder and conduct disorder) is suitable. The issue is not simply one of labeling. In some cases, at least, the two syndromes may have significant causal connections.

A related, largely unexplored question concerns the impact that treating the depression has on the symptoms of the conduct disorder. Puig-Antich (1982) found that effective treatment of prepubertal depression with imipramine improved not only the primary depressive symptoms, but also the concurrent conduct disorder behaviors. Furthermore, discontinuing the imipramine did not lead to a relapse of the conduct disorder, unless a relapse of the depression also occurred. When depression did recur, the resurgent depressive symptoms preceded the reappearance of the conduct disorder.

A broader, related question concerns the relationship of affective disorders to interpersonal relations and personality style. Although personality style clearly influences the clinical expression of depression (Akiskal et al., 1983), depression can have an equally marked effect on a child's personality and interactions with peers. Korenblum et al. (1988) found that many symptoms of personality disorder, which is usually conceptualized as involving enduring maladaptive traits, were in fact mood dependent and improved with recovery from depression. Similarly, Puig-Antich et al. (1985a, 1985b) found that the impaired social interactions of depressed prepubertal children partially improved with affective recovery.

Anxiety and depression also often appear together in children (Puig-Antich et al., 1978; Puig-Antich & Rabinovich, 1986; Ryan et al., 1987a; Woolston et al., 1989); whether the predisposition to these disorders is transmitted in families jointly or separately has been the subject of considerable research and controversy (Carey, 1987). Depressed children appear to have an increased incidence of anxiety disorders, especially if their parents also suffer from depression and an anxiety disorder (Weissman et al., 1984b). Attempts to elucidate such familial comorbidity lead to extremely complex methodological questions. A recent study suggests that genetic factors may determine the individual's *sensitivity* to environmental stress, whereas nongenetic factors determine whether the resulting psychopathology takes the form of depression, anxiety, or both (Kendler et al., 1987).

The Fate of Childhood Depression: Continuity versus Discontinuity

Little is known about the extent to which childhood depressions persist into or precede adult depressions. There is evidence, however, that childhood depressive symptoms can be quite enduring (Kovacs, 1985b).

Poznanski et al. (1976) followed into adolescence and adulthood a group of children who had been diagnosed as depressed 4 to 11 years earlier. On follow-up, 50% were still clinically depressed, although their symptoms now more resembled adult depression with more prominent dependency and lessened aggression; the remaining children showed other forms of psychopathology. Lasting depression appeared to correlate with ongoing parental deprivation and rejection. Kandel and Davies (1986) found that adolescents who reported depressive symptoms at ages 15 and 16 years were more likely at ages 24 and 25 years to report similar symptoms and to have difficulty establishing an intimate relationship with a member of the opposite sex.

Childhood and adolescent depressions may be quite persistent. Kovacs et al. (1984a, 1984b) prospectively followed a large group of school-age children with diagnoses of major depression, dysthymic disorder, or adjustment reaction with depressive mood. Earlier onset of depression predicted a more protracted course. Ninety percent of the depressive adjustment reactions recovered within 9 months; dysthymic disorders, however, were strikingly chronic with 90% recovered only after 7 years. Major depressive disorders required about 1½ years for 90% of the sample to recover. Recurrent depression was also very frequent in both the children with major depression and dysthymic disorder; 40% of children who recovered from a major depression relapsed within the 7-year study period, and 69% of the children with dysthymic disorder developed a severe major depression (Kovacs et al., 1984b). Strober (1985) found adolescent depression to be quite tenacious, with 14% still symptomatic 3 years after onset.

Similarly, in a 4-year follow-up of an NIMH cohort of children of hospitalized patients with affective disorders, Apter et al. (1982) found that of 12 children originally diagnosed as depressed, 7 retained a depressive diagnosis, 3 showed other psychopathology, and only 2 were asymptomatic.

Finally, Zeitlin (1986) studied the records of patients who had been seen at the Maudsley as both children and adults. At first glance there seemed to be little continuity between the diagnoses given to them as children and adults. However, a comparison of diagnoses based on reported symptoms of depression rather than on actual diagnoses given at the time showed a surprisingly high continuity with 84% of cases of childhood depression meeting the criteria for depression in adult life. The clinical diagnoses actually given in each epoch did not reflect this continuity in identified depression because nondepressive symptoms so often dominated the picture (Rutter, 1986a).

Manic-Depressive (Bipolar) Illness in Childhood

Although the peak period of onset for bipolar affective disorder is the early 20s, at least one-fifth to one-third of manic-depressive patients become ill before the end of adolescence (Ballenger et al., 1982; Loranger & Levine, 1978). Many cases of adolescent bipolar disorder are misdiagnosed (Carlson, 1985). Mild cases may be dismissed as adjustment reactions exacerbated by the normal moodiness of adolescence (Feinstein & Wolpert, 1973). Severe cases are often misdiagnosed as schizophrenia because psychotic symptoms (such as delusions, hallucinations, thought disorder, and paranoia) and signs of behavioral dyscontrol (such as assaultiveness and legal problems) are especially common in adolescent manic breakdowns (Ballenger et al., 1982; McGlashan, 1988). If the clinician follows these cases over time, however, the schizophrenic features become less prominent in subsequent breaks. Researchers have described several distinct clinical pictures of adolescents with bipolar disorder (Akiskal et al., 1985; Strober & Carlson, 1982). A clear-cut episode of depression, for example, may precede the manic episode. In a 3-year follow-up of adolescents hospitalized with depression, Strober and Carlson (1982) found that one-fifth subsequently developed a manic episode. Characteristically, acute onset, increased sleep, psychomotor retardation, and psychotic symptoms marked the depression of these adolescents; in addition, they came from families with increased loading for effective illness. In some of these cases, the patient's antidepressant medication precipitated hypomania. Chronic depression, sometimes complicated by drug or alcohol abuse (Akiskal et al., 1985), may also dominate the initial clinical picture.

Among prepubertal children, full-blown bipolar disorder with symptoms closely resembling the adult criteria is rare but does occur, especially among the offspring of manic-depressive parents (Anthony & Scott, 1960; Lowe & Cohen, 1980). Researchers have even noted the syndrome in toddlers and preschoolers (Weinberg & Brumback, 1976; Brumback & Weinberg, 1977). The offspring of manic-depressives appear to have an increased incidence of various pathological symptoms; during childhood, however, most do not meet the full adult criteria for bipolar disease. (See also section Children of Depressed Parents below.) As with depressive symptomatology, the younger the prepubertal child, the less clear-cut is the correspondence with classic adult manic symptoms (Carlson & Garber, 1986).

The diagnosis of early onset bipolar disorder is often missed because of the prominence of delusional ideation or antisocial and impulsive behavior (Gammon et al., 1983; Tomasson & Kuperman, 1990).

One source of diagnostic difficulty is that the disturbed behavior patterns of many such children are not sharply episodic or cyclical, but blend, as Kraeplin observed, into extremes of temperament (Carlson & Garber,

1986). Secondly, symptoms of hyperactivity may be difficult to differentiate from mania; however, the presence of irritability, rapid mood shifts, and cognitive disorientation may be useful in distinguishing childhood hypomania from attention-deficit hyperactivity disorder (Nieman & Delong, 1987). This similarity has prompted the suggestion that lithium-responsivity might be useful for identifying hyperactive symptoms that are the product of a bipolar diathesis. Lithium may ameliorate symptoms such as aggressiveness, emotional lability, and mood swings; whatever its therapeutic usefulness might be, however, the nonspecific nature of lithium's effects casts doubt on the diagnostic validity of such an approach (Campbell et al., 1985).

Lowe and Cohen (1980) have suggested that a genetic model of classification with a continuum of syndromes might best serve the study of childhood mania. The first syndrome would phenotypically resemble adult mania, presumably with a similar genotypic loading for bipolar illness. The second syndrome would include cases with a presumed genotype similar to adult manic depressives, but with a different phenotypic presentation (symptom pattern). The manifestations of this second syndrome might include the diffuse, multiple symptoms shown by the young offspring of bipolar parents. Recent genetic data indicate that although some forms of bipolar illness are heritable as an autosomal dominant, the penetrance is incomplete, so that only about 65% of persons with the gene will actually develop the full syndrome (Egeland et al., 1987). Finally, there is the syndrome of "secondary mania" (Krauthammer & Klerman, 1978), in which the patient presents all of the phenotypic characteristics of manic behavior but apparently lacks any genotypic similarity to adult bipolar disease. For example, manic symptoms can occur in patients who have taken phencyclidine (PCP), received high doses of corticosteroids, or been abruptly withdrawn from major tranquilizers (Akiskal et al., 1979; Lowe & Cohen, 1980).

ETIOLOGY

Loss as a Predisposing Factor

As already noted, loss of a parent can produce a depressionlike picture in the infant (Bowlby, 1980; Spitz, 1946). In reviewing the life histories of older depressed children, the therapist often finds the loss of a significant person, either through death or family disruption.

Loss plays a central role in most psychological theories of depression (Bowlby, 1980; Brown et al., 1986). It can act as a distant predisposing factor or as an acute precipitating event. What is lost may be another person or a cherished aspect or image of the self (Bibring, 1953). Yet such losses are ubiquitous; they are an inevitable consequence of living and growing

(Viorst, 1986). What determines why some losses lead to depression whereas others do not?

Any fully satisfactory model of depression must thus explain how loss leads not only to sadness, but also to the more complex symptomatology of depression. Besides the feelings of sadness, the affective component of depression includes a variable mixture of joylessness, guilt, worthlessness, fear, shame, tension, and anger and contempt (directed against both self and others) (Izard & Schwartz, 1986). In addition, depression includes cognitive and motivational elements such as hopelessness, helplessness, apathy, fatigue, and giving up (Beck, 1976). Finally, persistent physiological changes accompany depression.

As yet, no single theory adequately accounts for how these various aspects of depression come into being and maintain themselves. Tentative answers, however, are beginning to emerge from several quarters: studies of *normal and pathological grief* (Horowitz et al., 1980; Krupnick, 1984), human and animal studies of the behavioral and somatic effects of *early separation* (Rosenblum, 1984), conditioning studies utilizing the *learned helplessness paradigm* (Seligman & Peterson, 1986), and cognitive studies of *attributional style*.

As noted earlier, infants who have not formed ties to a principal caretaker or who have suffered a disruption of such ties develop a depressionlike picture of joyless apathy, withdrawal, disturbed sleep and appetite, and altered neurohormonal functioning. The impact of separation and social isolation can be studied experimentally in greater detail by observing infant monkeys who during their rearing were separated from their mothers or peers (McKinney, 1977; Rosenblum, 1984). Infant monkeys' responses to separation vary greatly with species, age, sex, environment, and preloss attachment; their reactions do not fit a simple, invariant sequence of protest–despair–detachment. Nonetheless, such studies confirm that maternal loss can produce profound behavioral and physiological changes in infant primates similar to those seen in human infants. For several days following separation from the mother, the infant monkey manifests active disturbance with increased agitation and distress vocalization. A period of persisting decreased levels of social interaction, locomotion, and environmental manipulation follows, along with increased huddling and self-clinging. Infants sacrificed at this point show altered hypothalamic neurotransmitters and adrenal catecholamine synthesizing hormones. During the phase of behavioral depression, body temperature and heart rate decrease, accompanied by electroencephalogram (EEG) spectral changes and alterations in physiological circadian rhythms and sleep patterns. Separation studies with nonprimate infants confirm the importance of the mother's presence as a key regulator of many of the infant's crucial physiological processes and rhythms; this regulatory function is quite independent of her function as a source of nutrition (Pipp & Harmon, 1987).

Animal studies also suggest techniques of systematically exploring the interaction of social and neurobiological variables in the genesis of depression. For example, drugs such as alpha-methyl-para-tyrosine exaggerate the infant monkey's response to peer separation. In animals who are not subjected to separation, the drug has quite different effects. In some circumstances antidepressants such as imipramine can alter the protest and despair components of the response to peer separation and modify the response to repetitive separations (Suomi et al., 1978).

Individuals differ in their organismic responses to stresses such as separation. Engel and colleagues (Schmale & Engel, 1975) postulated two basic patterns of biological response to stress. The first was the well-known activating *fight-flight* reaction described by Cannon (1932), which prepared the organism to confront, control, or avoid the source of the stress. The second pattern they termed *conservation-withdrawal*, characterized behaviorally by the triad of inactivity, quiescence, and unresponsiveness. The authors studied Monica, a 16-month-old girl with a gastric fistula and severe failure to thrive, caused in part by maternal deprivation and frequent separations. For a period of several months, Monica's fistula permitted direct observation of her gastric activity in response to various situations. Whenever a stranger approached, observers noted hypotonia and decreased gastric secretion as the physiological concomitants of a sad expression, decreased activity, and even sleep. Engel and colleagues speculated that such "conservation depression" might serve as a homeostatic mechanism to husband energy in the face of a loss or stress that the subject felt unable to manage.

Other observers have also noted individual infants who react to stress (especially the stress of separation) with a profound lowering of physiologic arousal and drowsiness or sleep (see Emde et al., 1986). For example, Tennes et al. (1977) studied the pattern of cortisol secretion accompanying separation in one-year-olds. Most of the infants became distressed and increased their cortisol secretion when their mothers left. However, 10% of the infants instead became drowsy and went to sleep, while their levels of cortisol secretion *decreased.* (See also Chapter 7, "Anxiety Disorders," and Chapter 15, "Psychosomatic Disorders," for a further discussion of individual differences in autonomic reactivity to stress.)

These primitive depressive states in infants and toddlers usually are responses to massive trauma involving separation. Such infantile disorders do not meet all the criteria for adult depression, although they do share some features, such as social withdrawal, apathy, and altered appetite and sleep. As a result, a number of authors have preferred to view these disorders as a basic psychobiological reaction to deprivation rather than a true analogue of clinical depression (Bemporad & Wilson, 1978; Sandler & Joffee, 1965). The extent to which these disorders are precursors of affective illness in later childhood or adult life is still unknown and must await adequate follow-up studies (Harmon et al., 1982).

Studies of the impact of loss during childhood have been less extensive than studies of the infant and toddler period. At one time researchers argued that before adolescence children were incapable of true mourning, in the sense of grieving, letting go of the lost person, and attaching unambivalently to a new one (Wolfenstein, 1966). In contrast, Bowlby (1980) argued that children are indeed capable of successful mourning, but, like adults, can become caught up in pathological mourning, particularly in response to family factors. Pathological mourning, Bowlby felt, can take several forms, the most extreme being either chronic, unremitting mourning or an absence of conscious grieving. Unresolved mourning in childhood, Bowlby suggested, leaves the child vulnerable in later life to pathological developments such as ambivalence and anxiety in relationships; compulsive self-reliance (which avoids the risks of intimacy or dependence on another person); and compulsive care giving (which simultaneously attempts to bind the partner while repudiating any potentially disappointed needs of the self).

The analogy between depression and pathological mourning is an old one. Normal grief differs from depression in at least two ways: (1) the mourner is aware of the cause of his dejection, whereas the depressive often is not and (2) although very sad, the mourner, unlike the depressive, does not necessarily feel hopeless and generally does not have a diminished sense of competence and self-worth (Freud, 1917/1957).

In his classic paper "Mourning and Melancholia," Freud (1917/1957) attempted to explain how loss could lead to depression rather than simple mourning. Depression, Freud suggested, occurs when there are intense but unacknowledged, ambivalent feelings toward a lost (or, later theorists would add, disappointing or emotionally unavailable) person. In one of the earliest accounts of the process of identification, Freud speculated that the patient himself takes on or (to use Abraham's, 1916/1927, metaphor of incorporation) "takes in" aspects of the lost person as a way of maintaining a tie. Freud (1923/1961) suggested that this kind of identification is a basic process in personality formation: "[T]he ego is a precipitate of abandoned object-cathexes and—contains the history of those object choices" (p. 29). Next, however, the previously repudiated angry feelings, originally directed toward the lost person, are redirected toward the self and, in this disguised form, become conscious reproaches against the self. Thus, Freud noted, many of the depressive's self-recriminations and reproaches were originally accusations against the missing person. As Freud (1917/1957) aphoristically put it, "Thus the shadow of the object fell upon the ego . . ." (p. 249). From a psychoanalytic point of view, ambivalence toward important others plays an important role in the genesis of depression; this ambivalence is the source of the anger turned against the self, expressed as self-reproach, lowered self-esteem, and guilt.

Melanie Klein (1948) formulated the role of aggression in depression somewhat differently (see Chapter 7, "Anxiety Disorders" for a further discussion of Klein's views). She also stressed the early, infantile origins of the predisposition to depression. Klein suggested that from infancy onward, "depressive anxiety" stems from the child's concern that his aggressive feelings toward his mother may destroy her. The child thus fears that his hatred will prove stronger than his love and that his angry impulses will destroy both the internal and external wellsprings of goodness in his life. The child may make various attempts to alleviate or defend against this depressive anxiety. The most significant methods are reparation (the child attempts to repair or ameliorate the damage he fears he has done to mother) and the "manic defense" (a grandiose, magical, and reality-distorting denial of any badness in the self or in relations with others). Although many would quarrel with Klein's specific developmental chronology, her theory has provided an evocative and clinically useful framework for thinking about the vicissitudes of depression and aggression throughout the life cycle (Jacques, 1965).

In contrast to earlier theorists who emphasized the role of aggression turned against the self, Edward Bibring (1953) was more struck by the sense of helplessness, hopelessness, and loss of self-esteem in most depressions. He suggested that depression is essentially " 'a human way of reacting to frustration and misery' whenever the ego finds itself in a state of (real or imaginary) helplessness against 'overwhelming odds' " (p. 36). The main characteristics of this depression are decreased self-esteem, intense feelings of helplessness, a painful affect of dejection, and inhibition of function. Bibring suggested that this occurs when the ego experiences itself as powerless to achieve certain "narcissistically significant" goals or to maintain crucial relationships (real or internalized). These vital aspirations, Bibring felt, were of three types: (1) the wish to be worthy, loved, or appreciated, along with the parallel wish not to be perceived as unworthy; (2) the wish to be strong, superior, secure, and not to be weak and insecure; and (3) the wish to be good and loving and not to be aggressive, hateful, or destructive.

Either external or internal events that shake the foundations of self-esteem may produce despair over the incapacity to achieve these goals. External events include helpless exposure to "superior powers," illness, unredeemable loss, "the seemingly unescapable fate of being lonely, isolated, or unloved," or unavoidable confrontations with "the apparent evidence of being weak, inferior, or a failure." These disappointments, however, may also be internal; it is what happens when, despite the struggle to be good or loving, a person becomes aware of his own hateful aspects. Furthermore, an external disappointment or loss (e.g., of a loved one) may have especially powerful depressive reverberations when the person experiences it as an inner failure (e.g., "she left because I was hateful or selfish").

Studies of adult depression suggest that in several different ways a key factor in depression is the loss of a significant person. Recent loss or threat of loss (i.e., occurring within a few months of the onset of depressive illness) is prominent among the stressful life events that frequently precipitate adult depressions (Finlay-Jones, 1981). Moreover, Brown and colleagues (1986) have suggested that the loss of a parent in childhood either by death or separation is an important predisposing factor in the vulnerability to adult depression. These investigators even hypothesize that early childhood loss by death of a family member may predispose adult patients to more severe and psychotic forms of depression.

Despite such assertions, the long-term effects of the childhood loss of a parent pose controversial and methodologically complex questions (Brown et al., 1986; Tennant, 1988). Recent data suggest that such a loss in childhood need not in itself produce adult depression (Ragan & McGlashan, 1986). Rather, it may be a vulnerability factor, predisposing the adult to development of various psychopathological symptoms including depression in the face of stressful life events. Parental loss, in fact, may not be the key vulnerability factor. Following such a loss, the surviving parent or surrogate's degree of affectionate involvement with the child and style of discipline are significant determinants of subsequent adult depression (Brown et al., 1986; Tennant, 1988). Social class also exerts a powerful influence on this process in ways that are not fully understood. Socioeconomic status, for example, may affect such factors as the frequency of stressful life events in adulthood, the availability of social supports, the incidence of premature pregnancy and early marriage, employment and income status, and the presence or absence of a host of ameliorative factors (Rutter, 1981).

The social and family circumstances and processes surrounding disruption of the parent–child bond (whether from death, divorce, or other separation) appear as crucial to predicting outcome as the loss itself (Bowlby, 1988; Rutter, 1981, 1987). In this respect, different types of parental loss may have quite diverse concomitants. Whether the loss of a parent is through death or divorce seems to have important prognostic implications (Tennant, 1988); lumping these disparate disruptions together under the rubric "loss" may obscure these distinctions.

Despite much theoretical speculation and retrospective investigation, relatively meager systematic, prospective data are available concerning the impact of childhood bereavement. This is a striking gap in developmental knowledge, because as many as 4% of children lose a parent by age 15. The short-term effects of parental death are serious. Weller et al. (1988) found that as many as 45% of bereaved children met the DSM-III-R criteria for

Major Depression in the weeks following their parent's death. Strikingly, 25% were self-depreciating and 37% had suicidal ideation. The most troubled children were those who had a prior history of psychiatric difficulty and those whose surviving parent was depressed. Parents were often unaware of the depths of their children's grief and upset; many children reported wanting to spare their bereaved parent further stress.

Unfortunately, large retrospective studies shed little light on whether those children who become depressed in later life appear depressed either at the time of their loss or later in childhood. Also unanswered is how those children who later develop adult depression may differ in childhood from other bereaved children who do not later become depressed.

Although it is natural that loss or other disappointments should lead to sadness and loneliness, it seems at first unclear how to account for the hopelessness, helplessness, and decreased sense of self-worth that characterize depression. Beck (1976) has observed that among the symptoms of depression the "cognitive triad" of pervasive negative attitudes—toward the *self*, toward the *outside world*, and toward the *future*—play a central role. The self appears to be defective and inadequate; the world becomes excessively demanding and uncontrollable; and the future seems to offer continuing, unchangeable frustration. Recent work with the experimental paradigm of "learned helplessness" suggests how such pervasive attitudes of helplessness and hopelessness may be generated (Seligman & Peterson, 1986). *Learned helplessness* refers to the acquired perception that aversive events cannot be altered by any response the subject feels capable of performing (even though this may not in fact be so). (The term has also been applied to a lack of perceived control over desired pleasurable events.) The shock avoidance behavior of two groups of dogs was studied by placing the dog in a box so designed that the animal could avoid a shock by jumping over a partition within 10 seconds of a warning signal (Seligman et al., 1971). The first group of dogs had had no previous experience with shock. When placed in the experimental apparatus, virtually all of this group learned to escape the shock within a very small number of trials. In contrast, the second group of dogs, during the previous day, had been given numerous, unsignaled, and inescapable shocks. Unlike the first group, most of the dogs in the second group were unable to learn that they could avoid the shock by jumping over the partition. When the shocks began, they stopped running around, whimpered, and "seemed to give up and passively accepted shock." Even those few dogs who on one trial managed to escape by jumping would revert to taking the shock passively on subsequent trials. This effect persisted for as long as a month, depending on how soon the experimental trial followed the experience with unescapable shocks.

Uncontrollable shocks administered to animals produce far-reaching psychobiological consequences including decreased food and water consumption, weight loss, decreased aggressiveness and motor activity, and disturbances of grooming, libido, and sleep (Siever & Davis, 1985). Alterations in various neurotransmitter substances accompany this syndrome; moreover, its behavioral manifestations are susceptible to influence by administration of antidepressant medication (Weiss et al., 1982).

Repeated separation or early unmitigated loss of a parent by death, divorce, or desertion may well induce learned helplessness in the young child. Bowlby (1980) suggests such losses are accompanied by a profound sense of being unable to control the most vital aspect of life, namely the availability of a parent's care and affection. The child also feels unable to control the painful and repeated shocks of unrelieved neediness, loneliness, and disappointment. This sense of helplessness gradually pervades the child's very sense of self. Other forms of overwhelming and persistent adversity, such as physical neglect or abuse, extreme poverty, or chronic illness may also induce learned helplessness. Nonetheless, the availability of an affectionate caretaker is one of the most important buffers against the impact of such adversity, and the absence of such a caretaker is an exacerbating risk factor.

The child sometimes finds it easier to view himself as bad than as helpless and may defensively cling to the fantasy that the loss was his fault. In effect he chooses to believe that had he only been a better child, he could have avoided the loss. Other factors too, such as an attitude of blame on the part of the remaining parent, may contribute to this belief. In one series of children who had lost a parent by death, 40% attributed the cause of death either to themselves or to the remaining parent (Arthur & Kemme, 1964). In conscientious children, a cycle can ensue in which unattainable perfectionistic strivings fail to achieve the fantasied reparation, leaving the child with an ever-renewed sense of failure, self-reproach, and helplessness.

Although controversy continues regarding the cognitive aspects of the learned helplessness theory, the concept itself has been heuristically fruitful (Seligman & Peterson, 1986). The corollary concept of "attributional style" (Abramson et al., 1978) has provided an intriguing approach to the deficits in motivation, cognition, and self-esteem that are part of the depressive syndrome. The theory of *attributional style* proposes that individuals have three characteristic ways of explaining the causes of good and bad events; these dimensions of attributions are *internal* versus *external, stable* versus *unstable,* and *global* versus *specific.*

Abramson and colleagues (1978) suggest that a depression-prone attributional style is one in which the individual perceives uncontrollable bad events as being caused by (1) his own actions or characteristics, (2) unrelenting factors that persist over time, and (3) global factors that occur in a large number of situations. When a person habitually attributes the cause of bad events to internal, unchanging, and global factors, the actual occurrence of bad events will lead to feelings of helplessness, hopelessness, and lowered self-esteem. The hopeless Charlie Brown on the pitcher's mound exemplifies this attitude: The team will lose, it has always been thus; it is somehow his fault, although there seems to be nothing that he can do about it; and he perceives the ignominy of his career in baseball as but one more sign of his general lack of efficacy. Yiddish idiom provides a pithy label for such a character type: a *schlemiel*.

Researchers have operationalized the theory of attributional style in questionnaire form and have applied it to various groups of subjects (Seligman & Peterson, 1986). Studies of children and parents suggest that children and mothers (but not necessarily fathers) share common attributional styles and that, in both mother and child, their attributional styles for bad events correlate with depressive symptoms. In the same studies, inconclusive data suggested that a "pre-existing insidious attributional style for failure" (p. 241) may predate the actual development of depression.

Studies of nondepressed individuals suggest that such subjects are prone to optimistic distortions; they see themselves as being more efficacious and in better control than they really are and distort the balance of their successes and failures. Compared with depressed subjects, nondepressed children and adults are more likely to attribute success to internal, stable, and global factors, while seeing failure as due to external, transient, and situation-specific factors. In an article provocatively titled "Positive Denial: The Case for Not Facing Reality," Lazarus (1979) suggests that optimistic distortions encourage endeavor and sustain hope.

Beginning as early as the second year of life, children manifest the capacity for critically appraising their competency and can anticipate failure (Kagan, 1983). Professionals are only beginning to understand what determines whether the developing child's self-appraisals lead to relatively optimistic, confident expectations of successful mastery or pessimistic feelings of inadequacy and expectation of failure (Garmezy, 1986).

Not all cases of depression involve a history of actual bereavement or separation. Instead a child may lose a cherished image of himself or special closeness with a parent. In such cases, the content of the child's lowered self-esteem will reflect the specific aspirations he feels helpless to achieve or maintain (Bibring, 1953).

Each epoch of childhood has characteristic aspirations: on the oral level, to be loved and cared for; on the anal level, to be good, clean, and loving; and on the phallic level, to be admired and triumphant (Anthony, 1975a; Bibring, 1953). Conflicts at each level may lead to a denial or exaggeration of its aspirations, for example, a grandiose assertion of independence or self-sufficiency; an inordinate need never to be bad, defiant, or dirty; or excessive modesty and self-effacement. Where the cherished and needed views of the self are challenged sufficiently from within or without, depression may ensue. Thus, a child conflicted over dependency needs may suffer depression when events, such as the birth of a sibling, painfully confront him with his dependency or perceived lack of lovability. Similarly, a child with strong concerns over control of impulses may go to great lengths not to be bad, defiant, or dirty. When such a child finds himself unable to control angry or sexual impulses as perfectly as his ideals demand, he may become depressed and experience overwhelming feelings of guilt and helplessness ("I'll never be able to be a nice enough boy"). Finally, the oedipal child's sense of worth may revolve around being the center of attention or triumphing over rivals. When such a child feels helpless to prevent the defeat, retaliation, or ridicule that he fears, depression may result.

Some parents may have very specific pre-conditions for loving. Such parents regard their children as idealized extensions of themselves, and extend their affection on very specific terms. For example, the child must be unusually accomplished, say in music or sports or school, or must be particularly pious, or must be especially close and caring toward the parent. The talented or unusually compliant child may initially be able to meet such parental demands and will experience a sense of special closeness with the parent, whereas the child who cannot do so will feel helpless and defective. In adolescence or in later life, however, even the previously successful child may become depressed, because he feels unable to continue being good enough or his achievements no longer bring the specialness that he seeks (Kernberg, 1975, 1984a; Kohut, 1977; Miller, 1981; Shapiro, 1979). This fall from grace may hit such children hard, rendering them especially prone to depression. These children often suffer from overprotection and an inappropriately prolonged perpetuation of a fantasied fusion with parental specialness and omnipotence. Unlike less coddled children, the "special" child may lack the ultimately strengthening immunization of experiencing losses, frustrations, and disappointment in "bite-size," manageable portions. (Chapter 11, "Narcissistic Disorders," discusses this group of children.)

Among the many depressed children, one poignant group comprises those who have depressed parents. Such a child often feels that he has a duty to relieve his parent's depression, and he reproaches himself and feels helpless at being unable to do so. In some cases, too, the depressed parent may project or "read into" the child hated aspects of the parent's self (or of the parent's own ambivalently regarded parent). As discussed later in greater detail, being reared by a depressed parent may be one of the most potent influences in the subsequent development of a depression-prone child (Anthony, 1983). (Of course, predisposing hereditary factors as well as pathological interactions with the depressed parent may also be at work.)

In summary then, the particular ways that children strive to be good, loved, worthy, strong, and secure vary with age, individual, and family. Where external events or unrealistic internal standards (relative to the child's capacities) lead to persistent inability to achieve these goals, depression results. Among the most powerful external factors is the loss or unavailability of a reliable, nurturant other. As Bowlby (1980) put it:

[T]he principal issue about which a [depressed] person feels helpless is his ability to make and maintain an affectionate relationship. The feeling of being helpless in these particular regards can be attributed, I believe, to the experiences he has had in his family of origin. (p. 247)

Psychobiological Factors

The principal biological hypotheses concerning the causes of affective illness center on the role of *biogenic amines*, abnormalities in the *hypothalamic-pituitary-adrenal axis*, and derangements of key *biological rhythms*.

The Biogenic Amine Hypothesis.

Before discussing the biogenic amine theory of depression, it is important to review the role of neurotransmitters in the nervous system (Young & Cohen, 1979). The functional unit of the nervous system is the nerve cell (or neuron). Each neuron receives impulses from adjoining neurons through a network of fine branches called *dendrites*. If the stimuli playing upon the dendrites reach a certain critical threshold, a self-propagating wave of electrochemical activity, called an *action potential*, spreads away from the dendrites and down an extended fiber, called an *axon,* until it reaches the fine branchings in which the axon ends. Neurons transmit nerve impulses in only one direction, from the dendrites toward the end of the axon. The junction between two nerve cells is called the *synapse,* from the Greek word *synaptein,* meaning "to join together." This is the region where the axonal ending of one cell, the *presynaptic* neuron, lies close to the dendrite of another cell, the *postsynaptic* neuron. The actual gap, or *synaptic cleft,* between the two cells is extremely small. Because of the many fine branchings of both the dendrites and the axon, each neuron can have an exceedingly large number (perhaps as many as 75,000) of incoming and outgoing connections with other neurons. The human cortex alone contains approximately 10^{14} synaptic contacts (Whybrow et al., 1984). This prodigious number of interconnections makes possible extremely intricate patterns of information transfer and processing.

Nerve signals moving along the axon of the presynaptic neuron can be transmitted across the synaptic cleft to the dendrites of the postsynaptic neuron by chemical substances called *neurotransmitters*. Although many neurotransmitters have now been identified, the commonest and most important substances are *monoamines*, which nerve cells synthesize from amino acids. One major transmitter, *serotonin* (5-HT), is synthesized from the amino acid tryptophan and is chemically classified as an indolamine, whereas two other transmitters, *dopamine* and *norephinephrine* (also called *noradrenalin*), are derived from tyrosine and are referred to as catecholamines. Following synthesis, the presynaptic neuron stores the transmitter in numerous small packets, called synaptic vesicles, located in the axonal ending, close to the synaptic cleft. When a nerve signal propagating along the presynaptic cell's axon reaches the nerve ending, these packets empty their load of neurotransmitter into the synaptic cleft, in close proximity to the dendritic membrane of the postsynaptic neuron. Presynaptic neurons are termed *serotonergic, dopaminergic,* or *noradrenergic,* depending on the transmitter released by the cell.

Molecules of the released transmitter substance bind onto specialized sites (termed *receptors*) located on the postsynaptic cell's dendritic membrane. Once bound, the neurotransmitter molecules initiate complex changes in the dendritic membrane's chemical and electrical permeability at that spot. Some neurotransmitters are inhibitory, that is, they decrease (or stabilize) the permeability of the postsynaptic membrane, whereas other neurotransmitters increase dendritic membrane permeability, thus exerting an excitatory influence on the postsynaptic cell. When the sum of the excitatory and inhibitory neurotransmitter influences playing on the postsynaptic neuron's dendrites reaches a critical threshold, the neuron fires, sending an action potential sweeping down the axon and on to the next set of synapses.

The nervous system has evolved several ingenious methods for regulating the short- and long-term impact of each release of neurotransmitter on the postsynaptic neuron. For example, to facilitate precise, rapid signal transmission across the synapse, some means of terminating the neurotransmitter's action after each release burst is necessary. Otherwise, the postsynaptic cell membrane would remain "jammed" on or off (depending on the type of transmitter). To prevent this, two processes rapidly clear the neurotransmitter substance from the synaptic cleft: first, active reuptake of the neurotransmitter back into the presynaptic nerve ending, which also conserves transmitter; and second, destruction of the neurotransmitter by two enzymes, catechol-*o*-methyl transferase (COMT) and monoamine oxidase (MAO). Other complex regulatory processes modulate the amount of neurotransmitter released by the presynaptic neuron and the sensitivity and number of postsynaptic receptors to the transmitter (Siever & Davis, 1985).

Various drugs can have potent effects on the regulatory processes. A group of antidepressants known as the *monoamine oxidase inhibitors* (MAOIs), as their name implies, block the degradation of neurotransmitter by MAO, thereby increasing its availability. In contrast, the *tricyclic antidepressants* increase neurotransmitter activity at the synapse by blocking the reuptake of these substances by the presynaptic nerve ending.

The original biogenic amine hypothesis suggested that the critical factor in the transmission of impulses was the amount of neurotransmitter available. Thus, researchers proposed that depression followed the decreased activity of key neurotransmitters at important synapses in the brain and mania resulted from increased activity. Evidence for the theory came from the observation that the drugs that deplete brain amines, such as reserpine, induce depression, whereas the drugs that increase neurotransmitter availability at the synapse (i.e., the tricyclic antidepressants and MAOIs) alleviate the symptoms of depression and, in some predisposed patients, induce mania. Conversely, the drugs that reduce transmitter activity at the synapse may be useful in mania but may precipitate depression (Whybrow et al., 1984).

Subsequently, researchers observed that the impact of neurotransmitter activity is determined not only by the amount of neurotransmitter available, but also by the number and sensitivity of postsynaptic receptors. Bunney (1977) for example, suggested that changes in receptor sensitivity partially determine the "switch" from one mood state to another in manic-depressive cycling.

The catecholamine and indoleamine transmitters may both play a role in depression. Individual differences in response to specific antidepressants have led to the suggestion that the different types of depression are associated with functional deficits of the different monoamine transmitters or the balance between them (Maas, 1975).

The biogenic amine hypothesis had a tremendous impact on subsequent investigations, providing the heuristic impetus for a vast body of research into the mood disorders. It now appears, however, that more sophisticated models of dysregulation of neurotransmitter activity must replace the initial simple conceptions of deficiency or excess. Current models propose that impairment in the homeostatic mechanisms regulating neurotransmitters result in a vulnerability to erratic or unstable neurotransmitter activity. Such dysregulation might result in erratic basal output; disruption of normal periodicities (such as circadian rhythm); or less effective buffering, with less selective responsiveness to environmental stimuli and a slower return to basal activity (Siever & Davis, 1985).

Severe melancholia and mania cause disturbances in many basic psychobiological functions regulated by the limbic diencephalic parts of the brain. In addition to mood disturbances, these include (Whybrow et al., 1984):

1. Disturbances of the sleep–wake cycle, including alteration in EEG sleep architecture.
2. Alteration in appetite and libido.
3. Changes in the ability to experience pleasure.
4. Disruption of normal body rhythms, ranging from the daily circadian cycle regulating wakefulness, body temperature, and circulating levels of cortisol and other hormones, through the monthly menstrual cycle, and including long-period adaptation to seasonal fluctuations in length of daylight.
5. Alteration in psychomotor activity.

6. Abnormality in the feedback regulation of corticotrophic, thyrotrophic, and gonadotrophic hormones.
7. Abnormalities of biogenic amine metabolism.

Neurobiologists are only beginning to understand how these complex disturbances in arousal, appetitive, psychomotor, circadian, sleep, neuroendocrine, and pleasure functions relate to each other. These core psychobiological functions are susceptible to influence by both internal factors, including affects, and external environmental influences, such as light and psychosocial stimuli. For example, some children, like adults, may be vulnerable to a seasonal affective disorder, induced by seasonal changes in the duration of daylight and treatable by appropriate supplemental lighting (Rosenthal et al., 1986). There is growing evidence, however, that the basic regulatory mechanisms for these functions are located in the midbrain and may be mediated in part by shared neurotransmitter mechanisms (Whybrow et al., 1984). Any satisfactory biological theory of depression and mania will have to explain how predisposing genetic, personality, and early experiential factors interact with precipitating biological, environmental, and life events to lead to the "final common path" of a fully expressed manic or depressive syndrome. How such multiple factors produce the particular constellation of psychobiological dysfunctions described above remains one of the great challenges of modern biological psychiatry.

Biological Markers

There has been far less study of the biochemical and psychophysiological aspects of depression in children than in adults. Researchers have found some interesting biological abnormalities in adult depressive patients, but it is unclear to what extent these factors reflect underlying causal processes and to what extent they are the consequence of the depressive state and its accompanying stress.

Researchers distinguish two types of associated biological features or *markers* for depression: *state markers* and *trait markers* (Puig-Antich, 1986). State markers are abnormalities that appear at the onset of an overt depressive episode and then normalize as the depression remits. In contrast, trait markers are abnormalities that are present long before the actual onset of depression in a patient and persist even after recovery. The search for trait markers is especially intense because they are presumably related to the underlying mechanisms of vulnerability to depression and would permit early identification of high-risk subjects.

In adults the best studied biological markers for major depressive disorders include sleep EEG, neuroendocrine regulation, neurotransmitter metabolism, and transmitter receptor sites (see reviews by Puig-Antich, 1986, 1987). Although their relationship to the pathogenesis of depression remains obscure, these markers are of interest because of their presumed link to central nervous system functioning. However, the impact of development on these measures, even in a nondepressed population is unknown, obscuring the significance of these markers for childhood depression. Many studies involve only a few subjects and have not been well replicated. Most measures have either proven to be nonspecific for depression or have returned to normal once the symptoms remit (e.g., Khan, 1987a; Puig-Antich, 1986).

Puig-Antich (1986, 1987) has proposed that abnormal growth hormone regulation may represent a stable trait marker for childhood depression. During episodes of major depression, prepubertal children secreted more growth hormone during sleep than did normal children or children with other psychiatric disorders (Puig-Antich et al., 1984b). In addition, certain depressed prepubertal children showed an abnormal pattern of growth hormone secretion when given an insulin-induced hypoglycemia provocation test, a procedure believed to test indirectly the functional status of hypothalamic neurotransmitter systems. These abnormalities persisted even after overt depression had remitted and antidepressant medication was discontinued (Puig-Antich et al., 1984a). Depressed prepubertal children also show abnormal patterns of growth hormone secretion in response to other challenge tests that probe the regulation of the hypothalamic neurotransmitter system (Jensen & Garfinkel, 1990). If replicated and demonstrated *prior* to the onset of actual depression, these findings may lead to a true trait marker for prepubertal depression that is perhaps linked to a functional deficit in hypothalamic serotonin regulation (Puig-Antich, 1986).

Researchers at NIMH who have found abnormalities in cholinergic receptors on the surface of fibroblasts cultivated from depressed patients have proposed another possible marker (Nadi et al., 1984). Ill first-degree relatives shared this abnormality, but not normal relatives or controls. These receptors have not been studied in depressed children, and the original findings remain to be replicated.

The Dexamethasone Suppression Test, a measure of dysregulation of hypothalamic-pituitary control of cortisol secretion, is a state marker that has been widely studied in adults. The specificity and sensitivity of this measure for childhood depression is less clear, because researchers have not adequately explored the effects of age, dosage, and diagnostic variables (Doherty et al., 1986; Khan, 1987a; Leckman, 1983).

Genetic Factors

Family studies of bipolar (manic-depressive) illness and unipolar depression (serious depression without mania) strongly suggest that genetic factors play a part in their transmission. These factors place the children of parents with affective disorders at risk over and above the deleterious environmental impact of such parents' possibly disturbed child-rearing practices.

In several studies of chronically depressed adult patients, monozygotic (MZ) twin pairs showed a higher concordance rate (76%) for depression than did dizygotic (DZ) twins (19%) (Tsuang, 1978); even when reared apart, MZ twins had a concordance rate for affective illness of 67%, a figure statistically similar to the overall concordance rate for MZ twins reared together (Tsuang, 1978). A recent study of a nonclinical sample of child MZ and DZ twins suggested that genetic factors accounted for about half the variance in the level and lability of subclinically depressed moods (Wierzbricki, 1987). Torgersen (1986b) concluded from his twin studies that important hereditary factors existed in both bipolar and major depression but were not apparent for milder forms of depression. Studies of adopted children reared away from their depressed biological parent have also suggested that genetic factors operate in addition to the psychological experiences of being reared by a depressed parent (Nurnberger & Gershon, 1982; Wender et al., 1986).

Although many older family studies reported in the literature suffer from serious methodological shortcomings, recent carefully designed studies confirm that first-degree relatives of patients with affective disorders have an increased risk for developing an affective disorder (Weissman et al., 1984a, 1984c). Gershon and his colleagues (1982) studied the lifetime prevalence of major affective disorder (including schizoaffective disorder) in first-degree relatives of adult probands (patients) with schizoaffective disorder, bipolar disorder, and unipolar disorder. The prevalence rates for affective illness in the relatives of these proband groups were 37%, 24%, and 20%, respectively (compared with 7% in the relatives of normal control). The most frequent disorder diagnosed in affected relatives was unipolar depression. The risk for major affective illness in adult offspring increased from 27% with one affectively ill parent to 74% with both parents ill.

Weissman and her colleagues at Yale (1984a) found similarly increased rates of affective illness in the relatives of both severely depressed adult psychiatric inpatients and less severely depressed outpatients when compared with normal controls. The frequency of affective disorder was equally high in relatives of both the milder and more severely depressed probands. Although alcoholism, drug abuse, and sociopathy have sometimes been considered "depressive spectrum" disorders, neither the NIMH nor the Yale study found an increased incidence of these disorders in the relatives of affectively ill probands. There is some indication that phenomenological subtypes of depression may breed true in families. For example, adult patients with delusional forms of depression seem to have relatives with a particularly high rate of delusional depression (Leckman et al., 1984).

Most family studies, such as the ones just cited, begin by looking at adult probands. In the nature of things, studies of *adult* probands leave unanswered many questions about childhood depression. Childhood onset of affective illness, for example, may represent a higher genetic loading of factors predisposing to depression, greater penetrance of any given genetic factor, or the presence of exacerbating environmental factors (including psychiatrically disturbed parents) (Weissman et al., 1987).

Unfortunately, family studies of childhood affective disorder have suffered from methodological problems (Cytryn et al., 1986). One of the few studies that examined the families of affectively ill *child* probands is that of Puig-Antich and colleagues (1989). The relatives of these children showed an increased incidence of depression and alcoholism. However, the degree of family aggregation varied depending on the probands' clinical picture. In contrast with other groups of depressed children, those depressed children who had made a suicide attempt or who had a comorbid diagnosis of conduct disorder showed lower familial rates of major depression. The study also suggests an inverse relationship between the age of onset in probands and the "affective density" of their pedigree (i.e., the proportion of relatives suffering from affective illness). Strober (1985) found a 21.7% morbid risk of affective disorder in the first- and second-degree relatives of adolescents with affective disorders, a strikingly higher rate than in the families of control patients with other psychiatric disorders. Strober also noted that adolescents with "endogeneous" types of depression were more likely than adolescents with other depressive syndromes to have affectively ill family members; they also showed a trend toward more bipolar relatives. Children with manic-depressive disorder also show a remarkably high rate of affective disorder in family members (Dwyer & Delong, 1987).

An unresolved debate is whether bipolar and unipolar illness are best conceptualized as genetically distinct disorders with independent familial transmission. Alternatively, Gershon and colleagues (1982) concluded that their data were compatible with a "multiple-threshold, multi-factorial model" (Reich et al., 1972), in which the different disorders could fit a single dimension of underlying vulnerability, with bipolar disorder representing a higher degree of transmissible vulnerability and unipolar disorder representing a lesser degree of genetic liability.

A further complication of this debate is that these disorders are probably genetically heterogenous. In recent studies of a large Amish family with three generations of bipolar illness, vulnerability for the disorder appears to be inherited as an autosomal dominant. However, penetrance of the gene is incomplete; of those who inherit the gene, only about 63% actually develop a major affective illness. Although most affected family members had manic-depressive illness, other relatives showed schizo-affective disorder (bipolar type), unipolar major depression, or mania only.

Linkage studies initially suggested that the responsible gene was on the short arm of Chromosome 11 (Egeland et al., 1987). More recent data from this pedigree, however, now call this conclusion into doubt (Kelsoe et al., 1989). However this issue is resolved for this large pedigree, other genetic loci appear to be at work in other families with affective illness. Thus, in several bipolar families, researchers have established that the Chromosome 11 locus was *not* involved (Detera-Wadleigh et al., 1987; Hodgkinson et al., 1987). Some families with a strong pedigree of bipolar disorder may carry the relevant gene(s) on the X chromosome, whereas in still other families X-linked transmission does not occur (Mendlewicz et al., 1979; Robertson, 1987). There are also pedigrees where polygenic mechanisms appear to be at work (Kidd et al., 1984).

Powerful new methods of linkage analysis, such as the restriction fragment length polymorphism technique used in the Amish study of bipolar inheritance (Egeland et al., 1987), open up vistas for research and prevention but also pose new ethical dilemmas. In pedigrees like the Amish one, these techniques will soon make it possible to determine at an early age which children are highly likely to carry the gene for bipolar illness. Since only about 63% of those individuals who carry the gene actually develop the condition by adulthood, researchers can now study more precisely how the gene expresses itself at various stages of development and what factors increase the child's risk or protect him from becoming symptomatic. Ignorance of what constitutes effective prevention, however, complicates the therapeutic imperative for preventive intervention with the children most at risk. Furthermore, although early identification enables preventive intervention, it also risks stigmatizing as yet asymptomatic children in their own eyes and in the eyes of others.

Children of Depressed Parents. One of the largest groups of children at risk for depression are the children of depressed parents. The children of parents with affective illness are at risk not only for developing affective disorders but for other psychopathology as well (Anthony, 1975b; Gaensbauer et al., 1984; Zahn-Waxler et al., 1984a, 1984b). A wide range of personality and conduct disorders, as well as depression, have been described in such children (Cytryn et al., 1984, 1986; Weissman et al., 1987). Compared with controls, the children of depressed parents also show an increased prevalence of suicidal ideation and acts (Weissman et al., 1984c). The psychopathology noted in many of these children as infants and toddlers cannot readily be assigned a DSM-III diagnosis although it places them at risk for future difficulties. Often it is not until they enter school that a diagnosable pattern of depression or other disorder emerges (Cytryn et al., 1984).

Beyond the presence or absence of specific diagnoses, the adaptational and interpersonal style of children of affectively ill parents has become an enlarging area of study (Anthony & Cohler, 1987; Beardslee, 1986; Cytryn et al., 1986), as has the broader concept of children's adaptation to the stress of parental illness. A growing number of cross-sectional and longitudinal studies demonstrate the multiple risks of having a psychiatrically ill parent. In addition to the possible influence of the genetic risk factors, the child must often cope with disturbed parent–child interactions, increased family stress, and in those families where the parent's illness requires recurrent hospitalization, parental absences (Kauffman et al., 1979). These studies also raise the crucial and still unanswered question whether the risk factors for children of affectively ill parents are specific and unique to the parent's diagnostic category, or whether they reflect nonspecific factors such as severity, chronicity, presence of psychosis, and parental absence through hospitalization.

Wynne and associates (Fisher et al., 1980; Harder et al., 1980; Kokes et al., 1980), who compared the offspring of various groups of affectively ill, psychotic, and nonpsychotic parents, concluded that factors such as the parent's overall functional impairment and the family's communication deviance were more closely related to outcome measures of the children's competence than was the parent's specific diagnosis. Other studies indicate that not only do the severity and chronicity of parental depression correlate with impaired adaptation and psychopathology, increased discord between the parents also has an exacerbating effect (Keller et al., 1986). Conversely, researchers are just beginning to identify the social, familial and individual factors that protect high-risk children from developing pathology (Anthony & Cohler, 1987; Beardslee, 1986; Rutter, 1987a; Weintraub et al., 1986).

The parent's depression (or mania) may affect the child through several mechanisms (Emde et al., 1986). These include contagion; early identification with a parent's depression (A. Freud, 1966); lack of emotional availability with consequent lack of positive reinforcement, interaction, or empathic attunement to the child's behavior (Stern, 1985); and parental deprecation of the child (perhaps through projective identification wherein the parent reads hated and denigrated aspects of himself into the child and then attacks or rejects the child for them) (Cytryn & McKnew, 1980; Scharff & Scharff, 1987). Maternal depression appears to have a more deleterious impact than paternal (Keller et al., 1986). Several factors disrupt and disorganize the ability of depressed mothers to care for their children (Anthony, 1983b), including feelings of inadequacy and helplessness, ambivalence toward the child as a competitor for supplies, increased self-absorption, and a hypersensitivity to criticism. These ongoing transactional consequences of depressed parents' relative emotional unavailability probably have as great an impact as actual parental absences due to hospitalization. In addition, the child of a parent with manic-depressive illness must cope with the parent's erratic and unpredictable behavior and mood swings (Anthony, 1975b).

Although retrospective studies demonstrate that the offspring of depressed parent(s) have a higher risk of being depressed in adulthood, prospective studies are just beginning to delineate how these at-risk offspring look in childhood. Cytryn, McKnew, and their colleagues at NIMH (1982) studied the offspring, ages 5 to 15 years, of hospitalized unipolar and bipolar adults. Compared with children of normal control parents, the children of these affectively ill patients showed an increased prevalence of depressed affect, major depressive disorder, and dysthymic disorder (as diagnosed according to the DSM-III criteria). Although the proband group of depressed parents included both bipolar and unipolar patients, at the time they were studied the affected children showed signs only of depression, that is, there was a striking absence of hypomanic symptoms in this age group. One teenager who at the time of this study had displayed only depression, 2 years later developed a bout of lithium-responsive mania (Cytryn, personal communication, 1985). By the ingenious use of comparison groups of nondepressed parents hospitalized for chronic medical illness, Cytryn and colleagues showed that having a chronically ill hospitalized parent could not solely explain the higher frequency of depressed offspring in the depressed parents.

More recently, the NIMH group (Cytryn et al., 1984; Zahn-Waxler et al., 1984a, 1984b) studied seven children of bipolar parents in a longitudinal fashion beginning at age 1 year. At the time of the study, the index parents (four of whom were mothers) were on lithium and in remission. During the second year of life, when compared with matched controls, these children showed more insecure, ambivalent attachment and less capacity for emotional self-regulation, especially of fear and anger. At age 2 years, psychological symptoms such as phobias, sleep disturbances, eating problems, excessive shyness and dependency, passivity, hyperactivity, social language problems, and tantrums were significantly more frequent in the proband children (Zahn-Waxler et al., 1984b). At age 2½ years, in a study of peer relations, the proband children revealed more inappropriate aggression toward peers following separation from mother. Additionally, the proband children showed less altruism, less sharing, and greater upset during a simulated argument between two adult observers (Zahn-Waxler et al., 1984a). Further follow-up of this sample is still in progress. Nonetheless, it is evident that from a very early age children of parents with a bipolar affective disorder show disturbance in attachment behavior, interpersonal relations, and regulation of affect.

Decina, Kestenbaum, and colleagues (1983) also followed a group of 13 children of manic-depressives for more than 5 years. They noted that almost half showed distractibility, poor concentration, impulsivity, transient rage reactions, and disturbances in academic achievement, as well as in affect such as lability of mood, hyperexcitability, and in some cases inappropriate elation. However, the proportion that showed only labile or depressed affect as opposed to hypomanic mood states is unclear from their report. Even when a child has a strong genetic predisposition toward a depressive disorder, his phenotypic behavioral expression can vary. The preventive implications of such studies are obvious: Clinicians treating seriously depressed parents must be alert for signs of depression in their children as well.

SUICIDE

American teenagers (ages 15–19) kill themselves at the rate of about 1,800 per year (Saltzman et al., 1988). In 1987, suicide was thus the third leading cause of death in adolescence, surpassed only by accidents and homicide; with an age-specific mortality rate of 12.9 per 100,000, suicide accounted for 13% of all deaths of young people ages 15 to 24 years (National Center for Health Statistics, 1989). Furthermore, many fatal accidents may be undetected suicides or may represent semideliberate, self-destructive accident proneness, as in taking increased risks or drinking while driving. In the United States, completed suicides are almost five times more common in adolescent boys than in girls; the suicide rate for white male youths is about twice that for other racial and ethnic groups (Centers for Disease Control, 1986).

The rate of reported completed suicides in prepubertal children is much lower than in adolescents. Among 5- to 14-year-olds, 251 suicides were reported in 1987, compared with 4,924 suicides among 15- to 24-year-olds (National Center for Health Statistics, 1989). Nonetheless, suicide was the sixth most common cause of death of 5- to 14-year-olds, with an age-specific mortality rate of 0.7 per 100,000, accounting for about 3% of all deaths in this age group. (These figures are largely for children ages 10–14, as national statistics usually do not include suicide as a cause of death for children under 10.)

During the past 35 years the dramatically high adolescent death rate from suicide has tripled in the United States, primarily because of the rising suicide rate in white males (Saltzman et al., 1988). During the same period, the number of attempted or threatened suicides reported in children and adolescents has also risen sharply. Despite many hypotheses, the reasons for the accretion are unclear. One line of speculation focuses on the high rate of divorce with its attendant stresses and the erosion of family and social supports for children. Another contributing factor may be increased drug and alcohol abuse; as many as 35% of suicides are associated with chronic substance abuse (Shaffer et al., 1988). Holinger et al. (1987) propose that the higher rates of both adolescent suicide and homicide are linked to the growing proportion of adolescents within the total population, which in turn leads to increased competition for limited employment, educational opportunities, and support services. Yet another train of thought suggests that suicide, long considered a sinful and forbidden act, has now become culturally legitimized (Shaffer, 1986a).

Teenage suicide has contagious features (Davidson & Gould, 1989; Shaffer et al., 1988). Children who attempt or complete suicide are more likely than controls to have had friends or relatives with suicidal behavior (Shafii et al., 1985). Attempted and completed suicides are sometimes followed by a cluster of other youthful suicides or attempts in the community. Such clusters may account for 2%–3% of adolescent suicides (Gould et al., 1990). Many but not all adolescents who become suicidal in response to the suicidal behavior of a peer have a prior history of depression or suicidality (Brent et al., 1989). Some studies have discerned increased teen suicides following prominent news accounts of suicidal deaths (Phillips & Carstensen, 1986) and fictional television melodramas on the subject (Gould & Shaffer, 1986). Other large-scale studies, however, have failed to confirm any significant association between television broadcasts and subsequent teen suicides (Kessler et al., 1988; Phillips & Paight, 1987). The contagion hypothesis is not new; Goethe's novel, *The Sorrows of Young Werther* (published in 1774), in which the fictional hero commits suicide, was widely banned for allegedly spawning a rash of romantic suicides in 18th-century Europe (Eisenberg, 1986). Recent Centers for Disease Control (1988) community guidelines for responding to suicide clusters emphasize the importance of not glamorizing suicide victims.

Psychological postmortems of child and adolescent suicides suggest common precipitants and vulnerability factors but do not definitively answer why such factors add up to suicide in one child but not another (Hoberman & Garfinkel, 1988; Shaffer, 1974; Shaffer et al., 1988; Shafii et al., 1985). Most adolescent suicides are impulsive and apparently are triggered by crises that are common in teenagers' lives (Hoberman & Garfinkel, 1988). Shaffer (1974) found the commonest precipitant was a disciplinary crisis; such episodes accounted for 37% of the child (under age 15 years) suicides that he studied from inquest records. Often, when the matter involved school or other authorities, the suicide occurred in the interval between the confrontation and the notification of the child's parents. Thus, anticipation of punishment, humiliation, and parental disapproval or disappointment may have played a key role. Not surprisingly, therefore, the next commonest precipitants were loss of face with peers (23%) and an argument with a parent (13%). Work-related disappointments, recent bereavements, interactions with a psychotic parent, or reading about a suicide appeared as the precipitant in 7% of the cases.

Children who commit suicide comprise a diagnostically heterogeneous group (King et al., 1991; Kovacs & Puig-Antich, 1989). Although depression is a major risk factor, not all adolescent suicides are depressed. Even in the absence of depression, conduct disorder and substance abuse are also important risk factors for suicide (Shaffer et al., 1988). Young white males who shoot themselves while intoxicated account for much of the past decades' increment in youth suicide (Brent et al., 1987). Shafii and colleagues (1985) found that a significant number of 12- to 19-year-olds who suicided had histories of drug or alcohol abuse, antisocial behavior, exposure to friends' or relatives' suicidal behavior, or parents who either had emotional problems or were absent or abusive.

The personalities of young suicides are also diverse (Frances and Blumenthal, 1989). The child suicides studied by Shaffer (1974, 1985a) fell into four personality categories; these children were generally (1) irritable and oversensitive to criticism; (2) impulsive, volatile, and erratic with a long history of school difficulties and substance abuse; (3) quiet, uncommunicative, and "difficult to get through to"; or (4) highly self-critical, perfectionistic children with intense fear of failure. In their postmortem series, Shafii et al. (1985) found that 65% of adolescent suicides had inhibited personalities and 70% manifested antisocial behavior.

Although the incidence of attempted adolescent suicides is difficult to estimate, they far exceed completed ones. The ratio of attempted suicides to completed suicides ranges from 30:1 to 150:1 (Jacobziner, 1965). In contrast to completed suicides, three to five times more female adolescents than male adolescents attempt suicide. Community-based surveys of adolescents elicit a surprisingly large number of self reports of suicidal thoughts and behavior. One high school survey found that as many as 9% of students had made at least one suicide attempt and, of these, nearly two-thirds made two or more attempts (Harkavy Friedman et al., 1987). Many attempts go undetected by parents or are not referred for help. What distinguishes the many adolescents in community samples from the small number who come to clinical attention is an important area for study.

Although completed suicide is uncommon in prepubertal children, suicidal ideation, threats, and attempts are surprisingly common. In a randomly selected community-based sample of schoolchildren, ages 6 to 12 years, about 9% reported suicidal ideas and 3% reported suicidal threats or behavior (Pfeffer et al., 1984). These suicidal tendencies are often persistent. In a follow-up 2 years later, Pfeffer et al. (1988) found about half of these children still had suicidal ideation, but only one child reported a suicide threat in the interim. Persistent suicidal ideation was associated with depression, death preoccupation, and general psychopathology. Among children seeking psychiatric help, suicidal thoughts and behavior are even more common. From 25% to 79% of preadolescent children seen in child psychiatry clinics and acute inpatient units displayed suicidal ideas, threats, or attempts (Pfeffer et al., 1979, 1982; Cohen-Sandler et al., 1982a).

Much investigation has focused on the degree of similarity between children who actually commit suicide and those who only contemplate, threaten, or attempt it (Brent, 1987; Pfeffer, 1986, 1988). Attempted suicides range from near-fatal attempts made with serious lethal intent through less dangerous attempts whose purpose is to communicate distress, to punish, or to coerce changes in the attitude or behavior of significant others (Shaffer, 1985a; Cohen-Sandler et al., 1982a, 1982b; Paykel & Rassaby, 1978). Although nonspecific suicidal ideation is common in adolescents (Kaplan et al., 1984), serious attempts become more likely with increasing hopelessness, intensity, and specificity (Brent, 1987; Robbins & Alessi, 1985). It is important not to dismiss talk of suicide or actual attempts as mere manipulative gestures. Of children who have made suicidal attempts, 20% to 60% do so more than once (Cohen-Sandler et al., 1982b; Pfeffer, 1988; Stanley & Barter, 1970). Lethality escalates with the number of previous attempts, even when the earlier attempts were judged to be nonlethal and "attention seeking" (Robbins & Alessi, 1985). In Shaffer's (1974) study, nearly half of the children who killed themselves had previously discussed, threatened, or attempted suicide.

Like children who complete suicides, suicide attempters are a diagnostically diverse group (Brent et al., 1986; Carlson & Cantwell, 1982; Khan, 1987b; King et al., 1991; Shaffer, 1982). Although many suicidal children are depressed, other suicidal children do not meet the criteria for depression. Instead, grievance and narcissistic rage may predominate, with little overt evidence of sadness or self-reproach. A review of 76 consecutive child psychiatric inpatient discharges showed that only 65% of the suicidal children met strict operational criteria for depression (Cohen-Sandler et al., 1982a). As a group, the suicidal children were more threatening to other people and less withdrawn than the comparison group of depressed nonsuicidal patients. Outward as well as inward rage, coupled with impulsive and coercive tendencies, is an important predisposing factor in many suicide attempts. Suicidal adolescents differ from nonsuicidal adolescents in their inability to cope with sad and angry feelings and their poorer capacity to think through the consequences of their actions (Khan, 1987b).

Certain teenagers are at particularly high risk for suicide attempts. It has been estimated that at least one-third of runaways or illegitimately pregnant teenage girls make a suicide attempt (Shaffer, 1985a). Repeated attempts are likely when family tensions or disorganization persist unabated (Cohen-Sandler et al., 1982b).

Some studies have suggested biological correlates of suicidal tendencies (Asberg, 1989; Stanley & Mann, 1988); for example, the very low spinal fluid levels of the serotonin metabolite 5-HIAA (5-hydroxyindoleacetic acid) found in some successful suicides may indicate very low brain levels of serotonin. However, in vivo studies suggest that such finding may be correlates of impulsivity or aggression rather than of depression or suicidality *per se*.

Suicidal children are often preoccupied with death, not only their own, but others as well, especially members of their family (Pfeffer et al., 1979, 1988). They do not necessarily see death as unpleasant or final but rather as an instrument of vengeance or coercion ("Then you'll be sorry you treated me this way.") Parents of suicidal children have an increased incidence of depression and suicidal ideation, threats, attempts, or completions as well as a high incidence of assaultiveness, impulsivity, frequent separations and remarriage, and drug or alcohol abuse (Pfeffer, 1989; Pfeffer et al., 1987). Such parents not only may provide a highly stressful home environment but also may model an impulsive, self-destructive coping style (Cohen-Sandler et al., 1982b; Tishler & McKenry, 1982).

Suicidal children suffer greater ongoing life stress than other child psychiatric patients, more often losing significant adults through death or divorce and more often acquiring new family members such as younger siblings and stepparents (Cohen-Sandler et al., 1982a). Despite suffering a greater number of losses, suicidal children in this study were more likely than other child psychiatric patients to have remained with at least one parent, and the suicide attempt occurred within the context of an intense, ambivalent, and coercive struggle with that parent. Thus, although suicidal ideation and attempt may represent a wish for surcease from pain or guilt or for reunion with a dead relative, they also often are active coping efforts by children caught in a stressful chaotic family situation. Such children may attempt suicide to express their rage, to counteract their helplessness in effecting changes, or to prevent further loss of significant persons or self-esteem.

Shapiro and Freedman (1987) contrasted two patterns of family and individual dynamics in certain adolescent suicides. For borderline adolescents, the motivation for suicide may be aggrieved or retaliatory sadomasochistic impulses, reflecting intense, unresolved ambivalent feelings toward the parents. In contrast, the adolescent enmeshed in a narcissistic family system may view self-inflicted death as the only avenue to individuation or reclaiming a sense of a separate, untrammeled self (Mack & Hickler, 1981). Perhaps Rilke had something similar in mind in his own epitaph, "Rose, oh pure contradiction, desire to be nobody's sleep beneath so many lids."

TREATMENT

Depression is a complex, multifaceted organismic response to loss or disappointment, involving psychodynamic, cognitive, and physiological components. In many cases, constitutional predisposing factors may intensify the severity of this condition. The treatment of depression requires attention to all of these elements and hence must also be complex and multifaceted (Petti et al., 1980). Although the recent "discovery" of childhood depression has led to a flood of papers on classification and description of this disorder, it is sobering to note that there has been no comparable attention to treatment (save perhaps in the area of psychopharmacology).

Psychosocial Interventions

Many depressions are reactive, the result of loss, deprivation, or ongoing stress. A careful evaluation of the child must include an assessment of the environmental events impinging on the child and the presence or absence of protective or exacerbating factors (Bowlby, 1988). The clinician must also explore the internal reverberations of these events, that is, their subjective meanings for the child.

Bibring (1953) formulated depression as a state of helplessness and hopelessness due to a perceived inability to achieve or maintain usual aspirations or relationships. Using this approach, he proposed that depression remits when its cause is reversed or mitigated in any of the following ways:

1. The important goals and objects seem once again to be within reach.
2. They become sufficiently modified or reduced to become realizable.
3. They are altogether relinquished.
4. Self-esteem is recovered by other means (without changing goals or objects).
5. The affect of depression is itself defended against (e.g., by hypomanic grandiosity or, in the case of children, by externalization and aggressive acting-out).

The following paragraphs explore the implications of this framework for treating childhood depression.

Identifying the Losses or Other Threats to Self-Esteem. If the child's depression is reactive to a specific identifiable loss, attention must obviously be given to identifying and ameliorating the pathogenic aspects of the loss. Hence, a major element in planning therapeutic interventions must be to identify the losses that a child may have suffered, the possible replacements or mitigation of the losses; and the internal or family factors that may interfere with attempted restitution. Unfortunately, any substantial depression is likely to be the outcome of a severe, prolonged loss with far-reaching ramifications, and such losses are not easily undone. Loss of a parent to divorce, death, or chronic illness is a common example. Nonetheless, the depressive consequences of such losses are not inevitable; much depends on the quality of care and attention available from the remaining (or new) adults in the child's life. However, even when there are adequate substitutes, the child's ability to mourn and to form new attachments may be impaired by factors that require therapeutic intervention. For example, family factors may interfere with mourning (Bowlby, 1980; Volkan, 1981). The constellation of tensions following a divorce often have just such an effect. A child needs to acknowledge and express grief or anger at the disruption of previous family relationships, the absence (relative or complete) of the noncustodial parent, and, often enough, the loss of home, friends, and neighborhood. In the wake of a bitterly contested divorce, the parents' mutual acrimony may leave a child without permission to do so. Similarly, unresolved mourning in the surviving parent may interfere with a child's grieving the death of a parent or may stir in the child feelings of disloyalty for wishing to find substitute figures. Finally, the child, depending on his developmental stage and dynamic makeup, may complicate the losses with fantasies of having been responsible for them (e.g., through angry, envious, or competitive feelings; through depletion of the lost person with demands; through having taken sides in a marital strife).

The threat to a child's sense of efficacy and self-esteem, however, may not be linked to a specific event; instead, external factors (such as chronic deprivation or ongoing parental hostility) or intrinsic ones (such as a physical handicap or a learning disability) may exert debilitating effects over time. Here again, the therapeutic goals are to ameliorate the impact of the condition on the child's self-esteem, perhaps through modifying the child's (and parents') unmeetable demands on himself and/or by finding alternative sources of self-esteem. These issues can be illustrated in the following example.

CASE EXAMPLE

Sam, a 17-year-old boy with moderately severe hemophilia, was referred by his hematologist for evaluation of family tensions. Interviews with Sam and his parents, Mr. and Mrs. T, revealed a likeable young man who both provoked and resented his parents' nagging him about schoolwork, chores, and the care of his illness. Despite being attractive, well-built, and personable, Sam was dejected, depressed, and had a low opinion of himself. His depression went well beyond what might be expected solely from the impact of his illness on his physical health and freedom of activity. His self-esteem was fragile and was additionally burdened by a complex network of family expectations and projections.

Although of average intelligence, Sam had done poorly in the elite, high-powered prep school where his parents had placed him. Mrs. T, who had been especially close and protective of Sam, was keenly disappointed in his mediocre academic performance. The mother's first love had been graduate work in history, which she had foregone for marriage and domesticity; she inwardly reproached herself and her husband for her sacrifice and looked to Sam vicariously to fulfill her academic aspirations. Sam sensed and suffered from her disappointment in him; despite their closeness—or perhaps because of it—he was also tormented by his inability to relieve his mother's marital unhappiness.

Mr. T, too, was bitterly disappointed in himself and in Sam. His own capacity for intimacy seemed to have been injured by the loss of his mother when he was 5 years old; she had succumbed to a hemorrhage for which he held her doctors responsible. Sam's frequent bleeds and the doctors' inability to cure the hemophilia were thus a source of constant rage and concern. Mr. T also felt he had compromised his own career goals in order to find employment, security, and adequate insurance for Sam's expensive medical bills. Nor was this all. Sam was an excellent athlete and a junior champion in a noncontact sport that did not risk internal bleeding or joint hemorrhages; nonetheless, Mr. T remained bitterly disappointed that Sam could not play basketball, the sport in which he had himself tried to excel.

Thus, the real limitations and renunciations imposed by Sam's chronic illness and average intelligence were magnified by their meaning within a family network of disappointments, losses, and only partially concealed resentments. The result was the frustration of Sam's attempts at individuation.

A year of weekly family and individual therapy clarified these issues, helping Sam and his family to take greater pleasure and pride in his substantial interpersonal and athletic skills, to mourn and accept better the renunciations entailed by Sam's illness and their own life courses, and to find alternative sources of satisfaction in their family and individual lives. Sam became less caught up in the passive-aggressive resistance to (and provoking of) what he experienced as his parents' simultaneously overprotective and excessive demands. With the decrease in conflict with his parents, Sam became better able to look after his illness and his schoolwork.

The psychosocial treatment of depression has several key elements, including the amelioration of losses, the ongoing availability and empathy of the therapist, and techniques of addressing the child's hopelessness and low self-esteem.

Ameliorative or Restitutive Measures.   It is often necessary to lessen the impact of losses or environmental interactions that beget a persistent sense of failure or inefficacy. Accordingly, treatment will often entail active environmental manipulations such as obtaining an appropriate school placement for a learning disabled school-age child or finding a nurturant, supportive day-care setting for a depressed preschooler with an overwhelmed mother.

The Role of the Therapist.   The therapist's continuing availability and interest are important existential presence, reducing the child and family's sense of isolation. The therapist's capacity for hope and his vision of the child as being worthwhile and possessing latent competencies are also powerful and crucial ingredients (Loewald, 1980).

The sad affects of many children threaten them with a sense of dangerous vulnerability; accordingly, the youngsters often push these feelings away and have difficulty acknowledging them. Within the context of a steady therapeutic relationship, the child may begin to experience and explore his griefs and discontents. Elvin Semrad, one of the great masters of psychotherapy, observed that the essential task of therapy is simple; it is to help the patient to share, to bear, and to put his life experiences (and losses) into perspective (Rako & Mazer, 1980). The therapist's steady, non-judgmental, and empathic interest and presence make it possible for the child to reveal and to bear his pain, his feelings of rejection, and his self-reproaches.

Careful attention to the patient's material (including play, dreams, fantasies, and artistic productions) and transference manifestations elucidates the idiosyncratic meanings that specific losses or failures have for the child and his family (e.g., Cohen, 1980a). This knowledge enables addressing and putting into better perspective guilty, shameful, and self-recriminatory attitudes that have exacerbated losses or frustrations; for example, a child's feeling that a sibling's death or a parent's chronic psychiatric hospitalization or abandonment of the family was somehow his fault. Although phase-specific dynamic issues (such as oedipal conflict) may give such notions their particular color and content, the basic mechanism is often the same: The child may prefer to feel guilty and responsible rather than to feel that he had no control whatsoever over momentous and overwhelming events. Helping the youngster to perceive the differences between thought and deed may provide significant relief from painful self-reproach. The child may come to understand that although he often wished his pesky sister would die or that he could have mother all to himself, that did *not* cause the sibling's death or the parents' divorce. Specific attention to such issues, as well as the child's gradual internalization of the therapist's noncritical, empathic attitude, mitigates the harshness of the child's own superego and condemnatory attacks on himself (Strachey, 1934).

Technical Issues in Dealing with the Child's Self-Esteem. The treatment of childhood depression must address the youngster's hopelessness and low self-esteem. The guilt and shame reducing elements of therapy have been discussed above. A powerful, ubiquitous element of therapy is the child's sense that the therapist likes and appreciates him, or to paraphrase Kohut (1977), has a gleam in his (her) eye for the child. In some children with profound narcissistic difficulties, however, this may be more than the therapist can manage. The child may controllingly demand the therapist's admiring subservience or preemptively repel him or her so as not to risk the perceived inevitability of painful rejection. In such cases, careful attention to the therapist's countertransference is essential in order to address these issues with the child (Anthony, 1975e; see also Chapter 11, "Narcissistic Disorders").

A major area of technical controversy concerns managing the vicissitudes of anger. A simplistic reading of Freud's equation of depression with anger-turned-against-the-self might erroneously suggest that the overt expression of anger diminishes depression. However, anger in itself begets a sense of wrongdoing; the depressed patient's guilt because he feels rage often contributes significantly to his sense of worthlessness. Voicing rage gives such a patient no cathartic relief, but merely reinforces the child's belief that he is not only a miserable wretch, but a wrathful one as well. Nonetheless, as the child reviews with the therapist his griefs, discontents, and self-reproaches, he may become better able to assess the responsibility for his various life circumstances. This, coupled with relinquishing the passive, helpless role of the victim, may lead to a more assertive, less masochistic stance that permits the child to voice disagreement and to defend his own interests more freely.

An important dimension of the management of depression is the need for parents not to be too giving and forgiving; the youngsters need a somewhat matter-of-fact, businesslike style of management; parents must set and maintain limits as well as requirements and expectations for reasonable performance. The low self-esteem of the depressed child does not respond well to the overly solicitous hovering warmth of the concerned caretaker; the child feels misunderstood in his badness and is driven to further extremes of dejection and self-abasement.

The above therapeutic components all implicitly address the depressed child's sense of helplessness, hopelessness, and worthlessness. To come to grips with these difficulties more directly, therapeutic approaches diverge in their use of suggestion and educative measures. Therapists vary in the extent to which they explicitly seek to bolster the child's self-esteem through complimenting skills and accomplishments, emphasizing the positive elements of the child's situation, or coaching and encouraging behaviors likely to enhance self-esteem. Similarly, therapists differ in how explicitly they attempt to teach problem-solving techniques or social skills.

Beck et al. (1979) have developed a *cognitive therapy* technique, based on a cognitive theory of depression. Beck postulates that depressives suffer from pathogenic, negative views of the self, the world, and the future—the "cognitive triad." They see the self as defective, inadequate, or unworthy; the world as overwhelming, demanding, or ungratifying; and the future as unalterably bleak, frustrating, and depriving. These attitudes are rooted in depressive cognitive schemata, stable patterns of organizing perceptions and events. Faulty styles of information processing that reinforce the depressive's systematic pessimism perpetuates these idiosyncratic schemata. Thus, the depressive is able to "snatch defeat from the jaws of victory," everywhere finding evidence to confirm his depressogenic assumptions. For example, a man may complain of being unloved and unlovable; when a women does seem attracted to him, he dismisses her because "Any woman who likes me can't be any good." The depressive thus selectively emphasizes, overgeneralizes, and personalizes events; things are absolute and dichotomized—either black or white (for the depressive usually the former).

Cognitive therapy directly addresses the depressed patient's personal paradigms, which produce and perpetuate his distorted views. Although Beck (1976) has speculated on the genesis of these "depressogenic schema," cognitive therapy concerns the here-and-now, rather than reconstructive efforts. The therapist and patient work collaboratively to identify and examine maladaptive assumptions and cognitive processes that reinforce the patient's sense of helplessness and worthlessness.

There have been few systematic applications of cognitive techniques to children (Lewinsohn et al., 1987). The developmental constraints imposed by the child's ability to reflect on his own cognition are unclear. Cohen-Sandler and Berman (1982) trained suicidal child psychiatric inpatients in nonsuicidal methods of interpersonal problem solving. The training appeared to increase the children's capacity for forethought, appreciation for the consequences of behavior, and ability to perceive alternative solutions for conflicts.

Treatment of Suicide Attempts

Clinicians must regard suicide threats and attempts in children as extremely serious although either parent or child, or both, may minimize and deny their importance. Ingestions and suspicious accidents should be carefully examined for self-injurious intent. Evaluation of suicidal risk and treatment planning requires careful assessment of the dynamics and interpersonal context of the suicidal symptoms; the persistence of suicidal ideation; the presence of psychiatric risk factors (such as depression or substance abuse) and personality risk factors (such as impulsivity); the availability of and capacity to use interpersonal supports; the degree of therapeutic alliance; family stability; and ease of access to lethal means (such as guns or medication). Therapy is almost always indicated and usually involves both the parents and child. In a situation previously inaccessible because of denial or avoidance, the crisis of a child's suicide attempt can provide a dramatic opening for therapeutic intervention. This opportunity, however, is often lost due to inadequate follow-up. In general, a child who has made a suicide attempt should be hospitalized when serious suicidal ideation continues, when the child seems affectively labile or severely impulsive, when the family cannot provide sufficient stability or supervision, or when there is difficulty in establishing an adequate alliance for outpatient treatment with the child and family.

Drug Treatment

Antidepressants and mood-stabilizing drugs such as lithium have been extensively studied in adults and play an important role in the treatment of adult affective disorders (Klein et al., 1980). There have been far fewer studies of these agents in prepubertal and adolescent affective disorders and, of these, only a few have been methodologically sound (Weller & Weller, 1984).

Antidepressants. The tricyclic antidepressants, such as imipramine, have been widely used in the treatment of childhood psychiatric syndromes such as enuresis, attention-deficit hyperactivity disorder, school phobia due to separation anxiety disorder; imipramine's efficacy in these conditions seems to be independent of its antidepressant action. In contrast, the usefulness of these drugs in treating the major depressions of childhood has been more difficult to establish. A confounding factor in children is the great interindividual variation in the absorption and metabolism of the drug; there may be a 15-fold difference in the plasma drug levels of different children receiving the same dosage of antidepressant (see Chapter 17). For both research and clinical purposes, it is usually essential to obtain plasma drug levels, because monitoring the mg/kg dosage alone may not be adequate to titrate a safe and effective dose. To prevent cardiotoxicity, current Federal Drug Administration (FDA) guidelines limit the total daily dose of imipramine to 5.0 mg/kg; for doses above 3.0 mg/kg the FDA recommends serial electrocardiograms (EKGs). In addition, high placebo response rates (up to nearly 70%) confound efficacy studies so that very high drug response rates would be necessary to be statistically significant (Puig-Antich et al., 1987).

Several studies (Weller & Weller, 1984; Puig-Antich et al., 1987) suggest that plasma drug level is a key determinant of therapeutic response to imipramine in prepubertal children. In their double blind study, Puig-Antich et al. (1987) found that, as a group, imipramine-treated children did no better than the 60% to 68% placebo response rate; however, those children with plasma levels of imipramine plus despiramine (its major active metabolite) above 125–150 ng/ml showed a 90% to 100% positive response rate. The authors speculated that many nonresponders might respond positively if they could attain these higher plasma levels; however, given the constraints of the 5 mg/kg FDA-mandated ceiling, they are unable to reach such levels. Whether other identifiable features distinguish responders from nonresponders remains to be seen.

Imipramine appears to be less effective in adolescents than in younger children; furthermore, unlike prepubertal depressives, adolescents with major depression show no correlation between therapeutic responses and plasma level (Ryan et al., 1986). Ryan and colleagues speculated that this may be due to high levels of sex hormones during adolescence. Where one antidepressant, such as imipramine, proves ineffective, other more serotonergic tricyclics (such as amitryiptyline), MAOIs, or newer bicyclic or heterocyclic antidepressants may prove effective.

Side effects of the tricyclics reflect their anticholinergic properties. These include dry mouth, constipation, blurred vision, increased diastolic blood pressure, orthostatic hypotension, tachycardia, and alterations in cardiac conduction; a lowered seizure threshold has also been noted (Klein et al., 1980; Campbell et al., 1985). If the therapist contemplates higher dose levels, he or she should consult the package insert carefully for FDA guidelines concerning EKG monitoring. The wide variability in children's absorption suggests that divided doses are prudent, particularly in younger children. Ryan et al. (1987b) have concluded from their EKG data that once adolescents have been titrated to a steady dose, a single evening dose of imipramine is safe. The potential toxicity of antidepressants requires caution when there is risk of a suicide attempt. (See Chapter 11 on attention-deficit hyperactivity disorder and Chapter 17 on enuresis for further information on the use of the tricyclics in children and adolescents.)

In addition to the tricyclic and MAOI antidepressants, several newer and structurally distinct antidepressants are now available. Fluoxetine, a tricyclic agent that specifically inhibits serotonin reuptake, has been widely used because it does not have many of the troublesome anticholinergic and cardiovascular side effects of the tricyclics. Common side effects of fluoxetine in children include restlessness and insomnia. A few children may become agitated while on fluoxetine with intensification of self-destructive behavior (King et al., 1990; Riddle et al., 1990).

Lithium. In adults, lithium has proven to be an effective treatment for bipolar affective disorder as well as for certain cases of schizoaffective and cyclic unipolar depressive disorders (Klein et al., 1980). The usefulness of lithium in the psychiatric disorders of childhood and adolescence has been less well defined. The FDA has not yet approved lithium carbonate as safe and effective in children under 12 years of age.

A major confounding difficulty is that bipolar affective disorder—the most lithium-responsive disorder in adulthood—often has only poorly defined, nonspecific prodromal symptoms in childhood. In the absence of hypomanic symptoms or a family history of bipolar affective disorder, lithium does not appear to be effective in hyperactivity or simple depression (Delong & Aldershof, 1987).

In childhood, lithium has been regarded as the best therapeutic agent for well-defined bipolar affective disorder (manic-depression). It also appears to be effective in several conditions that may be related to bipolar affective disorder such as "emotionally unstable character disorder," certain forms of hyperaggressive and explosive behavior, and behavior problems in children of lithium-responsive parents (M. Campbell et al., 1978, 1984; Delong & Aldershof, 1987). It is sometimes effective in aggressive or self-destructive behavior associated with mental retardation or pervasive developmental disorders (Campbell et al., 1985).

Delong and Aldershof (1987) suggest that, regardless of specific diagnosis, certain symptom patterns may warrant a trial of lithium; these include "cyclic affective extremes, especially hateful hostile anger, and manic over-excitement; a family history of affective disorder, especially bipolar; aggressiveness; and prominent neurovegetative disorders, especially hyperphagia, hyperdipsia, salt-craving, and encopresis" (p. 394).

Great caution is needed in administering lithium. Because toxicity occurs close to therapeutic serum levels, serum lithium levels must be carefully monitored (Klein et al., 1980). Side effects include nausea, weakness, tremor, polyuria, polydipsia, and fluid-electrolyte imbalances; long-term complications include renal and thyroid abnormalities (Campbell et al., 1985). Nonetheless, with adequate precautions, many children have benefited dramatically from taking lithium for lengthy periods, some for as long as 10 years (Delong & Aldershof, 1987).

Chapter 7

Anxiety Disorders:
Overview

> ... deep inside, in that silent place
> where a child's fears crouch...
>   LILLIAN SMITH

INTRODUCTION AND DEFINITION

This chapter and the two that follow deal with the anxiety disorders of childhood. This chapter summarizes current knowledge about normal and pathological anxiety as developmental phenomena, reviews psychological and biological theories concerning their nature and origins, and briefly surveys their current nosology in adults and children. Chapter 8, "Anxious School Refusal: School Phobia and Separation Anxiety Disorder," and Chapter 9, "Obsessive-Compulsive Disorder," deal with these two anxiety disorders in detail because of their clinical and theoretical importance. Finally, Chapter 15, "Psychosomatic Disorders," considers the closely related topics of hysterical conversion disorder, psychogenic pain, and the intricate relationship between stress, emotions, and autonomic arousal.

Anxiety is a complex emotional response to danger—a danger whose source cannot be identified, or, if identified, seems out of proportion to the emotion it evokes (Bowlby, 1973). In contrast, the term *fear* generally refers to the response to a known and specifiable threat or danger. Varied dangers elicit anxiety including threats to the person's physical or psychological well-being or to the availability of the people who assure and signify safety (Bowlby, 1973; Kandel, 1983). Like most emotions, anxiety has both a subjective aspect and an objectively measurable physiological component. The *subjective* manifestations involve both affective and cognitive symptoms (Beck & Emery, 1985). Thus, anxious children may describe themselves as "jumpy," "nervous," "tense," "scared," or "worried." Anxiety also affects thinking and perception: the subject may experience hazy or scattered thoughts with blocking, difficulty concentrating, and a sense of unreality that pervades his sensorium; on the other hand, the anxious subject may feel hypervigilant and jumpily alert. Repetitive frightening images or thoughts and fears of disaster may crowd into consciousness. The *behavioral* and *physiological* manifestations of anxiety involve the "fight-or-flight" pattern of autonomic nervous system arousal described by Cannon (1929). Perhaps "fight-flight-freeze-faint reaction" would be a more complete description of this primitive organismic response pattern (Beck & Emery, 1985). The physiological signs of anxious autonomic arousal include rapid heart beat, palpitations, rapid breathing, tremulousness and weakness of the extremities, restlessness and insomnia, loss of appetite, "hot and cold flashes," and sweating. The word *anxiety* may derive from the Latin *angere* ("to choke"), reflecting the tightening of the throat that often accompanies anxiety, or from the Latin *anxius* or *anxietas* ("troubled in mind"). In short, the person in the grip of an anxiety attack appears overalert, overaroused, and overprepared (Lader, 1980).

The anxiety response appears to have evolved as an essential biological adaptation, arousing the individual to anticipate and respond to signs of possible danger by avoidance or other active coping mechanisms (Kandel, 1983). Anxiety thus serves an adaptive function, helping the child to master difficult circumstances. In this light, the ability to experience and tolerate anxiety is a vital impetus to personality growth and development (Zetzel, 1949/1970a). On the other hand, anxiety is pathological when it becomes intense and persistent enough to incapacitate the individual or when it becomes unnecessarily restrictive because it occurs repeatedly in situations that hold no objective danger.

Developmental Aspects of Fear and Anxiety

Fears and anxieties are part of normal childhood. The situations that arouse fear change with the child's age and cognitive maturity; in addition, fearfulness and its expression are influenced by built-in (intrinsic) variables such as gender, cultural background, past experiences, and the security of the child's attachment to his caretakers, as well as by contextual factors such as the setting and availability of familiar persons (Bowlby, 1973). Work with human infants and animals suggests that important individual differences in the intensity and expression of anxiety persist throughout life and carry a substantial genetic component (Marks, 1987; Reznick et al., 1986; Suomi, 1986).

Spitz (1965) was among the first to note that crucial perceptual and cognitive developments in memory, anticipation, and object permanence are necessary before the infant can manifest certain types of anxiety. Thus, startle reactions, diffuse crying, and upset are common during the first few months of life in response to sudden loud sounds, pain, loss of support, or physical discomfort. At the same time, however, the very young infant does not manifest discernible signs of fearful apprehension. Beginning at about 4 months of age, the infant's growing ability to distinguish between familiar and unfamiliar faces and voices parallels early signs of wariness when he encounters the unfamiliar. Discrepant or unusual events cause the infant to pause and become alert, with attendant changes in heart rate. The infant orients himself to the novel stimulus and tries to make sense of it (in Piaget's terms the infant attempts to assimilate the new stimulus to existing cognitive schemata). If he succeeds, the infant may smile and appear to relax, again with characteristic autonomic changes. Otherwise the infant may remain wary, avert his gaze, or go on to a state of acute distress and crying.

During the second 6 months of life this apprehension at the unfamiliar is most apparent in the well-known phenomenon of "stranger anxiety." In the presence of strangers, the infant's somber, frowning wariness often progresses to full-blown tears, upset, and clinging. At this age infants also begin to show fear of strange objects (such as a jack-in-the-box), looming or rapidly approaching objects, and heights. By the end of the first year, the infant can recall and hence anticipate unpleasant experiences, as evidenced, for example, by crying when he sees the doctor with a hypodermic needle.

Normative studies of nonclinical populations have outlined the evolution of children's fears during the preschool and school years (Agras et al., 1969; Jersild et al., 1975; Lapouse & Monk, 1959; Lentz, 1985; Miller et al., 1972b; see reviews by Bowlby, 1973; Campbell, 1986; Orvaschel & Weissman, 1986). During the infant's first and second years, fears relate to actual events and objects in his daily life. Noises, heights, darkness, strangers (or familiar people in strange guise), doctors and shots, unfamiliar surroundings, and animals all powerfully elicit fear in toddlers. As the preschooler grows older, he develops the ability to anticipate and imagine harmful events. In addition to developing the capacity for symbolic thought, the child becomes familiar with the imaginary creatures, ghosts, and monsters typical of his culture, which can then give form to various fears, such as those of bedtime, the dark, or bad dreams. Young children, may not express anxiety directly, but may instead display motor restlessness, tantrums, aggressive behavior, and sleep disturbances. Somatic symptoms also frequently express anxiety in children: The most common symptoms are recurrent, diffuse abdominal pain; headaches; transient tics; and hyperventilation.

During the child's first 4 to 5 years of life many fears—for example, noise, novelty, and strangers—tend to attenuate. Indeed, the objects of early fear may even become the sources of pleasure or excitement. Other fears, such as those aroused by animals, storms, and darkness, decline only slowly with age. Global fears of monsters, ghosts, and bad dreams are widespread in preschoolers and decrease gradually during the elementary school years; they are replaced by more realistic and specific fears of bodily injury, physical danger, and death (Bauer, 1976).

One of childhood's most poignant and expectable existential crises is "death phobia," the realization of the irreversibility and universality of death (Anthony, 1975). This anxious realization of death as a personal possibility usually arises between 8 and 10 years of age; in bright children it sometimes appears earlier. The product of growing cognitive maturity, the anxiety stirred by this new awareness coalesces concerns about helplessness, abandonment, separation, punishment, and retaliation, all colored by the child's own hostile wishes.

From the age of eight or nine years, children also experience more fears about school (especially concerning teachers and tests) and social relationships generally. They worry about being ridiculed, embarrassed, or not fitting in, concerns that persist throughout adolescence.

Adolescence is a time of high anxiety. In a community sample of 14- to

16-year-olds, 16% met the DSM-III (1980) criteria for an anxiety disorder; almost 8% of the sample had enough impairment from their anxiety symptoms to be considered "cases" (Kashani & Orvaschel, 1988). The commonest disorders were overanxious disorder and phobias.

Normative studies thus indicate that childhood fears are commonplace (Jersild & Holmes, 1935; Orvaschel & Weissman, 1986). More than half of school-age children have multiple worries and fears that their parents are either largely unaware of or underestimate (Lapouse & Monk, 1959). At the same time, however, these fears are generally neither intense nor pervasive enough to interfere seriously with children's functioning (Agras et al., 1969, 1972; Rutter et al., 1970/1981). Although many fears are transient and soon outgrown, adults who suffer from fears of animals, storms, crowds, going out alone, or social situations often report that their fears began in childhood (Abe, 1972; Agras et al., 1969, 1972).

Many questions remain about the common fears of childhood. Why are they more intense in one child than another? In which children do these anxieties remain manageable or disappear, and in which children do they persist into later life, perhaps with disabling intensity? This chapter and the ones that follow attempt to address the little that is known about these questions.

NOSOLOGY—THE ADULT AND CHILDHOOD ANXIETY DISORDERS

Anxiety is a common component of many psychiatric syndromes. In certain patients, however, the principal symptom may be excessive anxiety, either diffuse and free-floating or specific to certain objects or situations. In such cases, the clinician speaks of an *anxiety disorder*. The anxiety disorders are defined as a group of conditions in which "anxiety is either the predominant disturbance, as in Panic Disorder or Generalized Anxiety Disorder or anxiety is experienced if the individual attempts to master the symptoms, as in confronting the feared object or situation in a Phobic Disorder or resisting the obsessions or compulsions of Obsessive Compulsive Disorder" (DSM-III, 1980, p. 225). Since the 1980 adoption of DSM-III, the anxiety disorders have been the subject of an explosive expansion of research. The latest revision of DSM-III (DSM-III-R, 1987) has reclassified the anxiety disorders to reflect some of the recent advances in the field.

Anxiety Disorders in Adulthood

DSM-III-R defines the following diagnostic varieties of anxiety disorder in adulthood:

Generalized Anxiety Disorder. Generalized, persistent anxiety with apprehensive anticipation of something bad happening to self or others, but without specific phobias, panic attacks, obsessions, or compulsions.

Simple Phobia. Fear of a specific object or situation that persists, that is recognized as irrational, and that results in a compelling desire to avoid the feared object or situation.

Social Phobia. Persistent irrational apprehension concerning, and desire to avoid, situations in which the individual fears others will scrutinize or embarrass him.

Panic Disorder with or without varying degrees of General Phobic Avoidance (Agoraphobia). Recurrent, brief, sudden attacks of intense apprehension and terror, often with feelings of impending doom, usually without identifiable precipitant.

Agoraphobia without Panic Attacks. Marked fear of being alone or of being in public places (especially busy streets or crowded stores). Avoidant behavior may increasingly constrict the agoraphobic's normal activities until he becomes a total recluse.

Obsessive-Compulsive Disorder. Recurrent obsessions or compulsions that are experienced as senseless or unwanted.

Posttraumatic Stress Disorder. A set of characteristic symptoms (including flashbacks, emotional numbness, trouble concentrating, insomnia, hyperalertness) following a severely disturbing psychologically traumatic event.

In addition, DSM-III-R (1987) defines an *Avoidant Personality Disorder,* characterized by social discomfort, fear of negative evaluation by others, timidity, and constriction of activities outside the home.

Anxiety Disorders of Childhood

The classification of anxiety conditions in childhood remains far from satisfactory. In addition to the anxiety disorders of adulthood, DSM-III-R (1987) recognizes two anxiety disorders of childhood or adolescence:

Separation Anxiety Disorder. Excessive anxiety concerning separation from those to whom the child is attached. Common manifestations include refusal to go to school (often called school phobia) and sleep difficulties.

Generalized Anxiety Disorder (formerly called Overanxious Disorder of Childhood). This disorder now has the same definition as Generalized Anxiety Disorder in adulthood (see above).

A third DSM-III diagnostic category, *Avoidant Disorder of Childhood or Adolescence,* was eliminated from DSM-III-R because it occurred only in the presence of, or as part of, other disorders. Anxiety symptoms also may figure prominently in *Adjustment Disorder (with anxious mood or mixed emotional features),* an acute and transitory maladaptive reaction to a recent, identifiable stressor.

Reliability and Validity of the Current Classification of Anxiety Disorders

Unfortunately, the interrater reliability of the DSM-III diagnostic categories for anxiety has been unexpectedly poor (Cantwell et al., 1979; Mattison et al., 1979; Werry, 1986). Some authors have argued that dividing anxiety disorder into subcategories (or even creating separate categories for anxiety and depression) is empirically unwarranted. These authors argue for a single broadly inclusive "internalizing" dimension that includes symptoms of anxiety, depression, and social withdrawal (Achenbach, 1980; Achenbach & Edelbrock, 1979; Quay & LaGreca, 1986; Tyrer, 1985). Although the relationship of the various anxiety syndromes to each other remains uncertain, researchers have had greater success in developing reliable rating scales and instruments to identify and quantify anxious symptoms in children, including general anxiety, test anxiety, separation anxiety, and obsessional symptoms. (For a review, see Gittleman-Klein, 1988).

An additional fundamental difficulty is that very little is known about the natural history of childhood anxieties or their relation to the adult anxiety disorders. McDermott (1985) has observed that research in the child and adult psychiatric disorders has proceeded like building a transcontinental railroad, with the two groups of researchers having separate starting points and working with different methods only to find that when they reach the middle, the tracks do not meet! Some adult conditions, such as simple phobias, social phobia, panic disorder, obsessive-compulsive disorder, and generalized anxiety disorder can (and often do) have their onset in childhood. Many adults with agoraphobia report a history of school refusal (separation anxiety disorder) in childhood, whereas others report active and independent childhoods (Klein, 1964). Thus, the relationship between the adult and childhood disorders remains uncertain.

CLINICAL FEATURES AND DEFINITION

Anxiety symptoms may take many different forms. As discussed earlier, anxiety has several facets: affective, cognitive, behavioral, and physiological. The relative prominence of these components differs from one case to the next. For some patients somatic symptoms of panic and feelings of dread predominate, with relatively little ideational content. Other patients may worry chronically with apprehensive expectations of various mishaps, yet may manifest relatively few observable behavioral changes. The intense avoidant behavior or the inability to leave home of still other patients may grossly constrict and compromise their ordinary daily activities. A full clinical evaluation requires carefully assessing the symptomatic contribution of each facet of anxiety (Wells & Vitulano, 1984; Barrios et al., 1981).

Anxiety symptoms may differ in their temporal patterning and object. Anxiety may be chronic and persistent (as in the case of generalized anxiety disorder) or acute and episodic (as in the case of panic disorder). Anxiety may also be relatively unattached and unfocused, in which case it is often termed *free floating*. Some cognitive theorists insist that anxiety is never without content; in their view careful investigation always reveals some ideation concerning personal danger or physical harm (Beck & Emery, 1985; Hibbert, 1984). In some cases, anxiety takes the form of general apprehension about a multitude of possible misfortunes, whereas in other cases, there is an irrational fear and avoidance of a single, specifiable object or situation (such as horses, plane travel, or bridges). The latter condition is termed a *phobia*, defined as "a persistent, irrational fear of a specific object, activity, or situation that results in a compelling desire to avoid the dreaded object, activity, or situation (the phobic stimulus)" (DSM-III, 1980, p. 225). The term phobia is derived from *phobos*, the Greek word for "flight." Phobos was also the name of the god of fear, a companion of Mars, who struck terror in the hearts of even the bravest warriors.

Generalized Anxiety Disorder

Generalized anxiety disorder (GAD) is characterized by persistent unrealistic and excessive worries of at least 6 months' duration (DSM-III-R, 1987). The anxiety is generalized and continuous, lacking the specificity of phobias, panic attacks, or obsessive-compulsive disorder. The predominant symptoms are constant apprehension, motor tension, autonomic hyperactivity, and hyperalertness.

DSM-III-R (1987) Criteria for Generalized Anxiety Disorder

A. *Unrealistic or excessive anxiety and worry (apprehensive expectation) about two or more life circumstances, e.g., worry about possible misfortune to one's child (who is in no danger) and worry about finances (for no good reasons), for a period of six months or longer, during which the person has been bothered more days than not by these concerns. In children and adolescents, this may take the form of anxiety and worry about academic, athletic, and social performance.*

B. *If another Axis I disorder is present, the focus of the anxiety and worry in A is unrelated to it, e.g., the anxiety or worry is not about having a panic attack (as in Panic Disorder), being embarrassed in public (as in Social Phobia), being contaminated (as in Obsessive Compulsive Disorder), or gaining weight (as in Anorexia Nervosa).*

C. *The disturbance does not occur only during the course of a Mood Disorder or a psychotic disorder.*

D. *At least 6 of the following 18 symptoms are often present when anxious (do not include symptoms present only during panic attacks):*

Motor tension
(1)   trembling, twitching, or feeling shaky
(2)   muscle tension, aches, or soreness
(3)   restlessness
(4)   easy fatigability

Autonomic hyperactivity
(5)   shortness of breath or smothering sensations
(6)   palpitations or accelerated heart rate (tachycardia)
(7)   sweating, or cold clammy hands
(8)   dry mouth
(9)   dizziness or lightheadedness
(10) nausea, diarrhea, or other abdominal distress
(11) flushes (hot flashes) or chills
(12) frequent urination
(13) trouble swallowing or "lump in throat"

Vigilance and scanning
(14) feeling keyed up or on edge
(15) exaggerated startle response
(16) difficulty concentrating or "mind going blank" because of anxiety
(17) trouble falling or staying asleep
(18) irritability

E. *It cannot be established that an organic factor initiated and maintained the disturbance, e.g., hyperthyroidism, Caffeine intoxication.* (APA, 1987, pp. 252–253)

As yet, few systematic studies have validated the concept of generalized anxiety disorder as a discrete diagnostic category. Some studies suggest that this syndrome may not be a valid separate diagnostic entity because it often overlaps other anxiety and affective disorders. Indeed, at some point in their lives, a very large proportion of those adults with generalized anxiety disorder have also experienced panic disorder, phobias, or major depression (Breier et al., 1985; Di Nardo et al., 1983).

There are few epidemiological studies using the generalized anxiety disorder criteria with children. Multiple fears and generalized fearfulness are common in childhood (see section Developmental Aspects of Anxiety); unfortunately, there is little systematic information about the subsequent course, severity, or functional impact of these anxieties. Many adult cases of generalized anxiety disorder appear to have had their onset in childhood.

The lives of sensitive children can be blighted by generalized anxiety. The works of many gifted writers—Rilke, Kierkegaard, and Proust to name a few—bear eloquent testimony to the misery that such children endure. E. B. White recalled:

> As a child I was frightened but not unhappy. I lacked for nothing except confidence. I suffered nothing except the routine terrors of childhood: fear of the dark, fear of the future, fear of the return to school after a summer on a lake in Maine, fear of making an appearance on a platform, fear of a lavatory in the school basement where the slate urinals cascaded, fear that I was unknowing about things I should know about. . . . (Elledge, 1984, p. 23)

> The normal fears and worries of every child were in me developed to a high degree; every day was an awesome prospect. I was uneasy about practically everything: the uncertainty of the future, the dark of the attic, the panoply and discipline of school, the transitoriness of life, the mystery of the church and of God, the frailty of the body, the sadness of afternoon, the shadow of sex, the distant challenge of love and marriage, the far-off problem of a livelihood. I brooded about them all, lived with them day by day. (Guth, 1976, p. 1)

Relatives often describe these anxiety-prone children as "oversensitive," "tense," "nervous" or "high-strung." Like E. B. White as a boy, such youngsters worry endlessly about grades, social acceptance, and all sorts of perceived expectations. Concerns about being humiliated, embarrassed, or publicly found wanting in some way are common. Although inwardly leading lives of "quiet desperation," outwardly these children may function quite competently, especially after they have gotten used to a new situation. Their high anxiety, in fact, may go hand in hand with perfectionism and unrealistically high self-expectations. These children's intense concerns about being embarrassed or scrutinized unfavorably may sometimes warrant the additional diagnosis of social phobia.

Panic Disorder

Although this clinical disorder is uncommon in children, considerable research has focused on it, remolding the current subdivision of the anxiety disorders (Klein, 1981). These intensive investigations of panic disorder promise to shed light on many of the biological mechanisms underlying anxiety.

Panic attacks are sudden intense experiences of overwhelming fear, terror, and sense of impending doom that usually last only a few minutes and often occur spontaneously, with no easily detectable precipitants, psychological or physical; they may even wake the patient from dreamless sleep. Massive autonomic overstimulation is reflected in prominent physical sensations, including palpitations, choking sensations, dizziness, sweating, tremulousness, faintness, and a fear of dying, losing control of the self, or going mad.

In contrast, anticipatory or generalized anxiety is more gradual in onset, more persistent, and less episodic than panic anxiety. In addition, there is usually an accompanying manifest content involving possible misfortunes to the self or others. Persons with simple phobias may have anticipatory anxiety about encountering the phobic object, or, if they actually encounter it, may experience a flare of intense fear.

Current research suggests that the distinction between panic anxiety and generalized (or anticipatory) anxiety is qualitative as well as quantitative. As discussed under Etiology, panic disorder has important genetic and physiological features that may distinguish it from other forms of anxiety.

DSM-III-R (1987) Criteria for Panic Disorder

A. *At some time during the disturbance, one or more panic attacks (discrete periods of intense fear or discomfort) have occurred that were (1) unexpected, i.e., did not occur immediately before or on exposure to a situation that almost always caused anxiety, and (2) not triggered by situations in which the person was the focus of others' attention.*

B. *Either four attacks, as defined in criterion A, have occurred within a four-week period, or one or more attacks have been followed by a period of at least a month of persistent fear of having another attack.*

C. *At least four of the following symptoms developed during at least one of the attacks:*
   (1) shortness of breath (dyspnea) or smothering sensations
   (2) dizziness, unsteady feelings, or faintness
   (3) palpitations or accelerated heart rate (tachycardia)
   (4) trembling or shaking
   (5) sweating
   (6) choking
   (7) nausea or abdominal distress
   (8) depersonalization or derealization
   (9) numbness or tingling sensations (paresthesias)
   (10) flushes (hot flashes) or chills
   (11) chest pain or discomfort
   (12) fear of dying
   (13) fear of going crazy or of doing something uncontrolled

D. *During at least some of the attacks, at least four of the C symptoms developed suddenly and increased in intensity within ten minutes of the beginning of the first C symptom noticed in the attack.*

E. It cannot be established that an organic factor initiated and maintained the distur-
    bance, e.g., Amphetamine or Caffeine Intoxication, hyperthyroidism.

Note: Mitral valve prolapse may be an associated condition, but does not preclude a
diagnosis of Panic Disorder. (APA, 1987, pp. 237–238)

Epidemiology of Panic Disorder.   Epidemiological studies suggest that
the lifetime prevalence of panic disorder is about 0.7% to 2.4% of the
general adult population (Robins et al., 1984). A survey of ninth graders
found that 11.6% reported having had spontaneous panic attacks (Hayward
et al., 1989). In all age groups, the disorder is more common in women than
in men.

The peak age of onset for panic disorder is 15 to 19 years (Black &
Robbins, 1990; Crowe et al., 1983; Moreau et al., 1989); however, it does
occasionally occur in younger children. Van Winter & Stickler (1984) described seven children, ages 8 to 17 years old, who suffered from panic
disorder; all had close family members who also had the condition, with as
many as four generations being affected in one family. In a study of 220
children of depressed and nondepressed parents, Moreau et al. (1989)
found 6 offspring with onset of panic disorder between 5 to 18 years; there
were no cases of panic disorder among the children of nondepressed
parents. All six children also had major depression and/or separation anxiety disorder. In their survey of ninth graders cited above, Hayward et al.
(1989) found that compared with their peers; the students who had experienced panic attacks were more depressed and more likely to have separated
or divorced parents. The strong evidence of a genetic contribution to this
disorder is discussed further in the section Etiology.

Clinical Features of Childhood Panic Disorder.   Children and adolescents with panic disorder may describe many of the same symptoms found
in adult patients. However, one possible alternate presentation of panic
disorder involves rapid, anxious overbreathing. Thus, many of the cases of
hyperventilation syndrome commonly reported in adolescence might in
fact be more accurately diagnosed as panic disorder (Herman et al., 1981).

Hyperventilation syndrome may be defined as overbreathing or hyperventilation in the absence of any evidence of an organic cause (such as metabolic
imbalance, cardiac or pulmonary pathology, drug toxicity, or neurological
disease). This syndrome can occur in individuals as young as 5 years or up
into adulthood; adolescence, however, appears to be the time of greatest
prevalence. Girls are affected about twice as frequently as boys. The patient
with hyperventilation usually presents in a dramatic state, pale, tremulous,
and with the rapid panting breathing that gives the syndrome its name. The
patient may say he is choking or is unable to catch his breath but, in fact,
usually does not actually complain about his breathing. Instead, he may

speak of dizziness, weakness, palpitations, or blacking out. Additional complaints include tingling or numbness of the hands and mouth, headache, chest or abdominal pain, and muscular trembling or shakiness. Although these patients appear very anxious, it is striking that only a few, perhaps 1 in 10, complain initially of anxiety.

Most of the physical symptoms are the direct physiological result of overbreathing, and once the hyperventilation is brought under control, the symptoms usually subside. Rapid breathing blows off large amounts of carbon dioxide, thereby producing a dramatic shift in the acid-base balance of the body. The resulting respiratory alkalosis in turn can cause "pins and needles" tingling or numbness; tetanic twitching, hyperirritability, or muscle weakness; and even abnormal EEG patterns or seizures. In rare cases, auditory hallucinations may occur. In such cases, the seizures or auditory hallucinations can be experimentally reproduced by asking the patient to hyperventilate deliberately.

Panic disorder can be severely disabling. As some sufferers grow older, they increasingly restrict their activities, remaining housebound or unable to leave the comforting presence of a secure figure such as a spouse or parent. Thus, agoraphobia may represent a possible outcome of panic disorder (Klein & Gorman, 1987).

An increased risk of suicidal ideation and suicide attempts is another recently noted concomitant of panic disorder and attacks. In a community-based epidemiological sample, Weissman et al. (1989) found that subjects with panic disorder or attacks had a markedly increased risk for suicidality, with as many as 20% of subjects with panic disorder reporting a history of suicide attempts. This increased risk appeared to be independent of the coexistence of major depression or substance abuse. Subjects with onset of panic disorder before age 16 years were at significantly greater risk than those with later onset.

Social Phobia

In the later elementary grades, children become acutely aware of their place in the social order and how they appear to their friends and classmates. Concerns about not fitting in are common. Having a physical problem (obesity, a lisp, even left-handedness), dropping the ball at sports, wearing clothes at odds with the group's fashion norms, or being the butt of a sarcastic gibe from a teacher or friend—all of these cause acute mortification to the adolescent or school-age child. The depths of their child's humiliation and embarrassment at a seemingly inconsequential episode may puzzle and dismay parents. In time most children with adequate self-esteem learn to take such contretemps in stride.

A few adolescents, however, remain haunted by persistent, irrational fears of being humiliated or embarrassed. Their avoidance of situations where they might be exposed to others' scrutiny may constrict their social life. Sometimes their social phobia is limited to a single fear, such as fear of eating or speaking in public, using public lavatories, or attending parties. In other cases, their social anxieties are multiple and pervasive involving, for example, fears of initiating a conversation, making a phone call, or dating (Liebowitz et al., 1985).

Either as a cause or consequence of their social phobia, many of these young people have low self-esteem and are hypersensitive to scrutiny. They perceive others (both in anticipation and in fact) as critical or disapproving (Nichols, 1974). Because anxiety may leave the social phobic fumbling, quavery voiced, or inarticulate, the phobia often feeds on itself, further adding to the phobic's fear of humiliation.

The subjective suffering and functional impairment caused by social phobias are often severe and may significantly compromise vocational advancement and the ability to enjoy the company of others. Depression is common, and alcoholism and drug abuse may result from the phobic's attempts at self-medication.

ETIOLOGY

The causes and underlying mechanisms of anxiety are only poorly understood. Knowledge concerning even normal fears and anxieties is sketchy, and the extent to which various forms of pathological anxieties require different explanatory models remains unclear. By and large, psychologically minded theorists and neuroscientists have approached the problem of anxiety from different sides of the mind–body dichotomy. In recent years, however, researchers have made increasingly ambitious attempts to integrate the models from these disparate realms (Kandel, 1983; Reiser, 1984).

This overview includes the principal psychological theories of anxiety: psychodynamic, ethological, and behavioral. Following that, it discusses the burgeoning research relating to the neurophysiological and genetic aspects of anxiety.

Psychodynamic Factors

In his later years, Freud (1926/1953) came to regard anxiety as central to both normal mental functioning and the genesis of neurosis. In his final formulation of how the mind worked, Freud saw anxiety not only as a pathological manifestation, but also as the key regulator of adaptive functioning (Brenner, 1955; Compton, 1972a; Reiser, 1984).

Freud postulated two types of anxiety—traumatic anxiety and signal anxiety. *Traumatic* (or *automatic*) *anxiety* was conceived as a primitive, powerful, organismic response that occurs when internal or external stimuli too great to be mastered engulf the psyche. It is the condition of a person caught in a tornado; the ego is overwhelmed. In contrast, Freud conceptualized *signal anxiety* as an attenuated form of anxiety that serves the adaptive function of signaling impending (or anticipated) danger so that defensive measures can be taken. It is the alarm felt before an examination or interview; it spurs preparation and coping.

In Freud's (1926/1953) view, automatic anxiety is characteristic of early infantile life, a developmental epoch when coping mechanisms are poorly developed. "[A]nxiety is seen to be a product of the infant's mental helplessness which is a natural counterpart of its biological helplessness" (p. 138). Freud regarded early experiences of separation as the paradigm of "traumatic situations" that cause intense, primitive automatic anxiety. "This anxiety has all the appearance of being an expression of the child's feeling at its wits' end, as though in its still very undeveloped state it did not know how better to cope with its cathexis of longing" (p. 137). Indeed, under the influence of Rank's notion of birth trauma, Freud suggested that the "primal anxiety" of birth might represent the earliest separation anxiety of all.

Although most of Freud's examples of traumatic (automatic) anxiety occurred in infancy or early childhood, overwhelming trauma in later life can also precipitate traumatic anxiety. Such conditions are currently termed Posttraumatic stress disorders; in earlier diagnostic schemes they were known as the "traumatic neuroses." These conditions occur after a person experiences massive trauma about which he feels helpless. Historically, the two world wars stimulated interest in this syndrome by focusing attention on the so-called battle neuroses (referred to as "shell shock" in World War I and as "combat fatigue" in World War II). The syndrome also appears frequently in children who are victims of violent crime, natural disaster, and other catastrophes (Eth & Pynoos, 1985; Terr, 1987). Symptoms of posttraumatic stress may be common in children from the inner city ghettoes who are chronically exposed to ubiquitous violence. The concept has also proven useful in understanding children's response to sexual abuse (Goodwin, 1985).

Freud believed that in the course of the infant's growth and psychological maturation anxiety is gradually transformed so that danger situations no longer produce a primitive, diffuse, overwhelming response. Instead, the anxiety elicited by anticipated danger becomes more finely tuned and modulated until it is ultimately transformed into a signal. A major function of this anxiety signal is to call into operation coping behaviors and psychological defense mechanisms.

It is important to note two points about Freud's signal anxiety model: anticipated dangers rather than actual traumatic situations ordinarily trigger its action, and the source of the anticipated danger may be either internal or external. Thus, the trigger for signal anxiety not only may be meaningful outside events but also unconscious inner wishes, fantasies, thoughts, or hankerings that, if acknowledged and acted on, would lead to a traumatic situation. Freud believed that as the child matures, the psychic meaning and content of the dreaded danger changes as well. There is thus a developmental hierarchy of potentially anxiety-producing situations. For the very young child, the mother's physical absence produces the greatest fear. Later, in sequence, fears of loss of mother's love, of genital injury (castration), or of the painful attacks by the child's own conscience (super-ego) come to dominate successive developmental phases. However, the fears characteristic of each developmental epoch also stir echoes of earlier fears. Even when none of the specific anxieties mentioned above are aroused, powerful sexual and aggressive urges can trigger anxiety automatically because of their perceived threat to the ego's organization (A. Freud, 1981).

Freud believed that the adaptive purpose of signal anxiety is to mobilize various coping responses. These include both realistic behavior to ameliorate external problems and unconscious psychological defenses to master internally generated sources of danger. These latter defense mechanisms might be regarded as internal coping behaviors or "mental equivalents of fight–flight behavior" (Reiser, 1984); they ward off inner (instinctual-affectual) sources of anxiety through repressing, displacing, or isolating the thoughts and impulses that threaten mental equilibrium. If all goes well, equilibrium is maintained. If the process goes awry, neurotic symptoms are generated. The bulk of Freud's clinical work was an elaboration of how manifest psychopathology results from such unsuccessful defensive maneuvers.

According to this model, signal anxiety performs its tasks of marshaling and directing coping behavior and mental defenses silently and without becoming conscious. For the most part we direct our thoughts and actions without explicit awareness of the dangers of a given external threat or troublesome impulse. Thus, for the most part people pay their taxes without thinking much about the punishment that might result if they failed to do so. Similarly, they repress, sublimate, or otherwise manage rageful and lustful impulses toward colleagues and acquaintances without consciously and anxiously contemplating the dangers of expressing their passions more directly. (Rado (1956) called this phenomenon "non-reporting fear.") Freud believed that it is only when coping mechanisms are inadequate that anxiety becomes conscious or disabling.

From this perspective, anxiety disorders could be divided into two main types. On the one hand, *phobias* would be regarded as symptomatic neurotic conditions in which defense mechanisms such as repression and displacement contain the anxiety stirred by inner conflicts and keep it relatively circumscribed, that is, limited to the presence (or anticipation) of the phobic object. On the other hand, in the *generalized anxiety disorders* (or anxious personality disorders), the various defense mechanisms fail to cope with and to structure troublesome instinctual conflicts. Instead, the stress provoked by the internalized conflicts spreads until it pervades the entire personality; the end result is chronic tension and fearful apprehension (Anthony, 1981).

During the past 70 years, Freud's theory of anxiety has undergone a great deal of criticism and revision (Compton, 1972b). Although later psychoanalytic investigators such as Bowlby (1973) and Mahler et al. (1975) also place a central emphasis on the role of separation in the genesis of anxiety, they differ from Freud in their explanation of *why* separation engenders anxiety (see the extensive review by Bowlby, 1973). Freud (1926/1953) hypothesized that the infant comes to experience the mother as the source of comfort and gratification for his various needs. In the mother's absence, unmet physiological needs build up tension that overwhelms the helpless infant. Freud suggested that each subsequent maternal absence recalls this prior state of helplessness to the infant; thus, separation produces anxiety by signaling the possible recurrence of an earlier traumatic situation.

Melanie Klein's (1952a) explanation for separation anxiety is more in keeping with her controversial emphasis on the vicissitudes of early aggression: "When [an infant] misses [his mother], and his needs are not satisfied her absence is felt to be the result of his destructive impulses" (p. 270). In Klein's view (1952b), anxiety "derives from the infant's apprehension that the loved mother has been destroyed by his sadistic impulses or is in danger of being destroyed, and this fear. . . contributes to the infant's feeling that she will never return" (p. 288).

Bowlby's (1973) cogently argued position, grounded in his ethological viewpoint, is that the infant's distress upon separation from his primary attachment figure is an intrinsic response, not reducible to other terms. Bowlby labeled his own theory of attachment and separation a "primary drive" theory; the infant's growing attachment to his mother (and his distress at separation from her) represent a primary drive toward attachment, which is not the by-product of other needs or instincts. Bowlby (1969, 1973) contrasted this theoretical viewpoint with Freud's, which Bowlby termed a "Secondary Drive Theory" of attachment (or more derisively a "cupboard theory of love"): Attachment to the mother and anxiety over her absence are secondary to her function as the gratifier of various needs, such as food. Mother is not important in her own right but rather as a gratifier of other needs.

Other theoretical revisions have involved emphasis. Melanie Klein (1952a, 1952b) shared Freud's notion that dangerous instinctual impulses are central to anxiety. Klein, however, emphasized *aggressive* wishes and their derivative sadistic fantasies as posing the greatest danger to the ego; it is against these wishes in particular that the various psychological defenses are directed. Klein saw primitive aggression as innate in the infant's psyche;

in her view, intense early aggression produces two forms of anxiety, each of which in turn gives rise to characteristic defensive operations (Segal, 1980). In the earliest epoch of life, the infant manages such aggression by projection onto the mother, which results in the infant's perceiving his psychological world as populated with dangerous, persecutory objects. He manages his resulting persecutory (or "paranoid") anxiety by splitting his images of mother and himself into idealized (and hence safe) "good" parts and dangerous, hateful "bad" parts. Because, in this theory, the predominant anxiety is of being destroyed by a bad persecutory object ("paranoia") and the principal defense involves splitting ("schizoid") operations, Klein used the term *paranoid-schizoid position* to describe this configuration of characteristic anxieties, defenses, and object relations. This paranoid-schizoid stage stood in contrast to a later phase that she termed the *depressive position*. During this latter phase, the infant's greater integrative powers lead him to accept that he is himself the source of the angry, hateful feelings and that his mother is in reality an admixture of both gratification and frustration, of good and bad. As a result, the infant's aggression now stirs his fears that he has damaged or destroyed his mother. Klein termed this guilty concern "depressive anxiety." She characterized the cluster of depressive anxiety and the corresponding reparational defenses as the *depressive position*. Although most contemporary thinkers reject Klein's very early and dogmatic chronology, her emphasis on the relationship between anxiety and the early vicissitudes of aggression has proven clinically very useful.

Ethological Factors

In the course of their evolutionary adaptation to their natural environment, humans, like other vertebrates, have developed inborn instinctual fears in response to certain "natural clues" that portend possible dangerous situations. In humans, these include darkness, loud noise, heights, rapidly looming objects, isolation, and even mere strangeness. Such instinctually based warning systems are essential for survival, especially to the young of a species; they cannot await cognitive appraisal because often by the time a predator or other danger is upon an individual, it is too late. In survival terms, an ounce of instinctual avoidance is often worth many pounds of painfully learned experience. In other species, stimuli associated with potential predators, such as a pair of staring eyes or specific shapes moving rapidly overhead, elicit innate fear responses (Bowlby, 1973).

In modern-day life such cues no longer signal mortal danger with the same urgency that they did during the long childhood of our species when we were vulnerable furless primates living in the forests and grassy savannahs of Africa. Nonetheless, our evolving behavioral instincts adapted us for the environment where we and our primate ancestors spent our first few million years. Of course, even in modern urban life, the state of nature, "red in tooth and claw" (as Hobbes put it) may still be only as far away as the nearest dark street corner.

Natural fears of noise, height, looming objects, and the unfamiliar are all present in infants by the end of the first year of life. Indeed, these fears persist to a considerable extent into adulthood. Bowlby (1973) cautions that although such fears are sometimes labeled "unrealistic" (in terms of the modern-day environment), it is a mistake to regard them as intrinsically pathological. He rejects the notion that only fear of "real danger" is healthy and that other forms of fear are somehow childish or neurotic. "[T]he assumption that mature adults are afraid only of real danger, plausible though it may seem, is profoundly mistaken" (Bowlby, 1973, p. 152).

Isolation powerfully increases fearfulness, even in adults. As Willam James (1890) observed succinctly, "The great source of terror in infancy is solitude." Freud (1905/1953) put it somewhat differently: "Anxiety in children is originally nothing other than an expression of the fact that they are feeling the loss of the person they love" (p. 224). Research in attachment in both humans and monkeys has demonstrated that the infant's bond to the mother serves not only as a guarantor of physical survival but also as an essential prerequisite and organizer for cognitive and interpersonal growth (Bowlby, 1969, 1973; Harlow, 1961; Parkes & Stevenson-Hinde, 1982). Thus, not only does the absence of the mother (or other secure attachment figure) cause distress in itself; it leads to a generalized fearfulness toward the larger world. Conversely, the availability of a secure attachment figure may permit confident exploration of otherwise alarming unfamiliar objects and situations (Ainsworth, 1982).

In his classic experiments, Harlow (1961) studied the behavior of infant rhesus monkeys who were separated from their natural mother and reared with the continuing presence of a terry cloth-covered dummy "mother." When confronted with an unfamiliar toy animal, the infant monkeys fled the toy, rushing toward the dummy to whom they clung tightly. Somewhat older infants, after retreating to the "mother," relaxed and then approached the toy, at first with caution and then with increasing confidence. They proceeded to explore and handle the fear-inducing toy, occasionally returning to touch base with "mother." If, however, the familiar dummy "mother" was absent, an unfamiliar object introduced into the cage caused the same infant to curl up on the floor, rocking and crying in apparent terror. Mahler et al. (1975) observed in the exploring ("practicing phase") toddler the same need to "refuel" by periodically checking in with mother before sallying forth again.

The presence or absence of a secure attachment figure may thus tip the balance between fear and pleasurable interest, not only with unfamiliar stimuli but with other potentially fear-inducing situations as well. Freud (1905/1953) told the story of a 3-year-old boy he overheard calling out in a dark room: "Auntie, speak to me! I'm frightened because it's so dark."

When the aunt teasingly replied, "What good would that do? You can't see me," the child answered, "That doesn't matter; if anyone speaks, it gets light." Freud concluded, "What he was afraid of was not the dark, but the absence of someone he loved . . . " (p. 224n).

As the child grows older, confidence may come to depend less on the actual physical presence or absence of the mother (or other attachment figure) than on the child's perception of his mother's physical and emotional availability and reliability (Bowlby, 1973; Sorce & Emde, 1981). In large measure, this perception is an expression of the child's past experience of the mother's availability and reliability.

Psychoanalysts speak of the child's internalized object relations (Greenberg & Mitchell, 1983). From this point of view, much depends on whether the child has an internal image of himself linked to an attentive, responsive, and protective parent or instead sees himself alone or tenuously linked to an indifferent, ambivalent, or otherwise unreliable parent. Bowlby (1973) used the term "anxious attachment" to describe the insecurity shown by children who have been reared by multiple, unreliable, or emotionally unavailable caretakers, or who have been subjected to frequent separations or abandonments. Abused or neglected children, children reared in institutions, and children of emotionally disturbed parents often show this pattern.

Even less dramatic disturbances in the parent–child relationship can produce anxious attachment. Ainsworth and colleagues (1978) developed a strange-situation paradigm in the course of which they carefully observed 1-year-olds experimentally placed in a standardized unfamiliar situation. On the basis of such observations, they developed a method for reliably discriminating "securely attached" from "anxiously attached" infants. In comparison with their securely attached peers, anxiously attached infants at 1 year had experienced less harmonious interactions with their mothers, who in turn appeared less sensitively and reciprocally responsive to their infants' communications. Furthermore anxious attachment at 1 year of age has been found to correlate at ages 3 to 6 years with difficulties in the emotional, behavioral, and interpersonal spheres (Sroufe et al., 1983). Experimental work with monkeys suggests that separation from mother in infancy can produce a similar behavioral syndrome that persists into adulthood (Capitanio et al., 1986; Suomi, 1986). Anxious versus secure attachment behavior in the Ainsworth Strange Situation, however, is the result of many factors in addition to the child's experience with the caretaker. Both temperament and prior socialization experiences seem to exert a strong influence (Kagan, 1987).

Michael Balint (1955) spoke of two contrasting personality types, originating in early childhood. The first is the *ocnophilic* child, who fears separation and dreads exploring the spaces about him, preferring instead to cling to mother (or other secure objects). The second is the *philobatic* child, who is eager to explore the unknown world about him, while avoiding too much proximity with mother (Anthony, 1981). Based on his clinical material, Balint believed that the risk-loving, independence-seeking philobat's behavior is rooted in a highly ambivalent attitude toward closeness to mother. In contrast, Bowlby, Mahler, and Ainsworth see truly confident behavior as being grounded in a secure primary attachment to the mother.

Some psychoanalytic theorists have suggested that the projection of the child's own angry feelings onto the parents is a major factor leading the anxious child to fear the parent's unavailability through death, abandonment, or anger. Thus, when angry at a parent, the child, by dint of his own defensive work, comes to expect and fear retaliation or abandonment rather than support from the parent. Bowlby (1973), on the other hand, deemphasizes these intrapsychic sources of concern over the parents' availability and stresses instead the impact of actual interpersonal experiences. In his view, real traumatic separations, such as losses through death or divorce or parental threats of abandonment, are the most potent causes of insecure or anxious attachment. For many children with school phobia due to separation anxiety disorder, a major disruption in the child's pattern of attachment, such as a move or the illness or death of a close family member, precedes the onset of symptoms (Gittleman-Klein & Klein, 1980).

Bowlby contends that, in the course of child-rearing and family struggles, parental threats of abandonment occur far more frequently than is generally supposed. These may range from threats of divorce, threats of suicide, and threats to send the child away, to such dire warnings as "You'll see; you're going to give your father a heart attack if you keep that up." Some critics have charged that in his view of the genesis of anxiety Bowlby is too concrete and overemphasizes the importance of actual experiences (or threats) of abandonment. Bowlby's more fundamental point, however, is nonetheless compelling: Anxiety is always rooted in the child's object relations; it arises out of them and influences their vicissitudes.

From the second and third years of life, the content and intensity of childrens' fears are strongly influenced by learned cultural cues. Researchers have long suggested that parents' own fears and anxieties have a powerful impact on their offspring. The transmission of anxiety (or other affects) between mother and child is often described evocatively as empathic "contagion" (Eisenberg, 1958; Escalona, 1953; Sullivan, 1953). It is also possible, however, to conceptualize the process as an example of what learning theorists refer to as vicarious or observational learning. To become fearful of a situation, the child need not actually be hurt or otherwise suffer adverse consequences; often it is enough for him to see an adult, sibling, or peer get hurt or frightened (Bandura, 1977). Observational learning thus potently shapes the child's attitudes as to which situations are dangerous and which are safe. Other primates and mammals also learn what to fear or avoid by observing members of their species (Hinde, 1970). In an experimental situation, monkeys initially played freely with an object. However, after witnessing another monkey apparently emit cries of fear upon touching it, they subsequently avoided it (Bandura, cited in Bowlby, 1973).

On finding themselves in perplexing or potentially fear-evoking situations, children as young as one year look toward their parent for cues about the safety of a situation (Schaffer, 1971; Zahn-Waxler et al., 1979). This phenomenon is known as *social referencing*. It illustrates that the mother's emotional responsivity is as important as her physical presence in determining the infant's sense of security (Sorce & Emde, 1981). Such a glance not only provides a reassuring link to the parent, it also gives the child vital data regarding his parent's assessment of the situation. The mother's response heavily influences whether the child proceeds with further exploration or becomes cautious and apprehensive (Sorce et al., 1985). Several studies have shown a high correlation between the degree of children's fearfulness and that of their parents toward objects or situations as diverse as dogs, insects, thunderstorms, dental work, or the wartime bombing raids on London (Bowlby, 1973; Windheuser, 1977).

Family theorists have speculated that families develop their own paradigm, or system of shared assumptions, about the social world about them; these assumptions orient family members and coordinate their actions regarding each other and the world at large (Reiss, 1981). Some families see the outside world as threatening and hostile; accordingly each new offspring is acculturated into an intense wariness in dealing with people outside the family. Other parents, themselves the victims of intense anxiety over separation, inculcate their children with a sense that the world is filled with danger. In her thought-provoking book, *Necessary Losses,* Judith Viorst (1986) has a moving chapter about the painful struggles of such parents. She quotes from a poem by Louis Simpson*:

> The lives of children are
> Dangerous to their parents
> With fire, water, air,
> And other accidents;
> And some, for a child's sake,
> Anticipating doom,
> Empty the world to make
> The world safe as a room.

Unfortunately, when fearfulness is a familial pattern, it is not yet possible to distinguish the relative contributions of social learning within the family

*From "The Goodnight," in *A Dream of Governors*, by Louis Simpson, 1959, Middletown, Conn: Wesleyan University Press. Copyright 1959 by Louis Simpson. Reprinted by permission of Wesleyan University Press.

from genetic factors, such as a genetically transmitted predisposition to fearfulness (Weissman et al., 1984b).

Behavioral Factors—Learning Theory

Learning theory has provided several useful theoretical and experimental paradigms for studying the acquisition of anxiety. A number of important similarities exist between psychoanalytic and learning theory approaches to anxiety (Shaffer, 1986b). Freud's theory of anxiety relies heavily on an implicit conditioning or associative learning model (see Reiser, 1984 for an ambitious attempt to synthesize the psychoanalytic and learning theory models). Both theories emphasize early (traumatic) experience in the development of anxiety and attempt to explain how one specific fear becomes the source of another. Psychoanalytic theory invokes the process of *displacement,* whereas the phenomenon of *stimulus generalization* serves as the explanatory mechanism in learning theory (Shaffer, 1986). To the extent that psychoanalytic theory utilizes high-level cognitive mechanisms such as displacement or symbolization, it seems to imply that anxiety is a uniquely human phenomenon. In contrast, learning theory places much less emphasis on mediating cognitive variables. Animal studies employing conditioning paradigms have provided useful laboratory models for the development of fear and anxiety. Such models have facilitated research into the basic cellular neurophysiology of aversive conditioning (Kandel, 1983).

Classical (Pavlovian) conditioning, operant conditioning, and social learning have all been proposed as explanatory models for anxiety.

Classical (Pavlovian) Conditioning.

In the classical conditioning paradigm, the subject is presented with a stimulus called the *unconditioned* (or reinforcing) *stimulus* (UCS), which automatically (i.e., without conditioning) produces an *unconditioned response* (UCR). In Pavlov's famous experiment, the unconditioned stimulus (UCS) was meat powder, which reflexively produced salivation (UCR) in the hungry dog. If a second stimulus, termed the *conditioned stimulus* (CS), is presented just before the unconditioned stimulus, the subject learns to associate the two. A cognitive psychologist would say that the CS comes to be distinguished as a reliable predictor of the UCS. As a result, the CS will come to evoke the same response as the UCS; this response is now termed the *conditioned response* (CR). Thus, Pavlov sounded a bell (CS) just before presenting the meat powder (UCS) to the dog; after several such pairings, the sound of the bell alone (CS) was sufficient to make the dog salivate (CR).

Although Pavlov's experiment is an example of conditioned *appetitive* learning, it is also possible to produce conditioned *aversive* responses. Watson and Rayner (1920) used such a paradigm with an infant to produce an experimentally induced fear that they termed a "conditioned emotional response." Albert, a hospitalized nine-month-old, was pretested by being shown a live white rat, a rabbit, and various furry and nonfurry toys; he remained tranquil. In contrast, a loud noise (UCS) produced behind his head would regularly produce crying (UCR). During several experimental sessions 2 months later, presentation of the rat (CS) was regularly paired with the loud noise (UCS), which again made Albert cry (UCR). Following this series of paired presentations, the rat alone (CS) was enough to elicit Albert's crying and distress (CR). In addition, other furry animals and objects now also elicited the same distressed response. Watson and Rayner suggested that the paired exposures to the rat and the aversive loud noise together had made the rat a conditioned stimulus (CS) that could then produce a conditioned fear response (CR) by itself. The rat's ability to elicit Albert's crying, without the noise, persisted for several weeks. Unfortunately for the experimenters (although perhaps not for little Albert), the child's mother removed Albert from the hospital before Watson and Rayner were able to study the extinction characteristics of Albert's acquired fear.

Watson and Rayner went on to hypothesize that neurotic anxieties might naturally arise in a similar manner. Serendipitous pairing of a neutral stimulus (CS) with a naturally frightening one (UCS) could lead to a conditioned phobia that would otherwise appear to be unexplainable and irrational.

Watson and Rayner's experiment in particular and the classical conditioning anxiety model in general have been subjected to various critiques (Delprato, 1980; Shaffer, 1986b). If serendipitous conditioning caused acquired phobias, most neurotic fears would have to be the result of single exposures to a traumatic situation coincidentally paired with a previously neutral stimulus (i.e., single-trial learning). Furthermore, the two stimuli would have to occur within a very short time of each other, an unlikely event. Yet, in most experimental situations, the classical conditioning paradigm usually requires numerous paired exposures to achieve effective conditioning. The sole exception might be extremely traumatic situations, which can produce avoidance behavior with a single occurrence (e.g., the fear of driving that a person sometimes experiences after a life-threatening crash). In fact, in most phobic patients' histories the therapist rarely can find evidence of accidental traumatic encounters with the future phobic object that seem sufficient to account for the onset of the phobia. Further, in the absence of ongoing paired exposures to the CS in the presence of the UCS, an unreinforced conditioned response extinguishes fairly rapidly. Clinically, however, phobias can persist over long periods and even intensify without the subject actually reencountering the phobic object or hypothesized original aversive stimulus. Finally, in its unmodified form, the Pavlovian model suggests that any neutral stimulus can serve as the object of a phobia as well as any other; yet, in fact, the bulk of clinical phobias arise from a relatively narrow range of objects, such as certain types of animals, heights, and enclosed spaces (Marks, 1987). Thus, although intuitively appealing, the classical conditioning theory of anxiety leaves many questions unanswered (Shaffer, 1986b).

The *operant conditioning paradigm* hypothesizes that anxious or avoidant behavior persists because it is rewarded or reinforced. From this point of view, for example, the persistence of the school phobic's avoidant behavior might be the result of covert or overt approval, encouragement, or reward from his mother.

The *social learning paradigm* suggests that the individual can learn fears or avoidance behavior vicariously (Bandura, 1977). In this hypothesis, conditioned anxiety may develop if a child observes a model (such as a parent or other child) being exposed to a traumatic event. (For a further discussion of the social learning paradigms, see pp. 721–723.)

The three conditioning models reviewed above seem most germane to phobias or relatively focused anticipatory anxiety. In contrast, the learning theory paradigm that best fits generalized anxiety disorders is *unsignaled aversive conditioning*. In this paradigm, the subject is repeatedly exposed to an aversive stimulus without any cue or warning (Kandel, 1983). Because no signal reliably predicts danger, safety is also unpredictable. As a result, the subject remains in a state of constant apprehensive arousal. The *learned-helplessness paradigm* produces a somewhat similar state, in which the subject is repeatedly subjected to an aversive stimulus that he is powerless to escape or terminate. Both paradigms produce a sense of helplessness.

Like psychoanalytic theories, learning theory approaches do not adequately explain individual differences (Shaffer, 1986b). The theoretical analysis of a given case may convey a certain post hoc plausibility, but it provides no basis for prediction, and the theory does not explain why one child rather than another will develop a given anxiety disorder. Nonetheless, learning theories have had immense heuristic value in suggesting new methods of treatment and further lines of empirical investigation.

Finally, the current psychological theories, both psychoanalytic and behavioral, fail to account fully for the nature of anxiety and the highly variable capacity of different individuals to bear it (Zetzel, 1949/1970a). Behavioral theories, for example, distinguish several components of anxiety: (1) physiological, (2) subjective feelings and thoughts, and (3) overt behavioral avoidance (Graziano et al., 1979; Wells & Vitulano, 1984). These components do not necessarily covary. Clinical judgments of severity and impairment usually reflect the degree of avoidance behavior and subjective distress. However, the degree of avoidance behavior may not simply reflect the intensity of the child's psychophysiological distress. Despite intense subjective feelings of anxiety, some persistent children may show little avoidant behavior, whereas other children with less apparent ability to tolerate anxiety show extensive avoidance (Morris & Kratochwill, 1983;

Shaffer, 1986b). Clinicians even encounter children who manage their intense anxiety by seeking out dangerous situations, thereby converting frightened passivity into counterphobic activity, as in the case of the hemophiliac adolescent who insists on riding a motorcycle and playing tackle football. The boy's parents (and therapist) are consumed with apprehension, while the youth rails against their worried nagging.

Much depends on how the child tolerates and copes with anxiety. Certainly there is a discrepancy between the very large number of children reporting multiple fears in population-based studies and the much smaller proportion who come to clinical attention as functionally impaired patients. Although the severity of subjective distress may be important in determining who receives a clinical diagnosis of anxiety disorder, individual differences in factors such as anxiety tolerance and parental response may also be decisive.

As yet, developmental researchers know little about the origins of the capacity to tolerate anxiety. More research is needed to clarify whether genetic-biological factors (Shaffer, 1986b; Suomi, 1986), rearing variables such the quality of early attachment (Bowlby, 1973), or fundamental individual differences in temperament (Thomas & Chess, 1977) best conceptualize this capacity.

Biological Subtypes—Anticipatory Anxiety versus Panic Anxiety

Research during the past 20 years suggests that there may be qualitative as well as quantitative distinctions between the different types of anxiety. Largely because of work by Donald Klein (1981) and colleagues, anxiety is no longer believed to be a unitary biological phenomenon. Instead, current thinking distinguishes between acute *panic anxiety* and the more chronic *anticipatory anxiety* (which includes both generalized anxiety and simple phobic anxiety); these two types of anxiety differ in their psychological precipitants, pattern of familial inheritance, psychopharmacological responsiveness, and underlying biological mechanisms (Anderson et al., 1984; Klerman, 1986; Lesser & Rubin, 1986).

Panic attacks are sudden, spontaneous bouts of overwhelming terror accompanied by symptoms of massive autonomic discharge such as palpitations, dizziness, sweating, tremulousness, and faintness.

In contrast, anticipatory or generalized anxiety is more gradual in onset, more persistent, and less episodic than panic anxiety and is usually accompanied by specific anxious apprehensions of possible misfortune. The physical symptoms accompanying generalized and anticipatory anxiety are usually milder than they are in panic attacks.

The distinctions between these two classes of anxiety, however, go beyond phenomenology. A large body of research suggests that the intravenous infusion of lactate can readily provoke panic attacks in panic-prone individuals, whereas the same compound will generally have little effect when administered to patients with other anxiety disorders (see review by Shear, 1986). Such findings have led to the suggestion that response to lactate might even serve as a biological marker of proneness to panic attacks. (For a skeptical dissenting view, see Margraf et al., 1986.) Similar findings with the administration of caffeine or yohimbine (an adrenergic agent) or the breathing of carbon dioxide suggest that panic patients may have a special sensitivity to these substances.

Numerous theories have been advanced to explain this pharmacologically triggered panic. One theory proposes that panic involves stimulation of central noradrenergic centers (especially a midbrain structure called the *locus ceruleus*) in patients with an underlying biological vulnerability. (See section on Autonomic Nervous System Regulation for further discussion of the role of the noradrenergic system in anxiety.)

Despite the current research findings that suggest possible biological and genetic components to panic disorder, dismissing the role of psychological factors out of hand is unwarranted. Many panic attacks do have dynamically determined psychological precipitants (Freedman, 1984), and there is evidence that a high prevalence of stressful life events may contribute to the onset of panic disorder (Roy-Byrne et al., 1986).

Patients with panic disorder have a four- to five-fold increased prevalence of a generally benign cardiac condition called *mitral valve prolapse*. Evidence is accumulating that alterations in the autonomic nervous system balance, which are in turn associated with the anxiety disorder, may cause this cardiac syndrome. In many cases, the abnormal cardiac findings disappear with successful treatment of the anxiety disorder (Ballenger et al., 1986).

Genetic Factors

Clinicians have noted that anxious children frequently have anxious parents (Reeves et al., 1987; Werry et al., 1987). Twin and family studies suggest that there is a strong hereditary component in some, but not all of the anxiety disorders (Marks, 1986, 1987). In general, these findings indicate that genetic factors influence the development of both panic disorder and agoraphobia with panic attacks; in contrast, generalized anxiety disorder does not appear to have as strong a hereditary predisposition. At the same time, however, the high discordance rate for anxiety disorders even between identical twins indicates the importance of environmental factors (Torgersen, 1983). Looking at clinically anxious children as a whole, the contribution of genetic influences is unclear. Although anxious parents are more likely to have anxious children, researchers do not know what proportion of the overall population of anxious children is accounted for by anxious families (Shaffer, 1986b).

Data comparing monozygotic (MZ) and dizygotic (DZ) twins of various ages from nonclinic populations suggest a substantial genetic influence on such traits as fear of strangers, shyness, timidity, fearfulness and inhibition, separation distress, and "constant worrying" (Goldsmith & Gottesman, 1981; Marks, 1986, 1987). Turning to the formal anxiety disorders, twin studies show that MZ twins are much more likely than DZ twins to be concordant for phobic symptoms, panic disorder, or agoraphobia accompanied by panic disorder; however, the concordance rate for generalized anxiety disorder does not differ between MZ and DZ twins (Carey & Gottesman, 1981; Torgersen, 1983). Similarly, family studies suggest a high familial prevalence of panic disorder, but not of generalized anxiety disorder. The morbidity risk for panic disorder among first-degree relatives of probands with panic disorder is 17.3% to 20% versus 1.8% to 4.2% for the first-degree relatives of normal controls (Crowe et al., 1983; Harris et al., 1983). Pedigree analysis suggests that in some families, panic disorder is transmitted as an autosomal dominant trait (Pauls et al., 1980). Simple phobia has been shown to be significantly more common among the first-degree relatives of individuals with simple phobia than among those of nonanxious controls; family members, however, rarely had the same phobic object (Fyer et al., 1990).

These data, of course, cannot directly distinguish between genetic and environmental transmission. The interactions between these two factors are complex (Marks, 1986), and researchers lack sufficient adoptive studies to disentangle the two. However, unlike panic disorder or agoraphobia, the presence of generalized anxiety disorder in a parent has little effect on the child's degree of risk for anxiety disorder (Breslau et al., 1987). If the family transmission of anxiety is primarily the result of the family culture, identifications, or child-rearing practices, it is difficult to explain why only certain types of anxiety (but not others) show familial clustering.

Family studies also indicate that the high frequency with which anxiety disorders and depression tend to occur together in the same patients may be more than coincidental (Carey, 1987; Kendler et al., 1987; Leckman et al., 1987c). Several authors have noted a greater number of anxiety symptoms and anxiety disorder in the children of patients with affective disorders (Moreau et al., 1989); the presence of both depression and anxiety disorder in a parent greatly increases the offspring's risk for anxiety or depression (Weissman et al., 1984). Several family studies (Breslau et al., 1987; Leckman et al., 1983) suggest a shared genetic diathesis for anxiety disorder and depression; other studies have failed to show a familial relationship between these conditions (Breier et al., 1985).

Linkage studies utilizing powerful new molecular genetic techniques are now underway in families with several members who suffer from panic disorder (Crowe et al., 1987). Such studies should soon shed more light on the genetic mechanisms that may underlie panic disorder, including mode of transmission, chromosomal locus, and ultimately gene structure and function.

An unanswered question concerns the extent to which children's anxiety symptoms resemble those of their parents. As noted earlier, the natural history and life course of the various anxiety disorders are as yet poorly understood. Many adult patients with panic attacks or agoraphobia report a childhood history of marked separation anxiety and difficulty adjusting to school (Berg et al., 1974; Gittleman, 1986; Gittleman & Klein, 1984). At least one study (Berg, 1976) indicates that the children of agoraphobic women carry an increased risk of about 14% for school phobia. If childhood separation anxiety is a possible early manifestation of agoraphobia or panic disorder, these offspring, as they grow older, may come to resemble their agoraphobic mothers ever more closely. Other studies of children with school phobia have shown a greater incidence of separation anxiety in the parents and of school phobias in the siblings (see Chapter 8, "Anxious School Refusal").

These considerations concerning familial predisposition to anxiety raise the question: Exactly *what* is inherited? Although animal models are imperfect analogues to human anxiety, they permit controlled breeding and adoption studies that are not feasible with humans. (For a review of animal genetic models of anxiety, see Marks, 1986, 1987; Weiss & Uhde, 1990.) Strains of monkeys (Suomi, 1986), mice (Broadhurst, 1981), and dogs (Dykman et al., 1969) have been bred that show genetically determined differences in reactive, nervous, or fearful behavior. The rhesus monkey studies conducted by Suomi (1986) are especially thought provoking. Suomi found that rhesus monkeys show stable individual differences in their degree of anxiety-proneness or timidity. Throughout their life span, certain monkeys tend to display fearful or anxious reactions in situations where their peers (of comparable social-rearing background) initiate exploration or playful social interactions. These situations involve exposure to novel stimuli or brief separations. In response to separation from family or friends, anxiety-prone monkeys show less positive coping behavior and greater depressive reactions than their nonanxious peers. These same monkeys are not only behaviorally highly reactive to stress or novelty, they are also physiologically more reactive in that they show more dramatic and prolonged activation of their hypothalamic-pituitary-adrenal axis. In the absence of stress or separation, the behavior of the anxious monkeys does *not* differ from their peers; it is only when they are confronted with obvious stress or challenge that the individual differences emerge.

Most pertinent to the present discussion, pedigree studies and cross-adoption experiments indicate that there is a substantial genetic contribution to these individual differences in stress reactivity. Suomi et al. (1981) found that siblings who from birth had been placed with different foster mothers and reared apart showed fewer differences in their physiological and behavioral reactivity to stress than did genetically unrelated individuals who had been reared together.

Like the young of many other species, children show stable individual differences in their tendency to manifest anxious inhibition in face of unfamiliar or discrepant stimuli. Kagan (1987) and colleagues studied a group of 21-month-old children and identified the 10% who responded to unfamiliar people, objects, or situations with the greatest signs of inhibition, withdrawal, and anxious distress. Inhibition in infancy was associated with increased morning cortisol secretion and a lowered threshold for autonomic arousal as reflected in various peripheral autonomic measures (Kagan, 1987; Kagan et al., 1988). Behavioral inhibition in response to the unfamiliar proved to be a highly stable trait. At age 7 years, these same children continued to be more inhibited with peers and in unfamiliar situations; approximately one-third of these children manifested clinical symptoms of anxiety or social withdrawal (Gersten, 1986, cited in Rosenbaum et al., 1988). A 30-year follow-up of the Berkeley Guidance Study Sample found that boys who were shy at ages 8 to 10 years were more likely than their peers to delay marriage, parenthood, and stable careers and attained less occupational success and stability (Caspi et al., 1988).

Data from twin and adoption studies suggest that these early constitutional differences are at least partially genetic in origin (Daniels & Plomin, 1985). The young children of parents with panic disorder and agoraphobia have a higher rate of inhibition to the unfamiliar than a matched comparison group of children of parents with other psychiatric disorders (Rosenbaum et al., 1988). However, Kagan and colleagues (1987) speculated:

> The actualization of shy, quiet, timid behavior at 2 years of age requires some form of chronic environmental stress acting upon the original temperamental disposition present at birth. . . . Thus, it is important to differentiate between those children and adolescents who are quiet and restrained in unfamiliar social situations because of the influence of temperamental factors and those who behave this way because of environmental experiences alone. (p. 171)

If the predisposition to maladaptive anxiety is genetically determined in humans, the question arises as to how such vulnerability is physiologically mediated. This raises the broad and complex topic of the biological mechanisms underlying the anxiety disorders. Are there biological markers that might identify people at risk for anxiety disorders? In the monkey studies noted above, excessive activation of the hypothalamic-pituitary-adrenal axis serves as a concomitant of anxiety-proneness (Suomi, 1986). Also as discussed earlier, researchers have devoted much work to lactate sensitivity as a possible marker for panic disorder (Margraf et al., 1986). The specificity of such markers is unclear, however, as is their relationship to the presumed mechanisms producing pathological anxiety. In an intriguing but as yet unreplicated study, Shaffer and colleagues (1985) found a significant association of anxiety disorders at age 17 with the presence of "soft" signs on neurological examination at age 7. In the absence of such "soft" signs, anxiety at age 7 was not predictive of later anxiety disorder; however, anxious dependent behavior at age 7 that was accompanied by soft signs greatly increased the risk of persisting difficulties with anxiety in adolescence. These findings suggest that neurodevelopmental factors may influence the development of anxiety disorders.

Autonomic Nervous System Regulation

The most prominent physical manifestations of anxiety are symptomatic of autonomic nervous system arousal, especially arousal of the sympathetic component. Consequently, one recurrent line of speculation has focused on the possibility that pathological anxiety reflects a disorder of autonomic regulation. Investigators pursuing this lead have looked for evidence that anxious people might have abnormal autonomic responses to various stimuli and have also sought differences in autonomic functioning between anxious patients and normals at rest (Gorman, 1984). Another hypothesis has been that anxious patients, rather than having higher levels of autonomic arousal, are simply more sensitive and hyperaware of their physiological processes (Schandry, 1981). Although patients with anxiety disorder do have greater awareness of their heartbeat than controls, these patients also have a faster basal heart rate, less cardiac deceleration after a stressful stimulus, and greater lability of cardiac rhythm (Gorman, 1984). In addition, under stress (such as public speaking), anxious patients show a more dramatic shift of blood flow away from the skin and viscera and toward the musculature than do controls. Similarly, compared with normals, the anxious patient's skin conductance (a measure of autonomic arousal) is higher and more labile. Although all subjects show an increase in skin conductance following stressful or novel stimuli, many (but not all) anxiety disorder patients are slower than normal subjects in habituating to repeated stimulation. Patients with various anxiety disorders do not react alike. For example, the habituation responses of patients with a simple phobia resembled those of normals more closely than those of patients with other anxiety disorders (Lader, 1967).

Researchers have devoted much investigation and speculation to determining which components and neurotransmitter subsystems are responsible for the autonomic symptoms of anxiety (Hoehn-Saric, 1982; Reznick et al., 1986). Although anxiety symptoms often seem to reflect sympathetic overresponsiveness, there also appears to be evidence for diffuse parasympathetic abnormalities. Clearly, no simple theory fits all the facts.

Despite these complexities, the search continues for the origin and nature of the autonomic arousal that characterizes anxiety. One of the most interesting lines of investigation concerns the role of the noradrenergic system in anxiety and the influence of the *locus ceruleus*, a small cluster of neurons at the base of the brain stem (Redmond, 1979; Foote et al., 1983). This nucleus contains most of the central nervous system neurons that use noradrenalin as a neurotransmitter; its central function is to serve as the origin of a large number of radiating fibers (called noradrenergic projections) that fan out to wide areas of the brain, especially to the limbic system, the hypothalamus, and the cerebral cortex. At the same time, the locus ceruleus seems to receive inputs from the major sensory (and pain) systems of the body, channeled through certain key pathways in the brain stem (Aston-Jones et al., 1986.)

Redmond (1979, 1982) and colleagues (Charney et al., 1984) have proposed that the locus ceruleus and its connections mediate the physiologic and behavioral components of anxiety. They observed that anxietylike behavior could be elicited in monkeys by electrical stimulation of the locus ceruleus; furthermore, drugs that increase locus ceruleus firing, such as yohimbine, provoked anxiety reactions in monkeys, in patients with anxiety disorders, and in nonclinical human controls (Redmond & Huang, 1979). The researchers could block these effects (at least temporarily) with drugs that diminish locus ceruleus firing, such as clonidine, or, in animals, by the electrical destruction of the locus ceruleus. Monkeys with experimental lesions of their locus ceruleus do not show the usual emotional response to threats, including the approach of humans or dominant monkeys.

A wide range of sensory and pain pathways indirectly innervate the locus ceruleus. The level of spontaneous locus ceruleus activity in awake monkeys fluctuates with the animal's level of vigilance and arousal (Foote et al., 1980). Noxious stimuli produce a sustained increase in locus ceruleus activity. Connections to and from the cortex may permit subjective awareness of the level of arousal as well as provide the means whereby the meaning or relevance of a stimulus influences the response (see Reiser, 1984).

Other researchers (Aston-Jones et al., 1984) have concluded that the locus ceruleus also performs inhibitory functions; inhibitory inputs to the locus ceruleus, they propose, lead to decreased discharge (or discharge of neurons that have inhibitory connections), thereby decreasing overall arousal and favoring "tonic vegetative behaviors."

These findings and others have prompted the suggestion that the noradrenergic locus ceruleus system serves as a "gating system" or modulator of autonomic tone, balancing the organismic orientation between external and internal environments (Aston-Jones et al., 1984). Further, this hypothesis suggests that the locus ceruleus may be a relay center for an "alarm" system regulating autonomic activity in response to fluctuating external stimuli. According to this hypothesis, stimuli that elicit increased vigilance and arousal might do so by moderately activating the locus ceruleus. These stimuli might include not only actual pain but also situations that lead to anticipation of pain. This mechanism might thus underlie the autonomic and subjective arousal accompanying anticipatory anxiety. Correspondingly, extreme anxiety or fear would result from intense activation of the locus ceruleus (Redmond, 1982).

In its current form, the locus ceruleus hypothesis leaves unanswered whether the locus ceruleus is the primary generator of pathological anxiety attacks (e.g., panic attacks) or whether the locus ceruleus produces anxious arousal in response to overstimulation from other neuronal systems. Although pathological anxiety may result from a persistent dysregulation of brain noradrenergic circuits, neurobiologists remain ignorant of the neuronal and molecular mechanisms that might account for this chronic functional hyperreactivity (Redmond, 1982). However, despite many contradictory and ambiguous findings that preclude uncritical acceptance of the locus ceruleus hypothesis, the theory remains heuristically important and a fertile ground for many valuable research hypotheses.

Other intriguing clues to abnormal brain functioning in anxiety disorders come from the positron emission tomography (PET) studies of Reiman and colleagues (1986). Patients with panic disorder who were vulnerable to lactate-induced panic showed an abnormal asymmetry of cerebral blood flow and oxygen metabolism in a region of the brain known as the right parahippocampal area. These same patients showed an abnormally high whole brain metabolism. Significantly, these abnormalities were present in the resting, nonpanic state and were absent in both normals and patients with panic disorder who were not vulnerable to lactate-induced panic. It is unclear whether these right parahippocampal PET abnormalities represent a local increase in neuronal activity, an asymmetry in neuronal structures, or some other local anomaly. The hippocampus and the structures with which it connects (known collectively as the "limbic system") are evolutionarily ancient structures at the base of the cerebrum that appear to be intimately involved in the expression of memory and affect. The hippocampal system receives abundant noradrenergic projections from the locus ceruleus and has been suspected of playing an important role in the neurobiology of anxiety (Gorman et al., 1989; Gray, 1979). Reiman and colleagues proposed that the parahippocampal abnormality determines vulnerability to panic attacks. Whether these PET abnormalities represent persistent markers of a genetically determined panic-prone disposition is still undetermined.

Benzodiazepine Receptors

The benzodiazepines are a class of antianxiety drugs, the best-known of which, diazepam (Valium), chlordiazepoxide (Librium), and alprazolam (Xanax), are among the most commonly prescribed of all medications. These structurally related drugs appear to have a specific "anxiolytic" or anticonflict effect, reducing subjective anxiety in humans and decreasing conditioned avoidance or conflict behavior in animals. These antianxiety effects occur at doses well below those that produce sedation.

Until 1977, the benzodiazepines' mechanism of action remained obscure. In that year, researchers discovered specific high-affinity receptor or recognition sites on the nerve cell membrane that selectively and reversibly bind the benzodiazepine molecule. The discovery of these benzodiazepine receptors has led to fundamental insights into the biochemical basis of anxiety.

The clinical potency of the various benzodiazepines correlates directly with each drug's affinity for binding with the receptor site. Subsequent research has revealed that binding of the benzodiazepine molecule to the benzodiazepine receptor triggers neurophysiological events that produce the antianxiety effect of the drug. These effects stem from alterations in the neuronal membrane's permeability to the chloride ion; these changes in permeability render the nerve cell less excitable. (Nerve signals are triggered and propagated along the length of the neuron by a cascade of electrochemical changes; these electrochemical currents are caused by transient changes in the nerve cell membrane's permeability to certain key ions.) Because the bulk of the benzodiazepine receptors lie in the neuron's synaptic region, these inhibitory changes can have a potentially far-reaching impact on the transmission of signals from one neuron to the next.

The benzodiazepines, however, cannot produce these effects by themselves. They require the simultaneous presence of another substance, gamma-aminobutyric acid (GABA), a major neurotransmitter whose intrinsic actions are basically inhibitory. Benzodiazepines greatly enhance these inhibitory properties. At the same time, GABA potentiates the binding of benzodiazepine by increasing the receptor's affinity for the drug. These findings have led researchers to hypothesize that the benzodiazepine receptor and the GABA receptor are part of the same large "supramolecular receptor complex" that binds both substances; in turn, the degree to which GABA and benzodiazepine molecules are both bound to this receptor complex regulates the flux of chloride ions through the cell membrane (Paul & Skolnick, 1984).

The possibility that the benzodiazepine-GABA-receptor complex is involved in the pathogenesis of anxiety has given impetus to the search for naturally occurring substances in the body similar to the benzodiazepines, whose existence might shed light on the natural functions of these receptor sites. This search resulted in the discovery of a class of substances called the beta-carbolines, which were extracted from human urine. At first the beta-carbolines were thought to occur naturally in the human body. Subsequently, however, they were shown to be chemical artifacts of the process that was used to extract them from urine. However, despite this initial misapprehension, the beta-carbolines have continued to attract great interest. Their significance lies in their ability to bind tightly to the benzodiazepine receptor site, thereby competitively blocking access to any benzodiaze-pine molecules present. Not only do the beta-carbolines counteract the action of the benzodiazepines, many of them produce intrinsic effects that are just the opposite of the benzodiazepines. Thus, when given experimentally, these beta-carbolines produce agitation, autonomic and adrenal arousal, and a subjective sense of extreme apprehension and "almost intolerable tension" (Dorow et al., 1983). Increases in arousal from small doses of beta-carboline may actually *improve* learning; in contrast, benzodiazepine drugs *lower* arousal and impair learning (Venault et al., 1986). Similarly, moderate levels of anxiety may enhance performance on a variety of tasks; extreme anxiety, however, is disruptive.

Other lines of evidence point to the importance of the benzodiazepine receptors in the genesis and regulation of anxiety. The benzodiazepine receptors occur in especially high density in parts of the limbic system, a structure intimately involved in regulating emotion. Electrical stimulation of these areas produces anxiety symptoms, whereas microinjections of benzodiazepine produce anticonflict effects. Individual differences in the density and distribution of benzodiazepine receptors may also shed light on individual differences in fearfulness (Insel et al., 1984). Conditioned anxiety in rats appears to alter benzodiazepine binding in the brain. Individual monkeys appear to vary in their behavioral sensitivity to the anxiogenic effects of the beta-carbolines. In this connection, Maudsely rats, a strain bred selectively for genetic predisposition to fearfulness, have much lower densities of benzodiazepine receptors, compared with nonfearful cagemates (Robertson et al., 1978).

How the benzodiazepine-GABA-receptor model of anxiety relates to the noradrenergic model of anxiety described above is as yet unclear (Freedman, 1984; Insel et al., 1984).

The Neuroanatomy of Anxiety. The diverse clinical phenomenology and pharmacological responsiveness of the various anxiety disorders suggest that anxiety is not a unitary phenomenon. For example, as Gorman et al. (1989) have observed, antipanic drugs, such as imipramine, block panic attacks but do little to relieve anticipatory anxiety. On the other hand, relaxation training and many benzodiazepines (such as diazepam) reduce anticipatory anxiety, but do little to prevent panic attacks. Phobic anxiety does not appear responsive to either class of medication.

Summary

As this lengthy review suggests, the anxiety disorders are a diverse group of conditions whose pathophysiology in all likelihood involves multiple neurotransmitter systems and brain structures. Attempts to develop a neurophysiological model for these complex phenomena are still highly speculative.

The recent hypothetical model of Gorman et al. (1989) suggests that three basic components of anxiety can be distinguished by clinical presentation and psychopharmacological responsivity: acute panic attacks, anticipatory anxiety, and phobic avoidance. Their model localizes these phenomena in the brain stem, limbic system, and prefrontal cortex, respectively. In support of this hypothesis, Gorman et al. cite a large body of neurophysiological evidence detailing the functional and anatomic connections between these areas. Their model in turn suggests a variety of hypotheses that can be empirically tested using new imaging techniques, pharmacological and neurophysiological studies, and careful trials of cognitive-behavioral treatments.

Clinicians and researchers alike are challenged by the need to integrate the many competing explanatory models of anxiety in both the psychological and neurobiological realms. These models have important implications for treating as well as understanding the various anxiety disorders. The following two chapters use these diverse paradigms to examine in greater detail two childhood anxiety disorders: anxious school refusal and obsessive-compulsive disorder.

Chapter 8

Anxious School Refusal: School Phobia and Separation Anxiety Disorder

INTRODUCTION AND DEFINITION

Historically, the term *school phobia* (or *school refusal*) has denoted a condition in which children repeatedly refuse to go to school and when pressed become anxious or panicked (Johnson et al., 1941). In certain cases, the child asserts that some situation at school (real or potential) makes him afraid; the perceived threat may be a harsh teacher, a bully, the locker room, ridicule from peers, and so on (Last & Francis, 1988). In many other cases, however, "phobia" is a misnomer, for close clinical investigation reveals that the child is not so much frightened of *school* as terrified of *separation* from his mother and home. Both these forms of anxious absenteeism must be distinguished from truancy, which is part of a broader conduct-disordered pattern of oppositional or antisocial behavior.

Because many school-refusing children fear the absence or loss of an attachment figure (such as the mother) or of familiar surroundings (such as home), some authorities have suggested the term *separation anxiety* for this condition (Bowlby, 1973; Estes et al., 1956). In DSM-III-R *Separation Anxiety Disorder* describes a broad category of children with a variety of difficulties and anxieties over separation. Many cases of anxious school refusal best fit under this rubric.

DSM-III-R Diagnostic Criteria for Separation Anxiety Disorder

A. *Excessive anxiety concerning separation from those to whom the child is attached, as evidenced by at least three of the following:*

(1) *unrealistic and persistent worry about possible harm befalling major attachment figures or fear that they will leave and not return*

(2) *unrealistic and persistent worry that an untoward calamitous event will separate the child from a major attachment figure, e.g., the child will be lost, kidnapped, killed, or be the victim of an accident*

(3) *persistent reluctance or refusal to go to school in order to stay with major attachment figures or at home*

(4) *persistent reluctance or refusal to go to sleep without being near major attachment figure or to go to sleep away from home*

(5) *persistent avoidance of being alone, including "clinging" to and "shadowing" major attachment figures*

(6) *repeated nightmares involving the theme of separation*

(7) *complaints of physical symptoms, e.g., headaches, stomachaches, nausea, or vomiting, on many school days or on other occasions when anticipating separation from major attachment figures*

(8) *recurrent signs or complaints of excessive distress in anticipation of separation from home or major attachment figures, e.g., temper tantrums or crying, pleading with parents not to leave*

(9) *recurrent signs or complaints of excessive distress when separated from home or major attachment figures, e.g., wants to return home, needs to call parents when they are absent or when child is away from home*

B. *Duration of disturbance of at least two weeks.*

C. *Onset before the age of 18.*

D. *Occurrence not exclusively during the course of a Pervasive Developmental Disorder, Schizophrenia, or any other psychotic disorder.* (APA, 1987, pp. 60–61)

The categories of school phobia (or school refusal) and Separation Anxiety Disorder are sometimes discussed as if they are synonymous; in fact, they are not identical. Some school phobics do indeed have excessive fear about some aspects of school and do not suffer from separation anxiety; conversely, although a large majority of children with Separation Anxiety Disorder exhibit school refusal, not all do (Last et al., 1987a). The children who avoid school due to fear of some aspect of school often meet the DSM-III-R criteria for another anxiety disorder, such as Simple Phobia, Social Phobia, Avoidant Disorder of Childhood, or Overanxious Disorder (Last & Francis, 1988; Last & Strauss, 1990) (see Chapter 7 for DSM-III-R diagnostic criteria for these disorders).

Unfortunately, much of the literature on anxious school refusal does not distinguish between these diagnostic subtypes. Following historical precedent, in the discussion that follows the term *school phobia* (or "school refusal") refers to nondelinquent, anxious school refusal, with the caveat that this syndrome may represent the outcome of a variety of causes and may occur in the context of a variety of psychiatric disorders (Hersov, 1985b).

EPIDEMIOLOGY

The precise incidence of school refusal is unknown. Especially in younger children, mild, transient cases may resolve with parental support, sometimes aided by the pediatrician's reassurance. The rate of detection varies with the awareness of school personnel and parents and the degree of surveillance of attendance. Estimates range from 3 to 17 cases per 1000 schoolchildren each year (Gordon & Young, 1976; Granell de Aldaz et al., 1984; Ollendick & Mayer, 1984). Apparently, the disorder is equally common in both sexes. The condition may occur more frequently in upper socioeconomic status (SES) groups (Hersov, 1960a); however, the gender and SES distribution appears to differ across diagnostic subgroups (Last et al., 1987a).

CLINICAL FEATURES

Transient symptoms, associated with the child's wish to remain cozily at home rather than go to school, can occur as a normal vicissitude of separation and individuation. This is especially likely after an illness, vacation, or family upheaval. The Monday morning or postvacation blues of adults represents a common equivalent of the same dynamics. The child's drive for autonomy and his investment in friends, learning, and outside interests are usually sufficiently strong and gratifying enough to get him off to school (albeit sometimes not without parental encouragement and firmness).

In contrast, the school-phobic child not only fears but misses many or all days of school, usually remaining at home during school hours. He complains of not feeling well, refuses to get dressed, and finds a multitude of excuses for not going to school each day. Not infrequently, the child elaborates vague complaints such as headaches, stomachaches, or dizziness that represent, in part, rationalizations and, in part, psychosomatic anxiety symptoms. Frequent trips to the pediatrician may not uncover any physical findings. If the parent challenges the child's complaints, his level of protest rises exponentially, the symptoms inflame, and he is in despair. Once the parent relents and the child is permitted to stay at home (or once school hours are over), the symptoms abate; the youngster rarely mentions his physical complaints on weekends (Waldfogel et al., 1957). In general, school-day mornings are the most difficult times of all. If forced to go to school, the child may panic, putting up violent resistance, hiding under the bed, or running from the car. Bribes, threats, reassurance, entreaties, punishments, and appeals to reason are all equally ineffective. Anxiety appears to be most intense just before the child leaves home or is on the way to school.

Some youngsters complain about unfair teachers, bullies, or the indignities of showers, the locker room, or gym. Addressing these issues with the school personnel may sometimes enable the child to return to school. These cases might accurately deserve the term *phobic* (or fearful) *avoidance of school*. In many cases, however, the apprehensions prove to be mere surface versions of a deeply rooted inner anxiety; in such instances, even elaborate environmental manipulations involving changes of teacher or school fail to secure the child's return to school.

The clinical course and presentation vary. Onset or exacerbations often occur after a brief illness, vacation, or weekend. School phobia may begin acutely following a trauma that raises the child and/or family's anxiety, such as a death or family loss or upheaval. It may also follow other anxiety-producing changes, such as a move or change of school. Many cases have their onset with the transitions from elementary school to junior high school or from junior high to high school. In acute cases where the clinician can identify clear precipitants, the degree of overall pathology in the child and family is often less severe and pervasive than in chronic cases of more insidious onset (Baker & Wills, 1978). In older children and adolescents, a gradual onset is more common and may represent the culmination of a progressive withdrawal from peer activities. In such cases, the school refusal is often part of an overall inability to deal with the demands for age-appropriate coping with peers or for independent functioning (Coolidge et al., 1957; Hersov, 1985b).

Close examination of the child and family usually reveals major problems outside the area of school attendance. Many such children are tightly bound to their families, and concerns about separation and ambivalence toward attachment figures often pervade the entire family's functioning (Bowlby, 1973). Along with school attendance, the child has often abandoned most friends and outside activities; there may be few remaining interests or pulls to lure him away from home. Unable to go to school, the child spends the day at home or accompanies his mother on her errands, serving as her companion and guardian. Unlike the truant who runs away from school to wander off and have fun, the school phobic avoids school to stay close to his mother and home.

School-phobic children often appear subdued and miserable, with little *joie de vivre*. Although they may be intellectually bright, the development of their autonomy is stunted, and their social interactions with peers are frustrating. Free-floating anxiety is common, especially concerning death and separation. These fears may manifest themselves as a fear of falling asleep or of sleeping alone, worries about burglars or accidents, and concern that death, illness, or abandonment will afflict their parents or themselves. Nightmares with much morbid content of similar character may be frequent.

Depression is a frequent concomitant of school phobia (Hersov, 1985b; Kolvin et al., 1984; Waldron et al., 1975). It may be difficult to distinguish the symptoms of anxiety from those of depression (Bernstein & Garfinkel, 1986). Some authors regard school phobia or separation anxiety as part of the natural history of childhood depression; from this perspective, the affective illness is the underlying disorder (Agras, 1959; Geller et al., 1985). On the other hand, Gittleman-Klein and Klein (1973) have argued that the depressive symptoms of school phobics represent demoralization, secondary to the limitations imposed by their primary anxiety disorder. This important question remains unresolved; in practice it is often difficult to distinguish between the primary disorder and the secondary disorder (Bernstein & Garfinkel, 1986). (Chapter 7 deals further with frequent co-occurrence and family aggregation of depression and anxiety.) Theoretical issues aside, the depression in these children can be severe and disabling. In Shaffer's (1974) psychological postmortem of childhood suicides, four of the children had suffered from school refusal.

Developmental Considerations

When first attending nursery school or a play group, preschoolers commonly experience initial anxiety; with parental and teacher support, most adapt rapidly (Slater et al., 1939). In the preschool histories of many school-phobic children, however, persistent separation difficulties with frightened clinging and weeping are apparent. The child's anxiety about separation may be magnified when the mother experiences corresponding and contagious anxiety about leaving the child. The young child, however, does not yet have an internal conflict between the desire for independent functioning and the fear of being apart. The clinginess is expressed openly and directly, and somatization is rare.

The latency-age school phobic is more ashamed of dependent longings. He does not express them overtly and may in fact deny them, even to himself. Instead, neurotic defenses, such as displacement, avoidance, and somatization help ward off direct awareness of the child's painful anxiety concerning the availability of his mother (or father) as an attachment figure.

Because in adolescence the developmental push toward separation and independence is normally extremely strong, school phobia during that epoch usually indicates serious underlying pathology and carries a more ominous prognosis than symptoms that appear in earlier childhood. Although school phobia may first be explicitly diagnosed in adolescence, a careful history often reveals a long series of frequent school absences with implicit collusion by the parents in the child's separation avoidance (Coolidge et al., 1960).

Differential Diagnosis

Delinquent Truancy. The truant usually avoids both home and school for the pleasures of friends and the excitement of the streets. Unlike the school phobic, he shows little anxiety about separation or conflict about school absences; rather, his school avoidance appears as part of a broader pattern of conduct disorder. In general, such truants are less passive, dependent, and academically proficient than the school phobic (Hersov, 1985b). Compared with the school phobic's family, the delinquent's family is less likely to be overprotective and anxiously hovering and is more likely to be large, poor, and indifferent.

Learning Disabilities. The child with learning disabilities often experiences school as an ongoing traumatic experience that constantly challenges his self-esteem and sense of competency. After many episodes of academic failure, the learning-disabled child may wish to avoid classroom activities. However, unlike the school phobic, he still takes pleasure in nonacademic school activities, such as gym and recess, and enjoys the companionship of peers. Moreover, excessive separation anxiety is not present. In contrast, school phobics are often bright and have less difficulty with the academic than with the social aspects of school.

Diagnostic Subtypes

At times school phobia has been treated as if it is almost synonymous with separation anxiety disorder. However, careful clinical examination of patients and a review of the literature suggest that the syndrome is heterogeneous in etiology, associated psychopathology, course, prognosis, and hence optimal treatment (Atkinson et al., 1985; Hersov, 1985b; Hersov & Berg, 1980; Last & Strauss, 1990; Waldron et al., 1975). Waldron et al. (1975) concluded that there are four overlapping types of school phobia.

Type 1. The "family interaction" type includes cases of school refusal due to separation anxiety in the context of a mutually hostile, dependent, clinging relationship between child and parent (most often mother).

Type 2. The "classic phobic type" includes phobias of school based on "the defenses of displacement, projection, and externalization"; these differ from other childhood phobias only in the child's greater need for his mother's presence.

Type 3. The "acute anxiety type" is characterized by the child's "overwhelming conscious concern" about a parent's safety in the child's absence; an actual danger exists in many such cases.

Type 4. The "situational-characterological type" involves "fear of real situations in school that threaten the child with failure, loss of self-esteem, or even bodily harm"; however, the child's sense of great vulnerability to these situations (which others may take in stride) often stems from long-standing characterological difficulties in autonomy and self-esteem.

Last and colleagues (1987a) have reemphasized the importance of distinguishing between separation anxiety and true social or simple phobias regarding school as causes of school refusal. Because anxiety about social evaluative/performance concerns is so common and severe in adolescent school phobics, many cases warrant a diagnosis of *social phobia* of school (Last & Francis, 1988). Last and Francis note that in contrast to separation-anxious children, the truly phobic children's fears reflect avoidance, are well circumscribed, and are limited to the school situation. When not in school, these children may not require the mother's presence or the security of home to feel comfortable. In a clinic-referred sample of anxious school refusers, Last and Strauss (1990) found 38% met DSM-III-R criteria for separation anxiety disorder; 30%, for social phobia; 22%, for simple phobia; and 10%, for other anxiety disorders.

Using a variety of measures, Last and colleagues (1987a; Last & Strauss, 1990) compared children with a phobic avoidance of school (based on a simple or social phobia) and children with separation anxiety disorder (three-fourths of whom also exhibited school refusal). Compared with separation anxious school refusers, phobic school refusers had later onset and severer school refusal. More children with separation anxiety disorder were female, prepubertal, and came from lower socioeconomic circumstances. Depression and other anxiety disorders were common concurrent diagnoses in both groups; however, the children with separation anxiety disorder appeared more severely disturbed. Depression and anxiety were frequent in the mothers of both groups, but, compared with the mothers of phobic children, the mothers of the children with separation anxiety disorders were significantly more likely to suffer from depression and to have a history of school refusal of their own.

ETIOLOGY

Family Factors

Anxious school refusal is often rooted in familywide concerns about separation (Bowlby, 1973; Eisenberg, 1958b; Waldron et al., 1975). Although in younger and less severe acute cases, these fears may be the result of an isolated trauma, such as a death or other loss, a long-standing pattern of family pathology is common (Coolidge et al., 1957; Malmquist, 1965; Waldfogel et al., 1957). Compared with matched psychiatric controls, parents and siblings of children with school phobias or separation anxiety disorders show a higher prevalence of depression and anxiety disorders (Bernstein & Garfinkel, 1988). However, anxiety and affective disorders appear to be more prevalent in the mothers of children with separation anxiety disorder than in the mothers of children with true phobias concerning school (Last et al., 1987a).

In the most common pattern, the child's anxieties about separation reflect the fears of a parent (usually the mother) about the hazards of independent functioning. When exploring the backgrounds of the mothers of school phobics, clinicians often discover a history of childhood school phobia or agoraphobia (Berg, 1976; Last & Strauss, 1990). These families, which Malmquist termed *phobogenic,* tend to convey an implicit or even explicit view that life outside the family is hostile and ungratifying. School phobics' mothers have a high incidence of depression and frequently have a history of unresolved, anxious, and ambivalent attachment to their own mothers, which they reenact in their relationship with their school-phobic child (Bowlby, 1973). Although the school phobic's mother views herself as providing much-needed protection for the child against the slings and arrows of a harsh and unsympathetic world, in fact, the child often serves as her companion and buffer. The school-refusing child may be the mother's closest confidant, to whom she unburdens her marital problems. At the same time, even though she has implicitly fostered the child's excessive demands, the mother may resent them. Many school phobics, although shy and passive outside the home, are domineering and bullying toward their mothers. This behavior, too, may recapitulate a dependent, yet resentful relationship between the phobic's mother and her own mother.

Marital problems are common in such families. At work, the fathers generally experience little trouble with their autonomous functioning. At home, however, they are often passive or distant. They thus leave the mother emotionally deprived and fail to provide the child with an available ally or model for differentiation and separation (Skynner, 1974). The child senses himself without an anchor against the powerful current of his own and his mother's dependent yearnings. Other aspects of family functioning are also disturbed. Using the Family Assessment Measure, Bernstein et al. (1990) found that, by the parents' reports, the families of school phobics had relatively poor role definition and lacked consistency between explicit and implicit family rules. The families of children with comorbid depression appeared more impaired in these areas than those of children with anxiety disorder alone.

CASE EXAMPLE

The therapist first saw David X, an obese 12-year-old boy, after he had been out of school for a year. Despite the parents' avowed concern, school officials found them to be unhelpful in returning David to school. Mrs. X complained that no one at the school understood David's special needs and that the school's insistence that he return to class was uncaring and insensitive. Mr. X was unwilling to set firm limits with his son. If pressed to go to school, David refused, complaining of "dizziness and headaches." Mrs. X, a housewife, had no outside interests or friends and was afraid of driving anywhere alone. When David remained at home, his mother cooked various delicacies for him and told him her sorrows. Although David was allegedly too ill to go to school, he and his mother would frequently go shopping together. The father, a government official and workaholic, spent long hours away from home at his job. The parents rarely went out together, and Mr. X would usually occupy his evening hours reading and working.

Clinicians often observe another pathological pattern of family interaction in this disorder involving the parent's and/or child's belief that something terrible will happen to one or the other of them while the child is away at school (Bowlby, 1973). The child thus remains (or is kept) at home to prevent the feared event. Indeed, the commonest explanation that school-phobic children give for their behavior is that they fear something might happen to mother in their absence (Hersov, 1960a, 1960b). For example, a 12-year-old boy confessed that he stayed home because, while in school, he worried that burglars might break into his house and shoot his mother "three times in the stomach."

The origins of these fearful fantasies vary. In some instances they appear to represent warded off and externalized hostile wishes whose magical fulfillment the child must guard against. The child unconsciously wishes that something bad would assail the parents and must then cope with the reactions of his conscience. Other authors have emphasized the importance of *actual* misfortunes that occur in the family such as death, separations, and accidents, or the impact of overt threats of abandonment used coercively by parents against the child (Bowlby, 1973).

CASE EXAMPLE

John D, age 9 years, was hospitalized on an inpatient child psychiatry unit because of long-standing school phobia refractory to all attempts at outpatient treatment. John refused to go to school; if physically carried to school by his mother and uncle, he would run away as soon as they left and would hide in an abandoned house across the street from home. There John would spend the day keeping an anxious watch on his house through the window.

On the ward John was a frail, chronically anxious boy, with constricted affect and many learning disabilities. He appeared homesick, whiny, and unhappy. Mrs. D, a depressed and overwhelmed cleaning lady, recounted the family's traumatic and painful history. John and his father, a kindly but limited man, had shared a close relationship. When John was 4 years old, Mr. D had been devastatingly disabled by an anoxic episode during minor surgery. After enduring a lengthy hospitalization, the father now functioned at a retarded level and showed many organic personality changes; he spent his days either at home or at a sheltered workshop. The following year, another catastrophe befell the family. While caring for John, his beloved maternal grandmother suffered a disabling and ultimately fatal stroke. Faced with these stresses, Mrs. D had felt doubly bereft and burdened, and she turned increasingly to John for consolation and support. When feeling overwhelmed with depression or upset about John's misbehavior, his mother would frequently complain, "I can't take it anymore" or "It's killing me." John resented his mother's demands on him but worried about her depression; he feared that she too would become ill or die, leaving him all alone.

In other cases, the child (or parent) may fear that something terrible will befall the child while away from home (Bowlby, 1973). Thus, following her parents' separation and the father's disappearance to another state, an 8-year-old girl refused to go to school. The child both feared and wished that her father might kidnap her from school and felt that she must keep her eye on her mother, lest she too disappear. Mother made only feeble efforts to send her daughter to school. She had felt bereft at her husband's departure and clung to her daughter for solace and comfort.

In summary then, the basic mechanism of school phobia due to separation anxiety is usually the anxious attachment of the child to his parents. This attachment develops because one or more family members believe that separation is dangerous or hurtful and that the family can maintain safety and caring only if the child abandons his autonomous strivings and remains close to home.

Most accounts of these family influences emphasize mutual patterns of anxious attachment, shared family assumptions regarding the dangers of separation and the perils lurking in the external world, and the intrafamilial communication of anxiety. Such factors may account for the observation that a history of anxiety, especially agoraphobia or school phobia, is common among the mothers of children who refuse school because of separation anxiety. As noted in the previous chapter, however, substantial evidence suggests that genetic factors are also at work in the familial transmission of anxiety (Marks, 1987). To what extent such shared biological factors play a role in the school phobic family's pervasive atmosphere of anxiety remains unclear. If genetic factors are at work, the exact nature of the inherited vulnerability is also unclear. Just as depression is very common in children with separation anxiety, so too is the co-occurrence of depression and anxiety in their mothers (Last et al., 1987a).

Extrafamilial School-Related Factors

Under certain conditions, the school refuser's complaints about school, classmates, and teachers may serve as externalizations or rationalizations of separation anxiety, but this is not always the case (Granell de Aldaz et al., 1987; Hersov, 1985b; Last & Francis, 1987; Last & Strauss, 1990; Waldron et al., 1975). The two factors often overlap in ways that may be difficult to disentangle. On the one hand, the presence of a trusted companion improves most phobias (Bowlby, 1973). Hence, clinging to mother may occur even when the origin of the fear is located at school. On the other hand, overprotected children, whose anxious parents see the outside world as fraught with danger, are more likely to worry about bullies, harsh teachers, unfamiliar surroundings, and the stress of locker rooms, showers, and gyms.

Although most of the literature on separation anxiety focuses on separation from the mother, separation from familiar peers may also cause significant anxiety. For example, Field (1984) studied a preschool class of 3- to 5-year-olds during the 2 weeks before and the 2 weeks after the transfer of half the children to another school. Before the transfer, the departing students showed considerable anticipatory anxiety, which they manifested in fantasy and drawings, absenteeism, toileting accidents, eating and sleep problems, fussiness, and increased aggressive behavior, physical activity level, and tonic heart rate. After their departure, this agitated behavior decreased in the children who left but increased for those children who remained in the original school.

Neurobiological Factors

As noted in the discussions of failure-to-thrive (Chapter 1), depression (Chapter 6), and anxiety (Chapter 7), a good deal of animal research bears on these syndromes. The profound behavioral disturbances produced by separating young mammals from their caretakers are accompanied by significant neurobiological and metabolic changes. The neurophysiological mechanisms underlying attachment, separation anxiety, and their disorders are still poorly understood. The extent to which individual or familial aberrations in these underlying mechanisms might predispose an individual to separation anxiety is also unknown.

Psychopharmacological evidence provides a few tantalizing clues concerning these theoretically and therapeutically important questions. Several strands of evidence suggest that endogenous opioid (endorphin) systems (perhaps in the limbic area of the brain) are important in creating, maintaining, and regulating the comfort derived from mother–child contact (and the anxiety attendant on its disruption). Thus, even in very small doses, the opioid agonists markedly decrease separation distress in various species, whereas opioid antagonists markedly increase it (Herman & Panksepp, 1981; Panksepp et al., 1980).

Iatrogenic school phobia as a side effect of neuroleptic drugs such as haloperidol and pimozide has been observed primarily during the drug treatment of patients with Tourette's syndrome (Mikkelsen et al., 1981); accordingly, the condition has been named "the neuroleptic separation anxiety syndrome" (Linet, 1985). These medications may precipitate the sudden onset of severe separation anxiety including school refusal, clinging behavior, fear of being trapped in school, and worries about parental death. The symptoms remit with discontinuation of the neuroleptic. There is tentative evidence that tricyclic antidepressants may counter this side effect (Linet, 1985). To what extent sensitivity to this neuroleptic side effect is specific to Tourette's syndrome is unknown.

TREATMENT

Most authors view school phobia as a true psychiatric emergency. They state that to avoid chronicity it is mandatory to initiate a concerted effort to return the child to school as soon as the pattern of school refusal is clear (Eisenberg, 1958a, 1958b; Leventhal et al., 1967). The longer the child stays home, the more difficult it becomes for him to return to school: Friendships and group ties attenuate, homework and exams accumulate, and the unconfronted fear of going to school burgeons in the child's imagination (Eisenberg, 1959). The clinician who permits the child to remain at home for a prolonged period while undertaking treatment often risks stagnation and a false treatment alliance. Until the child and family actively confront their separation anxiety and attempt school attendance, the conflictual meaning and affects concerning separation may not be available to therapy. Often, it is only in the attempt to return the child to school that the mother or father's ambivalence about the separation becomes apparent (Leventhal et al., 1967). The clinician must carefully scrutinize the parents' failure to act firmly and authoritatively with the child about attending school. Some authors, however, take issue with insisting in all cases on immediate return to school (Davidson, 1960; Greenbaum, 1964; Hersov, 1960a; Talbot, 1957). They argue that excessive pressure may precipitate panic or even suicide attempts. In their view, a period of compromise, including home tutoring, may be necessary to escape the tug-of-war about attendance and to permit initiation of treatment.

Effective treatment of school phobia usually requires a flexible combination of individual and family therapy, together with work with the parents as a couple. Treatment of the child alone usually cannot extricate him from the web of conflicted family interactions regarding separation. The clinician must pay considerable attention to restructuring the parents' attitudes and managing the child's nonattendance. Indeed, final outcome and degree of improvement in the child often correlate closely with the effectiveness of therapeutic work with the parents. Collaboration between the therapist and school authorities can help to reduce the parents' anxiety about school as a dangerous place and to support the parents in their efforts.

When school phobia remains refractory to outpatient therapy, hospitalization may be necessary to break the impasse. Frankly confronting both the parents and the child with this alternative often stiffens parental resolve and motivates the child to try to return to school. Cases that do not respond to less intensive measures or where the families are too disturbed to participate in outpatient treatment may indeed require hospitalization, which can help the family and child experience and master the separation that they so much fear (Hersov, 1980, 1985b).

Even after the child has returned to school, it is important to continue treatment. Relapses are common, or the anxiety may take some other symptomatic form. In some instances, unless the family's basic anxieties over separation have been adequately addressed, when the child's symptoms ebb, another sibling takes the place of the one who has apparently recovered and begins in turn to remain home with the mother (Granell de Aldaz et al., 1987). Some families may stage a collusive "flight into health" and break off treatment with the child's return to school. The return represents the price the child and parent are willing to pay to avoid deeper and seemingly more threatening examination of their mutual enmeshment.

CASE EXAMPLE (*continued*)

David was seen in both individual and family therapy. In his individual work, he was able to acknowledge his conflicting feelings. When he remained at home, he had the pleasure of being waited on hand and foot and did not have to suffer any of the ordinary difficulties of school, such as making friends and worrying about girls. David, however, felt burdened and irritated by his mother's constant presence, and he was troubled about what would become of her when (or if) he grew up and moved away.

In the concurrent family therapy it became possible to elaborate the ways in which David had become the symptomatic bearer of the entire family's separation and dependency problems. Mr. X's counterdependent involvement in work and avoidance of his wife and family recapitulated his earlier relationship with his own depressed, clinging mother. In the course of treatment it also emerged that Mrs. X had never mourned the death of her own mother 5 years earlier and had thus never worked through the intense, even suffocating, but ambivalent relationship the two women had shared. Because Mrs. X was able to talk about her disappointment in her husband, she was also able to acknowledge her profound longing for closeness, a need she had sought to satisfy by turning to her son. David had made some tentative moves out of the family orbit, such as his now-abandoned lengthy phone calls to friends. Mrs. X had treated these calls as betrayals, foreshadowing David's abandoning her, even as she felt Mr. X had done.

As these issues were worked on in treatment, Mr. X became more involved around the house, Mrs. X contemplated returning to work for the first time since her marriage, and the family's need for David to remain home with his mother lessened. With a less guilty and more united front between his mother and father, David was able to get back to school; he did, however, remain vulnerable to relapses in resonance with his parents' marital upsets and in reaction to difficulties with teachers or peers.

Behavior Modification

Learning theory suggests that for treatment to be effective, an analysis of current factors reinforcing the child's nonattendance is essential. Thus, Ross (1972) proposed that initially school avoidance is reinforced by its fear-reducing function; subsequently, however, the reinforcements available at home maintain it. Dynamic theories also suggest that the secondary gains of remaining at home, such as the mother's attention and implicit or explicit approval, are important in perpetuating the child's symptoms. The average child finds the company of peers and the pleasures of mastery at school sufficiently rewarding to maintain attendance; in contrast, the vulnerable child, whose overprotective family has supported the use of avoidance to cope with anxiety, easily withdraws in the face of school challenges (Hersov, 1985b).

Behavior modification techniques, such as systematic desensitization and operant conditioning, have been widely reported. They appear to be most successful with school phobia in acute cases with good premorbid histories (Hersen, 1971; Ollendick & Mayer, 1984; Pattersen, 1965). Traditional psychotherapy also utilizes many of the techniques described in this literature, albeit in a less systematic manner (Miller et al., 1972a). These interventions include identifying and altering parental behaviors that reinforce school avoidance and verbally rehearsing the return to school with the child to identify, titrate, and master his anxiety. In some systematic desensitization paradigms the therapist, in the course of several sessions, accompanies the child through gradually expanded segments of the trip to school. Where the child is actually phobic about some aspect of the school situation, he is progressively reintroduced into the phobic situation for increasing periods, accompanied by a parent, therapist, or close friend (Eysenck & Rachman, 1965; Talbot, 1957). A hazard of the purely behavioral approach, however, is that it may not adequately address pathogenic family processes and the related character problems of the child. Successful utilization of behavioral techniques requires the parents to collaborate effectively in changing behaviors that presumably have reinforced the child's nonattendance.

Medication

The observation that tricyclic antidepressants prevent the panic attacks of adult agoraphobics has led to the discovery that drugs of this class, such as imipramine, can provide a dramatically useful adjunct to the treatment of school phobia (Gittleman-Klein & Klein, 1973, 1980). In one study a group of school phobics had remained absent from school despite a fortnight's intensive therapeutic effort by a psychiatric team. At that point, either placebo or imipramine were randomly added to their treatment regimen. Psychiatric treatment continued with both groups, but by the end of 6 weeks 81% of the imipramine-treated youngsters had returned to school compared with only 47% of the placebo group. Furthermore, imipramine had a marked impact on subjectively reported separation anxiety. All of the children on imipramine reported feeling much better (even those who did not return to school) compared with only 21% of the children on placebo. This finding is of interest because, despite their improved attendance, many school-phobic children who return to school continue to suffer from marked separation anxiety. Imipramine may thus be a helpful adjunct to psychotherapy for such children.

Work with adult agoraphobics has led to the distinction between *panic anxiety* at times of actual separation, and secondary *anticipatory anxiety,* which may be a conditioned response to the panic attacks. Imipramine appears to be more effective in preventing the panic attacks rather than in reducing anticipatory anxiety. Although Gittleman-Klein and Klein (1973) regard imipramine as specific for school refusal caused by separation anxiety, it may also be equally helpful in cases of phobic anxiety associated with school-related factors (Last, personal communication, 1988).

Most children require doses of 75–200 mg/day of imipramine. Separation anxiety usually begins to lessen within 3 weeks, although return to school may take longer because of pathogenic individual and family dynamics and the persistence of anticipatory anxiety. (For details and precautions regarding the administration of tricyclic antidepressants, see Chapter 6, "Affective Disorders" Chapter 11, "Attention-deficit Hyperactivity Disorder," and Chapter 17, "Disorders of Elimination—I. Enuresis"; the upper limit of 5 mg/kg/day should not be exceeded.)

Treatment Outcome and Course of Illness

Following various lengths of treatment, two-thirds or more of treated school phobics return to school (Coolidge et al., 1964; Hersov, 1960a, 1960b, 1985b; Weiss & Cain, 1964). Measured by this criterion, success is greater with children who are younger, have less severe pathology, and receive early treatment (Eisenberg, 1958b; Rodriguez et al., 1959). The various follow-up studies indicate that it is easier to achieve success in returning the child to school than in helping him with ongoing emotional problems (Berg & Jackson, 1985; Berg et al., 1976; Weiss & Burke, 1970). Coolidge et al., (1964) found in a 10-year follow-up that although 47 of 49 children treated with psychotherapy had returned to school, more than 50% of them led "colorless, restricted, unimaginative lives, with delayed or absent heterosexual development, excessive dependency, [and] blunted affect . . . " (p. 683). Other studies also demonstrate that anxiety, over-dependence, constriction, and poor peer relations frequently persist in children after they return to school (Berg & Jackson, 1985; Warren, 1965; Weiss & Burke, 1970).

The many apparent parallels between the separation anxiety disorder of childhood and agoraphobia in adults have raised the question of whether school phobia is a common precursor of agoraphobia. The results of these studies have been equivocal.

Various retrospective studies are inconsistent as to whether a childhood history of school phobia is more common among adult agoraphobics than among other clinical comparison groups (Gittleman, 1986). However, agoraphobic women who *do* have a childhood history of school phobia have an earlier onset of their agoraphobia along with more severe symptoms. They are also more likely to have school-phobic children than are agoraphobic women without such a history (Berg, 1976). Thus, school phobics are apparently predisposed toward later anxiety and emotional difficulties but not to any specific diagnosis (Hersov, 1985b).

Chapter 9

Obsessive-Compulsive Disorder

INTRODUCTION

Obsessive-compulsive disorder (OCD) is a disabling disorder in which the child is repeatedly beseiged with unwanted thoughts or internal urges to perform seemingly senseless acts over and over again. The term *obsession* (from the Latin *obsidere*, "to beseige") refers to recurrent, unwanted thoughts, often repugnant in content, that intrude unbidden on consciousness evoking anxiety or discomfort (Insel, 1984). Intrusive mental images may accompany these thoughts; in addition, they often involve sexual or aggressive ideas that the patient regards as morally reprehensible. For example, an otherwise obedient and devoted child might be tormented by the thought, "My mother's a whore" or "I'm covered with shit." This sequence keeps recurring against the child's conscious desire and despite efforts to put it out of mind.

The term *compulsion* refers to repetitive acts that the patient feels internally compelled or pressured to perform, even though the act seems senseless or excessive; the patient can resist these intense urges only with considerable tension or discomfort (Insel, 1984). Performing these acts brings little pleasure, only relief of tension. The commonest compulsions are concerned with warding off contamination (e.g., repetitive hand washing) or involve some pathological doubt (e.g., repeatedly checking the stove to allay the recurrent and groundless fear of having left it on). These latter symptoms led Esquirol, an early observer of the syndrome, to call it *folie de doute*, "the doubting madness." To be diagnosed with this disorder, the child's symptoms must be severe enough to cause significant distress or to interfere with his daily life. Furthermore, the child must experience the thoughts or impulses as unwelcome and struggle against them (in which case they are termed "ego-dystonic").

Despite its rarity, OCD holds great theoretical fascination (aside from the obvious importance of finding relief for its sufferers). From a philosophical viewpoint, the disorder illustrates just how slippery and illusive is the concept of human will. The patient "thinks" his obsessional thought and yet experiences it as not his own; he wants urgently to perform his compulsive act and yet at the same time strives desperately to resist the urge. Historically, the illness was important in developing Freud's (1894/1962b, 1909/1955b, 1913/1958) thought, for it dramatically illustrated his central concept of unconscious conflict. In Freud's view, the obsessional patient suffers from anxiety-provoking internal conflict aroused by troublesome hostile or sexual impulses that he then handles in characteristic ways. Obsessive-compulsive symptom formation vividly demonstrates the characteristic defense mechanisms that such patients employ to ward off intolerable impulses from consciousness: denial, isolation, reaction formation, undoing, magical thinking, doubting, and intellectualization. (For a more detailed discussion of these mechanisms, see pp. 282–286.) As Anna Freud put it,

"No other mental phenomena display. . . with equal clarity the human quandary of relentless and unceasing battles between innate impulses and acquired moral demands" (Nagera, 1976, p. 9).

Many questions remain regarding the genesis of this disorder. Freud (1913/1958) speculated that constitutional or hereditary factors strongly influence the obsessional's choice of symptoms. In addition to psychodynamic explanations of its symptoms, researchers have invoked genetic and organic factors, child-rearing patterns, operant conditioning, and social learning theory to explain this condition. These debates have raised fascinating but still unanswered questions concerning the relationship of this disorder to a host of other conditions: anxiety disorders, depression, temporal lobe epilepsy, anorexia, schizophrenia, and Tourette's syndrome (TS). Perhaps of greatest concern, however, is the troublesome fact that the treatment of OCD remains controversial and frequently unsatisfactory. Without better treatment methods, many obsessive-compulsive children are doomed to become painfully suffering obsessive-compulsive adults.

DEFINITION

The pathological symptoms of true obsessive-compulsive disorder must be distinguished on the one hand from the broad range of mild rituals and obsessions that occur as part of normal development, and on the other, from the obsessive-compulsive character type historically associated with this disorder.

"Normal" Obsessions and Compulsions

Rituals, repetition, and a certain degree of compulsiveness are expectable and adaptive aspects of normal child development (Leonard et al., 1990). On a dynamic, as well as a descriptive level, obsessive-compulsive defenses are also part of everyday adult psychic life. To a greater or lesser extent, we all employ defenses such as intellectualization, isolation, reaction formation, magical thinking, and undoing to cope with the uncertainties and dangers of both our inner and outer lives. Furthermore, these concerns transcend the individual. Central features of many religious and cultural practices concern ordering the world into the clean and the unclean, the licit and the illicit, the sacred and the profane; along with these go means for avoiding dangerous contamination and taboos plus rituals for purification and expiation (Douglas, 1970). Such concerns are also the stuff of many superstitions (Leonard, 1989b). By these devices both the social group and its individual members seek to safeguard themselves from external disasters and the disruptive effects of untamed lust, greed, and aggression.

Transient obsessions and compulsions are a common, perhaps universal, experience. From time to time, almost everyone gets "hung up" on a melody or distracted by a bit of doggerel that repeats and won't go away, or is assailed by recurrently intrusive, distasteful, and unacceptable thoughts and impulses. In an intriguing comparison of obsessive-compulsive patients and nonclinical subjects, Rachman and de Silva (1978) found that the form, and to some extent, the content of both groups' obsessions were similar. However, the differences in frequency, intensity, and consequences were critical. Compared with the patient sample, the obsessions of nonclinical subjects were rarer, briefer, and more easily dismissed. Furthermore, these "normal" obsessions were less vivid, less ego-alien and discomforting, and less likely either to provoke efforts at neutralization or to be accompanied by compulsive acts.

Obsessive-Compulsive Disorder

To exclude these normal obsessional phenomena of everyday life, the DSM-III-R criteria for OCD require that obsessions or compulsions be of sufficient intensity or frequency to significantly distress or interfere with the patient's normal routine or social or occupational functioning. In addition, these criteria require that the subject regard the thoughts or impulses as senseless and try to resist them.

DSM-III-R Diagnostic Criteria for Obsessive-Compulsive Disorder

A. *Either obsessions or compulsions:*
   Obsessions: (1), (2), (3), and (4):
   (1) *recurrent and persistent ideas, thoughts, impulses, or images that are experienced, at least initially, as intrusive and senseless, e.g., a parent's having repeated impulses to kill a loved child, a religious person's having recurrent blasphemous thoughts*
   (2) *the person attempts to ignore or suppress such thoughts or impulses or to neutralize them with some other thought or action*
   (3) *the person recognizes that the obsessions are the product of his or her own mind, not imposed from without (as in thought insertion)*
   (4) *if another Axis I disorder is present, the content of the obsession is unrelated to it, e.g., the ideas, thoughts, impulses, or images are not about food in the presence of an Eating Disorder, about drugs in the presence of a Psychoactive Substance Use Disorder, or guilty thoughts in the presence of a Major Depression*
   Compulsions: (1), (2), and (3):
   (1) *repetitive, purposeful, and intentional behaviors that are performed in response to an obsession, or according to certain rules or in a stereotyped fashion*
   (2) *the behavior is designed to neutralize or to prevent discomfort or some dreaded event or situation; however, either the activity is not connected in a realistic way with what it is designed to neutralize or prevent, or it is clearly excessive*

(3) the person recognizes that his or her behavior is excessive or unreasonable (this may not be true for young children; it may no longer be true for people whose obsessions have evolved into overvalued ideas)

B. *The obsessions or compulsions cause marked distress, are time-consuming (take more than an hour a day), or significantly interfere with the person's normal routine, occupational functioning, or usual social activities or relationships with others.* (APA, 1987, p. 247)

Diagnosis of this disorder thus relies heavily on the patient's subjective accounts of his symptoms. For the clinical researcher, the objective measurement and quantification of complex mental processes such as resistance, interference, and ego-dystonia pose major problems. As a result, although various rating instruments have been developed for assessing obsessive-compulsive symptoms, much more work is needed, especially with children, to ensure their reliability and validity (Berg et al., 1988; Goodman et al., 1989; Towbin et al., 1987).

Obsessive-Compulsive Character Type

Historically, certain character traits have been associated with the propensity to employ obsessive-compulsive defenses (Freud, 1908/1959). Reaction formation and undoing may lead to a marked wariness toward instinctual expression on every level. The obsessive-compulsive personality eschews aggression and instinctual libidinal pleasures, whether oral, anal, or genital; hence, such individuals become extremely conscientious, orderly, clean, meticulous, and parsimonious. Intellectualization and isolation of affect may further heighten their appearance of intellectual precision and unemotionality. Within limits, these traits may be virtues, but in excess, they become disabling. Mistrust of emotionality may become emotional constriction and colorlessness; intellectuality may turn into pedantry; conscientiousness and meticulousness may become rigidity and scrupulosity or, when combined with extreme, poorly tolerated ambivalence, may lead to paralyzing indecision and fear of error. DSM-III-R calls the pathologically extreme form of this personality type *Obsessive-Compulsive Personality Disorder.*

DSM-III-R Diagnostic Criteria for Obsessive-Compulsive Personality Disorder

A pervasive pattern of perfectionism and inflexibility, beginning by early adulthood and present in a variety of contexts, as indicated by at least five of the following:

(1) perfectionism that interferes with task completion, e.g., inability to complete a project because [one's] own overly strict standards are not met

(2) *preoccupation with details, rules, lists, order, organization, or schedules to the extent that the major point of the activity is lost*

(3) *unreasonable insistence that others submit to exactly his or her way of doing things, or unreasonable reluctance to allow others to do things because of the conviction that they will not do them correctly*

(4) *excessive devotion to work and productivity to the exclusion of leisure activities and friendships (not accounted for by obvious economic necessity)*

(5) *indecisiveness: decision making is either avoided, postponed, or protracted, e.g., the person cannot get assignments done on time because of ruminating about priorities (do not include if indecisiveness is due to excessive need for advice or reassurance from others)*

(6) *overconscientiousness, scrupulousness, and inflexibility about matters of morality, ethics, or values (not accounted for by cultural or religious identification)*

(7) *restricted expression of affection*

(8) *lack of generosity in giving time, money, or gifts when no personal gain is likely to result*

(9) *inability to discard worn-out or worthless objects even when they have no sentimental value.* (APA, 1987, p. 356)

The relationship of this personality disorder to OCD remains a topic of ongoing debate and controversy (Marks, 1987) (see pp. 276–277).

EPIDEMIOLOGY

Obsessive-compulsive disorder rarely comes to clinical attention. Within the general population (both adult and child), most estimates of the overall prevalence of the diagnosed disorder are low, that is, about .05% (Elkins et al., 1980). However, a recent large-scale door-to-door National Institute of Mental Health (NIMH) epidemiological study using a structured interview suggests a remarkably higher lifetime prevalence in the general population of 1.2% to 2.4% (Karno et al., 1988). Unfortunately, these epidemiological data do not reveal the features that distinguish the small fraction of persons who actually become psychiatric patients from the much larger group reporting obsessive-compulsive symptoms (Insel, 1984). Complicating any such study is the reality, previously noted, that at one time or another almost everyone experiences intrusive, distasteful, and unacceptable thoughts (Rachman & de Silva, 1978). Considerable uncertainty remains about the ability of the various structured interviews and questionnaires to distinguish reliably and specifically between normal obsessions and compulsions and those that warrant a diagnosis of OCD.

Retrospective studies of adult cases suggest that about one-third to one-half of adult obsessive-compulsive patients had their first symptoms before age 15 (Beech, 1974; Black, 1974). Freud's (1909/1955b) famous obsessional patient, the Ratman, recalled that his symptoms first occurred when he was 6 or 7 years old.

Although OCD is uncommon in childhood, its true prevalence in the general child population is unclear. In their classic epidemiological survey of the Isle of Wight, Rutter and his colleagues (1970) studied the island's total population of 10- to 12-year-olds. Of the 2199 children screened, only 7 (0.3%) had prominent obsessive features; there were no fully developed cases of OCD. On the other hand, in a study of 5596 high school students in a New Jersey county, Flament and colleagues (1988) found that as many as 2% of students reported obsessive preoccupations or behaviors that were either great in number and/or interfered markedly with their functioning. Only 0.35% of the total, however, met the full criteria for OCD; 0.22% of the students met the criteria for compulsive personality disorder. As in surveys of the general adult population, this study of a nonclinical adolescent population revealed a surprisingly high frequency of "subclinical OCD," that is, individuals who did not meet the full criteria for OCD but who had "one or two obsessive-compulsive symptoms that had a definite date of onset but did not appear developmentally continuous or accountable by situation or personality, and was seen [by the subject] as abnormal or undesirable" (p. 766). The investigators concluded that OCD in adolescence is more common than usually supposed and is frequently underdiagnosed and untreated.

Studies of child psychiatric clinic records indicate that children and adolescents diagnosed with this disorder make up 0.2% to 1.2% of clinic populations (Hollingsworth et al., 1980; Judd, 1965). In adulthood, OCD afflicts males and females about equally (Marks, 1987). Prepubertal boys with the disorder outnumber girls by a ratio of 3:1 (Swedo et al., 1989a). Boys also appear to have an earlier age of onset (Rapoport, 1986). Studies from different parts of the world suggest that similar presentations of OCD exist in other cultures (Insel, 1984). The familial distribution of this disorder is discussed under Etiology.

CLINICAL FEATURES

Normal Developmental "Compulsiveness"

Rituals, rules, and repetition are important, reassuring themes for all children (Leonard et al., 1990). Most toddlers and preschoolers, for example, develop a bedtime pattern—a favorite stuffed animal arranged just so, a particular story or song, a glass of water precisely placed by the bedside, a goodnight kiss—which must be scrupulously observed before they can securely yield themselves up to the uncertainties of sleep. Other normal, transient rituals of the toddler period may concern food or dress, such as a maddening insistence on wearing the same T-shirt or eating nothing but peanut butter sandwiches for days on end. The normal rituals of anal-phase children may serve several important functions (Adams, 1973). They attempt magically to ward off uncertainty, especially about separation. As Adams (1973) puts it, through such rituals the child tries "to force object constancy, to make his significant people more static, more reliable, through enmeshing them in a transitory obsessional web" (p. 7).

Across a broad range of developmental epochs, repetitious play provides a gratifying sense of orderliness and mastery, as well as intrinsic excitement. Thus, the baby banging again and again at his peg table, the grade-school girls chanting endlessly as they jump rope, and the video-game enthusiast repetitively blazing away at alien spaceships all have much in common. During the latency period, the child's emphasis on order and repetition provides important stability to the newly forming personality and both parallels and facilitates the child's involvement in the task of education. These school years are also the prime years for elaborate collections (from snakes to stamps) and organizations, such as Cub Scouts or Brownies, with all of their rituals, rules, uniforms, and associated paraphernalia. Group play during this period of life is often highly rule-oriented (Piaget, 1965); school-age players debate purported violations of baseball or dodge-ball rules with a passion that would put a zealous lawyer or theologian to shame.

Yet, behind the familiar and seemingly frivolous childhood games and hobbies, it is often easy to spot attempts to deal with more serious impulses and dangers. In the titillating game of "cooties," grade-school boys excitedly flee the contaminating cooties that the pursuing girls threaten to inflict by touching them (Adams, 1973). The boys repeatedly foray into the girls' territory to harry them, then flee the dangerous cooties again. The youngsters thus simultaneously toy with and ward off strong currents of sexual excitement and avoidance. In other games, the balance may be tilted even further toward the control of unsettling impulses and away from disguised gratification. The old game of "step on a crack, break your mother's back" embodies the notion of preventing dangerous consequences of hostile thoughts or oedipal incestuous fantasies by precisely performing a ritual— walking so as never to step on a crack in the sidewalk. Superstitions such as the possession of good luck pieces or avoidance of the number 13 represent less playful attempts to control fate or the unknown. Thus, in their struggles against the inner and outer dangers of life, developing children may employ many of the same defense mechanisms that find more florid expression in the thinking of the true obsessional: isolation, magical thinking, reaction formation, intellectualization, and undoing.

Despite these similarities, there are several ways to distinguish manifestations of normal compulsivity and ritualization from pathological obsessions and compulsions (Judd, 1965; Leonard, 1989b; Leonard et al., 1990). Developmentally normal rituals are not experienced as ego-alien or incongruous. On the contrary, they are pleasant and enjoyable. They are usually transient, and under mild external pressure the child can abandon the rituals without anxiety; typically he feels no need to struggle against them. Moreover, this normal compulsiveness does not compromise the child's general efficiency or everyday functioning.

Pathological Obsessive-Compulsiveness

The commonest age for the onset of pathological obsessions and compulsions is around puberty; however, many children develop the disorder much earlier. Indeed, cases as young as 3 years have been reported (Rapoport, 1986). More than half the children in one sample first showed symptoms during the period from 10 to 14 years of age; another 33% had their onset by age 9 or younger (Swedo et al., 1989a). The onset of symptoms may be either acute or insidious. The duration of illness prior to coming to professional attention is variable, reflecting not only the waxing and waning of the symptoms but also the secrecy with which the child hides his symptoms and the degree to which he can inveigle his parents either into complying with his compulsive needs or participating in his rituals. Parents differ in the extent to which they are willing to conform their behavior (and deform their judgment) to accommodate to or accept their children's symptoms; the degree of such parental collusion influences not only the point of diagnosis, but the treatment alliance as well (Rapoport, 1985).

The symptoms of obsessive-compulsive children resemble those of adult patients (Riddle et al., 1990c; Swedo et al., 1989a). The commonest pattern is an obsessive *fear of contamination*, with compulsive washing, cleaning, and avoidance of "contaminated objects." Such a child might spend an hour brushing his teeth in the "right way" prior to going to bed or feel compelled to wash for an hour after having used the toilet. These washing or bathing rituals may have to be performed in a complex and rigid sequence, such as left side of the head four times, right side of the head four times, and so on. Sometimes the child can be specific about the feared or loathsome contaminant, for example, germs, semen, or toxins, even while acknowledging the unreasonableness of the fear. In most cases, however, only a vague presentiment about contact with "something bad" fills the child with fear or disgust. Intrusive mental images tinged with fear or repulsion, such as being covered with excrement, may accompany the anxieties.

Another common symptom is a recurrent gnawing *pathological doubt leading to compulsive checking*. The checking usually concerns warding off some violent danger either to the self or to family members. The child may be tormented by nagging doubts that he has left a sharp knife lying about, forgotten to turn the stove off, or left a back door unlocked through which a burglar might enter. He must check the kitchen again and again, often imploring his mother and father also to check; finally they do so, and all is momentarily well. Within a few minutes, however, the child begins doubting the thoroughness of the search, his anxiety mounts, and presently he must check once again. If the child is prevented from checking or attempts to restrain himself, he becomes increasingly anxious and preoccupied with the potential catastrophe and is ever more driven to prevent it. Insel (1984) observed, "Checkers live as if they are the guilty party perpetually in search of a crime" (p. 6).

A less common clinical picture is the *pure obsession,* a cognitive disturbance without associated compulsive behavior. Frequently, these repetitive, intrusive thoughts are sexual or aggressive, filling the child with guilt, shame, or loathing. The obsessions can be purely verbal, but vivid mental images often accompany them. In other cases, the obsessive thoughts may appear to be meaningless, such as when the patient counts a series of numbers or endlessly repeats words or phrases that do not make sense, at least until their associations are understood. Some children are compelled to count objects about them, perhaps in specific groupings, such as fours or eights. Frequently, the child fears that harm will come to someone else or himself if he does not think or do whatever the ritual demands. Although compulsive motor acts such as checking or washing may not accompany the obsessive thoughts, the child may struggle mentally to ward them off with cognitive rituals or counterthoughts (Insel, 1984). For example, in response to a recurrent and intrusive sexual thought that she found repugnant, one menarchal adolescent girl forced herself to run mentally through the elements of the *periodic* table. In effect, the person uses one group of thoughts to undo the presumed injurious impact of another. From a psychodynamic perspective, these patients regress to magical thinking, the belief that thoughts can do actual harm and that to think a deed is tantamount to doing it. If such a person has thought about something bad happening and a misfortune does in fact occur, then his thought was surely responsible and appropriate expiation is necessary. Some obsessional children with intrusive ego-dystonic thoughts must compulsively confess them to their parents for reassurance. For example, a 12-year-old boy repeatedly had to confess to his mother that cracks in the wall or the number two made him think of her genitals and breasts; a 10-year-old Quaker girl had to confess that she was plagued with thoughts that her highly principled father was "racially prejudiced."

Other common compulsions include arranging objects, hoarding, pacing, and making complex gestures that may involve common activities, such as walking through a doorway or getting up from a chair, either repetitiously or in a precisely specified manner. The individual may have to arrange actions or objects in a specific order or pattern, such as even numbers or pairs. The ideational content behind these behaviors may be obscure. Freud (1909/1955b) remarked that patients themselves "may not always know the working of their obsessional ideas" (p. 359). Some children fear a specific danger if they resist or fail to perform their compulsions ("The house might burn down if I don't make sure everything is unplugged.") Others are simply aware of vague anxiety or tension. In such cases, where there is no ideational content and the compulsion involves simple actions such as repetitive touching, hopping, or licking, it may phenomenologically resemble the complex motor tics of Tourette's syndrome (TS).

In their large child and adolescent series at NIMH, Swedo et al. (1989a) found the following distribution of major presenting symptoms: excessive washing or grooming, 85%; repetitive actions (e.g., opening and closing a door; going through a doorway), 51%; checking, 46%; decontamination rituals, 23%; fear of something terrible happening, 24%; touching, 20%; counting, 18%; arranging, 17%; religious scrupulosity, 13%; and hoarding, 11%. These symptom clusters do not constitute discrete syndromes; in most cases, they coexist or alternate with each other (Insel, 1984).

CASE EXAMPLE

Janet, a 13-year-old girl, was finally hospitalized when she developed the compulsion to walk across a busy highway precisely eight times. Her mother had not previously challenged Janet's elaborate rituals, such as her bedtime requirement that the mother walk about Janet's carefully arranged bedroom five times in a counterclockwise direction. Janet could not explain the purpose of these rituals, but, if thwarted, her sense of impending dread quickly turned into obstinate anger, agitation, and panic. Although Janet's symptoms had persisted, waxing and waning in intensity, for several years, the specific contents of the rituals changed every few months. For example, at one period, before she could enter or leave a room, Janet had to turn the light switch off and on a specified number of times. These difficulties were apparent only at home. At school, Janet's teachers did not notice any bizarre behaviors and were puzzled to learn of her hospitalization. They saw her as quiet and generally compliant, although they were periodically surprised by what seemed to be rare outbursts of obstinacy.

Two of the defining characteristics of OCD are the retention of insight and resistance to the obsessional thought or compulsion. Flament and Rapoport (1984) noted, "The most striking feature is the severity of the psychopathology in the absence of formal thought disorder. . . . [T]hese children's relatedness and sensible discussion of their problems is in almost eerie contrast with their incapacity" (p. 29). However, both insight and resistance may be variable and difficult to judge. In calm moments, a child with OCD can readily admit that his need to wash or to check the stove is senseless. Nonetheless, when thwarted, the same child may become desperate and furtive, going to almost any lengths to perform the compulsive act. Resistance may vary with time and context; thus, by great effort, a child may refrain from enacting a compulsion at school but yield to it readily at home.

The personality structure of obsessional patients and its relationship to their obsessive-compulsive symptoms have been matters of considerable debate (Black et al., 1989; Marks, 1987). At issue is the question: To what extent do patients with OCD have obsessive-compulsive personalities? Orderliness, stubbornness, perfectionism, parsimony, a preoccupation with rules, and lack of spontaneity characterize the obsessive-compulsive personality. The DSM-III-R description of Obsessive-Compulsive Personality Disorder includes, in addition to the character traits noted above, emotional constriction, excessive devotion to work to the exclusion of pleasure or interpersonal relationships, and indecisiveness due to an inability to order priorities for fear of making a mistake. Individuals with a compulsive personality disorder may experience considerable distress and depression because of their indecisiveness and frequent ineffectiveness. However, they generally do not experience their preoccupations, ruminations, or excessive scruples as ego-alien and do not struggle against them.

In general, these dynamics and character traits parallel the "anal character" that Freud (1908/1959) saw as providing the predisposition to frank obsessional symptomatology. Some clinicians (Adams, 1973; Salzman, 1968) see frank obsessive-compulsive disorder as the extreme end of a spectrum that extends from the normal use of obsessional mechanisms at one end, through a predominance of obsessional personality traits, to overt symptoms of obsession and compulsion at the other. In his rich and thought-provoking book, *Obsessive Children,* Adams (1973) lumps children with frank obsessions and compulsions together with those rigid, constricted, joyless children who have a predominantly obsessive-compulsive character style. For these authors, the patient with a symptomatic obsessive-compulsive disorder has developed such extreme reliance on obsessional techniques that it pervades every aspect of functioning.

In contrast, Anna Freud (1966) observed that childhood obsessional symptoms occurred in the context of a great variety of personality types:

> While in adults, the individual neurotic symptom usually forms part of a genetically related personality structure, this is not so with children. In children, symptoms occur just as often in isolation, or are coupled with other symptoms and personality traits of a different nature and unrelated origin. Even well defined obsessional symptoms, such as bedtime ceremonials or counting compulsions, are found in children with otherwise uncontrolled, restless, impulsive personalities. . . ." (p. 151)

Systematic clinical studies of children and adults with OCD raise questions as to the extent to which frank obsessions or compulsions (i.e., "state" measures) correlate with obsessional traits, either concurrently or prior to the onset of symptoms (Black et al., 1989; Flament & Rapoport, 1984; Insel, 1984; Marks, 1987). In their high school population survey, Flament et al.

(1988) found that only 17% of the students who met the full criteria for OCD also had a compulsive personality disorder. Similarly, in the NIMH cohort of children with OCD, very few have been meticulous, orderly, or overconcerned with cleanliness in matters unrelated to their rituals, nor did they display such traits prior to the onset of symptoms (Rapoport, 1985, 1986). Only 16% of these children met the criteria for compulsive personality (Swedo et al., 1989a). Typically, a child might be adamant about doing a homework problem in a ritualized way but was not otherwise excessively neat or attentive to details. Although many of the youngsters were studious, shy, and nonaggressive, not all were isolated or withdrawn. Neither had they been excessively "good" or compliant children; some, in fact, were considered to be impulsive with a mild conduct disorder. What one wag has termed the "obsessive-impulsive" may be more than a joke. Several authors (Bolton & Turner, 1984; Hoehn-Saric & Barksdale, 1983) have described a subgroup of patients with *both* conduct disorder and OCD. These findings suggest that OCD is not merely a severe form of the obsessive-compulsive personality.

The following case example illustrates some of the fluid symptomatic features of this disorder, as well as the frequent concomitance of other difficulties.

CASE EXAMPLE

Kevin, age 11, was admitted to an inpatient psychiatric facility following a suicidal gesture in the form of an aspirin overdose. Interview revealed that he felt desperate because of the obsessive thought and mental image that he was "covered with shit." In response, he had been showering 4 or 5 times daily and washing his hands until they were raw. In the course of several months' hospitalization he grew so afraid of swallowing germs that be began to spit out his saliva, refuse food, and, presently, to sustain a considerable weight loss.

Pertinent history included slow motor development, shyness, and easy upsets with peers. The patient had been a sickly preschooler and a seemingly vulnerable and fragile child. In managing him, his mother was often harsh and punitive. There was a history of psychosis in one grandparent.

Adolescence was stormy despite several brief and unsuccessful trials at psychotherapy. Kevin's washing symptoms largely disappeared, but he continued to be plagued by intrusive thoughts that he found repellent. For example, for a period of time Kevin was extremely pious and would attend church daily, saying his rosary frequently. His prayers were complicated, however, by recurrent intrusive obscene thoughts about God or the Virgin Mary that he felt necessitated beginning each set of prayers all over again. His anguished confession of these blasphemous thoughts to the priest, sometimes several times a day, finally drew an ecclesiastical diagnosis of "scrupulosity" (Greenberg et al., 1987).

Despite his above-average intelligence, Kevin did poorly at school. Indeed, apart from his obsessions and compulsions, he was neither orderly nor inhibited; rather he lived a life of noisy desperation. He thus lacked the modicum of adaptive obsessional character traits that would have been useful in school or later at work. Although he had periods of piety during which he was assiduously devout and considered a vocation as a priest, at other times he fantasied and boasted to friends about his plans to become a male stripper, admired and pursued by women for his virility.

The overall organization of Kevin's personality was that of a severe borderline personality disorder. The relationship between frank self-loathing and obsessive-compulsive concerns with contamination was an interesting feature. Treated prior to the introduction of serotonin-specific agents, Kevin's intrusive thoughts and mental images of being covered with feces, as well as his compulsive washing, disappeared with low doses of phenothiazine medication. However, he remained plagued by painfully low self-esteem and self-loathing, which often took the form "I'm nothing but a piece of shit." (Early on, Freud, 1896/1962, p. 169, had concluded, "Obsessional ideas are invariably transformed self-reproaches which have re-emerged from repression. . . .")

Nosology

Several caveats are in order about the diagnostic schemata in DSM-III. As a nosological convention, DSM-III (APA, 1980) defined obsessive-compulsive disorder as "*not due to* another mental disorder such as Tourette's Disorder, Schizophrenia, Major Depression, or Organic Mental Disorder [italics added]," (p. 235) thereby implying that the clinician could distinguish between primary and secondary forms of the disorder. Very many patients with OCD have additional psychiatric symptoms, however, such as phobias, depression, and personality difficulties that are severe enough to warrant additional concurrent diagnoses. Certain associated symptoms, such as depression, may reflect the disturbing impact of living with a chronic, disabling psychiatric condition; it is possible, however, that these symptoms may bear a more direct relationship to the as-yet-unknown factors responsible for OCD. The revised criteria in DSM-III-R allow the diagnosis of obsessive-compulsive disorder coexisting with other diagnoses.

Obsessions and rituals also appear as symptoms in many psychiatric disorders including Tourette's syndrome, autism, schizophrenia, psychotic depression, anorexia nervosa, and certain organic brain syndromes. Much more research is needed to determine to what extent the mechanisms responsible for the symptoms of the primary syndrome are the same as or different from those producing the secondary syndromes. For example, recent research suggests that the frequent concomitance of tics and obsessive-compulsive symptoms in the families of TS patients reflects alternative phenotypic expressions of a single, autosomal dominant gene (Pauls & Leckman, 1986).

Finally, it is important not to reify the diagnosis of OCD by thinking of it as a homogeneous entity. As noted earlier, there are several descriptive subtypes (e.g., checking, fear of contamination, pure obsessions, etc). Adams (1985) has stressed the importance of carefully studying the patient's subjective experience to distinguish whether the obsessive symptoms are driven by fear, guilt, or shame. Further research is necessary to ascertain whether such clinically derived subtypes have distinctive predisposing features or follow a different clinical course.

Associated Features

Phobias and the Question of Anxiety. Both phobia and obsessive-compulsive disorder are syndromes of "anxious avoidance" (Marks, 1987). Many patients with primary OCD have phobias, especially in the area of their obsession. Indeed, compulsive washers are often mislabeled "germ phobics" (Insel, 1984). Patients who fear contamination (and some compulsive checkers) resemble phobics in their anxiety to avoid irrationally feared objects. However, the obsessional patient is more inescapably haunted than is the phobic patient. Because the obsessive is driven by internal stimuli, he obtains only temporary relief from performing his rituals (Insel, 1984). In contrast, to the extent that phobias are associated with external stimuli, the phobic may obtain at least transient security by avoiding the object of his phobia. Of course, many phobias tend to "spread" beyond the original object; in addition, even in the absence of the phobic object, phobic patients often develop a high degree of anticipatory anxiety lest they encounter the feared object.

About 40% of children with severe OCD have a current or past history of another anxiety disorder (Riddle et al., 1990c; Swedo et al., 1989a). Separation anxiety is common in such children who are often preoccupied with fears or intrusive images of mishaps to their loved ones. Children frequently cannot ascribe any content to the anxious tension that threatens them should they resist or fail to perform a compulsive ritual. Often, the closest they can come to describing their apprehension is that "something bad" might happen to their family.

These factors raise the broader question of the general relationship of obsessive-compulsive disorder to the anxiety disorders (Marks, 1987). In DSM-III-R they are generally grouped together. Freud saw OCD as driven by anxiety. In the psychoanalytic view the patient's anxiety reflects a failure of repression that permits forbidden impulses to emerge into consciousness. Symptoms result from the attempt to contain the anxiety, either by isolating and transmuting the mental representation of the impulse into an obsessional thought or by attempting to undo its feared consequences through a compulsive act. Anxiety is also central to learning theories that conceptualize compulsive symptoms as conditioned responses to anxiety-provoking events, the responses being reinforced by the reduction of anxiety.

Other evidence casts doubt on the tendency to group obsessive-compulsive disorder with the anxiety disorders (Berg et al., 1986). Many obsessives feel driven by guilt, shame, or disgust, rather than by anxiety or fear (Adams, 1985; Insel, 1984). Nor are family studies helpful in clarifying this issue. In some families, the relatives of adult obsessive-compulsive probands have an increased incidence of anxiety neuroses; in other studies of childhood obsessives, the family loading for anxiety disorder (other than OCD) is not increased (Berg et al., 1986). Except for the anxiety associated directly with their symptoms, most obsessional patients do not meet the criteria for an anxiety disorder. In general, direct measures of physiological arousal in childhood obsessives suggest that high levels of autonomic activity are not of primary etiologic significance (Berg et al., 1986). Perhaps it is not surprising then that anxiolytic drugs provide little relief for the obsessional patient.

Depression. Depressive symptoms are extremely common in both children (Flament & Rapoport, 1984) and adults (Insel, 1984; Marks, 1987; Welner et al., 1976) with OCD. Depression, either current or in the past, can be diagnosed in about one-third of children with severe symptoms of OCD (Riddle et al., 1990c; Swedo et al., 1989a). In about half of these children, depression appeared to follow the onset of the obsessive-compulsive symptoms and may be secondary to the stress of the chronic disabling symptoms. In the remainder of cases with associated depression, the depression antedated the obsessive-compulsive symptoms. In adults, true obsessions or severe self-reproachful or somatic ruminations may follow the onset of a primary affective disorder (Fenton & McGlashan, 1986; Welner et al., 1976).

Differential Diagnosis

Schizophrenia. Obsessions and compulsions may be difficult to distinguish from delusions. By definition obsessions are recognized as being internal in origin and are resisted, whereas delusions are not. In actual practice, as resistance waxes and wanes, the distinction may be difficult to draw; for example, obsessional fears of being contaminated may blur into delusional fears of being poisoned (Insel, 1984). Unlike the schizophrenic child, however, the child with OCD usually shows well-preserved interpersonal relatedness, no formal thought disorder, and good reality testing (at least outside the area of the child's obsessional symptoms).

Despite their seemingly bizarre symptoms, only a very small number of obsessionals develop full-blown schizophrenia. When it does occur, such a transition may take place long years after the onset of the obsessive-compulsive symptoms. For example, beginning at age 5 years, one young man had developed rituals involving endless rearrangement of the shoes and clothing in his room (Fenton & McGlashan, 1986). At age 17 he developed florid psychotic symptoms and came to believe that he was now controlling national and world events through his long-standing rituals. During the next few years he continued to run a chronic schizophrenic course, accompanied by persisting obsessive-compulsive symptoms.

Autism, Retardation, and Other Developmental Disabilities. Children with retardation, brain damage, or autistic syndromes are often perseverative in both action and mental set and frequently show repetitive stereotyped movements (such as rocking or hand-flapping). Kanner (1943) characterized autistic children as having an "anxiously obsessive concern with sameness" that resulted in catastrophic upsets at any alteration in their surroundings or schedule. Many children with pervasive developmental disorder, schizotypal personality, or high-level autism have bizarre and compulsive preoccupations, such as a fascination with highway route numbers or unusual fanatically acquired collections. Bender (1954) coined the term "impulsions" to describe these circumscribed interests, fanatically pursued to the exclusion of other activities and relationships. In general, children usually experience the above symptoms as ego-syntonic; their lack of insight into the irrationality of the behaviors and the absence of any efforts to resist them distinguish these conditions from primary OCD (Rapoport, 1985).

Anorexia Nervosa. Anorexia nervosa may resemble OCD in terms of obsessional thoughts (either about food or being too fat) and compulsions (which may include driven patterns of exercising and/or eating rituals); the degree of insight and resistance in anorexia is highly variable. Anorexia nervosa may either precede or accompany a true obsessive-compulsive disorder (Insel, 1984; Welner et al., 1976). The preceding case example of Kevin is illustrative. As a preteen, his fear of swallowing germs led him to refuse food and lose considerable weight. However, he did not meet the criteria for primary anorexia in that he neither felt fat nor pursued thinness. In later adolescence, however, Kevin did develop a classic anorexia nervosa syndrome. He felt he was too fat (even as he lost over 25% of his body weight) and relentlessly pursued a weight-loss program with the fixed idea that thinness would gain him love and popularity. Common to both periods was extreme anxiety over his oral dependent longings, which he perceived as dangerous and weakening.

Tourette's Syndrome. The best-known symptoms of TS are motor and vocal tics, which may include compulsive verbal ejaculations. Although the movements involved in the motor stereotypies are fragmentary and meaningless, many Tourette's sufferers struggle constantly against the compulsion to perform more complex motor acts such as imitating others' gestures (echopraxia), touching people or things, hopping, licking, or biting. In addition, true obsessions or compulsions occur in well over half of TS patients (Grad et al., 1987; Pauls et al., 1986b). The subjective state of mind of the TS patient also resembles that of the pure obsessive-compulsive because both share a sense of constant, grueling struggle against a powerful, disturbing internal urge or thought. (For a further discussion of the inner world of the TS patient see Chapter 10, "Tic Disorders.")

Tourette's syndrome is usually distinguished from primary obsessive-compulsive disorder by the presence (or history) of chronic motor and vocal tics. In practice, the symptom overlap in the clinical presentation of these two disorders may be considerable (Pitman & Jenike, 1988). Many TS patients, especially as they grow older, have significant obsessions or compulsions, but careful study also reveals that as many as 20% to 24% of children who present with a diagnosis of OCD have odd motor "twitches" or a history of motor tics (Riddle et al., 1990c; Swedo et al., 1989a). Swedo et al. (1989a) found these minor motor tics were most common in males, in younger patients, and in acute cases.

Because both OCD and TS are disorders of inhibition and volition, the association between tics and obsessive-compulsive phenomena raises many intriguing etiologic questions. It suggests that similar genetic and neurophysiological mechanisms may be at work in both conditions. Furthermore, the close relatives of TS patients have an increased incidence of obsessive and compulsive symptoms (often without conspicuous tics). The analysis of TS pedigrees suggests that in these families, chronic multiple tics and obsessive-compulsive disorder are alternative phenotypic expressions of the genetic diathesis for TS, which is transmitted as an autosomal dominant gene (Pauls & Leckman, 1986).

ETIOLOGY

Psychodynamic Theories

Depending on their theoretical predilections, writers with a psychoanalytic orientation have approached obsessional phenomena from varying perspectives (Adams, 1973; Nagera, 1976). Most psychodynamic authors view the obsessional child's dilemma as a maladaptive defense against guilt, anxiety, and uncertainty; at the same time, they emphasize different elements of the obsessional diathesis. Like Freud himself, some authors have emphasized the specific instinctual dangers and conflicts that preoccupy the obsessive. Others, such as Sandler and Joffe (1965) and Shapiro (1965), have focused on the peculiarities of the obsessive's ego functioning. Still others, such as Salzman (1968), have stressed cultural, child-rearing, and interpersonal factors. (For a thoughtful critique and synthesis of these views, see Adams, 1973.)

Freud felt that the structure of OCD reflected the sufferer's unsuccessful struggle against unacceptable aggressive and sexual impulses, especially those related to the Oedipus complex. In Freud's (1913/1958) view, the obsessive's oedipal conflicts lead to a regressive intensification of anal-sadistic eroticism; that is, the patient retreats to an earlier level of affective and cognitive development characterized by heightened concerns about angry soiling, the need for omnipotent control of others, and intense conflicts between love and passive compliance on the one hand and rageful destructiveness on the other.

Rado (1959) believed that the obsessive's style reflects the parent–child conflict about autonomy and authority characteristic of this developmental period: enraged defiance alternating with guilty fear. Even at this level, despite extensive defenses such as reaction formation, undoing, or isolation, the patient cannot contain his conflicts. Although these defense mechanisms play a role in normal personality functioning, Freud felt that their excessive and unbalanced use gives obsessional disorders their characteristic quality.

Undoing represents the patient's attempt to make up for or to take back previous thoughts or actions that he regrets and feels to be dangerously hurtful. For example, a guilt-stricken 6-year-old who had accidentally killed his envied sister's gerbil by playing with it too roughly carefully put the dead animal back in its cage, changed the litter, and filled the food and water containers.

Reaction formation represents a parallel maneuver in the character realm, only here the individual is not so much undoing an act as reversing an attitude. In particular, he adopts a psychological stance diametrically opposed to an unacceptable impulse. Thus, in place of the wish to soil angrily, the nascent obsessive becomes fanatically neat. Similarly, the child replaces rebellious and hateful feelings and the urge to attack the parent with a compulsive, compliant meekness and a scrupulous repudiation of assertive anger; he converts sexual urges to asceticism along with a puritanical disdain for the pleasures of the flesh, and so on.

Isolation consists of dehiscing thoughts or behaviors from their affective context and associations, so that the idea itself remains in consciousness, but merely as a "thought" stripped of all feeling. Freud (1894/1962b) hypothesized that as a result, "[The] affect, which has become free, attaches itself to other ideas which are not in themselves incompatible; and, thanks to this 'false connection,' those ideas turn into obsessional ideas" (p. 52).

Clinically, the obsessive-compulsive pattern often has the quality of a last-ditch defense. Despite the obsessive's efforts to control the conflict between his impulses and his conscience, the tenuously contained impulses continue to generate constant anxiety, requiring unending exertions in the form of ever more stringent rituals and strenuous struggles against obsessive ideas. As Freud (1912/1953) put it:

> An obsessional neurotic may be weighed down by a sense of guilt that would be appropriate in a mass-murderer, while in fact, from his childhood onwards, he has behaved to his fellow-men as the most considerate and scrupulous member of society. Nevertheless, his sense of guilt has a justification: it is founded on the intense and frequent death-wishes against his fellows which are unconsciously at work in him. It has a justification if what we take into account are unconscious thoughts and not intentional deeds. . . . Whenever I have succeeded in penetrating the mystery, I have found that the expected disaster was death. (p. 87)

Child analysts also note that transient obsessional phenomena often appear during normal development. For example, in the face of strong parental pressure toward toilet training, cleanliness, and condemnation of aggression, preschoolers may show excessive orderliness, disgust with dirty hands, and repetitive behavior (A. Freud, 1981). Child analysts also view the normal latency child's emphasis on orderliness and rules as in part dynamically determined. In respect to this latency group, cognitive and psychodynamic theorists differ widely. The cognitive psychologist emphasizes the development of what Piaget (1954) termed "concrete operational" thinking—the ability to look at a situation from several perspectives and to conceptualize matter as subject to dynamic transformational processes that can be reversed in the child's mind. This achievement includes mastering classification and series formation—capacities that the child pleasurably and repetitiously exercises by accumulating and rearranging extensive collections (of everything from beer cans to fossils) and the enjoyment and elaboration of complex, rule-governed games (involving everything from playing fields to computers and video screens).

Psychoanalytic theorists concur that neuromaturation and the growth of autonomous ego functions are essential to the emergence of the rule-oriented, orderly behavior of latency (Shapiro & Perry, 1976). They also propose that such behavior helps the child cope with persistent instinctual pressures that by no means disappear with the resolution of the Oedipus complex (see Volume 1, Chapter 14, "The Grade-School Child"). The latency child struggles to control forbidden genital and pregenital impulses through repression, reaction formation, sublimation, and fantasy formation (Sarnoff, 1976). There may even be a regressive intensification of anal-sadistic drives. Obsessional defenses, such as reaction formation against these impulses, manifest themselves in a heightened emphasis on orderliness and cleanliness. The latency child's collections often illustrate both these regressive anal-phase instinctual impulses and the defenses against them: retentively accumulated hoards that, despite endless rearranging and ordering, never quite emerge from chaos or constantly threaten to spill over into an untidy mess.

The dynamic perspective thus emphasizes the conflictual and defensive aspects of obsessive-compulsive phenomena and implies a secret or disguised instinctual gratification behind the compulsive act or thought. In the context of the normal latency child, repetitive play and rituals may help bolster and serve as a displacement for the child's attempts to ward off masturbatory impulses. The relentless "itch" of a compulsion, repetitiously enacted, desperately resisted but equally desperately yielded to, has led some psychoanalysts to view compulsions as "masturbation equivalents" (Ferenczi, 1926).

According to psychoanalytic speculation, several predisposing factors, presumably constitutional, favor the formation of obsessional pathology. Although recent empirical work (Flament & Rapoport, 1984) fails to support earlier impressions that obsessional children are generally of above-average intelligence (Rachman & Hodgson, 1980), one such postulated factor is precocious ego and superego development. Anna Freud (1965) stressed that often "the incompatibility between relatively high moral and aesthetic superego demands and relatively crude fantasies and drive derivatives leads to the internal conflict by which in turn the obsessional defense activity is set in motion" (p. 125). Other hypothesized predisposing factors include "a constitutional increase in the intensity of anal-sadistic tendencies or a constitutional preference for the use of defense mechanisms such as reaction formation, intellectualization, isolation, etc." (A. Freud, 1966, p. 117). Such speculation does not help much because invoking early constitutional factors always raises the need for other explanations; among these Anna Freud (1966) included "the result[s] of inheritance combined with parental handling."

Psychoanalysts emphasize another cognitive feature that they consider to be a hallmark of the obsessional style—what Freud described as "over-valuation of thought" (Shapiro, 1965). The obsessive believes that thought has almost magical power over reality. He fears that his hateful or sexual thoughts will have the same real-world effect (and certainly the same moral onus) as action. The obsessive thus takes even one step further Jesus's admonition that "whosoever looketh on a woman to lust after her hath committed adultery with her already in his heart" (Matthew 5:28). The obsessive believes that thinking *is* the same as doing. In the case of pure obsessions, the same magical reliance on thought extends to the patient's reparational efforts. If only he can order his thoughts correctly, or ritually think the correct counterthoughts, he can avert disaster. As a consequence of overvaluating thought, many obsessional children become ruminatively preoccupied and virtually paralyzed; their overly cerebral, hairsplitting, punctilious approach leaves them always procrastinating and incapable of concluding projects. At the same time they half believe their endless rumi- nating has accomplished something. Thus, like Hamlet, their "native hue of resolution/Is sicklied o'er with the pale cast of thought,/And enterprises of great pitch and moment/With this regard their currents turn awry,/And lose the name of action" (*Hamlet,* Act III, Sc. 1, ll. 83–87).

Several authors have linked cultural factors and child-rearing practices to the genesis of obsessional difficulties; this is especially likely in children of parents with obsessional personalities. Kanner (1957) believed that such children suffered from "an overdose of parental perfectionism." Clinicians have also cited lack of parental empathy and intolerance for the child's negative feelings as crucial pathogens. Adams' (1973) study of 30 obses- sional children described their families as being highly verbal yet aloof and emphasizing conventional "correctness," cleanliness, and perfectionism. Rather than valuing spontaneity in their child, these parents "denied ag- gression and libido but vaunted precocity of the constraining ego" (p. 64). Salzman (1968) noted, "The consistent theme in all obsessionals is the presence of anxieties about being in danger because of an incapacity to fulfill the requirements of others and to feel certain of one's acceptance."

The notion of childhood acculturation to an obsessional family ethos of overconstraint and perfectionistic habits seems plausible. An alternative, or complementary, possibility is that heritable factors may partially determine family members' shared overmeticulous style. Unfortunately, researchers have little systematic data concerning the intergenerational transmission of cognitive and emotional styles. Reviewing the available findings, Rachman and Hodgson (1980) concluded that obsessional parents transmit to their children a general maladjustment manifested by timidity, overdependence, and anxiety rather than specific obsessional preoccupations.

Whatever the validity of hypotheses suggesting the intergenerational cultural transmission of obsessive-compulsive personality *traits,* their appli- cability to true obsessive-compulsive disorder is unclear. The view of Rapoport et al. (1981) that OCD is a distinct condition, "discontinuous from obsessional traits" casts doubt on the pathogenic environmental influence of an "obsessional" family style. Although the parents of children with OCD show a high prevalence of obsessive-compulsive symptoms, these symptoms are often quite different from those of their offspring, making it unlikely that the parents served as models for their children's ritual behaviors (Lenane et al., 1990; Swedo et al., 1989a).

If environmental influences do play a role, what factors besides an overmeticulous obsessional family culture might produce an offspring with OCD? Most likely a number of factors must converge. Perhaps particular environmental or constitutional factors render some offspring more vul- nerable than others to the expression of a genetic loading for OCD or to the toxic effects of an obsessional family tradition. Or perhaps the confluence of certain interpersonal tensions dooms vulnerable offspring to developing overt symptoms. Much more research into the genetic, neurological, and family determinants of psychopathology and cognitive style will be necessary to answer these questions.

Some of these inquiries were examined in an uncontrolled family study of adult patients with OCD (Hoover & Insel, 1984; Insel et al., 1983b). The prevalence of obsessional traits such as excessive cleanliness and perfectionism was very high among family members, but the authors found *no* additional cases of OCD among the many relatives of the proband patients. Although the authors found no additional cases that fit all of the DSM-III criteria for OCD, the supercleanliness and the overmeticulousness of several relatives were extreme. What distinguished these family members from the identified patients, however, was that their habits and attitudes did not interfere with their lives nor did they attempt to resist them; furthermore, these relatives neither held irrational beliefs about cleanliness nor did they endlessly multiply rituals.

Another characteristic of these obsessive families was the expectation of unusually strong filial devotion from generation to generation. These very tight, clanlike ties were maintained at the price of social isolation that deprived family members of possibly corrective contacts with the outside world.

Several other family dynamics seemed to converge on the proband patients (those who developed true obsessions and compulsions). Relations between their parents were disappointing and strained. As a result, at least one parent's intense unsatisfied desire for closeness focused on the child rather than on the spouse. The obsessive-compulsive symptoms served as protective barriers erected by the patient against the parent's (and perhaps the patient's) longing for symbiosis. For example, fear of contamination led several patients to bar access to their bedrooms, forbidding their parents' entry and precluding any physical contact or even dining together. The patients' symptoms often blocked any direct, tender involvement with the parents, yet these symptoms frequently enslaved the parents through endless supportive caretaking. Although the offspring preserved a superficial aloofness, their incapacitating rituals made them incapable of functioning in any environment that did not cater to them totally.

Neurobiological Factors

Several lines of evidence indicate that neurobiological factors may play a role in childhood obsessive-compulsive disorder (Behar et al., 1984; Elkins et al., 1980; Modell et al., 1989; Rapoport, 1989; Zohar & Insel, 1987). These findings include:

1. Overrepresentation of boys among prepubertal obsessive-compulsive patients.

2. High concordance rate in monozygotic twins.

3. Increased prevalence in patients with Tourette's syndrome and their relatives.

4. Therapeutic response to drugs such as clomipramine and fluoxetine, which act on the serotonergic neurotransmitter system.

5. Abnormalities of the basal ganglia and frontal cortex discerned by imaging techniques.

6. Positive response in some adults to neurosurgical lesions of the frontal lobe or cingulate gyrus.

Obsessive-compulsive disorder is associated with organic brain syndromes such as viral encephalitis (especially that associated with the post-World War I influenza epidemic), perinatal complications (Capstick & Deldrup, 1977), diabetes insipidus (Barton, 1976), Sydenham's chorea (Swedo et al., 1989b), and frontal lobe and basal ganglia strokes and neoplasms (Ward, 1988). In addition, adolescents with OCD show a high incidence of frontal-lobe abnormalities on neuropsychological testing (Behar et al., 1984b). Moreover, on neurodevelopmental examination, a large majority of OCD children show subtle neurological findings, the commonest of which are a choreiform syndrome or a syndrome of left-sided immaturities and soft signs (Denckla, 1989).

These various lines of evidence suggest that obsessive-compulsive symptoms may result from pathogenic factors that impinge on neurotransmitter (serotonin) regulation and on the functioning of the basal ganglia (Wise & Rapoport, 1989). In addition, hormonal factors (especially androgens) and other neurotransmitter systems (such as the dopamine pathways) probably play a mediating role (Swedo & Rapoport, 1990). Rapoport (1989) and Modell et al. (1989) have reviewed the rationale for these conclusions, and the discussion that follows draws on these reviews.

The antiobsessional efficacy of clomipramine, fluvoxamine, and fluoxetine (three antidepressants that increase serotonin activity at the synapse by blocking neurotransmitter reuptake) suggest serotonergic dysfunction in OCD (Fontaine & Chouinard, 1986; Zohar et al., 1988; Zohar & Insel, 1987). A high pretreatment level of platelet serotonin is a strong predictor of a positive clinical response to clomipramine (Flament et al., 1987). An additional clue to the importance of serotonin is the correlation between symptom severity and low levels of the major serotonin metabolite (5-HIAA) in the cerebrospinal fluid of patients with OCD (Leonard et al., 1988). However, the various neurotransmitter systems are intricately interrelated, and the role of serotonin is likely to be complex. For example, dopaminergic dysfunction appears to play a central role in Tourette's syndrome, which is strongly associated with obsessive-compulsive symptoms (see p. 282); in addition, high doses of dopaminergic stimulants such as amphetamine or methylphenidate can lead to both simple motor stereo-typies as well as more complex obsessions and compulsions (Swedo & Rapoport, 1990). These authors have suggested that the key defect may lie in the relative balance of serotonin and other neurotransmitter systems.

Neuroendocrine factors also may have a modulating role (Leonard, 1989a; Swedo & Rapoport, 1990). With puberty, the relative preponder-ance of boys over girls with OCD decreases from the 3:1 ratio in prepuber-tal children toward the equal gender distribution in adults. Symptoms may exacerbate during puberty or, in females, in the premenstrual or postpar-tum state. Antiandrogens may transiently ameliorate symptoms.

Researchers have suggested that dysfunction of the basal ganglia and their cortical connections plays an important role in OCD (Wise & Rapoport, 1989; Modell et al., 1989). Wise and Rapoport review the evi-dence implicating these structures. First, compulsive symptoms were fre-quent sequelae of the 1918 epidemic of viral encephalitis, which was prone to produce neurotoxic lesions of the basal ganglia. (For a moving personal account of disabling post-viral-encephalitic obsessional symptoms, see Hartnell, 1987). Second, the incidence of OCD is higher than expected in patients with Sydenham's chorea ("St. Vitus' dance"), a movement disorder that occurs as a complication of rheumatic fever when the immune system attacks the basal ganglia (Swedo et al., 1989b). Third, OCD can occur as a sequela of other neurotoxic insults that affect these structures (e.g., carbon monoxide poisoning or, in one case, a wasp sting). Fourth, quantitative CT scans of obsessive-compulsive patients have shown significant reduction in the volume of these patients' caudate nuclei (Luxenberg et al., 1988). Fifth, PET-imaging studies of obsessive-compulsive patients have found in-creased metabolic rates in the caudate nuclei and associated lateral orbito-frontal cortex (Baxter et al., 1988; Nordhal et al., 1989; Swedo et al., 1989c).

Wise and Rapoport (1989) and Modell et al. (1989) propose detailed neurochemical models of how abnormalities in the basal ganglia and the neurotransmitter systems regulating these cortical connections can cause the inappropriate release of fixed-action patterns in the form of obsessions or compulsions. Following Tinbergen's (1966) description of stereotyped grooming in male sticklebacks, naturally occurring stereotyped motor be-haviors have been studied in numerous species. Lorenz (1981) described "inherited drives of fixed behavior," relatively automatic behaviors that can occur without social learning. In various mammalian species, these fixed-action patterns may include self-grooming, nest building, food hoarding, danger avoidance, and courtship and mating behaviors. Typically, these behaviors are "released" in appropriate functional situations; many social and neurohormonal factors influence their amplitude and frequency.

One group of authors suggests that OCD symptoms represent an inap-propriate release of complex fixed-action patterns (Swedo, 1989; Swedo et al., 1989a; Wise & Rapoport, 1989). The same authors hypothesize that the basal ganglia are intimately involved in the storage and automatic execution of complex motor schemata and regulate the sensory control and release of these action patterns. Defects in the functional integrity of the basal ganglia and their cortical connections might lead to either the inappropriate release of fixed-action patterns or difficulty in appropriately terminating them. Such dysfunction may psychologically manifest itself as the OCD patient's pervasive doubt or inability to feel he has finally "got it right" in the realm of grooming, averting danger (or contamination), or completing a routinized sequential act (such as counting). The affected individual's response to this inner doubt and compulsion is reflected in his degree of resistance to or compliance with this repetitive urge.

Although such models remain speculative, they indicate a new field of inquiry, "neuroethology," which promises to enhance understanding of both human and animal behavior.

Genetic Factors

Family and twin studies of OCD suggest some inherited predisposition to obsessional behavior but also the importance of other unknown factors in the development of the full-blown syndrome. A study of obsessionals who were twins revealed that monozygotic twins had a higher concordance rate for full-blown OCD than did dizygotic twins. If concordance was determined from obsessional or phobic traits alone rather than from full-blown OCD, the concordance rate for monozygotic twins increased even further (Carey & Gottesman, 1981).

Close relatives of patients with OCD frequently have marked obsessional traits (Lenane et al., 1990; Riddle et al., 1990c); in many cases, however, these eccentricities (such as extreme cleanliness) are neither resisted nor viewed as troublesome (Hoover & Insel, 1984; Insel et al., 1983b). In direct interviews close relatives of obsessive-compulsive probands also indicate a higher frequency of OCD than expected from a general population. For example, Pauls (unpublished data, 1989) found that about 25% of the first-degree relatives of OCD probands met the OCD criteria. Swedo et al. (1989a) and Lenane et al. (1990) discovered a history of OCD in the first-degree relatives of 25% to 30% of children who had the disorder. In addition, most family studies also show higher than expected frequency of other psychiatric disorders in the relatives of OCD patients (McKeon & Murray, 1987). For example, in Flament and Rapoport's (1984) study, siblings of OCD patients showed a relatively high frequency of impulse control disorders and learning difficulties.

As noted earlier, TS patients often suffer from obsessive-compulsive symptoms severe enough to warrant the additional diagnosis of OCD. Furthermore, the close kin of TS patients show a strikingly high prevalence of obsessive-compulsive symptoms, often in the absence of prominent tics

(Pauls et al., 1986b). Such family studies suggest that OCD and TS represent alternative phenotypic expressions of the same genetic diathesis, which is transmitted as an autosomal dominant trait. However, phenotypic expression is sex-influenced in that female subjects with the gene are more likely to have obsessive-compulsive symptoms, whereas male subjects are more likely to have TS or chronic motor tics (Pauls & Leckman, 1986). These findings suggest that at least some cases of OCD represent an alternative expression of the factors responsible for TS (Pauls et al., 1986b).

It thus appears that at least one form of familially transmitted OCD is genetically related to TS. It is as yet unclear whether this form of OCD differs in its clinical features or pathophysiology from other forms of OCD apparently unrelated to TS. Also unknown is whether there are nonfamilial forms of OCD ("phenocopies") or other familial forms of OCD ("genocopies").

This unfolding story promises to be complex because many children with OCD have a history of tics (Swedo et al., 1989a). Furthermore, examination of the first-degree relatives of patients with OCD reveals that as many as 7% either currently have chronic tics or have had them in the past; these tics are most common in the families of probands who have both OCD and tics (Pauls, unpublished data, 1988).

TREATMENT

Psychotherapy

During most of the 20th century, psychotherapy constituted the principal mode of treatment for OCD. Nonetheless, there are no systematic studies of its efficacy. Nemiah (1984) has observed, "It is one of the ironies of clinical psychiatry that, although the obsessive-compulsive disorder illuminates the psychoanalytic concept of psychodynamic conflict perhaps better than any other psychoneurosis, its symptoms generally remain impervious to psychoanalytic treatment" (p. ix). This pessimism is not shared by those dynamically oriented child therapists who have reported favorable outcomes with psychotherapy (e.g., Adams, 1973; Anthony, 1975; Chethik, 1969). Adams (1973) recommends a flexible, interpersonally oriented approach, which produced "improvement universally" in those children who remained in treatment for more than 30 sessions. (These unquantified findings are difficult to evaluate as his heterogeneous sample included children with both true OCD and obsessional character traits.) Adams actively uses the therapist–patient relationship to help the child clarify his affects in the here-and-now, to encourage more spontaneous and direct communication as an alternative to overintellectual obfuscation, to support risk taking and a tolerance for uncertainty in place of an insistence on magical omnipotent control, and finally to foster growth of hedonic enjoyment both in interaction with the therapist and with peers. Adams cautions against nondirectiveness and an excessive emphasis on interpretation and analytic neutrality, which he believes tend to mirror and reinforce a sterile obsessional style.

Family therapy has been used to provide support and to address family interactions that may reinforce the child's symptoms. Some family approaches combine behavioral techniques with strategic, problem-focused interventions that collectively alter the functioning of the family system (Fine, 1973; O'Connor, 1983).

Behavioral Therapy

Foa and her co-workers in Philadelphia (Foa & Goldstein, 1978) and Rachman, Marks, and colleagues in England (Marks, 1987; Rachman & Hodgson, 1980) have extensively and systematically applied behavioral techniques to the treatment of obsessions and compulsions. Although these large, systematic studies were carried out with adult patient populations, their treatment principles are now being applied to younger patients (Bolton et al., 1983; Campbell, 1973; Friedman & Silvers, 1977; D. Green, 1980; Weiner, 1967). In general, the results of these scattered studies with children do not yet approach the 70% to 80% improvement rates claimed in the behavioral therapy studies with adults (Rachman & Hodgson, 1980).

A method derived from the approach developed by Victor Meyer and his collaborators (1974) combines exposure and response prevention (Foa & Steketee, 1984). The child is exposed to real or imagined contaminants or other feared objects to reduce his anxiety about them; furthermore, within the treatment situation, compulsive responses are blocked to increase his control of ritualistic behavior.

During history taking, the clinician elicits information about both the external cues (e.g., sharp objects, touching doorknobs) and internal cues (e.g., blasphemous thoughts) that trigger discomfort or anxiety. He or she also attempts to identify the dangerous consequences, physical or psychological, that the checking or the rituals are intended to ward off (e.g., catching a venereal disease from touching a doorknob; mother being killed by a burglar who enters through the unlocked door). As psychodynamically oriented therapy reveals, the chain of obsessional anxieties is often long and obscure; not only does contamination spread from one object to others, but also the "underlying danger" may be difficult to discern because of the multiple symbolic and associative displacements. The clinician notes the manifold avoidance behaviors, both passive and active, used by the patient to avoid discomfort (e.g., the child not only engages in compulsive washing but also avoids all restaurants for fear of germ-contaminated food).

With this information in hand, the therapist plans an individualized schedule of exposure and response prevention to take place in his or her presence. In vivo exposure to feared objects or actions may be combined with fantasy exposure to their dread consequences (which cannot be modeled in reality). For example, in early sessions, the therapist might join a compulsive checker in the kitchen where the patient views sharp knives left out for an hour at a time on a tabletop; the checker is also asked to imagine his brother cutting himself and bleeding to death, and then to visualize his own subsequent trial and imprisonment. In later sessions, the therapist might ask the checker to set the knives out himself or to handle them. Relaxation techniques may be woven into the exposure sessions to help the patient tolerate anxiety; however, relaxation training without exposure is generally ineffective (Marks, 1987). Response prevention might consist of limiting the checker to a single check of the kitchen each day.

Despite their efficacy with ritualistic compulsive patients, behavioral techniques have been difficult to implement in cases with pure obsessions, where the ruminations and cognitive rituals are limited to the realm of thought (Rachman & Hodgson, 1980).

Implementation of a behavioral program requires a great deal of motivation and cooperation from the patient; much support and careful attention from the therapist are also essential to maintain a positive treatment alliance. As many as 25% of adult obsessive-compulsives who approach behavioral treatment decide not to participate (Foa & Steketee, 1984). For children, it is often useful to involve the parents as cotherapists, in particular by having them help with the homework of such a desensitization program (Flament & Rapoport, 1984). This strategy also permits scrutiny of possible family overinvolvement in the child's ritualistic behavior. In cases of extreme parental collusiveness, hospitalization may be necessary to implement treatment.

Medication

Medication may be a useful adjunct for obsessive-compulsives who do not obtain relief with behavioral or psychotherapeutic interventions alone. The most carefully studied drugs have been the tricyclic and bicyclic antidepressants and the monoamine oxidase inhibitors. In addition, a panoply of other drugs including anxiolytics (such as the benzodiazepines), antipsychotics (such as the phenothiazines), lithium, and clonidine have been tried in small or uncontrolled studies. However, the methodological limitations of most of these studies make it difficult to draw firm conclusions from this body of literature. These limitations include the small size and diagnostic heterogeneity of many samples as well as unsatisfactory outcome measures (Towbin et al., 1987). Nonetheless, the following paragraphs attempt to summarize these findings.

In recent years, much investigative interest has focused on clomipramine (Anafranil). This chlorinated tricyclic antidepressant is closely related to imipramine, but is a much more potent blocker of serotonin uptake than other tricyclic antidepressants. Controlled studies, including several with children (Flament et al., 1985; Leonard et al., 1988, 1989c), indicate that clomipramine is effective against obsessive-compulsive symptoms in up to 75% of cases (Insel et al., 1983a; Insel & Mueller, 1984; Leonard, 1989a; Towbin et al., 1987). Effective dosages are comparable to those used in the treatment of depression. Improvement may not occur for 3 to 5 weeks after the onset of medication; discontinuation of the medication usually results in a recrudescence of symptoms within 1 to 2 months (Pato et al., 1988). Anticholinergic side effects are common (Flament et al., 1985). Although some studies have been inconclusive, the majority suggest that clomipramine is markedly more effective in ameliorating obsessional symptoms than other tricyclic antidepressants; despite occasional individual responders, the other tricyclics have not been shown to be superior to placebo (Leonard, 1989a; Leonard et al., 1988, 1989c). In a preliminary study, Swedo et al. (1989a) also found clomipramine to be superior to desipramine in adult women with trichotillomania, who repetitively pull their own hair, sometimes until they are bald. These researchers regard this condition as an OCD variant, perhaps involving inappropriately modulated grooming behavior.

Given the frequent co-occurrence of obsessive-compulsive symptoms, depression, and anxiety, Marks (1983) has suggested that the therapeutic efficacy of clomipramine and other antidepressants represents a nonspecific effect on mood and/or anxiety. However, most researchers have concluded that clomipramine has a direct and specific antiobsessional action not mediated by its antidepressant effects; their studies indicate that the magnitude of improvement in the obsessive-compulsive symptoms of individuals given clomipramine is independent of either the baseline degree of depression or any drug-induced changes in mood (Flament et al., 1985; Insel et al., 1983a; Leonard et al., 1988).

Clomipramine's specific and potent inhibition of serotonin uptake probably is responsible for its superior antiobsessional effect compared with other tricyclic antidepressants (Zohar & Insel, 1987). This effectiveness has encouraged the search for other nontoxic selective blockers of serotonin uptake. One such agent, fluoxetine, a bicyclic compound, has recently been marketed as an antidepressant under the trade name Prozac. In addition to having an antidepressant action, fluoxetine is effective for OCD symptoms (Fontaine & Chouinard, 1986; Turner et al., 1985). The FDA has not yet approved the drug for use in children, because research has not systematically established its safety and efficacy in this age group; however, anecdotal reports and uncontrolled open trials (Riddle et al., 1990a), suggest that fluoxetine has beneficial antiobsessional effects in children and adolescents. Double-blind controlled studies of its efficacy in children with OCD are now under way. The principal side effects of fluoxetine in children are insomnia and restlessness (Riddle et al., 1990b). Like other antidepressants, fluoxetine may have a disorganizing effect in a small number of children (King et al., 1990).

Fluvoxamine, another potent inhibitor of serotonin uptake, has also proven useful as an antiobsessional agent in double-blind studies of its efficacy (Goodman et al., 1990). In the United States this agent is currently only available for investigational use.

Monoamine oxidase inhibitors have also proved to be useful in some cases of OCD (Insel et al., 1983a), although their efficacy may be greatest when panic disorder or agoraphobia accompany the obsessive-compulsive symptoms (Towbin et al., 1987).

The ambiguous research data require the clinician to use trial and error in the practical pharmacological management of children and adolescents with severe OCD that has not responded to behavior therapy or psychotherapy. Clomipramine or fluoxetine is probably the first choice. On balance, fluoxetine appears to have fewer troublesome side effects; little is known of how the two agents compare in efficacy. If panic or agoraphobic symptoms are prominent, a monoamine oxidase inhibitor might be appropriate; such drugs are hazardous, however, unless the child's diet can be carefully monitored. If psychotic symptoms are present, antipsychotic medication is indicated. Finally, Goodman and colleagues (unpublished data, 1989) have observed that if fluoxetine alone is ineffective in relieving obsessive-compulsive symptoms, adding a small amount of haloperidol or pimozide may potentiate its effectiveness.

These unresolved psychopharmacological questions underline the need for better descriptive and outcome studies of OCD. Etiologically, obsessive-compulsive symptoms are clearly heterogeneous. A still unanswered question concerns the extent to which the coexistence of anxiety, depression, or thought disorder affects the presentation, natural history, or treatment response of the obsessive-compulsive symptoms. Jenike et al. (1986), for example, have noted that when obsessive-compulsive disorder occurs in the context of a schizotypal personality disorder, the symptoms are often resistant to drug treatment. It would be valuable to know whether family history, symptom pattern and course, or response to various drugs delineate subtypes with different prognoses or etiology (Towbin et al., 1987).

Pharmacotherapy is by no means a panacea for the obsessive-compulsive syndrome. Obsessive thoughts and rituals do not necessarily go away on medication. The patient does, however, experience them as less distressing; moreover, rituals seem to have less capacity to interfere in the patient's life and can be better resisted, with less accompanying anxiety (Flament et al., 1985a). Alleviation of obsessions and compulsions with medication does not by itself alter either the character pathology or the social withdrawal and isolation that so often accompany the core symptoms (Salzman, 1983; Thoren et al., 1980).

Prognosis and Treatment Outcome

The clinician must struggle to integrate the psychological and neurobiological paradigms proposed for OCD. The former emphasizes internal conflicts, anxiety regulation, and maladaptive defensive style. The latter stresses the predisposing genetic, constitutional, and organic factors. At present, the clinician has few established guidelines in coordinating psychotherapy, behavioral treatment, and medication. Unfortunately, without adequate outcome studies the choice of treatment method in any given case depends all too often on the therapist's theoretical predilections rather than on reliable indications for one modality or another.

Education, support, and general attempts to reduce anxiety and conflict in both the patient and the family are undoubtedly important. In children whose obsessional symptoms appear embedded in an overly perfectionistic or constricted character structure, these maladaptive personality traits deserve psychotherapeutic attention regardless of the other modalities employed.

The success of any proposed treatment can only be assessed against background knowledge about the natural history of the disorder including its long-term course. Existing long-term follow-up studies predate the use of specific serotonergic drugs or behavioral methods; most of these studies also suffer from various methodological problems. Follow-ups of adult obsessional patients suggest that OCD runs a chronic but variable course (Black, 1974; Goodwin et al., 1969; Kringlen, 1965; Rachman & Hodgson, 1980). Only a small number of patients ever experience a complete and permanent remission of symptoms, and about one-third of the patients run a deteriorating course. In between these extremes lie the majority of patients; their symptoms may wax and wane, but they are rarely symptom-free (Black, 1974). Patients with OCD do not appear to show greater proneness to schizophrenia, suicide, or substance abuse (Goodwin et al., 1969).

Follow-up studies of childhood obsessional patients present a rather pessimistic picture (Hollingsworth et al., 1980; Warren, 1960). Writing prior to the availability of the new antiobsessional drugs, Elkins and colleagues (1980) somberly concluded that "the disease is resistant to therapy and runs a dismal course in a great number of cases" (p. 514). The majority of these children continue to experience moderately severe obsessive-compulsive symptoms into young adulthood. By choosing careers where their obsessional symptoms are either useful or acceptable, some sufferers make an adequate occupational adjustment. Most of them, however, continue to have difficulty forming close interpersonal relationships. The patients in Hollingsworth et al.'s (1980) study were treated primarily with psychotherapy once or twice a week; those who participated in the follow-up study all felt that their symptoms were less disabling after treatment, but only 3 patients out of 10 claimed to be symptom-free. Bolton and colleagues

(1983) treated 15 hospitalized adolescent obsessive-compulsive patients with behavioral techniques combined with family and milieu therapy. Their approach emphasized "simplicity, clarity, and correct identification of feelings" as well as the toleration of distress and anger; in addition, clomipramine was used in four cases. As follow-up 9 to 48 months later, 7 cases (47%) remained free of obsessional symptoms; 3 were mildly incapacitated, 2 ran an episodic course, and 2 were severely incapacitated.

Most impressions of the natural history of obsessive-compulsive symptoms are drawn from patients with difficulties that are sufficiently severe and persistent to bring them to clinical attention. Much less is known about the many subjects who report obsessive-compulsive symptoms in community-based samples; many of these subjects never seek treatment. Berg et al. (1989) conducted a 2-year prospective follow-up of a community-based sample of high school students whom they had surveyed for obsessive-compulsive features (Flament et al., 1988). An initial diagnosis of OCD was generally associated at follow-up with either persistent OCD or "other psychiatric disorder with obsessive-compulsive features." At follow-up, about one-quarter of the adolescents previously diagnosed as having subclinical OCD or obsessive-compulsive personality now met the full criteria for OCD, whereas most of the remainder showed persistent obsessive-compulsive features. The study data suggested that even in nonreferred adolescents obsessive-compulsive symptoms may be both persistent and disabling.

Chapter 10

Tic Disorders

INTRODUCTION

Tics are recurrent, rapid, meaningless movements or sounds. Apparently purposeless, they are often repetitive and generally involve functionally related groups of muscles, in which case they are called *motor tics*. Tics may also consist of involuntary noises or words and are then called *vocal tics*. The person who manifests these behaviors is called a *tiqueur,* and the word is occasionally used as a verb: *to tic.* The most severe form, with both vocal and motor tics, is known as Tourette's syndrome (TS).

The tic disorders provide an interesting experiment of nature illustrating the complexity of volition. These stereotyped movements resemble voluntary motor acts in that they are the product of coordinated, systematic motor action; they are involuntary in the sense that they lack apparent purpose and occur without deliberate intent. Although the tiqueur, with effort, may suppress the tics for minutes or hours, sooner or later they will recur against his will. Common motor tics include eye blinks, grimaces, head shakes, jerking of the fingers or hands, shrugs, and shaking of the foot or leg. Common vocal tics include guttural throat-clearing noises, lip smacking, sniffing, chirping, or repeated syllables out of context. So many children tic at some point in their lives that most parents or teachers have been tempted at one time or another to shriek, "Stop that twitching" (or "Stop making that noise"). Fortunately, tics are usually a transient phenomenon, and only a small number of children show multiple tics that persist throughout life.

DSM-III-R (APA, 1987) describes three specific tic disorders: *Transient Tic Disorder, Chronic Motor* or *Vocal Tic Disorder,* and *Tourette's Disorder.* These conditions run the gamut of symptomatic intensity from the transient and merely annoying to the chronic and severely disabling. DSM-III-R descriptively distinguishes these three disorders in terms of the frequency, persistence, and variety of tics. However, the precise criteria employed by DSM-III-R to make these distinctions are arbitrary, rather than demarcating truly distinctive syndromes with different etiologies or clinical course. For example, growing evidence suggests that, in terms of etiology, chronic tic disorder and TS are most likely not separate entities; rather, they represent points on a continuum of severity of a single genetic disorder. Some transient tics may also represent a mild expression of the same genetic trait (Kurlan et al., 1988).

The tic disorders are of great interest to the clinical researcher—the transient tics because they are so prevalent and TS because it causes dramatic disability and offers elusive clues regarding the neurophysiological organization of volition and inhibition.

DEFINITION

DSM-III-R Diagnostic Criteria for Transient Tic Disorder

A. *Single or multiple motor and/or vocal tics.*

B. *The tics occur many times a day, nearly every day for at least two weeks, but for no longer than twelve consecutive months.*

C. *No history of Tourette's or Chronic Motor or Vocal Tic Disorder.*

D. *Onset before age 21.*

E. *Occurrence not exclusively during Psychoactive Substance Intoxication or known central nervous system disease, such as Huntington's chorea and postviral encephalitis.* (APA, 1987, p. 82)

DSM-III-R Diagnostic Criteria for Chronic Motor or Vocal Tic Disorder

A. *Either motor or vocal tics, but not both, have been present at some time during the illness.*

B. *The tics occur many times a day, nearly every day, or intermittently throughout a period of more than one year.*

C. *Onset before age 21.*

D. *Occurrence not exclusively during Psychoactive Substance Intoxication or known central nervous system disease, such as Huntington's chorea and postviral encephalitis.* (APA, 1987, p. 81)

DSM-III-R Diagnostic Criteria for Tourette's Disorder

A. *Both multiple motor and one or more vocal tics have been present at some time during the illness, although not necessarily concurrently.*

B. *The tics occur many times a day (usually in bouts), nearly every day or intermittently throughout a period of more than one year.*

C. *The anatomic location, number, frequency, complexity, and severity of the tics change over time.*

D. *Onset before age 21.*

E. *Occurrence not exclusively during Psychoactive Substance Intoxication or known central nervous system disease, such as Huntington's chorea and postviral encephalitis.* (APA, 1987, p. 80)

EPIDEMIOLOGY

Transient tics are common symptoms that appear more frequently in childhood than in adolescence or adult life. Surveys of large nonclinical populations show that at one time or another about 3% to 8% of children have tics (Zahner et al., 1988). Ages 6 to 11 years seem to be the peak frequency period for this behavior. Tics seem to occur more frequently in the families of transient tiqueurs (see Etiology) and to affect more boys than girls by a ratio varying from 2:1 to 4:1.

Tourette's syndrome is much less common than transient tic disorder. Until recently, TS was considered to be extremely rare. However, with increased lay and professional awareness, many more cases (including mild ones) are being identified. Researchers have estimated the prevalence of TS in children under 18 years at 9.3 per 10,000 for boys and 1 per 10,000 for girls (Burd et al., 1986). The prevalence rate in adults is much lower, about 0.5 per 10,000, suggesting that many cases remit after adolescence (Zahner et al., 1988). Epidemiological studies indicate that there are many mild, clinically undiagnosed cases. The Tourette Syndrome Association has compiled a registry of several thousand self-identified TS patients in this country. In most studies, males outnumber females by a ratio of about 3:1 to 9:1. Familial clustering occurs, with an increased incidence of both TS and multiple motor tics in the families of TS patients (Pauls et al., 1984).

CLINICAL FEATURES

Transient Tic Disorders

Isolated transient tics, especially eye blinks or other facial tics, are extremely common in childhood. Blinking or sniffing tics may initially be misdiagnosed as refraction problems or allergies. When the tics involve the rest of the body, it may be difficult, if not impossible, to distinguish them from habitual autoerotic manipulation or general fidgetiness. Transient vocal tics are uncommon.

Simple transient tics frequently appear at times of acute excitement, boredom, or chronic stress. Simple tics may wax and wane in intensity. To what extent the propensity to develop simple transient tics reflects a genetically transmitted vulnerability is unclear (see section on Etiology). Similarly it is not known whether children with simple transient tics are at increased risk for the attentional or cognitive difficulties that often accompany the tics of Tourette's syndrome.

Although Mahler (1949) left open the role of constitutional factors, she approached tics from a psychodynamic perspective and distinguished several types of psychogenic tic. In her view, many tics represented "transient tension phenomena," presumably discharging anxiety and muscular tension. Certain other tics, she speculated, had a more complex neurotic structure, representing a compromise or "symbolic expression of a conflict in body language." However, such tics may gradually lose their "obvious and clear connection with the original motivation" and occur seemingly at random.

Chronic Tic Disorder

By definition, tics are classified transient if they last less than a year and chronic if they persist beyond one year. Like other tics, chronic tics may fluctuate in intensity and are often exacerbated by stress, excitement, or fatigue. Although many children with chronic motor tics improve markedly by later adolescence, in a small number, tics persist relatively unchanged. The causal heterogeneity reflected by this varied outcome is unclear.

Gilles de La Tourette's Syndrome

Tourette's syndrome (TS) takes its name from George Gilles de La Tourette who in 1885 described what he considered its cardinal features: convulsive muscular jerks, inarticulate cries, and finally coprolalia (uttering obscene words) and echolalia (echoing others' words) (Gilles de La Tourette, 1885/1982). He recounted, among other cases, the tragic and exemplary history of the Marquise De Dampierre. When first seen by Itard, the Marquise, then 26 years old, was already confined to her estate by her illness. The affliction had begun at age 7 with jerking of the arms; these convulsive jerks later spread to the rest of her body. In later childhood unformed vocalizations appeared and finally repetitive obscene epithets. After a lifetime of seclusion, she was seen as an octogenarian by Charcot who noted the persistence of her symptoms. As Gilles de La Tourette gained clinical experience with the syndrome, which he speculated was hereditary, he noted that there was no mental deterioration and that the disease, although chronic, ran a waxing and waning course with periods of remission and exacerbation for the individual symptoms. Many people think of the florid, dramatic symptoms described by Gilles de la Tourette whenever they hear of the syndrome that bears in his name. In reality, however, most cases are far milder; many do not even come to clinical attention.

The initial symptoms of TS resemble the transient motor tics of childhood described above and appear between ages 2 and 16 years, with a mean of about 7 years (Bruun, 1988). Usually these motor tics appear first in the head and face and then, during the ensuing months and years, gradually involve the upper parts of the body and, ultimately, the trunk and legs (Jagger et al., 1982). The variety of these motor tics is virtually inexhaustible. They may consist of *simple motor tics*, which are quick, meaningless movements (blinking, rapid jerking of the head or limbs, grimacing, teeth grinding, shoulder shrugging, knee jerking, etc.), or *complex motor tics*, which are slower and more purposeful in appearance (biting, kissing, hitting, touching, clapping, sniffing objects, etc.) (Cohen et al., 1985).

In the early phases of the disease, when only one or two motor tics are present, differentiation from transient tic disorder may not be possible. Vocal tics, however, which usually appear after the motor tics, strongly suggest TS. Initially, these variegated vocal tics may be *simple* ones consisting of loud or soft noises such as guttural throat clearing, sniffing, clicks, and chirps. Later, vocal tics may become *complex,* consisting of inappropriately blurted words or phrases, often out of apparent context. Speech prosody may be altered with loss of fluency and overemphasis of certain words or syllables.

Coprolalia and echolalia, when present, tend to appear around puberty. For example, one boy with unformed vocalizations in early latency later began to shout out explosively at inappropriate moments "Easter!" or "Christmas!" and still later on "Puberty!" Finally, in adolescence he developed frank coprolalia (R. Gross, personal communication, 1980). Attempts to suppress scatalogical outbursts may result in the partial breakthrough of stuttered initial syllables (e.g., "sh-sh-sh" or "f-f-f") or substitutes ("Sugar!"). Although the lay public frequently associates coprolalia with TS, it occurs in only about one-third of individuals seen in specialty clinics (Bruun, 1988).

During preadolescence various complex motor tics and compulsive acts often make their appearances, including touching objects and tapping, kissing, biting, or touching self or others (especially sexual organs). Other striking symptoms include "mirror" phenomena, the compulsive imitation of what others have just said (echolalia) or done (echopraxia). Careful questioning may also reveal obsessive-compulsive mental phenomena such as recurrent, intrusive, and unwanted thoughts or images, often concerning injury, sex, death, or other emotionally charged issues. The compulsions consist of powerful impulses to perform various actions, such as counting or arranging objects, which can be restrained only with great difficulty, if at all. Classic compulsions, such as washing rituals may appear, as well as obsessive doubting and checking (Grad et al., 1987). By adulthood, these overt obsessive-compulsive symptoms may warrant an associated diagnosis of obsessive-compulsive disorder in as many as 55% to 90% of TS patients (Pauls et al., 1986). (See also Genetic Factors and Chapter 9, "Obsessive-Compulsive Disorder.")

The prevalence of these several symptoms varies from patient to patient, ranging from the ubiquity of motor tics through making loud noises (67%); touching objects, self, or others (50%–55%); tapping (43%); coprolalia and echolalia (37%); and echopraxia (21%) (Jagger et al., 1982). The frequency and intensity of symptoms also vary widely between individuals. Many patients, at least in public, may show only a few furtive motor tics or noises; others, a small minority, may be swept by constant storms of activity, almost convulsively hurling themselves about the room, hitting at themselves, or being unable to complete a sentence without a torrent of cries and noises. A few patients injure themselves seriously with the violence of their explosive tics. More deliberate self-destructive behaviors also occur, such as head-banging or poking self with sharp objects (Cohen et al., 1985).

Within the individual patient, the severity of any given tic or symptom also fluctuates. One tic will often disappear for a while, only to be replaced by another. Symptoms usually escalate with emotional stress or physical fatigue and decrease markedly during sleep. By dint of considerable effort, the patient can often suppress individual symptoms for short periods, albeit with increasing difficulty. Once he relaxes vigilance, there may be an explosive release. Thus, some children can completely or partially suppress their symptoms in school or church or while playing a musical instrument. Some patients attempt to disguise a tic as an ostensibly purposeful gesture (e.g., an arm twitch as a brushing back of the hair) or to substitute a more socially acceptable tic for a repulsive one.

Patients with earlier onset of tics often have a more severe and persistent course. The symptoms of TS are often most socially disabling in adolescence, when concerns over social acceptance are paramount. By later adolescence, however, many patients experience spontaneous improvement (Bruun, 1988), and a few show long-term remissions, perhaps with obsessions and inner compulsions as their only residue (Cohen et al., 1987b). In most cases, however, lifetime intermittent symptoms are the norm.

Joseph Bliss, a TS sufferer for 62 years, recorded his symptoms and sensations meticulously over several decades and gave an eloquent account of the inner life of the TS patient (Bliss, 1980). His account captures the half-voluntary, half-involuntary quality of his tics, as well as the subtle sensations that accompany the tics in many cases of TS:

> Each movement is preceded by certain preliminary sensory signals and is in turn followed by sensory impressions at the end of the action. Each movement is the result of a voluntary capitulation to a demanding and relentless urge accompanied by an extraordinarily subtle sensation that provokes and fuels the urge. Successively sharper movements build up to a climax, a climax that never comes. There really is no adequate description of the sensations that signal the onset of the actions. The first one seems irresistible, calling for an almost inevitable response. It is possible to apprehend it at this point, to recognize it, and to realize that it can be studied, modified, or even temporarily extinguished. . . .
>
> But the mind cannot forever be on the alert for this preliminary phase. Sooner or later the sensation appears when the mind is distracted by other things and/or has forgotten what can happen. Then the feeling appears, and the attempt is made almost as a reflex to be rid of the annoyance. A slight movement results and escalates instantly into sharper movements in the frenzy to get relief.
>
> [A] very rapidly escalating desire to satisfy the sensation with movements intended to free oneself from the insistent feeling ensues. . . . The TS movements are intentionally bodily movements. The intention is to relieve a sensation, as surely as the movement to scratch an itch is to relieve the itch. . . .
>
> When highly activated, the sensation immediately preceding a movement can be compared, inexactly, with a number of other types of feelings (1) a

compelling, though subtle and fleeting, itch; (2) the moments before a sneeze explodes; or (3) the tantalizing touch of a feather.

The end of a TS action is the "feel" at the terminal site of the movement, a feel that is frequently accompanied by a fleeting and incomplete sense of relief. The relief (if perceived at all) dissipates, to be replaced quickly with a new urge to repeat the action. . . . The sensation now is comparable in intensity and motivation, if not in character, to a flaming itch that seems to pull the fingers to fierce scratching for relief. This now kinesthetic sensory effect demands even more violent movement. . . . After some time and torment, exhaustion becomes a competing demand. Only sleep extinguishes the action. Or an orgasmic distraction. Or a calamity.

[T]he symptoms will constantly recur and need to be confronted and extinguished endlessly. The result is a kind of half-life in which there is constant vigilance and divided attention. (pp. 1344–1346)

The TS patient must deploy this constant vigilance not only against meaningless motor acts but against a host of other impulses: to curse, to touch, to hit, and to kiss. There are many fleeting thoughts and impulses (usually concerned with sex or hostility) that most unafflicted people permit only momentarily into consciousness before banishing them; the TS patient, however, is driven to shout them out (e.g., "nice tits!"; "Look at that fat guy!"; "Outta my way!") or put them into action (e.g., pinching, kissing, or touching).

Such a patient feels himself split in two—a shameful, chthonic, barely controllable half represented by the tics, which threatens constantly to burst into the open, and a constantly vigilant half, which must endlessly strive, with only partial success, to keep the daemonic element in check. The very boundaries of the self—the distinction between what is passively experienced and actively willed—is constantly in question for TS children, who encounter a relentless series of impulses, thoughts, and motor urges experienced partially as uncontrollable and involuntary and partially as willed (Cohen, 1980b). This divided inner life has a powerful effect on the TS child's developing sense of self.

The seemingly bizarre and sometimes obscene behavior of certain TS patients led early observers to equate the syndrome with severe character pathology. Although by no means synonymous with severe or psychotic psychopathology, the disease can profoundly affect development when symptoms are frequent or conspicuous. The social problems of such children, especially those with coprolalia, are obviously serious. Frequently teased by classmates, shunned by strangers, and reproved by teachers, these children lead the painful and sometimes lonely life of the pariah.

In addition, TS children have several difficulties that cannot be fully attributed either to social stigma and isolation or to inner turmoil. Even before tics first appear, many children later diagnosed as having TS are emotionally labile and irritable; parents often describe them as having a "short fuse." Difficulties with classroom learning and attention, as well as impulsiveness, are common and also frequently antedate the onset of tics. Although the distribution of TS patients' intelligence scores appears normal, many have subtle deficits on attentional and cognitive processing tasks (Golden, 1984; Hagin & Kugler, 1988). Difficulties in visual-motor integration and perceptual organization are common in those TS patients who also have attention deficits with hyperactivity (Dykens et al., manuscript submitted for publication, 1990). These children's school performances are often below their apparent ability, and their learning and attentional problems continue into adolescence. Not surprisingly, before the full panoply of TS symptoms manifest themselves, a large number of such children receive diagnoses of learning disability or attention-deficit hyperactivity disorder (ADHD). In at least 50% of children with TS, ADHD may be an accurate concurrent diagnosis (Cohen et al., 1985).

For many children with TS, their emotional lability and ADHD-like symptoms may be much more disabling than their tics (Stokes et al., 1988). No clear correlation exists between the severity of the tic disorder and these symptoms; children with mild tics may nonetheless be severely impulsive and inattentive.

ETIOLOGY

In recent years researchers have made great advances in elucidating the determinants of TS and related tic disorders. The emerging picture of TS may well serve as a model for other childhood-onset neuropsychiatric disorders: an apparently genetically determined vulnerability, age-dependent expression of symptoms (which may reflect maturational factors), sexual dimorphism, stress-dependent fluctuations in symptomatic severity, and possibly significant environmental influences on the phenotypic expression of the underlying genotype (Leckman et al., 1988b). These discoveries have important implications for treating and preventing this disabling disorder. Perhaps even more significant, advances in understanding TS provide "a useful paradigm for the integration of genetic, biological, and experiential factors in the emergence, natural history, and range of expression of a disorder" (Cohen, unpublished manuscript, 1989).

Genetic Factors

One of the most exciting recent advances concerns the genetics of TS. About 65% to 90% of TS cases have a positive family history of either TS or chronic multiple tics. In family studies in which chronic multiple tics are treated as a less severe manifestation of TS, the vulnerability to TS appears to be transmitted as an autosomal dominant trait (Pauls & Leckman, 1986, 1988). However, gender and other factors influence the phenotypic expression of the gene.

Twins show a marked discrepancy in the concordance rate for TS for monozygotic (MZ) twins (53%) compared with dyzygotic (DZ) twins (8%) (Price et al., 1985). When the criteria are broadened to include *any* tics in the cotwins, the concordance rates are 77% or higher for the MZ pairs and 23% for the DZ pairs. This discrepancy suggests a strong genetic component for TS and reinforces the likelihood that many milder forms of tics are related to TS. At the same time, the finding that a small number of the MZ twins are fully discordant for tics suggests that nongenetic factors also play a role.

Which nongenetic factors influence the phenotypic expression of the TS gene remains unclear. Differences in prenatal environment are one possibility, suggested by the observation that in the discordant MZ pairs, the twins with TS were significantly lighter at birth than their unaffected cotwins (Leckman et al., 1987a). Similarly, Pasamanick and Kawi (1956) found an increased rate of complications during the gestation of TS children compared with controls. A retrospective pilot study by Leckman et al. (1990) found that the severity of maternal life stresses and maternal nausea and vomiting during pregnancy were robust predictors of later tic severity. How these potential prenatal risk factors exert their influence is unknown. TS patients' symptoms often intensify with anxiety and increased stress; Leckman et al. (1987b) have suggested that stress may also play a role in the onset of symptoms in genetically vulnerable individuals.

Range of Expression of the TS Gene.   The family study data cited earlier suggest that chronic multiple tics represent a less severe phenotypic expression of the TS gene (Pauls et al., 1984). It is logical to ask to what extent genetic factors also play a predisposing role in the transient tics of childhood. Such tics appear to be a common developmental phenomenon; population surveys identify as many as 15% of school-age boys as having tics (Zahner et al., 1988). Clinicians have speculated about the possible role of anxiety, stress, and internal conflict in the genesis of transient tics. Unfortunately, there have been as yet no longitudinal studies to delineate the natural history of common tics or to assess the number of children in whom tics either persist or recur.

Kurlan et al. (1988), in their study of a large family with a high prevalence of TS and chronic motor tics, found two family members with a history of nonrecurrent transient tics (i.e., less than a year's duration). Although their geneotype could not be precisely defined, their pedigrees suggested that transient tic disorder may also represent a mild alternate phenotypic expression of the TS gene. Thus, in some individuals, transient tics are related to the TS gene; such individuals with transient tics may thus also transmit TS to their offspring (Kurlan et al., 1988). Further research is necessary to resolve whether other forms of transient tics exist that are not genetically determined ("phenocopies") or that have alternate genetic determinants ("genocopies").

Obsessive-Compulsive Symptoms. As discussed earlier, obsessive-compulsive symptoms are common in patients with TS. Conversely, a history of tics is often found in patients coming to clinical attention for obsessive-compulsive disorder (OCD). However, a more intimate relationship than comorbidity exists between these disorders. Family studies strongly suggest that TS and at least some forms of OCD are alternate phenotypic manifestations of the same underlying gene. Thus, the frequency of OCD in the first-degree relatives of TS patients is increased (Pauls et al., 1986; Pauls & Leckman, 1986). These relatives, especially females, may have OCD *without* any of the tic symptoms of TS. The equally high prevalence of OCD in the families of TS patients both with and without OCD suggests that the two disorders are not independently transmitted. Although this TS-related form of OCD may be less severe than that occurring without a family history of tics, the two forms of OCD seem otherwise clinically indistinguishable (Pauls & Leckman, 1986). (See also Chapter 9, "Obsessive-Compulsive Disorder.")

It appears that the families of TS patients do not specifically transmit TS, but rather a genetic vulnerability that can be variably expressed as either obsessive-compulsive disorder and/or a tic disorder ranging in severity from transient tics through chronic tics to full-blown TS. Studies at the Yale Child Study Center (Pauls & Leckman, 1988; Pauls et al., 1990) suggest that this vulnerability is transmitted as an autosomal dominant trait with very high penetrance (close to 100%) for males and somewhat lower penetrance (about 70%) for females. Thus, in families with the TS gene, males who carry the gene are extremely likely to manifest one of these disorders, whereas females are less likely to do so. Furthermore, the expression of the gene shows sexual dimorphism, that is, females, compared with males, are more likely to manifest the gene as OCD. The exploration of the possible hormonal, genetic, and/or neuromaturational factors underlying this sexual dimorphism is an important area for further research. Another uncertainty concerns the additional, nongender related factors that determine the diverse outcomes for genetically vulnerable individuals: tic disorder, OCD, or some combination of the two. Comings and Comings have argued that the phenotypic manifestations of the putative TS gene are even more protean and span a wide array of disinhibition disorders including anxiety disorders, attention-deficit hyperactivity disorder, and affective disorders. However, their methodology and conclusions remain open to question (Merz, 1988).

Utilizing new recombinant DNA techniques, linkage studies of large pedigrees afflicted with TS promise to reveal the specific genetic locus (or loci) responsible for vulnerability to TS (Pauls et al., 1990). This advance will permit sequencing of the gene and a more precise analysis of its function. In addition, the ability to determine which relatives of TS or OCD patients actually carry the TS gene will make it possible to learn more about the environmental factors that influence the gene's phenotypic expression. In conjunction with the ongoing search for the TS gene, long-term prospective studies of high-risk children (i.e., those who have a parent or sibling with either a tic disorder or OCD) are underway. Such studies should also help delineate the risk and protective factors that influence the developmental expression of the TS gene (Leckman et al., 1990).

Neurobiological Factors

Neurotransmitter Systems.   The pathophysiology of TS is still unknown. Recent investigations have focused on the role of disordered central nervous system neurotransmitter mechanisms (Chappell et al., 1990; Cohen et al., 1979; Leckman et al., 1988b). Alterations in the balance of the dopaminergic, serotonergic, noradrenergic, and endogenous opioid systems have all been suggested by different lines of evidence; knowledge is still tentative and fragmentary. The ability of dopamine agonists (such as dextroamphetamine or methylphenidate) to exacerbate or even precipitate the tic symptoms of TS suggests *dopaminergic* involvement. In many cases, dopamine-blocking agents (such as haloperidol and pimozide) markedly reduce TS symptoms. However, the reduced level of dopamine metabolites in the cerebrospinal fluid (csf) of TS patients does not fit a simple dopamine hypothesis (Cohen et al., 1979). *Noradrenergic* mechanisms in TS seem possible from several findings, including the ability of anxiety and stress to exacerbate symptoms and the apparent efficacy of clonidine (a blocker of central alpha-2 noradrenergic activity) in reducing some TS patients' symptoms. *Serotonin* is of interest because of its apparent role in OCD and the substantial reduction of its principal metabolite in the csf of TS patients (Cohen et al., 1979). The *endogenous opioid peptides*, especially the dynorphin group, have also drawn much attention. These neuropeptides interact with other transmitter systems. Tentative findings from csf studies (Leckman et al., 1988a) and postmortem studies of TS brains (Haber et al., 1986) suggest possible alterations in dynorphin regulation.

The balance and reciprocal relationships of the several neurotransmitter systems are exceedingly intricate. The possibility that TS may be a metabolically as well as clinically heterogeneous disease further complicates unraveling this complex skein of data. Thus, some TS cases are extremely sensitive to haloperidol, a dopamine antagonist, whereas other cases are refractory to even large doses but respond readily to clonidine (Leckman et al., 1988b).

Neuroanatomical Localization.   Neuroanatomical speculation about the pathogenesis of TS (as well as OCD) has focused on the midbrain structures known as the *basal ganglia* (Chappell et al., 1990; Swedo & Rapoport, 1990). These regions are rich in various neurotransmitters and are extensively connected to the sensorimotor and associational regions of the cortex (Albin et al., 1989). Furthermore, they play a role in various movement disorders including Parkinson's disease, Huntington's chorea, and Sydenham's chorea. Postmortem studies of a small number of TS brains suggest altered neurotransmitter levels in the basal ganglia (Anderson et al., unpublished data, 1989; Haber et al., 1986). In addition, a small pilot study of adult TS patients using positron emission tomography (PET) scanning found increased glucose metabolism in the basal ganglia and in the temporal and frontal lobes (Chase et al., 1984).

Stimulant Medication. Motor tics are a common side effect of stimulant medication; most often the tics gradually disappear following the medicine's discontinuance. However, in a small number of the many children treated for hyperactivity, stimulants such as methylphenidate (Ritalin) precipitate full-blown and sometimes irreversible TS (Golden, 1977; Lowe et al., 1982). It is unclear whether these hyperactive children were genetically vulnerable with unrecognized prodromal cases of TS in whom methylphenidate simply hastened the development of full-blown symptoms or whether these children might have remained tic-free were it not for medication. A study of six pairs of identical twins concordant for tics suggests the former possibility; even though only one twin in each pair received stimulant medication, both twins in each pair ultimately developed tics (Price et al., 1986). Stimulant medication, however, should be used only with extreme caution in hyperactive children with tics or with a family history of multiple tics (Golden, 1988).

TREATMENT

Transient Tic Disorder

Simple transient tics most often occur at times of emotional tension. The clinician should direct attention to identifying and relieving the underlying stresses in the child's life. The indications for individual psychotherapy and/or family therapy depend on the basic emotional difficulty. If this approach is taken, it is usually best not to focus psychotherapy too narrowly on the tic itself.

Behavior modification approaches that have been tried with some success include negative massed practice (deliberately and provocatively repeating the gesture), positive reinforcement for inhibition of the tic, practicing of competing movements and awareness training (Azrin & Nunn, 1973).

The transient natural course of most simple tics complicates the assessment of treatment methods.

Tourette's Syndrome and Chronic Tic Disorder

The first stage of treatment is a broad-based, comprehensive assessment of the child's psychological, social, and educational adaptation. Beyond evaluating the child's neurological status and TS symptoms, it is essential to explore the impact of the condition on the various spheres of the child's life. As noted earlier, the obsessive-compulsive symptoms and attentional, learning, and behavioral difficulties that often accompany TS may cause greater impairment than the tics themselves (Stokes et al., 1988).

Medication. Drug treatment may be targeted at the tic symptoms, attentional deficits, or obsessive-compulsive phenomena associated with TS. The indications and choice of medication are different for each of these symptom-realms.

A trial of medication for tics is indicated if the child's tics cause physical discomfort, interfere with classroom participation, or create social difficulties for the child. It is important to obtain an adequate picture of the child's baseline, premedication level of tics. Both the clinician's observations and parents' reports should be documented on standard tic rating scales such as the Tourette Syndrome Global Scale and the Tourette Syndrome Symptom List (Leckman et al., 1988c).

Haloperidol (Haldol) has been the most widely used drug, and many TS patients respond well to small doses. Side effects, however, are often substantial and may include sedation, cognitive blunting, depression, and, rarely, a dramatic pharmacologically induced upsurge of separation anxiety (Mikkelsen et al., 1981). These side effects are an especially severe problem in those patients who require large doses of haloperidol to control their tics. Habituation is a concern with many patients for whom even ever-increasing levels of haloperidol lose their effect. Rebound phenomena, with a catastrophic exacerbation of symptoms after withdrawing the drug, are a serious complication presumably due to drug-induced receptor supersensitivity. A few cases of Tourette-like tardive dyskinesias have been reported in apparently psychotic children after withdrawal of long-term neuroleptic medication. Because of potential cardiac conduction abnormalities, a base-line EKG should be obtained before beginning neuroleptic medication.

In recent years, pimozide (Orap), a neuroleptic with more specific dopamine receptor-blocking activity than haloperidol, has been made available in the United States for treating TS. Pimozide appears to be as effective as haloperidol in controlling tics. Although pimozide has been reported in some studies to have the advantage of less sedation and fewer dystonic reactions than haloperidol (Moldofsky and Sandor, 1988), pimozide may have potentially greater cardiac effects. As with other neuroleptics, extrapyramidal symptoms, tardive dyskinesia, depression, and sedation are also side effects of pimozide.

The complications of haloperidol and pimozide treatment have created growing interest in alternative medications. One such agent is clonidine (Catapres), an alpha-adrenergic blocking agent originally developed as an antihypertensive. Clonidine has found increasingly wide use as a drug of first choice because of its less severe short- and long-term side effects and its frequent beneficial effects on the ADHD-like side effects that often accompany TS (Cohen et al., 1980; Leckman et al., 1985). Clonidine is usually given in 3 to 4 doses daily to maintain tic control. It is most often begun as a single 0.05 mg dose in the morning with additional doses gradually added at noon, after school, and at supper time. Total daily doses above 0.3 mg usually lead to problematic side effects. Many TS patients on clonidine experience improvement of their tics and reduced tension (Leckman et al., 1988d, unpublished data, 1990). The principal side effects of clonidine are drowsiness, which is often transient, irritability, and hypotension. On a given dosage of clonidine, improvement may take several weeks or months to become fully apparent. Hence any clinical trial of clonidine must be of adequate duration and involve gradual titration of the dosage.

The attentional deficit and the impulsivity of many TS children frequently impair their social and academic development. Careful assessment of these symptom areas is important and should include systematic observations by parents and teachers on a standard rating instrument such as the Conners' Rating Scale (see Chapter 11, "Attention-Deficit Hyperactivity Disorder").

Clonidine's beneficial effect on the impulsivity, inattention, and emotional lability that are often part of the TS picture make the drug potentially useful for children who have both tics and ADHD. Many, but not all experts, consider the stimulant drugs to be contraindicated in such children (Golden, 1988). A trial of clonidine may be helpful in those children with TS who have only mild tics, but whose impulsivity, distractibility, and lability are major problems at home and school. The tricyclic antidepressants, such as desipramine, have also proved helpful for the ADHD-like symptoms of TS and appear to represent another useful alternative to stimulant medication (Riddle et al., 1988a).

In children with TS who are troubled by prominent obsessive or compulsive symptoms, a trial of fluoxetine (Prozac) or clomipramine (Anafranil) may be warranted (Riddle et al., 1988b, 1990a). As neither drug has yet been approved by the FDA for general use in children, such trials are best done as part of a carefully designed protocol.

Other Treatment Considerations. The dramatic impact of medication in many cases of TS should not obscure the need for establishing a long-term relationship with the child and family to assess and monitor the child's overall adaptation and to provide empathic support and treatment as needed (Cohen et al., 1988). Psychotherapy, parent counseling, and vocational and special education measures may all help manage the psychosocial and educational complications of the disease (Towbin et al., 1988). Particularly important functions of the clinician are to serve as the child's advocate and as a source of information and education to the child's school, which may have little experience with TS. Parents and children need much ongoing help and support in dealing with what is often a serious lifelong condition that influences psychological, educational, social, and vocational adjustment. Helping parents, child, and teachers understand the child's condition as a chronic, constitutional disorder, but a potentially ameliorable one, is important in destigmatizing symptoms that may otherwise be seen as willful, defiant, or crazy. The Tourette Syndrome Association, a national self-help group of TS patients and their parents, is a valuable source of support and information.

PART IV

Disorders of Learning, Attention, and Behavior

Chapter 11

Attention-Deficit Hyperactivity Disorder

INTRODUCTION

Attention-deficit hyperactivity disorder (ADHD) consists of developmentally inappropriate levels of *inattentiveness* and *impulsivity,* usually accompanied by *hyperactivity.* Frequently associated features include *emotional lability, irritability, learning disabilities,* and *aggression.* The syndrome is sometimes better known under its older rubrics, "minimal brain damage" or "minimal cerebral dysfunction." Such terms embody an implied etiologic hypothesis, whereas others, like "hyperkinetic syndrome," emphasize a particular symptom. However designated, it is one of the most frequently diagnosed behavioral disorders of children, and, as such, it is the object of great clinical interest and theoretical controversy. In some clinic samples, up to one-third of children carry this diagnosis (Weiss & Hechtman, 1979), and in the United States more than 600,000 children a year receive stimulant medication for its treatment (Barkley, 1981). At the same time, prominent critics of the concept have doubted the very existence of ADHD as a valid syndrome (Rutter, 1983a). Although they concede the existence of inattentive and hyperactive children, the critics maintain that these symptoms do not cooccur regularly, nor do they delineate a distinct group of children who are reliably distinguishable from children with other diagnostic labels (such as conduct disorder). Such critics point to the notable difficulties in reliably identifying and diagnosing the disorder, and they remain unconvinced that the current diagnostic criteria truly define a distinctive group of children who share the same underlying pathophysiology, clinical course, prognosis, or treatment response (see Appendix 11–1 for further discussion).

The history of attention-deficit hyperactivity disorder provides a fascinating, albeit humbling, example of the developmental vicissitude of a syndrome from initial description through theoretical elaboration to ultimate overextension and reification. A brief historical overview provides the best introduction to this disorder's conceptual complexity (Kessler, 1980).

Fidgety, impulsive, inattentive children have long caused their parents and teachers to despair. A notorious illustration is the boy immortalized by a physician, Heinrich Hoffman (1845), in *Struwwelpeter,* a collection of cautionary poems about naughty children:

> Fidgety Phil,
> He won't sit still;
> He wriggles
> And giggles,
> And then, I declare,
> Swings backwards and forwards
> And tilts up his chair . . .
> See the naughty restless child
> Growing still more rude and wild.

> Till his chair falls over quite.
> Philip screams with all his might.
> Catches at the cloth, but then
> That makes matters worse again.
> Down upon the ground they fall.
> Glasses, plates, knives, forks and all.
> (pp. 18–19)

One of the earliest *medical* discussions of the relationship of childhood behavior problems and organic factors is an engrossing article entitled "Some Abnormal Psychical Conditions in Childhood." Written in 1902 by George Still, the author focused his discussion on "defects in moral control." Still reported long-term observations on children whose defective self-control stood in striking contrast to their normal general intelligence and apparent good upbringing. In some cases, deterioration in the child's behavior was acute and coincided with a clear-cut organic illness. In other cases, however, the child's lack of self-control was lifelong and bore no relationship to any diagnosable disease (although minor congenital anomalies were sometimes present). Among his diverse case examples, Still noted a preponderance of boys (3:1) and the frequent presence of choreiform movements, impulsivity, emotional lability, and "a quite abnormal incapacity for sustained attention." For example:

> [One] boy, aged 6 years, with marked moral defect was unable to keep his attention even to a game for more than a very short time, and, as might be expected, the failure of attention was very noticeable at school, with the result that in some cases the child was backward in school attainments, although in manner and ordinary conversation he appeared as bright and intelligent as any child could be. (p. 1166)

After the great World War I epidemic of encephalitis, Ebaugh (1923), Hohman (1922), and others described postencephalitic sequelae in children consisting of persistent behavioral problems; the authors termed this condition *post-encephalitic behavior disorder*. The symptoms, which appeared suddenly in previously well-behaved children, included impulsiveness; unmanageability and failure to progress in school; unresponsiveness to discipline; and motor abnormalities such as restlessness, hyperkinesis, and choreiform movements. A major theoretical development equating hyperactivity and brain damage came in 1934, when Kahn and Cohen (1934) coined the term *organic drivenness* to describe children and adults with a "high degree of general hyperkinesis . . . and outstanding difficulty, approaching an almost complete inability, in maintaining quiet attitudes (be it only for a few seconds)" (p. 750). Kahn and Cohen not only postulated a defect in brain stem organization but further speculated that in many cases, the only manifest evidence of the defect might be the drivenness itself.

The next major impetus came from Goldstein's (1942) landmark work on soldiers with war-related brain injuries. In testing these patients, Goldstein documented various defects in abstract thinking and perception. In addition, he noted a host of behavioral and cognitive "sequelae to cerebral pathology" including distractibility, inflexibility, lack of self-observation, difficulty in planning ahead, and a "catastrophic reaction" to frustration or failure. Goldstein emphasized that these behavioral defects were a general effect of brain injury that occurred over and above any specific localizing signs.

Goldstein's concepts and assessment techniques heavily influenced Strauss and Werner's group at the Wayne County Training Center. These investigators worked with retarded and "brain-damaged" children. Strauss and Werner's primary interests lay in delineating the psychological deficits of these children and then in developing suitable techniques for remedial education. Their seminal work emphasized the large and educationally important individual differences between children with various cognitive and perceptual impairments. Unfortunately, however, the diagnostic perspective of Strauss's group was less sophisticated than their descriptive or remedial approach. Drawing on Goldstein and his own work, Strauss asserted: ". . . all brain lesions, wherever localized, are followed by a similar kind of disordered behavior. . . ." (Strauss & Lehtinen, 1947, p. 20). A critical concept suggested by Strauss was that even in the absence of positive neurological findings or contributory history, the diagnosis of brain injury could be derived solely from the presence of disordered cognition, perception, or emotional behavior. Thus, in a later work, Strauss stated: "We are justified in diagnosing on the basis of functional rather than neurological signs" (Strauss & Kephart, 1955, p. 42). So influential was this work that the "Werner-Strauss Syndrome" became a widely used eponym for those children with poor emotional control, "organic drivenness," impulsiveness, cognitive inflexibility, and various perceptual difficulties.

Two questionable hypotheses were thus elevated into dogmas that were to have a pernicious influence on the further development of the field. The first hypothesis, epitomized by the above quotation from Strauss, was that *all brain damage produces a similar behavioral picture.* The second hypothesis, its contrapositive, held that *hyperactivity means brain damage, even in the absence of demonstrable brain pathology.*

In 1957, Laufer and Denhoff described a "hyperkinetic behavior syndrome" whose essential symptoms included hyperactivity, short attention span and poor powers of concentration, impulsivity, irritability, poor schoolwork, and generally labile, fluctuating performance and behavior. They postulated that the syndrome came from injury or dysfunction of the diencephalon (thalamus, subthalamus, and hypothalamus) or their cortical connections and further suggested that the syndrome might be associated with many of the perinatal risk factors for cerebral palsy. Twenty years earlier, working in the same hospital as Laufer and Denhoff, Bradley (1937) had discovered that amphetamine (Benzedrine) produced calmness and a dramatic improvement in the school performance of a group of children suffering from various behavior disorders. Additionally, Bradley noted that the drug was most likely to be effective in those children who had abnormal electroencephalograms (EEGs). Laufer and Denhoff (1957) elevated this observation into a third dubious dogma—a positive response to amphetamine can confirm the diagnosis of an "organic behavior syndrome." As discussed later in this chapter, several studies suggest that there is nothing unique about the effect of stimulants in hyperactive children when compared with the response in normal children (Rapoport et al., 1978, 1980a).

By the mid-1960s, the etiologic hypothesis—"hyperactivity equals brain damage"—was embodied in a profusion of new labels. Because direct evidence of postulated "brain damage" was often difficult or impossible to find, researchers now proposed that such children suffered from "*minimal brain damage.*" As Gesell and Amatruda (1941) had put it, ". . . an entirely negative birth history and an uneventful neonatal period may nevertheless demand a diagnosis of minimal injury because of persisting or gradually diminishing behavior signs" (p. 231). In 1962, Clements and Peters noted the "considerable overlapping" of symptomatology between children with specific learning disorders, certain forms of childhood epilepsy, psychosis, aphasia, and other known organic syndromes. Clement and Peters maintained that many "borderline and equivocal cases of organicity and central nervous deviation" (p. 186) existed that prevailing diagnostic practice tended to treat too readily as psychogenic. Instead, they proposed the term "minimal brain dysfunctions" (note the plural) "to call attention to any central nervous deviation present and to emphasize the contribution of that deviation to the adjustment problems of the child" (p. 187).

The main thrust of this paper was the need to remain aware of possible organic factors at work in children's pathology; from this viewpoint, "minimal brain dysfunction" simply implied: "Caution! Possible brain factors at work" (Denckla, 1978). As Clements and Peters (1962) put it:

> It is our contention that an honest blank should be reserved in our thinking for the inclusion of as-yet-unnamed subtle deviations arising from genetic factors, perinatal brain insults, and illnesses and injuries sustained during the years critical for the development and maturation of those parts of the nervous system having to do with perception, language, inhibition of impulses, and motor control.

By 1966, however, this cautious and otherwise modest notion had become reified into an exceedingly broad *diagnostic* category: "minimal brain dysfunction" (MBD). As Clements (1966) defined it in a prestigious federal Task Force report:

The term "minimal brain dysfunction syndrome" refers... to children of near average, average or above average general intelligence with certain learning or behavioral disabilities ranging from mild to severe, which are associated with deviations of functions of the central nervous system. These deviations may manifest themselves by various combinations of impairment in perception, conceptualization, language, memory, and control of attention, impulse, or motor function.

DEFINITION

The most recent operational attempt to define this area of pathology is the DSM-III-R category of Attention-deficit Hyperactivity Disorder. DSM-III-R defines three subgroups: (1) Attention-deficit Hyperactivity Disorder (ADHD), (2) Undifferentiated Attention-deficit Disorder, and (3) Attention-deficit Hyperactivity Disorder (Residual State).

DSM-III-R Diagnostic Criteria for Attention-deficit Hyperactivity Disorder

Note: Consider a criterion met only if the behavior is considerably more frequent than that of most people of the same mental age.

A. A disturbance of at least six months during which at least eight of the following are present:

    (1) often fidgets with hands or feet or squirms in seat (in adolescents, may be limited to subjective feelings of restlessness)

    (2) has difficulty remaining seated when required to do so

    (3) is easily distracted by extraneous stimuli

    (4) has difficulty awaiting turn in games or group situations

    (5) often blurts out answers to questions before they have been completed

    (6) has difficulty following through on instructions from others (not due to oppositional behavior or failure of comprehension), e.g., fails to finish chores

    (7) has difficulty sustaining attention in tasks or play activities

    (8) often shifts from one uncompleted activity to another

    (9) has difficulty playing quietly

    (10) often talks excessively

    (11) often interrupts or intrudes on others, e.g., butts into other children's games

    (12) often does not seem to listen to what is being said to him or her

    (13) often loses things necessary for tasks or activities at school or at home (e.g., toys, pencils, books, assignments)

    (14) often engages in physically dangerous activities without considering possible consequences (not for the purpose of thrill-seeking), e.g., runs into street without looking

Note: The above items are listed in descending order of discriminating power based on data from a national field trial of the DSM-III-R criteria for Disruptive Behavior Disorders.

B. *Onset before the age of seven.*

C. *Does not meet the criteria for a Pervasive Developmental Disorder.* (APA, 1987, pp. 52–53)

DSM-III-R Diagnostic Criteria for Undifferentiated Attention-Deficit Disorder

This is a residual category for disturbances in which the predominant feature is the persistence of developmentally inappropriate and marked inattention that is not a symptom of another disorder, such as Mental Retardation or Attention-deficit Hyperactivity Disorder, or of a disorganized and chaotic environment. Some of the disturbances that in DSM-III would have been categorized as Attention Deficit Disorder without Hyperactivity would be included in this category. Research is necessary to determine if this is a valid diagnostic category and, if so, how it should be defined. (APA, 1987, p. 95)

The evolution of DSM-III's treatment of this syndrome reflects the ongoing debate concerning its core features and the nature of the fundamental deficits underlying the syndrome. The original DSM-III categories, adopted in 1980, were Attention Deficit Disorder with Hyperactivity (ADDH) and Attention Deficit Disorder without Hyperactivity (ADD). The reference to attentional difficulties in the name of the disorder reflected the influence of Douglas's work (1983, 1984). Douglas emphasized that defects in attention (as well as in motivation, arousal, and control of impulsivity) were as central to these children's difficulties as their hyperactivity. Indeed, from the perspective of the original DSM-III schema, hyperactivity was not even a necessary feature. Some children did not manifest it at all; in other children, overactivity seemed to disappear with age, although other symptoms, such as impulsivity or difficulty concentrating, persisted. However, various critiques of the schema (Barkley, 1981, 1982; Prior & Sanson, 1986; Rutter, 1983a) led to the DSM-III-R (1987) revisions.

A major criticism of the original DSM-III formulation was that ADD without hyperactivity appeared to be relatively uncommon. When attention deficits occurred in the absence of hyperactivity, it was unclear whether the deficits had the same clinical concomitants or represented the same underlying disorder as when hyperactivity was present (Lahey et al., 1987). Furthermore, the finding that ADDH children were overactive even in their sleep suggested that hyperactivity was not simply the product of a more fundamental attentional difficulty (Porrino et al., 1983b). As a result, DSM-III-R reemphasizes hyperactivity as a core component of the syndrome. Finally, critics maintained that the DSM-III concepts of ADDH and Conduct Disorder overlapped excessively (Sandberg et al., 1978, 1980; Shaffer & Greenhill, 1979). Therefore the items in the DSM-III-R index of symptoms for ADHD were chosen for their ability to discriminate ADHD from Conduct and Oppositional Defiant Disorder in an empirical field trial.

Many feel that the DSM-III criteria were not adequately evaluated and that the committee-based DSM-III-R revision has accordingly been premature (Werry et al., 1987). The revision compounds the already formidable difficulty of comparing studies that have employed diverse criteria. It is still unclear to what extent the children identified as hyperactive by the DSM-III-R ADHD criteria overlap those selected by the DSM-III criteria. Preliminary data suggest that the DSM-III-R criteria select a larger and less purely inattentive group than do the older DSM-III criteria (Newcorn et al., 1987).

EPIDEMIOLOGY

Depending on the population studied and the diagnostic criteria used, prevalence estimates for the hyperkinetic syndrome vary as much as a hundredfold. In the United States, the diagnosis of hyperkinetic syndrome is made very frequently. At one time, the label was applied to 5% to 20% of all school-age children and to 22% to 40% of psychiatric clinic patients (Stewart et al., 1966; Taylor, 1985). Utilizing more precisely defined criteria, however, the prevalence in this country appears to be much lower, about 1% to 6% (Lambert et al., 1978).

In contrast to the U.S. approach, in Great Britain, among nonretarded children, the condition is diagnosed only rarely. Rutter and colleagues (1970), in their general population survey of the Isle of Wight, found an incidence of only one case per thousand children. Restless, inattentive behavior, however, appears to be as common in Great Britain as it is in the United States. These wide discrepancies probably reflect methodological disagreements about diagnosis rather than any true cross-cultural differences in prevalence (Prendergast et al., 1986; Taylor, 1986; Taylor & Sandberg, 1984).

Estimates of sex ratios for diagnosed ADHD vary from 5:1 to 9:1 in favor of boys (APA, 1987). Problems related to inattention, however, appear equally prevalent in both sexes; there may be a higher level of diagnosis in boys because their aggressive or defiant behavior presents greater management problems (McGee et al., 1987).

CLINICAL FEATURES

The clinical picture of ADHD is changeable because the behavior of an afflicted child varies strikingly across situations. More than that, as maturation, development, and the changing social and cognitive demands of each stage of life modify the child's behavior, the symptomatic profile also changes.

Researchers know little about the infancy of ADHD children. Many mothers recall that their hyperactive child was very active in utero. Retrospectively, mothers of hyperactive children report a high prevalence of nonspecific difficulties such as colic, irritability, and sleep and feeding problems that is reminiscent of the "difficult" children in Chess and Thomas's (1984) schema of temperamental categories (Rapoport et al., 1979; Weiss & Hechtman, 1979). Some infants may also display minor congenital anomalies such as wide-set eyes, low-set ears, large head, and inwardly curved little finger (Burg et al., 1980; Waldrop et al., 1978). These findings have been associated with later hyperactivity, inattentiveness, and difficult behaviors. Such children may be labeled "Funny Looking Kids" by tactless adults, including many professionals. Although these nonspecific behavioral and temperamental difficulties may have some predictive value for later hyperactivity, they are also common among infants who go on to normal childhoods as well as those who develop other emotional problems.

As discussed in connection with mother–infant fit (see Chapter 1), because of their poor modulation, irritability, demandingness, and seeming insatiability, temperamentally difficult infants often get off to a troubled start with their mothers. Mothers who perceived their 3-month-old babies as difficult were not only less responsive at the time, but remained so even when, by 8 months, the infants' behavior had become indistinguishable from that of control infants (Campbell, 1979). Further evidence of enduring parent–child difficulties comes from retrospective analysis of the 18-year Fels Longitudinal Study data (Battle & Lacey, 1972). A persisting disharmony existed between boys and their mothers if the boys had ranked high on the motor activity dimension as infants. Throughout grade school, such mothers remained critical of their sons and showed them less affection than did mothers of initially less active boys. As these boys grew, they continued to be seen as noncompliant toward adults and lacking in achievement motivation.

Although toddlers are normally active and have a short attention span, parents describe the hyperactive toddler as a relentless human dynamo. With the onset of walking, some previously tractable infants become hyperactive. In any case, the hyperactive toddler will not remain in his playpen or crib but manages to climb out and prowl the house, even after his exasperated mother has added enough reinforcing bars for a cellblock. Sleep patterns are often disturbed (usually light and short, but sometimes stuporously deep), and the child may sometimes be found wandering the house before dawn, rummaging through cabinets or climbing on the furniture. Some of these toddlers show little healthy caution, darting out into traffic or climbing into precarious situations; as a result, they are accident-prone. When present, poor coordination may increase their vulnerability, and they seem to learn little from numerous injuries and lacerations. The clinician must distinguish this accident-prone pattern from that of the anxiously counterphobic child or the erratic behavior of the partially neglected child whose preoccupied or indifferent mother fails to exercise enough vigilance over her toddler. Toys seem to disintegrate in the hyperactive toddler's hands as he roams from activity to activity. At home, he is likely to be emotionally labile, difficult to manage, and unresponsive to discipline. As early as their nursery school years even bright, hyperactive children experience difficulties. Their impulsivity and short attention span make them disruptive and difficult to engage, cognitively or socially. They are unpopular with classmates because they can concentrate on mutual activities only for brief periods. The hyperactive child's aggression, low frustration tolerance, and seeming insensitivity to others further complicate peer problems (Campbell & Paulauskas, 1979; Pelham & Bender, 1982; Pelham & Milich, 1984).

In constant difficulty with parents, teachers, and peers, such a youngster soon begins to develop a poor self-concept that, without intervention, will become steadily more entrenched. Typically, parents who seek help are advised that their toddler is simply immature and "will grow out of it"; careful follow-up studies, however, suggest that this hopeful prognosis is seldom warranted (Campbell et al., 1977; 1978). Longitudinal studies of nonclinic children indicate that from $2\frac{1}{2}$ to $7\frac{1}{2}$ years of age, activity levels remain consistent. (Halverson & Waldrop, 1976). S.B.Campbell and colleagues (1977, 1978, 1984) found that preschoolers identified as hyperactive at age $4\frac{1}{2}$ years continued to show hyperactivity and conduct problems in second grade at age $6\frac{1}{2}$ years. They noted that many active, oppositional preschoolers are merely going through a stormy developmental phase—the proverbial "terrible twos" (and threes)—in which tantrums, defiance, and restlessness are common and that it was difficult to distinguish such children from those who showed early signs of potentially chronic difficulties.

The ADHD child's difficulties become most glaringly apparent in the first three grades of elementary school, when most hyperactive children are initially referred for assessment (Weiss & Hechtman, 1979). The primary grades impose new demands to remain on task and in place. For the ADHD child who cannot "stop, look, and listen," these expectations are difficult to meet (Douglas, 1983, 1984). Even when bright, the ADHD child has trouble attending to instructions and persevering to the end of assignments. His papers are sloppy and disorganized; he frequently forgets to do assignments or to bring needed books or supplies. He may jump quickly to obvious but incorrect conclusions; in class exercises, he may impulsively blurt out wrong answers. Easily distracted, he is prone to distract others. Not only does he have trouble completing his own work, he disrupts the ecology of the class and is a source of annoyance to teacher and peers. Specific learning disabilities, such as dyslexia, are often present, and the affected ADHD child finds himself falling further and further behind his peers. Because context strongly influences the deficits, the unevenness of his performance may further frustrate and puzzle his parents and teachers.

In a highly structured situation with close supervision and one-to-one attention, the child may achieve up to his potential. In the open classroom or in large group exercises, however, he does poorly, forgetting instructions and seeming to dawdle or daydream interminably. Issues of concentration and motivation may be difficult to disentangle. The child may be able to concentrate for some time on activities that interest him, such as video games, but can show little perseverance in geography. The hyperactivity, when present, is most glaringly apparent during sedentary activities that require concentration; in free-play situations such as recess, the ADHD child may be difficult to distinguish from his normal peers.

ADHD children are often unpopular and isolated, both by their own account and in the opinion of their peers (Pelham & Bender, 1982; Whalen et al., 1987a). Because they lack a sense of personal boundaries, they often unknowingly invade other youngsters' territory by touching or handling their possessions. ADHD children also have a penchant for noisemaking. They tap, hum, sing to themselves, or otherwise vocalize in a fashion that many others find distracting and often enough annoying. As the group activities of latency children become more complex, ADHD children's short attention span and impulsivity make it harder for them to join in the play. In almost any classroom, youngsters are able with considerable accuracy to identify, half scornfully, half pityingly, which classmates are "hyper-diaper."

Faced with seemingly unavoidable ostracism and scorn, the ADHD child may deliberately choose the persona of the class clown or rebel, hoping thereby to win acceptance from peers. The vicious circle of poor performance → disapproval and frustration → low self-esteem → worse performance becomes ever more extended; such children are often desperately unhappy. Without intervention, ADHD children feel more and more defeated by school and, in many cases, by the third or fourth grade, they have altogether given up. Outside of school, the child may have few friends his own age; instead, driven both by preference and necessity, he chooses younger children who can look up to him, and whose company makes fewer demands on him.

At home, such children often suffer in comparison with their better behaved, higher achieving siblings (Borland & Heckman, 1976; Cantwell, 1985). Spats may be frequent, because the ADHD child's behavior is as annoying to siblings as it is to peers. Parents complain of their child's restlessness, lability, disorganization, and seeming imperviousness to discipline. At home, as at school, the child is often bewildered at the scoldings he receives; despite his remorse or upset, however, punishments and admonitions may have little effect. Such children profit from a home situation with a patient, firm, nonpunitive structure; likewise, their problems are exacerbated when parents are lax, inconsistent, excessively perfectionistic, obsessionally rigid, or narcissistically achievement-oriented. At home, too, the same cycle of mutual frustration, with resulting anger on the parents' part and depression and low self-esteem on the child's part, all too often ensues. As time goes on, it becomes more difficult to disentangle the primary effects of the ADHD child's constitutional deficiencies from the accumulating reactive problems related to difficulties at school, at home, and with peers (Weiss & Hechtman, 1979).

At one time, clinicians believed that the ADHD child's symptoms tended to disappear as he entered adolescence (Laufer & Denhoff, 1957). It is now clear, however, that although motoric hyperactivity sometimes diminishes with age, many or all of the symptoms of ADHD can persist into adolescence and even into adult life (Bellak, 1979; Gittelman et al., 1985; Gittelman & Mannuzza, 1985; Wender et al., 1981). In later life, restlessness, impulsivity, and difficulties with concentration continue to be frequent complaints of ADHD patients (and their families). Problems with impulsivity, low self-esteem, and schoolwork also continue. When aggression has been present in middle childhood (a finding in some 25% of ADHD cases), delinquency and antisocial behavior are frequent in adolescence, especially in the presence of poor parent–child relationships (Weiss, 1984) and lower socioeconomic status (SES) (Loney et al., 1981).

As a group, hyperactive children show a broad range of adult outcomes. At one extreme, about 30% to 40% grow up to function normally in most spheres despite some continuing deficits. At the other extreme, 10% show serious psychiatric or antisocial disturbance, which may require psychiatric hospitalization or jail. Those 40% to 50% of children in between continue to experience a broad range of educational, vocational, and interpersonal difficulties due to persisting problems in concentrating, impulsivity, and emotional lability (Hechtman et al., 1981; Weiss et al., 1985; Weiss & Hechtman, 1986).

Several long-term prospective and retrospective follow-up studies of hyperactive children are now available, although only a few are well-controlled (for a comprehensive review see Weiss, 1983, 1985; Weiss & Hechtman, 1986). Different diagnostic criteria for ADHD may yield quite divergent samples; therefore, it is important to ensure that any given outcome results from the ADHD condition itself and not from a bias in the diagnostic group sample, such as low IQ or SES. Hence, a control group, carefully matched for age, sex, IQ, SES, and concurrent diagnoses, is essential.

Weiss and Hechtman (1986) at Montreal Children's Hospital have followed a sample of hyperactive children and matched controls prospectively for more than 15 years. A large number of significant findings have emerged in these 21- to 33-year-olds. These hyperactive young people showed persisting school problems. By the end of the study, they had, on the average, completed less education, earned lower grades, repeated more grades, and were more likely to have dropped out of high school than was true of the controls. The hyperactives also had significantly more car accidents. During the 5 years preceding the 10-year follow-up, the hyperactives had more court referrals and more illicit drug use. (Interestingly, none of the hyperactives abused stimulants.) However, these difficulties diminished with time, so that during the year immediately preceding the 10-year follow-up, no differences from the control group were apparent.

Other follow-up studies have drawn more pessimistic conclusions concerning the development of serious delinquency. In an 8-year follow-up, Satterfield et al. (1982, 1987) compared the arrest records of a group of hyperactive boys with those of their nonhyperactive brothers and normal controls. The hyperactive boys' treatment had consisted of medication only for an average of 2 years. Depending on SES, 25% to 45% of the ADDH boys had multiple arrests for serious offenses, compared with 0% to 6% of the controls. By age 18, compared with their own brothers, these ADDH boys had a markedly increased rate of multiple arrests for serious offenses (27% of the hyperactives vs. 5% of the sibling control group) and of incarcerations (27% vs. none of the sibling controls (Cantwell, 1985)). In another prospective study, Gittleman et al. (1985) followed a group of ADDH children into late adolescence and young adulthood. These investigators found that the full ADDH syndrome persisted in 31% of the study population. Young people whose ADDH symptoms persisted had a greatly increased likelihood of developing a conduct disorder (48%), compared with either the originally non-ADDH controls (8%) or the ADDH children whose symptoms lessened with adolescence (13%). In all, about one-quarter of the initial group of ADDH children had an antisocial or conduct disorder at follow-up (Mannuzza et al., 1989).

In the Montreal study, at the 10–12 year follow-up, both hyperactives and controls had similar job status and job aspirations (Weiss & Hechtman, 1986). A particularly interesting finding in that study was the persistence of variability in the hyperactives' behavior depending on the demands of the social setting. When rating scales containing almost identical items were sent to both teachers and employers, teachers rated the hyperactives as being inferior to the controls on all items, whereas the employers gave the two groups the same rating.

Longer term evidence, however, indicates that ADHD patients do not do as well vocationally. Borland and Heckman (1976) carried out a 20- to 25-year retrospective study of a group of hyperactive subjects, taking the subjects' brothers as their control group. They found that the majority of the men who had been hyperactive as children were steadily employed and self-supporting as adults. However, they had more emotional and work difficulties and had failed to attain as high an SES as had their brothers.

Not surprisingly, hyperactive children also appear at risk for developing personality disorders. The Montreal follow-up found that many former hyperactive subjects had diagnosable personality disorders, with the antisocial, impulsive, and immature-dependent personality types being the most common (Weiss et al., 1985). When seen in their 20s, about one-quarter of these young adults met the criteria for antisocial personality disorder. Generally, the hyperactive subjects showed lower self-esteem than controls. More hyperactive children than controls recalled their childhoods as unhappy. "Feeling dumb," "family fights," and "being criticized" were most frequently cited as having caused unhappiness. Poignantly, the subjects' commonest responses to what had helped the most were the following: a particular adult who had believed in the child, a teacher who had helped turn the tide of failure, or the discovery of a special talent (Weiss et al., 1979).

A major conclusion of the Montreal study was that the cumulative interaction of certain child personality characteristics and family factors most powerfully predicts outcome (Hechtman et al., 1984). The family factors included SES and the mental health of family members (Weiss & Hechtman, 1986), whereas the major personality predictors were IQ plus three other highly correlated traits—aggressivity, low frustration tolerance, and emotional instability. Other investigators have stressed that childhood aggression is a more important predictor of adolescent outcome than hyperactivity (Loney et al., 1981). Thus, in predicting outcome, many global factors may be equally or more important than the degree of hyperactivity or inattentiveness. In summary, although the clinical picture of ADHD shows great variation among children and over time, the problems of the ADHD child appear early and tend to persist into adult life.

Basic Psychological Defects

The variety of descriptive labels (i.e., "MBD" vs. "hyperkinetic syndrome" vs. "attentional deficit disorder") reflect the lack of agreement regarding what constitutes the basic psychological deficit of this syndrome. Although early observers were struck by the excessive, driven motor behavior of such children, subsequent interest has focused on defects in deploying and organizing attention and maintaining motivation. Douglas (1984) has concluded that the ADHD child suffers from "(1) an unusually strong inclination to seek immediate gratification and/or stimulation; (2) an unusually weak inclination to invest attention and effort in demanding tasks; (3) an impaired ability to inhibit impulsive responding; and (4) an impaired ability to modulate arousal or alertness to meet situational demands."

The ADHD child shows defects in investing, organizing, and maintaining attention. As is the case with younger children, "high-interest" stimuli such as TV, may passively capture his attention even for long periods of time. His ability to sustain active attention is poor, however, especially when the material holds little interest for him (such as homework). Unlike his peers, as the ADHD child grows older, he fails to develop more active, organized perceptual and cognitive search strategies to extract information from his environment.

The ADHD child is also handicapped by his difficulty in shutting out competing stimuli (such as what the classmate next to him is doing) while concentrating on the task at hand. Deficits in attention and impulse control may be difficult to disentangle. For example, what is labeled "distractibility" may stem not only from difficulty shutting out extraneous stimuli but also from failure to inhibit inappropriate responses. Distractibility may also reflect a stimulus-seeking tendency that leads the child to respond to highly salient, but task-irrelevant, features of a situation (Douglas, 1983). Outside the cognitive sphere, many of the ADHD child's social difficulties arise from failure to inhibit impulsive behavior.

Researchers have attempted to formulate the ADHD child's difficulties in terms of the regulation of arousal. Unfortunately, it is often unclear whether such theories refer to autonomic or some form of cortical arousal. The concept of arousal has been used to explain why these youngsters often seem to be either too excited or not excited enough. When dealing with dull or repetitive tasks, the ADHD child may appear insufficiently alert, whereas in other situations, he may easily become overexcited and find it impossible to calm down. Whether an operationally defined concept of general arousal can be derived that would differentiate ADHD children from normal ones is as yet unclear.

The ADHD child's motivation and responsiveness to positive and negative reinforcement have created much debate. The ADHD child seems to lack "intrinsic motivation"; he is a poor self-starter. How responsive he is to external rewards and punishments is open to question. Wender (1971) has contended that such children are less responsive to reinforcement than are normal children. Douglas (1983, 1984) has taken issue with this idea: she has concluded that, if anything, such children are unusually responsive, so much so that they may pay more attention to the reinforcer itself than to the particular behavior being reinforced. She has also concluded that such children are very sensitive to the loss of reinforcement and respond poorly to infrequent, irregular, or long-delayed reinforcement. Kinsbourne (1984) has stated, "The ADD child needs something solid and concrete or frequent and salient before he, too, can control his behavior the way the rest of us can under a much wider range of conditions. But then he can. The attention deficit in ADD is not invariant. The machinery for efficient behavioral control exists in the ADD child. Extra activation is needed, however, to enable it to participate consistently in controlling the way these children live" (p. 145).

Hyperactivity is not a consistent feature in children with attentional deficits (Lahey et al., 1980, 1987). When it is present, however, the motor activity appears to be different from that of the normal child, both quantitatively and qualitatively. The hyperactive child is not only more active, he is also more disorganized, frequently jumping from one activity to another. He is less able to adapt his activity level to the demands of the situation, to recognize, for example, that what is fine on the playground is not acceptable in math class. In a naturalistic week-long, free-ranging study using solid state long-memory movement monitors, Porrino et al., (1983a, 1983b) studied the activity levels of hyperkinetic boys and controls (classmates) at home and at school. The hyperkinetic boys showed generally higher activity levels than the controls across all settings and at all times (including weekends and sleep). The differences were most striking, however, during structured school activities.

Porrino et al.'s (1983b) demonstration that hyperactive children are pervasively more active than normals, even during sleep, challenges the suggestion that hyperactivity is a secondary phenomenon caused by the child's attentional difficulties and poor powers of concentration. Although in this study, performance on an attentional task was a good discriminator between hyperactives and normals, the degree of hyperactivity did not correlate with performance on the attentional task. Another observation suggesting that hyperactivity is not simply secondary to attentional difficulties is that caffeine increases motor activity, but at the same time improves performance on attentional tasks (Elkins et al., 1981).

The ADHD child's attentional, inhibitory, arousal, and reward-seeking deficits are interrelated in such complex ways that it is impossible to specify which is the most basic. The researchers' puzzlement is mirrored by the frustrated adults in the child's life who remain characteristically uncertain whether the child "can't" or "won't" pay attention and sit still (Douglas, 1983). What is clear is that these primary deficits lead to cumulative secondary deficits as the child fails to acquire information and, more important still, fails to develop effective learning skills. Cumulative ungratifying and frustrating educational experiences lead not only to low self-esteem but also to decreased motivation and apathy further exacerbating the child's cognitive and attentional difficulties.

Associated Features and Minor Physical Anomalies

There is a persisting suspicion that ADHD represents a biological variant or, perhaps more likely, a common phenotypic manifestation of a variety of genotypic variants. This belief has led to a search for distinctive physical abnormalities that might serve as diagnostic signs as well as etiologic clues. Certain abnormalities do appear with greater frequency among ADHD children than in the general population: EEG changes, minor congenital physical anomalies, and neurological soft signs. However, these findings are not limited to ADHD, are not found in all ADHD children, and are not as yet specific enough to clarify the underlying physiological mechanisms.

Several minor congenital anomalies occur with relative frequency among impulsive and hyperactive children, including large head circumference, wiry "electric hair," epicanthal folds, wide-set eyes, low-set or malformed ears, inwardly curved little finger, single palmar crease, and disproportionate or fused middle toes (Rapoport & Quinn, 1975). Prospective studies of newborns with such anomalies reveal an increased frequency of hyperactive, inattentive, oppositional, and aggressive behavior, at least in boys (Burg et al., 1980; Ferguson & Rapoport, 1983; Waldrop et al., 1978). However, these anomalies are not present in all ADHD children and can be the outcome of various genetic or environmental causes. The presence of these stigmata in Down syndrome and trisomy 13 as well as in families with histories of childhood behavior disorders points to potential genetic determinants (Rapoport et al., 1974b). When the method of genetic latent structure modeling is used to analyze familial patterns of ADHD and minor physical anomalies, the results suggest the existence of a single autosomal dominant trait that can manifest itself as either ADHD or physical anomalies (Deutsch et al., 1990). Such anomalies can also follow maternal use of certain teratogenic drugs during the first trimester. Rapoport and Quinn (1975) have therefore proposed a genotype-phenocopy model to account for the many factors that can lead to these anomalies, which are also seen with increased frequency among children with speech disturbances, autism, learning disabilities, and other behavioral difficulties, and are apparently nonspecific. Because of the large number of false positives and negatives, the anomaly score by itself is not a clinically useful predictor for later hyperactivity.

Associated Conditions. The symptoms of ADHD often occur concomitantly with other disorders including mental retardation, conduct disorder, specific learning disabilities, "childhood psychosis," Tourette's syndrome, and in later life, various personality disorders (especially the antisocial and borderline types). The extent of such comorbidity has led some to doubt whether ADHD can validly be a distinct syndrome.

Although the DSM-III-R criteria for ADHD exclude children with Pervasive Developmental Disorder (PDD), many children with PDD also have ADHD symptoms. In addition, many children at genetic risk for schizophrenia show attention deficits even prior to the development of overt schizophrenic symptoms (Nuechterlein, 1986). Children with psychotic features or PDD generally have a deleterious response to stimulants. How these various forms of attention deficit relate to those of the more typical ADHD child is uncertain.

Finally, many children destined to develop Tourette's syndrome (TS) show prodromal symptoms of hyperactivity, inattentiveness, emotional lability, and learning difficulties of sufficient severity to have received a diagnosis of ADHD. Debate continues whether the co-occurrence of TS and ADHD is due to common genetic factors or independent genetic transmission of separate disorders (Pauls et al., 1986a, 1987).

ETIOLOGY

The most useful approach to understanding ADHD continues to be a broad biopsychosocial disease model (Weiss, 1984). Although Clements and Peters (1962) coined the term *minimal brain dysfunction* (MBD) in reaction to what they considered the then-prevalent overemphasis on psychogenic factors, their caveat remains just as timely today:

> It is necessary to affirm again that psychiatry must take into account the full spectrum of causality from the unique genetic combination that each individual is, to his gestation and birth experiences, to his interaction with significant persons, and finally to the stresses and emotional traumata of later life after his basic reaction patterns have been laid down. (p. 195)

Although current research focuses heavily on genetic, neurophysiological, and biochemical factors, it is important not to exclude the impact of psychosocial factors on the origins, development, diagnosis, and treatment of ADHD.

Psychosocial Factors

Family and social factors strongly influence the ongoing development of the ADHD child, yet whether they can *cause* ADHD remains unclear. Anxious children are often restless, but the situations that trigger their restlessness differ from the ones that exacerbate the activity level of the ADHD child. Both the parents' child-rearing practices and the teachers' instructional style can influence the child's development of a reflective, as opposed to an impulsive, cognitive style (Yando & Kagan, 1968). As early as the toddler period, children of depressed mothers show poorer concentration in ways that parallel their mothers' impaired attention span (Breznitz & Friedman, 1988). Research has associated early maternal deprivation and institutional upbringing with later restlessness, distractibility, and social unpopularity (Tizard & Hodges, 1978). As discussed below, however, institutionalized children may also be at higher genetic and prenatal risk for ADHD.

Environment influences the components of the ADHD syndrome in different ways. Paternite and colleagues (1976, 1980) found that environmental factors (such as SES and parenting style) did not significantly predict the severity of the primary or core symptoms of the syndrome (i.e., hyperactivity, inattentiveness, fidgetiness). However, the social environment did significantly influence secondary symptoms, such as aggression, impulsivity, and low self-esteem. Most long-term follow-up studies suggest that family factors are major determinants of outcome, especially adolescent aggressive and delinquent behavior, but provide contradictory evidence concerning the influence of SES (Weiss & Hechtman, 1986). To the extent that SES effects are apparent, they appear to reflect associated factors such as urban residence or parenting style and attitude rather than SES *per se* (Paternite et al., 1976; Weiss & Hechtman, 1986).

Some aspects of parenting style may be the effect, rather than the cause, of the ADHD child's difficult temperament (Barkley, 1985). Nonetheless, overall family competence seems to strongly influence the hyperactive child's development, especially the evolution of antisocial behavior (Weiss & Hechtman, 1986).

Brain Damage

Early investigators postulated that brain damage of diverse types (e.g., head trauma, infection, perinatal hazard) produced a single basic symptom picture that included distractibility and hyperactivity. By extension researchers then proposed that when these symptoms occurred in a child without apparent neurological abnormalities, lesser (or "minimal") brain damage was at work. However, current research into the consequences of overt brain damage caused by trauma or perinatal stress fails to support the hypothesis that brain injury results in uniform behavioral and cognitive sequelae (see reviews by Rutter, 1981b, 1982, 1983c; Rutter et al., 1983). Although gross traumatic brain injury, without doubt, markedly increases risk of both intellectual impairment and psychiatric disorder, the behavioral sequelae are nonspecific and variable. The single exception is an increase in inappropriate, socially disinhibited behavior that resembles the general lack of regard for social convention in the so-called frontal lobe syndrome of brain-damaged adults. Hyperactivity and distractibility, however, are quite rare as new symptoms following brain injury. Because gross, overt brain damage generally fails to produce ADHD-like symptoms, it becomes difficult to argue that minimal (and otherwise asymptomatic) brain injury lies behind all hyperactivity and distractibility.

Perinatal Factors

Similar issues arise concerning the influence of perinatal factors. Historically, early interest focused on possible perinatal causes of "minimal brain damage". As early as 1908, Tredgold (cited in Nichols & Chen, 1981) speculated that hyperactive children without overt signs of brain damage might nonetheless have suffered mild brain injury at birth, the effects of which were apparent only with the onset of schooling.

The epidemiological work of Pasamanick and co-workers in the 1950s suggested a correlation between perinatal complications and a spectrum of later difficulties—"a gradient of injury"—extending from death, severe retardation, epilepsy, and cerebral palsy at one extreme to mild learning difficulties and hyperactivity at the other (Pasamanick et al., 1956). Pasamanick and colleagues therefore proposed "a continuum of reproductive casualty," with severe brain damage causing serious neurological sequelae and lesser insults milder, behavioral sequelae. Perinatal complications increase with lower SES complicating tests of this hypothesis because apparent sequelae, such as retardation or hyperactivity, could be caused by psychosocial factors rather than the brain injury itself (Rutter, 1983c). Once SES variables are controlled for, various recent longitudinal epidemiological studies suggest that perinatal complications in fact have a low correlation with later hyperactivity or learning difficulties (Nichols & Chen, 1981; Sameroff & Chandler, 1975).

Social factors also have a powerful impact on the outcome of perinatal complications. The Kauai study demonstrated that in high-SES children, the effects of perinatal difficulties were largely attenuated by school age, whereas in low-SES children, they tended to persist (Werner & Smith, 1977).

Maternal smoking and alcohol consumption during pregnancy appear to be major risk factors for hyperactivity, even after controlling for social class factors and birth weight (Nichols & Chen, 1981; Ross & Ross, 1982). The implications for primary prevention are obvious.

The preceding discussion makes clear that the notion of "minimal brain dysfunction" as a lesser variant, or *forme fruste*, of traumatic, infectious, or perinatal brain damage is not convincing. An alternative theory of such dysfunction postulates a neurochemical or neurophysiological defect, most likely caused by a genetic abnormality rather than by brain damage (Wender, 1971).

Genetic Factors

Studies of activity levels in nonclinical twin populations indicate that genetic factors play a role in determining these levels (Willerman, 1973); these findings, however, cannot be uncritically extended to the clinical phenomenon of hyperactivity (Rutter, 1987b; Scarr & Kidd, 1983). Unfortunately, adequate twin studies of clinical hyperactivity are not available.

Family and adoption studies point to the importance of genetic factors in developing ADHD. Unfortunately, methodological flaws and limitations make these studies less than conclusive (McMahon, 1980; Ross & Ross,

1982; Weiss & Hechtman, 1986). Furthermore, the studies leave open the question, *what* is inherited? Thus, hyperactivity in children, especially when accompanied by aggressive antisocial behavior, appears linked not only to hyperactivity in their adult relatives, but also to antisocial behavior, hysteria, and perhaps alcoholism in these relatives.

Morrison and Stewart (1971) and Cantwell (1972) found that adult relatives (especially fathers) of hyperactive children had a significantly higher prevalence of retrospectively diagnosed hyperactivity themselves than did relatives of nonhyperactive controls. The hyperactive children also had a higher prevalence of alcoholism and antisocial personality among their adult male relatives and hysteria (Briquet's syndrome) among their adult female relatives. Several methodological shortcomings (including lack of an appropriate control group and inclusion of many hyperactive children who may have had conduct disorders) marred these studies. Morrison (1980) underlined the importance of using *psychiatric* nonhyperactive patients as controls when he found that although antisocial personality and hysteria were more prevalent in the parents of hyperactive clinic patients, alcoholism was equally common in the parents of both hyperactive and nonhyperactive psychiatric clinic patients. Thus increased parental alcoholism was associated with attendance at a child psychiatry clinic rather than specifically with hyperactivity. On the other hand, the siblings of hyperactive boys, if compared with siblings of nonhyperactive controls, show a threefold increased risk of hyperactivity (Welner et al., 1977).

The adoption studies of Morrison and Stewart (1973), Cantwell (1975), and Alberts-Corush et al. (1986) have suggested the hypothesis that familial influences are genetic rather than environmental. The earlier studies examined the adoptive parents of hyperactive children who had been adopted at birth; they found that the adoptive parents had no higher rate of alcoholism, antisocial personality, hysteria, or history of hyperactivity in their own childhoods than did the parents of nonhyperactive controls; moreover, the prevalence of these diagnoses in the adoptive parents was significantly lower than in the biological parents of groups of known hyperactive children. Alberts-Corush et al. (1986) compared the biological and adoptive parents of hyperactive and normal control children on several attentional measures. The biological parents of the hyperactive children had greater difficulties than did the other groups of parents. It is important to note that these studies did not directly compare the biological and adoptive parents of the *same* hyperactive children. An additional confounding factor in adoption studies is the possibility that hyperactivity may be more common in adopted children (Deutsch et al., 1982). If so, it is unclear whether the increased incidence of hyperactivity among adoptees might be due to the *in utero* effects of maternal stress in unwed pregnant women contemplating adoption (W. Goodrich, personal communication, 1983) or to the possibility that parents who conceive out of wedlock might have an increased prevalence of genetically determined impulsivity.

Most groups of hyperactive children are heterogeneous, often including many children who also show features of conduct disorder. It is therefore not surprising that the genetic antecedents, as they appear in the biological parents of hyperactives, seem to include a diverse range of behavioral pathology. The inherited factor may prove to be a predisposition to a broad "impulsive-conduct disorder" syndrome (Ferguson & Rapaport, 1983) or to a constellation of "disinhibitory syndromes" (Gorenstein & Newman, 1980), rather than to hyperactivity *per se*. It is also possible that parental behavior disorders are linked to aggression and conduct disorder in the proband children rather than to hyperactivity. As a result, patterns of genetic influence may differ among different subgroups of ADHD children. For example, the prevalence of parental psychopathology (especially alcoholism and antisociality) is greater for boys who are both hyperactive and conduct disordered than it is for boys who are only hyperactive (Reeves et al., 1987).

New genetic techniques, such as linkage analysis, may soon provide more detailed information about the genetics of ADHD. Applying such techniques, however, will require being able to specify clearly the phenotypes for study; this in turn entails identifying relatively homogeneous subgroups of ADHD children.

Neurobiological Factors

Abnormalities in the metabolism of monoamine neurotransmitters were proposed by Wender (1973) as a possible origin for hyperactivity; two lines of evidence suggested this hypothesis. First, the post–World War I pandemic of viral encephalitis lethargica that caused many cases of childhood postencephalitic hyperactivity also produced Parkinson's disease in numerous affected adults. The symptoms of Parkinson's disease were associated with the destruction of dopaminergic neurons. Wender therefore speculated that a dopaminergic lesion caused by a virus with a known predilection for neurons containing catecholamines might also have accounted for the hyperactivity in these postencephalitic children. Secondly, the symptoms of hyperactive children respond to stimulants and tricyclic antidepressants, which increase the functional availability of serotonin, dopamine, and/or norepinephrine neurotransmitters at nerve endings. Wender cautioned, however, against inferring cause from treatment; pneumococcal pneumonia is not caused by a penicillin deficiency!

Neurotransmitter regulation has been an attractive area for investigators in pursuit of an etiology for ADHD. Alterations in neurotransmitter functioning have powerful effects on mood, arousal, motor activity, cognition, and many overt behaviors. Although neurotransmitter functioning is partially genetically determined, a wide variety of organic and experiential influences also affect it. Toxins, infectious agents, hypoxia, and malnutrition as well as stress, social experience, and aging can all modify neurotransmitter processes. In both normal and aberrant development, the fate of these substances can serve as a crucial intervening variable (Alpert et al., 1981).

Following these speculative leads, a vast amount of research has attempted to identify possible abnormalities in the synthesis or regulation of central nervous system neurotransmitters that might account for the diverse symptomatology of ADHD (see S. E. Shaywitz et al., 1983; Zametkin & Rapoport, 1987 for reviews). Because currently it is impossible to directly study neurotransmitter functioning in the human brain, several alternative strategies have emerged. Most investigators have had to confine themselves to metabolic studies using blood, urine, or cerebrospinal fluid (CSF) samples; inevitably this methodology has many serious limitations. Pending further advances in positron emission tomography or tissue culture techniques, these indirect measures provide only a hazy picture of what is actually going on in the brain.

Researchers have looked for elevated or lowered levels of the major monoamine neurotransmitters: norepinephrine, dopamine, and serotonin. However, because of constant rapid turnover, the levels of free transmitter are very low and labile. To be sure, these substances are also present in other body tissues, but measures of the neurotransmitters in peripheral body fluids give little evidence of what is going on in the central nervous system. A more promising approach has been to study the metabolites of these transmitters, as well as the enzymes that control their synthesis and degradation. These by-products or end products are more easily measured than the neurotransmitters themselves; because they are less ephemeral, these metabolites and enzymes may serve as better indicators of transmitter system functioning (B. A. Shaywitz, et al., 1977; S. E. Shaywitz, et al., 1983). Unfortunately, the many studies of monamine transmitters and their metabolites in blood, urine, and cerebrospinal fluid have yielded conflicting and ultimately disappointing results (Zametkin & Rapoport, 1987).

More convincing, albeit less direct, evidence for the possible role of neurotransmitters in ADHD comes from pharmacological studies. Several drugs are available that alter neurotransmitter functioning. Additional evidence linking ADHD and brain catecholamines comes from the metabolic and behavioral response of ADHD children to these agents. For example, both methylphenidate and dextroamphetamine have complex effects on catecholamines (Kuczenski, 1983). Among their many actions, they *increase* the availability of catecholamines, especially dopamine, at the synaptic junction both by stimulating release and by inhibiting reuptake at the presynaptic nerve endings (Clemens & Fuller, 1979); at the same time they may actually *inhibit* the firing of catecholamine-containing neurons. The predominant mechanism may vary with age and other factors, perhaps explaining developmental and individual variations in drug response (such as which children are responders or nonresponders) (Young et al., 1984).

The tricyclic antidepressants and monoamine oxidase inhibitors (MAOIs), which have a markedly beneficial effect on ADHD symptoms, also increase synaptic catecholamine levels via other mechanisms. However, the etiologic implications of these dramatic drug effects are limited by the observation that they are not specific to ADHD (Ferguson & Rapoport, 1983).

ADHD children show changes in transmitter metabolites that reflect the actions of these drugs, albeit in complex and as yet incompletely understood ways (Donnelley et al., 1986; Zametkin et al., 1985). In one study only those children who showed a positive behavioral response to dextroamphetamine showed a decrease in catecholamine metabolite levels (Shekim et al., 1983). Detailed pharmacodynamic studies of ADHD children who are nonresponders or who respond selectively to one agent but not another may provide valuable clues concerning neurobiologically distinct subtypes of ADHD (Zametkin & Rapoport, 1987).

At present, the fragmentary evidence offers little support to any simple notion of a single neurotransmitter defect at a specific site. The pool of transmitters substances is not static; complex homeostatic mechanisms involving regulation of transmitter synthesis and inactivation as well as fluctuations in receptor sensitivity and density maintain a complexly determined equilibrium. Thus, an alteration in the levels of a given substance does not indicate the precise locus of a regulatory defect. Neither do neurotransmitter systems function in isolation; here too pathology may involve not just a defect in a single system, but rather an imbalance between systems reflecting a failure of compensatory adjustment (Alpert et al., 1981). Even on the neurochemical level, the causal web is likely to be complex.

An additional major area of current ignorance concerns normal and aberrant patterns of developmental change in neurotransmitter functioning. What little we know suggests that the levels, distribution, and functioning of neurotransmitters and their receptors undergo considerable change in the maturing organism (Young et al., 1984). However, the implications of these maturational patterns are as yet unclear (Shaywitz et al., 1983; Young et al., 1984).

Further, environmental or biochemical influences that have profound and lasting effects on neurotransmitter ontogeny during early development may have quite different effects or no effect later in development. Progress in understanding the aspects of neurobiological maturation that underlie psychological development will greatly improve insight into the vulnerability to aberrant development.

A final strategy has been the search for an animal model in which either identifiable genetic or biochemical factors produce symptoms resembling those of the ADHD child (Shaywitz et al., 1978). A hybrid strain of dogs has been developed whose natural behavior and responses to medication are similar to those of hyperactive children. These dogs show lower levels of brain catecholamines than do controls, a finding that suggests a possible genetic influence over these important mediators of behavior (Bareggi et al., 1979).

A particularly promising model has been the dopamine-depleted rat pups studied by B.A.Shaywitz and his colleagues at Yale (Alpert et al., 1981). When the neurotoxin 6-hydroxydopamine (6-OHDA) is placed in the cerebrospinal fluid of the developing rat pup, a rapid and permanent reduction of brain dopamine occurs. This is the more striking because other catecholamine neurotransmitters remain unaffected. The behavioral development of these dopamine-depleted pups shows significant parallels to that of ADHD children (S.E.Shaywitz et al., 1983). Thus, during early life, the 6-OHDA pups are more active than their untreated littermates and show learning difficulties as well as impaired ability to modulate their activity level with changes in the environment. Like their normal peers, as the 6-OHDA pups get older they become less active, but their cognitive deficits, such as impaired maze learning, persist. Moreover, methylphenidate and dextroamphetamine ameliorate 6-OHDA pups' hyperactivity, whereas phenobarbital exacerbates it. A final parallel with important implications for children with ADHD is the finding that environmental manipulation as well as pharmacological interventions improved both the hyperactivity and the learning deficits of the dopamine-depleted pups. Raising the 6-OHDA animals with normal littermates, rather than solely with other 6-OHDA pups, led to substantial improvement in several areas of functioning. The predictable presence of a mother, even an anesthetized mother, also had important ameliorative effects.

Disrupting key neurotransmitter systems during critical early periods of development has long-lasting and far-reaching effects; because similar disruptions in adult life produce quite different results, developmental issues have key importance.

Arousal and Maturational Lag

An influential but ultimately inconclusive approach to unraveling the cause of ADHD has been to speculate about proposed abnormalities in the arousal mechanisms of the brain. Such an approach attempts to link motoric and attentional difficulties found in ADHD to some presumed disturbance in the brain's responsiveness. It is assumed that some fault exists in the central nervous system's regulation of the level of alertness and neurophysiological responsivity to both external and internal stimuli. Such theorizing has an obvious appeal. ADHD children often appear to be less than optimally aroused. At certain times they seem overexcited, whereas at other moments they are bored and insufficiently alert (Douglas 1983). Unfortunately, the concepts of "arousal" and "activation" are as elusive and poorly defined as "attention" (Ferguson & Pappas, 1979). Some investigators have examined peripheral autonomic indices of arousal such as skin conductance or cardiovascular reactivity (Porges, 1984); others have focused on presumed central indices of arousal such as cortical evoked responses and shifts in EEG patterns (Callaway et al., 1983).

Arousal models tend to focus on either of two extremes: overarousal and underarousal (Ferguson & Pappas, 1979). *Overarousal* theories propose that ADHD children have too much input because they have trouble selectively filtering incoming sensory data; the result is cortical overarousal and distractibility (Laufer et al., 1957). *Underarousal* theories suggest that low arousal and insufficiently activated inhibitory control mechanisms result in the ADHD children being distracted from within and from without by stimuli that the normal child would ignore (Satterfield et al., 1974). An attractive feature of the underarousal theories is that they explain the effect of stimulants in calming the hyperactive child.

The literature addressing these complex questions is extensive, difficult to reconcile, and ambiguous (Ferguson & Pappas, 1979). Physiological differences do exist between ADHD and normal children. A number of investigators have found differences in EEG spectrum and evoked potential responses (Callaway et al., 1983); the magnitude and direction of these differences, however, vary with age (Satterfield et al., 1984). When concentrating, normal subjects show decreased spontaneous fluctuations of their peripheral autonomic activity. Some studies have found a deficit in the ADHD patient's ability to suppress these spontaneous fluctuations of autonomic activity during attentional tasks; this difficulty may represent a physiological counterpart to faulty behavioral inhibition (Porges, 1984). At the present time, however, no simple unidimensional arousal theory fits the existing data. This line of inquiry awaits further theoretical and operational delineation of the different types of autonomic, behavioral, and neurophysiologic arousal and their complex interrelationships (Conners & Wells, 1986).

Neuroanatomical Hypotheses

There have been many speculative attempts to propose specific neuroanatomical lesions to account for the hyperkinetic syndrome (Conners & Wells, 1986; Zametkin & Rapoport, 1987). Viewed historically, the brain loci proposed have been those stirring the greatest speculative and research fervor at the time. In the early 1970s, interest focused on the arousal-regulating functions of the reticular activating system and the reinforcement-regulating functions of the limbic system (Wender, 1971). More recently, speculation has centered on the frontal lobes and on the role of the locus coeruleus in regulating noradrenergic and autonomic arousal. The multitude of potential loci reflects basic principles of brain function as well as the changing fads in neuroscience. As Conners and Wells (1986) put it:

... everything is connected to everything else. Hardly any part of the brain can be understood as the single locus from which some behavioral function emerges *de novo*. Since the time of Sherrington, it has been conventional to regard brain functions as being interlocked in an orderly, hierarchical cybernetic chain of influences.... Such an arrangement helps us understand how apparently quite different behaviors such as paying attention, aggressive behavior, and restlessness may be localized in specific parts of the brain, while at the same time depending upon common resources in several widely dispersed brain regions. (p. 53)

The frontal lobes are of particular interest because many symptoms of frontal lobe dysfunction resemble those of ADHD including attention deficits, low frustration tolerance, impulsivity, emotional lability, poor social judgment, and difficulty in planning (Mattes, 1980). Neuropsychological studies strongly implicate frontal lobe dysfunction in ADHD (Chelune et al., 1986). Furthermore, cerebral blood flow studies of ADHD patients (in comparison with normal controls) have found decreased blood flow to the frontal lobes, basal ganglia, and mesencephalon (Lou et al., 1984, 1989). Methylphenidate increased perfusion of some of these areas while reducing perfusion of the primary motor and sensory cortex, suggesting a possible functional inhibition of these structures that corresponds to clinically reduced distractibility and motor activity. Although CT scans of hyperactive children have not revealed significant abnormalities (B. A. Shaywitz et al., 1983), a study of young adults with a previous history of "hyperkinesis/ MBD" found evidence of cortical atrophy (Nasrallah et al., 1986). Recent advances in positron emission tomography promise to produce a wealth of data regarding localization of neurotransmitter functioning in the face of various cognitive and attentional demands.

Another research area of great interest concerns the relationship of ADHD to the attentional deficits seen in children at risk for schizophrenia (see Chapter 3). Recent work suggests that abnormalities in frontal lobe structure and function play a key role in the pathogenesis of many schizophrenic symptoms (Weinberger, 1987). How the functional and anatomic defects (if any) underlying ADHD relate to those of schizophrenia remains to be elucidated. Bellak (1985) has even postulated the existence of "ADD psychoses."

Toxic Factors

Lead poisoning has long been known to produce serious sequelae in the form of intellectual blunting, hyperactivity, and behavioral difficulties. In mice, elevated levels of lead intake during infancy produce later hyperactivity (Silbergeld & Goldberg, 1974). More recently, interest has focused on the possibility that more modest body-lead loads can produce cognitive and behavioral impairment in children (Needleman et al., 1979).

Aside from pica, the various sources of environmental lead contamination are not clear. Researchers suspect that elevated air lead levels from gasoline additives are an important factor, although its significance should diminish as lead-free gas becomes the norm. Having a low SES and living near heavy automobile traffic predispose to an increased body lead burden. Several studies show that such increased body-lead levels are statistically correlated with small but significant decrements in IQ and are tenuously associated with hyperactivity and behavioral problems (Graham, 1983). However, lead levels seem to be influenced by SES and pica, which in turn may result from disturbances in the parent–child relationship. It is therefore unclear whether these findings represent a true toxic effect of subclinical lead poisoning or failure to control adequately for psychosocial factors predisposing to *both* high lead intake and cognitive-behavioral difficulties.

Nutritional Factors

A number of theories postulate nutritional toxins or food allergies as the cause of hyperactivity (Conners, 1984). These formulations have attracted many devoted followers and enjoy a faddish popularity disproportionate to any supporting scientific evidence. The most popular and thoroughly studied regimen was proposed by Feingold (1975), who suggested that hyperactivity represents cerebral irritability induced by artificial food additives and naturally occurring dietary salicylates. Feingold claimed that a diet eliminating these substances would dramatically improve the behavioral and learning problems of most hyperactive children and thus eliminate the need for stimulant medication.

On the whole, these claims have not been substantiated by careful study, although some questions do remain about possible benefits to a very small fraction of hyperactive preschoolers.

Well-controlled studies of dietary effects on behavior are notoriously difficult to perform and require the same rigorous attention to placebo control, rater blindness, dosage effects, and duration parameters as psychopharmacological research (Conners & Blouin, 1983). A commonly used paradigm has been the diet-crossover method in which hyperactive children are randomly assigned to two different diet conditions, the Feingold diet and a defined placebo diet, similar in many respects but containing additives and salicylates. After a specified period, the children are switched from one diet to the other. One of the greatest difficulties in such studies is to ensure that parents and children are blind as to which diet is in effect, and that in any case, their views are not communicated to the raters. The most carefully controlled study of this sort showed no advantage from the

Feingold diet for school-age subjects (Harley et al., 1978). Positive reports were apparent in parent ratings, but not in teacher ratings or laboratory tests; further, the pattern of parent reports suggested nondietary explanations for the positive reports. In contrast to these essentially negative results for school-age children, when preschoolers were placed on the Feingold diet, the parent reports (but again neither the teacher reports nor the laboratory findings) were more consistently positive. The investigators concluded that while they felt confident that the cause-effect relationship asserted by Feingold was seriously overstated with respect to school-age children they could not completely rule out a possible causative effect played by artificial food colors in a small number of preschool children. Connors and colleagues (1976) found inconsistent improvement in some children on the Feingold diet, but again in a pattern suggesting methodological artifacts rather than a diet effect.

Because of the methodological difficulties of long-term dietary studies, another approach has been suggested. This is the *specific challenge method*, designed to study more carefully the small number of children who appeared to improve on the Feingold diet. In three experiments of this kind, Conners (1980) gave such children cookies that contained either food dyes or placebo, alternating these foods in a double-blind counterbalanced fashion. In the first of these challenge studies, ingestion of the food dye produced a transient deterioration in the performance of several children on a visual–motor tracking task. These acute, time-limited effects were also reflected in a second study; here parental reports gave a picture of behavioral deterioration during the three hours after food dye ingestion. A third, more rigorous study of a larger sample, however, could not confirm these findings; neither could other carefully controlled challenge studies (Harley et al., 1978; Mattes & Gittleman, 1981). On the other hand, a different set of challenge tests studies have affirmed the deleterious impact of food additives (Swanson & Kinsbourne, 1980; Weiss et al., 1980), although these investigations are open to serious methodological criticism (Ross & Ross, 1982). In the diet trials that had a nonblind portion, large placebo effects were apparent, bespeaking strong biases in the parents' ratings.

Reviewing the large body of often contradictory research, Conners (1980) concluded, "On the basis of all the evidence available at this time, in answer to the question, 'Is there anything to Dr. Feingold's hypothesis?' one might answer, 'Yes, something—but not much and not consistently' " (p. 109). Parental insistence on a dietary approach, to the exclusion of other modalities, may be the result of eccentricity or faddishness; more often than not it reflects the failure of clinicians and educators to provide the parents with an effective, comprehensive, and long-term treatment plan for their hyperactive child. Heavy emphasis on dietary treatment consumes a vast amount of energy, often isolates the child from his peers, and, because of its narrow focus, may distract attention from comprehensive treatment. The

National Institutes of Health (NIH) Consensus Development Conference (1982) concluded,

> Defined diets should not be used universally in the treatment of childhood hyperactivity at this time.... A defined diet should not be initiated until thorough and appropriate evaluation of the children and their families and full consideration of all traditional therapeutic options... have taken place. (p. 292)

Conners (1981) put it more strongly:

> That there may be a few hypersensitive children cannot be disputed; but for most children the Feingold diet represents at best a waste of time, and at worst a negative factor in correct therapeutics.

Other popular, but unsubstantiated nutritional theories of hyperactivity concern the impact of sugar or caffeine in children's diets. Although many parents believe that sugar makes their children temperamental, hyperactive, and easily upset, double-blind sugar-challenge studies have produced conflicting data concerning sugar's behavioral effects (Behar et al., 1984a; Conners et al., 1987). Based on a series of elegant experiments, Conners and colleagues (1986, 1987; Schwab & Conners, 1986) have concluded that the impact of dietary sugar is not due to *direct* effects of blood glucose on the brain. They suggest that the conflicting findings stem from the complex relationships between nutrients and brain neurotransmitter activity, mediated by the effect of food on the relative plasma levels of the amino acids that serve as precursors of neurotransmitter synthesis (Wurtman, 1987).

Two hours after either a high-protein or high-carbohydrate breakfast, normal and hyperactive children received a large amount of either sugar or placebo; they then participated in a variety of attentional, autonomic, and hormonal studies (Conners et al., 1986, 1987). Following a high-carbohydrate meal, sugar produced decreased attentiveness. However, this deleterious effect did not occur when a high-protein meal preceded the sugar challenge. The inattentiveness and drowsiness that follow the ingestion of carbohydrates (taken alone) is apparently due to an increased synthesis of brain serotonin (Wurtman, 1987). This in turn is caused by the increased brain uptake of tryptophan (the amino acid precursor of serotonin) secondary to high insulin-induced levels of tryptophan relative to other amino acids. In contrast, dietary protein produces large amounts of neutral amino acids that competitively block the brain's uptake of tryptophan and thereby prevent any serotonin-mediated deterioration in attentiveness.

Thus, provided they are part of (or follow) a well-balanced meal that includes adequate protein, carbohydrates (such as sugar) do not produce inattentiveness. These findings reinforce the importance of schoolchildren having well-balanced meals (especially breakfast) that contain a substantial amount of protein. Children with behavior problems frequently have abnormal food habits (Conners et al., 1987; Krieger, 1982). Especially, when their parents are lax, noncompliant, or impulsive, hyperactive children may be likely to consume large amounts of sweets and little else. Hyperactives seem especially sensitive to the deleterious cognitive effects that occur when sugar is ingested in the absence of adequate protein (Conners et al., 1986). Whether this sensitivity reflects underlying neuroendocrine or neurotransmitter imbalances requires further careful study.

Many children consume high levels of caffeine in cola, chocolate, and tea. Their daily consumption may be as much as 10 mg/kg, a level that produces jitteriness and anxiety in most people. The impact of caffeine on children's attention and motor activity is complex, leading to suggestions that it might cause hyperactivity in some children while serving as a helpful therapeutic agent in others. In normal children, low doses had little effect on activity and attention; high doses (10 mg/kg) *increased* vigilance, but also *increased* activity (Elkins et al., 1981). This finding is of considerable theoretical interest, because it is sometimes suggested that the hyperactivity of the ADHD child during sedentary tasks is secondary to his attentional difficulties, yet caffeine improves attention, while exacerbating restlessness. Some children's restlessness and irritability may be due to chronic consumption of excessive caffeine; assessment should therefore include a careful history of caffeine intake. There is some evidence, however, that the habitual high-caffeine consumption of some children may have a possible physiological basis and thus constitute a form of self-medication. Rapoport et al., (1984) found that when children who were regular high-caffeine users were given large amounts daily for two weeks, they showed none of the restlessness, moodiness, and irritability usually produced in children who were not regular high-caffeine consumers. Furthermore, when placed on a caffeine-free diet, the habitual high-caffeine consumers became *more* impulsive rather than less. The design of the study was such that these findings could not be attributed to tolerance or withdrawal effects.

TREATMENT

The ADHD child's multiple handicaps affect all spheres of his life: academic, social, and emotional. The assessment and management of such children must be equally multifaceted and requires the close collaboration of parents, teachers, and physician. During the past two decades, the pharmacological treatment of ADHD has attracted the bulk of research and popular attention. Despite dramatic short-term effects, however, the long-range benefits of drug treatment alone are disappointing. ADHD is a heterogeneous disorder: It does not have a single cause or a single symptom picture nor is there a single cure. Furthermore, ADHD children frequently lack crucial social and academic skills. Successful treatment must therefore include not only controlling symptoms such as impulsivity and inattentiveness, but also fostering normal development and acquiring age-appropriate skills. The consensus is growing that ADHD children benefit most from a comprehensive, multimodal treatment involving a judicious trial of medication in conjunction with special educational techniques, parent counseling, and (in many cases) group, family, or individual psychotherapy for the child, as needed (Satterfield et al., 1981, 1987). The most effective treatment coordinates the various modalities addressing specific problem areas, rather than applying different therapies globally and indiscriminately (Hansen & Cohen, 1984).

Assessment

The diagnostic evaluation of the ADHD child requires carefully assessing all areas of the child's functioning. In addition to ruling out other, correctable causes of inattention, a comprehensive assessment of the child's strengths and weaknesses is essential to careful treatment planning.

During such an assessment several points deserve special emphasis. First, the clinician must obtain a picture of the child's behavior in different contexts from multiple sources. Interviews with the parents, a playroom interview with the child, information gathering directly from the school, structured psychological testing, and a developmental pediatric examination are all vital.

From the parents, it is important to obtain both a careful developmental history and an account of the child's difficulties, including the situations that exacerbate his problems, an estimate of current stresses, and a description of the family's attitude toward the child and his problems. It is also important to assess the quality of parenting and overall family functioning. An impulse-ridden chaotic family style, intense marital conflict, parental preoccupation or parental psychopathology are all likely to intensify the child's symptoms and complicate the treatment.

A brief, structured interview with a child who is on his best behavior with a stranger is notoriously unreliable in diagnosing an attentional deficit. On the other hand, one or more leisurely interviews can clarify the child's characteristic behavior as well as the details of his cognitive style and emotional concerns. The ADHD child is not oblivious to his difficulties with teachers, parents, and peers. Given a sympathetic ear, he will often reveal his frustration, unhappiness, and low self-esteem. The interview can tentatively provide answers to several important questions. How readily does the child acknowledge his difficulties? How does he explain (or deny) them to himself? Does he cope with his problems with others by clowning, by compensatory grandiosity and entitlement, by withdrawal, by self-castigation?

As part of the diagnostic process, it is important to establish not only whether alternative diagnoses might apply (i.e., anxiety disorder, pervasive developmental disorder, schizophrenia, etc.), but also what concurrent conditions (such as conduct disorder, learning disability, or depression) must also be addressed in treatment.

The teacher is a primary source of information about the child's academic progress and social interactions. Furthermore, as treatment proceeds, the teacher can provide invaluable data about the impact of various therapeutic interventions. Although often annoyed and frustrated by the ADHD student, most teachers are eager and gratified to be consulted in planning treatment. A visit to the school to meet with the teacher and to observe the patient in his classroom setting is often essential. It is equally important for the clinician to become familiar with the school's machinery for providing special education and resource help to students who need it.

Structured psychological testing assesses both school achievement and cognitive and emotional strengths and weaknesses. Despite a normal overall IQ, the ADHD child may show considerable subtest scatter, with particular weakness in the Arithmetic, Digit Span, and Coding subtests of the WISC-R (Milich & Loney, 1979). Although at present no specific clinical tests of attention correlate satisfactorily with parents' and teachers' ratings, specialized tests of other cognitive and perceptual areas can elucidate particular learning difficulties that might be present. Well-standardized tests can assess visual and auditory perception, memory, and specific visual motor functioning (Taylor & Warren, 1984), whereas psychological testing can provide useful information about the child's approach to structured tasks.

The child's general health and physical growth should be assessed with a careful physical exam and history. A detailed review of medication is also essential to rule out iatrogenic causes of hyperactivity, such as barbiturates or other seizure medication. Medical causes of inattentive or fidgety behavior, including pinworms, hyperthyroidism, Sydenham's chorea, hearing loss or refractive difficulties, and petit mal or temporal lobe epilepsy should also be ruled out. A developmentally oriented neurological exam will assess the child's neuromaturational status. The exam tests neurological functions such as laterality, motor overflow phenomena, diadochokinesis (rapid alternating movements), choreiform movements, and other fine and gross motor tasks. Abnormalities may include either mild and subtle focal or localizing signs (e.g., asymmetry) or signs of developmental immaturity (Denckla, 1978). A standardized format for administering and scoring this exam has been developed by NIH (Denckla, 1985). The diagnostic implication of such soft signs is still unclear, because in some studies they appear to be nonspecific, perhaps correlating with IQ (Shaywitz et al., 1984). However, asymmetrical or lateralizing signs, when present, may provide valuable clues to localization, or they may suggest variations in cerebral organization that can predispose the child to hyperactivity and learning disability (Denckla, 1978). A standard EEG has little practical use unless evidence suggests a seizure disorder.

Parent Counseling

Work with parents is essential in treating the ADHD child. Educating parents about their child's difficulties can help shift their perspective from seeing their child as a "bad boy" to seeing his need for help. Such a change in view helps diminish punitive attitudes while emphasizing the child's need for structure and consistency.

Practical guidelines are often helpful to parents. For example, it is important to provide adequate outlets for the child's motor restlessness. Thus, before settling down to homework, the child may need some outdoor activities. Household routines should be consistent; the parents should develop a regular schedule with the child, post it on the refrigerator door, and review it frequently. Chaotic, overstimulating situations and tasks that require the child to sit still for long periods should be avoided. Parents should try to identify and encourage hobbies and activities at which the child can excel, thereby boosting his self-esteem as well as sublimating his energy and aggression. The activity will obviously depend on the child's capacities and interests. For one, it might be art; for another, karate lessons or organized sports. Activities that require concentration should be for periods he can handle; parents should learn how to "quit while ahead," by interrupting an activity on a positive note and resuming it later, rather than keeping the child at it till be becomes frustrated and falls apart.

Self-help books for parents, such as those by Stewart and Olds (1973), Gardner (1973), and Wender and Wender (1978), contain much useful advice, but clinicians must recognize the limitations of advice-giving alone. Increasing parental competence requires an ongoing relationship where the participants can review and discuss a full spectrum of issues. Such topics include not only the management techniques that the parents have tried, but also their feelings about the frustrating and taxing job of rearing a hyperactive child. At best, families have difficulty providing the structured daily routine and consistent discipline required by ADHD children. Chaotic, disorganized families or families where parental psychopathology or marital tensions interfere with child-rearing compound these problems. In such cases, family or marital therapy (or individual psychotherapy for the disturbed parent) may be a prerequisite to adequate treatment of the child (Ziegler & Holden, 1988).

Parents and teachers often employ formal and informal behavioral techniques to reinforce desirable behaviors and to diminish undesirable patterns (Sprague, 1983). The target behaviors should be specific and strategically chosen (e.g., getting homework done or being ready for school on time) rather than global (e.g., "being a good boy"). They should also be within the child's reach, so that he can have the pleasure of mastery, rather than the frustration and disappointment of another failed expectation. More ambitious goals can be approximated gradually.

Whenever possible, emphasis should be on positive reinforcement. The parents should provide reinforcement in close proximity to the behavior in question. For example, the child could receive a gold star or a check on a chart immediately after completing his assignment or household chore, with the payoff for the required number of accumulated marks following as soon as feasible. Using such a procedure is far more likely to be successful than promising some grand, all-or-nothing reward in a vague and distant future (e.g., "I'll buy you a bike if you get good grades this semester"). The method is most effective when the child participates at the outset in negotiating the reinforcers.

Behavioral programs most often succeed when they can be readily incorporated into the household or school routines. Behavioral techniques may diminish specific behaviors, such as aggression in the classroom, but may fail to influence other areas of deviance, such as attention and impulsivity (Abikoff & Gittleman, 1984). The practical considerations, pitfalls, and limitations of applying operant techniques to hyperactive children have been reviewed (Conners & Wells, 1986; Gittleman, 1983; Pelham, 1982; Ross & Ross, 1982; Sprague, 1983).

Although the failure of operant reinforcement procedures to produce lasting and generalizable effects on cognitive functioning has caused considerable disappointment, it has encouraged interest in what has been termed *cognitive therapy*. This approach focuses on metacognitive strategies involving planning and self-monitoring, the "stop, look, and listen" skills in which the ADHD child is deficient (Douglas, 1983, 1984). In one paradigm, the adult imparts self-control strategies by first modeling aloud the self-directed mediating commands used in approaching a task. Thus, in building a model airplane with the patient, the teacher or therapist might "think to himself [herself]" aloud: "Now let's see, how am I going to get this propeller on the plane? I'd better check the directions. I'm supposed to put the axle it turns on here. I think I'll try it before I glue it; I'd better go very slowly and gently, because it's pretty delicate. Now, is that right? Let me check it against the diagram. Something doesn't look right. Let me stop and see what's different about it. . . . " He or she then shows the child how to develop and finally how to internalize such self-directed commands.

Using the cognitive training approach to ameliorate the ADHD child's inefficient and impulsive cognitive style has considerable theoretical appeal. First, it would seem to develop crucial, generalizable skills. Second, by emphasizing internally rather than externally mediated control processes, the approach promises to enhance the child's sense of personal efficacy. Unfortunately, although rational, this promise is not always realized. In fact, systematic studies of self-control or cognitive training have yielded mixed or disappointing results (Abikoff & Gittleman, 1985a). Whether they represent inherent limitations of the method or the need for further refinements of technique remains to be seen (Whalen et al., 1985).

Moreover, operant behavioral or cognitive techniques cannot substitute for medication; indeed, many measures indicate that medication is superior to behavioral therapy alone. On certain outcome measures, however, combined medication and behavior therapy can be superior to either modality used alone (Gittelman, 1983; Horn et al., 1983).

The importance of involving the child's classroom teacher in the initial diagnostic assessment and the ongoing evaluation of any therapeutic interventions has been alluded to. Often, the knowledge that the parents are concerned and that other professionals are involved and eager to collaborate will bolster the teacher and increase his or her tolerance. Many (but not all) ADHD children require modifications in their school programs, especially when specific learning disabilities are also present. Such modifications may range from resource help or extra tutoring within the class setting to special remedial classes or special school placement. Instructional planning for the ADHD child should address the following elements: maintaining small class size, pacing work sessions to the child's shorter attention span, decreasing extraneous stimulation, minimizing disruptive transitions, and proximity to the teacher for close monitoring and reinforcing desirable behavior.

Medication

About 75% of ADHD children show a positive symptomatic response to the stimulant drugs dextroamphetamine (Dexedrine) and methylphenidate (Ritalin). When a positive response occurs, it is usually prompt, dramatic, and wide-ranging. Given an appropriate dose, within about 30 to 60 minutes the ADHD child shows decreased extraneous motor activity and impulsivity and improved concentration and cognitive functioning on a variety of measures. He becomes more cooperative and less aggressive, albeit sometimes less talkative and more withdrawn; overall, his social interactions generally improve. These effects peak between 1 and 3 hours after administration, are usually gone by 4 hours, and may leave in their wake a rebound of increased hyperactivity and difficult behavior. Pemoline (Cylert), a longer and more gradually acting stimulant, produces similar improvement; however, significant benefits may not be evident until the 3rd or 4th week of administration (Conners & Taylor, 1980).

The effects of the stimulants are multiple and complex. All four factors of the Conners Teacher Rating Scale (i.e., Conduct-Problem-Aggressivity,

Inattentiveness, Anxiety-Tension, and Hyperactivity) respond to some extent to stimulant treatment; however, the most reliable and consistent improvement occurs on the hyperactivity scale (Barkley, 1977). (See Appendix 11–1 for discussion of rating scales.) Just as researchers have not teased apart the cognitive, motivational, and attentional deficits that are most basic to the ADHD child's difficulties, so too they cannot specify which ameliorative effects of the stimulants are most basic. Rather than regarding these drugs as a magic bullet for a given symptom, the clinician should bear in mind how little is known about the interactions of the drugs' various effects.

Effects on Activity Level. Porrino et al. (1983a) conducted a 4-week placebo-controlled study of hyperactive boys. As they went about their daily activities each of the boys wore a long-memory activity monitor. The investigators were thus able to document convincingly the striking effect of dextroamphetamine. Administration of a morning dose of the drug led to a prompt, marked decrease in activity levels that lasted about 8 hours (longer than is clinically apparent in most cases); indeed, the hyperactive boys' levels of activity went down to that of normal matched controls. This monitor-measured decrease paralleled a marked improvement of scores on the Conners Teacher Rating Scale and the conduct and hyperactivity factors of the Conners Parent Rating Scales.

As noted in other studies that have explored the interaction between social context and drug response (Whalen et al., 1978, 1979a, 1979b; Whalen & Henker, 1980), the effect of the dextroamphetamine on activity varied with the setting. The greatest decreases in activity produced by the medication occurred in sedentary academic studies at school; in contrast, the medication actually *increased* activity levels during gym classes, apparently because of better on-task behavior, secondary to improved attention, motivation, and/or stamina.

The same investigators also noted that activity level showed a biphasic response to the drug. After about 8 hours, the therapeutic, that is, activity-decreasing, effect of the drug seemed to wear off, and the child became *more* active during the late afternoon and evening than he had been on placebo. This rebound effect persisted until the next morning, even during sleep. The effect on activity during sleep again suggests that the hyperactive child's increased kinetic levels are, at least to some extent, independent of attentional factors, which medication would not influence during sleep.

Effects on Attention Measures. The stimulant drugs have been shown to improve impulsivity and attentional deficits. Medication improves the child's performance on laboratory vigilance tasks (Rapoport et al., 1980a); in addition, on tests of simple and choice reaction times, both accuracy and response speed are better. Stimulants improve scores on the Porteus Maze

Test, which involves not only concentration, but also the ability to plan and control impulsive responding (Barkley, 1977). These laboratory improvements are reflected in the classroom where Whalen et al. (1978, 1979a, 1979b) found that unmedicated hyperactives were disruptive, inappropriate, and off-task more often than were normal controls. Hyperactives displayed more motor activity and spontaneous talking, made more noise, and initiated more social contacts than did normal controls. Methylphenidate reduced these behaviors to the point that the hyperactive boys were not significantly different from their normal peers. The experimental design included observing the hyperactive and control groups in several different classroom contexts: easy versus difficult material; self-paced versus externally paced tasks; quiet versus noisy conditions. Contextual factors strongly influenced differences between the hyperactives and their normal peers, as well as differences between responses while on placebo and on medication. Under self-paced conditions with easy materials, there was little difference between the hyperactives and normal controls' off-task behavior; not surprisingly, in this context, medication had little effect on the hyperactives' attention to task. In contrast, with difficult material under externally paced conditions, the hyperactives were much more frequently off-task than were the normal controls (who were also less attentive in this context than they had been in the first); correspondingly, in this context the hyperactive boys showed a striking response to medication, which reduced their inattentiveness to the same levels as those of their normal unmedicated peers.

Effect on Cognitive Measures. There is now a consensus that the stimulants have beneficial effects on activity and attention. Considerable doubt exists, however, about their impact on more complex intellectual functions, especially as reflected in educational achievements. Studies of stimulant effects on complex tasks have yielded inconsistent results. In some studies stimulants seem to have improved scores on the WISC Performance IQ, the Draw-a-Man IQ, the Frostig Test of Developmental Perception, subtests of the Wide Range Achievement Test (WRAT), paired-associate learning, tests of visual and auditory discrimination, and oral reading. In other studies, however, these gains have not appeared (Barkley, 1977; Barkley & Cunningham, 1978; Conners, 1985). The inconsistency of these findings has led most authors to doubt whether the improvements that occur are due to direct drug effects on higher cognitive processes. Instead, these positive changes probably reflect increased ability to attend to the task, increased motivation (including reduced boredom and fatigue), and improved ability to inhibit selectively and to plan (Barkley, 1977). During psychological testing, examiners rated stimulant-treated children as more cooperative, better motivated, with more interest in the tasks and possessing a higher frustration tolerance (Gittleman-Klein et al., 1976).

Douglas et al. (1986), however, found stimulant-induced improvements across a wide range of academic, learning, and cognitive measures. They concluded from their data that the beneficial effects of medication extended "beyond improving test-taking attitudes, increasing on-task behaviors or facilitating vigilance." Better organization of mental effort, more efficient information processing, and improved self-monitoring and correction of errors also seemed at work.

In light of these dramatic, laudable effects, it remains a disturbing paradox that, despite marked improvement in the classroom manageability of ADHD children (Abikoff & Gittleman, 1985b), researchers have found it difficult to demonstrate any beneficial long-term effects of stimulants on such children's academic achievement scores. Improved classroom behavior is, of course, neither a trivial benefit nor one to scoff at. In terms of the child's relationships with teachers, parents, and peers, such improvement may make a critical difference. Nonetheless, studies have failed to show that, in the long run, medication improves the *academic* performance of most such children (Barkley, 1977; Barkley & Cunningham, 1978; Gittelman, 1983; Gittelman-Klein & Klein, 1976). To a large extent these negative findings may be the result of methodological shortcomings such as poor drug compliance, failure to adjust timing and dose for optimal effect, lack of uniformity in the nature of the treatment sample's academic difficulties, and poor outcome measures (Conners, 1985; Douglas et al., 1986).

To the extent that these studies are valid, however, how can the lack of clear-cut long-term academic progress be reconciled with medication's striking beneficial behavioral effects? A possible explanation is that stimulants simply may not affect the basic causes of these children's academic difficulties (which, as discussed earlier, extend beyond the purely attentional sphere). A further suggestion is that the ADHD child develops ingrained negative attitudes toward school as well as cumulative deficiencies in substantive information and problem-solving strategies; what emerges is a complex of disturbances and deficits that medication by itself cannot reverse (Barkley & Cunningham, 1978). As a corollary, medication would be likely to have an impact on achievement only when combined with other remedial educational interventions. If this viewpoint were correct, clinicians might expect to see benefits by initiating both medication and appropriate remedial educational approaches at an early age. An additional complication in assessing the impact of medication is that optimal dosages for decreasing disruptive behavior may be excessive in their effect on inquisitiveness or cognitive alertness (Barkley & Cunningham, 1978; Charles et al., 1981; Sprague & Sleator, 1975, 1977).

Effect on Social Behavior. Medication also dramatically affects the social interactions of hyperactive children. Observational studies confirm the clinical impression that stimulants render hyperactive children more compliant and cooperative, less defiant, and less emotionally labile

(Barkley, 1985). For example, when children and mothers were observed at free play and working together on a structured task, mothers of unmedicated hyperactive children were less responsive to their children than mothers of normal peers (Cunningham & Barkley, 1979). When the mothers of hyperactives did respond, they were more negative and more controlling. In response to their mothers' frequent demands, the hyperactive boys were less compliant than were normal peers. Hyperactive boys have more difficulties complying with their mothers than with their fathers; even with fathers, however, they show more negative and noncompliant behavior than do normal children (Barkley, 1985). Unlike placebo, methylphenidate made a dramatic difference: The hyperactive boys became more compliant during the structured task, whereas their mothers became less commanding. During free play under the medication conditions, the mothers became more responsive and encouraging and the children spent more time playing away from their mothers (Barkley et al., 1985).

In clinical practice, it is not unusual for mothers to report spontaneously and enthusiastically that medication has dramatically improved their relationship with their child. It enables them both to escape from a mutually abrasive struggle and a grim pattern of harsh, exasperated, and fruitless parental attempts to control the child (Schachar et al., 1987). As with other beneficial effects of stimulant medication, it is unclear whether this positive behavioral effect is secondary to drug-induced improvements in attention or represents an independent action of the drug (Taylor, 1983).

Medication also affects social behavior in classroom and play settings. Whalen, Henker, and colleagues (1980, 1987a, 1987b; Whalen & Henker, 1984) have provided much thought-provoking data on the "social ecology" of ADHD and its treatment. In classrooms unmedicated hyperactive boys showed very high energy levels and rates of talking and initiating interactions (Whalen et al., 1979b). Medication eliminated these differences between the hyperactive boys and their normal, unmedicated classmates. In addition, medication reduced negative social behaviors in unstructured settings (Whalen et al., 1987b).

Although overall sociability in such settings was not decreased by medication, subtle dysphoric effects could not be ruled out. Thus, on a structured interactional task, despite improved actual performance, medication reduced the positive feedback hyperactive boys gave to classmates and increased their own self-derogatory comments. Other hints of dysphoria could be seen in peers' ratings of medicated hyperactives as moodier and more unhappy than unmedicated hyperactives (Whalen et al., 1987a). Whether these implied dampening effects are deleterious is not yet clear.

Peers are highly sensitive to the social deficits of hyperactive children and the impact of medication. Hyperactive boys taking placebo were perceived far more negatively than boys taking stimulant medication and normal comparison peers (Whalen et al., 1987a). Peers viewed unmedicated hyperactive boys as more hyperactive and as having more school and conduct problems than hyperactive boys on methylphenidate. In addition, peers saw the untreated hyperactives as messier, poorer at sports, less healthy, less likable and less desirable as classmates or companions. In contrast, medicated hyperactives were not seen as significantly different from normal peers, save in their lack of proficiency at sports and cruelty to animals. Thus, peers viewed the deficits of hyperactive boys and their medication responses as extending far beyond the core symptoms of inattentiveness and hyperactivity. Unfortunately, even with a positive behavioral response to medication, the popularity of ADHD children may remain low (Riddle & Rapoport, 1976). Furthermore, as Whalen et al. (1987a) noted, although medication can quickly reduce unpleasant behavior, it cannot provide the child with a repertoire of age-expected social skills whose acquisition requires both time and coaching.

Effects on Mood—Developmental Aspects. In most adults, stimulants such as methylphenidate and dextroamphetamine produce euphoria and reduce fatigue. Researchers formerly believed that the calming action of these drugs on hyperactive children was a "paradoxical effect" that was characteristic only of this group; they further believed that as the hyperactive child entered adolescence, this therapeutic effect disappeared. Both of these beliefs have now been questioned.

Normal and hyperactive children do not differ qualitatively in their response to stimulants. Rapoport et al. (1980a) found that neither group of children experienced euphoria with dextroamphetamine; indeed, both normal and hyperactive children frequently reported that the drug made them feel "funny" or "tired." These investigators speculated that these differences in mood response may reflect physiologically determined aspects of mood regulation that do not mature until puberty; for example, some frontal lobe dopaminergic pathways do not fully develop until the second decade of life (Mattes et al., 1984; Weinberger, 1987). In contrast to their divergent age-determined mood responses to dextroamphetamine, at moderate dose levels adults and children showed similar cognitive and attentional responses. These included improved vigilance, improved cognitive performance, and decreased motor activity during cognitive testing.

Many hyperactive children continue to show a therapeutic, noneuphoric response to stimulants well into adolescence (Klorman et al., 1987; MacKay et al., 1973; Varley, 1983). Rapoport (1977) reported a 16-year-old girl whose long-term stimulant medication had to be stopped because, for the first time, she developed a euphoric response. However, such responses seem to be uncommon. Although some cases have been reported (Goyer et al., 1979), the abuse of stimulant medications by adolescents who are receiving them for treatment of ADHD appears to be unusual.

Some studies (Wender et al., 1981, 1985) have concluded that adults with residual symptoms of ADHD (and retrospectively diagnosed histories of this condition during childhood) also continue to show a beneficial, noneuphoric response to stimulants; other investigators, however, have challenged the possibility of predicting adult stimulant response on the basis of childhood ADHD symptomatology (Mattes et al., 1984). Sadly enough, systematic longitudinal data from the same subjects do not yet exist; the only available information is anecdotal. Whether the presence or absence of euphoric response to stimulants is a significant biological marker, and whether it remains a stable finding throughout the life cycle continue to be fascinating questions. In depressed adults, the presence of an initial euphoric response to dextroamphetamine has been reported to discriminate between biochemical subtypes of depression. Patients with this response are the ones most likely to benefit from predominantly noradrenergic antidepressants, such as imipramine (Whybrow et al., 1984).

In children, the dysphoric effects of stimulants have considerable clinical importance. Despite dramatic social and cognitive benefits, children may dislike how they feel on medication, which could account for much of the ubiquitous noncompliance with treatment. A significant minority of children on stimulants appear sunken-eyed, withdrawn, and anhedonic; such children may feel sad and have crying jags. These symptoms may gradually disappear or may diminish with a reduced dosage or an alternate drug; sometimes, however, they necessitate stopping stimulant medication altogether.

Dosage Studies. The time- and dose-related aspects of stimulant effects have significant theoretical and clinical implications.

Following a single dose of methylphenidate, blood levels peak between 1 and 3 hours, with considerable variation among children in the timing, duration, and magnitude of the peak response (Gualtieri & Hicks, 1985; Kupietz et al., 1982; Shaywitz et al., 1982). Meals seem to have little effect on absorption.

Following a single dose of dextroamphetamine, plasma levels remain elevated considerably longer than with methylphenidate. Peak blood dextroamphetamine levels occur 3 to 4 hours after administration, with a half-life of about 7 hours (Brown et al., 1979). Strikingly, however, marked behavioral improvement begins as early as 30 minutes to 1 hour after administration and disappears by about the 4th hour, even though blood levels are still near their peak at that time.

The observation that significant behavioral and motor effects occur during the initial absorption phase and do not correlate with specific blood levels of dextroamphetamine or methylphenidate may reflect an initial release of neurotransmitter stores, which become depleted despite persisting high drug levels. This hypothesis would account for the failure of clinical response to correlate with drug blood levels. It may also explain the failure of time-release preparations of dextroamphetamine and methylphenidate to provide a sustained clinical response, despite sustained blood levels.

The pharmacokinetics of pemoline are less well known. Although substantial benefits often require 3 or 4 weeks' administration, improvement may sometimes be noted within 2 hours of the first dose (Zametkin & Rapoport, 1987). In addition, pemoline seems to produce a more sustained behavioral effect throughout the day than does dextroamphetamine or methylphenidate, a fact not entirely accounted for by its somewhat longer half-life.

A major issue in the field is to determine the differences between drug-responders and nonresponders (Halperin et al., 1986). It is not clear whether the failure to respond arises because these children do not achieve an adequate blood level. On this point, pharmacokinetic studies yield contradictory findings. Some studies (Shaywitz et al., 1982) have found a correlation between blood levels and clinical response, whereas other studies have not (Gualtieri et al., 1982). Blood levels are clearly not the whole story in explaining the lack of a therapeutic drug response. Kupietz et al. (1982) identified an adverse responder whose performance on a cognitive task deteriorated steadily with increasing methylphenidate blood levels.

Sprague and Sleator (1975, 1977) have cautioned that the optimal stimulant dose may differ with the target symptom (i.e., cognitive performance vs. social inappropriateness). They concluded from their data that a methylphenidate dose of 0.3 mg/kg produced an optimal effect on cognitive functioning but was less effective than a 1.0 mg/kg dose in controlling motor and social behavior. The 1.0 mg/kg dose, however, reduced cognitive performance to placebo levels. Thus, when titrating dosage levels against behavior changes, it is important to determine which behavioral symptoms have priority.

Sprague and Sleator's findings have also not yet been adequately replicated by others (Conners, 1985). Indeed Solanto and Wender (1989) found the performance of most children with ADHD on a task of cognitive flexibility *improved* with increasing dosages of methylphenidate (up to 1.0 mg/kg). Similarly, Conners and Solanto (1984) found a linear dose-response relationship, with higher doses of medication (up to 1.0 mg/kg) producing fewer errors of commission on a reaction-time task. Conners and Solanto (1984) cautioned that different behaviors (i.e., activity and attention) may have not only different dosage-response curves, but also different time-action curves. When autonomic, attentional, and activity measures were followed after administration of methylphenidate, the drug's effects on the variables had different time courses. For example, after about 4 hours improvement in vigilance (as measured by a reaction-time task) returned to predrug levels; in contrast, improvements in activity level and impulsivity (as measured by a continuous performance test) were still present at the 6-hour mark. Further, with alterations in dose the time-response curves for each measure showed distinctive changes. On the basis of such findings, Conners and Solanto speculated that different physiological systems, each with its own characteristic response to medication, may underlie the diverse effects of the drug. They also concluded that "there is no single dosage level . . . (such as 0.3 mg/kg of methylphenidate) that is optimal for *all* cognitive functions" (Connors & Solanto, 1984, p. 202). This conclusion underlines the need for careful ongoing monitoring of all aspects of the child's behavior in assessing medication response.

Use of Stimulant Medication throughout the Life Cycle. It is during the latency years that the effects of stimulant medication seem most dramatic and have been most widely studied. The current view of ADHD, however, is that the condition is a life-long, constitutionally determined disorder manifesting itself variably throughout the life cycle. This belief, in turn, has led to trials of the medication outside the grade school years.

Preschool Years. Despite some beneficial results, serious questions remain about the advisability of stimulant treatment for the preschool child; the FDA has not yet approved the use of stimulants for this age group as safe and effective. Although methylphenidate improved teacher ratings and test performances on motor and cognitive tasks, Conners (1975) found that hyperactive preschoolers were less responsive to stimulants than older children. Using carefully titrated doses, Schleifer and colleagues (1975) found that methylphenidate improved hyperactive 3- and 4-year-olds' behavior at home but not in their nursery school or on psychometric testing. More important, the medication very often deleteriously affected mood and social interaction, with the children exhibiting more solitary play, sadness, irritability, and excessive clinginess in addition to the usual side effects of insomnia and anorexia. Because of these side effects, at the end of the study, only 10% of parents opted to keep their preschoolers on medication despite their improved behavior at home.

Adolescence. Data are also scanty concerning the effects of stimulant medication in adolescence. Researchers have suggested several reasons for this neglect (Weiss & Hechtman, 1986). First, there was a mistaken belief that hyperactivity and attentional deficits disappeared with puberty. The corollary belief was that the beneficial effects of stimulants on hyperactive children also disappeared with adolescence. Concern about growth suppression, along with the fear of fostering drug abuse, further inhibited the use of stimulants after puberty. Finally, the recalcitrance of many adolescent patients made for poor cooperation and medication compliance, and the pervasiveness of their school and social problems made drug effects difficult to evaluate.

Despite these difficulties, a growing body of data suggests that stimulants have a useful adjunctive role in treating adolescent ADHD. Open trials with adolescent ADHD patients suggest that stimulants improve classroom behavior (as indicated by teacher ratings of restlessness, inattention, and aggression) and performance on some psychometric tests. Double-blind placebo-controlled studies (Coons et al., 1987; Klorman et al., 1987; Varley, 1983) have also shown clear beneficial effects of methylphenidate in adolescents. Patient, parent, and teacher ratings; global assessments of behavior at home and school; and performance on cognitive and attentional tests have confirmed these findings. In Varley's (1983) study, the adolescent subjects, all of whom had been responsive to methylphenidate earlier in life, showed clear symptomatic improvement with 0.15 mg/kg of methylphenidate, with slight further improvement on 0.3 mg/kg. As noted earlier, most adolescents with ADHD do not show euphoria in response to stimulants; indeed, they may show the same anhedonia or dysphoria as younger children. The mood response of such adolescents needs careful monitoring for it may change as they grow older (Rapoport, 1977). Most experts believe that despite the risk of drug abuse among ADHD adolescents generally, abuse of prescribed stimulants by these adolescents is rare (Weiss & Hechtman, 1986). Isolated cases of abuse do occur, however, and underline the need for great caution. Goyer and colleagues (1979) reported a 13-year-old boy who showed a marked improvement in restless behavior, inattention, and classroom uncooperativeness when on methylphenidate. Although the patient was carefully observed, neither positive nor negative mood changes could be detected at daily doses up to 80 mg. Subsequently, the patient was discovered to be stealing medication and taking up to 200 mg per day. Other distinctive features of this case, which may suggest relative contraindications for stimulants in at least some adolescents, included additional addictive behavior, a predominance of antisocial features that overshadowed his attentional difficulties, and a three-generation family history of substance abuse. Desipramine may prove useful in cases where the potential for abuse contraindicates prescribing stimulants.

Adulthood. Evidence is accumulating that residual symptoms of poor concentration, restlessness, irritability, and impulsivity persist into adulthood. This development has led to the concept of "Adult MBD" (Bellak, 1979; Mann & Greenspan, 1976) and to trials of stimulants in adults with life-long histories of ADD (Wender et al., 1981, 1985; Wood et al., 1976). These studies are difficult to evaluate because it seems likely that adults meeting the criteria of ADD in adulthood are an otherwise heterogeneous group; furthermore, although the nonspecific effects of stimulants on normal adults have not yet received systematic study, they are clearly wide-ranging. Wender's group treated a number of adult subjects with ADD-like symptoms and a childhood history of ADD (retrospectively diagnosed by interview with the subjects' parents). These investigators found that methylphenidate and pemoline (as well as MAOIs) produced dramatically beneficial effects on these patients' concentration, impulsivity, irritability, and interpersonal sensitivity (Wood et al., 1976; Wender et al., 1981, 1985). These subjects, most of whom had not come to psychiatric attention as children, showed a calming, noneuphoric response to stimulants that was quite unlike the excitement shown by stimulant abusers. In contrast, adult patients with ADD-like symptoms but without a retrospectively diagnosable childhood history of ADD did not show a similar therapeutic response. Wender interpreted this lack of reaction as evidence that stimulants do not merely induce a general euphoriant or antidepressive effect regardless of diagnosis, but rather offer a specific, therapeutic effect in "true" adult ADD. More recently, these findings have been challenged by Mattes et al., (1984). These investigators treated a number of adults with ADD-like symptoms by administering methylphenidate. Only a minority of such patients showed a positive response, and at best their improvement was mild. In contrast to Wender's findings, Mattes and colleagues found that a history of childhood ADD was *not* a useful predictor of response; in fact, the best responders were those subjects with a history of multiple drug use. The specificity and advisability of stimulant treatment in adult ADD thus remain controversial.

Side Effects of Stimulant Medication

Despite their frequent benefits, stimulants often produce behavioral and affective side effects that necessitate careful monitoring. Insomnia, loss of appetite, and mood changes are among the commonest side effects of stimulant treatment in childhood (Klein et al., 1980). In addition, abnormal movements, tics, and overfocused or compulsive behavior may occur at least transiently in a large proportion of children receiving stimulants (Borcherding et al., 1990).

As many as half of the children on stimulants have trouble falling asleep, especially if medication is given in the afternoon or if a long-acting preparation is used. Paradoxically, Chatoor et al. (1983) found that despite its causing lighter sleep (as measured polysomnographically), a calming bedtime dose of stimulant medication helped certain restless ADHD children get to sleep earlier and more easily. For these restless children, the motoric calming effects of stimulants seemed to help them settle down.

Loss of appetite also occurs in up to half of stimulant-treated children, although this effect often wears off toward evening when the child may even become voraciously hungry. A good breakfast, along with the morning dose of medication and parental flexibility about a late supper and beforebed snack can help maintain caloric intake. Careful monitoring of height and weight are important to avert or minimize growth inhibition (see below).

Stimulants can have dysphoric effects including depression, apathy, and crying jags; together, these serious side effects may sometimes require reducing or stopping medication. Even though children behave better on it, they may report that the medication makes them feel "funny," tired, or cranky (Rapoport et al., 1980a).

Complaints of headache and abdominal pain are common, especially early in treatment; fortunately, they are usually transient. Cardiovascular side effects, such as increased heart rate or elevated blood pressure are usually not clinically significant; these vital signs should be checked before stimulant treatment is begun.

Hallucinations and bizarre behavior occur rarely; they are most likely in misdiagnosed children who on closer inspection have a psychotic or pervasive developmental disorder (Klein et al., 1980).

A serious, controversial side effect of stimulants is the now well-documented exacerbation or precipitation of tic disorder (Lowe et al., 1982). When children with ADHD are carefully observed following initiation of stimulant medication, investigators have noted that a large proportion of the youngsters develop, at least transiently, abnormal movements, including oro-facial movements, tremors, tics, or stereotypies, such as picking at their clothes or fingers (Borcherding et al., 1990). In certain cases, stimulants appear to precipitate or hasten the onset of full-blown Tourette's syndrome (TS). It is unclear whether stimulants have this ominous effect only in constitutionally predisposed children, in essence hastening the appearance of symptoms that were destined to occur in any case. Studies of several identical twin pairs suggest this may be the case; in each of these pairs, although only one twin (perhaps the one most severely affected by ADHD-like prodromal symptoms) received stimulants, ultimately both twins developed TS (Price et al., 1986). Although children at risk for TS constitute only a small fraction of all ADHD children, a large proportion of children who eventually develop TS show ADHD-like prodromal symptoms, including hyperactivity, attention deficit, and learning difficulties. Thus, before prescribing stimulants to children with any signs of tic disorder, extreme caution and careful evaluation are necessary. Denckla (personal communication, 1982) even cautions against using stimulants in children with marked choreiform movements (elicited by having the child stand with eyes closed and fingers and arms outstretched).

Stimulants, especially dextroamphetamine, produce overfocused, perseverative, or compulsive behavior in a substantial number of children with ADHD (Solanto & Wender, 1989; Borcherding et al., 1990). These difficulties may be subtle or severe. For example, Borcherding et al. observed one boy receiving stimulants who played with Legos for 36 hours straight without food or sleep; others played video games or cleaned compulsively.

Decreased growth in height and weight are potentially serious side effects of stimulant medication. The conflicting reports concerning the existence and magnitude of stimulant-related growth inhibition reflect the considerable methodological difficulties involved in such studies (Greenhill, 1984; Mattes & Gittleman, 1983). The magnitude of growth inhibition appears to be related to the type of stimulant and the total dosage. Dextroamphetamine is the worst offender, suppressing the velocity of height growth by as much as 32% (Greenhill, 1984). Methylphenidate appears to be less growth-inhibiting than dextroamphetamine. Mattes and Gittleman (1983) found that for their sample group as a whole, during a 4-year period, the magnitude of growth inhibition from methylphenidate was small, with methylphenidate dosage accounting for only 2% of the variance in final height. Nonetheless, they cautioned that in any individual child the inhibition may be substantial. Other studies indicate that the height gains of children on methylphenidate may be decreased 0.4–0.9 cm per year, with a cumulative height deficit of as much as 7.5 cm less than expected growth (Mattes & Gittleman-Klein, 1979, cited in Greenhill, 1984).

Inhibition of weight gain also occurs with stimulant medication, averaging about 1.5 kg less than expected after the first two years of medication (Rapoport, 1983). Because weight can be made up later in life, inhibition of weight gain is less worrisome than height growth inhibition. Whether these growth lags in height and weight are fully made up for in adolescence is unknown, as are the effects on growth of stimulants given during adolescence. Drug holidays appear to be useful because significant, but incomplete, catch-up growth occurs during summer vacations and other drug-free periods (Mattes & Gittleman, 1983; Safer et al., 1975).

The causes of stimulant-induced growth inhibition are not known. Decreased caloric intake due to drug-induced appetite suppression is probably a major culprit. Although the stimulants do not seem to interfere with the most important bursts of growth-hormone secretion that occur during sleep, they do inhibit the sleep-related release of prolactin (Greenhill, 1984).

In light of these uncertainties, prudence demands careful baseline measurement of height and weight with trimonthly monitoring once stimulant treatment has started. The lowest clinically effective dose should be used with drug-free periods whenever possible.

Nonstimulant Drugs. Although the stimulants remain overwhelmingly the most popular drugs for treatment of ADHD, other drugs have been used effectively; in certain ADHD children, when stimulants are ineffective or are contraindicated, these alternative medications may be preferable. Tricyclic antidepressants ameliorate ADHD symptoms (Biederman et al., 1989a; Pliszka, 1987). Although the optimal dose continues to be a matter of debate, these drugs may be effective without the latency seen in the initiation of antidepressant effects. An interesting sidelight is the efficacy of the tricyclic antidepressants in ameliorating childhood conduct problems that are secondary to depression (Puig-Antich, 1982). How this relates to its efficacy in ADHD is unclear.

Whether the tricyclics are as effective as the stimulants is open to question. Somatic side effects may be more prominent than with the stimulants (Rapoport et al., 1974a). The tricyclics, however, have a smoother, longer action than stimulants and may be more effective in the evening without causing insomnia.

Desipramine has been the most intensively studied tricyclic for the treatment of ADHD (Biederman et al., 1989a, 1989b; Garfinkel et al., 1983). Although these clinical studies have found the drug effective and generally well tolerated, caution is needed in its use. Biederman et al. (1989b) found that desipramine produced small increases in diastolic blood pressure, heart rate, and electrocardiographic conduction parameters that were not clinically significant in healthy children. However, three cases of sudden death have occurred in children receiving the drug (Riddle et al., 1991; "Sudden Death," 1990). As with adults, tricyclics may produce disorganization, agitation, or hypomania in a few adolescents, perhaps those with a vulnerability to psychosis or mania. Despite the widespread use of tricyclics with children and adolescents, the pediatric use of these agents has not been approved by the Food and Drug Administration, save for nocturnal enuresis. (See Chapters 6 and 17 for additional information on the clinical use of the tricyclics.)

Clonidine, a noradrenergic agonist, has also proven useful for ADHD symptoms in a small double-blind study (Hunt et al., 1985). Widely used as an adult antihypertensive, this drug is of considerable interest. When administered to certain children with Tourette's syndrome, it not only reduces their multiple tics but relieves their concomitant inattentiveness, impulsivity, and irritability as well (Cohen et al., 1980). ADHD children with motor tics may be specially vulnerable to developing Tourette's syndrome if placed on stimulant medication (Lowe et al., 1982); clonidine may prove especially useful for such children.

Zametkin and his NIMH colleagues (1985) have found MAOIs effective in ADHD patients. Although this action is of considerable theoretical interest, the dangers of hypertensive reactions and attendant dietary restrictions limit the childhood use of this class of drugs.

Treatment Outcome—Pharmacotherapy

Despite the dramatic short-term impact of stimulants on the hyperactive child's behavior, the influence of medication alone on long-term outcome is difficult to demonstrate. Stimulants do not consistently produce either short- or long-term improvement in actual academic attainment (as opposed to classroom manageability). The Montreal follow-up study (Weiss & Hechtman, 1986) explored the outcome in young adulthood of a group of hyperactive children who had received stimulants during childhood for at least 3 years. The authors compared this population with a matched normal group and a group of hyperactive young adults who had received no stimulants. Not unexpectedly, in many areas such as school, work, and the frequency of serious psychopathology the hyperactives, even the treated hyperactives, fared worse than their normal counterparts. Nevertheless, medication did have some important meliorative effects. Compared with their untreated hyperactive peers, the hyperactive young adults who had received stimulants looked back on their childhoods more positively, had fewer problems with theft and aggression, had generally better social skills and self-esteem, and showed less need for current psychiatric treatment. The authors concluded that although stimulant treatment did not eliminate many difficulties, it appeared to lessen social ostracism and hence protect self-esteem.

Outcome of Multimodality Treatment

A series of outcome studies by Satterfield et al. (1981, 1982, 1987) highlight the superiority of a long-term multimodal treatment approach over brief treatment or the use of stimulant medication alone. In the first study, on the basis of a comprehensive assessment, hyperactive children were assigned to individually tailored treatment programs. All children received medication plus a combination of individual, group, family, and/or educational therapy. Parent work consisted of training in behavioral techniques, parent casework, and parent and/or conjoint parent–child groups.

Outcome was explored for two groups of children who did not differ on pretreatment measures. In particular, a group of children who remained in treatment for 2 to 3 years was compared with a group who received less than 2 years' treatment. Both groups showed significant improvement; children did not seem to drop out because they were initially more severely disturbed or because they failed to respond to treatment. Nonetheless, when compared with the group receiving less treatment, those children who remained in the program 2 to 3 years (average 35 months) showed less antisocial behavior, were more attentive in class, were better adjusted at home and school, and showed greater global improvement.

A recent study (Satterfield et al., 1987) examined the outcome 9 years after clinic entry for two groups of boys, one receiving multimodal treatment and the other stimulant medication only. Again, there were no significant differences on the pretreatment variables. By ages 14 to 21 years, 30% of the drug-treatment-only subjects had two or more felony arrests versus only 7% of the long-term multimodal treatment subjects. Other measures of delinquent outcome showed similar striking advantages to long-term multimodal treatment. On balance, these studies found an unusually good outcome for those receiving long-term multimodal treatment compared with other treatment follow-up studies.

APPENDIX 11–1
DIAGNOSTIC AND CONCEPTUAL CONTROVERSIES
SURROUNDING ATTENTION-DEFICIT
HYPERACTIVITY DISORDER

Many practical and theoretical controversies rage about ADHD involving several different issues and levels of challenge (Rubinstein & Brown, 1984; Rutter, 1983a).

One set of questions concerns *reliability*. Can clinicians reliably diagnose ADHD? Is it possible to operationally define and reliably measure its component symptoms—inattentiveness and overactivity? If a child is symptomatic in one setting but not in another, which is more salient for diagnostic purposes? Further, even given concurrence about a child's degree of activity and inattention, do sophisticated observers agree about whether the diagnosis of ADHD applies?

A second set of questions concerns the *validity* of the ADHD category, whether it is a "real" illness. First, there is the question of whether the syndrome has internal consistency. Do its constituent symptoms actually co-occur more frequently than would be predictable on a random basis? For example, within the older concept of MBD, do hyperactivity, learning disabilities, and neurological soft signs tend to occur in the same child? Or, using the more restricted contemporary category of ADHD, do hyperactivity and inattention appear together? Next do the ADHD diagnostic criteria define a clinically valid group? Do children diagnosed as having ADHD resemble each other in important ways (other than the selection criteria)? For, if ADHD is a meaningful diagnostic category, applying the diagnostic label to a child should assert something beyond the observation that he is inattentive and perhaps very active. Membership in a valid diagnostic group should make possible further inferences about etiology, associated clinical features, probable clinical course, or response to treatment (Ferguson & Rapoport, 1983; Rutter, 1983a). Equally important, can ADHD children be distinguished from children with similar problems but different diagnoses, such as conduct disorder or oppositional disorder?

Finally, can ADHD children be divided into useful subgroups? For example, is the original DSM-III distinction between ADD with and without hyperactivity a valid one?

Problems of Definition and Reliability

It is difficult to give the terms *attention* and *activity* rigorous operational definitions. The label of *inattention* is often applied to a variety of behaviors that might arise from inadequate motivation and impulsivity, as well as from defects in specifically cognitive areas such as impaired vigilance or ability to resist and exclude distractions (Douglas, 1983, 1984; Rutter,

1983a; Shaffer & Schonfeld, 1984). In addition, situational factors may be at work such as inadequate reinforcement or inappropriateness of the task. Similarly, the appropriate measure of overactivity is debatable: Should it represent the total amount of gross motor movement or the degree to which activity level fails to be appropriately modulated in the face of situational demands? Behavior reflecting dependency, anxiety, or aggression may also give the impression of inattention or overactivity in an otherwise on-task child. Because observers' attributions of inattentiveness or hyperactivity cast so wide a net, there is little assurance that all children so labeled have, even descriptively, the same defect in psychological functioning, let alone a common distinctive underlying physiological or psychopathological mechanism. Thus, definitional problems include many unresolved questions about reliability and validity. Playing the devil's advocate, Shaffer & Schonfeld (1984) have argued that "the problems of defining and hence measuring [overactivity and inattention] are so considerable that they call into question the wisdom of basing a clinical syndrome on their presence or absence" (p. 120).

Rating Scales.   Rating scales or laboratory measures have been suggested to objectively quantify and give uniformity to assessments of children's behavior (Barkley, 1982). Each of these techniques has its own difficulties.

The most widely used and best studied rating scale is that of Conners (Conners, 1973; Conners & Barkley, 1985; Werry et al., 1975). Using this 39-item scale, teachers rate children on items assessing classroom behavior, group participation, and attitudes toward authority. Conners (1973) has also developed an abbreviated 10-item teacher form and a parents' version.

The Conners scale has been extensively studied, and normative data have been gathered for several populations. Direct observational studies have validated the scale (Abikoff et al., 1980), which correlates highly with DSM-III diagnoses (Goyette et al., 1978). The scale has also proved extremely useful in assessing symptomatic responsiveness to medication. Factor analysis of the Conners scale yields four major factors: conduct problem, inattentiveness–passivity, hyperactivity, and tension–anxiety (Conners & Barkley, 1985; Goyette et al., 1978).

Despite their aura of numerical exactitude, rating scales have certain inherent difficulties. Basically, they summarize an individual's assessment of various checklist items, each entailing a subjective judgment. Rating-scale items such as "inattentive," "short attention span," "easily distracted," are not operationally defined. Further, the rater is not a precision instrument that assesses each behavioral item in isolation; rather the rater responds in global ways to all that he or she knows about the child, a phenomenon sometimes referred to as the "halo effect." On the one hand, a virtue of such scales in assessing children's adaptation to relevant, real-life situations is that parent and teacher ratings integrate a large amount of contextual data and judgments about the child's behavior; on the other hand, the lack of precise operational definitions means that different children may well be labeled inattentive or overactive for different reasons, thereby blurring the distinction between different clinical entities and blunting the scales' ability to discriminate between normal and significantly impaired children.

Although a scale may be reliable from a psychometric point of view, the impression of quantitative objectivity that such scales confer may be to some extent spurious. Conners himself has stressed that rating scales "are not diagnostic devices. They are simply measures, in a very crude way, of somebody's impression of the presence of a class of symptoms" (Conners [discussion of Shaffer & Schonfeld], 1984, p. 129). Although some critics, such as Barkley (1982), have decried the absence of agreed-upon quantitative diagnostic criteria for ADHD, a single score on a statistically derived scale cannot replace a broad-based clinical assessment that considers the total context of the child's development and history. Therefore, the clinician should not treat a high numerical score as though by itself it constitutes a psychiatric diagnosis.

Laboratory and Observational Measures. Various laboratory measures have been utilized as diagnostic aids to objectify and assess activity and attention. These instruments include actometers and motion detectors as well as tests of vigilance and impulsivity, such as the Continuous Performance Test. Researchers have used many of these same measures in attempting to delineate the precise nature of the ADHD child's deficiencies in regulating attention and activity. Because of expense and formidable technical difficulties, many of these techniques have limited applications in clinical practice; furthermore, the laboratory setting is likely to put the ADHD child on his best behavior so that one-shot, short-term measures may not validly reflect characteristic behavior (Kinsbourne, 1984). Indeed, ADHD children's performance on the Continuous Performance Test varies with the presence or absence of an adult (Draeger et al., 1986).

In their week-long naturalistic study of boys' free-ranging activity levels at home and at school (a study made possible by solid state, long-memory movement monitors), Porrino et al. (1983b) found good agreement with teachers' (but not parents') ratings of activity level on the Conners scale. Because earlier findings had yielded only inconsistent correlations between laboratory and clinical measures of activity, the authors concluded that short-term measures in restricted settings may yield misleading results. As for inattention, the relationship of various laboratory measures to observers' ratings of inattentiveness is even more complex and uncertain (Shaffer & Schonfeld, 1984). Evidently, specific laboratory measures do not yet exist that can quantify or replace observers' complex (and difficult to operationalize) contextual judgments of activity and inattention. Direct, time-sampling behavioral observations fail to correlate highly with teachers' ratings. Noting this, Whalen et al., (1978) commented:

> There will probably never be an observation schema that could capture the essence of a boy diving under a desk, scooting across an entire classroom to roll under a room divider, or tripping on a cord to bring a tape recorder crashing to the floor. Moreover, given the constraints of time sampling, these events are highly likely to occur during "off" periods on the observation schedule, leaving an indelible impression on the teacher's memory, but only blanks on the code cards. (p. 185)

How Much Is Too Much?   Even if clinicians or researchers agreed on the facets of activity and attention that are clinically relevant, they would still have to confront another knotty question: Above what level of activity or inattentiveness should a child be considered abnormal? Attentiveness and activity levels appear to be distributed normally across the general child population (Huessy, 1984). By definition, half of all children will be above the mode.

The question then is one of excess. Who is to be considered excessively active or inattentive? This question can be approached in several ways. The researcher who asks parents and teachers soon realizes that excess is in the eye of the beholder. For example, in one Buffalo study, 49% of the parents considered their children to be overactive (Lapouse & Monk, 1958), and in the Isle of Wight study (Rutter et al., 1970), of all the 10- to 11-year-old boys ultimately judged *not* to have a psychiatric disorder, as many as one-third were described as overactive or unattentive by the parents and teachers (Shaffer & Greenhill, 1979). Researchers have suggested that teachers are better judges of ADHD symptoms than parents because teachers see children in a setting that requires concentration and motivation. Presumably, teachers also have wider experience with a broad range of children as a basis for making comparisons. It is therefore of interest that in one questionnaire study in Urbana, Illinois, teachers rated 48% of a random sample of students as distractible, 30% as hyperactive, and 50% as restless (Werry & Quay, 1971).

If the clinician used the crude judgments of either these parents or teachers as the sole diagnostic criterion, he or she would have to diagnose an extremely large group of children as hyperactive. In other respects, many of these youngsters would be quite normal and would have little else in common. One solution is to select children whose scores on a well-normed measure are two or more standard deviations above the mean. Many research designs employ the 10-item Conners Abbreviated Teacher Rating Scale (Conners, 1973) and take a score of 15 or above on the hyperactivity subscale as their selection criterion for hyperactivity. Applied to the general population, such a procedure will identify about 5% of children as hyperactive (Trites, 1979). Where professionals draw the cutoff line for excessive activity and inattentiveness is more than a matter of convention; the decision has a powerful impact on the characteristics of the group of children so selected.

Variability across Settings. Diagnosis also becomes equivocal when adults in different settings have divergent opinions about a child's behavior. The DSM-III definition of ADD recognizes this problem, when it notes that the observer's standards and the setting in which the child is observed influence the identification of symptoms. Parents, teachers, and doctors often assess the same child quite differently, depending on whether the child is seen at home, in school, or in the office (Lambert et al., 1978; Schachar et al., 1981).

When two teachers observe the same child simultaneously or the same teacher observes the same child over time, the reliability of the Conners scale is quite good. However, when teachers rate the same child in different classrooms, their scale scores show only fair agreement. The agreement between teachers and parents rating the same child at school and at home is even lower (Rutter, 1983a). In Rutter et al.'s (1970) study of the entire 10-year-old population of the Isle of Wight, 9.9% of the children were rated high on a hyperactivity scale by their parents and 8.3% were rated high by their teacher. However, the agreement between parents and teachers was low, so that only 2.2% of the children in the total population were identified as hyperactive by *both* parent and teacher (Schachar et al., 1981). In part, these discrepancies reflect true differences in the child's behavior (depending on the novelty, structure, and demands of the different settings); in part, the discrepancies may also reflect differing explicit or implicit standards of judgment (Rapoport et al., 1986a). Cultural, professional, and idiosyncratic personal norms all influence the observer's standards of excessive activity or inattention in a child.

Several studies differentiate children who show "pervasive" hyperactivity (i.e., as judged by both their teachers at school and parents at home) from those designated as "situationally" hyperactive (i.e., as judged hyperactive in only one setting) (Campbell et al., 1977; Sandberg et al., 1978; Schachar et al., 1981). In general, pervasive hyperactives showed more severe hyperactivity and attentional difficulties; in addition, they were more likely than the situational hyperactives to display disturbances in conduct, marked cognitive impairment, neurological soft signs, earlier onset, and poorer prognosis. Thus, specifying the range of situations in which a child's symptoms occur defines not only quantitative but also qualitative aspects of his pathology and winnows out reactive upsets specific to a single context.

Problems of Validity

Researchers have proposed two strategies to assess the validity of the ADHD syndrome (Rutter, 1983a). The first is to ask whether the various components of the putative syndrome actually tend to occur together. The second is to examine whether children diagnosed with the proposed syndrome share other distinctive clinical features, such as etiology, biological or behavioral concomitants, prognosis, or response to treatment.

Do the Symptoms Co-occur? A fundamental question is whether the proposed criteria reflect the actual associations and patterning of symptoms in the child population. The notion of MBD, for example, postulates the co-occurrence of various symptoms such as perceptual and learning difficulties, hyperactivity, and neurological soft signs. Unfortunately most definitions of MBD do not include exact criteria specifying how many or which signs or symptoms must be present to make the diagnosis. Nichols and Chen (1981) analyzed the longitudinal data of the Collaborative Perinatal Project, which had followed about 30,000 children from gestation into grade school. Examining the distribution of children's ratings for learning difficulties, hyperkinetic behavior, and neurological soft signs, the authors chose cut-offs for each rating that selected the 8% of children most deficient with respect to that rating. Of the 8% defined by this method as having any one symptom, only 2.5% had *two* symptoms, and only 0.18% had all *three* symptoms. Although this last figure is about 3 times higher than would be expected from a chance distribution, it represents only a small fraction of the total child population. The association among hyperactivity, learning disabilities, and neurological soft signs is thus so tenuous that it calls into question the validity of any simple syndrome of MBD.

Building on the more restricted, better-specified DSM-III criteria for ADDH, various studies have tried to use different factor or correlative analyses to assess whether hyperactivity and inattention do co-occur. The results have been equivocal and, in the light of complex methodological issues, difficult to interpret (Lahey et al., 1980; Langhorne et al., 1976; Rutter, 1983a). Although the current nomenclature of Attention-deficit Hyperactivity Disorder (DSM-III-R, APA, 1987) presupposes the association of hyperactivity and inattention, the extent of this relationship still awaits empirical determination.

Do ADHD Children Have Common Clinical Features? Another strategy has explored whether ADHD children show unique clinical features, such as distinctive biological characteristics, prognosis, or treatment response. A major question raised by British critics of the ADHD concept is whether ADHD can really be distinguished from conduct disorder; they suspect that the overlap between the two diagnostic categories is so great that it invalidates ADHD as a separate entity (Sandberg et al., 1980; Shaffer & Greenhill, 1979). DSM-III-R acknowledges the many common elements of the two disorders by placing them (together with Oppositional Defiant Disorder) in the same subclass, Disruptive Behavior Disorders. However, the DSM-III-R criteria for ADHD were selected for their ability to discriminate among the three disorders.

The overlap is indeed considerable (Shapiro & Garfinkel, 1986; Werry et al., 1987). Stewart et al. (1981) examined consecutive admissions to a child psychiatry clinic and found that about half the children were diagnosed as hyperactive and about half were diagnosed as unsocialized conduct disorder; about one-third of the total sample carried both diagnoses. The overlap was such that three-fourths of the children with conduct disorder were also diagnosed as hyperactive, and two-thirds of the hyperactives also had a diagnosis of conduct disorder. On several measures, the children who were both hyperactive and conduct disordered resembled those children who had only a conduct disorder more than they resembled those who were only hyperactive. A general population study (Sandberg et al., 1980) found similar results and noted that children's hyperactivity scores correlated very highly with the same observer's rating of the child on conduct disturbance.

The methodological issues involved in this debate are many and complex; they include the nature and source of the ratings (Langhorne et al., 1976; Milich et al., 1982), sample characteristics, and the statistical analyses used (Laprade & Trites, 1985). A major confounding factor concerns the extent to which sample composition and ratings reflect children's "nuisance value" rather than actual hyperactivity or inattention (Campbell & Werry, 1986).

In contrast to the view that ADHD cannot be meaningfully differentiated from conduct disorder, several studies have shown that there is a subgroup of hyperactive children who do *not* have conduct disorders (August & Stewart, 1982; McGee et al., 1984a, 1984b; Stewart et al., 1981; Trites & Laprade, 1983, Werry et al., 1987). Despite the frequent co-occurrence of the two conditions, careful comprehensive clinical evaluation (going beyond rating scales alone) reveals many "pure" hyperactive children (Milich et al., 1982). Although these hyperactives do not seem to differ from "mixed" hyperactives-aggressives or pure conduct disorder children in terms of perinatal history, neurological soft signs, or minor congenital anomalies, the pure hyperactives may have fewer social disadvantages and more developmental delays and cognitive impairment (including a wider scatter on the WISC IQ subscales and lower verbal IQs) (August & Stewart, 1982; McGee et al., 1984a, 1984b; Szatmari et al., 1989).

Clinical experience and systematic long-term studies suggest that family and social factors strongly influence whether an ADHD child develops a conduct disorder (Weiss & Hechtman, 1986). The interaction of the ADHD child and his parent is characterized by noncompliance on the child's part and controlling and negative responses from the parent (Barkley, 1985).

These negative, conflictual, mutually antagonistic interactions are a fertile ground for reinforcing the child's coercive, aggressive behavior, especially when parents are lax, inconsistent, or aggressive in reaction to their taxing child.

The high rate of delinquency, substance abuse, and antisocial behavior in ADHD adolescents (Gittleman et al., 1985; Satterfield et al., 1982; 1987) has also raised a question: Does the clinical course and outcome of ADHD differ in any meaningful way from conduct disorder (Cantwell, 1981; Shaffer & Greenhill, 1979)? Outcome studies indicate that IQ, childhood aggression, and general family and social factors may be more important predictors of outcome than are hyperactivity or inattentiveness. With different initial sample characteristics, the various follow-up studies have drawn conflicting conclusions concerning hyperactives' risk of developing serious antisocial behavior or conduct disorder (Mannuzza et al., 1989). In some studies, depending on social class, the risk appears to run as high as 24% to 45% (Gittleman et al., 1985; Satterfield et al., 1982). In contrast, Weiss and Hechtman (1986) found in their 15-year follow-up that, of the many hyperactives exhibiting antisocial behavior in midadolescence, most did *not* continue such behavior into later adolescence and early adult life. Although by the end of this period three or four individuals had serious criminal records, as a group the hyperactives did not have significantly more antisocial behavior or substance abuse than the matched control group. Weiss (1983) has therefore suggested that the antisocial difficulties of the hyperactive child may be more transitory than those of the pure antisocial child. Whether this is a valid conclusion must await follow-up studies that compare hyperactives to suitable contrast groups of conduct-disordered children.

Another approach to validation has been to assess whether ADHD has distinctive causal factors or biological features. This strategy has so far provided only weak evidence for ADHD being a distinctive and unitary entity (Ferguson & Rapoport, 1983; Rutter, 1983a; Shaffer & Greenhill, 1979). Although genetic factors have been demonstrated for some hyperactive children, there is no evidence that the pattern differs from that seen in family history studies involving other psychiatric difficulties, especially conduct disorder (Ferguson & Rapoport, 1983). Although several biological factors (such as a history of perinatal complications or the presence of mild EEG abnormalities, minor congenital anomalies, and neurological soft signs) show some correlation with hyperactive behavior, these relationships are nonspecific; that is, the abnormalities are also correlated with other behavioral disorders (Reeves et al., 1987). More specific markers have not been found. Finally, there is little evidence that the response of ADHD children to stimulant medication is qualitatively different from that of other groups of children (Rapoport et al., 1980a; Taylor, 1983).

Reviewing the genetic, neurophysiological, and biochemical evidence,

Ferguson and Rapoport (1983) have concluded that there are general correlations between "biological alterations" and deviant behaviors, but that these correlations are not specific for hyperactivity or ADHD. These authors suggest that the weakness and nonspecificity of these associations may reflect the etiological and biological diversity of the hyperkinetic syndrome and the possibility that it is not a unitary disorder. Hyperactivity and/or inattentive behavior may represent the final common expression of various biological disturbances. Because there is so much still to be learned about the underlying mechanisms and their pathways of behavioral expression, it is possible, as Ferguson and Rapoport (1983) have speculated, that some new, more broadly defined diagnostic category, such as "impulse-conduct disorder," will provide a better fit for the emerging biological data than does the current category of ADHD.

The answers to these questions are obviously important. Unidentified or uncontrolled-for differences in the samples selected for study often create differences in findings between investigators. As emphasized elsewhere in this volume, progress in treatment and research depends on defining homogeneous groups of subjects for study and comparison.

Chapter 12

Learning Disabilities

Having made a strenuous effort to understand the symbols he could make nothing of, he [Gustave Flaubert] wept giant tears. . . .

For a long time he could not understand the elementary connection that made of two letters one syllable, of several syllables a word.

—Souvenirs Intimes
CAROLINE COMMANVILLE
(Simpson, 1979)

INTRODUCTION AND DEFINITION

One of the commonest problems for which parents seek help is a child's failure to make satisfactory academic progress. Academic failure has serious consequences for children. It can have devastating effects while they still attend school and can lead to long-range exclusion from full economic and cultural participation in their society. Characteristically, once the child becomes aware that he is lagging behind the others, such failure breeds a pervasive sense of isolation, shame, and low self-esteem that during school hours folds the child about like a cloak. Often such a youngster is up against a complex problem that neither clinicians nor educators fully understand.

Adequate learning depends on a child's innate cognitive capacities, motivation, unconscious fantasies, capacity to attend to tasks, familiarity with the language spoken at the school, and the degree to which the child's accomplishments match the expectations of parents, school, and community. And all of this has not yet taken into account the quality of classroom instruction. Working in collaboration with the parents and school, it then becomes the clinician's task to identify the degree, scope, and causes of the child's failure, and, where possible, to suggest the type of help necessary.

On a statistical basis, environmental and emotional factors probably account for the largest proportion of children who perform below their academic potential. Inadequate schools, impoverished, chaotic, or demoralized home conditions, and family and peer values that do not encourage learning take their toll of many children, especially those who are victims of the "culture of poverty." Primary emotional causes of school failure are manifold. Depression, anxiety, and other serious emotional disorders may interfere with the child's availability to learn. Oppositional and narcissistic character traits hinder the child's ability to cooperate with teachers and to produce academically. In some cases, unconscious needs for punishment or the wish to thwart parental expectations may also play a role. The academic performance of overstimulated or overindulged children may suffer from their incapacity to contain impulses, to defer gratification, or to sublimate adequately important drives that motivate learning. These include aggressive and competitive strivings, curiosity, and the wish to be loved and admired. Finally, school and learning may become entangled in specific neurotic conflicts. For a variety of reasons, the child may unconsciously perceive achievement, success, curiosity, or intellectual assertiveness as dangerous and therefore defensively inhibit these traits (Rothstein, 1982).

Many children's school difficulties stem from developmental dysfunction in crucial cognitive areas, including attention deficits, memory impairments, receptive and expressive language disorders, higher order difficulties with reasoning and abstraction, and organizational deficiencies (Levine & Zallen, 1985). In adolescence, such deficits may become increasingly apparent as the curriculum becomes conceptually more difficult and presumes a progressive automatization and ready availability of many rote skills that such students may not have mastered.

This chapter focuses on yet another group of learning handicaps, the *specific learning disabilities,* a broad group of cognitive deficits presumed to be neurologically determined and largely constitutional in origin. The delineation and the exploration of these disorders have proven to be of great scientific and practical pedagogic interest. At the same time, when evaluating individual children's school difficulties, it is important to keep a broad focus and not to choose too narrowly or exclusively between "organic" and psychosocial paradigms (Rothstein, 1982). Constitutional neurobiological factors undoubtedly exert a strong effect on the learning capacity and style of all children. At the same time, children with specific learning disabilities are even more sensitive than their normal peers to the influence of emotional, environmental, and instructional factors (Silver, 1989b).

The Concept of Specific Learning Disorder

The very construction of achievement tests ensures that half of all children will perform below grade level (defined as the level of difficulty at which half the children in a grade have mastered the material). A most important question is whether there is a discrepancy between a given child's overall intellectual potential and actual academic performance. Historically, IQ tests developed from the need to determine which children in the French public school system could or could not learn (Gould, 1981). Unfortunately, measures such as IQ inevitably tended to be taken out of context by many people, who treated them as though they really reflected a unitary element present in each child—intrinsic general intelligence. Their further assumption was that this general intelligence factor could be accurately and stably determined and given a numerical value. The experienced clinician knows that the IQ scores of a given normal child may in fact vary widely and that emotional, linguistic, and cultural factors heavily influence the degree to which a specific IQ score reflects any innate capacity to learn. A thoughtful study of the learning disorders raises important challenges to any simple notion of general intelligence as a single, indivisible factor.

Bearing these caveats in mind, it is important to note that in many academic areas achievement is highly correlated with measured IQ, especially verbal IQ. For example, reading achievement correlates 0.6 with full scale IQ scores (Yule & Rutter, 1985). Thus, one of the commonest causes of poor school achievement and inadequate learning may be low general intelligence; its effects may in turn be compounded by poor motivation, poor instruction, and, perhaps most serious of all, discouragement.

Despite the broad general correlation between reading and intelligence, there are many more poor readers than would be predicted from the normal IQ distribution curve of the general population. That is to say, superimposed on the predicted normal distribution curve of reading skills, a significant "hump" at the lower end of the curve represents an unexpected group of reading failures not explained by low general intelligence (Yule & Rutter, 1985). This finding is the statistical counterpart to the frequent clinical observation that there are children whose reading is seriously deficient despite apparently adequate schooling and normal or even above-average intelligence. It is, therefore, important to distinguish between *general learning (or reading) retardation* as a concomitant of low IQ and *specific learning (or reading) retardation* where, given both the child's age and IQ, the child is performing below the expected level.

The area investigated most intensively has been reading, and the terms *specific reading retardation, specific developmental dyslexia,* and *developmental reading disorder* are often used interchangeably. The concept of specific learning disorder is, however, applicable to other academic skills as well, such as spelling or arithmetic.

Defining Specific Learning Disabilities

The proper means of defining the specific learning disabilities has created much controversy (Adelman & Taylor, 1986; Rutter, 1978b; Wong, 1986; Yule & Rutter, 1985). One approach has been atheoretical and purely operational; for example, diagnosis of specific reading disorder is made if the child's achievement in reading is more than two standard deviations below that expected from someone of that chronological age and IQ (Rutter & Yule, 1975; Yule & Rutter, 1985). The other approach has been to use exclusionary criteria to delineate a group of children whose cognitive deficits are presumably neurologically based. Thus the definition of specific learning disabilities embodied in the federal Education for All Handicapped Children Act (P.L. 94-142, 1975) explicitly excludes children whose "learning problems. . . are primarily the result of visual, hearing, or motor handicaps or of mental retardation, of emotional disturbance, or environmental, cultural, or economic disadvantage" (Office of Education, 1976).

DMS-III-R Diagnostic Criteria for Developmental Learning Disorders
Developmental Reading Disorder
   A. *Reading achievement, as measured by a standardized, individually administered*

test, is markedly below the expected level, given the person's schooling and intellectual capacity (as determined by an individually administered IQ test).

B. *The disturbance in A significantly interferes with academic achievement or activities of daily living requiring reading skills.*

C. *Not due to a defect in visual or hearing acuity or a neurological disorder.* (APA, 1987, p. 44)

Developmental Arithmetic Disorder

A. *Arithmetic skills, as measured by a standardized, individually administered test, are markedly below the expected level, given the person's schooling and intellectual capacity (as determined by an individually administered IQ test).*

B. *The disturbance in A significantly interferes with academic achievement or activities of daily living requiring arithmetic skills.*

C. *Not due to a defect in visual or hearing acuity or a neurological disorder.* (APA, 1987, p. 42)

Developmental Expressive Writing Disorder

A. *Writing skills, as measured by a standardized, individually administered test, are markedly below the expected level, given the person's schooling and intellectual capacity (as determined by an individually administered IQ test).*

B. *The disturbance in A significantly interferes with academic achievement or activities of daily living requiring the composition of written texts (spelling words and expressing thoughts in grammatically correct sentences and organized paragraphs).*

C. *Not due to a defect in visual or hearing acuity or a neurological disorder.* (APA, 1987, p. 43)

The DSM-III (APA, 1980) regards these conditions as disorders of specific areas of development not due to another disorder. It adds, however, that "because (they) occur so frequently in conjunction with other disorders, they are coded on a separate axis (Axis II) to ensure that they are not overlooked" (p. 92).

There is much debate in the literature over how best to operationalize the definition of learning disabilities and how to specify the exclusionary terms. This debate has immense pragmatic, as well as theoretical importance (Eisenberg, 1978; Wong, 1986). Levels of funding and access to federally mandated special education classes depend on these definitions. The specific definition embodied in state educational regulations determines which children meet the criteria of learning disability and hence eligibility for special educational assistance.

A frequent criticism of the current federal definition of learning disabilities is that the exclusionary criteria may deny services to children who, in addition to specific learning disabilities, may also suffer from sociocultural disadvantage, emotional disturbance, or mental retardation (Eisenberg, 1978). Consequently, the federal Interagency Committee on Learning Disabilities (1987) has proposed the following new definition:

Learning disabilities is a generic term that refers to a heterogeneous group of disorders manifested by significant difficulties in the acquisition and use of listening, speaking, reading, writing, reasoning, or mathematical abilities, *or of social skills.* These disorders are intrinsic to the individual and presumed to be due to central nervous *system* dysfunction. Even though a learning disability may occur concomitantly with other handicapping conditions (e.g., sensory impairment, mental retardation, social and emotional disturbance), *with so-*cioenvironmental influences (e.g., cultural differences, insufficient or inappropriate instruction, psychogenic factors), *and especially with attention deficit disorder, all of which may cause learning problems, a learning disability* is not the direct result of those conditions or influences. (p. 222)

PREVALENCE AND EPIDEMIOLOGY

The definitions of the disorders will heavily influence any estimate of the prevalence of learning problems. In one instance, a study of *general* reading retardation revealed that 28% of all the public school sixth graders in Baltimore were 2 or more years below grade level (Eisenberg, 1978). According to U.S. Department of Education (1987) data, during the 1985–1986 school year 4.7% of all students were classified as learning disabled. The Centers for Disease Control, however, estimate that the true prevalence is even higher, perhaps 5%–10% of all school-age children (Interagency Committee on Learning Disabilities, 1987).

Difficulties with concentration, short-term memory, or sequential processing may interfere with the learning-disabled child's ability to participate successfully in complex latency-age games and play. Poor motor coordination may impair the child's athletic proficiency and enjoyment. Such children also have difficulty understanding the nuances of language, such as humor or irony, as well as the subtle pragmatics of conversation. As a result of these impairments, peers may ostracize or tease the learning-disabled child. In response to these frequent rebuffs, the learning-disabled child may become depressed, withdrawn, passive, suspicious, or hypochondriacal; a common maladaptive response is to adopt the role of the class clown (Silver, 1989).

Learning disorders show strong familial aggregation (Pennington, 1990). There is a higher prevalence of specific learning disabilities in the family members of learning-disabled children than in the general population, and identical twins show a high concordance rate for reading disabilities compared with fraternal twins (LaBuda and DeFries, 1990). In many cases, strong genetic factors appear to determine the appearance of these conditions. At the same time, environmental factors also have a powerful influence; the incidence of specific learning disabilities is higher in urban areas and in the later children of large families. A very careful British study of *specific* reading retardation (i.e., reading more than two standard deviations below the level predicted by both IQ and age) found the condition in as many as 10% of schoolchildren in urban London, but only 4% on the more rural Isle of Wight (Berger et al., 1975). These findings, which indicate that the environment evidently played a large role in the reading retardation, emphasize the influence of nongenetic factors.

Specific learning disorders are common after serious head injury and, even where intelligence is normal, in cerebral palsy (Yule & Rutter, 1985). General learning problems, like mental retardation, are associated with low birth weights, prematurity, or perinatal difficulties (including maternal smoking and heavy alcohol use) (Nichols & Chen, 1981; Shaywitz et al., 1980); it is less clear, however, to what extent *specific* learning disabilities are related to such difficulties. As will be discussed later, there is a high association of specific learning disabilities with attentional deficits and conduct disorder.

CLINICAL FEATURES

The decision that specific learning disabilities exist is usually arrived at by exclusion. Their assessment represents an attempt to eliminate environmental and experiential factors and to focus diagnostic attention on hypothesized intrinsic deficit factors within the child. It seems very likely that none of the specific learning disorders, such as developmental reading disorder, represent a single unitary condition; rather they are groups of disabilities with differing but related clinical features and etiology (Smith et al., 1990). Not enough is known about learning disabilities to have a causally based typology (such as is developing with the subtypes of genetically based mental retardation). At present, the best clinicians can do is to attempt to formulate a provisional descriptive typology by reviewing the child's functional strengths and weaknesses. This requires evaluating the various academic skill areas and assessing the child's perceptual motor, attention, mnemonic, and linguistic capacities.

Specific Reading Disorder

Reading is an extremely complex motor, perceptual, cognitive, and linguistic process. To read, the child must have an array of skills that are properly meshed and integrated with each other. Several basic language-processing skills are essential to would-be readers including ability to distinguish phonemes; adequate short-term language memory; ability to discern the syntactic structure of phrases and sentences; and understanding of the semantic meaning of words and sentences (Mann, 1986). Beyond these prerequisites, a reader must learn how to transform letters into sounds;

more technically, he must learn the phonological rules for translating lexical ("letter") representations into phonetic ("sound") representations. This skill, in turn, entails the following capacities:

1. Accurate perception of the shape, orientation, and sequence of letters.
2. Sufficient short-term memory to retain their visual content.
3. Ability to make accurate associations between letter groups (graphemes) and their phonetic equivalents (phonemes).
4. Memory for word length, outline, and complex letter configurations that do not fit general phonetic rules.
5. Ability to synthesize sound sequences into words.
6. Translation of spatially arranged sequences of words into syntactically and semantically meaningful sentences and, if reading aloud, into accurately vocalized and inflected sound sequences.

Reading failure can occur at any one (or more) of these processes or levels of integration.

The fluent adult reader, like a competent adult driver, performs and integrates a large number of complex tasks quite automatically; characteristically, the adult seldom remembers how difficult it was to learn to read. To carry the analogy further, the dyslexic child may be likened to the novice driver of a poorly responsive car. He is just learning to shift and to steer; at the same time he is unsure about what the traffic rules are, which side of the road to drive on, where he is going, and which roads will take him there. Add to this pressured state of mind a high level of anxiety over the glowering gaze of the traffic cop and the honking of the other drivers, and you have a general picture of the classroom experience of a severely dyslexic child.

Subtypes of Dyslexia

The criteria for developmental reading disorder do not define a unitary condition, but speak rather for a heterogeneous group of disorders. There is much debate about the most useful ways to define subtypes of reading disorders (McKinney, 1984; Senf, 1986; Smith et al., 1990). One approach is to classify dyslexics according to their apparent pattern of ability deficits. The works of Mattis (1978), Denckla (1972, 1978), Rourke and Strang (1983), and Spreen and Haaf (1986) suggest such a schema; their approach distinguishes visual-spatial, audio-phonological, and language disorder subtypes.

According to this schema, some children show a *visual-spatial type reading disability,* evidenced by reversals of letters (p-q, d-b) and words ("dog" for "god," "saw for "was") and by failure to discriminate between words that are similar in shape. These children tend to show a higher incidence of right–left confusion on body-schema tasks (such as an inability to carry out commands like "put your left hand on my right elbow") and may have mixed or incomplete laterality as indicated by hand preference. Such children may have poor visual memory of how a printed word looks (i.e., its sequential structure) beyond a crude notion of its length and outline. As a result, these youngsters are often poor spellers, especially concerning idiosyncratic aspects of spelling (e.g., double or silent consonants) that are less susceptible to phonetic analysis. However, as noted below, these same children often have excellent visual skills regarding holistic perception of spatial configurations. Their weakness is in the relatively specific area of sequencing and verbal association to visual stimuli.

According to the schemata of Denckla (1978) and Mattis (1978), another group of children have a more frequent kind of reading problem—*audiophonological type reading disability*. These children have difficulty deciphering words through phonetic analysis. The errors that dog these children's learning efforts (e.g., "evaporates" for "evacuates," "the Merchant Mary" for "the Virgin Mary") consist of phonemic substitutions and missequencing of phonemes within words, both when reading and when naming or repeating. Some of the children have problems in handwriting and mild disturbances in articulation, whereas others do not. Although these youngsters have no gross defects in their oral language comprehension, they have a "tin ear for language"; when stressed by rapid, lengthy, syntactically complicated speech, they may show subtle aural comprehension problems.

Yet a third group, which perhaps contains the largest number of dyslexic children, displays a more general *language disorder*. In addition to their reading problems, these youngsters suffer from (1) mild to severe dysnomia (an inability to name) on oral naming tasks, (2) diminished comprehension of complex spoken speech, and (3) poor discrimination of speech sounds. Language acquisition may have been slow for these language-disordered dyslexics, and, unlike the first two groups, their verbal IQs tend to be markedly impaired relative to their performance IQs. Outside of the verbal realm, the motoric, visual-spatial, and abstract conceptual abilities of these children are generally normal.

Developmental Dysgraphia

Poor spelling and reading usually accompany each other, at least in young children. As they grow older, dyslexic children with audiophonetic processing problems at times can compensate adequately for their reading deficit through growth in visual recognition skills but they still have difficulty in spelling. In addition to combined reading and spelling disorders, "specific spelling retardation" exists; that is, some children have serious spelling difficulties in the face of average or above-average reading ability (Frith, 1983).

Nondyslexic Learning Disabilities

Researchers have studied or defined skill areas other than reading much less intensively. Difficulties in some school areas, such as a lack of gymnastic or art skills, or the presence of tone deafness in music, are not even considered learning disabilities although much could be learned by studying them as such. The *nondyslexic* learning-disabled children, such as those with arithmetic problems, generally show more impairment in their spatial and sequential-configurational skills than in their language skills. On the WISC-R, they often show a lower performance IQ than verbal IQ score, whereas many of the dyslexic children show the reverse. The nondyslexics do poorly on constructional tasks such as puzzles and models; in addition, they are often clumsy, with a poor sense of direction and a history of slow motor milestones. Finally, these children may have subtle problems in understanding the metaphorical aspects of language and in developing flexible cognitive strategies.

Developmental Arithmetic Disorder (Dyscalculia)

Solving mathematical problems involves a complex chain of processes. Dyscalculia can occur because of failure at one (or more) of the links in this chain. Thus, defects in logic, organization, or procedural skills may be present, individually or in combination. Moreover, they can be independent of or associated with defects in simple calculation skills. Some of these processes are related to the same information-processing skills that are vulnerable in dyslexia; others depend more on spatial organizational skills.

Assessment

Children with learning problems require a careful developmental history and a thorough psychological study, as well as a skillful examination for developmental neurological defects. It is particularly important that testing be conducted by a psychologist (preferably one trained in neuropsychology) or special educator experienced in educational assessment. Hearing and vision should be tested to rule out gross deficits. The clinician should obtain and review school records and should gather a report on the child's school performance directly from the child's teachers.

In taking the history, the diagnostician should ask about perinatal problems, delayed motor or speech milestones, attentional problems, serious illnesses, and evidence of seizures or "absence" spells. Family background should be reviewed for a history of learning problems and for sources of possible emotional stress that may be impinging on the child. How the family views the child's school problems and what sort of emphasis the family places on academic achievement should be explored. Structured parent questionnaires, such as the Yale Children's Inventory (YCI) (Shaywitz et al., 1986, 1988) are useful in obtaining comprehensive, well-standardized information.

Direct examination of the child should assess the child's general level of emotional functioning and determine whether there is evidence of concomitant depression, conduct disorder, attentional deficit, or situational reaction problems. Hand, eye, foot preference should be noted. It is valuable to master the skill of examining for neurological soft signs, such as overflow, choreiform movements, and difficulty with rapid alternating movements. The diagnostician can conduct many simple tests of motor and perceptual coordination in a gamelike way and can easily incorporate them into the general child psychiatric or pediatric exam (Touwen & Prechtl, 1970).

In general, EEG or CT scan are not indicated unless there is evidence of seizure disorder or focal neurological disease.

Psychological testing should include well-standardized tests of cognitive abilities such as the Wechsler Intelligence Scale for Children-Revised (WISC-R) and/or the Kaufman Assessment Battery for Children (K-ABC), as well as a detailed evaluation of academic skills and achievement. Although it is important to see how well a child scores quantitatively on standard administration of these latter tests, it is equally necessary to analyze the types of errors and to assess the child's best level of functioning under optimal conditions (e.g., without time limit). Tests of reading ability should include not only single word recognition, but also reading aloud and silently and then checking for comprehension. In addition, detailed evaluation of the child's expressive and receptive language abilities, auditory skills, and visual-motor-spatial skills may be indicated.

Associated Disorders and Differential Diagnosis

Learning problems are often associated with attentional and emotional disorders (Gallico et al., 1987; McGee & Share, 1988; Thompson, 1986). As noted earlier, children with conduct disorder as well as children from urban settings and large families have an increased prevalence of both general and specific learning problems compared with their peers. At present it is unclear to what extent these associations are causal or represent common underlying mechanisms (Duane, 1989; McGee et al., 1986; Yule & Rutter, 1985). In some cases learning difficulties might be the result of inattention, emotional disorder, or impulsive, antisocial behavior; in others, the frustrations, alienation, and lowered self-esteem associated with academic failure might produce inattentiveness, emotional difficulties, or antagonistic behavior (McGee & Share, 1988). In yet other cases, common constitutional or sociofamilial factors might produce both the learning disorder *and* the associated psychopathology. Any one of these factors impacts powerfully and substantially on the others. The oppositional child, who resists out of a basic negativistic stance, or the narcissistic child, who cannot tolerate imperfection or critique, will avoid learning and will develop a pattern of defensive reactions that can radically impede skill acquisition. If these patterns occur in a context of primary difficulty in reading, writing, or calculation, the problems will enhance and exacerbate each other. To determine which is primary and etiologic is no easy matter, but it is their interplay that is disastrous.

The exclusionary approach to defining learning disability is heuristically useful. Clinicians and policy planners must remember, however, that the frequent occurrence of the disorder makes it likely that it will also afflict many children who coincidentally are also attentionally impaired, emotionally disturbed, moderately retarded, or culturally disadvantaged. Whatever the underlying causal mechanisms of dyslexia, these doubly vulnerable children will have even greater difficulty than the pure dyslexic in finding and utilizing remedial help or otherwise compensating for their dyslexic problems.

Attention Deficit

Many children with specific learning disability show attention deficits (often with hyperactivity), and vice versa (Halperin et al., 1984; McGee & Share, 1988). The apparent frequency of this association originally led to the concept of minimal brain dysfunction (see Chapter 13).

In assessing an underachieving child, it may be difficult to disentangle the relationships among attention deficit, hyperactivity and specific learning disorder. Teachers often describe children with specific learning disabilities as "daydreamers." It is important to determine whether the child's poor attention span is observable *both* at school and at home (in which case the diagnosis of attention-deficit hyperactivity disorder should be considered), or whether it occurs primarily in the classroom in connection with the child's cognitively weak subject areas. A dyslexic child in a regular reading class is not unlike someone watching a foreign language movie without subtitles; it is difficult for him to keep his attention from wandering. On the other hand, even in the absence of specific learning disorder, an attention-deficit hyperactivity disorder can cause learning failure. Within the classroom, the inattentiveness and restlessness of children with ADHD will vary more with the degree of structure and supervision than with the specific content area being taught. Children who suffer from a specific learning disorder *and* an attention-deficit hyperactivity disorder are impaired both in their participation in remedial programs and in their capacity to develop compensatory skills; they are thus doubly handicapped.

Although researchers often postulate common underlying constitutional or neurological factors, it is not yet clear why learning disabilities are so often associated with ADHD (Ackerman et al., 1986; Duane, 1989; Krupski, 1986; McGee & Share, 1988) and how children with pure dyslexia differ from those with dyslexia *plus* ADHD. The presence of a concomitant attention-deficit hyperactivity disorder greatly influences the likelihood of referral for special education (Sandoval & Lambert, 1984).

Conduct Disorder

Children with specific learning disorder often show conduct problems. In one epidemiological study, as many as one-third of children with specific reading retardation had conduct disorders, whereas one-third of children with conduct disorder had specific reading retardation (Rutter et al., 1970). Among serious delinquents, both general academic failure and specific reading disability are extremely common (Lewis et al., 1980). Here again, it is often difficult to establish a clear causal picture. Repeated frustration and failure in school due to learning disability readily lead to low self-esteem, anger, and a sense of resentment and isolation from school and society. Add to this an unempathic and chaotic family setting, and the resulting admixture may easily predispose a child to delinquency. In one sense the bad behavior may represent the youngster's effort to gain status and worth he lacks at school. On the other hand, the internal chaos and external disruptiveness of the conduct-disordered child make him less available for learning and classroom participation.

Emotional Problems

Learning-disabled children frequently show low self-esteem, discouragement, depression, and other emotional problems (Gallico et al., 1987). Cause and effect may be difficult to distinguish. School failure from any cause is usually extremely painful; such a youngster feels set apart, "dumb," or "crazy," and is likely to experience ridicule from peers (Simpson, 1979). As a result, learning disabilities often have a severe impact on the developing character of the school-age child and adolescent. Erikson (1950) considers the school years crucial for consolidating a sense of industry. This factor is a key element of identity formation, essential to the child's confidence in his capacity for worthwhile work; without it, he is left with a haunting feeling of personal and social inferiority. Unfortunately, the identity of learning-disabled children is too often organized around a sense of themselves as being inadequate, incompetent, and unskilled (Pickar, 1986). Such a child may become depressed or develop a total aversion to going to school. A careful investigation can usually identify the school-related aspects of the child's emotional reaction, which differs in character from the more general separation problems of the anxious child with a school phobia.

The implications of these children's neuropsychological vulnerabilities can extend far beyond the academic sphere (Glosser & Koppell, 1987; Pearl et al., 1986; Silver, 1989). The administrative process by which schools classify students as learning disabled is influenced by factors unrelated to children's ability and achievement. This selection bias may account for the strong preponderance of boys reported in clinic- and school-based samples of learning-disabled children. For example, an epidemiological survey of second- and third-grade students found that 8.7% to 9.0% of boys and 6.0% to 6.9% of girls met research criteria for reading disability. Among the same group of children, however, the school system had identified as learning disabled 10% to 13.6% of the boys but only 3.2% to 4.2% of the girls. Overactivity and behavioral difficulties likely to disrupt the class heavily influenced which students teachers referred for evaluation and special educational placement; teachers rated more boys than girls as problematic despite comparable levels of overall ability and achievement (S. Shaywitz et al., 1990).

Some learning-disabled children may also have social difficulties and interactional problems with their peers that cannot be attributed solely to discouragement, low self-esteem, or stigmatization caused by their poor academic performance. These difficulties may stem from deficient nonverbal reasoning abilities as well as from difficulty in reading nonverbal social cues such as facial expression, gesture, and body posture (Denckla, 1983; Duane, 1989; Rourke & Strang, 1983); such youngsters have been described as suffering from a learning disability that involves the rules of ordinary social interaction (Denckla, personal communication, 1985).

Children with primary emotional problems are also in frequent difficulties at school because of poor motivation, preoccupation, or anxiety. Thus, seriously depressed, borderline, psychotic, obsessional, or school-phobic children may all do quite poorly in school and lag academically. The child with a primary emotional problem, however, is unlikely to show the learning-disabled child's uneven profile of cognitive strengths and weaknesses. In particular, if a previously higher level of academic functioning has subsequently deteriorated, the clinician should suspect a diagnosis other than specific learning disability. Such a situation should also raise the question of a higher level organizational difficulty that has become manifest only with the demands of more advanced grades (Levine & Zallen, 1985).

Neurological Disease

Even when the child is of normal intelligence, learning problems often accompany such frank neurological disease as epilepsy, cerebral palsy, and head injuries (Yule & Rutter, 1985). Although these learning problems may be general, the affected children may show considerable unevenness in their academic functioning, with one cognitive area, such as reading, particularly affected.

Some experts would, by definition, exclude mentally retarded children from the ranks of the learning disabled. Indeed the definition of learning disabilities embodied in the federal special education statute P.L. 94-142 has often been so interpreted. However, many mentally retarded children have difficulties in reading (or in other academic skills) beyond that predicted by their general IQ; unfortunately these twice-burdened children may be arbitrarily denied needed remedial services.

If a child who is having trouble at school has a history of staring or "absence" spells, a seizure disorder such as petit mal or temporal lobe epilepsy should be considered. A history of acute onset of learning disorder with a progressively worsening course mandates a careful neurological evaluation to rule out a toxic, traumatic, infectious, or neoplastic process or a progressive degenerative disorder (Kandt, 1984). Severe headaches should always be carefully investigated. They may be erroneously attributed to tension, and the diagnostician will miss the rare progressive lesions, such as recurrent bleeds from a vascular malformation involving the temporal lobe speech areas (a finding that has been reported in dyslexics) (Geschwind & Galaburda, 1985).

ETIOLOGY

The causes of learning disabilities remain obscure. Indeed, clinical ignorance is encyclopedic. Methodological and definitional problems abound (Keogh, 1986; Swanson, 1988). The current inability to delineate homogeneous groups of children whose distinctive deficits can be adequately specified hampers research (Senf, 1986; Stanovich, 1986). There is also intense debate about which task performance measures are most relevant to identifying presumed underlying cognitive deficits and how to distinguish the manifestations of such presumed intrinsic deficits from the effects of poor instruction, discouragement, or academic learned helplessness.

It is often presumed that the learning disabilities reflect some neurologically based cognitive dysfunction, most likely constitutional in nature. Given the evident heterogeneity of children diagnosed with learning disabilities, however, it seems likely that no single mechanism is at work in all of them. Researchers are only just beginning to learn which elementary operations form the bases of human cognitive activities, how these elementary operations are localized and organized in the brain, and what biological factors can lead to their disruption (Posner et al., 1988). Furthermore, whatever biological determinants may exist, many socioenvironmental variables (both interactional and instructional) powerfully influence the development and expression of learning disabilities (Berger et al., 1975; Stanovich, 1988).

Even on a descriptive level, the learning-disabled child's functional deficits have given rise to controversy (Mann, 1986; Stanovich, 1986). Consider the example of dyslexia. For many years, the dominant theories suggested that deficits in visual processing (such as scanning or faulty visual sequencing) were basic to dyslexia. Other theories suggested that deficiencies in short-term memory or cross-modal integration of visual and auditory information were to blame. In recent years, however, the consensus has grown that dyslexia reflects deficits in basic linguistic capacities rather than deficits in nonlinguistic cognitive-perceptual processes.

In support of this view, Vellutino (1987) found that, compared with normal children, dyslexics do not appear to have difficulty scanning and recalling visual sequences. Dyslexics seemed unimpaired on tests involving matching or recalling complex wordlike sequences of visual symbols that had no verbal or phonetic meaning. However, when the task involved symbols that had verbal significance (i.e., were associated with phonemes or words), the dyslexics did much more poorly. Similarly, Vellutino (1987) found dyslexics had difficulty with associative and rule-learning tasks "only when the tasks required them to store and retrieve the auditory representation of words and syllables" (p. 39). Other studies similarly suggest that dyslexics' auditory perception and short-term memory for nonlinguistic material are also largely intact.

Poor readers appear to suffer from difficulties in spoken-language processing and lack of phonological sophistication (Mann, 1986). Using a timed naming task, Denckla and Rudel (1976) found that dyslexics were slower and less accurate than normal controls in naming not only letters, words, and numbers, but also common objects and colors. Poor readers also have difficulty in clearly discerning and recalling the phonemic sequences that make up words (Mann, 1986). These defects in phonetic perception and storage are apparent in spoken-language processing as well as reading.

Genetic Factors

During the past 80 years, the tendency for reading disabilities to run in families has been noted repeatedly (Pennington, 1990). Twin studies show a much higher rate of concordance for dyslexia between monozygotic twins than between dyzygotic twins; these data suggest a substantial genetic component in many reading disorders (LaBuda & DeFries, 1990). Large family studies, although confirming the familial nature of many cases of dyslexia, suggest that reading disability is a genetically heterogeneous disorder (DeFries et al., 1978; Lewitter et al., 1980; Smith et al., 1990). In one group of learning disability pedigrees, linkage studies point to an autosomal dominant gene on chromosome 15 (Smith et al., 1983; 1990). The complexity of the reading process raises the question of what is the heritable core deficit in familial dyslexia. New sophisticated genetic analytic techniques permit closer study of the "phenotypic core" of this disorder. For example, there is evidence that phonologic coding skills have a strong heritable component (Pennington, 1990; Smith et al., 1990).

Neurobiological Factors

Position emission tomography (PET) scan investigations have shed light on the localization of linguistic operations in the human brain and promise to advance understanding of the basic neurophysiology of reading (Posner et al., 1988). Researchers have hypothesized that the processing of individual words involves separate internal codes related to the visual, phonological, articulatory, and semantic analysis and representation of the word. Although understanding the word involves operations on all these levels, certain tasks selectively involve some codes more than others. According to this theory, for example, matching words by rhyme involves the phonological representations of the words, whereas rotating a letter to an upright position utilizes the visual code. PET data suggest the involvement of distinct neural systems in these diverse operations and suggest how and where these systems are localized.

A recurrent speculation suggests that dyslexia is linked to abnormalities in cerebral organization and lateralization (Annett & Manning, 1989; Duane, 1989). From early in fetal development the human brain shows anatomical and physiological asymmetries between its left and right sides. The cerebral hemispheres appear to be functionally specialized as well. The left hemisphere is usually dominant for language and motor skills whereas the right hemisphere is usually more involved in certain spatial and musical abilities (Geschwind & Galaburda, 1985). Unfortunately, many of the complex issues concerning the functional differentiation of the cerebral hemispheres have been oversimplified into grand dichotomies and sweeping generalizations about right- and left-brain styles of thinking.

Both during embryogenesis and postnatally, many factors influence anatomic and functional lateralization including genetic endowment and gender-related factors such as the degree of androgen activity and sensitivity. Gender-related factors are reflected in the finding that, on the average, adult women are superior in verbal skills whereas men tend to excel in spatial skills; however, these sex differences do not become fully manifest until puberty (Benbrow & Stanley, 1980; Feingold, 1988; Maccoby & Jacklin, 1974; Wittig & Petersen, 1979). Individuals with sex chromosome anomalies may have marked learning disabilities despite average intelligence. For example, girls with Turner's syndrome (XO) lack the usual second X chromosome; in addition to ovarian dysgenesis and lack of pubertal development, these girls show a specific disability in tasks requiring spatial perception and organization (Silbert et al., 1977). Early brain damage may also lead to anomalous cerebral organization with consequent cognitive deficits and an altered pattern of lateralization.

The relationship between handedness and the functional or structural specialization of the cerebral hemispheres is complex. Almost all right-handed individuals have left cerebral dominance for language; however, about two-thirds of left-handers also have left hemispheric language representation, whereas the remaining one-third have right or bilateral hemispheric language representation (Geschwind & Galaburda, 1985).

Several studies have suggested that compared with normal controls, children and adults with dyslexia (or other learning disabilities) are more likely to lack full right-handedness (Geschwind & Galaburda, 1985; Hiscock & Kinsbourne, 1987). (Interestingly, non–right-handedness may also be overrepresented in gifted individuals with high mathematical or visual-spatial abilities.) Non–right-handedness in itself does not cause dyslexia; rather it is likely to be a marker of altered cerebral organization and dominance. The altered lateralization and cognitive deficits in many learning-disabled patients who are non–right-handed may be the result of early brain damage or some other abnormality that disturbs cerebral organization during fetal development.

Many theories have attempted to explain how alterations in cerebral specialization might cause learning disabilities as well as the superior mathematical or visual-spatial skills of some left-handed individuals. One ambitious theory attempts to link increased prenatal testosterone activity both to delays in left hemisphere development and to alteration in immune functioning (Geschwind & Galaburda, 1985). However, pending further research, such theories remain highly speculative.

Direct evidence of structural and neurophysiological abnormalities in dyslexics is tentative but provocative (Duane, 1989). Postmortem neuropathological studies of a small number of dyslexics' brains have revealed abnormalities in the neuronal organization of the cortex and connected subcortical structures; these cortical anomalies were noted predominantly in the left hemisphere and appeared to reflect abnormalities in the embryonic organization of the brain. In addition, the usual asymmetry between the right and left posterior brain regions was absent (Galaburda et al., 1985).

In vivo imaging techniques also suggest anatomical and neurophysiological abnormalities in dyslexics. Computed tomographic and magnetic resonance imaging studies have reported that dyslexics lack the normal asymmetry of the posterior brain regions (Denckla et al., 1985; Rosenberger & Hier, 1980; Rumsey et al., 1986). New noninvasive techniques such as positron emission tomography, cerebral blood flow mapping, event-related potential, and quantitative EEG mapping have also been brought to bear on the problem (Duane, 1989; Lou et al., 1990). These provide data on dyslexics' brain functioning not only at rest but, more relevantly, during reading or other cognitive processing tasks. Although these studies have involved small groups of disparately defined dyslexics tested under differing conditions, they collectively point to significant differences between the brain processes of dyslexics and normal controls. These studies suggest that dyslexics show (1) alterations in the activity of the left parietal, midtemporal, and lateral frontal cortical regions and (2) a relative reduction in the frontal activation normally seen during attention-demanding tasks (Conners, 1987; Duffy et al., 1980; Rumsey et al., 1987).

TREATMENT

Children with learning disabilities need highly individualized special education based on a careful, ongoing assessment of the child's strengths and weaknesses (Lerner, 1989).

Unfortunately, there is little reliable systematic research to inform practitioners about the most effective remedial techniques for specific deficits (Gittleman, 1983, 1985). It is possible to outline broadly the required strategies. First, it is necessary to build on the child's existing strengths. In particular, individualized help must target the child's strongest perceptual and cognitive channels, helping him to utilize more than one sensory modality. A child who is weak in phonemic analysis may profit from learning phonemic units that are presented visually on flash cards. Similarly, in kinesthetic drill work the child traces out the morphemic units with his hand while sounding them aloud; this approach provides multisensory feedback for learning. Children can master rules and generalizations governing sound–symbol equivalents, and teachers can help them to utilize the intact areas of their intellect by learning contextual and semantic clues to a word's identity. Success and progress in areas of intact strength can help to maintain the vulnerable self-esteem of the learning-disabled child.

At the same time, carefully titrated remedial work must continue in the area of the child's deficits (e.g., auditory synthesis and sequencing) by using direct drill and linking weak skills to strong ones.

The various theories concerning the nature of the underlying deficit in dyslexia have given rise to corresponding remedial strategies. Visual-scanning, perceptual-motor, and motor dominance theories, for example, have led to oculomotor training, perceptual-motor remediation, and motor patterning exercises (Smith, 1986). Unfortunately, there is little evidence that skill training in these areas has had any appreciable carryover effect on reading performance. The current consensus is that there is no substitute for intensive instruction in reading itself (Gittleman, 1983). However, much remains to be learned about the relative merits of different strategies for teaching reading (e.g., the phonetic decoding method versus a whole word recognition approach). At present, there is no schema for subtyping dyslexia that would allow diagnostic selectivity of the appropriate remedial method.

Some children retain their reading deficits well into adult life; nonetheless they are able to use their often-superior skills in other areas such as spatial configuration for both pleasure and professional accomplishment. A history of childhood dyslexia is present in a striking number of successful artists and craftsmen. Other dyslexic children may remain weak in oral reading, but once they reach a "take-off" level of competency in word recognition, they utilize their general semantic and comprehension skills to become good silent readers. The notion that all dyslexics suffer from globally deficient language skills is belied by the presence in their ranks of eminent writers (e.g., Flaubert, Yeats, Hans Christian Andersen) and articulate politicians (e.g., Woodrow Wilson, Nelson Rockefeller) (Simpson, 1979).

Where an attention deficit disorder accompanies learning disabilities stimulant medication may improve attention span and handwriting. Such medication, however, appears to have little effect on the specific learning disabilities themselves.

Recent research suggests that piracetam (an analogue of the neurotransmitter gamma-aminobutyric acid (GABA)) has positive effects on dyslexics' reading accuracy and comprehension. In addition, EEG studies of visual evoked potentials indicate that piracetam may facilitate the information processing of visual linguistic stimuli, especially in the left parietal region of the cortex (Conners & Reader, 1987). More research is needed to confirm and expand these findings.

As with attention deficit disorders (see Chapter 13), there is little evidence that megavitamins, mineral supplements, or additive-free diets have a beneficial effect on learning disabilities.

The clinician must provide ongoing support and counseling to the family and serve as an active advocate for the learning-disabled child in dealing with the school system.

Parents often require considerable assistance in helping their child obtain the remedial instruction to which they are entitled under the federal Education for All Handicapped Children Act (P.L. 94-142 (1975)). The appropriate special education intervention depends on the degree and nature of the child's learning disability, as well as on the level of concomitant social, emotional, and attentional difficulties. For some children, regular tutoring at home by parents or by a competent tutor may bridge the learning gap. For others, a regular classroom placement with daily supplemental sessions of remedial help (either in class or in a "resource room") are sufficient. Finally, there are children whose educational needs require nothing less than a self-contained classroom or school.

When emotional and social difficulties are prominent, individual, group, or family psychotherapy may be indicated (Silver, 1989). Disorganization, low self-esteem, emotional lability, and poor interpersonal skills often make learning-disabled children as challenging to their families as they are to their teachers. Sibling rivalry is often intense; the learning-disabled child must frequently endure the humiliation of being surpassed in school achievement and popularity by a younger brother or sister.

In addition to much practical assistance in managing, caring, and planning for their learning-disabled child, parents need help to deal adaptively with the disappointment, anger, and guilt their child's difficulties expectably stir in them.

Helping the parent and child to maintain their self-esteem and sense of efficacy is one of the major goals and challenges of treatment. The development of hobbies, talents, and lesiure activities in which the child can experience a sense of competency and camaraderie helps to combat the pervasive sense of isolation and failure these youngsters too often experience. In adolescence, help in vocational planning and the encouragement of skills for independence are especially important (Schumaker et al., 1986).

At one time learning disabilities were a stigma that children and their families often suffered in isolation, believing themselves to be unique in their failings. Although these disorders remain a painful burden, support is now more widely available in parent and advocacy groups such as the Association for Children and Adults with Learning Disabilities, the Council for Learning Disabilities, the Council for Exceptional Children, and Parents of Gifted/Learning Disabled Children. Clinicians should strongly encourage parents to seek out and join such self-help groups. A variety of popular books are also available for the parents of learning-disabled children. Among the best are the books by Silver (1984) and Smith (1980). Eileen Simpson's (1979) *Reversals* is a moving and perceptive account of her struggles with dyslexia, undiagnosed until young adulthood.

Chapter 13

Conduct Disorder

INTRODUCTION

A striking phenomenon of our day is that delinquency and aggressive behavior, despite their ubiquity, remain theoretically elusive, poorly understood, and inadequately managed. Where understanding is absent, theories rush in to fill the vacuum, and there are, indeed, many theories. This chapter, in surveying some of the more important contributions to the field, attempts to distinguish merely ingenious and interesting ideas from theories that show some promise of becoming functionally relevant.

THE NATURE OF CONDUCT DISORDER

Conduct disorder is really action that violates a code. The code may be formal (in the legal sense) or informal; it may be familial, academic, or subcultural; whatever its character, the quality that distinguishes—and defines—conduct disorder is that there is an act of transgression. Loeber and Schmaling (1985, p. 338) quote a somewhat more behavioral version of this principle: "recurrent violation of socially prescribed patterns of behavior" (Simcha-Fagin et al., 1975).

DIAGNOSIS

The definition of this condition has long been problematic. Investigators have resorted to various clustering tactics, and one set of terms has succeeded another only to be replaced by yet another. Many investigators in the field prefer to create their own language, particularly if they are studying a special segment of the conduct disorders. Thus, when Wooden and Berkey (Wooden & Berkey, 1984) evaluated a large population of children who set fires, they called their groupings:

1. The *Playing-with-Matches* children.
2. The *Crying-for-Help* children.
3. The *Delinquent* children.
4. The *Seriously-Disturbed* children.

Again, when Offer et al. (1979) carried out their very sophisticated demographic study on a sizable population of delinquents with nonorganic disorders, their categories of classification were:

1. The impulsive delinquent.
2. The depressed borderline.

3. The empty borderline.
4. The narcissistic delinquent.

Quay arrived at yet another influential categorization by culling three clusters from the factor analysis of a population of institutionalized delinquent boys (Quay, 1964, cited in Achenbach, 1982). One group was called *socialized-subcultural* delinquency; the second, *unsocialized-psychopathic* delinquency; and the third, *disturbed-neurotic* delinquency. In contrast to this approach, if diagnosticians can be classified as either "splitters" or "lumpers," surely the ultimate lumpers are Yochelson and Samenow (1976, 1977; Samenow, 1986) who utilize a single classification: youngsters with a criminal mind.

Two additional problems merit mention. For one, conduct disorder is an omnibus term that embraces a great many diverse forms of action. Everything from operating a con game to committing armed robbery falls within its scope, so its symptomatology is protean, multiform, and complex (see Appendix 13-1). Another problem is that the appearance of conduct disorder may completely mask or represent some other condition. Depressive states, adjustment disorders, anxiety states, organic mental disorders, certain varieties of psychotic reactions, borderline conditions, certain compulsive disorders, and other psychiatric conditions can all find expression in disturbances of conduct. Hence, clinicians are often uncertain whether they are dealing with conduct disorder or with an expression of a different underlying condition.

DSM-III Diagnostic Categories

In the diagnostic language of DSM III (APA, 1980), the condition of Conduct Disorder was originally divided according to the degrees of aggression (the patient is either aggressive or nonaggressive), and the degrees of socialization (either socialized or undersocialized). A given youngster could thus fit into any of four subcategories—socialized aggressive, undersocialized nonaggressive, socialized nonaggressive, or undersocialized aggressive—depending on how well he met the criteria for that particular designation. Clinicians have now had enough experience with this approach to suggest that some of these clusters work, whereas others do not.

Metaanalysis

Recent years have seen a more empirical approach to developing subcategories of conduct disorder. The most extensive diagnostic exploration so far has chosen as its subjects not a population of delinquents but a population of populations. It is a metaanalysis of 28 studies (culled from 22 papers) involving antisocial behavior. This work by Loeber and Schmaling (1985) reviews data arising from 11,603 children. Because the analysis is, by far, the most wide-ranging undertaking of its kind, the findings are especially interesting.

The authors developed a list of 34 antisocial behaviors and then, by factor analysis, explored how these symptoms distributed themselves among the children in the various studies. Correlational matrices and ratios were developed to state the probability of one given behavior appearing with another, and at length, a one-dimensional solution emerged as the simplest and most powerful expression of their findings. At one end of this dimension were clustered the covert antisocial behaviors, and at the other end, the overt. The authors' account of the actual items is as follows:

> One end of the dimension was anchored by [such items as] alcohol and/or drug use, truant, in a gang, runs away, has bad companions, steals, and sets fires.... The other end of the dimension ... was anchored by hyperactive, screams, moody, stubborn, demanding, teases, poor peer relations, argues, impulsive, sulks, jealous, attacks people, temper tantrums, threats, loud or rowdy, fighting or aggressiveness, cruel, irritable, shows off, brags and boasts, swears, blames others, and sassy. (p. 346)

The overtness of behavior refers to the likelihood of its being enacted in the presence of observing adult authority figures such as parents or teachers. Although some adults became aware of covert behavior, they usually did so after the fact, typically because of dealing with the youngsters' lies, evasions, rationalizations, or justifications. Although the clustering was quite striking, a subgroup that included both overt and covert behaviors proved to be critically important because those youngsters who engaged in both aggressive assaults and covert depredations turned out to be the ones most likely to have confrontations with the police. Interestingly, the children displaying overt antisocial behaviors or an admixture of overt and covert elements were identifiable in the preschool years. Purely covert behavior was usually detected later in childhood, often not until late in latency.

In the distribution of these traits and behaviors along the great single dimension, midway between the two extremes was the item *disobedience*. It seemed to be a bridge, a shared quality linking both extremes. This finding suggests that disobedience is the key factor in both kinds of delinquent proclivity and tends to support the position advanced by Gerald Patterson (1982) that treatment must start precisely in the address to disobedience.

DSM-III-R Diagnostic Categories

The revised version of the DSM-III, the DSM-III-R (APA, 1987), is still too new to allow for adequate assessment of its utility or accuracy; before it was published, it had been tested in a nationwide survey; the categories that emerged reflect this experience. DSM-III-R includes several important conceptual changes from DSM-III. Conduct Disorder is now a subcategory within a larger, more embracing classification called Disruptive Behavior Disorders. The really new term is the word *disruptive*. Evidently it was selected to indicate that the primary character of the diagnoses under this rubric is the unpleasantness the patient generates for the people around him. Individuals with Disruptive Behavior Disorders are at best disturbing and, in many instances, may be intrusive, destructive, or, in some sense, antisocial. In any case, this larger category covers three formerly independent diagnoses: Attention-deficit Disorder with Hyperactivity, Conduct Disorder, and Oppositional Disorder, which are all now subsets of Disruptive Behavior Disorder. Moreover, there have been some changes in nomenclature as well; thus, the Attention-deficit Disorder with Hyperactivity has become Attention-deficit Hyperactivity Disorder (ADHD). Conduct Disorder is still designated as such in DSM-III-R although its subcategories have been changed, and Oppositional Disorder is now subsumed under Conduct Disorder and has been renamed Oppositional Defiant Disorder.

Because the Attention-deficit Hyperactivity Disorder is presented in Chapter 11, only the DSM-III-R descriptive material on the classification of the Conduct Behavior category and subcategories will be set forth here. Within the framework of DSM-III-R, the following material is culled from the larger category of Disruptive Behavior Disorders.

DSM-III-R Diagnostic Criteria for Conduct Disorder

A. *A disturbance of conduct lasting at least six months during which at least three of the following have been present:*
   (1) *has stolen without confrontation of a victim on more than one occasion (including forgery)*
   (2) *has run away from home at least twice while living in parental or parental surrogate home (or once without returning)*
   (3) *often lies (other than to avoid physical or sexual abuse)*
   (4) *has deliberately engaged in firesetting*
   (5) *is often truant from school (for older person, absent from work)*
   (6) *has broken into someone else's house, building, or car*
   (7) *has deliberately destroyed others' property (other than by firesetting)*
   (8) *has been physically cruel to animals*
   (9) *has forced someone into sexual activity with him or her*
   (10) *has used a weapon in more than one fight*
   (11) *often initiates physical fights*
   (12) *has stolen with confrontation of a victim (e.g., mugging, purse-snatching, extortion, armed robbery)*
   (13) *has been physically cruel to people*

Note: The above items are listed in descending order of discriminating power based on data from a national field trial of the DSM-III-R criteria for Disruptive Behavior Disorders. (APA, 1987, p. 55)

The DSM-III-R factors listed above group themselves along an axis that resembles Loeber and Schmaling's, with the more covert activities at one extreme and the overt transgressions at the other. Animal experiments also suggest that there are two quite different forms of aggression (designated by researchers as *affective* and *predatory* aggression). Evident biological differences distinguish the two, and the data are thus beginning to suggest that three typical forms of aggressive behavior characterize every careful schema, whether it is laboratory or clinical in nature. There is the *covert* or *predatory* form (Offer et al., 1979, call this group the *narcissistic delinquents;* Quay (1979) refers to them as the unsocialized psychopathic type); there is the *overt* or *active* form (Offer et al.'s *impulsive* delinquent; Quay's *socialized-subcultural* type), and there is the mixed group with characteristics of both the covert and overt forms (Offer et al.'s *depressed borderline* and *empty borderline* groups; Quay's *disturbed neurotic* delinquents).

DSM-III-R (APA, 1987) adds several subvarieties of Conduct Disorder that embrace a number of these characteristics. These are:

Solitary Aggressive Type
The essential feature is the predominance of aggressive physical behavior, usually toward both adults and peers, initiated by the person (not as a group activity). (p. 56)
Group Type
The essential feature is the predominance of conduct problems occurring mainly as a group activity with peers. Aggressive physical behavior may or may not be present. (p. 56)
Undifferentiated Type
This is a subtype for children or adolescents with Conduct Disorder with a mixture of clinical features that cannot be classified as either Solitary Aggressive Type or Group Type. (p. 56)

Criteria for Severity of Conduct Disorder
Mild: Few if any conduct problems in excess of those required to make the diagnosis, and conduct problems cause only minor harm to others.
Moderate: Number of conduct problems and effect on others intermediate between "mild" and "severe."
Severe: Many conduct problems in excess of those required to make the diagnosis, or conduct problems that cause considerable harm to others, e.g., serious physical injury to victims, extensive vandalism or theft, prolonged absence from home.

Within the larger province of the Disruptive Behavior Disorders, there is now included, as noted, Oppositional Defiant Disorder. The diagnostic criteria for this condition are as follows:

Oppositional Defiant Disorder
Note: Consider the criterion met only if the behavior is considerably more frequent than that of most people of the same mental age.

A. *A disturbance of at least six months during which at least five of the following are present:*
 (1) often loses temper
 (2) often argues with adults
 (3) often actively defies or refuses adult requests or rules, e.g., refuses to do chores at home
 (4) often deliberately does things that annoy other people, e.g., grabs other children's hats
 (5) often blames others for his or her own mistakes
 (6) is often touchy or easily annoyed by others
 (7) is often angry and resentful
 (8) is often spiteful and vindictive
 (9) often swears or uses obscene language (p. 56)
 Note: The above items are listed in descending order of discriminating power based on data from a national field trial of the DSM-III-R criteria for Disruptive Behavior Disorders.

B. *Does not meet the criteria for Conduct Disorder, and does not occur exclusively during the course of a psychotic disorder, dysthymia, or a major depressive, hypomanic, or manic episode.*

Criteria for Severity of Oppositional Defiant Disorder
Mild: Few, if any, symptoms in excess of those required to make the diagnosis and only minimal or no impairment in school and social functioning.
Moderate: Symptoms or functional impairment intermediate between "mild" and "severe."
Severe: Many symptoms in excess of those required to make the diagnosis and significant and pervasive impairment in functioning at home and school and with other adults and peers." (p. 57)

PREVALENCE

A number of epidemiological studies have attempted to assess how many young people are caught up in the disturbed and disturbing behavior patterns that define this diagnostic group. The very nature of the problem makes such an assessment difficult. Thus, I (JDN) was discussing this point with the director of an agency that for the most part serves inner-city children. I asked the director, "What percentage of the kids out there do you think are actually delinquent?" Without stopping to think, he answered confidently, "All of them!" As far as he was concerned, he was seeing only the children who got caught; he explained his view in this way: "A gang of kids are throwing stones at the streetlights and breaking the bulbs. A police car pulls up and the police get out, whereupon the gang members run off.

The police give chase and catch one or two children. They may have to face charges, but, in fact, all of the kids are guilty." From this view the statistics represent only those delinquents who are apprehended.

In DSM-III-R, however, the term *Conduct Disorder* is not designed for the occasional malefactor; it refers specifically to those youngsters who are in systematic difficulties on a more-or-less continuous basis for at least 6 months. Most clinicians would consider 6 months too short, because such a time span could suggest some sort of reactive condition—in the face of stress or trauma, the youngster has responded by acting aggressively. Clinicians who work in this realm are used to patients with histories that go back for years. Although this more extended view of the problem narrows the field somewhat, it still leaves many questions unanswered, such as, How bad is bad? And who decides? To pick a rather extreme example, for certain young men, group sex with a girl is just a robust and manly kind of fun; they may be genuinely surprised and profoundly chagrined when they presently face charges of gang rape. Their particular subculture and group ethos just did not define it that way.

Thus, another important variable is the role of subcultural factors. In the not-too-distant past the crime statistics did not reflect events within the black ghetto; those data simply were not recorded. People were wounded, people were killed, and no one took very much note; indifference to the plight of ghetto dwellers extended even to keeping records of the crimes that affected them. As cultural values changed, the statistics became more comprehensive. However, because a major sector of the low-socioeconomic-status (SES) population was now being reported and because low-SES children who become delinquent tend to prey on or lash out chiefly against the neighboring poor, it appeared that the situation had gotten much worse.

Yet another variable arises from shifting cultural values. As a society, we are far more sensitive to violence today than we were 100 years ago, or even 50 years ago. Child abuse was not even a crime 50 years ago, and what is today called *police brutality* was taken for granted as the natural way to manage criminals.

Yet another confusing factor, especially when diagnosing younger children, is the distinction between the pathological and the developmental norm. In effect, the prevalence of conduct disorder must be measured against the background of what normal children look like within given contexts. One sizable study based on teachers' reports gives a behavioral profile of normal children in school. In 1971 Werry and Quay surveyed a group of over 1700 youngsters in kindergarten, first grade, and second grade. These were mostly white, middle-class boys and girls. The distribution of reported behaviors for boys and girls, respectively, was as follows: disruptiveness—46.3% and 22.3%; disobedience—26.1% and 10.6%; fighting—31.3% and 6.2%; and hyperactivity—30.3% and 13.8%. This is quite a noisy background against which to measure conduct disorder. Some additional findings did not make things simpler: restlessness—49.7% and 27.8%; boisterousness—33.8% and 11.2%; and attention seeking—36.7% and 20.6% (quoted in Quay & Werry, 1986, p. 53).

As for adolescents, Cernkovich and Giordano asked the students at a large midwestern high school to fill out an anonymous questionnaire indicating the antisocial acts they had committed within a given time frame. The results, published in 1979, were illuminating. Thus, for boys and girls, respectively, the self-reported figures included the following: burglary of occupied residences—10% and 2%; burglary of unoccupied residences—17% and 4%; theft (less than $50.00)—34% and 26%; theft (more than $50.00)—13% and 5%; sexual intercourse (with opposite sex)—78% and 62%; sex for money—5% and 1%; carrying a weapon—34% and 17%; running away from home—16% for both sexes; use of hard drugs—15% and 19%; selling marijuana—35% and 20%; school probation/suspension/expulsion: 32% and 27%. Note again that these data were submitted by a nonclinical high school population (Cernkovich & Giordano, 1979, cited in Achenbach, 1982).

How then to speak meaningfully of prevalence? In fact, the relatively few substantial reports differ from one another in considerable degree. In their several studies, Rutter et al. (1975) found a prevalence rate of approximately 4% for conduct disorder; these figures arose within an essentially rural context. Using similar methodology, Graham (1979) arrived at a figure of 8% within an urban context (in each case this included both boys and girls). Quoting unpublished material by Glow, Quay and Werry added data from Australia showing that in a sizable survey, the overall rate of childhood disturbance was 12%, and the frequency of conduct disorder was 4% (Quay & Werry, 1986).

Offer, Ostrov, and Howard (1987) recently addressed the issue of prevalence among adolescents by approaching a population of high school students with a questionnaire that was designed to cull out psychiatrically disturbed students and to divide them into two categories: the quietly disturbed and the actively disturbed. To be in the quiet category meant that "by self-report had not received professional help more than once, had not been stopped or apprehended by the police, and had never committed any repetitive serious delinquent acts" (p. 85). Although the remaining active group could certainly have contained members who were disturbed in some fashion other than conduct disorder, the likelihood is that whatever else they may have manifested, there was a behavioral component as well.

The results of the study were as follows: 17% of all the boys and 22% of the girls were considered to be disturbed by the rather careful criteria of the study. Of these, 65% (of the 17%) of the boys and 38% (of the 22%) of the girls were actively disturbed. These figures yielded a conduct-disordered proportion of 11% for the boys and 8.4% for the girls. Because these data are based on the youngsters' self-report, the result is probably fairly accurate (Offer et al., 1987).

Some other figures may clarify the actual prevalence of the disorder. Of all the youths brought into court and adjudged to be delinquent, only 10% to 13% have engaged in violent behavior against persons, and of those, less than 5% will be involved in more than one such crime. All the others have been involved in offenses against property or against rules (Wolfgang, 1978).

Perhaps more relevant still is the informed opinion that of all the crimes actually committed, only 10% are detected and end up with indictments. Another relevant datum is that by age 20, 25% to 35% of all American youths have a court record for some sort of offense other than a traffic ticket. Perhaps the professional who said "All of them!" was not so far from the mark. And these statistics hold true not just for the impoverished inner city, but for society as a whole (Wolfgang, 1978).

COURSE

Because conduct disorder may indeed be a symptomatic expression of many other conditions, it is perhaps inappropriate to attempt to depict a particular course with which it is associated. Nonetheless, typical sequences of events have been described in at least a significant subgroup of those children who manifest the symptoms of this condition.

In considering the more general aspects of the condition, the work of Robins is of particular interest (Robins & Wish, 1977). Robins found a pattern common to many cases. It usually followed this sequence: Shortly after first entering school, the child would be repeatedly truant. Academic difficulties would follow, often culminating in school failure. Alcohol abuse would appear, accompanied or followed by sexual miscreance, typically in the form of promiscuity; then, in varying order, dropping out of school, drug abuse, and delinquency would follow. This account has important implications for both prevention and prognosis. At the same time, however, its overly general terms do little more than restate the forms of such deviance; it does not illuminate the underlying etiologic or temperamental factors that are so crucial to understanding a given case.

(To illustrate the richness of data available for the many subvarieties of the condition, Appendix 14.2 provides a detailed description of one subtype—firesetting. This material reviews the approaches of various investigators in attempting to explain this behavior. A similarly detailed exposition could be included for many other antisocial acts.)

Temperament

The long-term outcome report of the New York Longitudinal Study followed 133 subjects from early childhood. Of these, 45 were diagnosed as behaviorally disturbed and, for the most part, were called adjustment reactions. Two, however, were designated as conduct disorders, and in both instances, the onset of their symptomatology was observed between 3 and 5 years of age. The great bulk of the adjustment reactions were initially detected during that same interval (Thomas & Chess, 1984).

During early infancy it is difficult to determine clinically which children are likely to become behaviorally disordered. Although at the start of life the temperamentally "difficult child" poses problems for his caretaker, even he does not predictably go on to show symptoms of conduct disorder. Indeed, some evidence in the literature indicates that the quiet child may be more likely to develop the disorder.

In any case, aggressive tendencies in boys can be identified early and tend to persist throughout the life-span. Typically they can be perceived in the preschool years, and various studies have observed their stability well into adulthood (see Olweus, 1979, for a review). To be sure, the specific stresses that will evoke the aggressive response in a given individual are contingent on that person's world of meanings and personal experiences, but the general trend has been well documented.

Cloninger (1987) has offered a system for describing the structure of personality disorders that seems likely to influence the approach to conduct disorder. He has devised a "unified biosocial theory of personality," which views personality as having three basic patterns of adaptation: to novelty, to danger, and to reward. The patterns are designated as *novelty seeking, harm avoidance*, and *reward dependence*. These vary independently; a given individual may possess high, average, or low amounts of each trait. Biologically, these dimensions represent a variation in the brain's "incentive" or activation system (novelty seeking), in its "punishment" or inhibition system (harm avoidance), or in its ability to be conditioned (reward dependence). Cloninger proposes that a specific neurotransmitter system with its own biochemistry and its own anatomical distribution is associated with each personality dimension.

Behaviorally, each adaptive style produces a characteristic profile depending on whether the individual possesses the trait in high, average, or low degree. For example, the individual who is excessively high in harm avoidance is likely to be fearful, pessimistic, and inhibited, whereas the person with very low harm avoidance will be confident, unlikely to worry, comfortable with strangers, at ease in the face of danger, and ready to risk injury.

Pairing these several dimensions (e.g., average harm avoidance accompanied by high reward-dependence, or low novelty seeking combined with high harm avoidance) introduces variations. This approach creates six second-order clusters of personality traits (e.g., impulsive-aggressive, oppositional, opportunistic).

Finally, on a tertiary level eight third-order clusters arise from joining all three dimensions and produce profiles that strongly suggest many specific personality diagnoses. In particular, the antisocial personality (in a sense, the adult form of at least some kinds of conduct disorder) is characterized by high novelty seeking coupled with low harm avoidance and low reward dependence as primary elements; impulsive-aggressive, oppositional, or opportunistic traits as secondary elements; and the full-scale diagnosis of antisocial personality as the final tertiary cluster.

Perinatal Events

Nor are children with known biological difficulties the likeliest candidates for the diagnosis of conduct disorder. Although children with a history of prenatal problems, complicated deliveries, or even known brain damage are undoubtedly more vulnerable, a rather limited minority of them actually become delinquent. The island of Kauai studies (Werner & Smith, 1977) demonstrated that perinatal vulnerability was a significant predictor of later difficulties only if accompanied by stressed socioeconomic conditions; statistically, a middle-class child with fairly severe perinatal difficulties would be far *less* likely to develop a conduct disorder than would a low-SES child with minimal problems at birth.

Onset and Preschool Years

In the development of conduct disorder early object loss may be a far more telling event than perinatal trauma, especially if the loss occurs in the vulnerable second half of the 1st year of life; however, good confirming data are lacking. By the 2nd year of life, nevertheless, behavioral deviance is readily discernible. It may appear as hyperactivity, invasiveness, destructiveness, persistent biting, running away (some children begin to do this almost as soon as they can walk), tremendous power struggles, cruelty to pets, difficulty in being solaced by caretakers, aggressive behavior toward peers and other siblings, unusually intense and sustained tantrums, and a great readiness to cry with little capacity for self-comforting. When toilet training is successful, bladder control is sometimes achieved before bowel control (the reverse of the usual pattern); very often, however, training is not successful, and such youngsters tend to have a high incidence of enuresis and encopresis. The parents will remark on the child's disobedient, oppositional, negativistic, obdurate, destructive, obstinate, and willful behavior. They may comment that the child has a will of iron, will not mind, and insists on having his own way.

During the preschool years (ages 2½ years to 5 years) the more severe cases are likely to show high levels of malicious behavior, especially toward younger siblings. Such children have been known to set fires, engage in sexual seduction, injure siblings, learn to beg, become expert manipulators of family members, and engage in active stealing. Enuresis continues to be common, and cruelty to animals, which may not have been manifest earlier, may appear now. At nursery school these youngsters are beginning to be recognized as different, and other children may start to avoid and to exclude them.

In the island of Kauai study, Werner and Smith noted that among the large population of children whom they followed from birth through adolescence, a group of youngsters from low-SES families lived under chaotic conditions. A subgroup of the preschoolers growing up in these disturbed environments were extremely active, were difficult to manage, and seemed socially immature. As the study went on, the members of that subgroup were very likely to become delinquents. It is particularly important to note that when similar childhood behavior occurred within a better structured middle-class setting, it did not carry the same prognosis (Werner & Smith, 1977).

Other investigators have followed populations of children from an early age, although for shorter periods than Werner and Smith. Thus Richman and colleagues (1982) culled 94 problem toddlers out of a population of 705 children, and tracked these youngsters (along with an equal number of controls) until they were 8 or 9 years old. By the time they were 3 years old, about a third of the problem group were in the difficult-to-control, poor-peer-and-sibling-relations category. By age 8 years, a third of these acting-out children were still showing antisocial behavior. If, however, the severity of disturbance was considered, then it became evident that those who were severely disturbed at age 3 were much more likely (74%) to show evident antisocial behavior at age 8.

The Grade-School Years

The full array of the symptoms of conduct disorder becomes evident in the grade-school years. Even the milder cases, whose deviance was heretofore considered tolerable, now begin to sound loud social alarms. During the earlier years, the aberrant behavior may well have confined itself largely to the home, but sooner or later, as development advances, it spreads to the school. In more severe cases, it is likely to manifest at both home and school from the outset. In some instances, the full profile of the condition is much more evident in the school and is not perceived as a problem at home for a long time. This is perhaps most commonly the case with the more narcissistic children who have a certain pathological niche at home but who cannot get similar preferential treatment from teacher or peers, and who then act up. Learning problems are ubiquitous and affect most (not all) cases of conduct disorder; truancy is common. Commonest of all, however, are the complaints of disobedience, disruptiveness in class, and disrespect for authority; these are the true markers for this condition at school. Among their other problems, these children do not work well at academic tasks. They do not complete homework and projects; they read less well; they tend to get lower grades on achievement, IQ, and ordinary school tests; and they early commence a pattern of inattention and, presently, of nonattendance.

ETIOLOGY

Given the enormous variety of clinical syndromes that may have behavioral components, the etiology of conduct disorder is almost coextensive with the etiology of psychiatric illness (for a description of some of the varieties of conduct disorder, see Appendix 13–1). To keep some orientation among the plethora of theories and information, the classes of etiology will be divided into three main categories: biological, sociological, and psychological. This section cannot provide an exhaustive account of all the theories currently in vogue but will instead sample the best known or most promising theories.

Biological Factors

There is now reason to believe that an element of genetic predisposition is among the factors that make for deep-seated and persistent delinquent patterns. In general, two types of studies have attempted to clarify this point. One is the examination of adoptees. The basic structure of such studies is to find populations of parents who display a particular type of disturbance and to cull from them the parents whose children were placed out for adoption at an early age. The study then tries to determine how many of these adopted-away children, raised in a home environment where that syndrome does not exist, nonetheless develop a condition that resembles the syndrome of their biological parents. The work of Cloninger et al. (1987) and of Hutchings et al. (1974) demonstrates that a propensity for criminal behavior is clearly discernible under these conditions and leads to the conclusion that:

> Some factor transmitted by criminal parents increases the likelihood that their children will engage in criminal behavior. This claim holds especially for chronic criminality. The findings imply that biological predispositions are involved in the etiology of at least some criminal behavior (Mednick et al., 1984, p. 893)

Because these data are collected from adult records and do not describe the childhood and adolescent behavior of the subjects, the heritability of childhood conduct disorder remains to be demonstrated.

Twin studies are the other major means of studying possible genetic linkages. A recent report by Graham and Stevenson (1985) examined the degree of concordance for deviance (as rated independently by parents and teachers) between fraternal (dizygotic) and identical (monozygotic) twins. It turned out that if one identical twin was rated as deviant, then two times out of three, the other would also be rated as deviant. But if one fraternal twin was rated as deviant, then the chances were only one in three, or less, that the other twin would receive such a score. Although these results do not rule out a possible role for environmental influences, they do imply that the presence of a particular genetic constitution makes an important difference in the potential for deviance.

There is much to suggest a genetic predisposition toward conduct disorder. Just what is inherited that makes for the expression of such behavioral disturbance is, as yet, simply unknown. Studies of temperament suggest an early organization of personality that brings with it poor synchrony and inner regulation, a low threshold for stimuli, a consistently troubled mood, a considerable degree of intensity, and a high level of motility. These factors make for the "difficult child" from whose ranks later conduct disorders are all too likely to be culled (Thomas et al., 1968). The reported data, however, do not establish a very firm connection between an early history of difficult temperament and the later appearance of conduct disorder. Plomin, in fact, insists categorically that difficult temperament in infancy is not significantly associated with later clinical problems. Statistically, it does predict the appearance of certain kinds of behavior, but so far that has not risen to the level of clinical utility (Plomin, 1983). Others suggest that retardation, attention-deficit hyperactivity disorder, stimulus hunger with an accompanying quest for sensory input, and/or autonomic reactivity and passive avoidance learning may all play a role (Rutter, 1971, p. 179).

In any case, from an etiologic view, genetic factors alone are not enough. When, however, the inborn vulnerabilities combine with such elements as an upbringing that inclines a youngster toward narcissism, an undisciplined or inconsistently disciplined home life, and an environment that begets turbulence, tension, and chronic confrontation, these factors will forge the next link. Finally, if the social framework for all these elements offers delinquent models and promotes delinquent values, then the etiologic chain is complete, and the syndrome is likely to find its fullest expression. But the data are becoming increasingly persuasive that the genetic contribution to vulnerability is a real one.

Brain Damage/Child Physical Abuse. Anyone who examines a sizable number of delinquents will find that many of them have been victims of child abuse. Not uncommonly, it has involved severe head injury at an early age; indeed, a high percentage of these teenagers report that earlier in life they were knocked unconscious by their parents. Dorothy Lewis stresses that violence enacted by the adolescent is particularly likely to have been preceded by violence directed toward him during the vulnerable formative years. The youngster's deep-rooted, chronic rage at the mistreatment he has received often compounds the effects of the control-weakening organic brain injuries and the force of the powerful parental modeling. Together these factors create an intense pressure toward eruptive and dangerous behavior and thus reinforce the violent diathesis. In her recent work, Lewis emphasizes that such individuals need a great deal of protection, containment, careful diagnostic efforts, and intensive therapeutic work of eclectic character and long duration (Lewis, 1981a, 1981b).

Because the majority of battered children do not become delinquent, and no known mechanism explains how head injury would, in fact, cause violent behavior, some additional constructs would have to be added to demonstrate why only some of the victims of this style of upbringing pursue an antisocial course. Moreover, as Rutter has noted, the presence of the battering and head injury indicates disturbed psychosocial rearing conditions, and there is no way to distinguish how much of the damage is due to the head injury and how much to concomitant environmental stress. Rutter concludes that "brain damage (however assessed) is present in only a tiny minority of delinquents and it is likely that it is of negligible importance in the genesis of delinquent behavior in the population as a whole" (Rutter & Giller, 1984, p. 171).

Attention-Deficit Hyperactivity Disorder (ADHD). In England, most of the cases that American child psychiatrists diagnose as ADHD are considered to be conduct disorders. At best, the degree and the quality of the interrelationship between these two syndromes is ambiguous; at worst the diagnostic issue is chaotic. The chances are that clinicians are dealing with more than one condition, but that their surface appearances are similar enough to cause a considerable degree of overlap. This is specially likely to occur when the clinician relies on rating scales to distinguish among these several possibilities (see Chapter 11, "Attention-Deficit Hyperactivity Disorder").

Certainly much hard data indicate that the diagnosis of ADHD is all too often associated with conduct disorder and with later antisocial personality. Cantwell (1981) reports the connection in a variety of studies. Thus, retrospective accounts of the childhood of adults with known antisocial personality, as well as various kinds of follow-up evaluations of children once diagnosed as ADHD, all confirm that the childhood condition often precedes the later personality disturbance. About 25% of the cases of ADHD later develop conduct disorder, with a somewhat smaller percentage going on to actual delinquency. Some have speculated that the underlying mechanism binding the two together is the stimulus hunger that seems to afflict some ADHD children. Investigators hypothesize that at least a subgroup of such youngsters experience low arousal of the central nervous system. The hyperactivity then is interpreted as an attempt by these youngsters to obtain the necessary stimulation, which is otherwise barred to them. In a similar vein, Quay (1965) has suggested that the habitually antisocial individual is also engaged in stimulus seeking. Currently, some of the symptoms associated with ADHD have been relieved by stimulants; this result has been regarded as supporting such a concept. On the other hand, this form of intervention is clearly *nonspecific,* and the entire assumption is at best dubious.

Parental and familial factors apparently play a major role in determining which ADHD children move toward conduct disorder. On follow-up, the most antisocial youngsters come from homes where the father was himself a victim of learning or behavioral problems, or where there were a variety of evidences of failed parenting. Rutter (1971) considers family discord to be the strongest of all the family factors that contribute to antisocial behavior in childhood.

Rutter, too, offers what is perhaps the most widely held view about the connection between the two diagnoses. He suggests that the hyperkinetic syndrome makes learning difficult for the child and marks him as peculiar among his peers. Such a youngster thus operates at a constant disadvantage and is under continual social and academic stress. The resulting feelings of rage and exclusion incline the child to resentful retaliative behavior, and the conduct disorder appears (Rutter & Giller, 1984). The possibility that genetic influences or common neurological deficits play a specific role in linking the two conditions remains to be explored.

Neurotransmitters. In recent years, the exploration of central nervous system (CNS) functions has been vastly enriched by researchers' ever-deepening understanding of how individual neurons exchange information. Given an essentially intact anatomical structure, the nervous system in general and the brain in particular can be thought of as a huge switchboard with literally billions of messages flashing back and forth among the myriad elements. The way that messages are transferred among the neurons, or nerve cells, and anything that would facilitate or impede the transfer of information become matters of the most far-reaching import for the functioning of the entire system.

In current research, a key site for study has accordingly become the point of juncture between nerve cells, where the tendrils of one cell approach closely enough to the substance of another to allow a message to get across. Such a site of exchange is called the *synapse.* The commonest intersection of that kind occurs between the axon terminals of one neuron and the dendrites or cell body of another, but axon-to-axon transmission is also known. The actual transmitting agent is one or several of a group of chemical substances known as *neurotransmitters.*

These substances are relatively simple compounds. They are manufactured within the nerve cell itself, carried in vesicles to the periphery, and then ejected into the interneuronal space. They diffuse across this gap (the synaptic cleft), but, to be effective messengers, they must then find receptors (precisely designed receptacles made specifically for them) on the target neuron. If they can succeed in doing that, they fit into place, whereupon, like a thrown switch, they initiate a responsive pattern in the nerve cell to which they are affixed.

None of this process is haphazard; there are checks and modulating agents at every step of the way. The rate and quantity of the neurotransmitters' formation are under careful regulation within the neuron; the time during which these messenger substances can persist within the synaptic cleft is limited by several mechanisms (they can be reabsorbed back into the emitting neuron or they can be enzymatically destroyed within the space between the neurons); and the availability of receptors is also subject to several regulating forces. The presence of such a wealth of regulatory controls on the effectiveness of these neurotransmitters bears testimony to the extraordinarily powerful role they play in human affairs.

About 50 such neurotransmitters are known today, and more are being discovered every year; because each of them may have one or more types of receptor, the field of study becomes complex indeed. What is critical, however, is that neuroscientists are now able to identify and to measure these substances, and, in at least some instances, to discern circumstances when they are present in excess or when they are lacking in some measure. This has made it possible to design treatments based on this information. The many new antidepressants and antipsychotics, the great host of tranquilizers and mood-altering agents, and the entire science of neurochemistry are developing in large measure within the framework of the study of neurotransmitters and their clinical effects.

In particular, four neurotransmitters have been given special attention in relation to research in aggression. Most of the studies currently available have been carried out on animals (for obvious ethical and practical reasons). Nonetheless, certain generalizations can be made.

The animal researchers who have studied aggression tend to distinguish between *predatory* and *affective* aggression (Wasman & Flynn, 1962; also cited in Alpert et al., 1981). The affective type usually arises from frustration or pain; it expresses itself in the form of frenzied rage with a high level of autonomic arousal, in effect, a kind of outburst. By way of contrast, the predatory type tends to be a contained and focused stalking, a planned, deliberate behavior designed to accomplish some aggressive goal and accompanied by a much lower level of arousal. Predatory aggression terminates when the animal has killed its prey. The significance of the distinction between these two types of aggression is that the underlying neurochemical behavior in each instance is significantly different.

In a recent review, Alpert et al. (1981) emphasized the four neurotransmitters that have been the object of the largest portion of the available research. These agents are *dopamine, norepinephrine, serotonin,* and *acetylcholine.* Dopamine and norepinephrine are called the *catecholamines* and are both derived from an amino-acid precursor called *tyrosine.* A series of chemical steps convert tyrosine to dopamine and dopamine in turn to norepinephrine. The derivation is important because the factors controlling the chemical steps that transform tyrosine into the catecholamines are very much influenced by several specific enzymes that activate these steps. Medications that affect these enzymes and alter this rate of formation, for example, can have profound effects on the presence or absence of these vital substances.

One of the most readily demonstrable associations is the increased production and release of brain norepinephrine in states of affective aggression. Some findings suggest that norepinephrine may also inhibit predatory aggression. These findings, however, are by no means clear-cut and entirely convincing, and a good deal of work remains to be done.

The chemical serotonin is derived from the amino acid tryptophan. Serotonin is something of a chemical modulator, an inhibitory regulator of all affective expression. A fall-off in the level of serotonin seems to provoke or to release aggression; a higher level of serotonin inhibits aggressive activity. Accordingly, the various techniques for lowering the rate of formation of serotonin or otherwise depleting the brain of its presence have a distinctly provocative effect on both affective and predatory aggression. More important still is the finding that the ratio of serotonin to catecholamine, that is, the balance of inhibitory and facilitating substances, might well be the key to understanding some of the observed events.

Acetylcholine, another important neurotransmitter, is derived from a chemical called *choline,* which is present in many common foods. As with other neurotransmitters, this substance is manufactured by a series of steps, each of which is available for enhancement or inhibition. In addition, as it crosses the space between the neurons, acetylcholine is received on the other side of the synaptic gap by one of two classes of receptors, called the *muscarinic* and *nicotinic* receptors. Considerable evidence now suggests that when acetylcholine is present in quantity and when the muscarinic receptors are the active ones, then affective aggression is enhanced. Hence, any factors that inhibit acetylcholine formation, interfere with acetylcholine transmission, or block the muscarinic receptors from accepting this chemical messenger may diminish such aggression.

High levels of acetylcholine increase predatory aggression to the point that nonpredatory animals chemically treated in this way will attack and kill unaccustomed prey. However, in most behavioral sequences, it is the balance among the several neurotransmitter systems (with their various inhibiting and augmenting effects) that produces any given pattern of behavior.

Finally, much theorizing has focused on dopamine as the critical factor. An early theory advanced by Wender to account for the behavior of the hyperactive child illustrates this neurotransmitter's role in the thinking of the field. Wender noted that in animal experiments, an unresponsiveness to positive and negative reinforcers was associated with dopamine deficiency. Because stimulants tend to reverse this condition in animals, and stimulants are the most effective medication for the symptoms of hyperactivity in humans, might not the basic disturbance in these hyperactive children be one of relative dopamine deprivation? No direct evidence exists that this is, in fact, the case, and the theory remains unproven. But it does illustrate how such formulations are employed.

Quay and Werry (1986) offer a somewhat different view. They regard the delinquency-prone youngster to be, on the one hand, excessively inclined to seek immediate rewards, and on the other, simultaneously unable to inhibit impulse. In particular, the child with undersocialized conduct disorder "reflects an overactive reward system and an underfunctioning behavioral inhibition system resulting in impulsive, disinhibited, and reward-seeking behavior" (p. 51). They believe that these traits are linked to specific biological profiles. In particular, Quay and Werry quote evidence that dopamine is the agent principally associated with reward pathways, and norepinephrine with behavioral inhibition. That this evidence seems somewhat inconsistent with the former account reflects the many contradictory findings in this field. Quay and Werry cite research to the effect that the enzyme that would normally convert dopamine into norepinephrine (a substance called *dopamine-beta-hydroxylase*) is frequently deficient in cases of adult personality disorder who are rated as high in aggression. They argue that, in the relative absence of this important enzyme, dopamine would continue to form but would not be converted into norepinephrine. Accordingly, dopamine would tend to pile up (making for ever greater reward-seeking behavior) while, at the same time, the production of norepinephrine would be proportionately curtailed (with a corresponding diminution of inhibitory tendencies). Hence, in cases of aggressive disorder, the biologically based reward-inhibition systems are deviant and may reflect a genetic predisposition.

Although such theories remain highly speculative and investigations are in their earliest stages, the further study of neurotransmitters will undoubtedly open up new doors to the understanding of and the ability to influence human behavior. At present many contradictory findings and many isolated results defy explanation; more to the point, no dependable chemical way of regulating most cases of human aggression has as yet been developed. Nonetheless, this is an area of the greatest promise.

Seizure Disorders.   The association between seizure disorder and conduct disorder is too frequent to be coincidental and too vague to be definitive. The correlation is far and away highest in the group of seizure disorders that together make up the temporal lobe syndromes. To say the least, the findings in a sizable percentage of these cases tend to be of rather uncertain character. Dorothy Lewis in particular has emphasized the high prevalence of these temporal lobe syndromes in the population of antisocial youngsters; in the series that she and her colleagues studied (Lewis, 1981), 6% (1 child in 17) of a group of court-referred juvenile delinquents showed signs of such disorder. A still-more-striking finding emerged when a group of young people incarcerated for very violent behavior was studied; within that population, 26% (one youth in 4) could be characterized as displaying temporal lobe involvement. According to these investigators, the more dangerous and primitive the behavior, the more likely it is that this kind of brain disturbance will be present.

In respect to diagnosis of temporal lobe dysfunction, Lewis describes an array of diagnostic symptoms that include staring episodes, memory blackouts with inability to recall specific acts (whether violent or not violent), transient inability to understand what was said by others, dizzy spells, brief attacks of intense emotion without known cause, a temporary loss of thought control, blackouts of consciousness, perceptual disturbances such as micropsia or macropsia, repeated déjà vu experiences, recurrent patterns of automatic movements, and transient olfactory or gustatory hallucinations. When four of these findings occur together in a given individual, then a temporal lobe syndrome is presumed to be present. It is particularly important to note that in such cases, if antisocial acts do occur, they are not an expression or a consequence of seizure activity. If it occurs at all, the violence occurs *between* seizures and presumably is associated with the general state of the brain. Violent acts during a seizure are almost unheard of.

Practically speaking, the diagnosis of a temporal lobe syndrome implies a very detailed and painstaking exploration of what may, at times, be very uncertain data. An additional difficulty arises because the symptoms ascribed to this syndrome overlap with many other diagnoses; that is to say, a number of psychiatric and neurological conditions might display similar manifestations (including psychosis, conversion reaction, depersonalization syndrome, malingering and the several factitious disorders). How these behavioral symptoms relate to abnormalities in the EEG requires more systematic study. Nonspecific EEG abnormalities are common, and more work is required to identify *which*, if any, EEG deviations are diagnostically or etiologically significant. Nonetheless, a definite subgroup of delinquents convey an overall sense of a nervous system that gives way under stress, that cannot contain the buildup of tension, and that finds an action channel for discharge. Although there is little foundation for assuming that the violent acts perpetrated by individuals with temporal lobe syndromes directly express seizure activity, the possibility of an altered threshold for impulse control as a function of epileptic diathesis remains an elusive but tantalizing possibility.

In this connection, a syndrome called *episodic dyscontrol* has been introduced into the adult literature (Bach-y-Rita et al., 1971) and has subsequently been described for children (Nunn, 1986). Briefly, the syndrome describes a clinical state wherein the child is usually not aggressive but has periodic outbursts of violent and dangerous behavior that usually erupt without a clear-cut precipitant (or one without sufficient magnitude to provoke such an attack), and that are frequently directed toward a close family member. The patient is often fearful prior to the outburst, is inaccessible to influence during the episode, and is amnestic or filled with remorse after it has ended. The majority of such children have demonstrable brain lesions, and the syndrome is thought of as an expression of their organic brain damage.

This condition has not attained sufficient consensual validation among clinicians to be included as a formal diagnosis in DSM-III-R.

Anxiety and Delinquency. For many years, it was considered axiomatic that delinquents do not experience anxiety in the same way as do normals or neurotic patients. This view arose out of a group of experiments that subjected delinquents to aversive stimuli, measured their reactions, and compared these responses to the reactions of nondelinquents. As cited by Achenbach (1982), the original experiments were performed in 1957 by Lykken. The subjects included a population of institutionalized sociopaths, of institutionalized nonsociopaths, and of normals (all late adolescents and young adults). All had to complete a number of tests that measured their autonomic reactivity. In one instance, they had to learn their path through a maze, with an electric shock following certain kinds of mistakes; in another, to listen to sequences of buzzers where again shocks followed certain combinations. They were also asked to make choices between different hypothetical unpleasant tasks. The sociopaths emerged with characteristic profiles of response. In their choices of task, they preferred frightening to difficult undertakings; in their maze responses, they made more shocked than unshocked errors; and in their reactions to the buzzer test, they showed less galvanic skin reaction when they did get a shock. All in all, they showed poor avoidance learning, that is, they did not seem to learn from experience.

Some years later a further elaboration of this design included an additional dimension. Again the maze and the shocks were employed, but this time, half of the prisoners received an injection of adrenalin before they took the test, and the other half received a placebo. Characteristically, under placebo conditions, the nonsociopaths learned quickly to avoid the shocks whereas the sociopaths did not. Once the adrenalin was added, however, just the reverse took place; the nonsociopaths did more poorly on the test, whereas the sociopaths improved markedly. The conclusion drawn was that sociopaths do better with high arousal, whereas normals are disorganized by that much stimulation. This finding has led to much theorizing about the underlying nature of delinquency, for example, that one of the reasons for the delinquents' behavior is the pressing need for stimulation.

There are now many such experiments in the literature, but only one will be mentioned. When sociopaths were given the maze test under a variety of punishment-and-reward conditions, they regularly fell below normals except under one set of conditions. If the punishment meant a loss of money (they started out with a pile of quarters but lost one with each error), the sociopaths did better than the normals. They also experienced higher galvanic skin response and described as much anxiety as normals. Hence, according to one interpretation of these data, matters of values rather than inherent ability or inability to experience anxiety are at work here; what has meaning to the sociopath evidently differs from what is important to the normal (Schmauk, 1970).

Testosterone and Delinquency. A good deal of work has been done on the possible relationship of plasma testosterone level and antisocial behavior. In part, it was hoped that this might shed light on the marked increase of delinquent behavior at puberty. At best, however, an uncertain relationship has been described in the literature between testosterone levels in boys and delinquent behavior. This relationship was reexamined by Olweus et al. (1980) in a carefully designed study. They found only a weak, nonsignificant correlation between testosterone levels and the self-report of their subjects on such antisocial behaviors as petty theft, truancy, and vandalism. What did emerge, however, was a strong positive correlation between testosterone levels and the readiness of the youngsters (by self-report) to respond to provocation and threat with physical or verbal aggression. Another positive correlation was that between testosterone level and low frustration tolerance (or impatience). In any case, the presence of a close tie between this endocrine level and antisocial behavior in general is at best equivocal.

Sociological Theories

This section surveys several sociological theories that have played a large role in determining public policy. Two types of sociological theory stand out in terms of their influence and explanatory power: the *strain* theories and the *subcultural* theories. In many ways these were the dominant presences in the mid 20th-century formulations. Each of them actually subtends a wide area of research and theory building, and only representative examples will be reviewed.

Strain Theories. Toward the latter part of the 19th century, to explain certain aspects of antisocial behavior, Emile Durkheim, a French sociologist, formulated a theory of what he called *anomie.* Merton (1957) brought this theory to the attention of American social scientists in a famous article originally published in 1935 and republished in 1957. Many subsequent theoretical formulations derived directly from this concept, and it has been of seminal importance in the thinking of American sociologists. Because it describes the effects of social frustration, the group of approaches it has evoked are called the "strain theories." Although the literature on anomie is extensive, only one representative view will be described.

Cloward and Ohlin, perhaps the best known authors associated with this approach, based their ideas solidly on the concept of anomie. They regarded the major effects of deprivation as arising from the disparity between the upwardly mobile goals that society sets forth for underprivileged people and the realistic avenues that are actually available to allow such people ever to attain those goals. The goals include the full range of possibilities implicit in American society, whereas the legitimate avenues are littered with difficulties and, in most instances, altogether blocked. Anomie theory assumes that the result is enormous frustration. Accordingly, for Ohlin and Cloward, the solution to the social disintegration arising from racism and poverty became the pragmatic issue of finding concrete ways to provide disadvantaged people with the necessary opportunities to get ahead in life. In their book, *Delinquency and Opportunity* (Cloward & Ohlin, 1960), these authors construct a model of low-SES youth facing a choice. These young people may on the one hand seek their fortune within the structure of conventional society; on the other hand, their environment also offers them the path of criminal achievement. When a ghetto youth tries to get ahead in his life, to study, to work, and to rise in the system, he finds that a vast interlocking network of built-in cultural barriers keeps the doors of opportunity closed and simply does not allow entry of a lower class individual. His family cannot teach him polished and refined language, his school cannot compensate for his special educational needs, employers want him either for transient jobs, such as unloading a truck, or for dead-end jobs, such as janitorial work, and even where such overt factors are overcome, subtle exclusion on the basis of race enters in so that wherever he turns, there is no access.

The other choice available to him is to become a criminal. Here he has three possible routes. He can join what the authors call the *conflict subculture* and become a violent denizen of the street, robbing and mugging for whatever those activities may net him. He can join the *retreatist* subculture and withdraw from the whole frustrating business into the hazy world of addiction, getting money any way that he can to pay for his habit. Or he can find entry into the *criminal* subculture, learn to be an artful thief, try to earn his spurs within the rackets, and seek to rise in the lucrative world of drug dealing (or other antisocial "businesses"). In the face of the blocked official channels, if the youth wishes to better his lot and move upward in society, these antisocial subcultures become his sole opportunities, and he may eventually resort to them.

This theory achieved such a level of recognition that during the presidency of Lyndon B. Johnson from 1963 through 1969 (the era of the war against poverty), it served as a foundation for the entire concept of the Office of Economic Opportunity (funded at some 900 million dollars). Sad to relate, the war against poverty was not won, and the Office of Economic Opportunity is no more.

In fact, when a group of Chicago sociologists attempted to verify the existence of these subcultural groupings by studying Chicago gangs, they found little evidence of the delinquent specialization into subcultures that this theory postulated. If anything, most of the gangs represented "conflict" forms of adjustment. Fighting and assault were their principal characteristics, but they had certain social functions as well, such as sports and just hanging around (Short et al., 1963; also cited in Achenbach, 1982). Another study found little evidence for high aspirations among delinquent youth; many such youngsters wanted to pump gas or wash dishes, and it was difficult to fit their stated ambitions into the framework of a strain/anomie conceptualization (Rosenberg & Silverstein, 1969; also cited in Achenbach, 1982).

Subcultural Theories. Another great category of sociological approaches is the group of subcultural theories.

The classic explanation of many parents for their offspring's failings is to blame the trouble on bad company. If their child had not hung out with a "bad crowd," none of the problems would have happened. There may be something to this, or at least so think quite a sizable array of sociologists.

A leading theoretician in this realm has been Sutherland, whose theory of differential association says, in effect, that young people care profoundly about their acceptance and status within the social group available to them. If these peers exhibit delinquent behavior, then the young person is strongly influenced to keep up and to earn acceptance by meeting the expectations and the standards set for him by the group (Sutherland & Cressey, 1974). The underlying mechanisms of identification and intensive association with offenders are enough to account for the ensuing misconduct.

Yablonsky (1962) set forth a particular variant on this theme. He saw the gang as a near group, a loose, fluid, changing entity, expanding and contracting as circumstances altered. If a fight was shaping up, a great influx of sometime members would join in the excitement. Then, as things died down, the membership would fall off. The conduct problem was thus a matter of association, but far less consistently and in a much less certain fashion than Sutherland had described.

Sherif and Sherif (1964) also studied gang behavior and concluded that for many youngsters, the delinquent behavior actually is not a form of deviance at all. The professional cannot understand any youth without considering the context within which he lives; for many a deprived youngster his gang is his reference group, and his behavior is likely to exhibit a high level of conformity to peer group values. What appears to be antisocial activity relative to the larger society is, in fact, a form of compliance with the rules and expectations of the smaller but more significant social unit to which he belongs.

Considered together, the strain theories and the subculture theories might explain some cases of delinquency, but they suffer from a similar failing. They are unable to account for the self-evident fact that only some members of a given neighborhood or school population become delinquent, whereas many others, despite exposure to the same strains or the same subcultural influences, nonetheless do not.

Control Theories. Control theorists have put forward a contrasting set of ideas. These social scientists operate from quite a different group of basic assumptions. They take the position that, as temptable human beings, we are all subject to strains that would encourage delinquency; the remarkable thing is that there is not more of it. Why isn't there? The answer is that within the individual's personality makeup, an array of mechanisms make for control. People can resist the temptations or, in any case, restrain antisocial impulses because something stops them. The focus of study is then on that something.

The approach of the control theorists offers several advantages. For one thing, the role of the family is immediately present as an item of consideration. For another, these theorists are not necessarily bound to a focus on gang or social class concerns. There is room in their formulations for a wider spectrum of considerations, for looking at individuals and for weighing organic factors as elements that might influence impulse control.

A number of investigators have begun to ponder the meaning of deterrence as an element in the formation—or in the avoidance—of delinquent patterns (Briar & Pillavin, 1965). Some of the significant deterrents for young people are the good opinion of the family, the fear of apprehension, the desire to succeed at school, the fear of being categorized as a delinquent, and the desire to preserve chances for future success.

These factors can be genuine deterrents. Some of them have a socially constructive character in the sense of binding the youngsters to school and family and positive social values. Other factors deter by their negative valences—fear of apprehension and punishment, anxiety about possible social exclusion, concern about marring future opportunities, and the like. The fear of legal consequences may have both direct and indirect effects: The direct effect is to inhibit antisocial acts by the chilling anticipation of the ensuing punishment. The indirect effects, however, may teach the youngster to consider his actions, to weigh what is right and what is wrong and to distinguish between them, to instill within him respect for law, to make proper behavior habitual, and to give him a sense that conforming behavior is right, good, and reasonable.

Some of these propositions have been subjected to path analysis (Johnson, 1979), a mode of weighting various factors to evaluate their interactive influence on causing or restraining the delinquent act. Among the elements that the author considered were social class, parent–child relationships, school experiences, concerns about the future, delinquent associates, delinquent values, and the influence of threatened punishment. A sample of 734 tenth graders (two-thirds of the sophomores enrolled in three high schools in Seattle, Washington) were given a self-reporting questionnaire that took about an hour to fill out. In analyzing the results, the author found that social class and concerns about the future were of minor importance as etiologic influences. In the final analysis, delinquent associates had the greatest influence on law violations, with the adoption and expression of delinquent values being an important parallel factor. Curiously enough, parental attachments seemed to play only a minor role in the reporting of these adolescents, whereas school experiences were a good deal more prominent in their thinking.

Johnson concluded his analysis at this point, but it seems highly likely that the young people who were going the delinquent route had, in effect, already lost their parents as guides, models, and important sources of attachment. They had instead turned to the peer group to seek what they could not find or use within their homes and to make up for the failures and humiliations they were encountering at school. Faced with such stresses, some youngsters become depressed and others withdraw into a fantasy world. Johnson's study suggests, however, that there is a sizable group whose rage and hurt tend to be turned out on their world. In this sense they are quite different from many of their peers, but not from all. Inevitably they seek out those similar youths, band together for mutual support, and develop group attitudes in keeping with their defensive needs (a combination of arrogance, contempt, hostility, pugnaciousness, macho assertiveness, plus a devaluation of conventional values). The delinquent subculture is then well under way.

Another theorist who has attempted a path analysis of this sort is Olweus (1980). He worked with a sizable population of Swedish schoolchildren and studied two cohorts, 76 sixth graders and 51 ninth graders. Using peer ratings and intensive parent interviews as raw data, he focused his inquiries on a number of early familial and temperamental factors that might lead to aggressive reaction patterns in boys. In brief, he found that when boys were active and hotheaded during their early years, their likelihood of developing in an aggressive direction increased. If the mother did not set adequate limits and instead responded to aggressive behavior with a lax or tolerant attitude, this contributed substantially to the aggressive outcome. As a separate variable, the use of physical punishment or strong threats by the parents could also augment the aggressive tendency. Finally, the attitude of the principal caretaker was of paramount importance. "If the mother is negative, rejecting, or indifferent to the boy when he is young (and later), this is likely to result in the adolescent boy becoming relatively more aggressive and hostile toward his environment" (p. 651). In part, this negative attitude finds expression in the power-assertive disciplinary techniques (threats and corporal punishment) noted above. The extent to which a given child's temperamental stance drove the parents into the unloving, uncaring, and hostile position they eventually assumed does not emerge clearly from this study.

Television. Finally, in even a brief review of the sociological realm, it seems appropriate to refer to a much debated but suggestive dimension of influence: the media, and, in particular, television. Investigations have been carried on for decades in an attempt to demonstrate the ways that the media affect youngsters. Researchers have made the commonsense point that with many children spending anywhere from 5 to 6 hours a day watching the TV screen, the media cannot be a trivial factor in shaping their growth. The problem, however, has been to prove that this hunch is true, and this has turned out to be inordinately difficult to accomplish. Ultimately, the findings were pulled together by a group within the Department of Health and Human Services (1982). They noted that most of the research community believes that TV violence does lead to aggressive behavior on the part of the children and teenagers who watch the programs.

Of the many efforts to explore this point, two studies tend to demonstrate a direct connection between television viewing and violent behavior. An English study built on intensive interviews of boys and their mothers ultimately involved 1565 subjects. The findings that emerged suggested that where boys had a proneness toward violence, watching brutal scenes on TV led them to enact simple, primitive violent attacks in a sort of direct imitation of the behavior that they had so recently viewed. Control boys did not behave in this way (Belson, 1978).

The other study involved a 10-year follow-up of children who had first been evaluated at age 8 years. In several of these boys, a number of factors had predicted violent behavior; at follow-up at age 18 or 19 years, the aggressive behavior was indeed present. In sorting out the importance of the various elements that the author thought had contributed to this outcome, the predilection for viewing violence on TV emerged as a statistically significant factor with good predictive value (Eron, 1980).

In this connection, the following are important questions: Just how does watching TV actually effect behavior? By what means does television influence the viewers? Currently four chief mechanisms have been suggested.

OBSERVATIONAL LEARNING.　This is the "monkey see, monkey do" kind of influence, the classic modeling that underlies so much of children's social learning in their homes. They see behavior enacted before them, and they tend presently to repeat the patterns that they have thus encountered. If a great deal of the behavior to which they are exposed is violent in character, the tendency of all children—and in particular of the more vulnerable subgroup—to imitate what they have observed is bound to be considerable.

TELEVISION VIEWING AS JUSTIFICATION.　When vulnerable youngsters, who are already violent or, at best, violence-prone, watch TV, whatever inner controls they have established directly confront the image and the aura of violence that pervade so many media offerings. The displayed behavior can now be employed by the potentially violent youth as an excuse or a justification for perpetrating the violent behavior to which he is, in any case, inclined. From this theoretical position, viewing TV mayhem creates a predisposition to violence that vanquishes the superego, or diminishes the external inhibitions: "See, everybody is doing it so I am free to do it as well."

AROUSAL AS A FACTOR.　This somewhat physiological view assumes that the observation of violence has a stimulating effect on the observer. The theory goes on to assert such a degree of psychosomatic arousal will increase the predisposed individual's proneness to violence. This then is the mechanism by which viewing images is thought to increase aggressiveness; the bodily response to the stimulating images exposes the vulnerability through which the aggressive behavior can all too readily emerge.

INFLUENCE ON ATTITUDE FORMATION.　The various studies and surveys suggest that children who watch a great deal of TV tend to assume that violence is rampant in the world. Such youngsters are on the whole more suspicious and untrusting than their less involved peers. Although many other influences can affect their attitudes, the association is suggestive. In any case, this personality set is believed to increase the likelihood of violent behavior.

Professionals cannot as yet regard the association between TV and violence as finally proven, but the data are certainly provocative. The various hypotheses linking the time spent before the TV screen to increased aggressive behavior provide important potential links in the causal chain. Of course, time spent watching TV may also reflect parental attitudes and laxness.

Psychological Theories

A consideration of the individual psychological profile of these youngsters reveals a strange world. It is a different kind of environment in which conduct disorder is a syndrome, a symptom complex, and an illness of sorts in its own right. At the same time, it is even more likely to be an expression of or associated with a variety of other conditions.

Conduct Disorder and Mental Illness. The major mental illnesses, such as the psychoses, have some very definite tie-ins to these behavioral disorders. Lauretta Bender (1947) defined a form of childhood illness that she called pseudopsychopathic schizophrenia; the masking of psychotic syndromes of one kind or another by behavioral symptoms is not uncommon. At least two major studies indicate that a good many people who appear at clinics as hyperactive and aggressive children are later quite likely to be admitted to hospitals with adult forms of psychosis. Indeed, among the more dangerous and severely criminal youth (who presently become institutionalized), a sizable percentage turn out to be rather floridly psychotic with overt hallucinations, delusions, and thought disorder. To be sure, a number of different kinds of psychoses (drug-induced, depressive, manic, and schizo-affective, to name a few) may affect them, but many of this group are clearly schizophrenic, with the added qualification that a rather prominent paranoid component is present. The antisocial behavior appears when, unable to distinguish fantasy from reality, they begin to act on the basis of their persecutory delusions.

Of particular interest is the growing recognition that, in some instances, the appearance of antisocial behavior actually represents the precursor form of or the early expression of affective illness, in particular mania or hypomania. In these cases, the irritable, invasive, hyperactive patterns along with the highly disturbed judgment that characterize the condition are perceived as a form of behavioral disturbance. Nor is the distinction an easy one in the younger child before the classic cyclic pattern has taken form. A history of alcoholism or of major affective illness in a close family member is of crucial importance in helping at least to open up the possibility of such a diagnosis.

The majority of conduct-disordered youngsters, however, are not mentally ill in the usual sense of the word but suffer instead from personality disorders.

Borderline/Narcissism Theory. In recent years, within psychoanalysis, there has been a tremendous expansion of the theoretical constructs relating to borderline and narcissistic pathology. In particular, a number of authors have attempted to clarify the nature of borderline pathology, of narcissistic development, and of self-psychology. The literature is extensive and complex and for that reason, instead of trying to cover it all, the following material will be devoted to the work of one group of investigators, Offer et al. (1979), who have sought to apply many of these concepts to delinquents in a rational and methodologically sophisticated manner.

These authors have surveyed a population of delinquents who were considered to be severe in degree of disorder and nonorganic in respect to the etiology of their pathology. When the investigators used the appropriate statistical means to sort out the many factors that they had observed, the youngsters fell into four discernible and significantly different groups: impulsive delinquents, empty borderlines, depressed borderlines, and narcissistic delinquents. The authors pointed out that not one of the youngsters they studied represented a "pure" example of any of these types; usually the scores on the several instruments employed were mixed, with leanings toward a particular subgroup. Indeed, the authors state that there probably are no pure types. Nonetheless, certain aggregates emerge for the clinician, and the clustering in their study was evident and statistically valid. Each type will be briefly described.

IMPULSIVE DELINQUENTS.   The typical finding in these cases is impulsivity and poorly integrated controls in the face of yearning, frustration, or rage. The youngster is inclined to lash out at others when under stress, to carry out antisocial acts demonstrating manhood or satisfying needs, and to treat people in emotionally abrupt, unreflective, and thoughtless ways. Such a youth is likely to be anxious, distant, self-centered, self-serving, and lacking in empathy. The youngster's relationship life is shallow, and the fantasy life is severely limited. It appears as if impulses are enacted directly without the mediation of preliminary thought or of partial discharge in daydreams. The history is usually lifelong, and the child has often been in trouble from his earliest years.

In tracing the development of this condition, the authors turn to Kohut's (1971) reconstruction of the early development of impulse controls. According to this view, the baby develops the ability to inhibit impulse through the soothing and comforting interventions of mother. Using mother both as source and as model, the baby takes in the experience of being soothed, catches the trick of it, and so learns to self-soothe. But mother also frustrates in tiny, recurrent ways, comforting the infant each time so that he can endure the necessary delay or lack of immediate satisfaction. The baby internalizes the mother's ministrations and begins to help himself past the easier confrontations and privations. Tolerance of frustration develops from this sequence of experiences. Given a predictable and continuing relationship of this kind, bit by bit the child learns to cope with disappointment, with delay, with not getting his own way immediately. As soon as development permits, the child can utilize such alternatives as fantasy to help cope with his yearnings, and, if all goes well, in time, he will achieve the cognitive competencies of planning for long-range goals.

However, there are also situations where this kind of mother–infant interaction either does not occur, or, if it does occur, it comes in episodic, uncertain, and unpredictable fits and starts. In the face of such rearing patterns, the smooth emergence of the necessary control apparatuses does not take place. In rare cases, there may be a generalized panimpulsivity; more typically, however, there will be a variety of specific stimulus-sets in response to which the youngster will erupt, or "fall apart." The child will then strike out or lunge for immediate gratification, no matter how inappropriate or unearned. This then gives rise to the form of conduct disorder that Offer et al. (1979) call the *impulsive delinquent*. In a way this is the picture of the unreconstructed 18-month-old, untroubled by an as-yet-undeveloped fantasy life, wanting what he wants when he wants it, and ready to act up in order to get it.

NARCISSISTIC DELINQUENTS. The narcissistic youth is characterized chiefly by his grandiose and egocentric stance. He is likely to be extremely exploitative and manipulative; he has regard neither for truth nor fairness except when these ploys allow him to extract some advantage for himself, to justify his miscreance, or to put others on the defensive. His grandiose pretensions lead him to a pattern of demandingness and a sense of entitlement that brook neither reason nor any measure of compromise; certainly the youngster displays no deference at all toward the rights of others and shows no empathy whatsoever for their feelings. The sense of entitlement in turn permits guilt-free stealing and simple, unambivalent joy at achieving a successful swindle. Self-seeking dominates his relationship life; he judges people only according to their availability to gratify or to be exploited. Ultimately the youngster is capable only of a kind of idealized self-love. So oriented, he is not free from the basic human need for attachment; given this outlook, however, the child tends to seek an object as much like himself (or, more precisely, like his ideal notion of the self) as possible; as a result bisexuality and perversions are common. A contributing factor here is that so long as pleasure is forthcoming, the teenager is relatively indifferent about whom he turns to or what means he uses for gratification. Philosophically this outlook represents a classic inversion of one form of Kant's categorical imperative, that is, people are always ends in themselves, they may never be merely means to an end. To the narcissist, people are always means, and only the self is an end.

In many ways, this kind of pathology lies within the province of disturbances of ideal formation. The child's behavior may reflect such pathology in a variety of ways. The omnipotence and grandiosity that are so characteristic of the syndrome are often a kind of caricature of the ideal self that the youngster strives to realize. Of course, the idealization can go either way; it can be self-directed or can turn outward to others. Idealization reserved for the self can lead to many authority battles; after all, if the child is already ideal, who are all those others—peers, parents, teachers, or police—to tell him how to be or what to do? On the other hand, if the orientation is toward the idealized other, then much of the behavior will represent the quest for this perfect parent, with endless testing and discovering that people are unreliable and imperfect. Any or all of the various forms of flight behavior (escaping in daydreams, dropping out of school, joining a cult, running away from home, resorting to drugs and alcohol, and attempting suicide) are likely to ensue as the youngster pursues a reunion with an idealized other.

The child's pervasive sense that he is himself ideal or is involved with idealized others tends to beget characteristic social attitudes: hauteur, arrogance, and contempt for the nonidealized, denigrated others. Inevitably, such behavior evokes challenge, rejection, and limit setting of some kind. When frustrated or denied, a pressing need for revenge flares up readily within the narcissist; indeed, "getting even" can be the ruling passion in his life. Because the youth is, in fact, enormously self-centered and demanding, he is always encountering frustrations of what he sees as his perogatives, and is accordingly angrily aggrieved a great deal of the time. Moreover, each such frustration or wound leaves a deep trace; the child experiences all these slights as profoundly personal injuries. The feeling is not so much: How can you deprive me of this? It takes on more of the character of: How can you deprive *me* of this, how can you do this to *me*? When the wound is experienced in so personal a fashion, the only response that holds any promise of relief is the act of repaying in kind, of making the author of the wounding feel exactly the same personal pain. Only this kind of action offers a measure of surcease; hence the preoccupation with revenge. In most such instances, the youngster realizes the revenge primarily in the form of fantasy; where, however, the youngster takes arms against his troubles and seeks to repay the psychic wound in physical fashion, some very serious and pathological behavior may well ensue. In the extreme cases, the rage can be literally murderous. Offer et al. (1979) believe that this narcissistic type is perhaps closest to the description of the psychopath that recurs so frequently in the classic psychiatric literature.

Separate sets of observers working with altogether different populations have independently arrived at very similar conclusions. Yochelson and Samenow (1976, 1977, 1986) have written extensively about what they call the "criminal mind," whose description is exactly that of the narcissistic delinquent. They stress the cognitive dimensions of the condition, emphasize these narcissistic mechanisms as a distinctive way of thinking, and assert that, more than any other single factor, this special cognitive pattern defines the serious delinquent.

To return to narcissism in general, however, the underlying psychopathology can be regarded developmentally. The grandiosity that is so central to these youngsters is a derivative of very early relationship states, in particular, the affinities of the infant in the first year of life, whose awe-inspiring caretaker seems omniscient and omnipotent. For a long time the baby clings to her and feels so very close that in effect he is one with her, fused with her, a part of her. Eventually he begins to detach from her in greater or lesser degree and goes through a vulnerable and difficult time. To help in this transition, the infant may carry some of the mother's grandiosity with him, or, even as he succeeds in separating, the baby may carry away a special need to be attached to some object of adoration, to be forever seeking such a person. If the child's major adaptive tactic has been to carry forward the sense of the grandiosity as part of himself, then he may later become a vain, self-aggrandizing, demanding individual. If, on the other hand, the infant continues to crave the external ideal, then he will be a joiner, sharing the grandiosity of the delinquent gang or the cult leader. If the youngster's earlier experience with an idealized other was with a sadistic or a battering parent, then he may later be drawn to a sadistic leader of a gang whose members join together to commit battery on others.

THE EMPTY-BORDERLINE DELINQUENT.   These youngsters are distant, poorly related, and immature. They have never developed an adequate sense of self; they are isolated people who remain basically unattached to others; within themselves they experience a quality of profound emptiness left behind by a developmental course that has never allowed them a full sense of connection to a caring parent.

From a developmental view, a genetic loading may make these children very vulnerable so that at best they require rather special parenting. In the nature of things, some members of this fragile group will encounter parents who are themselves disturbed; these parents are remote, depressed, alcoholic, or inconsistent, or they otherwise fail to meet the children's needs. As a result, these youngsters' development is arrested at a moment of primitive and poorly organized ego structuring. Thereafter, when their impulses and inner yearnings become overwhelming, they continue to be threatened by the eruption of bizarre and psychoticlike experience.

When not under stress, these youngsters are passive, uncommunicative, relatively unrelated, and have little to offer in terms of engagement with a therapist. They have never had an adequate degree of intimacy or caring from a loving mother and lack the outlook or the techniques that make for a successful social encounter. They are psychologically poised over a vortex of unfulfilled and primitive yearning that ever draws them in, and that they can keep at bay only by maintaining the defensive emptiness as a distancing device; accordingly, they fear closeness. They show little evidence of empathy and form poor or fleeting alliances with peers. With adults, they tend to be needy, passive, and dependent. These youngsters may resort to sexual promiscuity, somatic complaints, or antisocial behavior to attract some equivalent of, or substitute for, the yearned for but deeply repressed sense of desired connection with others. The antisocial behavior comes into play in this connection; its mission is to establish a kind of pseudorelationship with others. The child's behavior is often based on violence and provocativeness, which are among the readiest ways to bring about a simulacrum of interpersonal encounter. This kind of behavior will certainly engage controlling adults, and in this curious fashion the youngster achieves a version of connectedness and is helped to contain the dangerous inner pressures. On the other hand, when incarcerated and limited from further antisocial enacting, such youngsters may go through brief episodes of delusional or psychotic thinking. In the nature of things, they will go to great lengths to avoid such terrifying experiences. Need frustration will tend to evoke psychotic thinking and may lead to temper tantrums or running away. Suicidal impulses are often expressed at such times. A basic theme is likely to be the fear of loss and abandonment; at some level there is a pervasive desire for union or reunion, but often the child cannot articulate it, and the predominant affect is a feeling of emptiness. Functionally, the emptiness is a major defense against the primitive thoughts and affects that might otherwise overwhelm these troubled young people. There is a haunting quality of amorphousness and impoverishment to their characterological makeup; at best they are very hard to reach. They probably share some of the characteristics that the DSM-III-R assigns to the Schizotypal Personality Disorder.

THE DEPRESSED-BORDERLINE DELINQUENT. These youngsters exhibit the clinging, defiant, fluctuating, object-seeking behavior of the borderline, but they do not display the quality of emptiness found in the empty-borderline delinquent. Instead, they have had enough early relationship to allow themselves to feel the hurt of object longing, and to suffer pain and rage because of these unfulfilled needs. They are less likely to exhibit bouts of psychoticlike thinking and the accompanying fear of loss of contact; instead, their painful issue is the always threatened loss of object attachment. Much of their antisocial behavior is in response to frustrations in their object-seeking behavior; thus, if they are in therapy, they will characteristically act up in the face of the therapist's missing an hour or going on vacation. Their basic relationship paradigm is likely to involve many symbiotic elements with anaclitic depression actively present as part of the struggle with differentiation and separation. Object seeking is the dominant psychological presence in their lives; emotionally, they are very expressive and highly reactive, especially to frustration or the threat of loss; the rage and explosiveness with which they may greet disappointment and frustration in their relationships can lead to major acts of vandalism, violence, or self-injury.

Psychopathologically it is likely that the condition of these children is more akin to the affective than to the schizotypal disorders. They often harbor feelings of profound worthlessness that accompany their object hunger and their sense of confusion of self and other. Their delinquent behavior has much about it of seeking punishment and degradation in an attempt to appease the bayings of the depression; often it precipitates flamboyant and bizarre antisocial patterns. The depression can pass over rather readily into overtly suicidal behavior. There is, however, a great propensity for attachment, which makes a therapeutic relationship a valuable and critical factor in treating such youngsters.

Social Learning Theory

Although this approach was originally introduced by Bandura and Walters (1963), its chief spokesperson today is Gerald Patterson (1982).

As noted earlier, Patterson considers the lowest common denominator of conduct disorder to be disobedience. Whatever else the parents may state about their problem child, they always say, "He won't mind." Despite its specific varieties and behavioral shadings, for Patterson, this disobedience is the basic core of the condition.

A second common factor in the behavior of conduct-disordered children is the quality of arrested social development. If an investigator studies normal development and measures at different developmental levels the degree of erupting, complaining, invading someone else's boundaries, and troubling of other children that occurs, a high titer of such behavior normally appears at about 18 months of age and continues thereafter. As the normal toddler grows older, however, the level of such behavior usually decreases, so that by the start of grade school, it is only minimally present. In the case of the child with conduct disorder this decrease does not occur; such a child continues to act socially as he did at a very young age. Patterson offers three possible reasons for this: the child may be temperamentally different, like Chess's difficult child; the parents may have failed to reward compliance; or, the parents may have failed to punish noncompliance. Of the three, the latter is the most common. As a result of this omission in the child's socialization, the child is retarded in learning to respond to social stimuli, both in terms of obedience and in terms of general deportment.

The consequence is a double-edged problem for the child; in fact, two major disturbances in social learning ensue. The youngster learns to respond in deviant fashion with all the symptomatology of conduct disorder and the inevitable troubles that follow from such behavior; at the same time he suffers from a serious lack of the elementary social skills necessary for negotiating the vicissitudes of ordinary childhood social exchange. In other words, the youngster is in trouble with the adult world because of his conduct, and with the world of his peers because he does not know how to get along with other children or to engage in the normal give-and-take of peer exchange. The ensuing syndrome is the simultaneous expression of this learned deviancy and failed socialization.

As the condition develops the child adopts a host of delinquent values such as resorting to immediate gratification at the expense of pursuing long-term goals; attributing responsibility for his actions to factors outside himself; and using pain to control others, to enforce compliance with his wishes, and to obtain gratification.

Patterson describes two varieties of such children: the *Social Aggressors* and the *Stealers*. The difference arises from the differential training received by each group. Thus, the parents of Social Aggressors are helpless in the face of the child's direct defiance, and they resort to empty verbalizations (nattering) and scolding without directly forbidding the undesired behavior. Or, at the moment, they may thunder forth with dramatic threats—"No TV for a month!"—that they might enforce for a day, but which in all probability they never fully carry out. This response is, however, restricted to defiance; these parents really would not tolerate stealing or some of the more covert destructive behaviors, such as vandalism. The parents of the Stealers, on the other hand, would not tolerate direct defiance and would scotch that out of hand; but they turn a blind eye at such covert behavior as theft and staying out late at night. In each instance, over time, the behavior is shaped in keeping with the paradigm of what is tacitly permitted and what is forbidden.

The developmental necessity of childhood discipline, the punishing of undesirable acts, receives solid support from a number of large studies. One of the most interesting was the Cambridge-Somerville Youth Study, an ambitious effort to prevent delinquency by targeting a number of grade-school boys and pairing them, so that one received the benefit of a treatment program and the other did not. This project was initiated during the 1930s with plans to treat 325 boys. Unfortunately, the outbreak of World War II interrupted the study, and it was never completely carried out. Nonetheless, the researchers gathered a great deal of information on the background of the boys and their families, and, in particular, about the child-rearing practices employed in their homes. From the point of view of intervention, the project was a failure; if anything, over time (so great was the interest in this undertaking that a 30-year follow-up was accomplished), the treated youngsters had higher rates of delinquency and longer adult criminal records than did the untreated (McCord, 1982, cited in Achenbach, 1982). But the mass of data accumulated by the investigators was revealing in a different way. It was possible to link the kind of disciplinary pattern in the home with the boys' degree of subsequent difficulties. Thus, *all* of the boys whose parents were at once quarrelsome, neglectful, and lax in discipline became delinquent. However, where parents who were otherwise similar (i.e. quarrelsome and neglectful) used withdrawal of love as a disciplinary measure, only 14% became delinquent. More than that, when all the different types of home were reviewed, the lowest rate of delinquency (21%) was found in the settings where consistently punitive discipline was maintained. Where a more loving kind of discipline was employed, the rate rose to 27%. Where, on the other hand, lax or inconsistent discipline prevailed, then rates of 50% and 56% were recorded. The various contributions of parental laxness, quarrelsomeness, deviance, neglect, inconsistency, and hostility could be factored out, and each in its own way encouraged a pattern of delinquent response. There was no single characteristic profile (McCord et al., 1959; also cited in Achenbach, 1982).

These findings, however, highlight the role of aversive stimuli, that is, of significant punishment. It is echoed in the findings of another major study. Lee Robins followed up 524 individuals who had been seen in a child guidance clinic 30 years earlier. Parallel with these subjects she studied 100 control subjects from the same neighborhood. The study was remarkably complete and thorough. It found that 80% of the former clinic patients had adult psychiatric difficulties; of these, the largest percentage (22%) were considered sociopathic. (By way of contrast, at follow-up, only 2% of the controls fell into this category.) Among other items of note, however, was the observation that good patterns of parental discipline were the best preventive for sociopathy. Regardless of other negative factors, it seemed that this very malignant syndrome could be prevented by adequate controls and limits during childhood. The clinician can appreciate just how malignant the condition is by considering that to make the diagnosis, each child had to have at least six kinds of antisocial behavior and four episodes of such behavior—or one episode serious enough to merit court referral. As adults, 98% of the sample had been arrested for nontraffic offenses (Robins, 1974; also cited in Achenbach, 1982).

The evidence to date seems to indicate that utilizing punishment to set adequate limits during the formative years is the single most puissant element in the struggle against severe patterns of antisocial behavior. It will not prevent all such syndromes from appearing, nor, by itself, will it make for happy or well-adjusted adults. Optimally it should be linked with the many other positive elements that parents offer children and should be part of a wide spectrum of interactive behaviors. Nonetheless, the key reality is that the omission of adequate, consistent, and effective disciplinary practices is a dangerous and potentially destructive factor in child rearing.

Psychoanalytic Views

Psychoanalysts have been interested in those cases of conduct disorder that appear to represent a form of neurotic character organization and to express the same psychic mechanisms found in other neurotic character problems. Hence the language and concepts that describe character structure and neurosis are appropriate to conduct disorder as well.

Id Theory. The id is the great repository of the instincts, and it follows (within the framework of this theory) that if the aggressive instincts are too powerful or are insufficiently contained, then aggressive behavior will inevitably erupt. The word instinct has been subject to a great deal of challenge, definition, and redefinition. In recent years it has fallen into disrepute and has been replaced by the notion of drive or motivation. One theory asserts that an excess of aggression may be an innate component of the individual's personality makeup. This constitutional hypothesis suggests that aggressivity is genetic in nature and implies that an individual may be born with more than the normal share of such inner pressures. An alternative postulate is that intense early frustration or unempathic handling have resulted in an excess of rage. By the same reasoning, within the id there are erotic as well as aggressive impulses, and in some instances, the erotic motivations will be ascendant. A moderate degree of motivation will incline the individual to relate himself to his world as a loving, affectionate, warm sort of person. If such pressures are excessive, however, then the individual may have to cope with all the vicissitudes of hypersexuality.

Because professionals employ the image of these instincts (or drives or motivations) pressing to erupt into action and hence needing containment, it is necessary to ask: What contains them? Analytic theory describes two general classes of structures: The first is a part of the id, and the second belongs to the adjacent systems of ego and superego. This theory postulates that within the id, the erotic and the aggressive motivations tend to come together, to fuse, and thus to neutralize one another. This fusion of aggressive and erotic urges does not cancel out the associated energy, but instead converts it into a neutral form. As a result, the individual has a great deal of neutral energy available to apply to constructive purposes of his own choosing. This fusion produces the tempered emotional life that most people experience. If, however, the neutralization fails, and the aggressive motivations are released untempered and unchecked, then a great thrust of aggressive energy floods into the ego, with potentially catastrophic results. Unless this energy can be channeled in positive directions, the way is open for serious behavioral disturbance.

Ego Theory. Ego theory has long been at the center of psychoanalytic thinking, and investigators have suggested many sequences and mechanisms within its framework to help explain aggressive phenomena. Many of these concepts continue to provide the essential context for numerous other theoretical positions. In particular, this is true for the structure of the ego's mechanisms of defense, or, more briefly, the ego defenses (Freud, 1937).

Essentially the defenses are internal mechanisms that operate entirely out of consciousness. Nonetheless, they continuously work within the child's mind to help him contain his drives and adapt to his world. Because the defenses are outside of awareness, however, operationally the trained observer can discern the traces of their activity only by applying a series of outlines or templates to the child's behavior to make sense of what is happening within his mind. Thus, if a youngster is very angry at his mother, and insists that it is she who is angry at him, the examiner will place the template "projection" against the boy's behavior and measure it for applicability. In general, these defenses comprise a series of internal operations, or techniques of thought, that make it easier for a child to cope with his drives, and with his world. A few examples might best illustrate these ideas.

A young man, Thomas, has met a young woman, Susan, whom he likes very much. One day, he is walking along beside her when he sees Jim, a good friend of many years, coming toward them. Jim, a very popular young man in his own right, has not previously met the young woman. Feeling called upon to make introductions, Thomas says, "Susan, I'd like you to meet, ugh, tell her what your name is will you?" Suddenly, at the last second, despite their many years of familiarity, Thomas has forgotten Jim's name.

The mental mechanism involved is called *repression*. It takes form as this kind of forgetting—an apparently incomprehensible slip of the mind, which on the surface is meaningless. If a therapist were to explore Thomas's lapse in detail, however, he or she would likely discover that Thomas has always felt a bit in awe of Jim's social presence and attractiveness to girls and feared accordingly that once Jim met Susan, she would at once turn to Jim and away from himself. Thomas really did not want to introduce them, and that feeling was represented by repressing (forgetting) Jim's name.

Other such defense mechanisms include displacement, reaction formation, isolation, denial, splitting, introjection, identification, doing and undoing, avoidance, conversion, somatization, and rationalization. All of these operations of the psyche are dedicated to coping with the inner and outer stresses while keeping anxiety at bay. The mechanisms are normal and universal; they become problematic when the individual addresses primitive operations to mature issues, or where excessive employment of a given mechanism dominates the psychic life of the individual.

A number of mental mechanisms tend most commonly to be associated with conduct disorder. There are, in particular, several that the clinician must keep in mind, because in clinical situations they reappear with striking regularity in association with disturbed and disturbing behavior. These tactics include the counterphobic defense, turning a passive role into an active role, identification with the aggressor, externalization, and projection. Other mechanisms that may play a secondary role are also described below.

THE COUNTERPHOBIC DEFENSE. This mechanism is concerned primarily with anxiety; it allows the inclined individual to cope with inner fears. The person who utilizes this mechanism has learned early that anxiety is extremely unpleasant; he tries to get away from the feeling as soon as it appears. The person prone to this defense will seek to quell anxiety by engaging in risk-taking behavior. That is to say, the individual unconsciously turns things about and pursues the threatening situation as though it were attractive. Behaviorally, he courts the dangerous and the frightening; for such a person, the hazardous is pleasurable and exciting— or if not pleasurable, it is nonetheless a challenge to which he must respond. Because risk-taking behavior does not necessarily imply abrogating the rights of others, clearly some other elements must be present to drive the pursuit of hazards in an antisocial direction. Properly contained and redirected, such a counterphobic tendency might incline a person to be a racing car driver, a mountain climber, or even a speculator on the commodities market. Whenever some heroic individual is driven to do some daring feat "because it's there," it is always possible that at least part of the motive was not just that it was there, it was also frightening. The danger, in particular, was a peculiar seduction for the counterphobic.

For this counterphobic tendency to take form as conduct disorder, however, the child must have to have some sort of problem with authority, some additional increment such as a need for revenge, or a disturbance in judgment. More specifically, the chief source of the anxiety in such cases is likely to be the fear of punishment (on an unconscious level, perhaps, the fear of castration) at the hands of some established authority, be it father, teacher, policeman, employer, and so on. Given such an additional factor, the youngster with counterphobic tendencies will be particularly provocative and challenging to authority. The message is "See what I'm doing? I am not intimidated by you. No matter how big you are, I don't care if you punish me!" Or it may take the form of "Go ahead and do your worst, you can't scare me, see if I care!" Such youngsters may engage in some very troubling and dangerous behavior indeed.

TURNING A PASSIVE ROLE INTO AN ACTIVE ROLE. One of the most elementary forms of mastery is to shift from the status of the victim to the role of the perpetrator. Almost anyone who has ever felt mistreated (and who has not?) has reversed things in fantasy: if only I were the tough guy on the schoolyard, boy, what I would do to him! If only I were the teacher and she was a pupil in my class, would I show her!

The wish to escape from the passive role of being helpless, vulnerable, and subordinate to take on an active and dominant position is a powerful motivator. On both a conscious and an unconscious level, it may be a guiding presence in the child's life, and he may focus much goal-directed behavior on achieving just that outcome: to reverse a formerly passive position by converting the self into an active agent.

During early childhood there is often little chance to cope successfully with various assaults and indignities. When the passivity has entailed deprivation of essential material and emotional nurturance, physical and psychological abuse, or any other serious mistreatment, then the need to reverse positions may become the dominant theme in the child's life. The result is a driven need to dominate sadistically or to mistreat others so that they now are forced into a subordinate, victimized role, and to play this out over and over again in an effort to efface the earlier pain, rage, humiliation, and sense of helplessness. Conduct disorder is a very natural outcome of some children's early experiences, and this mechanism is often the central hinge on which the behavior swings.

IDENTIFICATION WITH THE AGGRESSOR. First described by Anna Freud (1936/1946), this mechanism is really a version of the passive-into-active sequence, except that it seeks to undo the impact of a relationship with a particular individual. The element of specificity involved gives this behavior its unique character. It is basic to such phenomena as child battering, where the involved parent may be caught up in repeating with the child exactly what he or she experienced as a child at the hands of a particular caretaker. The explosion of violent behavior can come as a rush of response that the individual neither desires nor prefers, nor, in many instances, can control; in a sense it "happens" to the person.

Unlike the conversion of a passive role into an active role, this mechanism is not so much a general trend of character as a rather specific reliving of a given set of circumstances; the entire sequence is kindled by the appropriate triggering stimuli. It is a kind of remembering, not through recollection but through reenactment. The result can be cruel, violent, and destructive to an extraordinary degree.

EXTERNALIZATION. A more common kind of mechanism that does not necessarily give rise to troublesome behavior but is an accompanying defense in many aggressive sequences is called *externalization*. It involves a process not unlike projection. In brief, the child employing this mechanism will unconsciously (all these mechanisms are incomprehensible unless the reader keeps in mind that they are unconscious—and can never become conscious) take his inner fantasy of how people behave and turn it out on his external world, so that the youngster lives in an environment of his own creation. In a very real sense everyone tends to do this, but normally people have available the corrective capacity that comes with ego maturity and good reality testing. In the cases of conduct disorder, however, the corrective capacity is lacking or is insufficient. If a vulnerable child's parents and siblings have been jealous, manipulative, or noncaring and withholding, then he will see the people about him enacting just those attitudes and will manipulate relationships with them to bring about the mind-set that he seeks. The child will respond to their kindness with cynicism, to their bids for friendliness with mistrust, and to their attempts at cooperation with suspiciousness. As time goes on, the youngster will drive away those who approach, will evoke the worst in those with whom he works or consorts, and ultimately will recreate the whole tragic and traumatic environment in which he was hurt, thus proving to himself that that's the way people really are. It therefore follows for such a child that whatever a person does to get what he can or to keep what he has gotten is altogether justified. Although not inherently or necessarily a source of antisocial conduct, this orientation provides a fertile site for such behavior.

As a result, the child who is inclined to employ this mechanism is very much at risk. If he is brought up in a pathological household, he will continue to live that way forever, moving from one unhappy work experience to another, going through one bad marriage after another, and, in the more extreme cases, engaging in one antisocial act after another. The lives of such youngsters are marked by suspiciousness, provocativeness, mistrust, quarrelsomeness, and the same lack of respect for the boundaries of others that characterized the treatment they received in their own childhood homes.

PROJECTION. This mechanism allows the person to escape the onus of unwanted feelings. It differs from externalization in that *projection* is confined to specific affects; unlike externalization, projection does not imply expecting others to play given roles or to offer anticipated responses. It involves attributing to others the uncomfortable feelings and emotions that the child would otherwise have to experience as part of himself—and which he finds intolerable and rejects. Whatever the youngster experiences as distressing or unacceptable (e.g., hatred, the desire to torture or to kill, a homosexual yearning, a desire to dominate) is immediately and automatically attributed to someone else: It is not *my* feeling, it is *his*, or *hers*. This holds true for both erotic and aggressive feelings, and especially for such commonly rejected emotions as homosexual yearnings. The affected person might feel that others are looking at or gesturing to him in an erotic fashion; there is an accompanying conviction that the other person's feelings are the cause of the problem. Many degrees of disturbance are possible with this mechanism, and the majority of people who employ it are not dangerous and do not act on their concerns. They might worry or brood about them, or feel tormented or enraged; they might be endlessly suspicious of their lovers or spouses; they might feel picked on or mistreated by teachers or employers; and, all in all, life might be very hard for individuals with this paranoid attitude. From time to time, however, the affected youngster is so haunted by the resulting suspicions and feelings of threat, that he is driven to take action against people who he believes are offending or who are about to offend against him; violent behavior may follow. This very primitive mechanism stems from early development and is frequently part of psychotic disturbances. It is by no means confined to the severely mentally ill, however, and it is a common aspect of the psychic organization of many of the more serious conduct disorder patients.

OTHER MECHANISMS. Researchers have described a number of other mechanisms that have contributed in one way or another to shifting problem solving in the direction of inappropriate action. Thus, attempting to deny some painful reality by leaping into action, or trying to assert the reality of the self by enacting the impulse instead of merely thinking can serve as a sense of validation or proof of identity. Action seems to offer a kind of reassurance to some predisposed individuals. The child may use action as a bid to obtain much-needed controls; he may use it to indicate that he is about to lose control, in effect as a "cry for help." In each case inner experience becomes involved in an outward expression that may take form as antisocial behavior.

Superego Mechanisms. According to Freud's structural theory, the third great agency of mind is the superego, which is essentially the repository of the regulatory apparatus of personality—the conscience and the ego-ideal. The conscience acts to keep impulse at bay, to warn of potential transgressions, to forbid certain wished-for instinctual fulfillments, to inhibit the expression of even highly desired pleasure-seeking activities, and, where all this has failed, to punish the ego for its forbidden behavior.

The superego is also the bearer of the ideal part of the self, the so-called ego-ideal, which is the inner model of how the person would like to be, his sense of the perfect self. All people yearn to achieve to some goal, to live up to some model of ultimate wealth, wisdom, success, beauty, or achievement. Somewhere within is a sense of the ideal self, and, indeed, the child's feeling of self-contentment will often be a measure of how well he has approached this ideal state at any given point. The everyday sense of self-esteem that people experience is a function of how far away from or how close they feel to their ego-ideal.

Superego pathology takes many forms and usually has serious consequences. If the superego is too weak or is unable to resist impulse, then a major protector against troublesome behavior is not functioning, and the child is likely to be in social difficulties a great deal of the time. His personality makeup lacks the major instrumentality that keeps people socialized and civilized, and instead of controlling himself automatically and suitably, he will tend repeatedly to act inappropriately and impulsively until society looks at him askance. Indeed, failure of superego control is one of the major mechanisms at work in the organic brain syndrome; the old dictum used to be, for example, that the superego is soluble in alcohol. It appears as if certain types of organic insult tend to affect the higher inhibitory and regulatory mechanisms before they impinge on the impulses or the potential to act on them.

If a youngster's superego is not so much weak as awry, then he is woefully out of step with the society within which he lives and is dubbed a sociopath. Thus, a youth who has a reasonably good superego but who is taught criminal values from infancy will have a difficult time adapting to his larger society. Here the problem is not so much superego function as superego content.

SUPEREGO LACUNAE. A special form of superego defect was described by Adelaide Johnson (1952). She called the condition *superego lacunae* and described a state of affairs where, from early on, a hiatus has existed in the values conveyed to a child by a pathological family. Often the message is subtle and indirect; the mother says to the 3-year-old, "Johnny, bring me my purse and mind you, don't open it up and look into it." The child might have had no thought of opening the purse; however, once he perceives his mother's covert interest in having him do so, he complies. When she discovers what he has done, she becomes very angry, but somehow she conveys that, despite all the protestations, she is quite pleased with him, and the pattern is set.

A more recent view of this mechanism has arisen from family systems theory. According to this theory the parents are ridden with problematic impulses against which they struggle. Consciously they repudiate these erotic or aggressive wishes, and in the effort to control them, the parents project them into their offspring, who accept the assigned roles and enact them.

Particularly in the teens the tendency of youngsters to enact their parents' covert hints can be striking. A mother may tell her daughter before a date: "If you allow the boy to touch you here or here or there, you are lost; you will never be able to control yourself." Thus primed, the youngster gets into her boyfriend's car, and, indeed, in no time at all she is carried away. Later on, the mother protests to the doctor, "I told her, I warned her, but she wouldn't listen." The real problem is that the girl *did* listen and heard her mother's powerful covert message that she should not resist but should give in immediately and become sexually involved.

Johnson believed that such a child-rearing pattern created a sort of Swiss cheese superego with major gaps in its integrity. As the parents gave the youngster cues, the parental impulse would ride right through the superego defect and the youngster would comply by performing some antisocial act.

CRIMINAL FROM A SENSE OF GUILT. This mechanism was first described by Sigmund Freud (1957b) and is the source of much paradoxical antisocial behavior. The paradox arises because to all intents and purposes the perpetrator of the misdeed seems on some level to want to be caught. He may announce the intent to misbehave (or to commit a crime) in advance; he carries out the act in what is often a surprisingly public context; and he is likely to leave major and obvious evidence as to his identity at the site of the action. Not infrequently the youngster hangs around the scene and involves himself with the investigators, be they parents or police, hinting that he knows something about it, was a witness, or is otherwise involved. As a result, the child is frequently apprehended and punished, protesting all the while that he is innocent. To complete the picture, after the youngster is released or has otherwise paid his "debt to society," he proceeds to do the same thing again. Caretakers very quickly get the feeling that it is useless to punish such a youngster; it doesn't change anything, in fact, in the child's intrusively obstreperous way, he seems to want to be punished.

Exploring such cases is difficult. These youngsters can be endlessly provocative and, if pressed to explain their behavior, they have no interest in looking into themselves; if anything they ward off such attempts with considerable vigor. However, in the occasional circumstance where it is possible to achieve a measure of exploration with them, clinicians often discover that such children suffer from a profoundly neurotic process (no great surprise considering their inconsistent behavior) that seems at odds with the nature of their acts.

In brief, their problem is an excess of conscience. They are, in fact, a hag-ridden group, whose conscience is so severe, cruel, and unrelentingly sadistic that there is no enduring it. If allowed free play, this inner tormentor would drive them to self-mutilation or to suicide; at best it would plunge them into profound depression. This is an essentially unendurable state of mind, and the need to avoid it is immense. The affected individual is driven to blunt the agony and find relief from the danger.

By means of repression, the child first manages to mask the superego (the agent of conscience) so that it is out of sight albeit definitely not out of mind. This helps a little, but not very much. The voice of conscience may be stilled, but the sense of inner discomfort is not eased, and there is a terrible feeling of constant threat and inner wrongness. The youngster is tense all the time, often nervous and hyperactive. He feels troubled; perhaps there is a sense of impending doom; at any rate something is wrong. The unawareness is there because the conscience is masked, but the anxious nervous feeling remains because it is still pressing. The next step is therefore crucial, for at this juncture the person must accomplish a difficult trick. To relieve the inner discomfort he must externalize his conscience and turn it out on his world—and he must do so with no awareness that this is happening. If the child succeeds, he now is free of an inner burden, but he begins to experience the people about him as sadistic critics and inimical presences who want nothing so much as to punish and humiliate him. The youngster is infinitely more comfortable feeling spurned and despised, however, and can settle down. Faced with an external threat, he knows what is wrong and what to do about it. Accordingly, the child lashes back by provoking, attacking, and mistreating these hostile others and lives in a state of endless conflict and clash with his environment. Although emotionally the child may be relatively comfortable, somehow he cannot let well enough alone but must forever be getting into the kind of difficulty that leads to punishment. Life becomes a long litany of depredations and retaliations, of incessant friction and confrontation. Despite intelligence, talent, or lucky breaks, the child is forever a loser. Somehow his efforts always go wrong, and once again he faces catastrophe.

Withal, the youngster is making a good deal with himself. If he were to face his superego, he would be driven to die—emotionally if not physically—and perhaps physically as well. With the system externalized, the child can lie, hide, run away for a while, get a lawyer, put on an act, try to convince a judge; he has a chance to bargain or manipulate. With the inner voice of conscience there is no such recourse and no hope; it is all-seeing and knows the evil of the child's thoughts and intents, not to mention his deeds—he would simply be lost as the psychotically depressed are lost, with no way out. So the child's choice is in a way a sensible one, and he lives out Freud's formula: The child is a criminal from a sense of guilt.

TREATMENT

Inevitably, any discussion of treatment for so protean a condition as conduct disorder must consider the various etiologies and the allied disturbances that may underlie the disordered behavior. At the same time, at least a few general issues are indigenous to the diagnosis.

Of first order of importance is the site of treatment. The clinician must address two main questions with conduct disorder. The first question is, How dangerous is the child? The second question is, To what extent does the environment provoke and/or contribute to the disturbing behavior? These are always critical factors, and the would-be therapist has to carefully estimate how possible it would be to maintain the child in his "natural" setting (home, school, and neighborhood), as against removing him from some or all of these environments. To be sure, in many instances the question does not even arise; the child has made a serious suicide attempt, or has set dangerous fires, or is on some kind of wild rampage that is terrifying the neighborhood. Authorities then have no choice but to place the youngster somewhere, usually a hospital, where he can be safely contained long enough to allow for a meaningful evaluation.

The factors that determine the possibility of working within the home context fall chiefly within the considerations of dangerousness but reflect as well the psychosocial status of the parents, the child–parent relationship, and the ability of work to go on while the child continues to live within the sometimes fevered interactive broil of the pathological family process. Even where the child is not manifestly dangerous at a given moment, a meaningful diagnostic study might be impossible if frequent separations and episodes of running away characterize a particular familial milieu. Under such conditions it might be wise to hospitalize the youngster just to allow for a cooling-off period, as well as to give the evaluator a chance to see what the youngster looks like away from the family arena.

For milder cases, it may be possible to do the entire evaluation while the child continues to live at home. An outpatient study can also be conducted if the child has been placed in a foster home temporarily. In any case, choosing the site of treatment is a critical decision and must be made early; it is frequently the key to allowing an appropriate address to the issues.

Assuming, then, that the evaluator has a reasonably workable situation, some essential data must be amassed for each such case. Given the multiple syndromes that can find expression as conduct disorder, the workup must be unusually thorough (Lewis, 1981a, 1981b).

An exhaustive inquiry into biological factors is always in order, with particular attention to the evidence for or against drug use, ADHD, and any of the findings associated with temporal lobe syndrome; the diagnostician should give additional thought to the possible presence of unsuspected genetic, metabolic, and endocrine conditions. Neurological evaluation should be routine to rule out the possibility of an expanding lesion or of a degenerative disease, and genetic consultation may be indicated if the therapist detects any hint of unusual appearance (dysmorphism) or the presence of stigmata.

The direct interview with the child is likely to be a particularly rich source of diagnostic information. The evaluator should carefully screen for possible major mental illness and attempt to assess the youngster's affective state as well as to weigh any hints of possible thought disorder. In particular, he or she should rigorously examine the child's mental status and systematically explore each component (orientation, perceptual clarity, cognitive status, comprehension, information, short-term memory, long-term memory, ability to organize thoughts, thought patterns under stress, attunement to social nuances, interpersonal effectiveness, stability of level of consciousness, impulse awareness, impulse management, etc.). In addition, the interviewer should evaluate the child's status in the following areas: understanding of the issues that have brought them together; acceptance of responsibility for his actions; insight level; amount of observing ego that is present; character and degree of reliance on both normal and pathological defenses; type and quality of interpersonal attachments (with family members, neighbors, peers, and teachers); ideals and ethical standards, with a special exploration for the presence or absence of delinquent values; capacity for genuine remorse and concern for others; outlook on the future and on career possibilities. Finally, the interviewer should try to probe the nature of the youngster's fantasy and dream life (insofar as it is possible to obtain an in-depth view).

Along with the direct work with the youngster, considerable work is necessary with the parents. In particular, the examiner should elicit a full and meticulous developmental history with a specific search for the details of perinatal events and first-year-of-life experiences. To this should be added a complete health history with special stress on any history of accidents, ingestions, and previous hospitalizations. Moreover, information should be sought from school and other settings where the youngster may previously have been treated. Finally, the diagnostician should be in contact with a separated or otherwise absent parent if possible.

The direct study of the family is of particular significance for this syndrome, and a variety of contexts for family encounter are necessarily in order (the parents individually, the parents as a couple, the parents and child together, the parents and all the children together, home visits, etc.). From all this a working unit (some particular grouping of family members) should presently emerge as the most effective site for the focus of therapeutic energies. Whatever the context, the therapist needs to ascertain the ability of the family to keep appointments, to cooperate with suggestions, to implement recommendations, and to explore its own difficulties. This dimension of the study should be proceeding parallel with the psychiatric and psychological examinations of the child.

In that connection, it is safe to say that more than most disturbances, conduct disorder should be evaluated with the help of psychological testing. The possibility of some serious emotional condition masking itself as bad behavior is too well documented to allow for any degrees of freedom in the thoroughness of such a study. In the presence of educational problems, neuropsychological testing should also be included to assess the more subtle possibilities of learning disability that are so often present.

As the evaluation proceeds, the clinician begins to formulate a plan for therapeutic intervention. Most cases, by and large, require a combination of approaches because there is seldom only one problem that needs attention. Whatever the initial or the underlying difficulty, by the time the situation comes to therapeutic attention there is already a mix of issues. Schoolwork is in trouble; the family has hardened some of its attitudes and has ascribed a negative role to the youngster (the family pest, the troublemaker, the exception, the outsider, the cause of all the family's problems, etc.); the child's own self-esteem has usually come to ruin or is maintained at an unrealistic pitch of grandiosity; physical health problems are often present; the neighborhood is complaining; and the juvenile court may be involved and require a report. A host of secondary troubles are likely to be in the picture along with, and, indeed, as part of the conduct disorder syndrome.

Hence, from the outset, the clinician is generally working on a variety of fronts.

In addition to that, however, there is a synergistic interplay among the various interventions, and the usual experience is that each supports and enhances the effects of the other. Thus, the use of psychopharmacological agents goes well with individual psychotherapy, and the two together do better than either alone. Similarly, the child in individual therapy might benefit from simultaneous involvement with group treatment; the two together might move the youngster along a great deal more rapidly than either single modality. Family therapy might need some special evaluation along this dimension; some cases seem to do best if the work is confined to the family context, whereas others do much better if the child has at once family and individual work—but in separate contexts.

Because of the multiple etiologic forces at work and the complex and multifaceted symptomatology so often encountered, the evaluater's initial vision of diagnostic possibilities is often blurred. The delineation of a specific diagnostic picture is likely to emerge slowly. Somewhat paradoxically, one factor that investigators had thought would help sculpt the outlines of the condition was the child's response to psychopharmacological treatment. However, further research has made it clear that the response to stimulants, for example, is nonspecific; even normal children will show a discernible effect when given such medication. The key diagnostic information is likely to be obtained from detailed history taking. A prolonged history of violating the rules of social conduct and of overstepping the bounds of appropriate social behavior is the defining reality of the condition. In addition, the quality of the child's relatedness to parents, peers, teachers, and authority figures, and particularly to the examiner, is a major component of the profile that will emerge. The youngster defines the nature of the condition in a variety of ways: his quality of eruptiveness or even of menace, his smooth gliding over past misdeeds with glib justifications and rationalizations, his winning confession to minor misconduct while suppressing mention of far more serious misbehavior, his ready projection of responsibility on everyone about for whatever has happened. With conduct disorder, the child's own statements become a particularly important part of diagnostic thinking.

Both diagnostic and therapeutic decisions will hang on the quality of the family's functioning. The degree of defensiveness, denial, and rationalization to which the family normally resorts; the sense of preferring to turn inward and defend against the world, as against the readiness to turn outward and to cope with the world; the roles assigned to the various family members (in particular, to the index patient); the levels and forms of overt psychopathology of the various family members and the ways these affect interpersonal bonds within the family—all these will define the optimal form of treatment approach as well as the limits of therapeutic possibility.

Given the numerous school difficulties these youngsters characteristically display, the use of the school as a diagnostic sounding board as well as the availability of special educational resources are often key factors in sorting out the nature of the condition as well as in helping the particular child past his immediate distress. Close integration of the educational, diagnostic, and therapeutic efforts is a necessary condition for getting the best out of each.

Most conduct-disordered children probably have no discernible biological disturbance. They are borderline, narcissistic, or oppositional and, for the most part, manifest characterological psychopathology. This throws the major burden on the various psychological interventions and requires intensive work on the part of both the family and the therapist.

Where efforts at outpatient work do not succeed and the youngster's depredations continue, it is sometimes necessary to interrupt such therapy and place the child in the hospital (or other residential setting). Usually, the containment of the hospital structure as well as the separation from the parents results in at least a temporary subsidence of the disturbing behavior. Characteristically, hospital settings use many behavioral modes of intervention, such as restrictions of privilege, a token economy, a level system, time out, selective patterns of rewarding behavior, and seclusion rooms. Some of the settings that accept youngsters for long-term treatment also resort to wet-sheet packs and/or cuff restraints. Much creative thought has focused on the design of a therapeutic milieu, with such concepts as the life space interview (Redl & Wineman, 1957) introduced to describe some of the ongoing therapeutic tactics of this work. It falls to the staff to perform the necessary limit-setting, confrontation, empathic support, and external soothing that these troubled youngsters require. Marohn and colleagues (1980) have described perhaps the most sophisticated milieu design for this group. These authors specify an environment that focuses on a careful ordering of time, a recognition of the meaning of space, an evaluation of the psychological import of things and objects, a constant exploration and revaluation of the role of persons in the youngster's life, and a commitment to the idea that behavior and inner experience are understandable. The basic message permeating the milieu is that it is a place to do the hard work of gradually exploring and unraveling the dynamic messages concealed within the disturbing actions that characterize the patient's adjustment.

A number of settings have specialized in treating youngsters with drug problems. By and large, such agencies tend to emphasize the role of group confrontation, with the young patients being challenged, criticized, and "taken apart" by their peers as a mode of puncturing the defensive stances that maintain their pathology. Side by side with this, a spiritual revival kind of atmosphere is created as part of the milieu. Such settings typically employ recovered addicts as staff members because they can speak to the youngsters with singular authenticity.

No single form of psychotherapy has been put forward that is likely to help all such cases. Thus, Offer's four diagnostic types (Offer et al., 1979) would suggest the following therapeutic requirements. Dynamic, psychoanalytically oriented psychotherapy would be indicated in working with the depressed borderline. Such an approach, however, would probably be less predictably useful for the empty borderline, who would need at least some form of additional supportive or directive treatment. Similarly, the narcissistic patient could be approached by depth psychological means if the therapist could maintain the child in a safe environment for an extended period of time. But it will often take years to accomplish therapeutic goals with such a case, and the youngster might well require residential treatment for much of that time. The impulsive delinquent, on the other hand, would probably not respond to such tactics and would need a combination of ego-supportive techniques, such as a group approach within a tightly structured setting, plus a certain amount of directive individual guidance.

Not all families lend themselves to family therapy; there are situations that are so aberrant as to allow for only a spotty and fragmented kind of family work—if any. As a generalization, however, it seems fair to say that family psychopathology is so consistently a part of the background of conduct disorder that, regardless of whatever other modalities are being invoked, family work should always receive primary consideration. In particular, where the youngster is placed in a setting for an extended period, such continuing work with the family is critically important. Lacking this, whatever gains the therapeutic efforts directed toward the child achieve within the milieu are likely to be negated by the inevitable family efforts to restore the prior pathogenic equilibrium.

In this connection it is worth considering the suggestions advanced by Patterson (1982). He recommends that where possible, the clinician should institute a pattern of family management to address the specific etiologic sources of the difficulty, such as inadequate child-rearing skills, by utilizing a set of practices called *Systematic Common Sense*. The essence of the work is to have the families develop clearly stated house rules, to monitor actively the enforcement of the rules, to design and apply a defined and predictable pattern of punishments (contingent consequences) when a rule is broken, and to learn and carry through on a program of practical problem solving for the difficulties that do arise. The house rules spell out what is and what is not acceptable behavior. The monitoring refers to the parents' checking to make sure the rules are being obeyed, making sure as well that they know where the child is at any given time. Such a program often involves a great deal of effort. It requires teaching the parents the criteria of both acceptable and unacceptable behavior. In terms of punishment, it has been observed that strictness rather than happiness is the surest guarantor of good behavior (Rutter, 1979). The parents of antisocial children engage in a great deal of punishmentlike activity, but they do not confront the specific behavior at the time with a firm "no," and, if they do mete out a punishment, they do not carry it through. Instead they nag in a generally critical, complaining way, or they fly into a rage and become violent. To teach the proper forms of management, the therapeutic team must monitor the parents as carefully as they would have the parents work with the child.

Finally, with respect to problem solving, the parents have to learn how to set up a contract with their child. Whether or not it is written down, the point is to achieve sensible, agreed-upon, clearly stated expectations and specific consequences. If implemented, such measures can bring a modicum of order into the chaotic family life. According to Patterson, these elements are lacking in the way conduct-disordered children are reared, and the therapeutic work must correct the areas of specific deficit.

Kazdin et al. (1987) have found a combination of parent management training and problem-solving social skills training to be most effective.

Pharmacological treatment for conduct disorder is tentative and empirical; indeed, because of the lack of specificity (no available agent treats conduct disorder as such), there is a distinct quality of trial and error in undertaking such interventions. For example, the child with suspected temporal lobe pathology who has no overt seizures is likely nonetheless to be tried on carbamazepine (Tegretol). The clinician does this as a rule on the outside chance that it might help the child's state of general eruptive and irritable explosiveness. Enough cases appear to have responded to such treatment to make this a rather common procedure in attempting to deal with these often difficult and baffling therapeutic problems. There is no really good evidence that this medication helps much in the absence of seizures, but anecdotal accounts of success perpetuate the practice.

In a similar fashion, the neuroleptics are resorted to if a schizophrenic syndrome is suspected, and tricyclic antidepressants are likely to be administered where the patient meets at least some of the criteria for depressive disorder. In this connection, professionals in the field have now been alerted to the possible presence of manic or hypomanic conditions. A number of older teenagers come in with family histories of bipolar affective illness, and the teenagers themselves display recurrent episodes of eruptiveness or states of high irritability and chronic aggressiveness. Under such conditions, a good many of these patients are said to have been helped by lithium. At the same time, no consistent picture of the atypical cases who also respond to lithium has yet appeared.

In sum, as the nature of the problem begins to emerge from the accumulation of evaluative data, a number of primary diagnostic possibilities will suggest themselves. To the extent that some form of temporal lobe syndrome or a schizophrenic or affective disorder is suspected, or is clearly evident, the appropriate therapeutic intervention for that condition is a priori indicated.

To the extent that no specific therapy is indicated, then the therapist might resort to nonspecific therapy, for example, small doses of neuroleptics to decrease aggression.

Although a specific medication may be essential for treatment (e.g., in a case where a temporal lobe syndrome is, in fact, present), medication by itself does not begin to solve all the child's problems. The need to work with the environment, the home, the school, or the court continues to be a commanding presence in the therapist's calculations, and a site for major therapeutic investment. The use of multimodal therapy is the rule with such cases, and under ideal conditions the youngster will be engaged in a variety of ways. Group and family therapy alongside the individual work should be a routine consideration whenever treating such youngsters, and all this should parallel any psychopharmacologic approach.

There is today an uncertain quality to the approach to treatment for these youngsters. Nevertheless, the therapist's guiding principle must be to leave no stone unturned in seeking to provide relief for the child, the family, and society.

CONCLUSION

Whatever its form or its details, the ultimate outcome of a treatment attempt for conduct disorder can be assessed only over the long term. With any of the interventions referred to above, it is all too easy to obtain apparent short-term successes, with the child presently reverting back to miscreant behavior. It is important to follow through on treatment efforts, to carry the child past the residential placement, to stay with the case after a particular intervention has diminished the acting up, to keep in touch after the youngster has been placed in a special educational program. There is a stickiness to behavioral symptoms that probably reflects their early roots and long-standing presence before the child ever receives therapeutic attention. These factors, along with the disturbed familial patterns that maintain them and the social identities that such youngsters presently come to acquire, all establish and preserve the chronicity of the child's difficulties. Treating these conditions requires patience and dedication, but the pain and disability that the therapist can thus prevent make the effort worthwhile.

APPENDIX 13–1
DISORDERED CONDUCT: THE FORMS OF
ANTISOCIAL BEHAVIOR

Detailing some of the kinds of behavior that are usually subsumed under the rubric conduct disorder is not an easy task. Many different patterns of action, in various forms or under different circumstances, can become part of the conduct disorder syndrome. To give them a measure of organization, a distinction will be drawn (somewhat arbitrarily) between serious configurations of behavioral disturbance and merely troublesome aspects of enactment. The material to follow will therefore be divided into two sections. The first section is a list of some of the more common forms of disordered (antisocial) activity that are problematic in and of themselves. These will be designated as *direct*. Then there will follow a roster of some action patterns commonly associated with the basic expression of the disorder, yet which have a different, a less invasive, or at any rate a less dangerous or disturbing quality than do the direct behaviors. These will be described as *adjunctive*. The terms direct and adjunctive are not intended to convey any hint of etiologic force; they seek merely to clarify the distinction between figure and ground.

Direct Disordered Behavior

Although no attempt will be made to provide an exhaustive listing of the forms that conduct disorder can take, these examples will give some sense of the protean varieties and the many alternative dynamic factors involved in this group of disturbances.

Runaway. Running away is quite common and takes many forms: Some children run only to their grandmother's home to tell her how badly they are being treated by their stepfather; others take flight without any specific destination in mind but simply because the behavior has become erotized, and the initial moment of freedom carries with it a veritably erotic thrill. Some youngsters run away repeatedly and get arrested for antisocial acts as a regular part of the sequence; this is typical of children who begin a pattern of prostitution during such escapades. For many it is a preliminary attempt at suicide. When running away becomes habitual and when bad things start to happen during these episodes, the behavior should be regarded as a major problem.

The dynamics of the runaway are multiple and complex. Many children from all socioeconomic levels leave home because they are not wanted and are told this in so many words; they become the throwaway children who are cast forth by rejecting homes. Some youngsters become wanderers because they are in a state of extreme adolescent rebellion, and they either cannot abide the parents' assertions of authority or are bound and determined to get even with them. Others leave because they are being sexually or sadistically abused, and their mounting resentment of this treatment finally drives them away. Still others depart because they are mentally ill, and their voices tell them to go. Many children in poverty areas live amid highly stressful home arrangements where crisis-ridden and depleted parents have little to offer them; the youngsters may end up hanging around street corners and sleeping wherever they can to avoid a drunken father who wants to batter them, or they may find their way to pimps and a life of prostitution to obtain some simulacrum of care and affection.

One of the commonest underlying equations is the youth's attempt to master an early experience of object loss. The significant other ran out on the child when he was small, needy, and helpless; the traumatic impact of the experience has never healed; and now the youngster would master it by running out on those who hurt him (or those who stand in their place). The mechanism involved is turning the passive role into the active role, transforming the passive victim into the active perpetrator. It is one of the basic means of human coping, and underlies a great deal of antisocial behavior.

Gambling. Although gambling is typically associated with the difficulties and pleasures of adult life, some teenagers become enamored of slot machine play, pinball machine mastery, electronic game play, or of playing the "numbers," dice, and cards. The usual liking of children for fun and games becomes a point of fixation for a particular youth and appears to take over his life. The dynamics are not well known; there are probably a complex mixture of conscious and unconscious factors so that the pleasure in mastery of a particular technique blends in with some symbolic counterphobic equation of winning-equals-castration or winning-equals-averting-castration, as the case might be. The child battles the symbolic other, the unconsciously experienced ur-father, with all the excitement and emotional involvement to be expected from such an encounter. Often enough the unconscious goal is ultimately to lose. Some cases resemble variants of obsessive-compulsive disorder.

In DSM-III-R, there is a diagnosis designated as Pathological Gambling. It requires that two conditions be met; that the individual ". . . is chronically and progressively unable to resist impulses to gamble" (p. 324) and that the gambling must compromise, disrupt, or damage the individual's personal, family, or work life. A number of criteria are offered to define the presence of such damage. In the case of youngsters, the tendency does not often take full form, but it can be present in sufficient intensity to affect school and family life, and in some cases, it takes on disturbing dimensions.

Just as is true of drug use, the complications of gambling may give rise to more serious antisocial behavior than the game play itself. The complications are twofold. On the one hand, the gambling fraternity with which the youth associates often harbors dubious companions and expresses largely delinquent values; the admired models are typically con men or hustlers; and the overall atmosphere is often one of being part of an aristocracy that scorns and laughs at the poor, plebian, law-abiding fools who are caught up in going to school and working. The social climate does not reinforce the healthier kinds of behavioral adjustment.

On the other hand, if the player loses heavily, his temptation is to borrow or to bet on funds he does not have. The result is the sudden necessity for large sums of money, with no ready source available and with some very formidable creditors waiting impatiently. The youngster's credit and credibility with family and friends quickly become exhausted, and he is driven to seek alternative sources of money. The inclination to take someone else's money by force or by stealth becomes overwhelming, and various forms of criminal behavior characteristically follow.

Drug Use, Addiction. The youth of each historical epoch seem to have their own patterns of forbidden, regressive behavior, which they adopt as their preferred mode of defiance and self-assertion. In the 1920s it was carrying a hip flask; in the 1930s, it was climbing aboard a boxcar and riding the rails. In the 1960s and 1970s, drugs became a major means for adolescent self-identification and self-expression, and a host of agents were employed toward this end.

Some of the wilder and more flamboyant aspects of the so-called drug culture (e.g., the large musical festivals where drug use was rampant and part of the "experience") are now relatively rare, but the larger culture remains very much drug oriented. Adolescents as well as adults are deeply involved in the use of various agents. Because practically all such usage is illegal, the behavior falls under the rubric of conduct disorder (although technically DSM-III-R classifies this as "Substance Use Disorders").

Mention of drug use appears in two different places within DSM-III-R. The first (under the rubric of Psychoactive Substance-Induced Organic Mental Disorders) is within the overall diagnostic category of Organic Mental Disorders, where page after page of text is devoted to the several substances and their various effects. The second is Psychoactive Substance Use Disorders. Psychiatrists have learned to have a healthy respect for the capacity of these powerful agents to induce a host of severe reactions that pose impossible diagnostic problems unless the presence of the specific substance is at least suspected. Almost any other syndrome can be mimicked by the effects of these various chemicals, and the clinician may see anything from what seem to be acute schizophrenic breaks to suicidal depressions to panic attacks, each expressing the impact of a given substance on a particularly vulnerable youth.

For the diagnostician, it is worth noting that the DSM-III-R requires that the course of the condition be specified (continuous, episodic, in remission, or unspecified), and that the nature of the attachment to the substance be listed as either abuse or dependence. The abuser is the youngster who stays under the influence of the drug much of the time, and whose life comes to be dominated by this involvement. Dependency is signified by either tolerance or withdrawal, where tolerance means needing more and more of the agent to get the desired effects; and withdrawal means the psychobiological signs and symptoms of distress that follow the drug's cessation. These vary greatly with the agent employed, and the individual diagnosis depends on the substance. Specific mention is made of alcohol, barbiturate (or similarly acting sedative or hypnotic), opioid, cocaine, amphetamine (or similarly acting sympathomimetic), phencyclidine (or similarly acting arylcyclohexylamine), hallucinogen, cannabis, tobacco, and other mixed or unspecified substance abuse. Criteria are offered for abuse and/or dependence in each instance.

Among the other relationships between this group of conditions and conduct disorder, three elements merit special mention. The first is the behavior itself, that is, using the drug. In most areas this is prima facie illegal; it is a forbidden activity and whoever possesses the drug or uses it is by that act violating the law.

Second, the drug is often an intoxicant that has direct psychological effects on the central nervous system. One prominent consequence is that it frees the youngster from such inhibitions as might otherwise have been in place. A great many violent crimes are committed under the influence of alcohol, where the youngster draws on bottled courage to help him carry out the act. Other agents are also releasers in this sense, in particular phencyclidine. In addition to releasing, the intoxicating effects of the agent might induce a state of delirium so that judgment is disturbed, perception distorted, fantasies reified, and projected rage incarnated as terrifying, concrete threats. The uncontrolled and bizarre behavior that may ensue under such conditions can be very dangerous indeed. Finally, depression and apathy may result either as a rebound phenomenon (as with many stimulants) or as a side-effect of chronic usage (as with marijuana).

The third source of disturbed behavior flowing from drug use is the need to raise money to maintain the habit. As the drug becomes ever more the center of the drug-dependent young person's existence, all other values and relationships recede into a hazy limbo peripheral to the true heart of experience, the drug use. Because nothing else is as important, there is no incongruity in putting aside all other values such as honesty, sympathy, love, and trust; ultimately, the youth may resort to every manner of exploitation and chicanery, and even outright theft (with or without violence) to appease the inner need. This becomes altogether consuming and is experienced as overwhelmingly important. A good deal of street crime is the product of just such a chain of events.

Drug Vending, Pushing, Dealing.   For the addicted youth it is an all-too-easy step from confirmed drug use to the selling of such products to ensure his own supply. Many drug pushers are users who adopt the pushing as one sure way to continue their own habit; the money is good, and they occupy a position that carries a certain prestige within their chosen circle. At certain levels the procuring and marketing of drugs is a major aspect of organized crime, but for the most part, drug-dealing youths are independent entrepreneurs rather than members of a larger organization. From the view of the law-enforcement authorities, the selling of drugs is a far more serious crime than their abuse; the pusher keeps the market alive, and, not infrequently, in the search for new markets, he is the one who seduces ever younger children into the activity. Among teenagers, most of the selling is opportunistic, however, and the dynamics in such cases are not very different from those of the confirmed user.

Swindling, Conning.   This common form of deviance, unlike the more violent activities described above, is less the product of a particular subculture than it is the outcome of a style of child rearing that may arise in any stratum of society. The child is caught between parents who are at odds and who use the youngster as a source of vindication, as a spy, and as a target for their feelings about the other parent. In this way, they create a situation where survival for the child becomes a matter of how well he can play his parents off, one against the other. Many children thus learn early how to manipulate, how to deceive, how to tap into the weaknesses of this one and that one, and how to gain advantage for the self by deceit and by adroit and evasive behavior.

The older child becomes a con man; he is the youngster who appears at someone's door with a big smile and a glib story and within 30 seconds has gained access to the house and sold the person expensive subscriptions to a number of unwanted magazines that, in any case, probably will not be delivered. This sort of artful manipulation of people is the stock-in-trade of many narcissistic individuals who have learned the hard way that they have no hope of achieving an affectionate relationship by usual means. As they perceive their world, they must settle for some alternative, such as the exploitative possibilities that their talent for deception permits. They are curiously sensitive to the feelings of others and can "read" other people with exquisite accuracy, yet they lack all compassion or empathy for the affects they discern so well. But such a child has learned to read his caretakers' affects with precision and dispatch to obtain favors, head off an explosion, or avoid abuse; and these were caretakers who ignored the child's feelings. The child was a means to an end. And so, too, are the con man's victims a means to an end, with no trace of personal feeling for the exploited victim except perhaps scorn.

Forgery.   This is not a very common delinquent activity because it involves a degree of professionalism usually encountered somewhat later in the life cycle. However, a fair number of older teenagers do engage in this practice with someone else's checks or credit cards. In some cases at least, it is associated with identity problems. The youngster becomes somebody else for a while—in the service of illicit gain, to be sure—but nonetheless he directly assumes another's identity. Given the serious problems so many of these teenagers have with their self-definition and individuation, this behavior seems to be overdetermined (i.e., to be the product of the work of unconscious forces as much as, or more than, the outcome of conscious decision making).

Threatening, Terrorizing, and Extorting.   Not infrequently the behavior of older children or tougher children toward their smaller, weaker, or more peaceful peers consists of bullying and harassment, a demand for possessions, or a shakedown for lunch money. Occasionally it involves an even more serious dimension such as a requirement for sexual submission. Sometimes this is mere pretense; if the intended victim proposes to fight back, the bully withdraws. However, the potential victim has no guarantee that this is what will happen, and it may take a good deal of courage to stand up to a threatening opponent. Nor is it always pretense. A number of youngsters have been severely injured under these circumstances. In the face of such extortion some vulnerable children become so terrorized that they refuse to return to school. This form of bullying is, in fact, an expression of sadistic impulse, the desire to gain pleasure from forcing another person into a state of abject obedience. Over and above the actual deprivation of goods or money, the psychological consequences for the victim can be quite serious.

Olweus (1980) systematically studied the phenomenon of bullying. He examined a sizable population of such aggressive youngsters and described the typical bully as fearless and tough, not given to anxiety, and with a positive attitude toward himself. These aggressive tendencies were highly stable over time and, when present in the preadolescent years, predicted later antisocial behavior.

Assault, Battery.   Many mechanisms may contribute to this pattern. There are frequent accounts of youngsters attacking someone, not for personal gain in any financial sense, but because of jealousy, revenge, fear of attack, need to show off, preservation of "territory," or any of a host of other motives not connected with theft. To some extent this may be a response to social pressures; the youngster lacking this behavior would lose face in his peer group or in the general subculture. A Corsican youth participating in vendetta behavior is driven by powerful motives that may not be easily grasped by someone who does not share the youth's traditions.

Often enough, however, peaceful alternatives are available to address whatever the problem may be. The person in question nonetheless chooses the violent course and may be quite merciless and destructive toward his opponent. There is a readiness for assault, an inner gearing for the exchange of blows and the drawing of blood. Sometimes the underlying mechanism is the youngster's own castration anxiety. The need to conceal this and disprove it—the counterphobic stance—may override all other concerns and precipitate attacks on dangerous opponents. Sometimes it is the gambler's need to take on the (figurative) father, and sometimes the search for self-destruction lies at the heart of assaultive behavior. And finally, the chronic rage of the battered or the deprived child provides a fertile breeding ground for the growth of violence; here the lashing out is random and might be turned toward anyone.

Fighting. Schoolyard or neighborhood fighting was for many years considered part of growing up. It was a proper activity for a young boy, calculated to teach him manhood and to inculcate the essentials of getting along in the world. The tomboy girl might also seek to prove herself by beating up the toughest boy around and thus earn her coveted place in the boys' society. However, as cultural attitudes have changed, the expectation for, indeed the freedom for, fighting has shrunk to a corresponding degree. As a result, what would have once been considered ordinary rough-and-tumble is now a fairly serious form of misbehavior.

Children who fight are definitely problems by modern standards, even though the developmental forces within the child have not changed appreciably.

Many subcultural factors play a role here, and in certain tough neighborhoods, the unwillingness or the inability to fight might be an enormous handicap. At least one group of investigators believes that all adolescents need some kind of puberty rite, some sort of test or ordeal through which they must pass in order to feel fully mature (Bloch & Niederhoffer, 1958). They regard this lack as a root cause of delinquency; that is, because our society does not provide for an appropriate rite, the adolescents create their own, all too often in the form of defiantly deviant, and hence delinquent, behavior.

Schoolyard fighting has to be sharply differentiated from gang fighting. The pitting of organized groups against one another is a major source of lethal behavior among the young. The group dynamic tends always to encourage regression to more primitive levels of conduct, and the fantasy of leading troops into battle stimulates grandiose and dangerous fantasies. The result is a pattern of behavior involving guns, knives, chains, automobile antennae, and all manner of dangerous instruments. Death or maiming is a common outcome of such pitched battles. These are definitely group events, and the youngsters who participate might otherwise never be involved in violence. Indeed, as Yablonsky points out, the gang might undergo a rapid swelling of its ranks just before a "rumble," because some teenagers join in just to participate in the excitement of the whole affair (Yablonsky, 1962). There is a pleasure component to fighting that is largely overlooked, but it is apparent, for example, in the large attendance at hockey games and boxing matches.

Vandalism.   This is a common expression of chronic childhood rage. It involves the destruction or the defacing of property for no visible reason other than the sheer pleasure of doing it. The classic example is a group of young boys who break into a school building at night and go on a rampage, smashing, smearing, and breaking things in a random and "meaningless" fashion. They may destroy many thousands of dollars worth of goods and materials in a relatively brief period. The activity is a specific attack on the orderly and the organized; the wish is to bring it all to chaos and to disarray.

Under particular cultural conditions the vandalism may be directed toward specific groups, e.g., a right-to-life group may attack an abortion clinic, a nazi group may attack a synagogue, or one religious group may attack another that it considers ungodly—as with all conduct disorder the motives can be complex and multidetermined. But much of this kind of behavior is far less organized. Sometimes the mere existence of unguarded property can invite such attention from a predisposed youth population. An abandoned house or car will fall prey to a host of violent acts, sometimes for no discernible reason except that it is there and is vulnerable. Where the child population is particularly disturbed, any property that is not specifically protected may be selected as a target, bedeviling the lives and defeating the budgets of many institutional caretakers.

Aside from the more obvious kinds of emotional disturbance, certain restless, hyperkinetic children seem ever to be disassembling their world; wherever they are, they pick at the wall or the curtain, or they handle things—and presently the wall has a crack, the curtain is torn or is beginning to unravel, and whatever they have touched falls and shatters or comes apart in their hands. In some instances these results may be a by-product of the hyperactivity; they handle so many things and are in such constant and poorly integrated motion that some actions are bound to turn out this way, on a statistical basis so to speak. But in a great many cases an underlying deep-seated, chronic rage is also at work. In such instances, what gives the activity its particular color is the nature of the target rather than the underlying dynamics; the violence is directed toward property rather than toward a person.

However, as noted, most vandalism is the product of children acting in concert rather than an outcome of the restless manipulation of the poorly integrated hyperkinetic youngster. When large groups are involved, it is called a riot, and the destruction of property can then reach such proportions that the police stop trying to interrupt the behavior and simply stand aside until the worst of it has run its course. More typically vandalism is a form of covert antisocial behavior, carried out under circumstances where it is presupposed that no one will ever know who perpetrated the destruction.

Stealing, Theft. This form of misbehavior has innumerable varieties and can occur very early in the life cycle. Once a child has learned to distinguish between "mine" and "not mine," the possibility exists for the child to engage in the essential quality of theft, to take surreptitiously for himself what he knows is not his. Preschool stealing is by no means rare, and in deprived situations, many children become expert thieves by the early gradeschool years. It is probable that all children steal some time during their growing up, and the management of such incidents has a good deal to do with how the child later deals with temptation.

The dynamics of theft can range all the way from oral incorporation and the restitution of object loss through sadistic anal acquisitiveness and hoarding to the actualization of a castration fantasy (the thief symbolically castrates the victim by taking possession of what is his or hers). Ultimately, the fulfillment of the oedipal wish is a form of stealing. Narcissistic individuals, with their immense sense of entitlement, have no trouble rationalizing to themselves that they have more right to the stolen booty than did the original owner.

Although the kinds of stealing shade off into all the many types of white collar crime, such as embezzling and the manipulation of trust funds, this list is confined to two main subgroups: covert stealing and overt robbery.

COVERT STEALING. The varieties of stealing include both the efforts of the loner and the depredations of the gang. Where stealing becomes habitual, the youngster often develops a measure of skill along with a sense of pitting himself against an adversary and outwitting or besting that person at some sort of contest. Among all the patterns of conduct disorder, this is one of the few that can take the form of a genuine neurosis. Kleptomania, a compulsive need to steal in order to relieve anxiety, is an uncommon syndrome, but it does occur. For the most part, however, the primary motive for stealing seems to be the acquisition of goods to satisfy a material desire and/or a symbolic need without the permission of the rightful owner.

Some forms of stealing do have additional motivational sets beyond the merely acquisitive; they are perhaps most commonly seen in the relationship of the adolescent to the automobile.

• *Car Theft (joy-riding).* Perhaps the commonest form of adolescent car theft is joyriding. This is generally a group phenomenon, although it is by no means rare for a lone youth to engage in the activity. In any case, a car is broken into, car keys are stolen, or a car is located with the keys left in. One way or another the youngsters get the car started and proceed to drive around the community until the fuel is exhausted, the car is immobilized by an accident, or they simply get tired of it and walk away. Sometimes they return the car precisely to where it was located before the start of the adventure and make every effort to conceal that it was taken at all (other than replacing the gasoline). More often than not, however, the car is considerably the worse for wear, and the police often locate it in a ditch in undrivable condition.

The motives for this behavior are usually adolescent adventurism—a sort of test of the child's prowess—to force entry where he is not invited, to obtain a forbidden key, to start a car without a key, to drive about without a license, to exhibit bravado and flash in the possession of a forbidden vehicle, and thus, however transiently, to live out some grandiose fantasy. The underlying idea might well be of phallic character: the child takes possession of his father's penis and castrates him in a manner that is half play and half serious. For a time the youngster assumes the mantle of adult power and omnipotence, overrides the restrictions of the conscience, and does the exciting and the forbidden.

Group process plays a part as well; many youngsters who participate do so to be part of a set where issues such as group excitement, displays of daring, maintaining face, and earning status are powerful motives. The authorities who apprehend the youngsters usually regard this behavior as quite different from that of the more professional car thief, who takes the vehicle in order to sell it or to harvest the parts. Joyriding is often classified as an adolescent prank; typically the youngsters are given warnings or are put on probation.

The psychological picture of the professional car thief who makes money as a result of the theft is dissimilar. In particular, the motivational set of the habitual criminal here comes into play. There is usually a state of underlying chronic rage that is deeply buried. The thief carries out the procedure coldly and dispassionately; the behavior is calculated, planful, and is often performed with considerable technical expertise. The basic mind-set is predatory; there is a characteristic guilt-free indifference to the victim's plight, and the only conscious emotion may be a sense of triumph at having gotten away with the behavior.

- *Pickpocket.* This very common form of theft is typically part of the skills-profile of the practiced delinquent. Frequently the mental health professional learns that the youngster acquired the skill at an institution for delinquents where he spent some time. In any case, this form of deviance requires a good deal of competence and calculated intent. Pickpockets often work in pairs or groups; someone sets up a diversion while someone else accomplishes the actual theft. From the view of the practitioner, it is a business. The youngster goes to an event that brings people together and works the crowd. Skillful thieves can go for long periods without being caught. However, predatory but incompetent individuals who attempt this form of theft to obtain ready cash are more likely to be apprehended.

● *Housebreaking.* Adolescent delinquents frequently break into a deserted or a currently unoccupied house and pilfer it or vandalize its structure. Empty residences act as a magnet to certain vulnerable young, and these teenagers work out all sorts of feelings about their own homes by attacking the undefended and passive presence thus afforded them. This is psychologically a very different form of behavior from breaking and entering currently occupied homes and apartments, which is likely to be engaged in only by the more criminally oriented antisocial young (see discussion under Overt Robbery).

● *Shoplifting.* Of all forms of theft, this is far and away the most common. The opulence of the many store counters in the United States offers a continuing temptation to the vulnerable. Whether motivated by need, greed, adventuresomeness, neurotic compulsion, or the living out of some angry revenge fantasy, the concealed theft of the attractive item does have one characteristic that gives it a fatal lure: It seems easy. And, in fact, it often is; the aggregate loss of commodities to shoplifting amounts to a staggering figure. More than that, for a long time it was customary for the shop owner to relent upon apprehending such a shoplifter and merely to recover the purloined articles without formally charging the perpetrator.

Currently a new spirit seems to have pervaded the retail establishment, and many store managers have taken a far more vigorous approach.

Curiously, for a long time, shoplifting had been considered to be the province of puberty girls. Many of the things these youngsters prize most highly are relatively easy to take including makeup, clothing, and jewelry. In addition, the sense of being cheated out of what belongs to them is likely to be a common facet of the feeling life of many pubertal youngsters. In some cases this attitude might be due to a sense of castration engendered by the developmental events of puberty. Other girls might feel that in their families or their communities boys have all the advantages. In any case, many youngsters all too readily accept shoplifting as a reasonable, necessary, or even fun part of life. It is quite commonly enacted in pairs or groups. Sometimes teenagers tell of having to steal something in this fashion to earn membership into a particular clique. In the light of more recent figures, it is probable that boys and girls engage in this behavior to approximately the same extent.

OVERT ROBBERY

● *Armed robbery.* Many of the most serious crimes associated with the young fall into this category. The notion of acquiring and wielding power is a vital element in the fantasy life of many disturbed young people, and much of their energy is diverted into activities that pit them against the established order of things. In some ways they resemble unreconstructed 2-year-olds—negativistic, unrealistic, provocative, constantly seeking confrontations, and given to violence and tantrums. In a great many cases, organic problems impede such children's cognitive processes and thus their ability to make appropriate judgments. Often enough, this particular variety of biological difficulty also impinges on the impulse control apparatus, so that the ability to delay action and to think things out may not be available to that particular youth. Where such a state of affairs is superimposed on a personality structure beset by primitive fixations and inadequate superego formation, then a potentially violent person emerges.

The urge for power and domination in particular tends to encourage the use of weapons; the sadistic wish to reduce the target other to abject fear and submissiveness plays a large part in many of these crimes. So fantasy dominated is this behavior that at times the victim is shot or stabbed "for no reason at all," that is, for no logical reason rationally inherent in the situation. This type of behavior evokes the hue and cry about crime in the streets. There are in general two main varieties: mugging and breaking and entering.

● *Mugging* is the classic street crime that terrorizes the citizen who walks down the city block at night. In its mildest form it involves merely the attempt to grab the money and run—to seize a woman's purse, to snatch off a necklace, to grab a shopping bag. A more serious version is the assault on a man or woman that is accompanied by some level of physical violence, for example, by knocking someone over and grabbing a wallet, or by punching them repeatedly until they are reduced to helplessness and then robbing them. Finally, the most dangerous form of this behavior involves using some kind of weapon—a club, a knife, a gun, a chain, brass knuckles, and the like. Often the thief is satisfied merely to threaten with the weapon; the terror this is likely to engender and the rapid compliance with the demands for possessions suffice. Sometimes, however, the thief must injure or kill the victim to fulfill the fantasy thus set in motion and to placate the need for total dominance.

Many violent persons have themselves been victims of violence, and sometimes what they do on the street reenacts what happened to them when they were small and helpless and at the mercy of a sadistic adult. Through constant repetition they seek to overcome the traumatic quality of their own memories; they identify with the aggressor and live out the experience once again.

Quite another variety of motivation is that of the professional who may kill a victim quite dispassionately to reduce the likelihood of later identification. Most professional killers, however, are able to earn a much better income than that associated with the rather uncertain return of street crime, and the streets tend to be left to the impulsive, the primitive, the traumatized, and the unskilled.

● *Housebreaking.* The thief who breaks and enters in the night is the terror of the homeowner everywhere, and with good reason. Thieves who enter occupied homes by stealth tend on the whole to be a much more professional and serious type of criminal than the casual vandal of empty residences. Many, but not all, are armed and can be very dangerous if surprised and confronted. A goodly percentage are quite young and have learned the trade from older and more experienced criminals.

Firesetting. Despite a number of careful investigations, no specific dynamic formulation for firesetting has been discovered. The probabilities are that the impulse for this very dangerous and destructive behavior stems from all levels of psychosexual development. Fire is a perfect depiction of raging primitive oral devouring; it eats up everything. Fire is both a means of torture and the ultimate mess maker; as such, it personifies the quintessential tantrum of the rampaging anal sadistic impulse. Fire is the erotic passion that consumes and bears everything before it in the heat of its intensity; it is the height of unthinking phallic sexual ardor. The classic psychoanalytic formulation that viewed fire as representing the urethral impulse has little to recommend it beyond its ingenuity; certainly there is no mass of clinical evidence to make this a very convincing position.

Fire is attractive to children; at some time during toddlerhood there is a fascination with the phenomenon, and practically every child wants to light matches or to study fires. But the willful initiation of fire to satisfy some impulse for gain or for revenge is a highly pathological act that is a severe form of conduct disorder.

Cruelty to Animals. Certain disturbed sadistic children express the depth of their difficulties by displacing some of their rage onto small and usually helpless animals. Not infrequently such children have a rather poor grasp on their impulses and cannot distinguish reality from fantasy, at least at moments. Torture fantasies are by no means rare, but as a rule, children do not live them out in concrete terms. Those who do enact such behaviors tend on the whole to be of borderline or fully psychotic status.

Where this behavior is pursued and there is no disturbance of reality contact, then the likelihood is that the youngster is a severely narcissistic personality who lacks any empathy with his victim's suffering and enjoys only the sense of total dominance that he thus achieves.

Murder. The child as murderer is not a common phenomenon, but the adolescent who murders is by no means unheard of. Such crimes pose society some formidable questions. A sizable percentage of these murders involve immediate family members. Thus, the professional must seek to understand not merely murder but patricide or matricide. Many of the youngsters involved have serious mental illnesses, such as chronic brain syndromes, schizophrenia, or borderline conditions. With or without the presence of such syndromes, many of them have a severely narcissistic character makeup. Moreover, the nature of these syndromes is such that recurrence is likely.

The characteristic profile of youthful murderers involves a number of elements. These young people have often been the victims of parental violence; emotional deprivation has marked their early experience; they tend to perceive themselves as physically weak or inadequate in some way; they often have sexual problems of considerable degree; and their emotional life varies from the shallow and blunted to the wildly sadistic and violent. Miller and Looney (1974) subdivide adolescent murderers into three groups. The youngsters in the first group are at highest risk for murderous behavior and are characterized by a tendency totally to dehumanize their victims. Unable to make any kind of genuine object attachment, they accept violence as an appropriate way, perhaps the only way, to resolve tensions and frustrations. When balked (e.g., if someone catches them in the act of theft), such youngsters will act to remove the impediment with brutal and final directness. Children in the second group are prone to partial dehumanization; they do not ordinarily dehumanize persons about them, but in the face of frustration, especially during bouts of episodic dyscontrol, they become very dangerous. When under stress, these youngsters suffer from powerful inner conflicts. To resolve these conflicts, they externalize the hated part of themselves and project it onto the victim—whom they then turn on with unmitigated ferocity. Members of the third group experience moments of dyscontrol when under the influence of group pressure. Such youngsters may then join the group members and participate in the most violent kinds of behavior. Given the validation of the group accord, they are fully capable of torture and slaughter.

For the most part, such cases are currently being remanded to adult courts for disposition. Where the basic condition allows for hospitalization, this is often—but not always—the preferred route. In the case of the severe narcissistic disorder, the hospital will often do an evaluation and state that there is no treatable mental condition, and it is likely that the youngster will then enter the penal system.

Sexual Delinquency

SODOMY. Although used for almost any kind of sexual act other than heterosexual coitus, the usual sense of the term is to refer to anal intercourse. In particular, this form of behavior becomes conduct disorder when a larger older boy forces a smaller younger one to submit to penetration. It is less frequently used for enforced fellatio with either a boy or a girl.

EXHIBITIONISM. The two forms of this behavior that are commonly seen are public masturbation and flashing. Public masturbation is not uncommon among younger pubertal boys; the type of exhibitionistic exposure called flashing usually begins later in the mid or late teens.

PROSTITUTION. This very common form of sexual delinquency was traditionally confined to females. In recent years, increasing numbers of young boys have been making money as homosexual prostitutes. A sizable percentage of the young people involved have themselves been the objects of sexual exploitation in their own homes. However, the motives that bring teenagers of both sexes into this way of life are many and complex. Not the least of these is the special relationship offered the young woman by the pimp, a tie that combines masochistic degradation and exploitation along with assurances of being specially loved and valued.

RAPE. This behavior comes in many forms. It is frequently part of a larger pattern of violence that may start out as theft and then acquire the sexual dimension because the perpetrator has a helpless and frightened victim in an isolated place. It can be a solitary form of assault, or a number of youths can attack a girl, the so-called gang bang. Investigators have argued that this is not properly a form of sexual behavior at all, but is a pure and simple variety of aggressive or sadistic activity. Terms such as *anger rape* and *power rape* have been introduced to express this aspect of the behavior (Groth et al., cited in Vinogradov et al., 1988). Given the diversity of the circumstances under which it occurs, some rape behavior undoubtedly has this exclusively aggressive quality. But other patterns evidently involve erotic elements as well: The enactor seems to treasure a grandiose notion that the victim must love what he has done and desires more contacts of that sort. Such behavior probably represents one of the many disturbances to which erotic expression is so prone, that is, where the themes of power and domination become intermixed with sexuality and passion.

In any case, Vinogradov et al. (1988) has suggested a distinctive pattern of teenage rape. The rapist usually makes the attack in the victim's home or in a vehicle. Often enough the rape is incidental to some other crime such as theft. Although the majority of instances involve individuals of the same race, many rapes do cross racial lines, and most of the victims are unknown to the rapist before the act. As a rule, nothing in the deportment or dress of the victim provokes the rape, and the rapist is typically under the influence of drugs or alcohol.

VOYEURISM.   The peeping Tom is a well-known presence in many communities. Often the activity is sheerly opportunistic, that is, a young boy stumbles onto an occasion to spy on an unclothed woman and, thinking he can get away with it, proceeds to watch. When, however, this pattern of behavior becomes habitual and it becomes necessary for that boy to seek opportunities to peep, then a pathological state is present that may be relatively difficult to contain.

Adjunctive Disturbing Behavior

In certain problematic aggressive behaviors the target of the behavior is not the social surround but is instead an inward-turning injurious activity; as far as the outer world is concerned, it wears a nonaggressive facade. Although the behavior is typically part of a conduct disorder syndrome, in itself, it could not readily be classified as antisocial conduct. The following are examples of some of these behavior patterns.

Skin Cutting.   A great many disturbed young people display this form of deviant behavior. It tends to be seen with particular frequency among institutionalized youngsters, and the behavior frequently occurs in waves that spread through the institutional population and then die down, only to recur at a later date. The actual nature of the cutting is highly variable. It extends all the way from a series of impulsively administered parallel or crisscross slashes on one's arm to painstaking and elaborately labored efforts to draw a picture or depict a face on the forearm or the dorsum of the knee. Sometimes the youngster burns the skin with a cigarette tip, forming a series of dots in some sort of pattern. Occasionally it is part of a larger organization of self-destructive behavior and indicates increasing suicidal preoccupation, but for the most part, it seems to occur in individuals where suicide is not a clear and present danger and where the behavior subserves other purposes.

Although both boys and girls engage in skin cutting, it is far more common among girls. This might reflect a greater tendency for girls to respond to stress in masochistic ways because of some inherent gender-determined pattern; at best, the evidence for such an assertion remains inconclusive. It might express the social patterning and the image of femininity that girls receive from early childhood; again there is no convincing evidence one way or the other.

The behavior can also occur in groups, and as noted, in certain institutions it is endemic among the inmates. Sometimes it is part of the ordeal of joining a particular group; the youth must undergo a ritual of cutting the group's monogram into his skin. This is reminiscent of the German university student clubs where a facial saber scar was essential as a badge of manhood. However, it can also occur as the personal and solitary behavior of an otherwise unremarkable person.

Many different diagnostic labels apply to the various practitioners of this kind of self-molestation. Three important ones are the masochistic pattern, the sequence that turns rage against the self, and the narcissistic attack on a self-object by injury to the self.

MASOCHISM. Where masochistic pleasure is the predominant motive, the skin cutting is actually a form of masturbation. The child is fixated at an anal level of development, where the maximal sensuous pleasure is likely to be along the sadomasochistic axis. The expected and the sought-for qualities that dominate the child's attachments are therefore the opportunity to hurt, or to be hurt. In the course of growing up, there are bound to be major difficulties in interpersonal relations. The youngster, according to his disposition, tends to hurt others, or to provoke them into hurting him; he teases, needles, and bullies, or he is a cat's paw, a patsy, or a scapegoat. None of these approaches to making friends is likely to be very rewarding. In the face of the inevitable rejections, the youngster may lash out, seek revenge, have a tantrum, fall apart in some other way, withdraw, or attack some substitute other. The skin cutting comes about in connection with these latter choices. For withdrawal means to seek a solution within the self, and under such circumstances many youngsters will masturbate. Because, however, the fixation is at an early pregenital level, the masturbation is also expressed at that level; the youngster seeks pleasure through masochistic means rather than through genital stimulation, and the skin cutting follows.

TURNING AGAINST THE SELF. A similar but not identical tactic is the readiness to deal with the experienced rage of childhood by diverting it from its original target and redirecting it against the self. Although it sounds rather unlikely, it is one of the most common human practices and accounts for a great many behavioral disturbances. As noted earlier, it is easily observed in some toddlers who respond to upset and frustration by slapping or striking their own faces. Sometimes they will beat their heads against the wall in the intensity of their vexation.

Psychologically, what appears to happen is that they are angry at someone, perhaps at their mother or father. In the enormity of the infantile passion of 2-year-olds, they experience the impulse to attack, assault, destroy, obliterate the cause—and target—of their frustrations. But they are already old enough to contemplate this with fear; what if they should indeed destroy mommy, who would love them, who take care of them? She is so important, they need her so much, and yet, what to do about the rage? The solution of this particular group is to redirect it, to protect the important object by shunting the flood of anger and rechanneling it to the self. Better for the child's own body to suffer than to risk anything bad happening to mommy.

This behavior may be one of the early precursors of conscience; this crude, direct turning against the self may be a preliminary version of what the child will later experience as feelings of guilt (where some form of self-flagellation is so often the form of the experience). In any case, the compromise between killing the mommy and preserving her and her love for the child is to turn the rage against the self.

It is easy to see how in a disposed individual this turning against the self can take the form of skin cutting. Here too the rage is felt against caretakers or even society in general, but it is too dangerous to enact this directly. The feelings loop back to the self, and some form of self-injury follows. This is not identical to the masochistic pattern; it is not so much the erotic pleasure that dominates the behavior as it is the relief afforded by the opportunity to discharge rage without danger.

An additional element frequently appears in connection with this behavior. The parent who sees the child beating his head against the wall is likely to react strongly by trying to interrupt this behavior. Within such a context, many children learn very quickly the enormous leverage they can achieve by initiating a pattern of self-harm, and in the suitably attuned child, this can become a powerful behavioral means to achieve control of parental responses and even to dominate a household. Although it is a secondary gain, it is an important element in creating and maintaining such patterns.

NARCISSISTIC RAGE. Certain youngsters never successfully accomplish the process of differentiation from the primary caretaker. They are caught up in complex sequences of idealization and grandiosity that bind them to the important other, and at times of great emotion, they literally do not know where the self ends and the other begins. Given such a condition of boundary diffusion, the readiness to seek revenge on the other by attacking the self makes a kind of sense, at least to the involved children. Thus when they carve their own skin, they are also getting even with the primary caretaker.

Accidents. Many of the youngsters caught up in conduct disorder have an impulsive streak in their makeup deriving from the predictable mix of biological and sociopsychological factors. They may have irritable nervous systems, and they may be vulnerable to seizures or outbursts of rage and explosive behavior. They may have violent parents inclined to strike out at the child or at one another. They may be the outcome of child-rearing patterns that allowed and encouraged them to expect gratification of every impulse, or that, at any rate, failed to instill an orientation toward working for goals and delaying gratification. Instead a sense of entitlement was built in. Any of these patterns, or, as frequently happens, their combination, make for an individual who is prone to excesses of emotion that can trigger abrupt and violent action. It is a breeding ground for accidents, and these youngsters have many.

Those with convulsive potential or with poorly patterned nervous system integration have the inherent problem of often not being in good command of their movements. The presence of such integrative failures and loss of physical control can lead to behavioral slips such as falling off bicycles or swerving a car into the wrong lane. A different kind of difficulty arises from the psychological problem of turning the poorly mastered rage against the self. To be sure, this motivational set is less visible than skin cutting, but it becomes all too evident by exploring the dynamics of specific events.

If the clinician keeps in mind the role of accidents as a major contributor to childhood mortality statistics, the serious nature of this problem becomes painfully evident. Where such a turning-against-the-self element comes through prominently in the account of the patient's behavior, it merits special attention.

Enuresis. The high incidence of enuresis in delinquency was noted long ago and was studied in particular detail by Joseph Michaels (1938), who attributed the bedwetting to the generally poor patterning of impulse management that characterizes these disorders. He likened the dyscontrol of this biological function to the inability of so many of these youngsters to manage their emotions in an adequately modulated fashion. In each instance there was a failure of inhibition, and symptomatic behavior followed. There are a great many more enuretic children than there are conduct-disordered children, but the relatively high incidence of this finding in the behavioral dyscontrol group suggests again a biological element common to these conditions.

Promiscuity, Don Juanism. High levels of sexual activity are not a universal characteristic of conduct disorders. For all too many of these youngsters, successful sexuality is really beyond their capacities; what they do enact is likely to be crude, inadequate, and unrewarding. Both frigidity and impotence are common clinical occurrences. In many instances, however, the general lack of good impulse control along with the basic anger at all superego limitations make the average youth caught up in these behavioral syndromes particularly prone to respond to temptations and to violate moral precepts. In occasional cases the clinician finds a dramatic pattern of tempestuous and flamboyant sexuality.

Promiscuity is a common form of behavior. Much of it is less inherently sexual than it is an expression of pathological organization of the individual's relationship life. The analogy that comes to mind is the story of the man who was walking along outside the wall that surrounded a large orphanage. Suddenly a bottle came sailing over the wall, landed at his feet, and shattered. Inside the bottle was a note. The man retrieved the note, opened it up, and read: "Whoever you are, I love you."

This then is the essence of a common form of promiscuity, particularly as it is experienced by young girls. The relationship need is at once so catastrophically overwhelming and so distorted in its reality configuration that the individual turns to anybody, literally any body, and offers whatever will attract or invite to achieve some measure of or some simulacrum of attachment. This underlying dynamic dominates some types of the primitivized object seeking called promiscuity. It is by no means the only type: there are oedipally disoriented girls who are compulsively and repetitiously reenacting their own seduction at the hands of their fathers or older brothers; there are narcissistic children glorying in the grandiose fantasies of their sexual attractiveness and needing to demonstrate again and again that they can "get" any boy or girl they go after; there are abandoned psychotic or retarded children who find some sort of care within the deviant subculture of the pandering world. In short, a host of mechanisms can underlie this as well as other forms of female conduct disturbance.

Obviously the boys' Don Juanism, a parallel type of activity, can have similar origins. The clinician must note the additional presence of stressful castration concerns as a common factor in determining behavior. The boy's goal is to prove, against the background of a profound inner uncertainty, that he is not castrated. In counterpoint to the Don Juan behavior and the multiple enactments are the anxious and repetitious inner assertions: I tell you I'm not inadequate, I'm not castrated, see, I prove it, I'm successful. The castration threat, however, has an inner unconscious source, so no amount of external effort can really alter its clamor. Each "success" merely increases the fear and drives the individual to "prove" it yet again.

Pregnancy. This is a common and troublesome aspect of conduct disorder for many of the reasons already mentioned: It is a surpassingly successful form of rebellion and defiance; it often challenges the parents' most fundamental values; it asserts all sorts of claims to independence and precocious maturity; it is exhibitionistic; and it is a marvelous backdrop for the living out of numerous fantasies. Among the other factors at work are the subtle but profoundly influential subcultural values that are shaping the youngsters' behavior. In many instances, the girl was the product of her mother's teenage out-of-wedlock pregnancy and is continuing a family tradition. A common dynamic is for the young woman to see herself as, for the first time, having someone who is all hers and who will love only her; she will now correct and overcome all previous relationship deficits by having this blissful, ideal, and perfect union with a baby; she will undo all the damage and deprivation she has experienced by offering perfect care to the new baby; she will assert and underline her gender prowess and clear up any uncertainty about her femininity or attractiveness; and so on and on for a host of similarly unrealistic but powerful configurations. Sometimes the most powerful expressed motive is jealousy; a friend may have boasted that she had persuaded a certain highly esteemed youth to get her pregnant and the girl feels a great need to show that she can do as well. Typically these deeply held attitudes will often lead such a young woman to insist on having and keeping a baby when every one about her is counseling either abortion or adoption as the only viable alternative.

For the young man, an array of attitudes also collectively act to perpetuate the pattern. The need to assert his manhood, the need to bind the girl to himself, the need to deny feelings of inadequacy or castration, and the need to achieve status among his peers all play their roles in prompting the youngster to avoid contraception and to seek actively to impregnate his partner. Along with these more narcissistic motives there is frequently a mingling of both pride and caring in the attitudes of such young men, but they usually have a poor earning capacity and are not emotionally prepared to assume the responsibilities of fatherhood.

Venereal Disease. This is a common element in the lives of many teenagers with the predictable sequelae of chronic inflammatory conditions of one sort or another. Venereal disease then becomes part of the pattern of ill health that is so often an important dimension of conduct disorder; it is colored by the special emotional overlay that genital illness always involves, a sense of shame, a quality of profound anxiety, an even more troubled feeling about closeness and intimacy, and an awareness of yet another heavy cloud over the future. Under certain circumstances, where for example, rage, revenge fantasies, and counterphobic elements are particularly prominent, there may be an explosion of sexual activity: "If I've got it, let everybody get it! If a man did this to me, I'll give it to as many men as I can!" For the most part, however, the knowledge of a venereal infection merely adds to the already pervasive feelings of depression, low self-esteem, and sense of victimization—the feeling of being put upon by everything and everybody. The spread of AIDS into the adolescent population has made this problem even more serious and lethal.

Associated Character Traits

A very large variety of personality traits tend to be found in clusters of various kinds among the children and teenagers with conduct disorder. Sometimes these personality characteristics, rather than the disturbed (and diagnostic) behavioral patterns, are the most difficult for the parents to live with or are the most upsetting to teachers. Not all conduct disordered children display such behaviors; indeed, when Hewitt first tried to classify the delinquents that Jenkins had described, he came up with a group he called "Inhibited Children." Other investigators called these children

"Overinhibited" (Jenkins, 1973, pp. 14, 15). At any rate they were not obviously troublesome, and they carried out their antisocial acts quietly and without noisy dramatics. But these more inhibited youngsters are a distinct minority among this diagnostic group; in addition to their antisocial behavior, the large majority of such youngsters manifest a great many disturbing character traits that make life difficult and tumultuous for their families and schools.

Diagnostically, these behavioral tendencies will sometimes group themselves in a sufficiently systematic fashion to allow affixing a particular personality disorder label. More often than not, however, the aggregate is nondescript and not readily classifiable except as one of the characteristics of the basic behavioral pathology. A conduct-disordered child may exhibit any one or several of these behaviors. The following list, then, simply gives a sense of some of the behavioral variants that tend to be associated with this diagnosis.

Disobedience
Defiance
Rebelliousness
Demandingness
Negativism, oppositionalism
Provocativeness
Explosiveness, bad temper
Rudeness, sarcasm
Sullenness
   Surliness
   Tendency to pout
Spitefulness
Vengefulness
Crudity in word and gesture
Profanity, given to obscenity
Continual blaming and
   accusations
Mistrustfulness
Paranoid suspiciousness
Manipulativeness
Dishonesty, given to lying
   Deceitfulness
   Sneakiness
   Pseudologia fantastica
Trouble-making
   Fomenting group discord
   Tale bearing
Invasiveness

Arrogance
Boastfulness
Sadistic teasing
Bullying
Restlessness
   Tenseness, high-strung
      personality
   Inability to tolerate boredom
   Chronic irritability
Impulsiveness
Destructiveness
Stubbornness
Uncooperativeness
   Dawdling
   Procrastination
   Forgetfulness
School failure
   Inattentiveness
   Distractiblility
   Failure to do work
   Disturbance of other children
   Failure to respond to the
      usual disciplinary measures
   Leaving class without
      permission
   Cutting class without excuse
   Truant

Associated Personality Disorders

Generally speaking, the personality disorders are not considered to be childhood diagnoses. They imply a certain fixed and stable pattern of organization of personality elements that is the outcome of developmental work and that cannot be said to be in place much before mid to late adolescence. Nonetheless, in any number of situations it is all too evident that a particular configuration has taken form relatively early, and the clinician has no doubt about the personality organization with which he or she is dealing. Indeed, the authors of many prospective studies that have followed cohorts of children into young adulthood remark uniformly that childhood aggression tends to be one of the most stable configurations identified. Once present, it tends to persist into adolescence. Neurologists warn that a sudden outburst of aggression in adolescence without prior appearance during the grade-school years should arouse suspicion of some organic or psychotic process.

Twelve personality disorders are listed in the DSM-III-R and several of them are particularly relevant here. The listings are:

Paranoid personality disorder	Avoidant personality disorder
Schizoid personality disorder	Dependent personality disorder
Schizotypal personality disorder	Compulsive personality disorder
Histrionic personality disorder	Passive-aggressive personality
Narcissistic personality disorder	disorder
Antisocial personality disorder	Atypical, mixed, or other
Borderline personality disorder	personality disorder

Any of these might conceivably apply to a given case of Conduct Disorder as an axis II inclusion in DSM-III-R. The Narcissistic, Borderline, Antisocial, or Passive-aggressive categories would undoubtedly fit a great many of the young people who fall into the Conduct Disorder column, and where they seem to be appropriate, such diagnostic statements should be made. (Antisocial conduct disorder is applicable only to persons 18 years of age and older.) Because so little is known about personality formation, the diagnosis is an admission of ignorance as much as a description of the patient's pathology, but it does try to state somewhat more precisely what the clinician sees, and the clustering of traits to which he or she would give the most weight.

APPENDIX 13-2
ILLUSTRATIVE SYNDROME: FIRESETTING

This appendix describes one syndrome—firesetting—in some detail. Theoretically, each form of disturbed conduct could be treated in similar fashion, but that would detract from the primary thrust of this work, which is to survey the field rather than to explore all of the facets of conduct disorder in depth.

Introduction

There is a twofold reason for selecting firesetting as a model syndrome. First, it is not well understood, and the theoretical work on its conceptualization is just now getting under way. In that sense firesetting reflects general truths about the whole area of conduct disorder; many degrees and kinds of confusion and obscurity still prevail in attempts to comprehend it. Second, firesetting is one of the fastest growing and most serious crimes committed by children and adolescents. This is particularly true in the United States, which has the highest arson rate in the world. The total damage from firesetting each year runs into the billions of dollars. At the same time, it is so easy to carry out that many fires are set by preschool children, and it is so dangerous that even unintentional fires take many lives. It therefore merits special attention by every sector of society.

Description

The intentional setting of fires on the part of youngsters who have at least some sense of what they are doing is called *firesetting* or *torching;* legally, the intentional destruction of life or property by fire, or, more specifically, the willful and malicious burning of property is called *arson.*

Prevalence

In 1979, 42% of the nation's fires were set by destructive youths, essentially as a form of vandalism. In 1981, 38% of those actually convicted of arson were under 18, a higher percentage of juvenile involvement than for any other indexed crime. The large majority of firesetters were white, middle-class males (89% were males and 78% were white). Currently, the incidence of arson is increasing, and it is said to be one of the fastest growing crimes in the nation. Thus, according to recent statistics, children and adolescents are responsible for setting approximately two out of every five fires in the United States.

Types of Firesetters

The recent work of Wooden and Berkey (1984) provides one of the more thorough studies of this syndrome. Using a clustering technique, the authors sorted out four types of juvenile firesetters. These include:

1. The *playing-with-matches* type.
2. The *crying-for-help* variety.
3. The *delinquent* group.
4. The *severely disturbed* firesetters.

These types represent somewhat different age groups with distinct motivational sets and different approaches to the firesetting activity. In particular, the *playing-with-matches* children are the youngest, seldom being more than 10 years of age; often they are preschoolers. Because they do not, for the most part, seek to set fires other than the small conflagrations that fascinate them and seduce them into play, they do not properly represent cases of conduct disorder.

The *crying-for-help* children are somewhat older and may include early adolescents. Their behavior is an attempt to demonstrate their pain and to signal their need for succor and relief from some problem that besets them. Generally speaking, they cannot otherwise voice the problem or they have tried and no one listens.

The *delinquent* firesetters are usually in mid or late adolescence and are manifesting the classic lashing-out behavior of the angry and vengeful youth. These youngsters are concerned with power and vengeance, and setting the fire is typically an act of willful vandalism.

Finally, the *severely disturbed* cohort are youngsters who are apparently responding to some deeply neurotic or psychotic prompting when they kindle a conflagration.

Diagnosis

In the DSM-III-R, the term firesetting does not appear in the index, and the behavior is listed under Pyromania. This condition is one of the "Disorders of Impulse Control Not Elsewhere Classified." It has two primary features, the inability on repeated occasions to resist the impulse to set a fire, and an intense attraction to looking at fires and seeing them burn. A preliminary tension builds up prior to setting the fire, which is relieved by the actual fire. A good deal of pleasure accompanies this tension release and the further experiencing of the conflagration.

The DSM-III-R recognizes that the setting of fires may be part of many other syndromes, specifically, Conduct Disorder, Antisocial Personality, Schizophrenia, or Organic Mental Disorder. The diagnostic criteria include the recurrent failure to resist the impulse to set fires, the mounting tension before starting the blaze, the pleasure or relief experienced once the fire is under way, the absence of an alternative motive, such as the seeking of economic or political advantage, and the absence of any of the other diagnoses mentioned.

Actually, only a relatively small percentage of the firesetting activities of young people have any such origin. (The figure is probably somewhere in te range of 13%.) The large majority of fires are probably set as a result of adjustment disorders, conduct disorders, borderline or paranoid or narcissistic or antisocial personality disorders, attention-deficit hyperactivity disorder, or occasional cases of major affective disorder.

Etiology

In the majority of cases of firesetting, the reason(s) for the behavior is(are) never completely understood. There are some obvious exceptions, for example, where a youngster has committed a crime (such as a burglary) and is seeking to conceal the fact or the evidence that might implicate himself, or where there is an attempt to get insurance money. Under such circumstances, the motive is straightforward and self-evident. The same is true when the fire is set with some political motivation in mind, for example, to destroy police files or to strike a blow against some hated authority. But again, albeit an important group, these incidents are still a relatively small part of the total array of fire episodes.

The dynamics of firesetting form an area of considerable uncertainty. Small children are fascinated by fire and need to learn about it and to master the feelings that it evokes. Most families do not teach fire management very well, and much of what they teach comes down to an attempt to keep children from playing with matches. Even this instruction is often so perfunctory or ambivalent that many fires are set each year by preschoolers playing or experimenting with a small blaze that gets out of control. Where parents smoke, children may early learn about lighters and matches by blowing out the flames when their parents light up cigarettes. This action scarcely prepares the youngsters for all the consequences of fire. Folkman and Siegelman (1972) reported that of a group of 47 five- and six-year-olds, about two-thirds of the boys and one-third of the girls had played with fire, but only two children had actually caused fires that did any damage. All this certainly confirms that children are interested in fire, but it does not explain what draws children to this activity.

Freud (1930/1955a) published an article called "The Acquisition of Power over Fire" that sought to establish a connection between interest in fire and phallic-urethral drives. He proposed that the heat of the fire was analogous to sexual excitement and that men used the stream of urine as a means of mastery over fire. The fire itself was visually suggestive of the phallus in motion giving it a sexual symbolism.

Clinically, under certain circumstances, some firesetting has a clearly erotic element. Cumulative experience, however, suggests that this is but a single mechanism of the many at work and merely pushes the question back one place: Why should this particular form of eroticism dominate in the psychological framework of a given individual? Indeed, it seems likely that aggressive impulses are as much at work as erotic drives.

Current understanding does not allow a truly etiologic statement. It is possible, however, to note some of the correlates of firesetting. These do not identify the source of the firesetting, but they do clarify some of the conditions for its appearance.

Clinical Picture

In their book, Wooden and Berkey (1984) report on a study of 104 youngsters in San Bernadino County, California, who were known firesetters and who were matched against a group of nonfiresetting controls. The authors describe as well their findings with a different population of 536 juveniles who were caught setting fires on school property in that area over a 7-year period. The investigators also studied a group of firefighters in the same region.

Within the framework of the primary study, a consistent and robust finding prevailed throughout: The family constellations of the firesetters were appreciably more disrupted and disturbed than was the case with the controls. In 61% of the index subjects, the disruptions had been recent (28% of controls had such family problems); these disruptions included a recent divorce, a remarriage, a death, a new baby, or some other significant change. In 62% of these cases, the parents of the firesetters spoke of their child as being under severe stress for the preceding 6 months (whereas only 10% of the controls were so described). These findings are backed up by other reports in the literature that speak variously of desertion, alcoholism, abuse, parental psychosis, broken homes, adoption, illegitimacy, family disorganization with accompanying absence of father, and severe parental psychopathology (Kaufman et al., 1967; Lewis & Yarnell, 1951; Nurcombe, 1964; Siegelman, 1969).

In addition, the families reported that the youngsters were often adopted, were runaways, and/or did not respond to discipline. Furthermore, all of the firesetters had been in trouble with the authorities, and some of them frequently played with fire. All this stood in marked contrast to the control group.

The authors tried out a list of 84 behavioral-problem characteristics on the two populations; of these, 33 emerged as significantly different for the two groups. In particular, many more firesetters were given to stealing and truancy. There were behavioral and learning problems in school that were meaningfully different for the two cohorts; other researchers also have found that firesetters have serious school problems. By and large, these young firesetters do not like school, do poorly in school, and, as adolescents, often attack the school they attend.

Another major problem area was in peer relations. The parents of firesetters repeatedly observed that their children frequently played alone and, when with others, were easily led by peers. The firesetting children tended to be hyperactive. They were given to lying, impulsive outbursts, fighting, impatience, and jealousy. They were not infrequently shy, out of touch with reality, likely to stutter, violent, and poor losers.

Other investigators have reported similar findings and have correlated firesetting and severe rage reactions with chronic hyperactivity (Vandersall & Wiener, 1971). Other prominent findings that paralleled hyperkinesis were stealing, sadistic behavior toward siblings, running away, destructiveness, and aggression (Nurcombe, 1964). Showers and Pickrell (1987) studied 186 children who were psychiatric inpatients or outpatients by matching their demographic findings against a group of nonfiresetting patients who served as controls. The authors found that the firesetters were more likely to have been abused, to have a stepparent or other nonrelated adult in the home, and to have a mother with a drug or alcohol problem than were the nonfiresetting controls. Moreover, the average firesetter displayed almost twice the number of aberrant social behaviors as the controls. The overwhelming impression of all observers is that firesetting is almost never an isolated symptom; in most cases it occurs as part of a complex pattern of disturbing behavior within a highly aberrant family matrix.

Some attempts have been made to cluster these characteristics. Thus, Siegelman and Folkman sorted their youngsters into two groups: the first comprised restless, antisocial children who were hostile toward peers; the second included youngsters who also had poor peer relationships but who were anxious, withdrawn, and self-devaluing. A widely cited, earlier attempt at clustering (Hellman & Blackman, 1966) grouped firesetting with enuresis and sadistic behavior toward animals, but these results were not confirmed.

To be sure, in Siegelman and Folkman's study the younger group of firesetters did tend to be cruel to pets, but the older age group did not. As might have been expected, there was more enuresis among the younger children. Indeed, it is possible to list a number of additional behaviors that tend to characterize younger as contrasted with older, and less serious as compared with more serious groups of firesetting children. In particular, the younger firesetters, who were for the most part between 4 and 8 years old, tended to attack elements in the immediate family environment, such as siblings, pets, and toys. Many symptoms of immaturity were present, such as thumbsucking, bedwetting, or stuttering. In contrast, the older (late grade-school age) firesetting children (who were between 9 and 12 years old) would lash out at their peers. They would frequently be in fights, were poor losers, and were easily led into difficulties. Not uncommonly, their inner tensions found expression in nightmares and tics. These children tended to set fires in the morning, close to home or on their way to school. Finally, the oldest group, the 13- to 17-year-olds, were likely to show classical forms of psychiatric symptomatology. They manifested overt depression, displayed bizarre ideation, and verbalized in odd and disturbing ways. They were more prone as well to classical psychosomatic symptoms, such as vomiting and bowel problems. By and large, they set fires late in the day, at some distance from home, perhaps at school or on the way home from school. In aggregate, the available studies indicate that firesetting is part of a pattern of deviant activities that together form a larger picture of disturbance. The degree and the kind of associated behaviors vary with developmental level and with the severity of the overall condition, but firesetting will seldom occur in isolation; and the diagnostic problem will always be to discern the larger dimensions of the disturbance. Notwithstanding all that investigators have learned, the dynamic meaning of firesetting for these children, and the reasons it plays so large a role in their symptomatology remain elusive.

Having said that, it seems appropriate to describe the four types of firesetters in greater detail. The *playing-with-matches* youngsters are, on the one hand, merely curious about or are experimenting with fire and are as likely to injure themselves as anyone else (a far less common outcome among the other three categories). On the other hand, this type of firesetting occurs far more frequently in homes where divorce has taken place, or where family life has been otherwise disrupted. Whether this represents merely a lack of supervision or is a direct response to the emotional stress of family disturbance is not altogether clear; that it does occur has been substantiated (Kafry, 1978).

The *crying-for-help* youngster is best understood as the victim of some major pattern of stress, and the firesetting is part of the stress response. In this sense, the arson is directed in large measure at drawing attention to what is going on and summoning help. In general, the clinician can understand the character of the stress only by empathically grasping the nature of the child's experience (e.g., a bereft and solitary child who loses a pet may be deprived of the one unambivalently positive attachment in his life and may thus experience the loss as catastrophic). In other instances, however, the character of the stress is inherently overwhelming (e.g., sadistic or sexual abuse). In either case the child may, in sheer helplessness, send out a distress signal by kindling a fire. Not surprisingly, this is usually a solitary act performed by a younger child and is directed against some element of the immediate environment that clearly symbolizes the current conflict (e.g., a child might set fire to his mother's bed).

Where no relief is forthcoming, or where the child receives a paradoxical response in the form of some measure of reward for the firesetting behavior (e.g., evident parental delight at the child's clever trick, or some element of sensuous arousal at the visual aspect of the fire, or the excitement of fire engines and all the panoply of fire fighting), the pattern may take root, flourish, and become a recurrent theme in the child's life.

In Wooden and Berkey's study (1984) many of these calling-for-help fires were set by children who had recently been through a parental divorce or whose parents had separated. Frequently the firesetting occurred when for some reason attention was focused on another child; occasionally this behavior followed the death of a significant relative. A sizable percentage of this group were adopted children, and many were enuretic. Overall, these were a deeply hurt, and sometimes an angry and vengeful, group of children who were struggling to master overwhelming emotions.

The *delinquent* group were operating on the basis of quite a different set of motives. They were older than the members of the first two clusters, and there was often a quality of calculated intent, the classic form of "malicious mischief," associated with their behavior. The typical member of this group would be very much under the influence of a peer group with whom he was trying to prove himself or to maintain status. Such a child was likely to come from a fragmented and disturbed family environment, to evidence considerable emotional disturbance in his own right, to convey a sense of sexual immaturity, to have a long list of prior aggressive acts on his record, and to have done poorly in school. Characteristically, the firesetting would be a group phenomenon, sometimes associated with other crimes (and intended to cover up what had been done), and typically executed with some plan in mind for outwitting the authorities and enjoying the experience. Occasionally the behavior had the character of aimless destructiveness, the product of boredom and restlessness, with an underlying tone of defying authority and seeking some sort of hedonic outlet. By and large, the youngsters who perform these acts have long histories of delinquency, which usually include firesetting.

The fires set by this group are most likely to be ignited in or near school. It has been estimated that this kind of willful arson costs the public schools of the United States millions of dollars a year ("Arson," 1976). The commonest form of firesetting is the setting off of fireworks or explosives of some kind on the school grounds. Where the behavior involves arson directly, getting even with a teacher is the commonest motive. The worst fires come when the youth plots revenge, sneaks into school at night or on a weekend, and carries out the plan.

The authors felt that the last group, the *severely disturbed* firesetters, divided itself naturally into two subgroups. One was the impulsive neurotic type where the youngsters were inclined to steal, to sleep poorly, to act impulsively, to be unable to delay gratification, and to destroy their own possessions. The other subgroup included youngsters with borderline or psychotic characteristics; these cases ran the gamut from bizarre and explosive behavior to extreme emotionality accompanied by much phobic symptomatology, recurrent bouts of violence, and peculiar speech. Again, the presence of considerable family disturbance was almost universal among these young people. A common finding (and one that the authors considered predictive) was the distressed quality of the relationship between mother and child. How accurately this could predict arson per se rather than conduct disorder in general was not made clear.

Course of Development

In light of the complex clinical pictures described above, it is evident that firesetting can appear at many different points in the course of development, and is not restricted to a single dynamic sequence. Hence, it is not likely to have any single or even characteristic course. In describing children who begin to set fires in adolescence, however, Wooden and Berkey remark (1984) that the typical firesetter reaches his teens after "first feeling isolated, then wandering around, beginning to steal, disobeying and withdrawing from parents and teachers, and finally setting fires" (p. 4). This echoes the observation of Patterson (1976) who regarded defying, wandering, lying, and stealing as preconditions for the setting of fires.

Etiology of Firesetting

A great many theories have been offered to explain the motivations for firesetting behavior. The large majority of these etiologic constructs are overly general; often they seem merely to state the obvious without really explaining much. Thus, the formulation that regards firesetting as a means of lashing out against the environment is accurate enough but does little to clarify why the lashing out takes that particular form. In a few instances, the cognitive component evidently prevails; for example, a youngster commits a theft or a murder and then sets a fire to conceal any implicating evidence, or a youth is paid to set a fire so that someone can collect insurance. It is also relatively easy to understand that someone would set fires if that were his primary means of obtaining sexual gratification (i.e., the immediate impulse and its enaction become reasonably understandable, but why firesetting of all things should have come to occupy such a unique position in anyone's life is still a mystery). A child can deal with motives such as revenge and retaliation in many ways, however, and the reason(s) for the choice of firesetting continue(s) to remain elusive. And explanations that say the youngster did it out of boredom are really no explanation at all.

Wooden and Berkey (1984) assert that the lack of exposure to fire in the home and the accompanying lack of early instruction about its dangerousness and appropriate management allow the younger child to become curious without being informed. Fire becomes mysterious and consequently attractive, and playing with matches or experimenting is likely to follow. Experiencing the color, excitement, and pleasurable thrills associated with fire trucks and sirens may also lure the younger child to set more fires. So far the explanation makes sense, but the consequence should be that all children would then play with fire and very likely set fires—and that is simply not the case. In fact, as noted above, a number of psychosocial conditions, such as recent parental separation or divorce or other forms of family stress, seem to predispose even preschoolers to such patterns. Whether the firesetting represents a direct failure of parental supervision or some more obscure response to relative neglect (the parents are consumed to a large extent by their own travail and have relatively less affective investment available for the child), or whether some other dynamic is at work is currently unknown.

Wooden and Berkey (1984, pp. 34–35) offer the theory that in their experience, firesetters differ from nonfiresetters in their need for "power enhancement," that is, the firesetting children feel a lack of power or control both at home and in their interactions with other people generally, and they then begin to set fires as an expression of their helpless rage and as a response to parental abuse or neglect. This is true of all the more serious types of firesetting (the crying-for-help, the delinquent, and the seriously disturbed).

Fineman (1980) suggests that three conditions have to be met before a child deliberately sets a fire. First, the child must be characterologically vulnerable (as manifested by the many behavioral difficulties noted above); second, a significant stress must occur (in the form of family disruption, loss, or other crisis); and finally, some kind of positive reinforcement for the act of kindling has to be present (i.e., parental attention, pleasure, and excitement associated with the fire itself, or peer approval).

Within this framework, the crying-for-help firesetters may be unconsciously seeking relief from inner tension and trying to bring about some change in the family environment.

The delinquent youngsters may be seeking the thrills associated with the fire experience; they may get a direct sadistic pleasure in the destruction they cause and the feeling of power that this affords them; they may be proving themselves to their delinquent companions; they may set the fires in association with other crimes in an effort to conceal evidence; or they may set fires to challenge the authorities by escaping punishment. The severely disturbed children set fires in response to odd and discrepant impulses of irrational character such as psychotic prompting, paranoid ideation, narcissistic power struggles, or the rage engendered by overreaction to some life crisis.

A large number of firesetters have a history of sexual abuse. When boys have been homosexually abused, the rage thus engendered is often of monumental proportions, and the fires that they set thereafter have about them the quality of "total eradication of the offending object" (Wooden & Berkey, 1984, p. 102).

The clinician occasionally encounters the true pyromaniac, where the perverse goal of the firesetting is to achieve erotic arousal and orgasm. There is a sexual thrill for these youngsters in watching flames, and they may masturbate as part of the experience. Paradoxically, they sometimes use the masturbation to defend themselves against the impulse to set fires. In such cases, there is an intimate connection between the two acts, and in predisposed individuals, they can be linked forms of sexual expression.

There is at least some reason to believe that children who are institutionalized for setting fires have a higher-than-normal rate of chromosomal abnormalities (Barlett et al., 1968). Youngsters who are institutionalized in settings for delinquents and who share a history of firesetting have a number of other traits in common. They are said to be generally weaker than other inmates, with a vaguely bizarre physical appearance; to impress their caretakers as being socially inadequate and lacking in healthy aggressivity; to become sexual targets for the more assertive males; to convey a sense of being anxious, immature, and passive; and to manifest an inability to play. It has been proposed that these individuals experience the world in distinctive visual ways that differentiate them from the other delinquents. When they close their eyes, they frequently see fire or red. Images of fire are soothing to them or otherwise rewarding. If indeed this were to prove out as a testable hypothesis, it would be a beginning formulation of a rational explanation for symptom choice. Another notion is that the children are deprived of adequate warmth and sensory stimulation during their growing-up years; as a result they experience sensory deprivation and severe stimulus hunger, and they then attempt to compensate for the deficiency by turning to fire.

Heretofore, the discussion has centered largely on boys who are firesetters. Girls too set fires, however, and the dynamics in such cases may be somewhat different from those that are characteristic for boys. For one thing, as a group, girls are generally older than boys when they engage in firesetting. In contrast to the boys, they tend to set fires away from school, and they are less inclined to utilize fireworks. When they do set fires at school, the motive is usually to gain attention or to avoid a test rather than to achieve revenge.

Researchers have surmised that with the current change in sex-role behavior, the fires set by girls are beginning to take on some of the same characteristics that have been typical for boys' fires. Assertive and competitive issues are playing a part in both the frequency with which girls become involved in fire-related episodes and their choice of this form of miscreance. In the past, fires set by girls have tended to be directed against their own possessions or residence, a pattern suggestive of self-destructive tendencies (Lewis & Yarnell, 1951). Currently this may be changing.

In Wooden and Berkey's (1984) study, one-third of the girls who set fires had been victims of sexual abuse in childhood (a figure estimated as probably low), and the group of girls as a whole had more problems related to sexuality than did a control group of nonarsonist girls.

Treatment

Professionals have developed a number of measures to address the therapeutic needs of the different age levels and the several types of firesetting children. For the younger group, particularly the playing-with-fire and some of the less troubled crying-for-help youngsters, the most widely employed modality is some kind of *educational program*. Parents who have a preschooler must bear the greatest share of the responsibility for teaching the child about fire and protecting him from ready access to dangerous materials. When the child is of kindergarten or grade-school age, the educational effort might include asking the child a series of questions about what is dangerous, what different materials are for, how to help people hurt by fire, and so on. The teacher could offer a sequence of pictures to color (draw the dangerous things in red, the helpful ones in green, etc.) or could ask the child to connect the dots of an instructional picture to learn how to get out of a smoke-filled room.

Teachers have also used educational films, have assigned fire safety responsibilities for children when at home, have taught methods for recognizing if someone is playing with fire, and have engaged the child in fire-prevention tasks, such as caring for ashtrays. Assignments have been developed that require the child to devise queries for firefighters, to join with his parents in checking home safety devices, to draw pictures of self and family in connection with fire, or to complete a self-learning program and turn it in.

With the older and more troubled youngster, a common educational modality is to engage the child in some form of research about fire, for example, writing an essay, interviewing a firefighter, or earning a scout merit badge in fire fighting. Study allotments followed by a test have been devised (the "Learn Not to Burn" Knowledge Test) and are widely used.

A second general approach has been the use of *aversion therapy*. The child might be assigned to light 200 matches in a safe place, an undertaking that presently becomes boring in the extreme.

A third tactic is *positive behavior modification*. This involves getting the youngster to handle threatening material and rewarding him for maintenance of good control. Thus, within a structured safe area, the child is given toys and play materials that include concealed matches and lighters. The clinician then observes the child handling these objects and supports coping efforts.

One project pairs individual children with a history of firesetting on a one-to-one basis with a firefighter who has been trained to work with a troubled child. The result is a sort of Big Brother arrangement with a primary focus on firesetting (Holstrom, 1983).

Institutional placement is necessary for the more delinquent and the severely disturbed youngsters, both to protect the community and to try to help the young person. Where there is a considerable component of emotional disorder, the standard psychiatric treatment techniques are applicable and are vitally important. These include milieu therapy, individual therapy, and group approaches as well as other appropriate techniques. Generally speaking, however, the emphasis for this group falls on individualized attention. For the child who seems primarily conduct disordered, behavior modification, assertiveness training, anger management techniques, and group therapy are likely to be the basic program components. Overall, it appears that the clinician who makes a good effort can accomplish a great deal of successful preventive work with the younger, the more neurotic, and the more approachable youngsters. For the older and the more severe firesetters, however, treatment efforts are at best uncertain in their outcome.

Chapter 14

Narcissistic Disorders

INTRODUCTION

Only within the past decade have professionals seriously addressed the problems of childhood narcissism. Indeed, a definitive involvement with narcissism in general is a relatively recent phenomenon. For years, despite its prominence in the etiology and phenomenology of delinquency and other characteriological problems, the issue had received little attention from psychiatrists, psychologists, or sociologists. Then the work of Kohut & Kernberg gave the subject a salience and immediacy that aroused great interest; currently, the study of the narcissistic disorders is a leading clinical preoccupation.

DEFINITION

The term *narcissism* derives from the Greek myth of Narcissus, a splendidly beautiful youth who loved nothing so much as studying his own reflection in the surface of a pool. So lost did he become in this image that one day he leaned too far forward, fell in the pool, and was drowned. When Freud began to write about the powerful and compelling self-love that he so often noted in his patients, he turned to the tale of Narcissus to name this extraordinary form of human adaptation.

In his original formulations, Freud recognized *primary* and *secondary* narcissism. *Primary* narcissism is the basic and necessary self-regard that makes a person care about self-growth, self-care and self-preservation. As development proceeds, these interests form the core of what eventually becomes feelings of self-assurance, self-confidence, and self-worth.

After the child has attempted attachments with others, a different phenomenon may emerge—*secondary* narcissism. This involves the feelings a person gets from the regard of significant others. Not all such attachments are going to be fortunate; there will be moments of pain and rejection. Then, as a defense against an ungiving or unappreciative world, the child can turn his energies back to the self and nurse his own image at the expense of other relationships. Many pathological forms of narcissism are likely to be expressions of secondary narcissism, but the really serious disorders involve defects in forming the primary narcissistic structures.

In understanding narcissistic pathology, the key concept is *grandiosity*. This sense of the self as being superior, better than, more deserving than—in some sense—more important than others is a persistent theme that runs through the descriptions and the pathological behavior of the narcissist. It translates into a host of symptomatic behaviors: arrogance, selfishness, envy, boasting, overweening pride, intrusiveness, conceit, demandingness, refusal to accept social limits or norms, refusal to submit to group rules, demands for being made an exception, and insistence on having more than others have. When the narcissist does not attach the grandiosity to the self, he attaches it to some external source with special associations—belonging to a superior family, having greater wealth, living in a prestigious neighborhood, following a world-famous guru, or being a member of a cult with transcendent values. At the least, the narcissistic state involves extravagant daydreams and the expectation of special treatment by others. The narcissist who is frustrated in achieving demands and expectations may experience great pain and respond accordingly. He might pout and withdraw, sulk and accuse, or go off on a tangent of enormous rage, perhaps with overt tantrums or with silent fantasies of domination and plots of revenge. All too often the individual bitterly retaliates for having received narcissistic wounds.

In many milder cases, the narcissistic character pattern takes on a superficially appropriate and socially adaptive style. Only intimates—parents, spouse, or close friends—become aware of the person's enormous self-centeredness and grandiose stance within these important relationships. Sometimes the individual is so demanding that he can keep no friends at all and speaks dolorously of others' selfishness and conceitedness. Some narcissistics, on the other hand, have enough skill, wealth, talent or sheer intelligence to gain acceptance, admiration, and even indulgence from the world about them.

Many narcissists are very vulnerable people. Because they are keyed to external response, they need extraordinary recognition, appreciation, and regard from their environments to maintain even an elementary level of good feeling. Such a continual influx of attentiveness, praise, and appreciation is not likely to be forthcoming from most people, and so the narcissist is forever being hurt by someone. Such a person is like Lewis Carroll's red queen, who had to keep running in order to stay in place; if she stopped, she would begin to go backward. And so with the narcissist who, to avoid feeling hurt, requires constant reassurance of being loved, admired, and valued. The end result is considerable suffering; narcissists, despite their assumptions of grandeur and the pain they often cause others, are chronically distressed much of the time.

HISTORY

In one of his great theoretical papers, "On Narcissism," Freud (1914/1957d) asserted the clinical centrality of this issue, but his description was not altogether clear, and it was not immediately evident to what extent narcissistic problems played a role in everyday life. Although referred to repeatedly in psychoanalytic writings during the ensuing years, narcissism did not become the central theme of theory and debate until the work of Heinz Kohut and Otto Kernberg began to appear in the late 1960s. These two thinkers approached the issues from very different standpoints, and their research in effect created two schools of thought. Current thinking is derived from the dialogue between these two approaches.

An emerging interest in the problems of the borderline patient paralleled these developments. In particular, Melanie Klein's view of the borderline gained many adherents, and the use of the term *splitting* became ubiquitous. The reigning psychoanalytic approach was *ego psychology*, which involved attempting to understand and to explain symptomatic behavior in terms of conflict and the derivative disturbances of ego function. This perspective in turn focused on the defense mechanisms of the ego, both as theoretical constructs as well as sites for technical address. As a result, the ensuing decades saw a primary emphasis on defense or character analysis. In other words, with the advent of ego psychology, the focus shifted from the *content* of the oedipal experience to the *defenses* and *character structures* associated with it. To deal with these conflicts, the analyst worked with defenses such as displacement, reaction formation, repression, and isolation. The analyst analyzed the defensive component of dreams, and made forbidden wishes conscious by working with the mechanisms that kept them out of consciousness.

When psychotherapists began to emphasize borderline pathology, the focus shifted to the earlier, more primitive defenses, such as projective identification, introjection, denial, and splitting. More and more studies centered on the strange world of the infant during the first two years of life: his larger-than-life ur-figures (sometimes called imagoes); his extraordinary needs for attachment to these awesome presences; his problems with boundaries (when does the baby become able to distinguish self from other?); his primitive, overwhelming emotions; and his inherently inarticulate propensity for action. In particular, Margaret Mahler and colleagues (Mahler et al., 1975) set about establishing some order among these somewhat chaotic conceptions; Mahler developed the powerful approach that is tied uniquely to her name. She based her theory on the observed reactions of infants and toddlers to separation. Her ideas, which came to be known as the *separation–individuation theory*, demarcated a series of stages of psychological birth. This process begins with a fused conception of infant and mother; then, in a sequence of steps, the infant gradually and sometimes painfully starts to demarcate boundaries between himself and the significant other; finally, the baby acquires the capacity to discern and develop the lineaments of self as an autonomous presence in the social world.

These powerful conceptions gave substance and solidity to the search for a language and a way of thinking about the symptomatic expressions and behavior of the borderline, and, at the same time, paved the way for the study of narcissism. Researchers were now coming to see this personality configuration also in terms of early infantile adaptation, and the work of both Kohut (1971) and Kernberg (1975) rested on such early formulations.

Meanwhile, yet another theoretical development, the *object relations theory*, was gradually taking shape and gathering force within depth-psychological thinking. In the original Freudian model the psyche was a closed system, comprising the id, the ego, and the superego. The id gave rise to drives and yearnings that were constantly stoked by the biologically rooted instincts. Thus the desires for pleasure, nurturance, closeness, sex, elimination, sleep, and tension relief all came from the id. The ego defended itself from the eruption of these crude id drives into consciousness, tempered their expression and mode of their discharge, and made satisfying these inner drives adaptive and socially acceptable.

The ego did much of its work by using a series of mental mechanisms—inborn tactics of ordering the energy of the id drives—to redirect them toward appropriate targets, to parcel them out into suitable channels of discharge, to fractionate them in various ways that contained their intense expression, or simply to keep them locked away from consciousness. Crude and primitive yearnings could thus be refashioned into the nuances and the subtleties of civilized comportment. Freud felt that civilization was based on such sublimation.

Finally, the superego was the agency of mind that acted as the conscience, bearing the ethics and mores of the individual's culture. It subserved two main functions: to warn against, forbid, and inhibit antisocial behavior; and to contain the model, or ideal, of what the individual was to strive for. It thus regulated both guilt and self-esteem, and it was a major contributor to happiness or depression.

Freud's model was a self-contained system; there was no place within such an arrangement for other people as real presences. To some extent others could be taken into the system as representations or images; but the model could not describe the interaction of the id-ego-superego of the child with the mother as a real presence, and there was no concept of *reality* on the same level of abstraction as the id-ego-superego complex. Therefore, the child could not interact with the mother, but only with the mother's image as it appeared within the ego. Indeed, to achieve logical consistency, there was no way that the ego could interact with the image of the mother; a separate function of the ego had to be defined to do that. Hence, it was necessary to develop a complex language within which the self-representation interacted with the object-representation (*object* here meaning the generalized other). In effect these theorists took a Kantian approach, an individual could not know the *Ding an Sich*, "the thing in itself"; the person could know only its representation in his or her mind. Logically, even knowing the self was impossible; only the representation of the self existed in the individual's mind.

To deal with this difficulty, the object-relations theorists applied a kind of Occam's razor. They asserted that the primary reality was the actual presence of significant others. Individuals thus responded directly to their feelings and needs for this presence and to the pleasure or pain engendered through social interactions. The baby needed the mother in a primary way, not as a presence within a psychological matrix, but as an actual holding, supporting, nurturing entity who was there to give to baby. The mother's immediate presence or absence was a matter of the utmost import, evoking extremely strong emotional reactions. This kind of theorizing then talked about the sense of connectedness, or bond formed between the self and significant others. Carried to its extreme, as Kohut did, diagnosis would depend on the quality of this relationship, as recreated by the patient with the therapist (the transference paradigm). Accordingly, treatment would then be a matter of resolving these relationship issues.

Another great construct that had long been known was necessary to formulate a theory of narcissism: the notion of *idealization*. It was evident that people had ideals that were vitally important in determining the pattern of their lives and social adaptation. The classical theorists, particularly the Kleinians, spoke about the inner presence of idealized images of others (objects) and idealized images of the self. Presently, Kernberg was constructing a theory of psychopathology on the model of an ego that harbored at once a self-representation, an object-representation, an idealized self-representation, and an idealized object-representation (Kernberg, 1975).

Kohut's theory, on the other hand, tended to encompass a view of objects (other people) that was subject to distortions. These distortions were the result of privations (the early caretakers' failures of empathy), which left their traces within the ego. The patient looked to the therapist as a source of the missing empathy (a *self-object* in this terminology), or as an ideal, and reacted accordingly. This theory led to rather different sets of formulations and therapeutic measures.

Current Nomenclature and Diagnostic Formulations

Narcissistic Personality Disorder is included within the framework of DSM-III-R as one of the Personality Disorders. As such, it is a diagnosis of adulthood but, in fact, there is no stipulation as to the age of onset. Considerable clinical evidence suggests that this condition is commonly present in childhood and that its earliest symptoms or, at any rate, its precursors are recognizable in the preschool years.

The DSM-III and DSM-III-R Categories

The transition from the DSM-III to the DSM-III-R is interesting. The DSM-III provides four major distinguishing characteristics along with two of four possible disturbances in interpersonal relationships. The four principal features are:

1. *Grandiosity: Self-importance, uniqueness, exaggeration of one's capacities, a focus on one's specialness*
2. *Fantasies of one's own greatness and centrality in the larger order of things; a preoccupation with dreams of one's glory*
3. *Exhibitionism: a tendency to show off, a need to be the center of attention, a craving for constant admiration*
4. *An inability to tolerate criticism, a vulnerability to feelings of shame, a profound sense of humiliation and emptiness when feeling ignored or defeated, an unusual degree of rage in the face of such negative or wounding experience.*
5. *Finally, at least two of the following kinds of disturbance in interpersonal relations:*
   a) *A sense of entitlement and expectation that one merits special treatment—with corresponding dismay and exasperation if that is not forthcoming*
   b) *An assumption that one's own needs and desires matter whereas those of others do not, with a feeling of justification in one's right to exploit others for one's own ends*
   c) *A tendency to oscillate between attitudes of overidealizing significant others and devaluing them*
   d) *A lack of basic empathy with the feelings of other people so that the sufferings and concerns of others do not really register.* (APA, 1980, p. 317)

When DSM-III-R appeared, there were three essential characteristics that had to be present: a pervasive pattern of grandiosity (in fantasy or behavior), a lack of empathy, and hypersensitivity to the evaluation of others. The criteria further stipulated that these characteristics had to be evident in many contexts and provided a choice of 5 out of 9 possible descriptors:

(1) reacts to criticism with feelings of rage, shame, or humiliation (even if not expressed)

(2) is interpersonally exploitative; takes advantage of others to achieve his or her own ends

(3) has grandiose sense of self-importance, e.g., exaggerates achievements and talents, expects to be noticed and "special" without appropriate achievement

(4) believes that his or her problems are unique and can be understood only by other special people

(5) is preoccupied with fantasies of unlimited success, power, brilliance, beauty, or ideal love

(6) has a sense of entitlement; unreasonable expectation of especially favorable treatment, e.g., assumes that he or she does not have to wait in line when others must do so

(7) requires constant attention and admiration, e.g., keeps fishing for compliments

(8) lack of empathy; inability to recognize and experience how others feel, e.g., annoyance and surprise when a friend who is seriously ill cancels a date

(9) is preoccupied with feelings of envy. (APA, 1987, p. 351)

Although this listing of traits may be sufficient for diagnosing a narcissistic disorder later in life, its expression during childhood may take a somewhat different form. Usually the diagnosis is not a matter of uncertainty; the child is seldom an object of concern unless the degree of personality disturbance is quite extreme. For the troubled youngster, once this form of maladjustment is present, the basic issues do not change over time, and narcissistic adjustment continues (although perhaps it is ever more effectively concealed) throughout development.

The Forms of Narcissistic Behavior

The distinction between normal and pathological narcissism is a vital diagnostic issue. Up to a point, narcissism is normal. For good mental health, an adequate amount of self-love must be present; that is, the feelings toward the self must be essentially positive in quality and adequate in amount. The sense of basic trust that emerges at the end of the first year of life carries with it a feeling of worthwhileness; the child feels valued and hence valuable. This means that the infant has learned to have faith in the significant other and, at the same time, has gained confidence in his own lovableness and positive merit.

This expression of healthy narcissism provides the basic groundwork for optimism and a sense of feeling at one with the world. As the child grows older, the positive sense of the loved and lovable self continues to develop. In the toddler, it takes form as an ability to accept a reasonable amount of frustration without being overwhelmed by catastrophic rage and/or a sense of abject worthlessness; even in the face of upset, the youngster can be readily comforted because the narcissistic nucleus within is sturdy enough to reconstitute quickly, to regain, and ultimately to maintain the good feelings.

With further development this wholesome narcissistic presence allows for adequate self-assertiveness and, if necessary, for self-defense against the inroads of other youngsters. To some extent it takes on grandiose forms in play, but the child maintains a clear distinction between the play role and the real self. Thus, at three or four, the youngster who plays being the cowboy or the queen can give up the play cheerfully when it is time to wash hands before dinner. Later still, when the superego forms, the grandiose elements largely withdraw from the self-representation within the ego and become confined to the ego ideal. This leading presence grows and matures along with the rest of ego and superego so that, in time, the more fanciful and megalomanic elements give way to appropriate ideals. These in turn serve to lead and to inspire the individual's inner life. Gradually, the narcissistic elements evolve into realistic ambitions and aspirations, into goals and values, and, ultimately, into compassion, humor, and wisdom.

There is a gradual shading from normal to disturbed narcissism. The mild forms of the condition would not require diagnosis, let alone intervention. Indeed, the mildest cases may be rather characteristic of a great many people (although, to be sure, not the norm).

The range of narcissism is in some sense comparable to obsessive-compulsive tendencies. Normal people have a certain amount of compulsiveness; indeed, they need some of this trait to balance a checkbook and to maintain order in their affairs. However, a researcher studying the distribution of compulsiveness in a sizable population, is likely to find a gradual shift in the degree and quality of this proclivity; the curve will identify people with more and more of the characteristic, finally isolating a subpopulation whose lives have been taken over by the obsessive-compulsive trait. These are the individuals who become diagnosed as having an obsessive-compulsive disorder. Narcissism is probably distributed in the population in somewhat the same way.

Mild narcissistic tendencies are a concern here only as an exclusionary boundary. What this chapter deals with, then, is the true Narcissistic Personality Disorder, as defined in DSM-III-R. The condition implies a massive quantity of narcissistic disturbance, meriting both diagnosis and treatment.

There is a central difference between narcissism and many other extreme psychopathological conditions. Unlike severe compulsives, for example, individuals with truly pathological narcissism, may not be easy to identify. Indeed, their symptoms may initially be highly disguised, so much so that the therapist must invest considerable effort merely to make the diagnosis, and more effort still to reveal all the details of the problem.

Another notable distinction of narcissism is that its cluster of traits may be present in different degrees of seriousness. Some can occur with overwhelming force and give the personality its definitive hue, whereas others may be present only as a trace, a mild tinge, or a peripheral intrusion.

Narcissistic Symptomatology

Paulina Kernberg (1984) has delineated some of the symptomatic findings in narcissistic children. Obviously these findings will vary with the child's constitution and development as well as with the degree of severity of the particular syndrome. Yet, in aggregate, they convey some sense of the inner quality of the narcissistic problem in childhood. Here are some of the patterns she reports:

Poor and brittle self-esteem.
Inability to love others or to receive love.
Inability to depend on others.
Inability to experience fulfillment and gratification.
Chronic feelings of boredom and emptiness.

A grandiose sense of self.

Ambitious fantasies of success, power, beauty, or an ideal life.

Loneliness.

A transient pseudoidentity in response to admiration.

Feelings of emptiness in the face of a lack of admiration.

Attempts to demand, control, and exploit others.

Incapacity to experience the world as nurturing.

A feeling of intense, destructive envy because others can feel a sense of nurture.

A tendency in the child to establish coercive control over peers: a sense of entitlement that justifies exploitativeness.

Inability to tolerate friends other than as clones.

The transient attachment to friends who are fleetingly overidealized as the perfect person the narcissistic child would like to be.

The ready devaluation of friends if they become a source of envy.

Hypochondriac or somatic symptoms that result from the fear of projected envy.

A contradictory school record showing ambitious expenditures of effort side by side with inexplicable failures. This pattern may develop because the child insists on either being the best or devaluing the fields in which he cannot triumph.

Symptomatic depression (related to school failure) that arises from feelings of defeat and shame at not having triumphed. In addition, the child shows a ready tendency to devalue any reward that is not immediately forthcoming.

Difficulty in accepting the status of being a beginner.

Maintenance of an apparently easygoing, superficially friendly quality. The child may seem to portray an innocently charming hedonism; his attachments to others are shallow; and he has no long range investment in values or goals other than self-aggrandizement.

Malignant narcissism, a transition that some youngsters make from minor dishonesty to full-fledged antisocial narcissism, accompanied by ego-syntonic sadism and involving a pattern of aggressive self-affirmation.

Suicidal tendencies, possibly involving an omnipotent triumph over the usual human fear of pain or death.

Paranoid ideation associated with a projection of sadistic superego precursors.

This partial list gives something of the flavor of the condition. In clinical practice the major problems that bring the youngsters to attention include, first, the ubiquitous problem of poor school performance, followed closely by difficulties with peers. Another common precipitant of referral is the kind of rage some of these youngsters display; they are capable of extraordinary outbursts in the face of wounds to their fragile self-esteem and/or frustrations of their towering and grandiose expectations.

The chief complaint frequently involves unendurable behavior within the home. Such actions may include vicious attacks on peers, obscene and devaluing language toward parents, endless imperious, impossible demands directed toward parents, gross chronic disobedience, and eruptive and uncontrolled behaviors within the household. A particularly troublesome pattern is the lying that so often characterizes these youngsters. In their lives, the important thing is to be the center of attention, to be grand, to make an impression; such outcomes have far more valence for these children than any petty concerns about the truth of what they recount. Sometimes their families remark that the youngsters seem to tell stories when they have no evident need and apparently gain nothing from the telling. The child can even exhibit a state referred to as *pseudologia fantastica,* that is, a complete departure from any attempt at veracity. There is a constant outpouring of tall tales and sometimes very obvious lies, with the most vigorous and aggressive defense of these outlandish statements and every evidence of mortal wounding should anyone impugn their veracity. In such cases, the entire organization of personality is seemingly dedicated to making a sensation.

School difficulties arise from the inability of these youngsters to deal well with frustration and delay. If they happen to be bright and catch on quickly, they will often do well, glorying in their competence and often boasting of their achievements. But if the material does not come easily, they cannot endure the narcissistic hurt of not knowing and may devalue the class, fail to attend or to hand in assignments, and speak to the teacher in a critical, depreciating way that shortly gets them into trouble.

Because they look to peers as sources of admiration or as objects of manipulation, these children become rather solitary after a while and are unable to understand why no one seems to like them. Occasionally schoolmates tease them, and they may then resort to school refusal. Much depends on the degree of their disturbance and on their compensatory ego competencies (such as high intelligence, unusual talent, or a gift for being winning with people). The youngster who is not too handicapped by narcissistic configurations may even become a leader. Just acting in such a superior, knowing, and self-centered manner will attract some insecure peers, who wish that they could be as sure of themselves as the narcissistic child seems to be.

The more disturbed narcissist is not likely to do well socially. Sometimes the youngster learns early to conceal the grandiose feelings and basic attitudes lest they get him into trouble. He may then present at school as a daydreamy child who has little to say and whose work is spotty and uncertain.

One of the most salient characteristics of this disorder is the amount of suffering it entails. In a sense the grandiose stance is deceptive. The youngster seems to rise above the possibility of pain and is arrogant, superior, and domineering; he is exploiting and manipulating others, and is demanding special treatment. If anything, the child seems to be creating pain rather than suffering from it.

Nonetheless, such children are usually a mass of raw psychological wounds. Although they harbor all sorts of unrealistic expectations and inappropriate attitudes, to them these beliefs are very real and emotionally charged. When they do not get the special treatment they seek, they are deeply, mortally wounded. They feel profoundly misunderstood and grossly misused. They cannot understand, and they ask the same questions again and again: "How about *me*? How could you do that to *me*?" Narcissistic children experience every slight as a deep personal injury; they are forever not talking to one peer or feeling certain that another one dislikes them because of a social gesture so trivial that the other child was scarcely aware of committing it. But the action has poured acid on the narcissist's soul; the child is really in pain; and the only relief he can find is either to drift off into a grandiose haze, or, if he is prone to anger, then to plot some complicated revenge. Revenge and narcissism are peculiarly related, and it is natural and comforting for the affected youngster to imagine, and, not infrequently, to seek to act on such a revenge fantasy. For many children it is truly the only relief they know.

A narcissistic pattern in conjunction with an antisocial bent is often a serious combination. The arrogance, grandiosity, and single-minded self-centeredness of these youngsters render them particularly cruel and unfeeling, and they may inflict much suffering and deprivation on their victims. They can become ruthless, guilt-free, and self-justifying predators who feel entitled to whatever strikes their fancy, and who can act with a cold-blooded abandon that is disturbing indeed to those who encounter them clinically.

No single pattern of behavior will suffice to diagnose this condition. Instead, the clinician must study the life history, attitudes, and fantasies of the patient to tease out the critical data that determine the narcissistic profile. In the more extreme cases, the diagnosis is simple and straightforward. From the moment the child steps into the therapist's office, his patterns of dominating the situation and outmaneuvering the interviewer are the most prominent aspects of his adjustment; from the outset the character of the problem is all too self-evident. Sometimes, however, the narcissistic nucleus is much less obvious, and not until the diagnostician has tried several unworkable interpretations does it become evident that things are not what they seem.

PREVALENCE

Demographers have seldom employed this diagnosis, and as a result, few prevalence data are known. Normal narcissism is universal, and the minor elements of excessive or disturbed narcissism that glint through the interstices of both healthy and disturbed forms of character structure are probably almost universal. Certainly they are very common. But the full-blown syndrome, albeit frequently encountered, is scarcely commonplace. The likelihood is that a goodly percentage of delinquents fall into this category. (Chapter 13, "Conduct Disorder," discusses the narcissistic subgroup of delinquents. The major study that deals with this issue is by Offer et al., 1979). A crude estimate might be that 25% to 35% of delinquents fit this character type. Because the bulk of the cases of narcissistic personality disorder are not delinquent, however, these numbers do not contribute much toward a demographic estimate.

COURSE

Significant narcissistic pathology begins very early in life. In theory, it is initiated by disturbed infant–mother interactions within the first months of the first year of life; there are no criteria, however, for distinguishing such characteristics during the first year of life. Clinically, the evidence suggests that in severe cases, such youngsters show the following significant characteristics by the second year: They are unusually demanding, hard to console, given to tantrums when frustrated, hungry for the exclusive and undivided attention of the caretaker, and often unhappy. These tendencies are not so deviant as to excite comment; for the most part the children appear to be unusually needy, but normal, infants.

In the later toddler years these children may start learning how to use manipulative tactics, how to be consciously cute, and how to win the attention they crave without getting into trouble. Paradoxically, some of the children learn to gain attention precisely by getting into trouble; this skill may launch a long career of social difficulties. Temperamental factors play a vital role in determining the balance struck. Thus, a child with counterphobic adaptations may seek attention by taking risks, for example, climbing up on dangerous perches to show off; another child of more internalizing makeup may simply drift off into fantasies of grandiose wish fulfillment.

The preschool teacher may first identify the concrete problems. The school report may describe a constant need to be the center of attention, exhibitionistic behavior, an insistence on being special or first or an exception, an inability to endure correction—in short, any of the gamut of behaviors that typify the syndrome. In particular, the teacher may remark on how prone the child is to having hurt feelings; the narcissist's curious sensitivity is present early. Again, in predisposed individuals, a readiness for outbursts of rage and an insistence on getting back at another child for real or fancied slights may already be evident.

In grade school, some of these youngsters seem to drop out of sight for a while only to resurface with problems at puberty. During latency the more internalizing narcissists are likely to be dreamers rather than doers. Even under the best circumstances, however, such children are not likely to be well integrated into their peer group and would probably be described as shy, or as loners. The more externalizing representatives of the syndrome, who are most likely to be in trouble, often fall into one of these categories: class clown; class bully; teller of tall tales; chronic show-off; noisy, disrespectful distracters; or slavish followers of some flamboyant, negative leader. Paradoxically, they can sometimes be the teachers' pet (where the teacher is idealized, and the child ignores all other values in attempting to be most obedient and helpful, closest to, and noticed by the teacher). In short, one way or another, they seek to fulfill the mandate of their pathology, either by maintaining a position of grandiose centrality vis-à-vis all the others, or by finding someone else to idealize and attach to with cloying intensity.

Puberty often intensifies the symptomatology of these youngsters. Within the framework of normal development, the early adolescent shows a universal tendency to move toward a more narcissistic, self-preoccupied position as he encounters the changes in his body, intellect, and emotions. The youngster may spend hours staring into the mirror, writing in a diary, or fantasying dreams of glory. How much more, then, will this self-centered attitude become part of the adaptive mode of the predisposed youth. This probably accounts for the explosion of eruptive behavior that sometimes seems to come with the teen years. A quiet and otherwise nonexceptional child who reaches the age of 12 or 13 years, may suddenly discard a previous pattern of good behavior and become imperious, uncooperative, and altogether impossible. The usual explanation is that the youngster is "going through a stage." To be sure, that is true, except that the majority of teenagers do not become anywhere nearly as difficult; they may become more emotional, but they are not eruptive (Offer, 1969). Where florid symptomatology was present during latency, adolescence often tends to intensify its expression. The oppositional child becomes overtly rebellious; the demanding youngster becomes impossible; the show-off takes to freakish garb and bizarre self-ornamentation; the withdrawn idealizer joins a cult; the liar of yore now becomes the exemplar of *pseudologia fantastica;* the manipulator matures into a swindler; and the youth given to lashing out can develop into a violent and dangerous predator. As we noted, narcissistic problems form a major sector of the spectrum of conduct disorders.

It is important to keep in mind that the problem here is character pathology. Structural elements will take form during the developmental years to give personality its distinctive flavor and will probably persist thereafter as integral components of the person's adaptive apparatus. Maturational processes do not stop, and so modifications in such structures are possible. But, once set, many basic elements that cling to their earlier forms will continue to play a role in determining the interpersonal adaptive style of the narcissistic personality. Additional years and experience can modulate some of the vulnerable person's sensitivities and give him a measure of cognitive control over some of the distorted attitudes. With enough time and some good luck, it is possible to blunt the sharp edge of narcissistic difficulties and modify their intensity. But the basic problem does not easily go away.

ETIOLOGY

Narcissistic pathology is quintessentially psychological in nature, and to date, no research has tied this condition in a clear-cut way to any form of biological disturbance. Some investigators have suggested various biological links that are mentioned below; however, no very strong case has been made for any of these possibilities.

Most of the current consideration of narcissism takes place within the framework of psychoanalysis where (as noted) currently two principal theories—Kernberg's and Kohut's—seek to explain the phenomenology of the condition, ascribing its onset to two somewhat different factor-sets. Within the larger social realm, a strong current of opinion would relate the widespread prevalence of this form of symptomatology to major sociological changes in our time (Lasch, 1978).

Organic Factors

Although there is no known biological substrate, the manic's characteristic state of grandiosity in some ways suggests the symptomatology of certain kinds of narcissistic disturbance. Because of its demonstrable genetic component, manic-depressive illness is usually considered to have a biological basis (although the exact nature of the associated brain disturbance is still uncertain). As researchers come to understand the biology of this kind of affective disorder, their findings may clarify the mechanism of narcissistic grandiosity as well.

A suggestion that has appeared in the literature states that narcissism in humans may correspond to the territorial instinct in animals. The assumption here is that our species does have a territorial instinct that takes the form of the *self-as-territory*. The individual thus stakes out a self-terrain that is thereafter held to be inviolable. If this instinctual striving gets out of hand (e.g., the self-terrain extends to an impossibly wide perimeter), then the individual becomes preoccupied with defending this territory, and the character disturbance follows. Because there is no locus known in the brain for any such instinct, the point is really moot (Noshpitz, 1984).

Cloninger (1987) hints at another biological connection. This investigator offers a theory of personality based in part on the specification of certain core character traits that are under the influence of specific neurotransmitters. Because these neurotransmitters are associated with known anatomical patterns of brain organization (e.g., the locus ceruleus with the noradrenergic brain system and the substantia nigra with the dopaminergic system), the role of biological factors is clearly defined. High levels of a given neurotransmitter are associated with one group of behavioral tendencies; low levels with more or less opposite characteristics. When two of the neurotransmitter systems are involved (e.g., one system is present in excess whereas the other is relatively lacking, or both are in excess, or both are lacking), a second-order personality organization is present. And if all three systems are involved, then the full diagnosable personality disorder ensues. Thus, the various kinds of personality are viewed as arising from mixtures of these neurotransmitter-determined traits, and these, in turn, reflect genetically ordained high or low levels of the particular transmitters.

The basic personality traits Cloninger offers are *novelty-seeking* (high, average, or low), *harm-avoidance* (high, average, or low), and *reward-dependence* (high, average, or low). Within this framework, the narcissistic position is seen as a second-order emergent and is associated with high novelty-seeking and high reward–dependence. It involves patterns of excessive attention seeking, prodigal self-indulgence, excessively demonstrative and affectionate emotional expression, and much preoccupation in fantasy and imagined experiences (possibly involving dissociative states).

Although this is an ingenious and arresting approach, it is unclear whether Cloninger's definition of narcissistic adjustment is quite the same as the one that has been alluded to in this chapter. One the face of it, it would seem that a good deal of work remains to be done to reconcile these views.

Sociological Factors

Some trenchant observations have been made on the extraordinary consequences of the intense individualism and success orientation of our culture. Members of U.S. society are informed that they have many rights, that they can and should set ambitious personal goals, that their most vital imperative is to realize themselves and live up to their potentials, that they should seek maximal pleasure as part of good living, and that whatever seeks to limit their self-realization ane enjoyment is a form of undemocratic dehumanizing unfairness and they are morally justified in opposing it. Sociologists believe that this outlook, part of the current zeitgeist, has contributed to a national tide of narcissistic disorder, causing it to become a common disturbance for psychiatric referral.

Certainly the suggestion that self-centeredness in parents will beget children who are needy and who might themselves develop narcissistic adjustment patterns makes eminently good sense. It may very well be, however, that the social factors that make for this particular symptom or syndrome choice are still not entirely understood and that it will be some time before all these connections will be established.

Psychological Factors

This section addresses the thinking of Kohut and Kernberg in somewhat greater detail.

Kohut (1971) would have it that there is in all people a separate developmental line of narcissism that unfolds parallel with but distinctly different from the usual path of object relatedness. Individuals whose narcissistic development goes awry cope with different needs, pursue different goals, and experience different stresses from those whose development is more evenly balanced between narcissistic and object-related courses. Narcissistic children are less concerned with the instinctively dominated psychosexual and ego-developmental issues of anality and phallic oedipal realization and are more attuned to narcissistic yearnings, such as needing praise, being the center of attention, making an impression, being an exception, and being attached to an ideal. These imperatives pervade and alter their development from the time they are infants.

In describing the etiology of this development, Kohut regards the quality of mother–infant interaction as critical. The key phenomenon is empathy. The very young infant, in Kohut's view, looks to his mother not only for food, physical contact, and creature comforts, but for his sense of security and validation as well. The baby seeks assurance that he is valued, loved, and pleasing. He studies the gleam in his mother's eye as she dandles him and handles him; he looks for his reflection in her facial expression, the timbre of her voice, the gentleness of her touch. There is a critical mass of response elements in the mother's continuing interaction that cumulatively conveys to her baby a sense of being valuable. It involves a sense of the mother's delight in contemplating her baby, in interacting with, communicating with, playing with, and appreciating the very existence of the baby. These feelings are not yet communicable in words, hence, the recurrent emphasis on empathy. The aggregate of nonverbal messages about the mother's feelings conveys to the baby his mother's basic disposition toward him. From this matrix the sense of self as valued and valuable builds into the infant's consciousness. He absorbs the quality of his mother's feeling, adopting it as his feeling about himself. The infant's sense of being lovable, valuable, and inherently worthwhile, as well as the ensuing feelings of self-confidence and the capacity to trust others, blend together in an overall quality of self-esteem and security. This is the core of normal narcissism—a feeling of self-love built upon the sense of outer empathic acceptance and valuation.

In particular, empathy plays a role at two levels: *mirroring* and *idealization.* The earlier interaction is mirroring. The mother acts as mirror to the infant, initially as the symbiotic mirror, then as a sort of twin image, and finally as a separate figure who, nonetheless, responds in admiring, valuing fashion to the child's behavior. Empathy is critical, for it is precisely the mother's empathy that tells her what about the infant needs mirroring. In what way, and at what time. And it is the sensitivity and the accuracy of her mirroring that give the child the feeling of being understood and accepted. This is a vital function, and its importance to the child's self-esteem does not end with infancy.

A second dimension of empathy involves idealization. The baby passes the developmental level of needing mirroring and begins the work of separation–individuation. Now he looks to the mother as his all-knowing, all-powerful external source of supply and gratification. To the infant, his mother is larger than life, a supernal being. The baby views her in idealized terms, and as he separates from her, he absorbs some of her grandeur within himself. At moments the infant, too, is larger than life, autocratic, demanding, imperious. This idealization is the source of the grandiosity that typifies the narcissistic syndrome; it is the unresolved and continuing self-aggrandizement of the infant who has never given up the adaptive stance of this moment of development.

Where empathy is lacking, however, and the message that comes through from the mother expresses distaste or disinterest, or nonengagement; where the sense of a powerful outer presence who understands and accepts and cares for the baby is absent, then an adequate measure of self-love cannot grow. Instead, the infant has doubts about his worth, devalues his inherent lovability, and develops basic feelings of low self-regard. Because the essential feeling of self-love does not develop, there is an ensuing inner sense of worthlessness, emptiness, or inner ugliness. Under such conditions, the infant cannot value himself, and the core of a state of narcissistic vulnerability is established.

The lack of self-esteem is likely to be matched by a state of distrust of others. After all, from the outset the baby has learned that he cannot rely on others for obtaining good feelings: they do not feel what he feels, do not like what he is, and do not know his needs nor meet them. The child's only recourse is to cling to the infantile state of grandiosity. He substitutes self-love for the failed maternal caring; instead of exchanging affection, he seeks external praise; instead of forming a sharing relationship, the child can only continually attempt to repair what has gone awry and to obtain from an unwilling world constant demonstrated approval. This circumstance initiates the eternal search for the praise, attention, and admiration that signify acceptance and appreciation. Only in this way can the child allay the unending inner whisperings of self-devaluation.

Kernberg's (1975) stance in some respects resembles but in other ways differs noticeably from Kohut's position. In brief, Kernberg considers the inner psychological position of the baby. As the youngster differentiates, he develops a self-representation based on his concrete experiences of using his body and interacting with his caretakers. At the same time, however, the child is also elaborating an ideal sense of self derived in part from his caretakers' messages and in part from his own wishes and yearnings. Meanwhile, the baby's contacts with significant others lead to the construction of two images. One is a realistic sense of what these others (objects) are like. The baby, however, is also forming an image of the idealized other, in particular, an image of the idealized mother, and of the perfect union he would like to achieve with her. These thronging images from time to time give rise to fantasies; under normal conditions, however, the real images and the ideal versions maintain their integrity and distinct outlines, remaining clearly separate from one another.

Where the child encounters traumatic frustrations and deprivations, however, he will call powerful defensive maneuvers into play. At this point, the child will begin to break down the boundaries between his images. Thus the ideal self and the ideal other will begin to blur together into a single self–other unity, and this in turn will fuse with the self-representation so that the child's sense of self begins to take on an idealized cast. Thus, instead of feeling rejected and devalued by the mother's frustrating behavior, the youngster can turn to himself and begin to feel grandiose and elated. Instead of feeling like a child, he feels like an exaggerated personage, a blend of child and adult, a full-fledged adult, or a superpowerful adult, as the case may be (depending on the child's level of disturbance and the stress with which he is striving to cope). Kernberg considers the fusion of the self-representation, the idealized self, and the idealized object-representations to be the central pathological process, producing what he calls a *grandiose self*. It is the child's investment in, valuation of, and clinging to such a pathological structure that gives the narcissistic condition its basic character. In essence, the narcissistic stance is inherently defensive. Unlike Kohut, Kernberg does not regard narcissism as a separate line of development with its own way of unfolding and its own inner structure. Instead, the defensive formation follows trauma in the same manner as a neurotic formation, only in this instance, the trauma occurs far earlier in development than the oedipal period (the usual source of neurotic defensive structuring). The child's defense, accordingly, involves unique elements of ego structure that go awry in specific ways. The defining characteristic of the narcissistic organization is the child's creation of and attachment to the grandiose self as a primary defensive position.

Regardless of the professional's preferred theory of etiology, certain patterns of early experience tend frequently to result in narcissistic trends in children. Paulina Kernberg (1975) has delineated some of these vulnerable children as follows:

The child of a narcissistic parent.
The adopted child.
The deprived child.
The physically or sexually abused child.
The child of divorced parents.
The anorectic child.
The overgratified child.

Early traumata of severe or overwhelming character, such as deprivation and abuse, are a possible source of a narcissistic clinical syndrome. However, other important channels of onset, such as parents who overgratify or parentify the child, do not necessarily involve trauma in any simple sense.

The Child of a Narcissistic Parent.   The child of a narcissistic parent faces particular stresses. The parent cannot really consider the child as a separate entity; the youngster is always an instrument of the parent's ambition and is expected to be perfect in order to compensate for the felt shortcomings of others in the family or for devalued parts of the parent's self. Thus, from birth on, the child may be given a role to play. This is particularly true if the parent has experienced some early narcissistic injury, such as the loss of a sibling, the unlooked-for failure of a previous pregnancy, or the death of a young infant. For the narcissistic parent this is more than just a loss; it is a personal slight that life has visited on him or her, which must be made up for. And the new baby is given the task of accomplishing this goal; he is assigned the role of the substitute. This forces the child's development into an artificial mold that may have little to do with the youngster's natural proclivities; the end product is a distortion of development that can produce a variety of results—among them narcissism is a prominent likelihood.

Bleiberg (1984) makes the point that children reared under such circumstances lack any inner core of secure self-identity. They are geared entirely to the outside world, permanent role-players seeking external cues as to how to be "good." They are schooled in the firm knowledge that they must put aside whatever they naturally want to be in favor of what the parent expects them to be; they are acceptable only through a proper performance. Accordingly, they adopt a false self; they become actors, forever playing roles on the interpersonal stage with no inner core of a valued self on which to depend. It is a brief step from this to permanent dissimulation, lying, tale-telling, manipulation, and opportunistic exploitation of others as a way of life. At the same time the child feels a pervasive inner emptiness and chronic dissatisfaction with whatever he has, along with a sense of fundamental unlovability for whatever he truly is. Accompanying these feelings is often a pressing drive for constant display, in part to distract attention from the inner emptiness and in part to obtain reassurance of being valued, at least for the moment. Such a child is forever looking to the world of others for praise and approval because it is the only way he can reassure himself, from moment to moment, that he is acceptable; as a result the youngster is always performing. Ultimately, all this behavior translates into a deeply rooted rage toward the larger world of people for the sensed difference and the feeling of lacking something that others seem to possess.

A particularly undesirable situation occurs when a parent gradually reverses roles with a child; the parentified child is then pressed constantly to make decisions and to give praise, comfort, and reassurance to the needy parent. Certain children rise to such a requirement and seek with all their inner resources to fulfill the assignment thus thrust upon them. The grandiosity that follows is in a sense necessary to carry out the assumed role. At the same time, a deep underlying resentment usually accumulates and presently emerges as chronic rage. At some level, the child cannot help but react to the combined lack of need fulfillment, the deprivation of childhood gratifications, and the unfair burdens he has carried from an early age. Some youngsters carry it off successfully; they become managers, leaders, and assertive caretakers because their native endowment combined with the strictures of their circumstances to force the early expression of these potentials. At best, however, it is a precarious arrangement that often has lasting repercussions on the child's life.

Parentifying a child begets certain skill developments that can be quite striking. Thus, the narcissistic child, so dependent on outer cues, becomes expert in reading people's emotional signals. The youngster becomes adept at discerning emotional needs and at playing the role of the perfect fulfiller of whatever these needs might be. Often this effort takes the form of precocious behavior, and the child seems wise beyond his years—a miniature adult. Such actions play into the grandiose tendencies already encouraged by the child-rearing style of parentification. In effect, the child renounces the essence of childhood, which is to be cared for, and takes on instead the natural opposite: It is the child who does the caring. Because the child must care for himself, his personality presently acquires the characteristics of an arrogant, noninstructible, uneducable, and unregulated youth. Being a practiced role player, he can use his charm to sell magazine subscriptions, or can con an attendant into letting him break the rules, or can convince a judge that the police are lying. But if the depredations continue, the youth will earn an extraordinary reputation among the school teachers, police, or treatment personnel, a mixture of awe, profound distrust, and sometimes outright hatred. Often the authorities' negative responses are mixed with an unwilling and grudging admiration, and even the admission, "You can't help liking the person."

The Adopted Child. Adoption can cause a severe identity crisis in certain more vulnerable children. The notion that their biological parents gave them up causes an unresolvable narcissistic dilemma. Such children experience the idea of their placement (or, as they may come to feel about it, abandonment) as a primary and unhealing injury: "How could my [biological] parents have done this?" Or, with even more intensity, they ask: "How could they have done this to *me*?" The child who is prone to narcissistic problems has a curious thin-skinned quality—every issue comes down to the valuation of the self. Anything that challenges the sense of *me-ness* produces an unhealing wound that cannot be comforted or eased. And regardless of the care and attention lavished by the sometimes oversolicitous adoptive parents, the fact of having been adopted is like a painfully embedded arrowhead. Such a child can only explain his biological mother's abandonment by thinking that somehow he was not good enough to win or to hold her love. The majority of adoptive children, who do reasonably well, evidently do not develop this belief; where it does occur, however, it is a striking phenomenon. In its less severe manifestations it probably explains the quests of some adult adoptees for their biological parents.

The Deprived Child. Emotional deprivation from any source tends to throw children back on their own resources. Obviously in any given instance a host of variables will determine symptom choice. The child's genetic endowment and basic temperament are crucial. The kind of stress and its degree of severity, the child's developmental status at the time of the experience, subsequent encounters with additional stress factors, the presence of intercurrent health problems, the particular caretaker(s) involved, the nature of any subsequent compensatory management or therapeutic intervention, and the possibilities for sublimating the associated tensions can all influence the outcome. Nor is this a complete list: Multitudinous factors can play a role.

For certain predisposed children, however, early emotional deprivation seems to trigger a ready turn to the narcissistic position. Evidently this response is largely compensatory and defensive. In the face of abandonment and neglect, the youngster says in effect: "I do not need others, I have myself. Since I have learned that I can expect no one to care for me, I have decided that I don't care about them; I don't need them, and I don't want them." This attitude is commonly (albeit, not necessarily) accompanied by chronic anger.

As the youngster grows up, he becomes arrogant, self-centered, lacking in all feeling for others, self-serving, and thoroughly predatory. Because no one took adequate care of him, the child has had to learn to live by his wits; he reads others' signals accurately, dissimulates effectively, and can provide glib excuses and explanations. A definite subgroup of delinquents fall into this category. Where the developmental events have induced a state of constantly venting rage in the youngster, he can often be violent and dangerous. This situation is particularly likely if abuse has figured in the developmental course.

The Child of Divorced Parents. For a great many children, particularly preschoolers, divorce serves as a serious narcissistic injury. The children's sense of personal involvement in the divorce causes continual and unrelenting stress. Occasionally the parents unwittingly advance this process by turning the child into a pawn in their efforts to injure one another, or by making him the go-between as they battle for advantage. Sometimes a woebegone mother turns her small child into a confidant or a substitute companion. Or a father clings to and overgratifies a child to compensate for the deprivations that he feels the child is enduring. The child may see himself as the reason for the parents' breakup, or he may feel a responsibility to bring them together again. Sometimes the child chooses between the parents and feels that he has participated in these guilt-laden events. A host of elements can catch up the emotional life of any child in these contexts, and some youngsters respond by moving in a narcissistic direction and becoming inordinately difficult and demanding, accusatory and provocative, grandiose and arrogant. Sometimes the child's behavior is so deviant that it poses major management problems.

On the other hand, where the narcissistic organization is already present when the divorce threatens, the therapist may encounter quite a different sort of reaction. This is exemplified by a bright but very narcissistic 12-year-old's outburst to his parents: "How dare you consider divorce? You came together to create me and that makes your union sacred and special; to consider breaking it up is the greatest of personal insults to me, and I will not tolerate it!"

The Anorectic Child. No single psychodynamic sequence is associated with anorexia nervosa. Many of these children, however, do show the grandiose and demanding traits that define the narcissistic condition and seek actively to dominate their households in respect to food purchases, preparation, and usage, and in particular, the management of their own dietary intake. Where the narcissistic component is particularly marked, a monumental power struggle ensues; this tendency can seriously complicate the treatment of anorexia.

More than that, many of these youngsters have lived perfectionistic lives prior to developing their anorexia, striving to be straight "A" students, to perfect themselves in ballet or gymnastics, or to be flawlessly behaved. In a sense, the narcissistic trait was already in evidence but was still expressed in relatively sublimated form. With the onset of the overt eating disorder, the perfectionism grows excessive and unreal and is directed at the child's own body (although it may extend to many details of daily life as well). The anorexic child aspires to an ideal form that is beyond any rational discussion, and this desire presently becomes a monomaniacal passion that dominates the child's thinking and feeling life. It appears as if the small, flat latency body becomes an ideal, and the child strives for it with all the ardor of the totally committed.

The Overgratified Child. Finally, in considering the sequences that encourage narcissistic development, the clinician should remember the ubiquitous experience of *spoiling*. This common, garden-variety pattern of overgratification leads a child to grandiose expectations because, in fact, his idolizing, overgiving parents take every whim as a mandate and create a totally unreal state of expectation and self-valuation. From early on the child asks for a thing and is given it; then it asks for something else and receives it; then it requests the other and gets the other. Until one day the child asks for the moon. Such a child will presently be bitterly enraged at his excessively solicitous parents and feel cheated and deprived because of wanting something they could not afford, could not obtain, or finally perceived as dubious. The therapist who talks to such a youngster hears only complaints about all that he deserved and did not receive; the common observation of the overgratified child is, "I never got anything I really wanted." In a very real sense he may not have; parents who are significantly blocked in their capacity to perceive a child's needs and to meet a child's needs commonly resort to such child-rearing patterns. Sometimes they are unable to give to their child emotionally and compensate by giving material things instead; more often than not they are vaguely aware that their behavior is unwise, but they find it too gratifying to resist. In any case, the sense of entitlement and of expecting the gratification of all wishes ill prepares the child for the rigors of peer adaptation, school requirements, or, indeed, for socialization in general. Some rather severe narcissistic syndromes have come about through this route.

TREATMENT

The therapy for narcissistic disorder is essentially some form of psychological management on either an inpatient or an outpatient basis. In more eruptive cases small doses of neuroleptics may sometimes be indicated as nonspecific tranquilizers of frenetic emotional situations. The medication in no sense aims to relieve the narcissistic disturbance; it merely helps the involved child and family survive the current crisis. Certain hypomanic adolescents mimic the symptoms of narcissistic disorders but respond well to lithium carbonate, which treats their basic condition.

Psychotherapy

Some narcissistic children have responded to child analysis (Egan & Kernberg, 1984). However, the majority are probably treated by child therapy. In general, treatment must be rather intensive; in most instances at least two sessions a week are necessary. Therapy is likely to be prolonged, and it would be unrealistic to expect a good result in much less than two years. The problems are profoundly characterological, the treatment is often stormy, and the work takes a great deal of sustained effort.

The Kernberg and Kohut Approaches. The psychotherapeutic tactics employed will vary depending on the therapist's theoretical school. The Kernberg approach sets particular priority on interpreting the negative transference and the narcissistic defenses. Thus, the clinician might speak to the grandiosity in terms of its protective quality: "It's better to think of yourself as the powerful guy than to face the feelings that you are small and weak and could be hurt." Or the denial can be challenged with confrontation; "You'd like to feel you can put things over on everybody and not face the fact that in this situation you can't really control much that goes on." Similarly the defenses of devaluation and idealization have to be addressed, particularly as they manifest themselves within the patient–therapist relationship. The therapist's goal is to pinpoint how the patient strives to live out the grandiose stance within the therapeutic relationship and thereby to distinguish the several components of the grandiose self. During this effort, there must be constant tactful address to the defenses that protect this psychic organization.

Thus, in a variety of ways the therapist can interpret and, in effect, analyze the several aspects of the narcissistic defenses. In particular, this requires confronting the patient's various attempts to disparage the therapist, to exercise dominance, or to control the therapeutic situation. Obviously this work cannot always start immediately because many patients are not ready for such confrontational stress until the relationship has developed a sufficient degree of attachment and trust. Sooner or later, however, the therapist has to deal with these issues.

The long-range goal of the interpretive work is to help the patient separate out the self-concept from its fusion with the inner representation of the ideal self and the idealized object. As the therapist works steadily with the defenses, the patient gradually tends to begin perceiving the self and the other in more discrete and realistic terms, and thus to dissolve the pathological structure of the grandiose self.

For the Kohutian therapist, the work is likely to proceed rather differently. In particular, the clinician is not working so much with a defensive stance as addressing a deprivational syndrome that in turn has led to a characteristic style of relating. The key is the lack of adequate empathy in early mothering; the treatment is to recreate the early situation in the transference and to supply what has been omitted. Hence, it is important at the outset to determine the kind of transference paradigm the patient is creating. Is it one of the mirror transferences: symbiotic (the patient tries to fuse with the therapist), twin (the patient recognizes the therapist is a discrete, separate individual but tries to view the therapist as another version of the self), or reflective (the patient can accept the separateness of the therapist but seeks the therapist's admiration and total acceptance)? Or is it an idealizing transference, with the therapist being assigned the ideal role and the patient demanding acceptance as the favored child? The way the therapist conducts the work will be a function of the way the patient constructs the relationship. If the patient needs reflecting, then it is important for the therapist to act as the good mirror and fill in the function that may have been omitted or inadequately accomplished during early development. If the patients needs to regard the therapist as an ideal presence, the therapist can try to help the patient reconstruct the past and recapture the memory of someone who did play this role, or of a time when the patient needed someone to play this role and that person failed to help the child. Where things go well, gradually, with the combination of reflection and reconstruction, the patient can master the early traumatic experiences that confined development to the more regressed forms of narcissistic adjustment. The patient can then allow narcissistic tendencies to mature in a healthier fashion, and even move toward more appropriate kinds of object attachment.

In a typical example of a mirror transference, from the outset the child will not allow the therapist to speak or will direct what the therapist is to say. Thus, the child may start the therapy by organizing a school game in which the child is the teacher and the therapist is a rather troublesome student who is forever being criticized and punished. In effect the therapist is allowed no lines of his or her own, the therapist/student can say only what the patient/teacher permits. This confirms and reassures the child in the youngster's chosen role, as fragile and unrealistic as that may be. The Kohutian therapist plays the game as long as the child needs this form of transference, occasionally reflecting the child's feeling of needing to be in charge. The therapist constantly seeks an empathic sense of what the child has experienced in order to reflect it back, perhaps by remarking, "How important the teacher is, and how much the teacher knows!"

The Kernbergian, on the other hand, begins, at some point, to note that the child is making himself feel big by trying to make the therapist feel small. In one way or another the therapist directs the comments toward the grandiose self and addresses the defensive components of the behavior. In particular, the patient's anger and envy are prime targets for interpretation, because these affects form the glue that binds the elements of the grandiose self together. As these feelings are recognized for what they are and are reattached to their proper sites of origin, the self-representation will begin to emerge distinctly from the grandiose self and the grandiose object representations, and a healthier self-organization can follow.

The Aichhorn Approach. An earlier style of approach achieved a certain recognition, although it was never much emulated. This form of therapy was the work of Aichhorn (Eissler, 1949), in which he "deceived the deceiver." As a therapist, Aichhorn (1935) had the knack of sensing quickly what his patient might idealize and then of moving rapidly to play that role. This tended to set up an idealizing transference within which, from the very outset, the patient looked up to the therapist with awe and admiration. Aichhorn achieved this by demonstrating that he knew more about the delinquent way of life—about theft, swindling, and skullduggery in all their varieties—than did the youth. This generally captured the interest and respect of the young offender and initiated a good patient–therapist relationship. Although occasional attempts have been made to adapt this style to current therapeutic practice, it has never become a consistent tool in the psychotherapeutic armamentarium.

Family Therapy. Where the chosen mode of approach to a narcissistic problem is family therapy, the Kohutian therapist concentrates on striving to make the family more empathic. The goal is to treat the family rather than the child, and this requires working on the family attitudes in considerable depth. In effect, the therapist creates a therapeutic milieu in the child's home. In this view such children do not need interpretation, but rather "the empathic responsiveness of their environment in order to overcome their disturbed and disturbing behavior" (Ornstein, 1984). Because the syndrome is regarded as the fruit of failed empathy, it follows that it can be relieved by restoring the empathic potential of the parents.

In general, the therapist needs to address those aspects of family function that have served to beget or to maintain the child's narcissistic position. The child's seemingly incomprehensible difficulties often drive the parents into a stance of chronic exasperation and rejection. In the face of this, the therapist can carefully clarify the child's subjective world for the parents: the envy, emptiness, vulnerability, recurrent wounding, unallayable hunger for praise, and, ultimately, the covert depression at the failure of all these adaptive tactics. If some of the child's problems have arisen because of the parents' narcissistic use of the child, the therapist must explain the warping effects of such patterns (e.g., using the child to replace a lost object, to fulfill some parental ideal, or to act as parent to the parent). The parental resistance to recognizing the significance of such child-rearing practices can be of monumental proportions.

Finally, the basic task of so much family work—to normalize the hierarchical structure within the family—is very much in order in these situations. Often, the young pubertal boy is asked to show his mother special consideration because she is having her period; the pubertal girl is made privy to the mother's aversion to the father's sexual preferences; or a daughter may be the object of her father's scorn or sexual teasing. Sometimes the parents regard the child as a true oedipal rival and behave accordingly. In any case, it is necessary to reestablish the privacy of the parental lives, to exclude the child appropriately from both the knowledge of and the power over parental intimacy, and to restore the role of the parents as parents.

Inpatient Care

Closed ward care is necessary for violent or dangerous narcissistic patients. Occasionally such patients are prone to suicide as a tormented means of controlling and punishing the significant others in their environment. More often than not, however, their domineering and arrogant behavior, together with their sense of entitlement, has overflowed into physical exploitation of their environment. They may steal, extort, or use their manipulative skills to swindle people; they are often unmanageable at school ("No one can tell me what to do!"); and they are abusive and destructive at home. The inpatient service is likely to receive the full brunt of this behavior, and it is critical from the outset to set clear, firm limits and to enforce them systematically. Because these youngsters tend to engage in wily and deceptive tale-telling as naturally as they breathe, an unusual degree of staff coordination is necessary, and the simplification and systematization of life on the ward is essential for group survival under these circumstances.

Staff members often need special help to deal with the arrogant and provocative stance of these youngsters, and much staff backup and support are sometimes necessary. The milieu these youngsters need includes a staff who can be realistic and consistent without being retaliatory. Sensible limits are essential; controls have to be in place; and the staff must be able to take the challenges that young narcissists are likely to throw out. Intensive psychotherapy is an essential element in the patient's treatment, and intensive support and supervision are equally essential for the staff. Such treatment is likely to be lengthy, involving anywhere from 18 months to 3 years in an inpatient setting, with additional outpatient care necessary after release.

Inpatient Group Therapy

In some programs, the basic treatment tactic is one of group confrontation. In essence, this amounts to a direct assault on the grandiose components of the narcissistic position. The group gathers around the particular young-ster under discussion, and in the most direct and unvarnished way chal-lenges his pretensions, evasiveness, dishonesty, manipulation, arrogance, tale-bearing, adaptive strategies, relationship tactics, lack of feeling, at-tempts at dominating others, and any other behavior elements that have contributed to his symptomatic identity patterns. These traits are often excoriated, ridiculed, jeeringly mimicked, vehemently denounced and con-demned, held up to rigorous and searching public scrutiny and criticism, and made public property and the object of public shaming. Originally this approach characterized special programs for the treatment of substance abusers. The point of the work was to create a sort of mystical in-group to which the patient obtained access through the ordeal of being thus con-fronted, humiliated, and stripped of defenses in public fashion; after having endured this humiliation and shaming, the individual belonged and could join in visiting such treatment on the next applicant for help. The program created a rather special context within which some addicts could maintain themselves drug-free for extended periods. From these begin-nings a basic style of confrontational dynamics has evolved that has been used variously at such residential settings as Elan, and at various wilderness and survival programs. Although not designed for the narcissistic patient, the techniques seem curiously specific to identifiable narcissistic compo-nents. An analogous effort of quite different character was depicted on a television documentary called "Scared Straight." This approach attempted to scare or shock youngsters out of their delinquent status by taking them into penitentiaries where major criminals lectured and hectored the chil-dren on their inadequate adjustment and confronted them with the proba-ble outcome of their chosen paths. It was evident that a major component of the effort was to penetrate the assumed grandiose position of the delin-quents and to reach the frightened and infantile person within. The results have been dubious.

Overall, it is fair to say that many of these patients can be helped. Because, however, the therapist cannot know from the outset just how deeply into the character structure the pathology extends, the result is always uncertain. In the course of treatment runaways are rather frequent, and episodes of acting-out are the norm. The relationship paradigm of these patients is inherently pathological, and so the attachments they do form to staff are likely to be unusually demanding and complex. Enormous jealousy, wildly inappropriate blaming, exorbitant expectations, and towering rage when such expectations are not met are commonplace. Occasionally this behavior translates into permanent runaways or violent physical assaults. These factors always lend uncertainty to the therapeutic enterprise, because the patient's behavior may make further retention in the program impossible. Because of these uncertainties, the initial period of treatment should always be a trial undertaking.

PART V

Disorders of Body-Mind Integration

Chapter 15

Psychosomatic Disorders

> Soul and body, I suggest, react sympathetically upon each other: a
> change in the state of the soul produces a change in the shape of the
> body, and conversely: a change in the shape of the body produces a
> change in the state of the soul.
> —*Physiognomics*
> ARISTOTLE
> (quoted in Popper & Eccles, 1977)

INTRODUCTION

This chapter explores the hypothesis that social and psychological factors
play a role in the inception and course of certain childhood diseases and
physical complaints.

The relationship of body to mind has puzzled philosophers and scientists
for millenia. The study of psychologically mediated illness dramatically
underscores the current lack of knowledge about how these twin aspects of
human nature—the psychological and the somatic—interpenetrate each
other. During the centuries since Descartes, scientists have grown accustomed to thinking of a physical, neurobiological substrate to psychological
phenomena. Although the precise pathophysiological details remain unclear, clinicians and researchers are ready to accept the notion that organic
factors can codetermine mood (as in bipolar affective disorder), cognitive
style (as in attention deficit disorder), and even language and thought (as in
the aphasias and schizophrenia). However, the converse phenomenon of
psychologically mediated changes in bodily functioning remains strangely
puzzling and controversial. This chapter then considers aspects of various
childhood physical conditions that may be influenced or determined by
psychological factors as well as different theoretical attempts to elucidate
what Deutsch (1959) termed the "mysterious leap from the mind to the
body." The following chapter will illustrate the application of these concepts
by detailing their relevance for a specific disease—bronchial asthma.

Psychological and family factors powerfully influence the growing child's
coping responses and adaptation to physical illnesses of whatever origin.
They thus help determine the degree of resulting disability as well as
compliance and attitude toward treatment. Conversely, physical illness has
a significant impact on the child's emotional life and psychological development. These themes are also illustrated in the chapter on Asthma (see
Chapter 16).

DEFINITION

The term *psychosomatic* has had a checkered career, going in and out of
fashion, carrying first one connotation and then another. At one time,

certain diseases as well as their sufferers were considered to be psychosomatic: bronchial asthma, essential high blood pressure, peptic ulcer, rheumatoid arthritis, ulcerative colitis, neurodermatitis, and hyperthyroidism. Current thinking questions whether emotional factors alone can cause structural physical pathology. As a result, the denotation "caused by emotional factors" has fallen out of favor. At the same time, however, in some diseases and individuals, psychological factors may influence the course of illness and interact synergistically with certain physical causal factors. Thus, in its broadest current usage the term psychosomatic now describes an investigatory approach that seeks to understand how social and psychological factors influence the predisposition, inception, and course of various diseases (Weiner, 1977).

This approach to illness, as Weiner (1977) defines it, poses certain characteristic questions. Why and how is a person predisposed to develop one disease and not another? Why does the disease appear at one particular time in a person's life and not another? What determines the exacerbations and remissions of illness? In some cases, known genetic, infectious, immunological, or metabolic factors may explain much of the variance. In other cases how the individual feels and thinks, and how he experiences and responds to past and present events in his life may play a determinative role.

The ongoing debate about the proper classification of psychologically induced physical disorders reflects the continuing limitations of knowledge in this area. Most observers recognize two clusters of illness, dividing the spectrum according to the degree of identifiable physical pathology and the ease with which the symptoms convey psychological meaning. Thus, representing one extreme might be the paralysis of a limb or loss of sensation for which no physical cause can be found and whose pattern of functional loss does not correspond to the anatomy and physiology of the nervous system. More than that, the loss of function seems to be congruent with some psychological construct (e.g., a loss of sensation that stops exactly at the midline or is confined to a "glove" distribution). Further, the condition often provides the patient with important benefits, either intrapsychically or from his environment. Additional evidence for a psychological vector rather than a physical cause is that the loss or alteration of function seems to possess symbolic value or to represent an identification with someone who is important in the patient's life.

At the other end of the nosological spectrum stands such an illness as peptic ulcer, where many known physical factors are at work (genetic predisposition, a large mass of acid-secreting mucosal cells, high levels of pepsinogen, etc.) and physical pathology is clearly visible in the form of a large ulcerlike erosion of the stomach lining. However, the proximate cause of the patient's current bout of bleeding might be the stress surrounding a change of school.

This broad dichotomy is enshrined in the current DSM-III-R (APA, 1987) classification as follows:

I. *Somatoform Disorders*
    A. *Conversion disorders*
    B. *Somatoform pain disorders*
    C. *Somatization disorders.*
II. *Psychological Factors Affecting Physical Condition*

SOMATOFORM DISORDERS

In this group of conditions there are "physical symptoms suggesting a physical disorder (hence, Somatoform)" (APA, 1987, p. 255); however, upon appropriate investigation, no organic pathology or known physiological mechanism can be found. The condition looks like a physical illness and the patient may feel that it is; in fact, however, nothing is physically wrong. The disturbance is not under voluntary control in that "the individual does not experience the sense of controlling the production of a symptom" (APA, 1980, p. 241). Nonetheless, there is "positive evidence, or a strong presumption, that the symptoms are linked to psychological factors or conflicts" (APA, 1987, p. 255). DSM-III-R further subdivides the somatoform disorders into:

1. *Conversion Disorders.* These involve a loss or alteration in physical functioning. The condition usually takes form as a single symptom that cannot be explained by any physical disorder or known pathophysiological mechanism. Instead, the symptom appears to be an expression of psychological conflict or need. The symptom may simultaneously symbolize the conflict while helping to keep it out of conscious awareness. In addition, the symptom may also help the patient gain support from significant people in his life. Classical conversion symptoms include paralysis, local anesthesia, disturbance of vision, difficulty in swallowing, the occurrence of fainting or seizures, and inability to walk or talk.

2. *Somatoform Pain Disorders.* This consists of the presence of pain in the absence of any identifiable physical cause. The onset or exacerbation of the pain may be related to psychological conflicts or needs, to an experience of stress, or to some identifiable situational gain for the patient.

3. *Somatization Disorders.* This consists of recurrent, multiple somatic complaints of several years' duration not adequately explained by known physical disorders and involving the patient heavily with phy-

sicians, medication, and alterations in his or her life style (APA, 1987).

Conversion Disorders

Conversion disorders take their name from the notion of a psychological conflict being converted into physical symptomatology. The concept of conversion is of great historical as well as clinical interest, for the study of just such symptoms led Freud, as a young neurologist, to the theory of unconscious conflict. Ultimately, his investigations led him to invent psychoanalysis as a therapeutic technique.

As far back as Hippocrates, physicians had been puzzled by patients, usually young women, who showed a bewildering variety of fluctuating symptoms with no apparent cause. Plato (1889), like many of his Greek contemporaries, favored the hypothesis that the womb, "desirous of procreating children and when remaining without fruit long beyond its proper time, gets disconnected and angry and wandering in every direction through the body, closes up the passages of breath, and, by obstructing respiration, drives them into the utmost difficulty, causing all varieties of diseases." From this theory came the term *hysteria,* from the Greek *hystera,* meaning "womb."

Through the succeeding centuries investigators debated the relative contributions of physical and psychological factors. The giants of 19th-century French neurology, Charcot and Janet, studied hysteria closely (Havens, 1973). In their day hysteria included not only inexplicable paralyses, loss of sensation, and strange seizures, but also dissociations of consciousness, such as multiple personalities and fugue states of which the patient later had no memory. The patients were predominantly female, and they tended to be vivacious, dramatic, and highly suggestible.

Until recent decades, the terms *conversion symptom* and *hysteria* were used almost interchangeably. Current diagnostic thinking distinguishes more carefully between the physical symptoms and the personality features that may or may not accompany them (Chodoff 1954, 1974; Chodoff & Lyons, 1958). DSM-III-R recognizes that the overly dramatic, highly reactive character traits of these "grand hysteric" patients tend to cluster together in a distinct profile and labels them "Histrionic Personality Disorder." Patients with this personality type (which has been described as "a parody of femininity") are said to be colorful, frequently seductive, and alternately coy and demanding. Beneath their superficial charm, they are dependent, egocentric, and manipulative and given to melodramatic gestures. Conversion symptoms are not limited to histrionic personality disorder, however, but can occur within the context of almost any personality type (Chodoff & Lyons, 1958).

Charcot observed that the hysteric's paralyses and anesthesias could be

induced or removed by hypnosis. Together with a few of their contemporaries, Charcot and Janet believed that the hysteric's symptoms were "ideo-
genic"—that is, they were caused by the patient's ideas and experiences
rather than an organic lesion (Havens, 1973). Further, Janet and Charcot
reported that at least during the patient's normal waking life, he was usually
unaware of the ideas that determined his symptoms. Indeed, it was striking
that in the face of their dramatic physical symptoms such patients often
showed a puzzling lack of concern, *la belle indifference*. The patients' symptoms thus appeared to be controlled by a

> ... group of coherent associated ideas that become *fixed* in their minds as a
> sort of parasite, which remains *isolated* from everything else, but which can be
> projected externally in the form of related motor phenomenon. ... (This)
> group of ideas is guarded in its isolation from the control of that great
> collectivity of personal impressions that have been accumulated and orga-
> nized for a long time and that constitute the conscience or, more properly, the
> ego. (Charcot, quoted in Havens, 1973, p. 79)

As Charcot and Janet viewed it, this division or "splitting" of consciousness was due to a hereditary or traumatic weakening of the nervous system
or mental apparatus, a "sleep of reason." This allowed the formation of a
sequestered *condition seconde*—an organized group of ideas that controlled
the symptom but remained disconnected from the patient's waking
thoughts.

In 1893 Freud (Breuer & Freud, 1893–1895/1955) first made the epochal
suggestion that the physical symptoms of hysterical patients were the product of psychological conflict. He proposed that such a patient suffered from
impulses that were unacceptable to her (conscious) standards. Because she
could not acknowledge these "inadmissible" impulses, the patient could not
permit herself to become aware of her internal conflicts. Instead, she
expressed these tensions symbolically in the form of a symptom that represented in body language both the unacceptable impulse as well as the
prohibition against it. "In hysteria," Freud (1894/1950) wrote, "the unbearable idea is rendered innocuous by the quantity of excitation attached to it
being transmuted into some bodily form of expression, a process for which
I should like to propose the name of *conversion*" (p. 63).

Freud's contention was that the split in the patient's consciousness was not
the passive product of a weakened ego or impaired nervous system (as Janet
and Charcot had maintained) but the active product of an inner struggle
pitting one part of the personality against another. Perhaps, for example,
there was some sexual attraction or hostile impulse toward a parent or a
sibling, along with a strong inner taboo that forbade the act and condemned
the thought. Keeping this conflict out of consciousness spared the patient
all the anxiety entailed by awareness. But, she had to pay a price, namely the

constrictions that the symptoms imposed on her life. Freud termed this avoidance of conscious anxiety the *primary gain* of the symptom.

However, such limitations and handicaps obviously have social implications as well as individual rewards. The extra benefits that the patient derived because of her illness included extra sympathy, care, special deference, and attention from those about her. Together these factors constituted the *secondary gain*. Freud speculated that the hysteric's *belle indifference* reflected both the anxiety-binding function of the symptom and the secondary gains derived by the patient.

As a young neurologist, Freud had been shocked but intrigued by Charcot's contention that there was a sexual element in hysteria: "Dans ces cas pareils, c'est toujours la chose genitale, toujours, toujours, toujours [In such cases, it's always the genital element, always, always, always]" (Freud, 1914/ 1957, p. 14). In time, however, Freud came to agree that the unacceptable impulses that the hysteric warded off through conversion symptoms were most often sexual in nature. However, aggressive and competitive strivings, which revived oedipal conflicts, played a role as well. As discussed later in this chapter, dependent strivings also provoke childhood conversion symptoms; in such cases, the secondary gains of receiving extra attention and care in ways that are otherwise unavailable or unacceptable to the child may be especially important.

Freud took his first radical steps toward developing a new form of therapy during his studies (Breuer & Freud, 1893–1895/1955) of hysterical conversion symptoms. His mentor, Charcot, had used hypnosis to "suggest away" the hysterical patient's physical symptoms. Freud's colleague Breuer had used hypnosis to circumvent the patient's defenses and uncover the repudiated memories associated with the onset of the symptoms. Abandoning hypnosis, Freud discovered the technique of free association (Freud, 1914/1957), which allowed him to help the patient rediscover both the disavowed impulses and the revulsion against them that had precipitated the conversion symptom. The therapist had but to make the patient conscious of her previously repressed conflict, Freud contended, and the symptom would disappear.

DSM-III-R Diagnostic Criteria for Conversion Disorder

A. *A loss of, or alteration in, physical functioning suggesting a physical disorder.*

B. *Psychological factors are judged to be etiologically related to the symptom because of a temporal relationship between a psychosocial stressor that is apparently related to a psychological conflict or need and initiation or exacerbation of the symptom.*

C. *The person is not conscious of intentionally producing the symptom.*

D. *The symptom is not a culturally sanctioned response pattern and cannot, after appropriate investigation, be explained by a known physical disorder.*

E. *The symptom is not limited to pain or to a disturbance in sexual functioning.* (APA, 1987, p. 259)

Within the context of DSM-III-R the definition of conversion disorder is unique in that it includes an etiologic hypothesis as a defining criterion. Despite much intense, often ideologically tinged debate, the authors of the diagnostic manual could not develop an acceptable phenomenological definition of conversion without including implicitly the notion of unconscious motivation for the symptom.

Epidemiology. Estimates of the incidence of conversion symptoms in children vary widely with the criteria and populations studied. Studies of inpatient and clinic populations suggest an incidence of 8% to 13% of psychiatric referrals, but estimates from epidemiological studies and primary care settings suggest an overall incidence of less than 1% (Goodyer, 1981; Shapiro & Rosenfeld, 1987). In most, but not all studies, girls are more frequently affected than boys, at least from puberty onward. It is unclear whether this reflects the true sex distribution of the disorder or the likelihood that emotional factors are either more apparent or more frequently suspected in girls. Occurrence before age 5 is rare. Anna Freud (1926), however, described a convincing case of transient arm pain and paralysis in a boy of 2 years 3 months who had been frightened by observing a mishap with a dangerous well bucket that he had been tempted but forbidden to touch.

In the century since Freud began his work, conversion symptoms seem to have become less frequent; some hold that such symptoms now appear most commonly in certain ethnic groups, in rural settings, and in patients of lower socioeconomic status (SES) (Forbis & Jones, 1965). Although objective data are lacking, this shift in prevalence is often attributed to two factors: the general increase of sexual (and perhaps aggressive) permissiveness in middle-class child-rearing practices, and an increased sophistication about psychosomatic illness (so that the symptoms no longer provide so good a "cover").

Although outside the scope of this discussion, cultural and sociological factors obviously play a large role in conversion symptoms (Hollender, 1972; Rabkin, 1964). Familial clustering does occur but is usually considered to be evidence of modeling rather than genetic transmission.

Clinical Features. The most frequent conversion symptoms manifested by children are hysterical seizures, paralysis of a limb or gait disturbance, and visual disturbances. Less common manifestations include cough, dysphagia (Koon, 1983), aphonia, and other sensory disturbances (Shapiro & Rosenfeld, 1987). It is debatable whether psychologically induced autonomic reactions such as fainting, vomiting, or hyperventilation should be considered conversion symptoms or should instead be regarded as direct physiological concomitants of anxiety. The diagnosis of conversion hysteria is most appropriate when there is a clear symbolic meaning to the symptom (as in the example below); most cases are, in fact, equivocal. The syndrome of hysterical hyperventilation is discussed separately in Chapter 7, "Anxiety Disorders."

CASE EXAMPLE

Mary, a 16-year-old high school student, was seen for psychiatric evaluation of recurrent, upsetting, and apparently involuntary vomiting. A gastroenterological workup had been unrevealing. The symptom had begun several weeks earlier following a practical joke; in the cafeteria, an envious girlfriend had put curly hair clippings in Mary's sandwich. On discovering the hair by biting into it, Mary had become nauseated and vomited. The vomiting now recurred whenever she ate meat, but at no other times.

During the interview, Mary described her difficulties with her boyfriend, who had been putting a good deal of pressure on her for sexual favors. Thus far she had resisted his importunings because of her strict religious scruples and her fear of pregnancy. In addition, Mary had serious doubts, which she hesitated to acknowledge to herself, about his fidelity. Additional associations to the prank and the vomiting included pubic hair, friends' teasing her about morning sickness, and Mary's difficult family situation. Her mother, with whom she was both protective and competitive, was again pregnant but on the verge of leaving the father because of his numerous extramarital affairs. As Mary exclaimed how "fed up" and "sick and tired" she was of his behavior, it became difficult at times to tell of whom she was speaking, her father or her boyfriend.

In terms of intervention, a behaviorally oriented clinician might have approached the vomiting as a conditioned response in need of extinction (perhaps by desensitization). In Mary's case, the therapist took a psychodynamic approach. During three sessions, Mary and the therapist carefully explored her conflicts—her resentment (and longings) toward her boyfriend and father, as well as her feelings about her girlfriend and pregnant mother. The vomiting promptly disappeared, and Mary was better able to confront both her father and boyfriend with her grievances.

In true conversion disorder, no known physical disorder can account for the symptoms. The clinician should strongly consider the diagnosis of conversion disorder in cases where the symptoms "do not make medical sense." For example, sensory or motor impairments in such cases often fail to correspond to the anatomy and physiology of the nervous system; instead they correspond to a notion in the patient's mind. Thus, on careful examination, sensory loss may have a stocking or glove pattern or stop exactly at the midline. In hysterical gait disorder, the gait may be bizarre and the disability disproportionate to any objective evidence of muscle weakness or joint pathology (Dubowitz & Hersov, 1976). Stevens (1969) described a girl who could only walk backward. Furthermore, the patient's description or demonstration of the pathology may be vivid and exaggerated. When asked to stand or hop on one leg, the patient with hysterical paralysis may be unable to raise his foot off the floor (almost as though it were glued); exaggerated contortions accompany the attempt (Dubowitz & Hersov, 1976). (For details of diagnostic tests for conversion symptoms as part of the neurological exam, see Weintraub, 1983, and Gould et al., 1986.)

The exclusion of organic pathology is more difficult when the symptoms are not frankly incompatible with known neurologic processes. The clinician then faces a dilemma. The relentless, often fruitless pursuit of diagnostic procedures (frequently of more and more invasive character and increasing costliness) only further entrenches the conversion symptoms. Yet, the inability to find an organic cause is intrinsically unsatisfactory as a *positive* diagnostic criterion; in any given case, the failure may reflect only current ignorance or the limitations of diagnostic techniques. Indeed, as good determinists, clinicians must note that even a psychologically determined paralysis or sensory loss must have some central, perhaps cortical, neurophysiological manifestation as part of its final expression.

Because they are dissatisfied with diagnosis by exclusion, some authors have insisted on the presence of various proposed positive criteria to make the diagnosis of conversion disorder (Friedman, 1973). Among these purported criteria are a history of somatization disorder, associated psychopathology, the existence of someone in the child's acquaintance who serves as a model for the symptom, emotional stress preceding the onset of the symptom, a discernible symbolic meaning or primary or secondary gain from the symptom, hysterical personality, or *la belle indifférence*. However, these criteria have only limited validity; they range from the suggestive to the completely equivocal (Lazare, 1981).

A history of *somatization disorder* or a previous history of *conversion symptoms* lends weight to a diagnosis of conversion rather than organic illness. Similarly, since 35% to 50% of patients with conversion symptoms have serious *concomitant psychopathology* (such as depression, personality disorder, or schizophrenia), the presence of such pathology also makes the diagnosis of conversion disorder more likely (Lazare, 1981). However, such evidence is only probabilistic. The availability of a *model* whose symptoms the patient may unconsciously imitate is a more convincing finding. The illness of a significant person in the patient's life or a previous illness experienced by the patient might provide such a model. A frequent clue to conversion is the occurrence of considerable emotional *stress* shortly before the onset of symptoms. Children with conversion symptoms have a very high incidence of recent family stress and unresolved grief reactions concerning recent losses (Maloney, 1980). Unfortunately, because stress is so ubiquitous, a causal rather than a coincidental association is often difficult to establish. Furthermore, emotional stress can precipitate organic illness as well (Heisel et al., 1973).

Freud regarded the presence of *symbolic meaning* attached to a symptom as the central feature of conversion phenomena; unfortunately, this too is not a completely reliable diagnostic criterion. The unconscious symbolic meaning of a symptom is often difficult to discern upon brief evaluation, especially if the diagnostician does not proceed in a rote-interpretive fashion. Furthermore, the symptoms of organic illness will also take on personal and symbolic meaning to a patient, just as they provide secondary gain by evoking sympathy, attention, and extra care (Raskin et al., 1966). In a similar fashion, the presence or absence of hysterical personality traits such as suggestibility, seductiveness, or overly dramatic behavior are not reliable diagnostic indicators; conversion symptoms can be found in patients of any personality type.

Finally, the classic finding of *la belle indifference* occurs with equal frequency in patients with organic illness and conversion symptoms (Raskin et al., 1966). In fact, only a minority of children with conversion symptoms appear indifferent to their disabilities (Goodyer, 1981). Even the presence on neurological exam of variable insensitivity to pain, give-away weakness or a pattern of sensory loss that does not correspond to the neuroanatomy of the sensory system may be misleading. Although often considered pathognomonic evidence of conversion disorder, such signs are often apparent in the careful examination of patients with acute structural brain diseases (Gould et al., 1986).

The differentiation of conversion disorder from organic illness is complex, and the hazard of missing subtle or incipient organic pathology is always present. Diagnostic humility seems appropriate in the face of several long-term (1 to 11 years) follow-up studies of adult patients diagnosed with conversion disorders. In 13% to 62% of the patients, clear organic illness emerged that appeared to account for the symptoms initially diagnosed as conversion disorder (Lazare, 1981; Slater & Glithero, 1965). An unpublished study (Caplan, 1974, cited in Rivinus et al., 1975) found that when a group of children initially diagnosed as having "conversion hysteria" were studied longitudinally, as many as 46% were found to have proven organic disorders that explained their initial symptoms. Rivinus and colleagues (1975) reviewed a sample of children who had received initial psychiatric diagnoses 2 months to 6 years earlier. On follow-up they were found to have a variety of neurological diseases. The majority of these cases had presented with such physical symptoms as gait and posture disorders or visual difficulties. Final diagnoses included dystonia musculorum deformans, Fredrich's ataxia, retinal degeneration (Batten's disease), polymyositis, and spinal neoplasms. Close, ongoing surveillance and periodic reassessment are clearly indicated when unusual physical symptoms persist or progress.

Strictly speaking, the diagnosis of conversion disorder requires that the symptoms cannot be explained by known physical disorders. Nonetheless, conversionlike mechanisms frequently appear to be at work in patients with known organic illness. Creak (1938) thus distinguished between "true conversion hysteria" and "hysterical prolongation of a symptom originally part of an organic predetermined disease". Such psychogenic prolongation of organically determined symptoms provides a frequent diagnostic challenge; this problem is specially notable in the epileptic child who also has hysterical seizures and the school-phobic child who has a bout of flu and never gets over it. In such cases secondary gain is significant. These children draw important advantages from what sociologists have termed "illness behavior" or the "sick role" (Mechanic, 1962; Rabkin, 1964). Such youngsters accept the restrictions of illness with unusual compliance and even cheerfulness; as they begin to recover, they resist the removal of measures such as bed rest, bandages, or crutches from which other children are eager to be freed. The anxiety of both parent and child about the child's physical illness may reinforce this invalidism. Later in this chapter, as well as in Chapter 16, the discussion of "psychosomatic family" dynamics returns to these themes (Minuchin et al., 1978). Finally, for reasons that are still obscure, certain neurological conditions, such as multiple sclerosis, head injury, frontal lobe lesions, and encephalitis, predispose patients to concomitant conversion symptoms (Lazare, 1981).

Behavioral theorists have heavily emphasized the importance of secondary gain in developing and maintaining conversion symptoms. From this theoretical point of view, such symptoms are learned defenses against anxiety-producing situations, further reinforced by the gratifications of extra attention and care (Delamater et al., 1983; Laybourne & Churchill, 1972). The gains might include avoidance of school or conflict-laden home situations. These authors do not consider dynamic repression to be a significant factor, because the child may be aware of the anxiety involved in these situations. Indeed, this approach minimizes distinctions between conscious and unconscious, and even between conversion symptoms and malingering. For these authors, determining such distinctions is both clinically difficult and irrelevant to the therapeutic task of changing reinforcers in order to extinguish the symptoms. Accordingly, this viewpoint sees little significance in the degree of the patient's consciousness of volitionally producing the symptoms.

Conversion Paralysis and Other Motor Disorders. Limb paralysis and disturbances of gait and posture are the commonest childhood conversion symptoms. The difficulties may range from a postural disturbance such as torticollis to a total loss of the ability to walk. Variable amounts of pain or parasthesias may accompany the motor symptoms (Goodyer, 1981).

Blocq (1888) coined the term *astasia-abasia* to describe "a morbid state in which the impossibility of standing erect and walking normally is in contrast with the integrity of sensibility of the muscular strength and coordination of the other movements of the lower extremities" (cited in Hammer, 1967, p. 671). Severe stress may coincide with the onset of these symptoms, as in the

West Point plebes reported on by Hammer (1967). In other cases, onset follows a period of bed rest or reduced mobility that occurs during treatment for viral illness or minor injury. The children often complain of muscle or joint pain and may hobble or crawl about dramatically. In addition to joint and muscle pain, some children may show objective laboratory or clinical evidence of mild muscle or joint inflammation. However, when their mobility disturbance remains out of proportion to these objective findings or persists after their resolution, such cases properly fit Creak's (1938) category of "hysterical prolongation of a symptom originally part of an organically predetermined disease". If hysterical paralyses persist for months or years, actual physical sequelae such as disuse atrophy, contractions, or trophic changes may occur, further complicating both diagnosis and treatment. When the clinician observes such complications, it is usually in the context of reclusive families who sequester the child in a sick role, rejecting medical attention (Stevens, 1969).

Hysterical Seizures ("Pseudoseizures"). Hysterical seizures (often called "pseudoseizures") represent one of the commonest forms of conversion reaction. These attacks are often dramatic and bizarre, with uncoordinated flailing of the limbs rather than the characteristic tonic-clonic motions of the true grand mal seizure. During, and immediately after, a hysterical seizure, the EEG is normal; this stands in marked contrast to the true epileptic seizure, which is accompanied by a rhythmic paroxysmal EEG discharge and is usually followed by postictal slowing of the tracing. Tongue biting, incontinence, and postictal confusion are all usually absent in the hysterical seizure as are eye deviations, autonomic overreactivity, and altered reflexes such as the Babinski sign (Fenton, 1986). Despite dramatic falls and much thrashing about, physical injuries rarely occur. The patient with hysterical seizures is responsive to pain during the attack and may recall events that happen during the seizure. Pseudoseizures tend to occur in the presence of an audience, and appropriate suggestion can often dramatically terminate the attacks.

Pseudoseizures were a common component of the syndrome of hysteria that was seen so frequently toward the end of the nineteenth century. Charcot and his colleagues thus spoke of "hystero-epileptics." As they observed, pelvic thrusting was often a prominent feature of these seizures, which often had a strong sexual flavor.

Despite these differential features, distinguishing between true seizures and hysterical attacks may be extremely difficult. Such hysterical seizures are not infrequent among epileptic patients who also suffer from bona fide ictal attacks, and this association compounds the difficulty (Fenton, 1986). And to still further complicate matters, situational stress can precipitate or increase the frequency of true seizures in epileptic patients. Activation of EEG by strong emotion has been reported in epileptic patients, especially those with psychomotor sensory epilepsy. Furthermore, environmental stress can precipitate seizures in several types of seizure-prone laboratory animals. Finally, anxious hyperventilation can culminate in epileptic seizures. Differential diagnosis requires the careful collaboration of both neurologist and psychiatrist. Only a negative EEG during a seizure provides ironclad evidence of its hysterical origin. Although the EEG tracing between seizures may produce evidence that the patient does have a seizure disorder, it is inconclusive as to the cause of any given attack. At times, only hospitalization on a special diagnostic unit equipped with videotape and 24-hour EEG telemetry equipment can determine definitively which seizures are real and which are hysterical (Holmes et al., 1980).

Unless children with pseudoseizures receive careful diagnostic scrutiny, they often end up on lengthy courses of anticonvulsive medication that can entail potentially toxic side effects and even exacerbation of their hysterical seizures. Identifying pseudoseizures is diagnostically and therapeutically important even in the child with well-established epilepsy (Williams et al., 1978, 1979). In such cases, psychological interventions such as psychotherapy, hypnosis, relaxation techniques, and biofeedback may help to eliminate otherwise uncontrollable seizures. These techniques may also be useful in controlling true seizures although many such studies are questionable because they fail to clarify whether the treatment is controlling true seizures or is diminishing hysterical pseudoseizures in the same patient (Williams et al., 1978, 1979).

Hysterical seizures are more common in adolescents than in younger children. Such pseudoseizures can occur in response to acute stress, especially of a conflictual nature. The seizure may both discharge anxiety and enable the adolescent to get away from the conflict via dissociative "passing out" (Gross, 1979). The patient with hysterical seizures may be aware of experiencing anxiety or inner turmoil immediately before the attack. On the whole, however, these youngsters are largely unconscious of the processes producing the symptoms (Gross, 1979; LaBarbera & Dozier, 1980). In fact, it is not always possible to determine the precise degree of the patient's self-awareness or volitional input into the hysterical symptoms.

Initially, Freud asserted that incestuous sexual abuse in childhood was the cause of later hysterical symptoms in his female patients. Subsequently, he altered his emphasis, suggesting instead that persisting childhood sexual (unresolved oedipal) fantasies rather than real sexual molestation determined the genesis of hysterical symptoms (Freud, 1905/1953). Although Freud never underestimated the impact of actual traumatic experience, more recent authors have reemphasized the pathogenic effects of incest and sexual abuse in childhood, including dissociative phenomena (such as fugue states and multiple personality disorder), hysterical seizures, and other conversion disorders (Goodwin, 1987; Putnam et al., 1986; Shapiro & Rosenfeld, 1987).

To bring the historical wheel full circle, several authors have recently reported on pseudoseizures in adolescent girls as a response to sexual exploitation (Goodwin et al., 1979; Gross, 1979; LaBarbera & Dozier, 1980). Several of the girls actually had been abused; others, with very religious upbringings, felt extremely guilty about their sexual experimentation with boyfriends. In psychotherapy, the latter girls displayed marked ambivalence concerning their own sexual urges and showed considerable mistrust of men, including their male therapists. Their pseudoseizures appeared to represent an escape from extreme conflictual feelings as well as "a compromise between inhibition and gratification of censored wishes" (LaBarbera & Dozier, 1980).

Other conversion disorders may also occur in the aftermath of sexual trauma. For example, in two-thirds of the conversion reactions reviewed by Volkmar et al. (1984), there was evidence of a sexual stressor, most often involving a close relative.

Visual Conversion Reactions

CASE EXAMPLE

John, a quiet well-behaved 12-year-old boy came to the clinic with a chief complaint of blurred vision; he complained that it interfered with his seeing the blackboard at school. At home, John would sometimes dramatically bump into walls or furniture, claiming that he hadn't seen them. In crowds, he would sometimes attempt to get his mother to lead him by the hand. The onset of his symptoms coincided with the appearance of severe family stress surrounding the breakup of his parents' marriage. John felt he was the guilty instrument of his parents' divorce because he had inadvertently discovered and revealed evidence of his father's infidelity. He was an ardent baseball player, however, and on his weekend visits with father he was still able to field and to hit the ball normally. Ophthamological examination revealed tubular fields (tunnel vision), the presence of fluctuating visual acuity, and no refractive abnormalities.

Visual conversion reactions are common in children and are usually characterized by just such fluctuating visual acuity and/or tubular visual fields. These symptoms are often susceptible to change upon suggestion or in response to operant conditioning techniques (Brady & Lind, 1961; Rada et al., 1969, 1973, 1978). Initially, the child's complaint often focuses on trouble with schoolwork, but stress and conflict at home are usually present. Family tensions are typically covert with a characteristic family style that suppresses conflict and fears impulsivity. Rada's group (1978) commented on the frequency of ill-concealed "family secrets" and the resulting bewilderment in the affected children. They cited one girl with visual conversion symptoms, who, perplexed about her parents' fighting, remarked, "Maybe if I had glasses, I could understand better."

It is sometimes possible to uncover specific conflicts about whether or not to look or to know, but in many cases such dynamics are not conspicuous. What the clinician sees instead are various nonspecific conflicts at work within the child. Moreover, among these children no particular personality type predominates. Concerns about vision are likely to be present in some family member with a history of eye troubles, or the child himself may have been plagued by previous visual difficulties such as strabismus. Such prior events offer a model for the new symptom.

Prognosis is variable. In a 2-to-3-year follow-up study (Rada et al., 1973) about 30% of the children showed no further psychiatric or ophthalmological difficulties. At the other end of the spectrum, 10% of the children showed no improvement in either sphere. An intermediate 35% showed either psychological or visual symptoms that persisted or recurred episodically.

In the recurrent cases, secondary gains seemed particularly important. Some children learned to use their recurrent visual symptoms as a barometer of psychological stress. A particularly serious aspect of this study is that with continuing surveillance, 15% of the children were found to have organic eye disease such as macular pathology. A number of signs should particularly alert the physician including persisting, progressive, relatively nonfluctuating visual problems, especially if they interfere with activities the child enjoys, such as sports. A persistent central scotoma (blind spot) should also raise the suspicion of incipient organic eye disease.

Somatoform Pain Disorder

Introduction. Vague recurrent childhood pains of obscure origin constitute one of the commonest problems to plague both parents and pediatricians. Abdominal pains, headaches, and limb pains are common in childhood, whereas back pain (a frequent adult complaint) is rare. In the large majority of cases, no organic causes can be found. Instead, emotional factors frequently appear to be at work.

Definition. The DSM-III-R definition of somatoform pain disorder closely parallels the DSM-III-R definition of conversion disorder.

DSM-III-R Diagnostic Criteria for Somatoform Pain Disorder
A. *Preoccupation with pain for at least six months.*
B. *Either (1) or (2)*
   (1) appropriate evaluation uncovers no organic pathology or pathophysiologic mechanism (e.g., a physical disorder or the effects of injury) to account for the pain

(2) *when there is related organic pathology, the complaint of pain or resulting social or occupational impairment is grossly in excess of what would be expected from the physical findings.* (APA, 1987, p. 266)

Epidemiology. Most epidemiological studies have not utilized the DSM-III-R definition of somatoform pain disorder. However, various pediatric studies of recurrent pain give a rough estimate of the problem's potential magnitude (Apley et al., 1978; Oster, 1972). Using strict criteria for inclusion, namely, at least 3 months of recurrent pain of sufficient severity to interfere with activities, Apley and colleagues (1978) summarized the various estimates of recurrent pain in schoolchildren as follows: Recurrent abdominal pain affects from 11% to 16%; limb pain, 4% to 20%; and headache, about 14%. Of course, not all of these pains were psychogenic. Nonetheless, in a majority of cases, no organic causes could be identified. Thus, with the caveats to be noted later, diagnosticians could find organic causes in only 7% to 20% of the cases of children with recurrent abdominal pain. Similarly, only in about 4% of children with recurrent limb pains could a positive organic factor be found. In cases of headache, convincing physical causes were found in only 5% of the cases of recurrent headache (excluding migraine which itself affects about 4% of children).

Various pain syndromes often coexist. Thus, about 40% of children with limb pains also have abdominal pains or headaches (or, as a child in Apley's study put it, "Sometimes I get my tummy ache in my head"). Pediatricians have coined the term *Periodic syndrome* to describe the pentad of headache, fever, abdominal pain, limb pain, and recurrent vomiting that apparently occurs as a reaction to stress; this reaction pattern tends to run in families. Children who complain of recurrent pains often belong to pain-prone families. As many as 50% of children with recurrent abdominal pains have a parent with a history of functional gastrointestinal complaints. The parents, especially mothers, of children with headaches or recurrent limb pain more frequently give a history of similar pains (currently or during childhood) than do parents of a controlled group of children (Oster, 1972). Uncontrolled studies also suggest an increased family incidence of migraine and allergies (Liebman, 1978).

Clinical Features. Recurrent abdominal pains illustrate many features of the psychogenic pain syndrome as well as the methodological difficulties inherent in studying such disorders.

Recurrent abdominal pain affects as many as 1 schoolchild in 9. The pain is usually vague and periumbilical. In attempting to differentiate between organic and nonorganic pain, the precise location of the pain is usually an unreliable guide. Bouts of discomfort bear no consistent relationship to meals, bowel movements, or diet (with the possible exception of milk products, discussed below). School attendance is usually poor, and in about 25% of the cases the clinician can identify excitement, punishment, or school and social events as exacerbants (Liebman, 1978). Adler and colleagues (1982) reported abdominal pain due to pressure from highly competitive (but personally frustrated) parents concerning the child's participation in organized sports. The physical exam is usually negative except perhaps for pallor and mild diffuse abdominal tenderness. Headache, nausea or vomiting, limb pain, fatigue, and loss of appetite often accompany the attacks of abdominal pain. Neither diarrhea nor constipation are consistent findings. When constipation does occur, treatment of the constipation does little to relieve the distress (Galler et al., 1980).

Even after extensive workups, most studies report successful identification of organic causes for the pain in only 5% to 20% of the cases (Apley et al., 1978). The most common organic causes of recurrent abdominal pain are regional enteritis, ulcer disease, and urinary tract disorders, especially chronic urinary infections. These statistics apply only to Western industrial societies; in much of the Third World endemic intestinal parasitic infections afflict many children.

A common condition that the diagnostician must rule out is lactose intolerance. This malabsorption syndrome results from a maturational decline in lactase, the intestinal enzyme that digests lactose, the principal sugar in milk. This decline is probably genetically determined. It begins in the preschool years and, if the affected child continues to ingest significant amounts of milk or milk products, can cause gas, diarrhea, and intermittent abdominal pain. About 10% to 15% of Caucasian schoolchildren and a much larger percentage of noncaucasian children suffer from this condition.

Studies employing a sophisticated breath-hydrogen test (Barr et al., 1979; Liebman, 1979) found that as many as 25% to 43% of children with otherwise inexplicable recurrent abdominal pain showed lactase deficiency. Most of these lactase-deficient children showed improvement of their pain on a milkfree diet, and a reexacerbation of their symptoms when they resumed their regular (milk-containing) fare. Unfortunately, neither dietary history nor the presence or absence of pain symptoms in response to a lactose load accurately predicted the children whose pain was due to lactase deficiency.

Other investigators have cast doubt that lactase deficiency causes recurrent abdominal pain. Lebenthal and colleagues (1981) found the same prevalence of lactase deficiency in children with recurrent abdominal pain and in a matched control group. Further, after a year's trial of a lactose-free diet, the overall frequency of improvement in abdominal pain was the same for both the children with and without lactase deficiency and did not differ significantly from the group of children who remained on an unrestricted diet.

Both controlled and uncontrolled studies have concluded that children with recurrent abdominal pain tend to be depressed, anxious, sensitive, and eager to please (Galler et al., 1980; Wasserman et al., 1988). Internalizing symptoms, including perfectionism, frequent worrying, and low self-esteem are also common (Garber et al., 1990; Liebman, 1978). In other controlled studies both these children and their mothers have shown high anxiety levels (Garber et al., 1988). However, no specific personality type is pathognomonic; indeed, these traits are also present in many other children including those with organic abdominal illness (Garber et al., 1990; Raymer et al., 1984).

Many children with abdominal pain have difficulty expressing their feelings verbally about frustrating situations (Galler et al., 1980). Many such children seem to come from a background of serious family problems where the family adaptive style encourages the children to suppress their feelings and hide conflict.

Other recent epidemiological and controlled studies of children with abdominal pains have not found an increased incidence of depression or overcompliance (Hodges et al., 1985). One epidemiologic study found children with abdominal pain were more likely to be temperamentally difficult (Davison et al., 1986). Another study of the same population found an increased incidence of antisocial and hyperactive symptoms. This study also suggested an interaction of temperament with environmental stresses; in contrast to children without pain, children with recurrent abdominal pain were more likely to be having trouble settling into school, to live in public housing, and to have mothers who were less likely to turn to their husbands for support (Faull & Nicol, 1986).

In studying a series of children who had been hospitalized for evaluation of their recurrent abdominal pain, Hughes (1984) observed overt signs of major childhood depression. The hospitalization probably reflected both the intractibility of their symptoms as well as the relentlessness of their parents' pursuit of physical causes. Family histories were replete with past and present illnesses, deaths, or threatened losses. All the children met the full DSM-III criteria for a major depressive episode; they were preoccupied with family problems, especially their mother's health and depression. The mothers in turn were anxiously overprotective. Hospital staff experienced these mothers as "sad, watchful, hovering, critical, and needy." Children and mothers shared an anxious concern about bodily functioning and loss. These mothers rejected medical reassurance about the absence of physical abnormalities and continued an "anxious, pessimistic pursuit of medical solutions."

The assessment of recurrent abdominal pain thus requires careful medical management. Several authors have outlined a diagnostic approach involving a few basic laboratory studies that should exclude the vast majority of organic causes (Apley et al., 1978; Galler et al., 1980; Stickler & Murphy, 1979). Weight loss and anemia in particular should heighten suspicion of organic illness. If, however, initial laboratory and physical findings are unremarkable, the physician must make a careful psychosocial evaluation of the child and his family, with special attention to current stresses and the family style of handling tensions. A relentless pursuit of invasive tests runs the risk of perpetuating invalidism. Through well-meaning but never-ending efforts to find a "physical cause," the physician can risk iatrogenic perpetuation of the illness (Weiss, 1947). All too many such children (and adults) end up enduring unnecessary exploratory surgery.

The presence of clear organic pathology does not obviate its need for careful psychosocial evaluation because children with organically determined abdominal pain also have a high prevalence anxiety and depression (Garber et al., 1990).

Etiology. The physical processes that link emotional factors to the perception of pain are unknown. Researchers have explored various hypotheses. Although patients with recurrent abdominal pain were once thought to have generally lowered pain thresholds, direct testing has failed to support this possibility (Galler et al., 1980).

In some cases a bout of viral gastroenteritis appears to be a precursor. By interacting with personality characteristics, environmental stresses, and psychophysiological constitutional factors, such an infection may establish a cycle that perpetuates the pain syndrome long after the virus is gone.

Researchers have suggested that autonomic dysfunction links recurrent abdominal pain and emotional disorders in childhood. Abnormalities in autonomic reactivity have been reported both in children with recurrent abdominal pain and in their parents (see review by Galler et al., 1980). Autonomic imbalance may also underlie abnormalities of intestinal motility in such children. Many children with recurrent abdominal pain appear to have prolonged intestinal transit times and an excessive response to parasympathetic drugs. It appears that there is a relationship between emotional upsets and style of autonomic functioning, but how they are connected remains a major area for psychosomatic research.

Familial factors also play a role in recurrent abdominal pain in childhood. Approximately half of children with this disorder have a first-degree relative with somatization disorder (Routh and Ernst, 1984). As noted earlier, depression and anxiety are common in the parents of such children.

There are several possible explanations for these familial patterns, beyond the impact of parental distress on parent–child interactions, including modeling, genetic transmission, and enculturation to a family style that favors somatic complaints rather than the direct expression of affect (Garber et al., 1990).

Treatment of Somatoform Disorders

The diversity of treatments for somatoform disorders parallels the broad range of etiologic theories. The history of such treatment could, in fact, serve as a gloss of the history of psychiatry. In the past, depending on whether the clinician's viewpoint was organic, psychoanalytic, socioenvironmental, or behavioral, treatment would focus on a weakened nervous system, unconscious intrapsychic conflict, disordered interpersonal relations and modes of communication, or learned maladaptive patterns of anxiety avoidance reinforced by secondary gains.

A review of the treatment literature for children (e.g., Schaefer et al., 1979; Shapiro & Rosenfeld, 1987) reveals a wide range of therapeutic modalities ranging from psychoanalytically oriented psychotherapy; family therapy (Liebman et al., 1976a, 1976b; Minuchin et al., 1975, 1978); hypnosis (Williams & Singh, 1976); abreactive drug interviews (Stevens, 1969; Weintraub, 1983); relaxation training and biofeedback (Conners, 1983); behavior modification (Laybourne & Churchill, 1972; Delamater et al., 1983); cognitive-behavioral techniques (Sanders et al., 1989); and placebo. As early investigators noted, suggestion has a particularly powerful (although not necessarily long-acting) impact on somatoform symptoms. Thus, nonspecific treatment effects, plus the tendency for conversion symptoms to fluctuate even when untreated, make treatment outcome particularly difficult to assess.

The physician's approach to evaluating and treating the patient and his family is of great importance (Apley et al., 1978). M. Green (1967) emphasizes that the physician must bear in mind the following questions concomitant with any physical diagnostic procedures: Why did the patient and his family come in now? Whose idea was it to come? How did the symptom start? When does it occur? What does the parent think is wrong? What are the conscious gains from the symptoms? Why was *this* symptom selected? What do the parents expect of the doctor? Lazare (1981) described this as a somewhat oblique approach that involves: "inquiring about the situation of the patient's life while listening for possible symbolic meanings in the symptom, the unbearable affects against which the symptom defends, and the social communication inherent in the symptom" (p. 748).

Treatment must not only restore the patient's normal functional level through symptom removal but also identify and ameliorate the underlying psychological stresses that cause the symptom. The tactics and priorities for achieving these goals vary with different treatments.

Often, it is sufficient merely to help the patient identify and put directly into words the seemingly intolerable feelings that the symptoms are defending against. Once the patient does this, the clinician can then help the child cope with and bear the painful repudiated emotions that he previously could express only in body language (Lazare, 1981). However, a concurrent active rehabilitative effort aimed directly at symptom removal may also be necessary, especially when these maladaptations severely constrict the child's activity. Delamater's group (1983) and others have argued that effective exploration and change in underlying individual or family dynamics may not be possible until the symptom is ameliorated.

The same view is implicit in the opening phases of Minuchin and colleagues' structural family approach (Liebman et al., 1976a, 1976b). There, the family therapist's opening interventions are highly directive and are intended to alleviate the patient's symptoms in order to decrease the use of the patient as a detour for family conflicts. As these family therapists view it, only then are the necessary "freedom and flexibility available to promote change in the family." In the case of the child with abdominal pain, for example, the initial maneuvers might include having the child keep a daily diary record of pain and its context (Liebman et al., 1976a). Each evening, the child, the less involved parent, and the therapist review this record by phone. The parents reward the child for gaining sufficient control of the pain to attend school regularly. The parents are assigned the task of supporting the child in attending school, with the less involved parent again taking the lead and the other parent acting as backup. These tasks become a vehicle for examining and changing the functional structure of the family; in attempting them, the family members highlight the patterns and conflicts that perpetuate the symptom. Only then can further interventions promote lasting disengagement of the child.

Learning theorists see the child's symptoms as often representing partially conscious attempts to avoid anxious situations. Behavioral therapists thus acknowledge the importance of identifying the anxiety-producing (or otherwise aversive) situations that the child seeks to avoid through his symptoms and providing alternative coping modes for the child. In behavioral treatment, however, direct symptom discouragement involves two primary tasks: to eliminate the positive (often inadvertent) reinforcers that maladaptively reward the child's incapacity, and to find effective reinforcers that will systematically reward successive steps toward restoration of full physical function.

For example, in treating a 10-year-old boy with astasia-abasia, Delamater et al. (1983) confined the boy to his room without social interaction or entertainment. The patient had to earn various specified entertainments and enjoyable social interactions according to a "step-by-step" behavioral program. The boy's rewards were contingent on successfully completing each level of his program; the steps specified a sequence of behaviors that successively approximated normal walking. Initially, maintaining a kneeling position without collapse for 5 seconds earned a star (10 of which had to be earned in order to receive a reward). Later, crawling 2 feet earned 2 stars; still later, standing with support of an object earned 3 stars, and so on. In this way the program gradually shaped walking behavior. (Dubowitz &

Hersov, 1976, and Delamater et al., 1983, have reviewed this rehabilitative approach to hysterical motor problems in detail; its applications to visual problems are described by Rada et al., 1978.)

Delamater and colleagues commented on the ward staff's initial resistance to shifting their own behavior so that it rewarded the patient's progress rather than his helplessness. Minuchin's family therapy approach addresses these issues in the "psychosomatic family," where the child controls the parents with his sick behavior, while they in turn reward his incapacities (Liebman et al., 1976a, 1976b; Minuchin et al., 1975, 1978). Sperling's (1968) contention that some psychosomatic children could be successfully treated only after their mothers were in treatment might thus have been an early, albeit less explicit and complete, approach to reordering the environmental reinforcers that maintain the child's illness. Such mothers, Sperling maintained, were nurturant only when their child was sick; when he was well and was making strides toward autonomy, they rejected him.

Perhaps the historical wheel has also come full circle with the use of hypnosis in children with conversion symptoms. Williams and Singh (1976), who found such children to be ready hypnotic subjects, have used hypnosis as a facilitating therapeutic adjunct. Their rationale for hypnosis, however, went beyond its 19th-century uses for suggestion and abreactive recall of the symptom's onset. They taught the children self-hypnosis to facilitate relaxation and to help the child incorporate a new and more autonomously adaptive outlook toward his tensions. For example, a child with hysterical blindness would repeat while in a trance state, "When people are very scared and upset, they may stop being able to see. By relaxing (with this exercise), I can overcome my scared and upset feelings." The therapists thus employed hypnosis to focus on the presumed causes of the child's symptoms and his capacity to alter his own contribution to it. They also observed that the child who has cornered himself with a well-entrenched conversion symptom may need a palatable route to "escape with honor."

Hypnosis, like other symptom removal techniques, should be used only after a careful diagnostic assessment and as part of an overall treatment program for both the child and family. It is a grave disservice simply to strip away a symptom that serves an important defensive function without helping the child and parents cope with the tensions that have driven the child to such a desperate extremity.

Without treatment, children with recurrent abdominal pain associated with stress do poorly as they grow older. Apley and Hale (1973) found that 8 to 20 years later, only one-third had lost all their symptoms and remained well. In another third, the abdominal pains ceased but were replaced by other symptoms including headaches, anxiety, and other somatic symptoms. And for a final third, the abdominal pain persisted, usually accompanied by additional symptoms. In this study, even with very long-term follow-up, previously overlooked organic causes emerged only rarely.

Outcomes of treatment for abdominal pain vary. In Apley's long-term follow-up series, informal psychotherapy by the pediatrician did not cure the pain. Nor did it alter the proportion of patients with persisting abdominal pain at follow-up compared with an untreated control group. However, in adulthood, the treated patients were reportedly better adjusted with fewer headaches and more rapid recovery from bouts of pain.

Other researchers report more optimistic findings about the impact of treatment, albeit in uncontrolled studies. Berger and colleagues (1977) used a family conference technique to enlist the family's support for a psychosocial approach to the child's symptoms. About 40% of the children in this series required ongoing formal psychotherapy. After 18 months, all but 10% of the patients showed enough reduction of abdominal pain to allow them once again to engage in normal daily activities, with a concurrent marked improvement in their school attendance and peer relationships.

The outcome for children with conversion disorder is likewise variable. (The high incidence of missed organic disease has been discussed above.) Estimates of outcomes for childhood conversion disorder range from poor, with many hospitalizations and operations in later life, especially in untreated cases, through excellent, with good recovery from the presenting symptom and good emotional adjustment at long-term follow-up (Goodyer, 1981). As yet, researchers have not determined why some children remain monosymptomatic or recover completely, whereas others develop a full-blown somatization disorder with successive symptoms, ongoing incapacitation, and constricted activities due to multiple somatic complaints.

In adult conversion disorder, Lazare (1981) concluded that good prognosis was associated with three factors: acuteness, recent onset, and definite precipitation by stressful events. Prognosis also appeared to be related to premorbid adjustment and the degree of major concomitant psychiatric disorder.

PSYCHOLOGICAL FACTORS AFFECTING PHYSICAL CONDITIONS

Psychological and social factors profoundly affect the susceptibility to illness and influence both the onset and course of disease. Early workers often placed excessive weight on psychological factors as *causes* of disease. With the possible exception of the conversion disorders, however, psychosocial factors are rarely necessary and sufficient conditions for the development of physical illness. Rather, in most illnesses, the symptomatic manifestations result from a complex interaction between somatic and psychological components, with each factor varying in its relative contribution to the final clinical picture.

Historically, interest focused primarily on seven diseases often termed *psychosomatic:* asthma, essential hypertension, peptic ulcer, ulcerative colitis, rheumatoid arthritis, neurodermatitis, and hyperthyroidism. Franz Alexander (1950) postulated that each of these diseases could be correlated with specific unconscious conflicts, although he acknowledged the necessary presence of additional biochemical and physiological predisposing factors. Alexander felt that the symptoms of these autonomically innervated organ systems did not symbolize conflict in the same way as did conversion symptoms, which usually appear in organs or muscles controlled by the voluntary nervous system. Instead, these "conflict constellations" sensitized the individual and made him vulnerable in some unknown fashion. As a result, life experiences that reactivated the conflict could then lead to prolonged emotional and autonomic arousal, which in turn resulted in organ pathology. Alexander believed these conflict constellations could be embedded in many personality types. However, other investigators, such as Dunbar (1943), postulated a causal association of specific personality patterns with specific illnesses. Numerous papers were written about the possible psychosomatic profile of the asthma patient, the diabetic, the ulcer patient, and so on.

In the past 30 years, however, empirical validation of such hypotheses has proven difficult, and there has been a good deal of disillusionment with too exclusive a focus on individual psychodynamics. Furthermore, a factor limiting the heuristic value of such theories was their tendency to link causally "variables at very different levels of abstraction. . . without due regard for intervening psychophysiological variables" (Lipowski, 1977, p. 235).

Today there is an ever-wider realization that the biological, psychological, and social factors in determining health or sickness interact on many levels and are extremely complex. Engel (1977) has emphasized the need for a biopsychosocial model. Contemporary psychosomatic theorists attempt to struggle with this multitude of variables; at the same time they remain wary of premature closure because the lack of knowledge about mediating mechanisms is still considerable. Accordingly, the current DSM-III-R definition of what used to be termed *psychosomatic disorders* is an exceedingly broad one.

Definition

DSM-III-R Diagnostic Criteria for Psychological Factors Affecting Physical Condition

A. *Psychologically meaningful environmental stimuli are temporally related to the initiation or exacerbation of a specific physical condition or disorder.*

B. *The physical condition involves either demonstrable organic pathology (e.g., rheumatoid arthritis) or a known pathophysiologic process (e.g., migraine headache).*

C. *The condition does not meet the criteria for a Somatoform Disorder.* (APA, 1987, p. 334)

A thoroughgoing review of current concepts in psychosomatic medicine is beyond the scope of this work; the interested reader can turn to several excellent reviews (Kaplan, 1980; Knapp, 1980; Lipowski, 1977; Reiser, 1984; Weiner, 1977).

Stress and Adaptation

Current psychosomatic approaches suggest that social and psychological events can potentially influence biological processes on a multitude of levels—neurological, hormonal, immunological, and so on—and can thus influence reactions all the way down to the cellular level. A seminal way of conceptualizing the impact of the environment has been the notion of *stress*. Selye (1974) defined stress as the nonspecific response of the body to any demand made upon it. Psychosocial stress has been defined as "external and internal stimuli that are perceived by and are meaningful to the person, activate emotions, and elicit physiological changes that threaten health and survival" (Lipowski, 1977, p. 237). Note the ambiguity of usage; at times *stress* refers to the challenging stimulus, whereas at other times it describes the organismic response. What is key, however, is that "social situations and events as well as such psychological states as conflicts and frustrated strivings may disturb homeostasis and impose adaptive demands on the organism" (Lipowski, 1977, p. 237).

Stress can produce many autonomic and hormonal changes in both humans and lower animals, hence Selye coined the term *general adaptation syndrome* to describe the pituitary-ACTH-mediated stimulation of adrenocortical hormones induced by stress. In addition, this generalized stress response also mobilizes the norepinephrine system controlled by the locus ceruleus (Gold et al., 1988). These changes constitute the body's normal adaptive mechanisms; when they occur within homeostatic limits they help to mobilize the organism to cope with the adaptive challenge confronting it. If, however, these normally adaptive mechanisms become poorly modulated, fail to function, or operate in an excessive manner, perhaps because of too frequent or inappropriate elicitation, illness may result. Normally, a complex series of feedback ("counterregulatory") mechanisms restrain the stress response to prevent it from becoming excessive. Under certain circumstances, as in melancholic depression, these brakes appear to fail.

Some investigators have dealt with stress as a nonspecific quantitative factor, implying that stresses differ from each other primarily in degree of magnitude and that their cumulative impact can be summated arithmetically. Thus, Rahe (1975) and Holmes and Masuda (1974) attempted to predict the statistical probability of the occurrence of illness as well as its severity by counting the number of recent life changes, to which they assigned differing predictive weights. Surprisingly, events generally considered pleasurable or fortunate, such as vacations and promotions, took their toll as stressors alongside unfortunate events, such as loss of job or illness in a family member. Similarly, Coddington and co-workers (Heisel et al., 1973) found that, when compared with a control group of healthy children, the children admitted to a hospital's general pediatric and surgical services had an unexpectedly high incidence of major life changes in the year before hospitalization. However, even in studies with statistically significant correlations between life event and illness, the correlations are small, generally on the order of 0.3, thus accounting for only a small part of the variance in the occurrence of illness. Some of the implications and serious methodological difficulties of such studies are discussed by Hurst et al. (1978), Kasl (1983), Miller (1989), and Rabkin and Streuning (1976).

In contrast to this quantitative approach, other investigators have emphasized the importance of the specific qualitative aspects of stress in determining illness. Engel (1967) has particularly emphasized the role of object loss, whether real, anticipated, or fantasied, as an antecedent of illness. Throughout the life cycle, loss and bereavement take their toll in increased morbidity and mortality. An earlier chapter discussed the often fatal marasmus of the institutionalized infant, whose physical needs are met but who has no stable and secure attachment figure (see Chapter 6, "Affective Disorders").

Following the classic studies of Parkes and Brown (1972), numerous studies of widows and widowers (Jacobs & Ostfield, 1977) have shown that in addition to the many expected psychological sequelae, the death of a spouse is often followed by poorer health and fatal illness in the bereaved partner. Still other studies have implicated loss as a contributing factor in childhood diseases ranging from cancer (Jacobs & Charles, 1980) through diabetes (Stein & Charles, 1971), to peptic ulcer (Ackerman et al., 1981) and thyrotoxicosis (Morillo & Gardner, 1979). Engel (1967) has concluded that when feelings of loss or bereavement cannot be coped with, a sense of helplessness and hopelessness ensues that results in the "giving up—given up complex." This theoretical perspective sees the state of "psychological impotence" accompanying loss as providing the affective context for the onset of many diseases and emphasizes the need for a "psychobiology of bereavement" (Weiner, 1977).

These two approaches to stress, the qualitative and quantitative, are not mutually exclusive. In more sophisticated life-events research, the number of life changes are not merely added up; rather, they are weighted according to the degree of accommodation each demands from the subject. In general, changes that receive the most weight involve loss, such as the death of a spouse, or, in the case of a child, the loss of a parent through death or divorce.

Life changes do not tell the whole story, because not all individuals who suffer major upheavals become sick. A key concept in Engel's model is failure of adaptation. It is not the loss itself, but the individual's failure to *cope* with loss that produces a sense of hopelessness. The first to emphasize this adaptational framework was Wolff, who maintained that disease is not a *direct* consequence of stressful life situations, but rather of the failure to adapt to such situations (Garmezy & Rutter, 1983; Weiner, 1977; Wolff, 1950). An important mitigating variable is the availability of social supports to serve as buffers (Cobb, 1976; Haggerty, 1980; Rabkin & Streuning, 1976).

Although the concept of stress has semantic ambiguities, it remains a far-reaching, heuristically useful concept that integrates the impact of social factors, the individual's evaluation of such factors, and the resulting psychological and physiological outcomes.

Affect and Expressive Style

In considering possible intervening variables between perceived stresses and the body's physiological responses, emotions appear to be a significant factor set. As early as 1694, William Harvey recognized "the signal influence of the affections of the mind. . . . [What] indeed is more deserving of attention than the fact that in almost every affection, appetite, hope, or fear, our body suffers, the countenance changes, and the blood appears to course hither and thither[?]" (quoted in Apley et al., 1978).

Although the psychophysiology of emotion is a burgeoning field of study, it still remains a bewildering realm. Undoubtedly, however, emotions have major autonomic and physiological concomitants in addition to registering in consciousness. These physiological components differ from one emotion to another, even in the same individual. Thus, when experimenters asked subjects to relive past emotional experiences involving happiness, sadness, anger, fear, disgust, and surprise, each affect produced a qualitatively different pattern of autonomic activity (Ekman et al., 1983; Schwartz et al., 1981). Interestingly, researchers obtained similar results when they gave actors muscle-by-muscle instructions (without any reference to emotional state) to make a face corresponding to each affect.

Little is yet known about the physiological manifestations of various emotional coping mechanisms—to what extent, say, repressing or consciously suppressing a feeling decreases or augments accompanying autonomic and hormonal manifestations. Shakespeare asserted, "Sorrow concealed, like an oven stopped/Doth burn the heart/to cinders where it is" (*Titus Andronicus*). In affect-arousing experimental situations, several studies suggest that subjects who either verbally deny their feelings or show low facial expressiveness experience the *greatest* physiological autonomic arousal, whereas subjects who readily express their feelings verbally or facially show the *least* autonomic reaction (Anderson, 1981; Malatesta et al., 1987). It is even possible that the availability of or propensity toward different emotional coping or defensive styles may be intimately connected with constitutionally determined aspects of limbic system and autonomic regulation.

The relationship of coping style to hormonal response is also still obscure. No clear pattern emerges from studies of coping styles in the face of acute or chronic stress (Rutter, 1983d). Studies of parents who were anticipating, and then mourning, the death of their leukemic children demonstrated that those parents who displayed their upset most openly showed the highest corticosteroid levels (Hofer et al., 1972a, 1972b). On the other hand, different findings emerged from a longitudinal study of the incidence of various psychosomatic symptoms in Finnish adolescents (Rauste-von Wright & von Wright, 1981). In this study, students who showed the *least* strain-induced increase in adrenalin and cortisol exertion during university matriculation exams experienced the *highest* levels of habitual somatic discomfort and trait-anxiety scores. These students also tended to show the lowest self-esteem and highest dissatisfaction with their home situation. Finally, Knight and colleagues (1979) studied the relationship of cortisol secretion to the effectiveness of ego defenses in children hospitalized for elective surgery. Children with rigid defensive styles relying heavily on denial or projection tended to adjust poorly to the hospital and to have high cortisol secretion. Children with more flexible coping styles adjusted better and secreted less cortisol.

Individual Response Specificity

The hypothesis that social and psychological factors can produce physiological changes mediated by the individual's affectively toned subjective evaluation of such events raises the further question of why individuals differ in their responses to given stresses. Further, why do certain individuals (but not others) develop specific diseases? These problems belong to the poorly understood realm of *individual response specificity* and *predisposition to illness*.

Individual response specificity refers to an individual's "enduring psychological and physiological tendencies to react to specific stimuli with individually specific patterns of cognitive, emotional, behavioral, and physiological responses" (Lipowski, 1977, p. 236). Here then are several crucial points at which individual differences may have an influence. Not only do different people confront different stressful events, but the impact of even the same class of events differs from person to person. The affective thrust of any given event, be it a move, a final exam, or parental divorce, obviously varies from child to child, depending on the child's past history; his ethnic, family, and social class position; the conscious and unconscious significance of the event to the child; and the child's personality type and characteristic style of coping.

Individuals also differ considerably in their characteristic patterns of somatic responses to stress. Lacey (Lacey & Lacey, 1958; Lacey & VanLehn, 1952) experimentally studied the autonomic reactions of both children and adults to physiological and psychological stressors. Measures included heart rate, blood pressure, and skin conductance (a measure of sweat gland activity). Lacey found that with repeated exposures to a single stressor as well as to different types of stressors, subjects showed a characteristic and reproducible pattern of response. In some subjects, increases in blood pressure were the most striking; in others, acceleration of the heart rate was the most prominent change; in still others, increased sweating predominated. Whether certain patterns of autonomic response stereotypies characterize those children prone to psychosomatic symptoms or anxiety disorders remains a critical unanswered question.

The origins of individual psychophysiological response characteristics remain the focus of much current study. To explain variations, researchers have invoked genetic and constitutional factors, early experience, unconscious conflict, personality style, social learning, and operant conditioning history (Weiner, 1977).

Genetic-Constitutional Factors. Primate studies have found that there exist intraindividual differences in infant monkeys' behavioral and hormonal response to stress (including separation); these differences in response style are stable from infancy to maturity but are apparent only in the face of actual stress or separation (Suomi, 1986). Thus, when challenged with a stress, some monkeys consistently display fearful behavior; throughout their life-span these highly reactive individuals show more prolonged and dramatic elevations in plasma cortisol level than do less reactive peers. Even when infant monkeys are reared by a foster mother, their response style tends to resemble that of their biological relatives, rather than that of their adoptive kin, suggesting that these constitutional differences may be genetic in origin.

Family Factors. Cultural and family coping styles are also important determinants of response to stress. To date, most family theories of coping style implicitly postulate intrafamilial *environmental* influences as the means by which coping styles are passed from one generation to the next. However, the primate studies just cited suggest that genetic influences may also account for family members' similarities in physiological response style or tendency to somatization. Thus far, twin and adoption studies have been inconclusive regarding the relative roles of genetic and environmental factors in somatization (Torgersen, 1986).

One of the most influential theories of how family functioning might shape a predisposition to psychosomatic illness is that of Minuchin and colleagues. From their studies of refractory diabetic, asthmatic, and anorexic patients, Minuchin and colleagues (1975, 1978) concluded that the transactional patterns of some families render them *psychosomatogenic*. Minuchin proposed an *open systems model* to explain the powerful reciprocity of the child's symptoms and the family's functional organization.

The importance of Minuchin's open system model lies in the attempt to go beyond a model of linear causality, in which specified family stresses lead to emotional arousal that in turn produces symptoms in the vulnerable child. The open system model suggests instead that the child's illness is embedded within an interpersonal and family context. The family system thus both shapes and is shaped by the child's symptoms.

Specifically, Minuchin speculated that certain predisposing characteristics cause these families to respond pathologically to the stress of an ill child. These pathological responses in turn exacerbate the child's illness. Minuchin assumed a "predisposing physical dysfunction" in the case of the diabetic and asthmatic children, but not the anorectic ones. The transactional patterns however, were common to all.

Among the predisposing characteristics that, according to Minuchin, render these families vulnerable are enmeshment, overprotectiveness, lack of conflict resolution, rigidity, and pathological use of the sick child. In these families the members are intrusive as well as overinvolved, overresponsive, and overprotective toward one another. They avoid conflicts, especially concerning issues of autonomy, which results in chronic tension that is hidden but unresolved. Poor boundaries exist between the generations and among family members. Hence, the parents' bond as a marital couple is weak in comparison with their parental roles or their alliance with one or more of the children. At the same time, these families are rigid; they find it difficult to adapt to change and growth. This stress-inducing family context gives the child's physical symptoms special significance. It permits the child's illness to become involved in the family's conflict in ways that perpetuate both the child's symptoms and the family's pathology.

Few empirical studies have attempted to confirm Minuchin's hypotheses concerning the families of children with psychosomatic illness (Kog et al., 1987), and one of the few independent studies failed to replicate Minuchin's findings in asthmatic children (Burbeck, 1979). Nonetheless, Minuchin's formulation remains an important theoretical influence and heuristic basis for treatment. The next chapter examines some theoretical implications and specific therapeutic applications of this model to the asthmatic child.

Alexithymia and Expressive Styles.   After many decades of debate, the role of individual personality style as a predisposing factor in illness remains a complex and still unanswered question. As discussed in the next chapter, many studies are marred by the failure to consider the extent to which personality deviations can be the *result* of chronic illness, rather than the cause. Early analytic thinkers suggested an inverse relationship between the open expression of affect and the appearance of psychosomatic symptoms. The theoretical assumption was that displacement of a conflict into a somatic symptom saved the ego from consciously experiencing anxiety or other disturbing affects. The clinicians interpreted the absence of conscious affect to be a result of an (unconsciously motivated) defensive operation, somewhat akin to repression or denial. However, clinical and psychophysiological data are still equivocal as to whether somatic arousal is greatest or least in individuals who openly express their feelings.

More recently, investigators have studied patients whose inability to verbalize their feelings appears to result from a presumed defect rather than from defensive inhibition. Sifneos coined the term *alexithymia* to describe patients who have "no words for feelings." Such individuals show "a relative constriction in emotional functioning, poverty of fantasy life, and inability to find the appropriate words to describe their emotions" (Sifneos, 1973, p. 255). Sifneos further proposed that such patients are predisposed to somatize their emotions. The alexithymic patient can describe endless physical symptoms, but not his psychological discomfort. In such cases, traditional insight-oriented psychotherapy is often unproductive and taxing for both the patients, who frequently drop out, and the frustrated therapists, who tend to regard such patients as "emotional illiterates" (Neill & Sandifer, 1982).

A host of studies have examined the prevalence of alexithymia in patients with various physical disorders. Some studies have claimed an increased frequency of alexithymia in certain illnesses; such findings are shaky, however, because the instruments used to diagnose this condition lack satisfactory reliability and validity (Lesser & Lesser, 1983; Oxman et al., 1985). Conceptually, alexithymia has not been sufficiently distinguished from the preoperational thought found in younger children, various primitive cultures, or patients of low socioeconomic status. Clinicians must also differentiate the condition from depression or the psychic numbing seen in severe psychic trauma (Neill & Sandifer, 1982). Despite these difficulties, however, the concept has had useful empirical applications. For example, the degree of asthmatic patients' alexithymia correlated well with the number and length of hospitalizations (Dirks et al., 1981). Various authors have speculated about the constitutional neurological defects that might underlie this state; in the light of inadequate data such hypotheses seem fanciful. More than that, they risk premature reification of a still-evolving concept. There has been little clinical application of the alexithymia concept to child research.

Physiological Mediating Mechanisms

The most significant gap in psychosomatic knowledge is a detailed accounting of how psychological and affective phenomena are translated into pathogenic physiological changes. In addition to the central role played by the autonomic nervous system, the production of illness may involve endocrine and immune factors as mediators.

Endocrine Factors. Psychological stimuli profoundly affect the regulation of many hormonal systems both on a short- and long-term basis (Rose, 1980). Although the work of Selye pointed to the adrenocortical hormones as the "stress hormones" par excellence, stress can also alter the levels of norepinephrine, beta-endorphin, thyroxine, insulin, prolactin, growth hormone, and testosterone. The magnitude and direction of these changes depend in still poorly understood ways on the duration of the stress, adequacy of coping, and individual variation.

These stress-induced endocrine changes may have far-reaching impact. For example, in diabetes, stress leads to increased levels of cortisone, glucagon, and free fatty acids, all powerful insulin-antagonists, which in turn bring about a rapid rise in blood sugar (Jacobson & Leibovich, 1984). Stress can thus trigger a deterioration in diabetic control. Because several measures can quantify diabetic control, diabetes has provided a useful model for psychosomatic research. Minuchin et al. (1978) studied a small group of frequently hospitalized young diabetics. Their blood sugar could be easily controlled in the hospital, but despite careful adherence to medication and diet, they recurrently and rapidly developed ketoacidosis at home in response to family conflict. Minuchin termed these children "psychosomatic diabetics." In experimental family interviews, free fatty acids were measured in the psychosomatic diabetic children. For this group, family conflict produced a more exaggerated and sustained rise in these substances than it did in other diabetics whose exacerbations were less severe and apparently unrelated to family conflicts. The observation that, in the short run, beta-adrenergic blocking agents acted to block the exaggerated mobilization of free fatty acids suggested the contribution of autonomic mechanisms.

Immune Factors. Psychosocial factors also affect immunological responsivity. In a group that has been exposed to an infectious agent, stress and other psychological factors play a role in determining which individuals develop clinical illness (Ader, 1983; Rogers et al., 1979). (Pasteur allegedly lamented on his deathbed, "The germ is nothing, the terrain everything.") Meyer and Haggerty (1962) and Haggerty (1980) followed 100 members of 16 families for a year and concluded that the occurrence of acute family crises as well as the level of chronic family stress significantly influenced the incidence of streptococcal infections.

Much current research focuses on how psychosocial factors influence immunological competency (Calabrese et al., 1987; Stein, 1986). The area is of great potential import, because altered immune activity may underlie not only susceptibility to infectious diseases, but the emergence of autoimmune and malignant processes as well. For example, stress greatly influences the development and spread of tumors in mice innoculated with tumor cells or oncogenic viruses (Rogers et al., 1979). Experimentally controlled stress has been shown to alter both cell-mediated and antibody-mediated immune functioning. For the most part stress depresses immune activity, but, under some circumstances, it has caused augmentation. Bereavement and depression also alter lymphocyte activity (Linn et al., 1984).

How such changes occur is still unclear. Stress-induced alterations in cortisone, thyroxine, growth hormone, and even endorphin levels have all been suggested as potential mechanisms. Many lines of evidence point to an intimate but complex connection between the immune and neuroendocrine systems. Both cell-mediated and antibody-mediated immune activity fluctuate with the body's circadian rhythms. Hypothalamic lesions are known to alter immune reactions. The autonomic nervous system may also influence immunological activity via direct innervation of the major lymphoid tissues. In addition, lymphocytes have recently been shown to have beta-adrenergic receptors whose functions are still unknown. Also, as will be discussed in Chapter 16, autonomic nervous system transmitters influence important immunological processes such as the release of chemical mediators from sensitized mast cells (the phenomenon partially responsible for allergic symptoms). Finally, recent classical conditioning experiments that produced alterations in immune response provide intriguing clues as to the potential extent of nervous system regulation of immune functioning (Ader et al., 1987; MacQueen et al., 1989).

The outlines of a new field—*psychoneuroimmunology*—are gradually becoming clear. This area of research focuses on the neuroendocrine mechanisms that mediate the reciprocal effects of behavior and immune function (Ader & Cohen, 1985). Progress in this field holds out the hope that in time, the "mysterious leap from the body to the mind" may come to seem a smaller one.

Chapter 16

Asthma

INTRODUCTION

This chapter will examine asthma as a model psychosomatic illness. Asthma serves as an excellent paradigm of psychosomatic illness in at least two ways.

First, asthma illustrates the heterogeneous forms that a psychosomatic illness can assume and the complex interactions of psychological factors with immunological, neurochemical, and genetic mechanisms that determine the course of illness.

Second, the historical evolution of psychological theories about asthma epitomizes the intellectual history of psychosomatic concepts. Early psychosomatic theories of asthma often invoked either specific personality types and dynamic conflicts or global notions of autonomic system dysregulation. Writing in 1963, Knapp observed:

> Investigations of asthma reflect many of the strengths and weaknesses of the psychosomatic field. They consist of a melange of observations, frequently from widely different viewpoints, evolving slowly from the anecdotal to the systematic stage, but seldom, to date, experimental in the true sense, and they are strewn with the wrecks of premature, explanatory theories. Often ... these follow an implicit model of the germ theory and try to find, in one or another facet of the syndrome, a *bacillus asthmaticus psychosomaticus*. (p. 235)

In more recent years, increasingly refined studies have revealed the complexity of asthma's pathogenesis. It has also become clear that not only can psychological factors influence the clinical manifestations of asthma; like any chronic illness, severe asthma can deleteriously affect the psychological development of both the child and the family. Studies of treatment compliance and health-maintaining behavior illustrate the large role psychological factors play in determining treatment utilization and efficacy. Future progress in the field will no doubt require more complex, multivariate models capable of integrating the new, interactive data that have become available with increasingly sophisticated measures of genetic risk, immune status, autonomic reactivity, and adaptive style (Knapp & Mathe, 1985; Mrazek, 1986).

DEFINITION

Asthma is a diffuse lung disease characterized by bouts of labored breathing, accompanied by wheezing, difficulty in exhaling, and coughing. Spasms of the smooth muscle lining of the bronchi cause these symptoms. In asthma, the bronchial muscle is "twitchy" (*Lancet*, 1982) or hyperreactive, clamping down in response to a wide variety of stimuli—allergens, infectious agents, irritants, and psychological influences. Once bronchoconstriction has taken place, edema follows; inflammation of the airway lining and increased mucus exudation then further impair breathing. In mildly affected patients the attacks are sporadic and transient, but all too often the asthma is chronic and persistent, leading to secondary progressive structural damage to the lung tissue. In general, the spastic obstruction of the airways that occurs during an asthma attack is reversible, either spontaneously or with treatment; at the same time, the underlying hyperreactivity and irritability of the small bronchial passageways persist. These traits can be detected in former asthmatics, even when they have been asymptomatic for decades (Ellis, 1983).

EPIDEMIOLOGY

Characteristically, asthma begins in childhood, affecting about 1% to 5% of all children. Less than 50% of these children are sufficiently ill ever to require hospitalization. Nonetheless, asthma is responsible for about 25% of all school days missed because of chronic illness (Weiss et al., 1972). The death rate is about 1.5 deaths per 1000 asthmatics per year. The peak age of onset occurs prior to, or at age 3 years; 40% to 60% of all patients have their initial attack before age 5 years. In childhood, asthmatic boys outnumber girls by about 2 or 3 to 1; by adolescence, the sex distribution becomes more nearly equal.

Studies of social class distribution are equivocal. A positive family history for asthma is found in about 50% of asthmatic children's first-degree relatives. A positive family history for other allergic diseases such as hayfever or eczema is also common.

CLINICAL FEATURES AND COURSE

The course and severity of asthma are highly variable. Childhood asthmatics frequently manifest illness early in life—39% by age 1 year and 57% by age 2 years (Ellis, 1983). About 30% to 50% of asthmatic children, however, are free of their illness by middle childhood, and a still larger proportion recover by adolescence. Thus, in itself, early onset does not portend a serious prognosis; on the other hand, those children who do develop severe, intractable, life-threatening asthma usually have a history of very early onset.

For some children, bouts of asthma may be infrequent or seasonal; they remit spontaneously or respond readily to bronchodilator medication. These children tolerate exercise well and have good school attendance. For other less fortunate children, asthmatic attacks are more frequent and persistent; even between exacerbations they commonly experience bouts of coughing and mild wheezing. Sleep is difficult, school attendance impaired, and exercise poorly tolerated; all of these problems adversely affect their social and emotional adjustment. These children require higher and more continuous levels of theophylline and adrenergic bronchodilators, with their attendant "coffee nerves" side effects. Ultimately steroid therapy, with its own serious complications, both physical and psychological, may be essential (Bender et al., 1988). In the management of difficult steroid-dependent cases, to avoid exacerbations, withdrawal of steroids may require a most careful and prolonged weaning process; sometimes it is impossible to effect such a withdrawal. These severely ill children often develop barrel-shaped chest deformities secondary to chronic hyperinflation and emphysema.

It appears likely that a necessary factor in asthma is a basic constitutional predisposition toward bronchospasm. The immediate precipitant of a given attack may be any one of a wide variety of stimuli including viruses, allergens, irritants, or psychological factors acting singularly or in concert. Methodological difficulties abound in distinguishing among these possibilities and making specific determinations; in most cases several factors converge with no one element emerging as the primary cause (Weiner, 1977). Although there is sometimes a particular precipitating agent, it nevertheless interacts with less obvious factors. In addition, the cause of an attack varies from patient to patient or with the same patient at different times. A study of asthmatics of all ages (Williams et al., 1958; cited in Weiner, 1977) found that in 29% of cases, extrinsic allergens played a predominant precipitating role; in 40%, respiratory infections; and in 30%, psychological factors. Yet, in more than 65% of the cases multiple factors, all actively working at the same time, brought on the attack. Thus, psychological determinants played a contributing role in 70% of the patients but proved to be the sole precipitant in only about 1%.

Allergic Factors

A large proportion of asthmatic children and their close relatives have a strong history of allergic diseases such as hayfever, hives, and eczema. As many as 25% of children with infantile eczema develop asthma later in life (Weiner, 1977). Many children have attacks following exposure to dust, pollen, dander, or food; in such instances the clinician may note a positive skin test to these allergens, together with increased concentrations of both total immunoglobulins of the IgE type and specific IgE antibodies against these allergens. Asthma that is related to hypersensitivity to a foreign substance is termed *extrinsic*. A few asthmatics may have apparently negative skin tests and a normal IgE; researchers have speculated that psychological factors may play a greater role in these *intrinsic* cases (Mrazek & Strunk, 1984). Other authors, however, believe that the distinction between extrinsic (allergic) and intrinsic (nonallergic) forms of asthma is invalid (Burrows et al., 1989).

Infectious Agents

In general, viruses appear to be the most serious infectious causes of asthma. The most frequent viruses are respiratory syncytial virus, parainfluenza, or rhinovirus; it is uncertain whether they achieve their asthmatogenic effect by stimulating the parasympathetic nervous system (through the vagal nerve receptors that are present in the bronchial lining) or by stimulating production of the increased IgE, which characteristically is elevated in patients with viral-induced wheezing (Ellis, 1983).

Other Physical Factors

Diffuse irritability of the bronchial lining is characteristic of asthma, and attacks may be triggered by strong odors and irritants such as smoke, paint fumes, or cold, dry air. Exercise often precipitates asthmatic attacks, although the physiology of this reaction is still obscure.

Emotional Factors

Many observations indicate that emotional factors play a strong contributing role in initiating some asthmatic attacks and determining the course of the disease. For this reason asthma is included under the rubric of psychophysiological disorders.

The Role of Affect. Hippocrates (quoted in Knapp, 1975) is reputed to have observed, "The asthmatic must guard against anger." Many asthmatic children and their parents report that a powerful emotion experienced by the child can trigger an attack (Graham et al., 1967; Purcell, 1963). The evocative emotion is often unpleasant, taking form as fear, anger, depression, or anxiety; but it may also be a positive feeling, such as pleasure or excited anticipation of some wished-for event. Even in the absence of overt motor expression of this emotion (e.g., laughing, crying, racing about), wheezing may thereupon occur, usually within a few minutes. In the laboratory setting, it is possible to induce wheezing in some asthmatic patients by discussing personally painful topics (Tal & Miklich, 1976; Weiner, 1977). In addition, many child asthmatics report that they can think themselves into an attack by brooding on an upsetting experience or feeling.

Methodological Considerations. Early attempts to define the emotional bases of asthma focused on the search for a specific asthmatic personality type, the delineation of paradigmatic internal conflicts, and the character-ization of certain mother–child relationships as asthmatogenic (Weiner, 1977). Several words of caution are in order regarding these hypotheses.

First, even when asthma and emotional disturbance coincide, the direction of cause and effect is often difficult to disentangle. A severe asthmatic attack, of whatever origin, is a terrifying experience for both parent and child; either of the two participants may feel overwhelmed with helplessness, desperation, and fear of death. Anyone who has suffered an attack of asthma or has seen the anxious desperation of a hunched-over, coughing, gasping child caught in a paroxysm of wheezing has some idea of the catastrophic panic and claustrophobic fear of suffocation that such attacks evoke. In addition, growing up with severe asthma entails absence from school and peers, restriction of age-appropriate activities, long-term medications with substantial psychological side effects (Bender et al., 1988), and frequent hospitalizations accompanied by frightening medical procedures. Serious asthma has a profound impact on the child, the parents, and their relationship. The outcome of such cumulative trauma depends on many factors, including the adaptive capacities and preexisting psychological strengths and vulnerabilities of the participants. In this connection, individual and family adaptation to illnesses is an ongoing developmental process. Findings gleaned from the studies of older, severely asthmatic children who have lived with illness for many years may not simply be transferred and regarded as causal factors in younger or less severely ill children.

Next, it is important not to generalize beyond what is known. Data from the study of severely ill children in residential treatment or from the in-depth psychoanalytic study of a relatively few patients may not be generalizable to all asthmatics. Nor do checklist screens of psychopathology applied to large samples guarantee validity. Such responses may not reveal many of the more subtle but salient psychological features and can obscure the role played by denial and reaction formation in such families (Knapp, 1975). Finally the clinician must always keep in mind that asthma is a complex, heterogeneous, and multidetermined illness.

Psychodynamic Hypotheses. Some psychodynamically oriented clinicians have postulated that asthmatic children have a common personality profile or a specific nuclear conflict (French & Alexander, 1941; Sperling, 1978). The youngsters in their studies were said to be typically anxious, passively dependent, self-effacing, and insecure, with difficulty in expressing strong feelings such as anger or grief. They showed basic conflicts between strivings for autonomy and fears of engulfment or abandonment; extreme and poorly modulated separation anxiety heightened the intensity of these feelings. Such emotional difficulties, in aggregate, were seen as characteristic of asthmatic children and of central, presumably causal, importance. Sperling (1978) postulated a psychosomatic type of mother–child relationship:

> The child is rejected by his mother only when he is healthy and evidences
> strivings of independence but is in fact rewarded for being sick and helpless by
> the special care and attention given to him at such time. (p. 180)

Sperling further hypothesized that the appearance of asthma in early
childhood coincided with the toddler's anal-phase struggles to abandon a
passive dependent role and strive for self-assertion. Because the asthmatic
child perceives danger in expressing his independence or aggressive impulses, she concluded that these impulses are discharged instead through a
somatic symptom. Knapp and Mathe (1985) hypothesized that many asthmatics had an early defect in personality development that left them
strongly attached to a parent figure, yet prone to powerful primitive
aggressive impulses, often strongly sadistic, which they struggled to keep
well hidden. Knapp (1975) observed that as asthmatic attacks become less
frequent in response to psychotherapy, an asthmatic child will sometimes
become freer in expressing overt aggression. In the early phases, however,
even hints of aggression may lead to guilty, depressed feelings and an
intensification of wheezing. In a similar vein, French and Alexander (1941)
postulated that the asthmatic has powerful, primitive longings for help,
along with a parallel array of aggressive impulses that he must repress
because he fears being repudiated by his mother. Asthma, in this view,
represents a conversion symptom, the symbolic equivalent of a suppressed
cry for help. In the view of Jessner and colleagues (1955) the asthmatic child
is motivated by profound separation anxiety and an unconscious dependent longing to be protected and engulfed by the mother even though he
remains fearful and wary of being enmeshed in too much closeness.

Empirical Studies. More recent work has questioned the general applicability of these hypotheses and the etiological conclusions to be drawn
from them (Weiner, 1977). Studies (e.g., Neuhaus, 1958) have compared
hospitalized asthmatics to other chronically ill children and to well children.
These studies demonstrated the presence of as great a level of anxiety,
dependency, and insecurity in the other chronically ill children as in the
asthmatics, a finding that suggests these personality traits may be the consequence rather than the cause of illness. Again, some typical dynamics of
severe asthmatics may merely express their adaptation to prolonged illness
and may not apply to less seriously ill patients. Some investigators (Graham
et al., 1967; Mrazek et al., 1987) have maintained that when sampling is not
biased toward the severely ill, recurrently hospitalized population, asthmatic children as a whole do not show any greater psychopathology than
the rest of the population. Attempts to demonstrate specific areas of conflict
such as difficulties with the overt expression of anger have also yielded
equivocal results (Weiner, 1977). Some studies (McNichol & Williams,
1973a, 1973b), indicate a tendency for behavioral disturbance in the asth-

matic and psychopathology in the mother to correlate with the severity of illness. In other studies (Block et al., 1964; Dubo et al., 1961) no such correlation was detectable.

It is possible that particular psychological factors are most salient in certain subgroups of asthmatics, and might not be apparent in studies of larger, more heterogeneous samples (Renne & Creer, 1985). Consequently, considerable research has focused on attempts to define such subgroups. Investigators have speculated that psychological factors might be more heavily at work in an asthmatic population where allergic factors are less important. Working prior to the availability of quantitative IgE measures, Block (1968; Block et al., 1964) divided a group of asthmatic children on the basis of scores on the Allergy Potential Scale, which arithmetically summated indicators of allergic propensity such as skin tests, blood eosinophil counts, family allergic history, and known allergens. In addition, there was a control group of children with congenital heart diseases or diabetes.

The high and low allergy potential scores (APS) group had comparably severe asthma, but the low-APS group children showed psychopathological features significantly more frequently than did the high-APS or control group. As rated by their mothers, the low-APS children were more rebellious, clinging, whining, nervous, and jealous and less self-confident than the other two groups. On projective tests they were more pessimistic, angrier in response to frustration, more preoccupied with orality and aggression, and appeared to derive more secondary gains from their illness than the other two groups. Given the relatively low levels of psychopathology found in the high-APS and control groups, Block felt these differences were not simply attributable to long-standing illness. Furthermore, compared with the high-APS group, the low-APS mothers appeared more frequently to "overinvest and overidentify with the child, on whom they are overly dependent for satisfaction of their own needs" (Block et al., 1964). The low-APS families showed more marital conflict along with more ambivalent and less satisfying mother–child relationships.

Effects of Separation from Family. Another historically important line of investigation concerning the apparent impact of emotional and family factors stemmed from the observation that when certain asthmatic children were removed from their homes and separated from their parents, their symptoms often promptly improved. At one time, many asthmatic children were sent to residential treatment centers in the desert or mountains to profit from the supposed beneficial effects of the clean, dry air. Physicians soon concluded, however, that it was the removal from their parents that so often produced the improvement. The same phenomenon is also apparent in children whose wheezing improves immediately upon admission to the ward, even before treatment is initiated, and whose asthma flares up promptly upon returning home.

Systematic studies at the Jewish National Home for Asthmatic Children by Purcell and colleagues (1962, 1969a, 1969b, 1972) attempted to explore further the effects of "parentectomy." Of course, removing a child from home alters many environmental factors beyond the emotional. Some skeptics argued that it was not the distance from the parents but from the dusts and allergens in the home that provided the relief. Two striking experiments attempted to control for allergen exposure, in order to demonstrate that the therapeutic effect of separation was indeed due to changes in the child's emotional atmosphere rather than to physical removal from home allergens. Unfortunately neither study controlled for possible changes in treatment compliance, a powerful confounding variable in any such experiment (Renne & Creer, 1985).

In the first experiment, rather than removing the child from his home, Purcell and colleagues (1969a) had a research caretaker provide home-based care for each of several asthmatic children while the parents and siblings went away for 2 weeks. The experimenters controlled as much as possible for allergenic factors such as diet, dust, and smoke. They studied two groups of children: those with a strong positive history of frequent attacks caused by emotional precipitants, and those for whom emotionally induced attacks were rare. The two groups were otherwise generally similar in respect to the severity of the asthma, allergic sensitivity, and so on. The children's past history enabled Purcell and colleagues to predict with striking accuracy that the patients with a strong history of emotionally induced asthmatic spells would (1) show a dramatic improvement in symptoms and pulmonary function tests during their parents' absence and (2) demonstrate a corresponding dramatic reexacerbation upon their return.

Those children without such a history did not show any improvement during the separation. Although separation anxiety (as distinct from actual separation) had often been postulated as a potential trigger for asthmatic attacks, the emotion-sensitive asthmatics showed no such effect. During the baseline period, when the parents' departure was imminent but had not yet occurred, the children did not have more frequent attacks or show deterioration in pulmonary functions, despite clinical evidence that many of these children and families had strong feelings about their separation.

In a second interesting experiment, Long et al. (1958) attempted to demonstrate that the impact of home allergens was not simple or invariant. Several asthmatic children were hospitalized with consequent improvement in their symptoms. Most strikingly, however, the children's wheezing did not recur when, without their knowledge, the experimenters pumped dust from each child's home into his or her hospital room. The investigators speculated that hospitalization reduced wheezing by relieving the child's anxiety concerning a close, mutually ambivalent tie to his or her mother.

In an effort to determine which asthmatics improved with "parentectomy," Purcell (1963) studied the differences between two groups of asthmatic children in residential treatment. One group consisted of rapidly remitting (RR) children, who within 3 months of admission to residential placement had their symptoms disappear without recourse to steroid treatment. The contrasting group was comprised of steroid-dependent (SD) children, who required ongoing steroids to prevent asthmatic attacks. Each of these two groups included about one-third of the residential patient population. The remaining third formed an intermediate group whose symptoms persisted in residential placement, but not severely enough to require steroids.

Studying the contrasting SD and RR groups, Purcell and Weiss (1970) concluded that asthmatic symptoms in the RR groups appeared to be "more intimately associated with neurotic and affective reactions," and the asthmatic symptoms of the SD children appeared to be more regularly linked to allergic and infectious factors. The differences were relative rather than absolute. For example, the RR children reported more often than did the SD children that strong, mostly negative, emotions triggered their attacks. On the basis of parent reports, the RR children had more "neurotic" symptoms such as headaches, constipation, and nightmares than did the SD children (Purcell et al., 1961). Psychological test data, however, showed no substantial differences between the groups in gross behavioral disturbance (Purcell et al., 1962). Parents of the RR group appeared to be more punitive and authoritarian than the SD parents (Purcell & Metz, 1962).

In addition, Purcell and Weiss (1970) observed that, away from home, even many severely steroid-dependent children required less medication and had fewer attacks. They concluded that emotional status and family interactions strongly influenced the course of asthmatic illness and modified the impact of known physical factors.

Because the RR children frequently reported that strong emotions triggered their attacks, Purcell's group (1962, 1969a, 1969b) developed a "psychological precipitant interview" that can be used to identify children in whom emotional factors play an important role in triggering or exacerbating asthma. These children also show altered psychophysiological reactions to stress, with more abnormal respiration and less vasoconstriction (a measure of sympathetic arousal) than those asthmatics without a history of emotional precipitants (Miklich et al., 1973). Such a history of emotional initiators has important treatment implications (Conners, 1983). When separated from their parents, these children tend to show symptomatic improvement, and in this group, relaxation training procedures are more effective in improving bronchial air flow than they are in other asthmatics (Alexander, 1972; Tal & Miklich, 1976).

Renne and Creer (1985) provide an interesting historical footnote to the Jewish National Home for Asthmatic Children's four decades of experience with "parentectomy" and residential treatment. During this period the proportion of rapid remitters fell from an initial majority of admissions to less than 12%. This decline may have reflected several factors. Initially, the Home largely admitted children from intact families; Renne and Creer speculate that many of these children may have used their symptoms manipulatively in an overprotective family context. During the ensuing years, however, the Home came to admit more behaviorally disturbed children, with severer asthma, almost half of whom were from single-parent homes. This patient population was much less responsive to parentectomy and rarely showed a dramatic improvement simply by coming into residential treatment.

The Role of Family Dynamics. Early psychosomatic theories suggested that conflict concerning dependence and autonomy in early childhood played a central, causal role in developing asthma (Weiner, 1977). This assertion, however, has been challenged by the thought-provoking longitudinal studies of Gauthier and her colleagues (Gauthier et al., 1977, 1978). These investigators engaged in a prospective study of a group of asthmatic toddlers and their mothers. In more than half of the children, the onset of their asthma had occurred by age 6 months. When the toddlers ranged from age 14 to 31 months, the authors began to follow the subsequent vicissitudes of the disease and also tracked several allergic, pulmonary, and psychological variables. They followed the children through ages 4 to 6 years and the beginning of school. The investigators paid special attention to the children's autonomous strivings, capacity for socialization, reaction to separation, and expressions of oppositionality, and evaluated each mother's reaction to her child's manifestations of opposition.

At ages 4 to 6 years, most of the children were doing very well, both physically and psychologically. Although their bronchi remained overly labile to beta-adrenergic stimulation, during the preceding year, most of the children had remained free of true asthmatic attacks, with the remainder showing less and less frequent bouts of wheezing. Similarly, in the areas of autonomy and oppositionality, the majority of the children continued to develop "very adequately," and they appeared to be happy and thriving at home, at school, and in social relationships. Mother–child interactions continued to be generally harmonious.

The most recent data showed a small increase in the few mothers who (out of either overprotectiveness, preoccupation, or depression) ignored the child's strivings for autonomy. However, these children's development of independent and oppositional strivings did not appear to be impaired. Thus, even in that small cohort with evidence of mother–child conflict, the children themselves were often developing well. This suggested that some mothers may experience difficulty without necessarily influencing the child's development. Furthermore, the relatively few children who still had severe asthmatic symptoms tended to have harmonious relations with their mothers. Where conflicted relationships did occur, it was among the symptomatically mild cases.

In contrast to Block's (1968) finding of an inverse correlation between allergic factors and the presence of emotional difficulties, Gauthier et al. found that the allergy potential score tended to be higher in the cases with some indications of troubled mother–child relations.

Gauthier and colleagues (1978) concluded:

> A disturbed mother–child relationship does not appear to be as frequent and manifest in childhood asthma as originally thought, nor does it appear to be primary. Rather, our results suggest that some mother–child dyads may be particularly vulnerable to the appearance of an illness such as asthma. However, this vulnerability which may lead to pathogenic or pathological mother–child relationships does not necessarily lead to a more severe asthmatic illness. (p. 691)

The asthmatic children studied by Gauthier et al. had relatively mild illness. In contrast, severe illness may take a greater toll of young children. Severely ill asthmatic preschoolers (with multiple hospitalizations) appear more likely than controls to show insecure attachment and various behavioral difficulties (Mrazek et al., 1987; Mrazek, 1986).

Looking beyond the mother–child dyad, the impact of family factors on both the child's asthma and emotional health has been the focus of as much research. On the one hand, studies such as Horwood et al. (1985), McLean and Ching (1975), and Dubo et al. (1961) have failed to find significant relationships between disturbed family dynamics and either the presence of asthma, its severity, or its degree of improvement at 10-year follow-up. On the other hand, for asthmatic children, family and parent–child factors do seem to serve as potential risk or protective factors for the development of significant psychopathology (Mrazek et al., 1987). Thus, Steinhausen et al. (1983) found that older asthmatic children's psychopathology was much more powerfully determined by family factors than by the severity of their asthma. Not surprisingly, many of these same family factors also correlate with the degree of psychopathology in medically well children. Similarly, Meijer (1978) noted that the degree of dependency found in asthmatic 6-year-olds was highly associated with their family relationship patterns rather than with their severity of asthma.

In contrast, Minuchin and colleagues (Liebman et al., 1974; Minuchin et al., 1975, 1978) concluded that for some asthmatics, family functioning and disease severity were intimately related. These investigators studied and treated a small uncontrolled group of severe chronic asthmatics whose illness appeared intractable to medical management short of residential treatment. In keeping with their general theory of psychosomatic family functioning, these investigators observed that not only did the family's functioning profoundly affect the asthmatic child's symptoms, the child's illness and treatment also characteristically affected the family organization (see Chapter 15 for a more detailed discussion of Minuchin's theory).

In the asthmatic families studied, Minuchin and co-workers noted that the parents often felt helpless and ineffectual. They tended to relinquish too much of the care of the child to the pediatrician in an overdependent fashion. One parent or the other would often become overinvolved in the care of the patient to the neglect of the spouse and other siblings. To avoid upsetting the patient, the family members submerged resentment about this neglect but then acted out in covert ways. The parents maintained dietary and athletic restrictions and avoided allergens in an overprotective fashion; this behavior isolated the asthmatic child from his peers and experiences of mastery while binding him ever more tightly to his family. Both the parent and the asthmatic child used the illness to exempt him from discipline and responsibility, conferring on him a unique status: simultaneously special, yet sick; weak, yet powerful; deprived, yet overindulged.

In summary, these authors concluded that "the patient's role in the family depends on the presence of his symptoms, and he has tremendous power to manipulate the family through his illness" (Liebman et al., 1974). Other family systems theorists have drawn similar conclusions (Onnis et al., 1986).

This family system view implies that the entire family must be the focus of any psychotherapeutic intervention. To confirm this view, Minuchin cited the allegedly striking success of their family therapy in reducing asthmatic attacks and hospitalizations. However, in light of the uncontrolled nature of their study and the lack of correlation between severity and family pathology in the other studies referred to above, it is unclear how far Minuchin's findings can be generalized (see discussion of family treatment below).

ETIOLOGY

Asthma is a complex disease in which immune, autonomic, infectious, and psychological mechanisms interact, most likely in varying fashions within different individuals, to bring about an attack (Ellis, 1983; Weiner, 1977). Most likely a necessary but not sufficient precondition is an innate tendency to broncho-constriction, the physiological basis of which is, as yet, unknown. When a predisposed individual is exposed to these various factors, either alone or in combination, wheezing results.

Genetic Factors

For monozygotic asthmatic twin pairs, the concordance rate for asthma is 19% versus 4.8% for dizygotic twins (Edfors-Lubs, 1971). This suggests that a genetic factor is at work, but one with apparently low penetrance. At present, investigators know little about the expression of this genetic factor. For example, does it control immune factors (such as specific IgE production), or does it regulate the chemical mediators of the immune response? In animals, both of these factors appear to be under specific genetic control; in humans, the propensity to produce IgE in response to commonly inhaled antigens appears to be under the control of a single gene locus, perhaps as an autosomal dominant trait (Cookson & Hopkin, 1988). Or perhaps is the sensitivity of smooth muscle receptors to various autonomic transmitters genetically determined? Neither do researchers know, as yet, which factors, psychological, physiological, or environmental, modify the expression of inherited genetic factors.

Allergic Factors

Most patients with allergically precipitated asthma have elevated levels of antibodies composed of IgE, a specific type of immunologically active globulin (Burrows et al., 1989). IgE has the important property of binding itself to the surface of highly specialized cells called *mast cells*, which are found throughout the body, including the lungs. The mast cells contain granules that are packed with powerful substances collectively called *mediators*. These mediators include histamine, serotonin and a whole host of other substances (for details, see Kaliner et al., 1987). When an allergic individual becomes sensitized by repeated exposure to an allergen, he or she develops an IgE antibody tailored specifically to engage and combine with that allergen. Of telling importance is that in allergic asthmatics, these IgE antibodies appear to cling preferentially to the mast cells of the lung tissue. When the sensitized individual is exposed yet again to the allergen, the IgE antibody seizes upon the allergenic molecules that have made their way into the body. This reaction in turn triggers a sudden destabilization of the previously quiescent mast cells to which the IgE was bound. The mast cell then releases the potent chemicals in its storage granules and spews them out into the surrounding tissue. Either via direct action or by stimulating the autonomic nervous system, these chemical mediators produce powerful contraction of the smooth muscle lining of nearby bronchi. Thus, IgE-mediated allergic reactions appear capable of producing an asthmatic attack.

In a general population study, the prevalence of asthma was closely related to age- and sex-corrected levels of serum IgE (Burrows et al., 1989). The story is complex, however, because factors not related to IgE can also induce mast cell activation or bronchospasm. Finally, animal experiments indicate that autonomic nervous system activity and various hypothalamic and brain stem centers influence both levels of antibody and mediator activity (Kaliner, 1982; *Lancet*, 1982). Indeed, psychological factors can influence mediator release. A dramatic recent experiment in rats demonstrated that the mast cells' release of mediators is susceptible to classic Pavlovian conditioning (MacQueen et al., 1989). When exposed to egg albumin, the mast cells of rats who had been sensitized to albumin released allergic mediators. For several training sessions, the rats' exposure to albumin was associated with a flashing light and humming fan. Subsequently, even in the absence of albumin, exposing the rats to the light and noise cue alone could induce their mast cells to release mediators.

Autonomic Factors

The autonomic nervous system is a major regulator of airway smooth muscle tone. Like most human organ systems, the airways are under opposing neurogenic controls (Kaliner, 1982). Stimulation of cholinergic or alpha-adrenergic receptors on the smooth muscle cells of the airway produces constriction, whereas stimulation of the beta-adrenergic receptors produces relaxation. Much research has focused on the suggestion that the bronchial hyperreactivity of asthma reflects an imbalance in autonomic control of the airways' smooth muscle caused by either an increase in excitatory (constricting) factors or a decrease in inhibitory (relaxing) factors (Kaliner, 1982; *Lancet*, 1982). This hypothesis is attractive because autonomic nervous system transmitters also modulate allergen-induced release of mediators from IgE-sensitized mast cell granules (*Lancet*, 1982). Finally, because strong emotions can powerfully activate the autonomic nervous system, this seems a probable link whereby feeling states can influence bronchial tone.

Several investigators have found suggestive evidence of altered autonomic responsiveness in asthma and other allergic diseases. (*Lancet*, 1982, and Kaliner, 1982, review these data.) Hahn (1966), for example, found that asthmatic children differ from nonasthmatic controls in skin temperature and heart rate responsiveness.

Cause and effect are often as difficult to disentangle in the physiological sphere as in the psychological. As yet, it is impossible to determine the extent to which observed abnormalities in asthmatics' autonomic responsivity represent a primary defect, a secondary effect of some more fundamental defect, or a side effect of long-standing illness and its pharmacological treatment. Much remains to be learned about whether asthmatic children more frequently have dysphoric affects, whether they have greater or more labile activation of the autonomic nervous system in response to a given affect, or whether their airways respond aberrantly to such stimulation.

Psychological Factors

Psychological factors have long been known to influence the bronchial musculature. As early as 1886, Sir James MacKenzie, by using a paper rose under glass, was able to precipitate asthmatic symptoms in a young woman who suffered from "rose asthma." Owen (1963) showed that the tape-recorded sound of their mother's voice produced abnormal respiratory responses in asthmatic children, but not in normal controls. This reaction was independent of the content of what the mother said. Under laboratory conditions, emotional arousal experimentally induced by a stressful math text, upsetting film, or deliberate recall of incidents of rage or fear measurably decreased pulmonary flow rate. Conversely, relaxation techniques decreased bronchial constriction. Interestingly, the degree of this bronchospastic lability correlated with a positive history of emotionally precipitated asthma; there was no correlation with the degree of allergic sensitivity (Tal & Miklich, 1976). On the basis of this pattern, the experimenters speculated that "the same phenomenon underlies emotional-bronchoconstriction, relaxation-bronchodilitation, and emotionally triggered asthma" (p. 190).

Psychological expectations also influence the impact of psychological and therapeutic agents. When asthmatic subjects were told that they were being administered an allergen, inhalation of a saline solution produced an increase in bronchoconstriction (often with wheezing). The identical solution in a different nebulizer then reversed the constriction when the subjects were told it was a medication that helped asthma (Luparello et al., 1968). Similarly, the response to the inhalation of true bronchodilators or constrictors varied in magnitude depending on the subjects' experimentally induced expectation (Luparello et al., 1970). The mechanism whereby suggestion acts physiologically is unclear, but it appears to involve the autonomic nervous system, most likely via the cholinergic innervation of the airways. In these experiments atropine, an anticholinergic drug, blocked bronchoconstriction in response to suggestion (McFadden et al., 1969). These observations confirm the major role suggestion plays in some asthmatics' response to treatment, a factor that confounds assessment of many treatment methods in the absence of adequate controls.

Current theory thus sees emotional arousal, rather than specific conflicts or psychopathology, as the psychological trigger for asthma in a physiologically vulnerable child (Purcell & Weiss, 1970). The evidence suggests emotionally induced autonomic arousal may serve as a final common pathway whereby psychological stresses might precipitate an asthmatic attack in a predisposed child. The specific content might vary from child to child—for one child, rage; for another, separation anxiety; for yet another, performance anxiety. Individual psychopathology of varying types and degree might well produce strong emotional arousal in a child. Family-induced upsets or expectations of a wheezing response to a given situation might similarly trigger such a response.

Psychological Influences on Coping Style and Involvement in Medical Treatment

As Minuchin and colleagues (1978) have noted, chronic illness can become a way of life for both the afflicted child and his family. Asthmatic children may malinger (i.e., consciously fake an attack) or deliberately induce an attack (often by hyperventilation). Asthmatic attacks that the child deliberately precipitates to avoid stressful situations, such as school exams, may be clinically difficult to distinguish from involuntary anxiety-triggered attacks. Many motives, including the wish to return to a caring and gratifying hospital setting, may prompt an asthmatic attack.

Asthmatic patients also dramatically illustrate the general proposition that personality is a powerful determinant of an illness's impact on an individual. Dirks and colleagues (1977, 1980) classified asthmatic children and adults according to the amount of panic and fearfulness they experienced during an attack. This measure correlated well with the patients' general propensity to fearfulness even between attacks, as assessed by the Minnesota Multiphasic Personality Inventory (MMPI) (Dirks et al., 1977). This panic-fear propensity was unrelated to the objective severity of the patients' asthma. Nonetheless, the degree of panicky fearfulness was a powerful predictor of rehospitalization rates, amounts of medication prescribed, and the patients' assessment of how much asthma interfered with normal life.

The patient's personality style interacted with the physician's style so that regardless of the actual severity of illness, panicky asthmatics had more medication prescribed, especially by more psychologically minded physicians (Kinsman et al., 1977). It is equally interesting that patients who scored extremely *low* on the panic-fear measure had as high a rehospitalization rate as those who scored extremely *high*. It seems likely that, on the one hand, panicky helplessness and subjective oversensitivity to somatic symptoms leads to frequent rehospitalization. On the other hand, denial and inattentiveness of early prodromal symptoms also represents a maladaptive coping style that may prevent a patient from taking appropriate steps early in an attack to mitigate its course. Continuing studies promise early identification of patients for whom psychological interventions may be particularly important (Dirks et al., 1981).

Finally, psychological risk factors also appear to play an important role in the case of those severely asthmatic children who subsequently die of their illness (Lewiston & Rubinstein, 1986; Strunk et al., 1985). Family disturbance, poor self-care and noncompliance, manipulative use of asthma, depression, and suicidal ideation all place the child at increased risk of death. For example, a manipulative asthmatic 13-year-old girl, desperately distraught about her parents' impending divorce, threatened to die if they preceded with their plans. On the courthouse steps, immediately following the final decree, she had an asthmatic attack from which she died the next day.

TREATMENT

As with all treatment modalities, the clinician needs to identify clearly the indications for and goals of psychological interventions. As Conners (1983) put it, "The aim of [comprehensive] treatment is not only control or elimination of the asthmatic symptoms but also development of patients into autonomous, competent, self-managing individuals" (p. 163). The psychological management of asthmatic children seeks to reduce the emotional exacerbants of the illness, the psychologically determined obstacles to optimal compliance with medical treatment, and the adverse impact of chronic illness on the child's personality development.

Psychotherapy

Asthma alone is not an indicator for psychotherapy or other psychological treatment. Psychological intervention can probably reduce asthmatic attacks only in those children with emotional factors that provoke attacks or interfere with treatment compliance. A specific inquiry such as the psychological precipitant interview developed by Purcell and colleagues (1969a, 1969b) (see above) may help identify such children. Severe psychopathology in the child may be an indication for psychotherapy addressed to such pathology, but this treatment is unlikely to affect the severity of the child's asthmatic attacks unless they are emotionally triggered. From this point of view, psychopathology is not asthmatogenic in itself but may predispose the child to frequent strong affects which, if his bronchi are sensitive to emotional arousal, trigger wheezing. It may also exacerbate asthma by interfering with treatment compliance. In such cases psychotherapy is "a means for reducing one portion of the sufficient stimuli responsible for the eruption of clinical asthma" (Purcell & Weiss, 1970). Unfortunately, despite much anecdotally recounted clinical experience (Jessner et al., 1955; Sperling, 1968), no adequately controlled studies demonstrate or refute the efficacy of individual psychotherapy or psychoanalysis in reducing the severity of asthma. There are somewhat more systematic data regarding family therapy and various relaxation, biofeedback, and behavior modification techniques.

Family Therapy

Clinicians have frequently suggested family therapy as a treatment modality in asthma. Again, although family pathology may require treatment in its own right, asthma per se is not an indication for family treatment. Careful assessment is necessary to determine the impact of the child's symptoms on family functioning and how family factors influence the course and management of the child's symptoms (Masterson, 1985; Renne & Creer, 1985). No clear correlation has been demonstrated between severity of family pathology and asthmatic symptomatology (Dubo et al., 1961; McLean & Ching, 1973). However, where family pathology and severe asthma coexist *and* there is reason to believe they exacerbate each other, family approaches may be helpful in treating asthmatics.

Sperling (1978) recommended treatment of the parents to "loosen the asthmatic tie" before attempting to engage the asthmatic child in individual treatment. Based on their theory of psychosomatic family functioning, Minuchin and colleagues (1975, 1978; Liebman et al., 1974) utilized a structural family approach in treating intractably severe asthmatics. The focus of their approach was to redefine "family roles away from the scapegoating, conflict detouring processes" that reinforced and gave central prominence to the patient's asthmatic symptoms. The family instead was helped to examine interpersonal issues within the family while progressively attempting outside activities in the world of school and peers. The first step was to help the family teach the patient deep-breathing exercises that produced relaxation and permitted the child to abort wheezing attacks. Most important, however, the authors assigned the task of teaching the child these exercises to the more peripheral parent (usually the father). This technique helped change the structural relationships within the family system. The parents were also instructed in the emergency treatment of wheezing spells and were equipped with epinephrine and syringes. Again, the authors assigned the less involved parent the task of administering the medication and contacting the pediatrician if wheezing persisted. The more involved parent was instructed to support the other parent in these tasks, but not to preempt or undermine him or her. This arrangement loosened the coalition between the overinvolved parent and the asthmatic child and increased the involvement of the more peripheral parent.

A major goal of the treatment was to disengage the patient from marital conflicts while shifting the parents' relationship onto a more mutually supportive, goal-directed level. As a corollary, parents were encouraged to plan activities of their own as a couple, whereas the patient was simultaneously encouraged to participate in activities with siblings and peers. The therapist confronted the parents about special treatment of the asthmatic child that permitted avoidance of household responsibilities and discipline. The therapy sessions encouraged parental problem solving about siblings' difficulties to remove the asthmatic child from a central position as the family's sole symptom-bearer and to stimulate the parents' ability to work together effectively as the joint heads of the family without being split apart or manipulated. As they tried to carry out these tasks, the family's pathological coalitions, struggles for control, and other dysfunctional sets became apparent. Long-standing but submerged marital conflicts emerged; now, however, the parents could address them directly rather than detour them through overinvolvement with the asthmatic child's symptoms.

Minuchin's group claimed dramatic success for this approach. Weekly sessions during a period of 5 to 10 months spectacularly reduced the frequency of attacks, eliminated rehospitalization, and drastically reduced the level of other medications. Unfortunately, these dramatic findings in a small group of patients are difficult to evaluate without a larger sample or adequate control group. As with individual therapy, there is a dearth of adequately controlled studies of the outcome of family therapy. The sole exception is a controlled trial of family treatment of asthmatics (Lask & Matthew, 1979). Treatment was much less intensive than in Minuchin's group but nonetheless demonstrated positive, if less dramatic, results.

Lask and Matthew treated a group of asthmatic children with six hour-long sessions of family therapy during a 4-month period. The focus of the family therapy was how the child's symptoms were influenced by and fed back upon the general family system of interaction. The therapists helped the family explore attitudes toward the illness, doctors, and medication as well as the themes of fear of death and painful and frightening emotions. Compared with an untreated control group receiving similar medical care at the same hospital, the asthmatics in the family treatment group showed significant improvement in daily wheezing and lung overinflation, although not in the forced expiratory rate as measured in the laboratory. Even this study, the authors noted, failed to control for a nonspecific "attention effect"—that is, the possibly beneficial effect of extra attention from the treatment team, regardless of the content of the therapy.

Other Treatment Modalities

In addition to more global family and individual psychotherapeutic techniques, clinical researchers have explored more specific, time-limited treatment modalities in asthma including relaxation training, systematic desensitization, hypnosis, biofeedback, and behavior modification; Conners (1983) has recently reviewed these techniques. Relaxation training improves laboratory measures of pulmonary functioning and bronchial relaxation, although in many patients not to a sufficient degree to bring about symptomatic improvement (Alexander, 1972; Alexander et al., 1979). One study has suggested that facial muscle relaxation training may be particularly beneficial (Kotses & Glaus, 1981). Conners (1983) speculated that high panic-fear levels or high scores on the anxiety-tension scales of behavioral checklists may identify patients likely to benefit from psychophysiological treatment techniques that are designed to reduce an antistress response style. Because relaxation training appears to be more effective in patients with a history of emotionally triggered asthma and demonstrable emotionally induced bronchoconstriction in the laboratory, some investigators have postulated a common mechanism underlying such bronchoconstriction and the therapeutic effect of relaxation training (Tal & Miklich, 1976).

How relaxation exerts a therapeutic effect remains a mystery. Relaxation is usually conceptualized as involving a decrease in sympathetic and adrenergic tone with perhaps an increase in parasympathetic cholinergic tone (Alexander et al., 1979). Because beta-adrenergic drugs help asthma and cholinergics exacerbate it, there obviously is still much to learn.

In addition to aiding in relaxation training, biofeedback techniques employing sophisticated monitoring equipment have been used to condition specific changes in airway resistance. Even in brief training periods such techniques can produce a marked improvement in bronchial airflow that is comparable to the improvement produced by bronchodilator medication (Feldman, 1976). How to expand such laboratory findings into a long-term treatment program capable of producing significant symptomatic relief remains a clinical challenge.

Behavioral techniques have been useful in other areas of asthma management. Operant conditioning techniques have been used to restructure reinforcers and decrease attacks in cases where parents or hospital staff powerfully reinforced and thus unwittingly encouraged asthmatic attacks (Creer, 1970; Lukeman, 1975). Therapists have also employed operant conditioning techniques to teach children the often-difficult task of using inhalation therapy equipment (Renne & Creer, 1976). As part of a multifaceted parent- and patient-education program, behavior modification techniques have also improved medication compliance (Richards et al., 1981). Several centers have developed self-help group programs for asthmatics and their families that combine education, exercise, and mutual support (Clark et al., 1981; Selner & Staudenmayer, 1979). Such programs have successfully promoted greater self-reliance and self-care among the children while encouraging more positive family attitudes.

Chapter 17

Disorders of Elimination

Enuresis

INTRODUCTION

Control of bowel and bladder is one of the toddler's greatest achievements. In his own eyes, as well as in the regard of significant others, the accomplishment sets him apart from babies. When the child loses or fails to develop such control, no matter the cause, his self-confidence and sense of self-mastery suffer seriously. This chapter and the one that follows will discuss disorders of urinary and bowel control, termed respectively *enuresis* and *encopresis*.

Through the centuries enuresis has offered a plaguing and perplexing problem to children and parents alike. To this day it remains a considerable mystery. Its causes appear to be manifold. Many cases apparently have a genetic or constitutional basis, whereas others seem to be transient expressions of emotional upset. Regardless of cause, however, the symptom usually has a serious emotional impact on the child. As seems true of psychophysiologic disorders in general, this condition appears to involve a complex interaction among physiological, developmental, and emotional factors.

The normal "physiology of dryness" is complex. Mature bladder function involves filling, sensing fullness (experienced as the desire to void), postponing voiding to a socially appropriate time and place, voluntarily initiating sphincter relaxation and bladder contraction, and maintaining both until the bladder is empty (Gross & Dornbusch, 1983; Yeates, 1973). During sleep, the sensation of bladder fullness normally awakens the continent individual, prompting him to get up and void.

Cultural influences, general child-rearing variables, and specific training factors all shape the development of socially appropriate voiding behavior (Cooper, 1973; Gross & Dornbusch, 1983; Sears et al., 1957). For training to be effective, however, the child must be adequately mature. Toilet training looms large in the concerns of parents, clinicians, and developmental theorists. Both psychoanalytic and behavior learning theories see the child's continence as learned behavior, shaped by the parents' love, praise, and disapproval. Yet the relative roles of maturation and training in acquiring continence are unclear (MacKeith et al., 1973). It is sobering to realize that without apparent training, newborn piglets will move away from the nursing area to the edge of the sty to deposit their feces and urine. On the basis of both ethological and human developmental data, some experts have concluded that dryness at night probably comes from maturation and not by training (MacKeith et al., 1973). From their perspective, the problem of enuresis entails identifying factors that facilitate or interfere with the emergence of this expected behavior.

DEFINITION

In general, wetting decreases with age; specifically, however, opinions differ as to the age at which wetting becomes abnormal (Verhulst et al., 1985).

DSM-III-R Diagnostic Criteria for Functional Enuresis

A. *Repeated voiding of urine during the day or night into bed or clothes, whether involuntary or intentional.*

B. *At least two such events per month for children between the ages of five and six, and at least one event per month for older children.*

C. *Chronologic age at least five, and mental age at least four.*

D. *Not due to a physical disorder, such as diabetes, urinary tract infection, or a seizure disorder. (APA, 1987, p. 85)*

EPIDEMIOLOGY

Between ages 1 and $3\frac{1}{2}$ years, dryness becomes increasingly more frequent. Most often, bowel control is attained first, followed by daytime bladder control, with nighttime bladder control coming last.

Data from the comprehensive general population National Health Examination survey, as shown in Table 17.1, detail the prevalence of enuresis by age and sex (Gross & Dornbusch, 1983). In this study enuresis was more frequent in boys, blacks, later born children (compared to only or firstborn), and in families of low socioeconomic status or with three or more children.

Using the more stringent criteria of wetting at least once weekly, the epidemiological study of the children of the Isle of Wight (Rutter et al., 1973) found the following lower prevalences:

Age in Years	Boys (%)	Girls (%)
5	6.7	3.3
9–10	2.9	2.2
14	1.1	0.5

Studies of selective service recruits and college students show enuresis to be a persisting problem in 0.5% to 4% of young adult men (Forsythe & Redmond, 1974).

Enuresis is referred to as *primary* if the child has never been dry for a period of at least 6 months, and it is termed *secondary* if wetting occurs after the child has been successfully dry at some point for at least that long. About 80% of enuretics are primary cases. Relapses are common, occurring in 25% of previously dry children; such relapses are commonest between the ages

Table 17–1. Percentage Enuretic by Age and Sex

	Age in Years											
	6	7	8	9	10	11	12	13	14	15	16	17
Males (white)	24.8	17.8	18.9	16.6	12.8	12.6	8.4	9.1	6.0	4.6	2.9	1.3
Females (white)	14.9	13.9	14.2	11.3	8.8	7.4	4.1	4.2	3.7	2.1	1.1	1.0

of 5 and 7 years, especially in boys (Oppel et al., 1968a, 1968b). Many secondary cases are reactive in character; these tend to be transient phenomena, in effect, brief regressions in response to stress. Another important distinction is between *nocturnal,* or night wetting (which occurs when the child is asleep or in bed), and *diurnal,* or daytime wetting (which takes place while the child is up and about). About 74% of wetters are nocturnal only, and 10% wet only during the day; the remaining 16% wet both day and night (Hallgren, 1956). About one out of a thousand cases of enuresis also shows associated encopresis.

Aside from their symptom, enuretics appear to be a very heterogeneous group. Different investigators, studying differing populations by a variety of means, have implicated a wide range of emotional, physiological, and familial factors.

ETIOLOGY AND ASSOCIATED CLINICAL FEATURES

Familial Factors

Enuresis tends to run in families. About 75% of all enuretic children have an immediate family member who also has or has had a history of this problem (Bakwin, 1961). This strong family association has even been found on an Israeli kibbutz, where the children predominantly sleep and are toilet trained away from the parents (Kaffman & Elizur, 1977). There is a markedly higher concordance rate for enuresis in monozygotic twins (68%) compared with dizygotic ones (36%) (Bakwin, 1973). Thus, beyond the impact of the dynamics and child-rearing practices of such families, genetic factors exert a strong influence.

There appears to be no consistent correlation between enuresis and toilet-training practices (Gross & Dornbusch, 1983; Sears et al., 1957). In considering individual cases, the clinician is sometimes impressed either by excessively early or coercive toilet-training practices or by a rather remarkable degree of laxity and indifference to the child's habitual wetting.

Enuresis is more common in large, disorganized, poor families with frequent disruptions of maternal care. Children in institutions also show a consistently higher incidence of this condition (Stein & Susser, 1966). Both are adverse rearing conditions that can deprive children of adequate social learning opportunities (Shaffer, 1985b). In one study, enuretics were more likely than other children to have had stressful experiences during the preschool years, including hospitalizations, moves, accidents, separations from the mother, births of younger siblings or family breakup due to death or divorce (Douglas, 1973). Such stressful life events may reflect generally disadvantaged family circumstances (Shaffer, 1985b); they can also interfere directly with acquiring bladder control.

Following hospitalization, fights or reprimands, the start of school, the birth of a sibling, or sleeping away from home, transient loss of bladder control frequently occurs in otherwise dry young children. Often it accompanies other symptoms of regression. Although such regression most often represents a nonspecific response to stress or to decreased maternal availability, more specific dynamics such as envy of a new infant sibling may also be at work. In the preschool years, urination is often linked in the child's mind with themes of sex and aggression. Conflicts about aggressive and sexual issues can trigger apparently involuntary as well as quite deliberate wetting; thus, the jealous or excited 4- or 5-year-old little boy may deliberately urinate in his parents' bedroom. Even popular usage notes this literal confluence of anger and urine in the phrase "to be pissed off."

Another subgroup of situation-specific reactive enuretics are young, timid children who have recently begun school and wet only at school (Shaffer & Ambrosini, 1985). In these children, the problem usually involves anxiety about using the school lavatory or asking for permission to leave class; tactful intervention by the teacher is usually curative.

Most studies, however, have been unable to link enuresis to any characteristic personality type or dynamic (Achenbach & Lewis, 1971; Rutter et al., 1973). In some children enuresis seems part of a larger mosaic of passive-aggressive protest behaviors; in others, it appears to be one of a host of manifestations of poor impulse control (Oppel et al., 1968a; Stein & Susser, 1965, 1967). On the one hand, some studies show enuretics to be more dependent, compliant, retiring, immature, and lacking in self-confidence than other children (Kaffman & Elizur, 1977; Shaffer, 1973). On the other hand, a disproportionate number of juvenile delinquents are enuretic.

Enuresis correlates with an increased incidence of psychopathology, although again not consistently with any specific type. About 20% of enuretic children do show other signs of emotional disturbance, a rate significantly higher than the general population (Rutter et al., 1973). Certain subgroups of these children have an even higher incidence of emotional disturbance: girls, older enuretics, and children who wet during the day. In depressed enuretics, wetting may vary with mood. However, what emerges most clearly in most epidemiological studies, is that the majority of enuretics do *not* appear to be psychiatrically disturbed. Where psychiatric problems and enuresis occur together, it is unclear to what extent the psychiatric problems cause or result from the enuresis or, indeed, to what extent they are both the outcome of common familial, emotional, or organic factors.

In some children enuresis can be correlated with neurological soft signs; developmental delays in walking, articulation, or language; late puberty; and shorter stature and lower bone age; in such cases maturational factors are undoubtedly at work.

Sleep Factors

Wetting is most likely to occur between midnight and 3 A.M. (Rapoport et al., 1980b). In recent years, sleep-related causes of enuresis have been much debated. A popular lay theory is that children wet because they sleep too deeply to rouse themselves when their bladders are full. However, enuretics are no more difficult to arouse than controls in response to calling or shaking (Boyd, 1960). Various studies have failed to find abnormalities in the sleep patterns of most enuretics and have reported that wetting can occur during any stage of sleep (Mikkelsen et al., 1980). When it happens during REM sleep, the dream content often concerns urination.

Urinary-Tract-Related Factors

Urinary tract infections may be present in as many as 5% of enuretic children, with a markedly higher incidence among girls (Shaffer, 1985b). Even though antibiotic treatment does not always stop the enuresis, the diagnosis and treatment of such infections are important to prevent long-term kidney damage. Indeed, it is possible that enuresis, especially in girls, may itself predispose to ascending urinary tract infections (Dodge et al., 1970).

Even when awake, many enuretics urinate more frequently than normal with a smaller volume to each voiding. These enuretics have bladders that distend less readily and show a sharper increase in pressure at relatively low volumes, producing an earlier urge to void than does the normal bladder. It is unclear whether this physiological pattern is due to greater bladder sensitivity or faulty inhibition of sphincter tone, or, for that matter, whether these physiological differences are themselves the product of frequent urination (Shaffer, 1985b, 1985c). Shaffer speculates that when other developmental delays are present, initial learning of bladder control may be more difficult and predispose to persistent incontinence.

In those enuretics referred to urological clinics, some studies have reported the presence of subtle bladder neck or urethral obstruction. For a time, there was a certain enthusiasm for the surgical treatment of such conditions. However, the current view is that for uncomplicated nocturnal enuresis, the clinician should view surgery with extreme caution, and should give precedence to more conservative procedures such as behavioral training and/or pharmacological measures.

Classification of Enuretics

Shaffer and colleagues (1984) studied a group of 126 enuretic children with respect to psychiatric and neurological status, functional bladder volume, and environmental circumstances. They found that in general, children with an associated psychiatric disorder had significantly smaller bladder volumes and more developmental delays. The distinctions between primary and secondary enuresis and between familial and nonfamilial enuresis were of little practical value. No classification predicted response to treatment.

The Impact of Enuresis

Whatever the origins of enuresis in any particular case, the symptom is a source of great shame and humiliation to the incontinent youngster. Even without the almost inevitable history of parental reproaches, exhortations, or dismay, enuretic children feel bad and helpless in the face of a symptom they feel unable to control. Such children live in dread of being discovered or teased; they either avoid overnight camp and sleep-overs or anxiously anticipate them as potential ordeals rather than as pleasures.

For most enuretic children, wetting carries the stigma of babyishness. Beyond the feared taunts and barbs of peers, the enuretic child's confidence and sense of self-mastery are shaken. Besides these general concerns, the symptom may take on other more specific or symbolic meanings (again, without regard to the symptom's initial origins). Thus, the wetting may carry sexual connotations, both exciting and shameful. The lack of control over a part of the body so intimately associated with the genitals may leave children ashamed of their identity as a boy or girl and concerned that something is wrong with this vital, secret part of their anatomy. They may also feel uncertain of their mastery of sexual or aggressive impulses. Especially in the phallic oedipal phase, prowess in urination is source of pride to boys. (Indeed, contests matching the range and duration of their urinary stream are common.) For the enuretic boy, experiencing himself as the passive victim of nocturnal wetting may stir fears of being weak or feminine.

TREATMENT

Through the centuries, treatments for enuresis have been as numerous as the proposed causes (Gross & Dornbusch, 1983). In fact, the effectiveness of various treatment modalities is hard to evaluate. To begin with, there is a high rate of both spontaneous improvement and relapse (Oppel et al., 1968b). Then, regardless of the means employed, there are strong placebo or nonspecific treatment effects (Werry & Cohrssen, 1965). Many children seem to improve, at least transiently, merely from the increased attention paid to them or to their symptom. Prophylactically, a noncoercive, non-punitive approach to toilet training is desirable (Brazelton, 1962a, 1973). This entails waiting until at least the second year of life when the child has sufficient cognitive capacity to understand what is being requested, sufficient linguistic competence to indicate his wishes, enough motor competence to sit on the potty unaided, and adequate sphincter control and physiological maturity to comply. It is also wise to defer training if the child is coping with some significant stress (e.g., a move, a new baby, a parental crisis). The child's most important recompenses for giving up the pleasures of unbridled elimination are a sense of his parent's love and pleasure and his own pride in self-mastery.

On their own initiative, parents with a young enuretic child often restrict fluids in the evening or awaken the child at night and take him to the bathroom. These measures may well be effective in the large number of enuretics who remit before ever reaching the doctor's office; however, controlled studies (Shaffer, 1985b; Fournier et al., 1987) cast doubt on their efficacy in cases of well-established enuresis. Where such home remedies are of no avail, children with enuresis need a careful pediatric evaluation, including a clean-voided urine specimen for urinalysis and culture. Medical conditions to be ruled out include causes of polyuria such as diabetes or proteinuria, congenital malformations, urinary tract infections, and seizure disorder (which may cause sporadic incontinence). A careful medical and developmental history and a psychosocial evaluation of the child and family are also important.

Several areas of the history deserve specific attention (Shaffer, 1985c). First, the nature of the incontinence should be carefully noted, including its duration, frequency, and pattern of fluctuation. Second, a careful history will usually reveal whether the enuresis is a relatively fixed, ongoing problem or a transient regression in response to a current conflict or to some situational stress such as the birth of a sibling, a move, or a parent's absence. In cases of secondary enuresis, the diagnostician should carefully scrutinize traumatic or other circumstances surrounding the relapse. Third, a family history of enuresis is important not only in terms of its possible genetic implications but also in terms of how it influences the parents' attitude toward the child's symptoms. Fourth, the diagnostician should thoroughly evaluate the overall quality of the parent–child relationship, the parents' attitude, and any previous attempts to deal with the enuresis. Parents may be excessively punitive, blameful, inconsistent, or lax. Previous unsuccessful attempts at treatment may have left both parent and child feeling helpless and discouraged.

As noted earlier, many cases respond well to nonspecific measures. (Shaffer, 1985b, 1985c provides an excellent overview of the principles of managing enuresis as well as a detailed review of the literature.) An important supportive element of the treatment is to reassure the frequently discouraged parents and the embarrassed child concerning the commonness of the symptoms and its favorable prognosis. When warranted, the clinician should emphasize that the wetting is not willful or under the child's conscious control (Shaffer, 1985c). Reduction of shaming and excessive punitive measures is important because it prevents further damage to the enuretic child's low self-esteem.

Baseline Data

In many cases, a simple star chart is an effective means both for gathering data and for treatment. With his parents' help, the child keeps a prominently posted chart (usually at the foot of the bed) on which the parents enthusiastically place a star for each dry night; lapses are not reproached, but they do not receive a star. After 2 weeks of charting, this heightened attention to the symptom and prompt systematic positive reinforcement for dryness, combined with the physician's reassurance, are sufficient to control the symptom in as many as 10% of enuretic children (Shaffer et al., 1968).

Psychotherapy

If there is evidence of emotional disturbance more pervasive than that expressed by the enuresis alone, family and/or individual psychotherapy may be indicated. When the enuresis is clearly a response to a recent stressful event (e.g., a move, birth of sibling), the therapist should address attention to the child's overall adaptation to the change. Thus, the focus of psychotherapeutic intervention is often on problem areas much broader than the enuresis. Nevertheless, such psychotherapy should not preclude the concurrent use of other appropriate treatments for the enuresis. It is often in the course of trying to implement a course of medication or to initiate a training program for the child's enuresis that the parents' collusive or punitive involvement in the child's wetting or their inconsistent attitude toward the symptom becomes apparent.

For unselected cases of uncomplicated enuresis psychotherapy alone is not indicated (De Leon & Mandell, 1966; Doleys, 1977). Whatever ancillary benefits may occur, psychotherapy has not been shown to be more effective than placebo in controlling enuresis. In one controlled study, "psychodynamic psychotherapy" was judged no more effective than "no treatment" and significantly less effective than the "bell and pad" method described below (Werry & Cohrssen, 1965).

Bell and Pad Training

A widely used and very effective remedy for enuresis is the bell and pad apparatus, which wakes up the child as soon as urination occurs. The child sleeps on two special mats that are separated by his bottom bed sheet. The two mats are connected to a battery and bell in such a way that if the child wets, a circuit is completed, the bell rings, and the child is awakened. The child is then instructed to go to the toilet to finish voiding, the sheets are changed, and the device is reset.

In different studies the bell and pad method produces a cure rate (defined as 2 weeks of continuous dryness) of 60% to 90%, usually within the first 2 months of treatment (Kolvin et al., 1972). To employ this method, a good deal of parental supervision and cooperation are necessary. The caretakers must set up the device properly; they must further ensure that the child does not sleep through the bell, dislodge the device, or turn off the alarm. As a result, treatment dropout is common as are suboptimal results due to failure to use the apparatus appropriately. (For a detailed account of the practical and theoretical aspects of this method and its common pitfalls, see Dische, 1973; Schmitt, 1982; Shaffer, 1985c.) Within a year following completion of treatment, relapse occurs in about one-third of cases (Turner, 1973).

The bell and pad's mode of action is not clear. Placebo effect, aversion, classic or operant conditioning, and social learning paradigms have all been proposed as explanations (Shaffer, 1985b). The method is much more effective than random night awakening and appears equal to or more effective than drug treatment (Fournier et al., 1987). Moreover, it has fewer potential adverse side effects and a lower relapse rate after termination of treatment.

A current theory asserts that enuresis may be due to decreased functional bladder capacity. Its proponents have accordingly advocated systematic daytime training to increase bladder capacity. This involves having the child increase fluids and attempt to delay urination by increments of several minutes each day after feeling the impulse to void. In controlled studies such training has shown about a 50% cure rate.

For many enuretics, tricyclic antidepressants such as imipramine have been found helpful, enabling about 30% to 40% of the patients to become completely dry within 2 to 4 weeks (Fournier et al., 1987; Rapoport et al., 1980; Shaffer, 1985b). However, as soon as the drug is stopped, a very high percentage of children relapse. Even in those still on the medication, tolerance may develop, with enuresis recurring (Jorgensen et al., 1980; Rapoport et al., 1980). The drug's mode of action is unclear and does not appear to be due either to imipramine's anticholinergic properties or its effect on sleep (Shaffer, 1985b). Improvement in wetting does not seem to relate to the drug's antidepressant effects; indeed, its antienuretic effect occurs at lower doses and more rapidly than does its antidepressant effects and is independent of the degree of pretreatment psychopathology (Rapoport et al., 1980).

Although all of the tricyclics are reportedly equally effective in treating enuresis (Shaffer & Ambrosini, 1985), imipramine has been the most widely studied. Absorption and excretion of imipramine are more variable in children than in adults; different children given the same dose may vary as much as 15-fold in the resulting serum concentrations of the drug (and its principal metabolite, desipramine) (Rapoport et al., 1980). Hence, no uniform dosage recommendation is possible. Optimum improvement seems to occur with combined imipramine-desipramine serum levels of 50–60 ng/ml (Jorgensen et al., 1980). To clinically titrate the dose, the physician might begin with one nightly 25-mg tablet of imipramine for 3 nights, increasing by one tablet every night if there is a wet episode, up to a maximum of 3 mg/ kg of body weight per day (Fournier et al., 1987). Depending on the dose level and anticholinergic properties of the specific tricyclic used, side effects may include orthostatic hypotension, hypertension, dry mouth, blurry vision, and constipation. The most serious side effects are cardiotoxicity and, rarely, seizures (Riddle et al., in press). A baseline EKG and blood pressure should be obtained and the EKG repeated for doses over 3 mg/kg per day, with 5 mg/kg the maximum. Drug holidays are recommended every 4 months or so to ascertain whether continued medication is necessary. Medication should be tapered, rather than stopped abruptly, in order to avoid flulike withdrawal symptoms. (For these and other practical aspects of medication management, see Shaffer and Ambrosini, 1985.)

Regardless of the treatment method employed, improvement in the child's enuresis usually results in markedly improved self-confidence and self-esteem (Moffatt et al., 1987).

Chapter 18

Disorders of Elimination

Encopresis

INTRODUCTION

Although rarer than enuresis, failure of bowel control stirs far more shame in the incontinent child and greater disgust and reproach from those about him than does bladder dyscontrol.

The age at which bowel control is expected (and usually attained) varies widely from culture to culture and even from family to family. Within our own country some families begin toilet training when the infant is between 12 and 18 months old, often with surprising success. In England, more than half of all children achieve bowel control by 18 to 24 months. Two large epidemiological studies, one in England (Stein & Susser, 1967) and the other in Sweden (Bellman, 1966), found that in both those countries most children are trained by age 4 years. In contrast, in some primitive cultures, children are not expected to achieve full bowel control until age 6 years (Whiting & Child, 1953). During the past 50 years, there has been a trend in our own culture toward later and more relaxed methods of bowel training (Brazelton, 1962a; Prugh, 1983).

DEFINITION

The term *encopresis* was originally coined to suggest a fecal parallel to enuresis. A controversy exists concerning the definition of encopresis, with some authors drawing distinctions based on the consistency of the stool, on the presence or absence of concomitant constipation, or on where the stool is deposited. The discussion that follows will adhere to the DSM-III-R criteria, which emphasize the repeated, age-inappropriate deposition of feces in culturally inappropriate places, with an absence of any apparent primary organic etiology.

DSM-III-R Diagnostic Criteria for Functional Encopresis

A. *Repeated passage of feces into places not appropriate for that purpose (e.g., clothing, floor), whether involuntary or intentional. (This disorder may be overflow incontinence secondary to functional fecal retention.)*

B. *At least one such event a month for at least six months.*

C. *Chronologic and mental age, at least four years.*

D. *Not due to a physical disorder, such as aganglionic megacolon.* (APA, 1987, p. 84)

EPIDEMIOLOGY

Epidemiological studies of the general child population suggest a prevalence rate in the 7- to 12-year age group of 1.3% to 1.5% for boys and 0.3%

to 0.7% for girls (Bellman, 1966; Rutter et al., 1970). Predictably, the prevalence of this condition is higher in pediatric and psychiatric clinic populations, namely about 3% to 6%, with boys again markedly outnumbering girls (Levine, 1975). Prevalence decreases noticeably with age, disappearing, with rare exceptions, by age 16 (Bellman, 1966). Enuresis is about 5 to 6 times more common than encopresis; about one-third of encopretic children are also enuretic.

Bellman's epidemiological study (1966) found that 16% of encopretics had a parent (in all but one case a father) with a history of childhood encopresis; about 9% of encopretic boys' brothers had a history of encopresis.

CLINICAL FEATURES

Various subtypes of encopresis are usually distinguished, although the usefulness of these distinctions is unclear. The term *primary* (or continuous) encopresis is used to describe the child who has never been fully bowel trained and whose lifelong history of fecal soiling has never been interrupted by any substantial period of continence. The term *secondary* (or discontinuous) encopresis is used to describe the child who was fully bowel trained at one time, but subsequently began soiling again. The onset of encopresis may be as late as 6 or 7 years of age.

Alternative subclassifications of encopresis include several clinical subtypes based on the consistency of the stools, the apparent precipitant of the soiling, and the pattern of where the soiling takes place (Bemporad, 1978; Hersov, 1985a; Rutter, 1975). These subtypes, however, should be regarded as tentative paradigms, rather than as reflecting the full complexity of clinical syndromes. As Levine (1982) has cautioned, in long-standing cases the symptoms often fluctuate: Normal movements may be interspersed with watery or rocklike stools, and although some children continue to show incontinence, they may proceed into and out of periods of fecal retention and constipation. Levine also suggests that the dichotomy between primary and secondary encopresis may not be as clear-cut as the traditional classification suggests, because many partially trained encopretics are difficult to classify.

Stools of Normal Consistency

About half of all encopretics have never been fully bowel trained (primary encopresis). These children usually have stools of normal consistency. Some primary encopretics, however, may show the abnormal stools characteristic of retention and megacolon (see below). Apparently these children have superimposed retention over an earlier pattern of infantile incontinence (Levine, 1975).

Another group of children with stools of generally normal consistency are those secondary encopretics who were previously trained, but who lost control in the face of stressful circumstances. Especially in younger children, illness, hospitalization, separation from mother, or the birth of a sibling may lead to a regressive loss of bowel control. Fortunately, in most cases this loss of control is transient. However, many chronic cases of secondary encopresis also have a history of onset associated with a stressful event (Bellman, 1966; Levine, 1975). In addition, some children with ongoing encopresis show a pattern of incontinence in response to upsets or overexcitement; such precipitants are often nonspecific.

Stools of Abnormal Consistency

Stools of abnormal consistency characterize a large number of encopretics. Many such children frequently stain their underwear with small amounts of liquid feces, punctuated infrequently by enormous, painful defecations of massive toilet-stopping stools. This pattern is due to chronic fecal retention, which, surprisingly, is a common symptom of encopretic children. Indeed, some authorities believe that it is a nearly ubiquitous feature of the condition (Levine, 1982). The rectum and lower colon of such children become distended with feces, often to massive proportions; Richmond and colleagues (1954) termed this condition *psychogenic megacolon.* Because of this stasis, increased water absorption leads to ever harder and more massive stools. The resulting painful defecation, as well as the anal fissures or hemorrhoids that may ensue, discourage the child still further from attempting a bowel movement. The stretched rectal wall and increased luminal volume render muscle contractions both weaker and less effective, thereby impairing further the child's ability to empty his rectum completely; at the same time the stretching of the anal canal compromises the efficacy of the sphincter muscles, permitting the leakage of watery stools that have percolated through, or around, the hardened, impacted fecal mass. Some children with liquid stools secondary to retention and megacolon are, in fact, misdiagnosed and treated by their parents for diarrhea (Davidson et al., 1963). Even those children who defecate daily may nonetheless fail to empty the rectum completely, leading to persisting megacolon. A plain X ray of the abdomen may be necessary to reveal otherwise occult retention (Barr et al., 1979).

Pressure on the bladder from a massive megacolon that fills the pelvis can cause enuresis (due to decreased bladder capacity) as well as the more serious consequences of urinary blockage, such as hydronephrosis and other obstructive uropathies. Chronic urinary tract infections are also common due to obstruction and—in the case of girls—constant perineal soiling. The section on Etiology discusses the possible psychological or physical factors leading to chronic retention.

Chronic, intermittent abdominal pain, poor appetite, and lethargy are all common in encopretic children, especially in combination with chronic constipation.

Patterns of Defecation

Most encopretic children defecate in their underwear although they will occasionally choose other inappropriate places when they cannot make it to the toilet in time. Many are ashamed of their soiling, deal with it furtively, and hide their soiled underwear in some secret cache, where their mother eventually discovers it, much to her dismay and undisguised disgust. This guilty furtiveness stands in contrast to the bizarre defecations of a small number of severely disturbed children who, seemingly deliberately and defiantly, pass stools of normal consistency in studiously selected wrong places. (Anthony, 1957, recounted the case of a child who defecated in the family piano.) A goodly proportion of such children may either be psychotic themselves or have psychotic parents. In some cases, revenge appears to lie behind the bizarre but provocative pattern of defecation.

Episodes of incontinence happen most frequently toward late afternoon and early evening. About half of the cases have occasional episodes of incontinence during the night; unlike enuresis, however, exclusively nocturnal encopresis is rare (Levine, 1975).

Encopretic children often protest that they "did not feel the stools coming" (Bellman, 1966). Typically, such children may be caught up in play and then make a last minute, unsuccessful dash for the bathroom; many children may not even be aware of needing to go to the bathroom until they actually feel the stools in their underwear. For some children, this inattentiveness to internal cues may be part of an overall attention deficit disorder; in others chronic bowel distention secondary to retention may lead to attenuation of bowel sensation. Similarly, although the encopretic's chronically foul odor may repel peers and family, the child's nose may have accommodated enough that he is unaware of his persistent unsavory aroma. A few encopretics even enjoy it.

Most encopretic children are unhappy and isolated. They are humiliated by what they and others regard as a shameful and infantile inability to control their body. Their symptom stirs reproach and revulsion in their parents, invites merciless ridicule and taunting from siblings and peers, and often precipitates depression and low self-esteem.

ETIOLOGY

Normal Development of Bowel Control

The normal development of bowel control involves both voluntary and involuntary reflexes. Defecation occurs as a result of the contraction of the rectum's smooth (involuntary) luminal musculature, accompanied by the relaxation of the anal sphincter. Distention of the rectum with feces normally produces a sense of fullness and usually initiates reflex contractions of the rectal musculature. Reflex contractions of the rectum and a corresponding urge to defecate are also produced by distention of the stomach with food, the so-called *gastrocolic reflex*, whose functioning is often conspicuous in infants. The process of expelling feces may also be initiated or facilitated by voluntary bearing down with the abdominal musculature.

Just as the propulsive force in defecation is under both voluntary and involuntary reflex control, so too is the anal sphincter subject to dual control. The anal sphincter consists of an internal smooth (involuntary) muscle portion and an external striated (voluntary) muscle portion. The internal sphincter, which is under the control of the autonomic nervous system, is maintained in a state of tonic contraction, thereby preventing the leakage of feces. This sphincter relaxes when the rectum is distended and defecation initiated. Together with other perianal muscles, the external sphincter, which is under voluntary control, can be deliberately contracted to resist the pressure of a wave of rectal contraction until it passes. Whether abnormalities in sphincter tone and responsiveness predispose some children to abnormal "defecation dynamics" and constipation has been the topic of much debate and study (Loening-Bauke & Cruikshank, 1986).

Infants less than 12 months old can achieve a semblance of bowel control by being regularly placed on the potty after each meal when the operation of the gastrocolic reflex appears imminent. True bowel control, however, is a complex skill involving the ability both to inhibit defecation and to initiate it voluntarily under appropriate social conditions. Such control involves a complex interplay of maturational, cognitive, and interpersonal factors. On a purely physiological level, it requires the presence of adequate involuntary peristaltic activity, an ability to discern sensations of rectal fullness, and full voluntary control over sphincter constriction and relaxation (Hersov, 1985a; Nixon, 1975). On a psychological level, toilet training involves an intricate interplay of social learning and more or less unconscious interpersonal motives.

Anna Freud (1965) described the process of toilet training in terms of a *developmental line* from unfettered wetting and soiling through autonomous control of bowel and bladder; she viewed the process from the view of both the child's intrapsychic development and his interactions with his mother. To summarize this approach, the child passes through several stages of bowel and bladder function. In the first stage, before the mother places any demands on the child, he has complete freedom to wet and soil. At the second level, the mother's beginning efforts to train the child encounter two conflicting attitudes in the child. To the extent that there is a positive, secure relationship between mother and toddler, the child, who regards his body products as precious, is inclined to surrender them to his mother as loving "gifts," in return for her praise and affection. On the other hand, the toddler who is beginning to assert his autonomy "stiffens his opposition to any interference with concerns that have become emotionally vital to him" (p. 73). Especially if the mother presses her demands in a harsh, uncompromising, or untimely fashion, a battle of wills is likely to occur. The child's excreta may thus become charged with aggression and wielded by him as weapons of rage, anger, revenge, or as an expression of disappointment against his mother.

In the third phase, according to Anna Freud, as the child initially achieves toilet training, he accepts and takes over the mother's attitudes toward cleanliness, making them his own on the basis of identification. From this point forward, the imperative for cleanliness becomes internal, rather than external. This self-responsibility, however, is vulnerable, being dependent on the mother's availability and the stability of the child's positive relationship with her. It is only much later, in a fourth phase, that control becomes secure as the child's concern for cleanliness becomes independent of his relationship with his parents.

Implicit in the classic Freudian perspective elaborated above is the notion that the child views training as a frustrating renunciation of an instinctual pleasure; from this view, the child finds only vicarious gratification in his continence (at least initially), based on his mother's pride and approval. Chess and Thomas (1984) have argued that this perspective discounts the significance of advances in task mastery and social competency, which are important autonomous sources of satisfaction to the child.

Much depends on the timeliness and the manner of the mother's promptings and demands. Anthony's (1957) work on "the potting couple" focused on the interactional system of mutual cues and communication between the mother and infant around elimination. When all goes well, the mother reads the infant's physiological cues and responds in such a way that the child becomes alert to his own internal sensations and learns how to respond to them. The process goes awry if the mother is not alert to or misinterprets the infant's cues or if she responds to them inappropriately or inconsistently. As with many developmental issues, the "goodness of fit" between the mother's approach and the child's temperament are often the decisive factor in determining the success or failure of training attempts.

Anthony (1957) proposed that most cases of primary encopresis were due to lack of adequate toilet training among children of chaotic poor families. In contrast, he felt that most cases of secondary encopresis reflected more serious psychopathology, the outcome of a "battle of the bowels" between the child and compulsively neat parents.

As with enuresis, there is marked disagreement in the literature regarding the extent to which encopresis indicates psychiatric disturbance. A number of psychiatric authors share Bemporad's view (1978) that "fecal soiling is rarely the sole symptom but rather the surface expression of an entrenched personality disorder often complicated by organic problems and reinforced by disturbed family relationships" (p. 161). Many pediatricians, however, see encopresis as a developmental disorder, based on organic constitutional factors, but with serious emotional sequelae in terms of lowered self-esteem and impaired interpersonal relationships. These differing conclusions regarding the relative contributions of social, constitutional, interpersonal, and personality factors may be artifacts of the different populations or subgroups seen by pediatricians and mental health professionals (Hersov, 1985a; Levine et al., 1980).

Maturational Factors.   Numerous developmental difficulties have been noted in encopretics, such as poor coordination, slow language development, hyperactivity, withdrawal, and social immaturity (Bellman, 1966; Bemporad et al., 1971; Olatawura, 1973).

Personality Factors.   Despite a higher than expected prevalence of behavioral difficulties and school adjustment problems, encopretics do not show a characteristic personality type (Achenbach & Lewis, 1971). Bellman (1966) found that encopretics were less likely than controls to have shown defiance at ages 2 to 3 years; also, in later childhood encopretics were more likely than controls to be anxious, to lack self-assurance, and to manifest difficulty in handling their aggression; an excessive number were overly inhibited in expressing aggression although a smaller subgroup of encopretics showed explosive, undercontrolled aggression. Bellman found no significant differences between the personality traits of primary and secondary encopretics. Although Anthony (1957) concluded that the secondary encopretic was characteristically the overcontrolled "compulsive child of a compulsive family," Levine (1975) found no significant differences between the primary and secondary group in compulsive neatness or hoarding behavior. In fact, such behaviors occurred in less than 30% of encopretics. Thus, the orderliness and parsimony that Freud (1908/1959) saw as typifying the "anal character" are not ubiquitous features of encopretics' personalities.

Sociocultural Influences.   Cultural factors play a major role in families' toilet-training practices; consequently there has been much speculation (but little hard data) concerning cultural and class influences on the genesis of encopresis.

Anthony (1957) concluded that the primary encopretic largely resulted from the lax and indifferent training children received in disorganized homes of low socioeconomic status (SES)—"A dirty child coming from a dirty family, burdened with every conceivable sort of social problem" (p. 157). Bemporad (1978), on the other hand, was impressed by what he perceived as the tendency of low-SES inner-city parents in this country to train their infants quite early.

In middle-class families, the move away from coercive toilet-training practices reflects a major historical impact of psychoanalysis on child-rearing practices; in the past 40 years or so the trend has been toward later initiation of toilet training (Brazelton, 1962a; Caldwell, 1964; Prugh, 1983). Although the effect probably has been generally salutory, occasionally families carry the policy to extremes. Most pediatricians have seen the infrequent, but strikingly misguided, "trendy" middle-class parents who neglect to train their preschooler because of ostensible concerns about prematurely traumatizing the child or constraining his freedom.

Reliable epidemiological data concerning such matters are difficult to come by. An early American study (Havighurst & Davis, 1955) noted significant differences in bowel-training practices among various cultural and socioeconomic groups. On the other hand, a more recent British study (Stein & Susser, 1967) found no impact of social class on the age of attainment or degree of success of preschoolers' bowel control. The Isle of Wight study (Rutter et al., 1970) found no relationship between social class and incidence of encopresis. In contrast to what he felt were the origins of primary encopresis in disorganized low-SES family life, Anthony (1957) saw the secondary encopretic as a "compulsive child of a compulsive family." Levine (1975) and Olatawura (1973), however, found a large number of secondary encopretics among welfare or low-SES families, whereas Bellman (1966) noted that the children whose parents had totally neglected to train them were often from middle-class homes.

Mother–Child Interactions. The relationship among cultural influences, parental toilet-training attitudes, and consequent predisposition to either eliminative pathology or particular character traits is complex and incompletely understood (Anthony, 1957; Sears et al., 1957; Whiting & Child, 1953).

Sigmund Freud (1908/1959) speculated that severe toilet training produced what he termed "the anal character," a personality type whose hallmark was the triad of orderliness, obstinancy, and stinginess (see also Chapter 9, "Obsessive-Compulsive Disorder"). Freud acknowledged, however, that the relationship was not simple because it seemed plausible that anal fixation might also result from overgratification and neglectful training. Finally, he proposed, constitutional factors might also play a significant role. Normative studies of the impact of toilet training on personality development have failed to show clear-cut links between toilet training experience and particular character traits (Hetherington & Brackbill, 1963).

Several early studies found a prior history of the use of severe, punitive training methods in a significant number of encopretics (Bellman, 1966; Huschka, 1942; Pinkerton, 1958). Bellman found that although mothers of encopretics did not start training earlier, they used coercive training methods more often than control mothers. They were more likely to deal punitively with early lapses during training, and they expected (and got) earlier full completion of training from their subsequently encopretic children. She also found that in matters apart from toilet training, mothers of encopretics tended to be anxious, emotionally unstable, unreliable, overprotective, and indulgent. This last finding is puzzling in light of Sears and colleagues' (1957) observation that mothers who were severe in toilet training tended to be demanding and restrictive about other aspects of the child's behavior including orderliness, sexual activity, and aggression. However, a history of coercive training is not a constant feature of secondary encopresis; Olatawura (1973) found that in his sample, the large majority of secondary encopretics had *not* been coercively trained.

Harsh or punitive training techniques seem to increase the likelihood of avoidance, withholding, and later difficulties. However, the overall affective context of the mother–child relationship may be of far greater importance than the specific techniques used. Prugh (1954) found that constipation, with or without fecal soiling, was twice as common in children who had been subjected to early bowel training compared with those trained at the usual time. However, he concluded that mothers with warm and close relationships with their infants could engage in premature or even coercive training without serious risk of subsequent difficulties. This parallels the results of Sears and colleagues' (1957) study of enuresis, which found that mothers' strictness (vs. permissiveness) was a less important determinant than maternal warmth (vs. coldness). Incontinence was more likely to develop in the children of mothers who were *both* strict and cold. Prugh (1954, 1983) and Pinkerton (1958) compared children with simple constipation (but no soiling) to those with soiling (with or without megacolon). They found a lower incidence of coercive toilet training and generally less family disturbance in the children with simple constipation.

However, the relationship between training and bowel difficulties is complex. As Anthony (1957) pointed out, not all children who receive coercive or neglectful toilet training develop bowel dysfunction; nor, do all children with bowel difficulties have a history of abnormal toilet training. Chess and Hassibi (1978) emphasize that a given child-care practice, such as a particular style of toilet training, can have markedly different outcomes when employed with temperamentally diverse infants. As an example, they cite the likelihood of failure when early reflex training methods are used with an active, temperamentally intense, physiologically irregular 1-year-old. Such a child is unlikely to be able to sit still long enough for his unpredictable gastrocolic reflex to produce a bowel movement in the pot; furthermore, if he is forced to sit still, his protests are certain to be intense. For such a child, training is likely to be stressful unless deferred until 2 years of age or later. On the other hand, a temperamentally less active and more tranquil, regular infant may indeed be capable of being readily and happily trained at 1 year by the same method that is catastrophic for his less well-modulated peer.

Family Influences. Bemporad et al. (1971, 1978), Hoag et al. (1971), and others have stressed the nature of the family context within which encopresis occurs. Bemporad conceptualizes encopresis as a hostile communication on the child's part in the context of a hostile–dependent power struggle between the child and his parents. From this view, although the encopresis may begin in a variety of ways, it becomes entrenched as a transactional behavior involving the entire family. The child's soiling thus serves as both a response to and an elictor of deviant parental behavior. The encopretic child's soiling punishes and provokes the depriving mother, while ensuring her continued attention and involvement with him. This conceptual formulation is similar to the ideas of Minuchin and colleagues (1978) regarding the functioning of psychosomatic families (see Chapters 15 and 19).

Bellman (1966) found that compared with families of controls, encopretics' parents were more likely to experience marital discord and to have had a history of psychiatric hospitalization. Bemporad and colleagues (1971) were struck by two common pathological features of encopretics' families. In many cases, the encopretic's mother lacked empathy for and would alternately infantilize and coldly reject her child. In addition, these investigators were particularly impressed by the high prevalence of fathers who were emotionally and/or physically absent from the home. Using an ingenious experimental design, Achenbach and Lewis (1971), found that the mothers, rather than the fathers, of encopretics dominated their families more commonly than was the case in the families of psychiatric controls; these authors were, however, unable to confirm other hypotheses concerning the correlates and antecedents of encopresis and enuresis.

A Developmental Perspective

We share Levine's (1982) view that encopresis is the product of multiple factors interacting in various ways during the early years of life. Levine stressed the contribution of numerous predisposing and risk-potentiating factors during infancy, toddlerhood, and the early school years. For example, early constipation may predispose the infant to later retention, especially if dealt with overaggressively by means of frequent suppositories or enemas. Perianal irritation or fissures due to constipation may further intensify withholding. Certain parents are strongly "bowel-oriented," with marked concerns about the regularity and consistency of the infant's bowel movements. In such families, when the infant has had early bowel difficulties, the stage may be set for a struggle for control around bowel functioning even before toilet training has begun (Prugh, 1983).

When training starts, it may exacerbate earlier difficulties or precipitate new problems. A variety of fears, both reality-based and irrational, may cause the toddler apprehension about use of the toilet or the act of defecation. Children most commonly fear loud flushing, falling in and being flushed away, and the cold seat and height (when trained on a full-sized commode). Many children also fear a snake or a monster in the toilet that can strike back. Bellman (1966) noted that the mothers of encopretics more frequently reported an early history of "pot fear" for their child than did the mothers of controls.

Other fears relate to the child's animistic and fantasy-filled notions about his stools and body. Using a Piagetian approach, Anthony (1957) traced the stages of what he termed *intestinal animism*—the young child's notions that his feces are alive and endowed with feelings. Anthony observed a correlation between the type of toilet training the child received and the valence of the animistic fantasies concerning his feces. Children with a history of coercive training had a strikingly high prevalence of fearful or hateful feelings toward their feces, whereas children with neglectful or cooperative training were more likely to express affectionate or even erotic feelings toward their feces. For some children, defecation may be associated with fantasies of losing part of their body or sending their feces away to die.

Erikson (1963) gives a dramatic and poignant account of a 4-year-old boy whose massive fecal retention began abruptly following the loss of a cherished nanny, who left to have a baby of her own; in the course of a perceptive home interview, Erikson uncovered the boy's mistaken notion that babies are born rectally and his identification with the pregnant nanny and the baby he used to be. By retaining his feces, he protected these figures who would be damaged by letting go. Erikson's exploration of these multiply-determined "cloacal" concerns led to prompt resolution of the boy's symptoms. In our experience, however, pursuit of sexual fantasies underlying the encopretic symptom is often unrewarding; the problematic affective issues are more often interpersonal ones concerning an aggressively tinged struggle for autonomy.

When toilet training begins during one of the periodic surges of negativism characteristic of the toddler period, elimination can get caught up in the child's more general struggle for independence and autonomy. The bathroom is especially likely to become a combat zone when there are already intense parent–child conflicts concerning control in other spheres of life.

Finally, even when bowel control has been established in apparently satisfactory fashion, during the early school years new stresses may cause predisposed children to become encopretic. The onset of secondary encopresis may coincide with changes that include illness, the birth of a sibling, the beginning of school, or the mother's return to work. The noise, smell, and lack of privacy in the school bathroom may lead some children, previously regularly trained at home, to begin withholding defecation, thus setting the stage for obstipation and overflow incontinence (Levine, 1982). Children with attentional deficits who are busy playing while away from home may miss their internal cues that it is time to go to the bathroom. In addition, their lack of persistence may lead to incomplete bowel movements, with gradually increasing constipation and, ultimately, incontinence.

Once established, encopresis becomes a source of great shame and humiliation to the offending child, who is frequently withdrawn and socially isolated and who experiences poor self-esteem. Ultimately, ongoing encopresis, of whatever origin, has a powerfully noxious and deteriorative effect on the relations between the child and his parents. As with many other psychosomatic conditions, in long-established cases it may be difficult to differentiate between the psychological factors that are antecedent causes of the disorder and those that are its secondary consequences.

Although encopresis almost always disappears by adolescence, rare, unusually refractory cases persist. In such instances, the symptom may become entrenched as a secret activity that the child both hates and prizes, drawing from it a perverse pleasure and sense of power (Bemporad, 1978). Bemporad sees the intractability of the symptom in adolescence as related to this shift in the soiling's function from being a form of transpersonal hostile communication to becoming a fixed source of intrapsychic gratification.

TREATMENT

Evaluation and Management

In most cases, the family pediatrician can best carry out the initial evaluation of encopresis with psychiatric consultation reserved for those cases that prove intractable to routine pediatric management or in which there are marked concurrent personality or family difficulties.

Physical examination, including abdominal X rays when needed, should establish the degree of stool retention and megacolon. Physical causes of constipation such as hypothyroidism, spinal cord lesion, or chronic Crohn's disease should be ruled out. Although Hirschprung's disease is frequently cited as part of the differential diagnosis of megacolon, it is improbable in a well-nourished school-age child with secondary encopresis, especially if there was no history of serious bowel problems in infancy (Levine, 1982). Concurrent urinary tract infection should be ruled out.

The pediatric management of encopresis with retention and constipation involves several elements: (1) initial education and demystification of the problem, (2) initial catharsis of impacted stools, and (3) establishment of an ongoing training routine with regular follow-up and monitoring.

In the protocol used at Boston Children's Hospital Medical Center (Levine, 1982), the initial counseling focuses on removing blame, reducing isolation (by letting the patient know that other children have the same problem), and explaining to the child with diagrams what goes on in his bowels. A treatment alliance is established around the notion of the pediatrician as a "coach" who will help the patient build up the muscles that control his bowels. This metaphor is well suited to the school-age child because it stresses the progressive, masterful, and autonomous aspects of his bowel control rather than the regressive and compliant aspects. The pediatrician explains to the child that they will clean out the "rocks" that block the intestine and prevent the formation of new ones so that the bowel can regain its strength, size, and feelings.

Adequate initial catharsis with enemas and Dulcolax (bisacodyl) is necessary to disimpact the child completely. When the retention is very severe or when it seems inadvisable to have the parents administer the enemas, the initial catharsis may need to be done in the hospital.

Any retraining program requires ongoing facilitation of defecation with a high-bulk diet, stool softeners, and, in severe cases, laxatives. Maintenance doses of mineral oil, 2 to 3 times daily, are the mainstay of most protocols, with the addition of oral laxatives when needed.

Retraining and Behavioral Techniques

A variety of retraining programs have been described in the literature (Ashkenazi, 1975; Ayllon et al., 1975; Azrin & Foxx, 1974; Levine, 1982; Plachetta, 1976; Schaefer et al., 1979; Wright & Walker, 1978; Young & Goldsmith, 1972). A central goal of many approaches is to reestablish the child's ability to sense rectal fullness and to use it as a cue for elimination in the toilet. Most plans entail setting aside one or two regular intervals each day during which the child sits on the toilet for 10 minutes and attempts to defecate, whether or not he feels the urge to do so. The child receives positive reinforcements for these regular attempts, with larger rewards for the actual production of feces. In the protocol used extensively and successfully by Wright and Walker (1978), a suppository is given if the child's morning attempt produces no results, with an enema added if the suppository is unproductive. In addition, the child receives no positive reward for the results. The authors claim that these measures are necessary only infrequently. (No doubt these intrusions act as much by means of their aversiveness as by any physiological mechanism.) A self-charting program with stars and other positive reinforcers for days without soiling is also often used. Opinion is divided about the advisability of mild negative reinforcement (e.g., "time-outs," loss of television privileges for the day, or an extra chore) for soiling lapses.

As part of his Full Cleanliness Training protocol, Doleys insisted that the child clean himself and wash his soiled clothes; the purpose, in this view, is both to teach responsibility and to motivate the child to remain clean by providing a negative consequence for any soiling (Doleys, 1983; Doleys & Arnold, 1975). Because the angry, mutually punitive struggle between parent and child is usually already intense, many clinicians, however, prefer using only positive reinforcers to shape and reinforce continence.

Although behavioral therapies are sometimes described as though they can be applied indiscriminately to all encopretics, it is important to distinguish (to the extent possible) among etiologically distinct subgroups. Ashkenazi (1975) differentiates between phobic and nonphobic encopretics. He uses the term *phobic* to describe young encopretics who cry, cling, and are afraid to approach the toilet. Ashkenazi hypothesized that these children had been traumatized by either painful bowel movements or very coercive training practices. The author suggested a gradual desensitization procedure for such children, with positive reinforcement of incremental approaches to the toilet until they are finally able to sit on it. Azrin and Foxx (1974) distinguished children who had never developed appropriate toileting behavior and described a training program for shaping these skills.

Presenting the training as a muscle-building regimen rather than as a punishment helps to foster a positive alliance with the encopretic child (Levine, 1982). The general consensus is that the successful implementation of any such program requires ongoing supervision and support in the form of regular phone calls and office visits.

Course of Treatment

In implementing a retraining regimen, serious family pathology often becomes apparent in the form of inability to follow through with the plan, inconsistency, inability to refrain from excess punitiveness, and even active sabotage. Active monitoring and follow-up by the pediatrician are essential, for it is only against the backdrop of a good working relationship between the doctor and family that it is possible to distinguish between simple discouragement and parental complicity in noncompliance. Some children and families become noncompliant when the treatment program appears to be unsuccessful. Levine and Bakow (1976) caution: "It is essential . . . to determine whether a child fails in treatment because of noncompliance or becomes non-compliant because the treatment is failing him" (p. 851).

In a significant number of cases, either treatment failure or serious concurrent individual or family psychopathology necessitates psychiatric referral. In such cases, depending on the locus of difficulty, a combination of individual psychotherapy, parent counseling, and/or family therapy is usually necessary. Even (or perhaps especially) when a child and family enter psychotherapy, ongoing close collaboration between the therapist and pediatrician is essential.

Treatment efficacy is difficult to evaluate rigorously against the known natural history of both relapse and resolution with time (Bellman, 1966). Wright and Walker (1978) claimed that their behavioral protocol was "virtually 100% successful if properly applied"; however, their follow-up was only 6 months and as many as 10% to 15% of families refused to enter the program. A more typical prognostic picture is that of the large Boston Children's Hospital cohort treated under the pediatric protocol outlined above (Levine & Bakow, 1976). Of the patients for whom one-year follow-up data could be obtained, 51% were in complete remission; 27% showed marked improvement with only rare incontinence; 14% showed some improvement; and 8% were essentially unchanged. Thirteen percent of the initial treatment group were lost to follow-up. Perhaps as some evidence of their refractoriness, 30% of the original sample had had previous psychiatric or psychological therapy and many of the children had a history of previous unsuccessful treatment by their family pediatrician. Not surprisingly, poorer outcome was associated with severe constipation; severe incontinence (especially those children who had frequent accidents during school or in pajamas); nocturnal encopresis; and multiple behavioral, developmental, and academic problems. Children who were excessively moody, disobedient, and fearless were more likely to have a negative outcome. Better compliance with treatment and a more internal locus of control (as assessed prior to treatment) were correlated with better outcome (Rappaport et al., 1986). Of 11 cases referred for psychotherapy at the end of the initial treatment year, 10 were still in psychotherapy a year later.

Isolated anecdotal case reports (Balson, 1973; Young & Goldsmith, 1972) have described symptom substitution in children successfully treated for encopresis. These authors reported that, as the encopresis resolved, aggressive behavior emerged in previously meek, overinhibited children. They suggested that this emergence was due to removal of the encopresis, which defended against the child's aggression. In contrast, Levine and colleagues' (1980) larger cohort showed that as encopretic children's soiling resolved during a pediatric treatment program, dramatic, but generally positive, changes emerged in their behavior and attitudes. While admitting the possibility of a "halo effect," Levine found less anxious, moody, and depressed behavior and decreased social isolation in the children who had been cured of their symptoms.

Although the majority of children with encopresis can be managed successfully without formal psychotherapeutic intervention, a hard core of treatment-refractory, multiproblem encopretic children require comprehensive psychiatric and pediatric management. The treatment of such children is often arduous. As noted earlier, psychotherapeutic intervention does not mitigate the need for ongoing coordinated pediatric treatment. Psychotherapy alone cannot restore normal bowel functioning in a massively impacted child.

The psychological management of encopresis entails identifying and altering the intrapsychic and interpersonal processes that trigger and maintain soiling (Bemporad, 1978; Levine, 1982). Bemporad advocates a family-oriented approach in which the therapist's prime task

> ... is to determine what is lacking in the child's everyday life, what is causing him to feel frustrated and angry, what is blocking an appropriate expression of his feelings—in short, the causes of his having to resort to soiling as a method of expression—and then to attempt to rectify these sources of discontent. (p. 167)

Bemporad sees a lack of empathic understanding as common in encopretic families; in his treatment vignettes, he describes how the symptom may be embedded in a perfectionistic and sterile family context that fails to provide the child with adequate structure or security or enmeshes the child in covert, unresolved family conflicts. Adequate treatment of such cases necessitates involving the entire family. Bemporad remarked that improvement of the encopresis often goes hand-in-hand with the reengagement of a previously emotionally distant father with the child and family.

As always, it is important not to take a blameful, exclusively parentogenic view. The encopretic child is often immature, withholding, and difficult to engage and understand by parent and therapist alike. Treating such children is often extremely taxing. In the case of one 9-year-old girl, her encopresis ultimately yielded to combined individual and family therapy and vigorous pediatric management. Although therapeutic intervention accomplished much useful work during the course of a year's individual play therapy sessions, this otherwise garrulous girl never uttered a word; at termination, despite her marked improvement, her only audible acknowledgment as she shook the therapist's hand in parting was to pass flatus loudly.

Chapter 19

Eating Disorders
Anorexia Nervosa and Bulimia

INTRODUCTION

Anorexia Nervosa

Anorexia nervosa is a dramatic, often life-threatening syndrome occurring most frequently in adolescent girls who intentionally starve and exercise themselves into a state of emaciation. Not all anorectics are girls; however, the preponderance of females to males is so great (about 20 to 1) that the feminine pronoun will be employed throughout this chapter in referring to sufferers of the disease. Although historically well-entrenched, the term *anorexia* (loss of appetite) is actually a misnomer, for these young women have not lost their hunger. Instead, their "relentless pursuit of thinness" (Bruch, 1978) represents a desperate attempt to assert their wills so that they can dominate their bodies, their physical appetite, their parents, and ultimately the very processes of time and adolescent growth. On the one hand, the anorexic's deliberate self-starvation is a declaration of independence from her mother with whom she is tightly enmeshed. By repudiating her passive and dependent longings, the young teenager hopes to delineate the previously blurred boundaries of her self and to relieve her overwhelming sense of ineffectiveness and lack of self-sufficiency. On the other hand, the anorexic's self-starvation returns her body to a childlike state, undoing the changes of puberty by halting her menses and transforming her new womanly curves into gaunt, skeletal angularities. Further, her obstinate dieting and rejection of sustenance soon precipitate a battle with her increasingly desperate parents who beg, cajole, insist, and threaten in a fruitless effort to get her to eat.

Especially in adolescence, the body is often the stage on which cultural and psychological conflicts are played out (Ritvo, 1984). Anorexia represents an extreme form of the ascetic mode of defense by which many adolescents attempt to quell the unsettling clamor of their body and its instinctual life (Blos, 1962; Mogul, 1980).

Anorexia also provides a striking example of how cultural forces help define an illness and influence its prevalence (Brumberg, 1988). At one time the disease was rare; today, however, the incidence of anorexia nervosa appears to be much higher than 30 years ago (Jones et al., 1980). Once confined almost exclusively to the children of the wealthy and the middle class, the condition has now acquired a social and literary cachet. Sours (1980) suggested that the anorectic, in her narcissistic preoccupation with achieving absolute separateness and autonomy, seeks to guarantee security. Sours perceived a common thread running through today's athletic fads, such as jogging, and the anorectic's efforts to achieve an ideal state of self-sufficient perfection by controlling and mastering the body and self. As hysteria was emblematic of the cultural and instinctual tensions of its era, anorexia has become a symbol of the narcissistic preoccupations of our epoch (Bemporad et al., 1988; Lasch, 1978).

DSM-III-R Diagnostic Criteria for Anorexia Nervosa

A. *Refusal to maintain body weight over a minimal normal weight for age and height, e.g., weight loss leading to maintenance of body weight 15% below that expected; or failure to make expected weight gain during period of growth, leading to body weight 15% below that expected.*

B. *Intense fear of gaining weight or becoming fat, even though underweight.*

C. *Disturbance in the way in which one's body weight, size, or shape is experienced, e.g., the person claims to "feel fat" even when emaciated, believes that one area of the body is "too fat" even when obviously underweight.*

D. *In females, absence of at least three consecutive menstrual cycles when otherwise expected to occur (primary or secondary amenorrhea). (A woman is considered to have amenorrhea if her periods occur only following hormone, e.g., estrogen, administration.)* (APA, 1987, p. 67)

Bulimia

Some anorectics (usually designated as *restrictors* or *fasting anorectics*) maintain relentless control of their self-inflicted starvation. Others are unable to clamp such an iron grip on their intake and periodically succumb to massive eating binges. This condition of periodic uncontrollable gorging is known as *bulimia* (from the Greek for "ox hunger") or, in DSM-III-R (APA, 1987) terms, *Bulimia Nervosa*. Accordingly, anorectics who periodically interrupt their self-starvation and binge in this fashion are termed *bulimic anorectics*. These binges are frequently followed by intense self-loathing and guilt. Bulimics often make themselves vomit after meals or purge themselves with laxatives. In addition to bulimic anorectics, a large and growing number of young women indulge in this same vicious *binge/purge* cycle (Boskind-White & White, 1983) but, despite frequent, wide weight fluctuations, do not lose sufficient weight to be considered anorectic. The boundaries between this condition, which is termed *normal weight bulimia,* and anorexia are still unclear. In addition to Bulimia Nervosa, the terms *bulimarexia* (Boskind-White & White, 1983) and *dietary chaos syndrome* have also been used to describe cases with mixed symptoms of dieting, bingeing, vomiting, weight fluctuation, and preoccupation with food.

Although known in affluent cultures as far back as ancient Rome, the incidence of bulimia appears to have risen markedly during the past two decades (Kaye & Gwirtsman, 1985). Bulimia (with or without weight loss) now seems to be far more common than "fasting anorexia." Prevalence estimates among high school and college-age girls suggest that as many as 3% to 12% of these young women engage in periodic bingeing and then practice self-induced vomiting to prevent weight gain. The practice is well recognized in the teen culture, even giving rise to the briefly fashionable slang exclamation, "Gag me with a spoon!" It is said that on any given evening in any large women's dorm a visitor will usually find at least one young woman throwing up in the bathroom.

DSM-III-R Diagnostic Criteria for Bulimia Nervosa

A. *Recurrent episodes of binge eating (rapid consumption of a large amount of food in a discrete period of time).*

B. *A feeling of lack of control over eating behavior during the eating binges.*

C. *The person regularly engages in either self-induced vomiting, use of laxatives or diuretics, strict dieting or fasting, or vigorous exercise in order to prevent weight gain.*

D. *A minimum average of two binge eating episodes a week for at least three months.*

E. *Persistent overconcern with body shape and weight. (APA, 1987, pp. 68–69)*

The current revision of the *Diagnostic and Statistical Manual of Mental Disorders* (APA, 1987) changed several criteria that had been included in the earlier DSM-III (APA, 1980) definition to associated features. These include "Termination of such eating episodes by abdominal pain, sleep, social interruption, or self-induced vomiting"; "repeated attempts to lose weight by severely restrictive diets, self-induced vomiting, or use of cathartics and/or diuretics"; "frequent weight fluctuations . . . due to alternating binges and fasts"; and "depressed mood and self-deprecating thoughts following eating binges" (APA, 1980, pp. 70–71). In addition, under DSM-III-R, anorexia and bulimia are no longer mutually exclusive disorders.

EPIDEMIOLOGY

Accurate estimates of incidence and prevalence of anorexia nervosa are hard to come by. There is a general impression that the absolute incidence of the disorder in Western industrialized societies and Japan has doubled several times in the past 10 to 20 years (Jones et al., 1980; Kendall et al., 1973; Sours, 1980), although Williams and King (1987) have presented evidence to the contrary. Crisp et al.'s study (1976) of English schoolgirls, ages 16 to 18 years, found an incidence as high as 1% in upper-class private schools and about 0.2% in the more economically heterogeneous public school system. The same authors estimated that in London the overall prevalence of severe anorexia nervosa was 1 case for every 200 girls 12 years and older. If mild, spontaneously remitting cases are included, the prevalence of anorexia may be as high as 1% of bright middle-class teenage girls.

Most cases of anorexia occur in girls between the ages of 11 and 18 years. Anorexia, at least in its classic form, is usually described as rare outside the middle and upper middle classes; however, reports of sporadic cases and community studies suggest that the prevalence in the nonwhite population and lower socioeconomic classes may be higher than previously believed (Pope et al., 1987; Pumaregia, 1986; Pumaregia et al., 1984; Yates, 1989). Multiple cases have been noted in certain families, and the incidence of anorexia found in the sisters of anorectic girls is about 6.6% (Theander, 1970).

Although many bulimics are reluctant to divulge their bingeing or vomiting, epidemiological studies suggest a high prevalence of bulimic behaviors, at least in the young female population (Halmi et al., 1981; Hendren et al., 1986; Pope et al., 1984; Pyle et al., 1983). These studies found that from 4.5% to 19% of female high school and college students admitted to bingeing. Self-induced vomiting, however, is much less frequent (Schotte & Stunkard, 1987). Thus, in the above population, self-induced vomiting (occurring at least weekly) in conjunction with binge eating had a prevalence rate of 0.5% to 1.7%. Males appear to represent about 5% to 10% of identified bulimics; in college-age men the prevalence of binge eating is about 0.4% to 4% (George et al., 1985); the prevalence of binge eating and vomiting that meets the DSM-III or DSM-III-R criteria for bulimia is 0.1% (Schotte & Stunkard, 1987).

These studies indicate that the symptoms and attitudes characteristic of persons with a diagnosable eating disorder are also remarkably common in nonclinical populations. The findings suggest that eating disorders may represent the extreme end of a continuum on which disturbed attitudes toward weight, eating, and body image are common. For example, surveying the population of two private girls' schools in the Washington, D.C., area, Hendren et al. (1986) found that more than 18% of the girls reported one or more major symptoms of an eating disorder. Thus, 7.5% to 14.6% of the students said that they thought about food or weight "all of the time"; 6.1% to 12% induced vomiting to control their weight; 2.2% to 2.4% used laxatives as a method of weight control; and 7.4% often fasted or starved to achieve the same goal. Even among the girls who did not admit to any of these major eating-disorder symptoms, 23.5% responded that they were never satisfied with their current weight and 44% admitted that they went on frequent eating binges. Schotte and Stunkard (1987), however, have warned not to accept uncritically weight-preoccupied respondents' self-reports. For example, some respondents characterized skipping breakfast as fasting or bolting a bag of potato chips as bingeing.

The development of standardized eating disorder surveys such as the Eating Disorder Inventory of Garner and colleagues (1983b) have aided both clinical studies and epidemiological surveys of nonclinical populations.

CLINICAL FEATURES

Anorexia Nervosa

The distinguishing feature of anorexia nervosa is emaciation due to a deliberate and willful refusal to eat that is carried out in the service of a "relentless pursuit of thinness" as a desired end in itself (Bruch, 1973, 1978). The anorectic has a morbid fear of being fat and resists weight gain by fasting and exercise, and, in some cases, by vomiting and use of laxatives. The anorectic's angry resistance against eating represents her intense struggle with her parents regarding control and autonomy, and it is fought out on the battle ground of her body. Throughout the course of the illness the anorectic shows a fervent and ambivalent preoccupation with food.

Primary anorexia nervosa must be distinguished from two other groups of conditions. The first group—so-called *secondary* anorexia—includes the many other forms of psychogenic food refusal (Bruch, 1973; King, 1963; Sours, 1980); the second group involves those cases where loss of weight and appetite is due to organic illness (Sours, 1980). Most of these conditions do not show the motoric hyperactivity, the stubborn single-minded pursuit of thinness, and the fear of weight gain that characterize the patient with primary anorexia nervosa. Thus, the schizophrenic patient with delusional fears of being poisoned may eat warily and fussily but does not seek deliberately to lose weight. Neither the phobic patient with a fear of swallowing germs nor the hysterical dysphagic have as their goal losing weight or altering their body image. Psychotically depressed patients may have little appetite for or interest in food; however, they lack both the driven physical activity and the energy of the primary anorectic and do not manifest the latter's fascinated preoccupation with food. Differentiation of anorexia from physical disorders producing eating disturbance is discussed in the section Physical Manifestations.

Because girls and young women constitute about 95% of the cases of primary anorexia nervosa, this section will refer mainly to females; a discussion of anorectic boys can be found in the section Anorexia and Bulimia in Males.

Although anorexia can have its onset anywhere from puberty to young adulthood, most cases have their onset between 13 and 20 years of age (Halmi, 1974); the distribution of age of onset has peaks at about $14\frac{1}{2}$ years and 18 years, that is, at about the beginning of high school and the beginning of college (Halmi, 1985a). For males, the peak onset is apparently younger, between 9 and 12 years of age (Wiener, 1976; Bruch, 1971a). Anorexia nervosa may appear before or after menarche; usually it appears after the pubertal changes have begun. For some anorectics, menarche comes relatively early and hence at a time of less fully developed psychological readiness.

The onset of the condition is often insidious, with a prodromal period of several months before dieting and weight loss begin in earnest. Usually, the anorectic was previously regarded as a docile and compliant child; during this period, however, the youngster may become reclusive, testy, and less tractable at home. She may throw herself into solitary activities such as studying or practicing the piano with new-found intensity and energy. Anorectics are often physically hyperactive, perfectionistically pursuing repetitive activities such as running, ballet, or calisthenics without apparent fatigue. Anxiety, depression, and diffuse irritability may be apparent, particularly in retrospect. There is a gradual withdrawal from peers, and any budding heterosexual interests disappear. In about half the cases an ostensible precipitant is present, such as a move, a loss, or a disappointment (Sours, 1980). These events, however, do not usually appear to fall outside the usual range of adolescent experience. When such a precipitant is present, the key factor is a feeling of disappointment either in herself or in a previously cherished other. Rejection by a boy, loss of a close girlfriend, or criticism from a favorite teacher may stand out in the anorectic's mind as the moment at which her conscious decision to lose weight began.

Such a youngster may have entered adolescence somewhat on the chubby side and usually starts dieting with an eye to losing a few pounds because someone has observed that she is "too fat." She may begin by becoming vegetarian, macrobiotic, or strictly kosher. The anorectic may embark on her diet (which quickly sets her apart from her family) with an air of spiritual purity and a "holier-than-thou" dietary superiority. Foods high in carbohydrates are among the first to go.

Unlike her normal peers who find dieting an unpleasant burden, the anorectic throws herself into her increasingly restrictive diet with relish. As she sees her pounds melt away, she comes to feel a heady sense of power and triumph. At the same time, however, she remains acutely interested in food, often cooking elaborate gourmet meals that she urges on her friends and family. While plying them with viands, however, she secretly scorns their gluttony and lack of self-discipline. In short order, the anorectic will have acquired an encyclopedic knowledge of calorie contents, a database that many a dietician would envy. However, she displays a quirky and idiosyncratic pattern of food aversions and narrowly circumscribed food preferences based on texture, taste, and appearance. She dawdles and fools with her food, maddening her tablemates who may have to endure 20 minutes of such "oral foreplay" as her splitting peas into fourths or carefully peeling and cutting a lima bean into tenths and then consuming only half of these bits. What eating she does do is anxious and joyless. When the anorectic's parents push her hard to eat, she may hide food in her pockets or take a mouthful, only surreptitiously to spit it out into a napkin to dispose of later. Increasingly tumultuous fights and confrontations with her parents are typical.

As her weight plummets, it becomes clear that the ideal figure and thinness that she pursues are no ordinary goal. Unlike the normal teenager who may go on a diet at least partly in the service of increased popularity and attractiveness, the anorectic becomes more socially isolated and loses whatever tentative interest in boys she might have had. Her dieting is directed toward mastering her body, her longings, and her sense of needy incompleteness and imperfection. She sees her gauntness as an outer manifestation of inner spiritual grace and superiority. The anorectic's cherished ideal is of an incorporeal "light and airy girl-to-be who [is] free of desire" (Galdston, 1974). Others are horrified by her increasingly skeletal appearance, which comes to resemble that of an Auschwitz survivor. Even at this point, the anorectic may complain of feeling fat; any weight gain terrifies her because it threatens her iron control over her body and appetites.

Despite the youngster's intense preoccupation with her body, she seems indifferent to the physical damage that she is doing to herself, even when she faces possible death. Some experts see the anorectic's denial of her emaciation as a cardinal diagnostic feature, representing a "disturbance in body image and body concept of delusional proportions" (Bruch, 1973). The anorectic may feel curiously estranged from her body and experience its emaciation as happening to something not part of herself; on the other hand, some anorectics feel that, for the first time, they are claiming their bodies as their own and are wresting control away from their mothers.

Paralleling the distortion of body image and body concept is another cardinal feature of this syndrome: "an inaccurate and confused perception and cognitive interpretation of stimuli arising in the body" (Bruch, 1973). Anorectics often complain of feeling bloated and distended after even the smallest food intake. Gastric motility studies show no abnormalities in the gastric activity of anorectics or in their awareness of contractions; under study conditions, however, these patients usually deny feeling hunger and are markedly inaccurate judges of the amount of food introduced into their stomachs. It is unclear to what extent the hunger sensations of the anorectic are truly altered, and to what extent, in the triumph of her asceticism, she denies her hunger pangs. What is clear is that the anorectic has lost the normal capacity for feeling hunger and satiety and can no longer eat in moderation. Many of these youngsters fear that if they relax their guard and permit themselves to eat, they will be unable to stop; this is, in fact, true for those whose iron control is punctuated with massive binges. In about half of the cases, the youngsters periodically gorge themselves, with ensuing feelings of disgust, sometimes relieved by deliberate vomiting or massive doses of laxatives (Hsu et al., 1979). Such bulimic anorectics may show wide, erratic fluctuations in weight. Other anorectics may relax their control only for fluids, but they then proceed to drink themselves into a dilutional, hyponatremic coma.

In her interpersonal relationships, the youngster often appears withdrawn from her peers and from those outside her family. With her family members, however, the anorectic is demanding, manipulative, and disgruntled. When hospitalized, such patients are superficially compliant but furtive and covertly manipulative. Intensely legalistic, they may quibble and split hairs about rules as minutely as they chop their food. Evasion and manipulation are common concerning weight, eating, compulsive exercising, and contact with their families. Such patients show little guilt about deceiving staff; they justify their breaches as legitimate rebellion against what they experience as the staff's repressive, coercive control. Although the anorectic's misery and emaciation initially evoke strong protective concerns, her haughtiness and secret sense of superiority and disdain (as well as her penchant for power struggles) soon exasperate both family and staff (Galdston, 1974).

In most instances, the youngster's mood is anxious, depressed, and irritable. Despite their frequent obsessional and perfectionistic rituals, these patients find it difficult to concentrate, in part because of their preoccupation with food and control and in part because of their state of advanced starvation. Many aspects of the anorectic's mental life may be the direct effect of starvation and are similar to those observed in nonclinical subjects of experimental and wartime starvation studies (Keys et al., 1950; Sours, 1980). For example, the sense of time, space, and body boundaries may be altered, with ensuing feelings of unreality, disassociation, and depersonalization. The anorectic's mental content is markedly constricted with a paucity of feelings, thoughts, or fantasies save those related to food and dieting. Depressive concerns focus largely on dissatisfaction with her efforts to achieve absolute control of her body and food intake. Such effects of starvation as irritability, dysphoric mood, sleep disturbance, social withdrawal, decreased libido, and difficulty concentrating may be difficult to distinguish from the syndrome of depression (Hudson et al., 1983; Swift et al., 1986). There is a shift toward more primitive mental operations such as projection and denial, obsessive rumination, and confusional states (Sours, 1980).

These physiologically determined features make it extremely difficult to engage the anorectic in insight-oriented psychotherapy while she is still in negative metabolic balance. Under such conditions, the evaluator is not even likely to arrive at an accurate picture of the patient's underlying personality structure. Several experts have commented on the almost monotonous uniformity of these clinical features across cases in the starvation phase, with individual differences emerging only during recovery. A striking and telling difference between starving anorectics and other victims of starvation is that the latter usually show apathy, lethargy, and fatigue. In contrast, the anorectic, in a relentless denial of the claims of her body, continues her frenetic hyperactivity even to the point of physiological collapse (Casper & Davis, 1977).

Physical Manifestations. Anorectics show many of the expected physical and physiological changes of starvation (Sours, 1980). The heartbeat slows and blood pressure and body temperature fall. Peripheral circulation is poor, and fingers and toes may show acrocyanosis and Raynaud's phenomenon. As a consequence of these changes, as well as reduced subcutaneous fat, anorectics have very poor tolerance for cold. Their skin coarsens and lanugo similar to that of the infant may appear. Blood changes include hypoproteinemia and mild anemia. An interesting difference between the anorectic and other victims of starvation is the anorectic's comparatively early loss and late recovery of menstruation. (Other endocrine changes are discussed in the section Etiology.)

As the anorectic's emaciation progresses, her vital signs may become increasingly unstable, and hypotension, syncope, and hypothermia may appear. She becomes ever more vulnerable to sudden, overwhelming infections or cardiovascular collapse. Congestive heart failure and cardiac arrhythmias are serious hazards, the latter often due to hypokalemia. Anorectics who vomit are particularly prone to serious electrolyte imbalances.

Clinical Course. Anorexia is a deadly disease with a mortality rate of 1% to 10% (Bruch, 1971b; Crisp, 1979; Sours, 1980; Swift, 1982). Even at the point of death, however, the anorectic may not relent, either denying her vulnerability and mortality or seeing in her death the ultimate apotheosis and triumph of her will. Suicide is also a risk, occurring in about 1% of cases (Eckert & Mitchell, 1986).

The clinical course of anorexia is highly variable. At one end of the spectrum lie a group of mild, transient cases (Herzog et al., 1988a). These may remit readily either spontaneously or following reassurance and firm confrontation from a respected figure outside the family. At the other end are those malignant cases that run a chronic or recurrent course well into adulthood or that end in death. About half of hospitalized anorectics require rehospitalization, many of them three or more times (Dally & Gomez, 1979). Furthermore, although many apparently successfully treated anorectics abandon their emaciation and even achieve normal weight, difficulties, such as preoccupation with weight, restrictive eating patterns, or bulimia with vomiting, often persist for years. Many are chronically depressed and socially impaired. Recurrences may be precipitated by the stress of separations, such as graduation or parental illness, as well as by such psychosexual turning points as engagement, marriage, or childbirth.

The most important prognosticator of adult adjustment is probably the youngster's underlying personality type (Goetz et al., 1977); however, investigators have also proposed a large number of other predictors of outcome. Onset after adolescence, male gender, chronic course or previous hospitalization, the presence of vomiting, persistent denial of illness, long-standing premorbid obesity, and enduring misperception of body size have all been associated with poor outcome (Herzog et al., 1988a; Sours, 1980).

Subtypes of Anorexia. Primary anorexia nervosa can occur in the context of diverse psychodynamics and a wide spectrum of underlying personality structures ranging from the neurotic to the psychotic. Although Bruch (1973) saw the near-delusional distortion of body image and of inner perception as suggestive of a borderline or schizophreniclike psychological organization, only a few anorectics show other overt symptoms of schizophrenia.

On the basis of interpersonal and intrapsychic factors, Sours (1979) delineated two paradigmatic groups of anorectics. Members of the first and less severely disturbed group have an essentially neurotic character structure and suffer from difficulties centered on oedipal-level sexual conflicts (although these are often superimposed on earlier difficulties in achieving autonomy from parents). Members of the second group of anorectics show a borderline personality organization with more pervasive disturbances in the sense of self and greater defects in ego functioning and relationships with others. As might be expected, in actual clinical experience many cases lie between these two poles.

Anorectics making up the first (neurotic) group are often younger adolescents who may be stressed by an early onset of puberty (Sours, 1979, 1980). These girls are relatively unprepared for the rapid maturational changes in their bodies' external appearance and the upsurge of sexual and aggressive feelings that accompanies the endocrine changes within. Such an adolescent feels that her body is only in tenuous control; she fears both her sexual feelings and her passive longings, whether directed toward men or toward her mother. The pubescent kindling of heterosexual drives reignites unresolved oedipal conflicts that had remained quiescent during latency. She experiences incorporative longings and elaborates fantasies of taking in food, of sinking into her mother's care, of being receptive to a penis or to a child developing within. Such ideation especially threatens her fragile sense of separateness, and so she wards off these feelings with hyperactivity, weight loss, and strenuous self-denial. Notions of oral impregnation, belonging to a much earlier period of childhood, may be apparent. Father, brothers, and boys in general may be seen as voracious, dirty, and disgusting.

For girls in the neurotic group, anorexia halts and even turns back the clock of sexual maturation, turning their bodies into either an asexual neuter object or a lean, tough body-phallus. Despite these concerns and conflicts, however, these girls have relatively intact egos and can utilize high-level defenses such as sublimation, reaction formation, and intellectualization. Accustomed throughout childhood to delaying and controlling pleasure in the service of high achievement, such a girl finds in this augmented self-denial and hypertrophied asceticism a ready and familiar mode of coping (Blos, 1962). Under the stress of adolescence she relates both to other people and to her own body in a regressive fashion. Defensively, she retreats to what might be termed an *anal mode* (Erikson, 1950) characterized by an all-or-none "sphincter morality" and a stubborn willful struggle concerning control. Albeit vulnerable, her sense of self is intact, and her object relations are not as primitive or disturbed as are those of the second group of anorectics. Compared with the borderline anorectic, the neurotic anorectic does not experience as much fear of self-fragmentation or primitive merging with an archaic, threatening evil image of her mother. In Sours' (1980) view, although the girls in this first group were compliant as children, they nonetheless negotiated some degree of separation and individuation from their parents.

Anorectics in the second (borderline) group are distinguished from their neurotic counterparts by their serious defects in ego organization, the primitivity of their object relations, and the prominence of their strong pregenital and aggressive impulses. As Sours (1980) put it, "Food substitutes for object relationships. Their primary disturbance is the perception of the self, not simply that of the body" (p. 343). In many areas of their lives they are high achievers; nonetheless, these young women have no sense of identity separate from that of their parents. Although they experience their pubertal changes as deeply disturbing, the core issue for these girls lies not so much in sexual concerns as in their fear of merger or surrender to a mother whom they perceive as powerful and threateningly intrusive. Such anorectics self-punitively castigate themselves both for their dependent longings, which threaten loss of autonomy, and for their independent strivings, which both they and their mothers perceive as hostile and dangerous. Their stubbornly cruel treatment of their own bodies simultaneously asserts their independence from their parents and masochistically expiates their rebellion. The borderline anorectic thus identifies with the mother whom she perceives as sadistically controlling, while at the same time she treats her own body as harshly as if it were a bad, threatening, intrusive object that she must defeat and subjugate.

Selvini-Palazzoli (1965) characterized anorexia as a form of "intrapersonal paranoia" in which the girl projects the image of a sadistic mother onto her own body; this, in turn, she must savagely master and subdue because she perceives it as "threatening, gnawing, indestructible." (A recovering borderline anorectic remarked that she began to permit herself to eat when she came to realize that it was really *her* body she was starving, not her mother's.) Like other borderline patients, the borderline anorectic has poor ego boundaries and a penchant for low-level defenses such as magical thinking, primitive identification, and projection; these defenses are deployed against her fear of attack and loss of self through merger or surrender to a bad object.

In addition to the above two groupings, certain very thin young women, typically models and dancers, have anorectic attitudes and behavior that are syntonic with their professional subculture. Many such young women maintain control of their symptoms; they keep themselves at a low but stable weight and hence do not come to clinical attention (Garner et al., 1984; Garner & Garfinkel, 1980; Sours, 1980). Another related group consists of those "obligatory runners," both male and female, whose extreme commitment to athleticism resembles the anorectic's preoccupation with dieting (Yates, 1987a). Similarly preoccupied with input and output, these runners aspire to an ever-elusive state of bodily perfection and spiritual grace, which they seek to achieve through mortifying the flesh. Like anorexia, this addictive form of running represents a disorder of asceticism.

Bulimic Anorectics. Another important subgroup of anorectics are those who engage in periodic eating binges or bulimia. About half of all anorectics have such spells of compulsive uncontrollable gorging, which abdominal discomfort, sleep, or vomiting bring to a halt; these binges are associated with feelings of self-loathing and guilt (Casper et al., 1980). Many of these bulimic anorectics gorge themselves several times a week and may spend large amounts of money or even steal food in order to support their food addiction. Most bulimic anorectics vomit after meals, usually deliberately. In addition, a few use laxatives or diuretics or purge themselves after bingeing. In contrast to the bulimic anorectics, nonbulimic "fasting anorectics" are less likely to resort to self-induced vomiting, diuretics, or laxatives to help control their weight. Although in some cases it may be conspicuous from the beginning, bulimia usually appears about 1 to 2 years after the onset of dieting.

Bulimic anorectics differ from fasting anorectics in other important ways (Casper et al., 1980; Garfinkel et al., 1980). Those with bulimia admit more readily to hunger feelings and show a higher degree of emotional distress and somatic complaints. Unlike the anorectic, whose eating disorder is usually egosyntonic, the bulimic often feels guilty and ashamed of her behavior (Herzog, 1987). As a consequence, she is less likely to deny her illness and more readily accepts hospitalization and treatment. Prior to the onset of the illness bulimic anorectics generally weigh more than fasting anorectics (they may even be obese) and rarely reach the same degree of extreme emaciation. A large number of bulimic anorectics' mothers also have a history of obesity. Bulimic anorectics are generally less emotionally constricted and have more outgoing personalities and more active heterosexual interests and experience than the pure fasters. Bulimic anorectics also show more labile affect and manifest greater anxiety, guilt, depression, and interpersonal sensitivity. In addition, they are more impulsive, make more suicide attempts, show a greater tendency to steal (usually food), and make greater use of alcohol and street drugs. They also tend to have more food fads.

Bulimia

Normal-weight bulimics constitute another important group of eating-disorder patients. A large and apparently growing number of young people, predominantly female, have severe, recurrent, ego-dystonic eating binges, usually followed by self-induced vomiting, guilt, and depression. Despite their frequent weight fluctuations, they do not lose sufficient weight to meet the criteria for anorexia, and hence are called normal-weight bulimics. These young women, who may furtively practice their bingeing and vomiting in secret for years before seeking help, are usually older and better functioning socially, professionally, and heterosexually than fasting anorectics. However, like bulimic anorectics, normal-weight bulimics also show a greater prevalence than expected of impulsive behavior, such as stealing food, abusing drugs, and attempting suicide (George et al., 1985). On self-report symptom checklists, normal-weight bulimics score higher than normals on such symptom dimensions as somatization, obsessive-compulsive traits, depression, anxiety, anger-hostility, phobic anxiety, paranoid ideation, psychoticism, and interpersonal sensitivity (Johnson et al., 1982; Weiss & Ebert, 1983).

Bulimics binge in order to relieve intense and intolerable feelings of boredom, loneliness, guilt, or anxiety (Johnson et al., 1982; Johnson & Larson, 1982; Kaye & Gwirtsman, 1985; Weiss & Ebert, 1983). As with the ruminating infant (see Chapter 1), their disordered eating appears to be a substitute for a missing object relationship. In gorging, the binge eater hopes to find the relief from tension or the soothing that she fantasizes she would achieve through merger with an idealized mother or lover. Afterward, in her ensuing guilt, depression, and self-loathing, the bulimic fears fatness and loss of control and seeks to purge herself not only of her now-hated food, but also of the badness within her.

Like the fasting anorectic, the bulimic is preoccupied with food and weight. Some bulimics have a prior history of being overweight and begin bingeing and vomiting during one of their intermittent attempts at dieting (Fairburn & Cooper, 1984; Halmi et al., 1981). Thus, although at any given moment a patient may carry the diagnosis of one eating disorder, over time many patients shift in their symptom pattern to meet the criteria of a different eating disorder (Herzog et al., 1988a; Vandereycken & Pierloot, 1983). For example, some girls evolve from obesity, through anorexia, to normal-weight bulimia; in contrast, others may develop bulimia first and then become fasting anorectics (Yates, 1989).

In some series, over half of the bulimics report binge-eating and vomiting at least once daily (Johnson et al., 1982; Mitchell et al., 1981; Pyle et al., 1981). It is not clear how representative these studies are, as the bulimic patients who volunteered may be the more severe cases. During these binges, which average about an hour, the bulimic may consume as many as 3,500 to 20,000 calories (Mitchell et al., 1981; Russell, 1979). Many bulimics have favorite binge foods, such as ice cream, peanut butter, or cake, that require little preparation or chewing and can be easily regurgitated. While a binge is going on, the bulimic feels driven and out of control. Normal meal patterns are lost as the bulimic alternates spells of binge eating and vomiting with prolonged periods of compensatory fasting; frequent weight swings are common. Once established, the habit of alternately binge eating and vomiting takes on a life of its own. Often the bulimic withdraws from social interaction and devotes an increasing amount of her time, energy, and money to this furtive practice. She comes to rely more and more on binge eating and then vomiting to relieve feelings of boredom, anxiety, depression, or tension. In this respect, the frequently drawn analogy to an addiction seems apt. (Occasionally, in some school settings, binge eating may be a group activity.)

Physical Manifestations. The medical complications of bulimia stem from bingeing and purging rather than from starvation (Halmi, 1985b; Mitchell & Bantle, 1983). Thus, repeated vomiting or diuretic abuse can result in dehydration, electrolyte imbalance, EKG changes, and potentially fatal cardiac arrhythmias. The regurgitation of acidic stomach contents may result in a metabolic alkalosis, detectable as a lowered serum bicarbonate level. Clinically, serial bicarbonate levels are often useful in monitoring the extent of clandestine vomiting. Acidic vomitus is also responsible for the dental problems and perhaps also the salivary gland enlargement so often found in vomiting bulimics. Knuckle and pharyngeal abrasions may result from inducing vomiting. In addition to arrhythmias, other potentially fatal complications include esophageal tears and acute gastric dilatation and rupture, with consequent hemorrhage, shock, or sepsis. Cardiomyopathy leading to fatal cardiac failure has been reported following repeated ipecac abuse to produce vomiting.

Metabolic abnormalities and disturbed modulation of cortisol, thyrotropin, and gonadotroprin secretion have been reported in normal-weight bulimics (Devlin et al., 1990; Gwirtsman et al., 1983; Mitchell & Bantle, 1983). Menstrual abnormalities are frequent in bulimic women, even in the absence of substantial weight loss (Hudson & Pope, 1987; Kaye & Gwirtsman, 1985).

Anorexia Nervosa and Bulimia in Males

Anorexia nervosa in boys is relatively rare; males make up only 5% to 10% of all cases of anorexia (Bruch, 1971a; Crisp et al., 1986; Halmi, 1974; Hay & Leonard, 1979; Scott, 1986). Males also constitute about 10% to 15% bulimics (George et al., 1985). As with girls, it is important to distinguish between *atypical* cases (in which weight loss is secondary to other psychiatric disorders) and *primary* anorexia (with relentless pursuit of thinness as an end in itself, hyperactivity, and misperception of body size). When primary anorexia nervosa occurs in boys, it usually appears in prepuberty. Like their female counterparts, superficially these boys seem to be functioning well; on close inspection, however, they are perfectionistic, overcompliant, and experience deep concerns about their passivity and lack of self-direction (Bruch, 1971a). Generally pudgy, these boys equate their fatness with passivity, femininity, and surrender to parental control. The immediate precipitant of their dieting is often some blow to their self-esteem that threatens regressive feelings of helplessness, passivity, and inefficacy. Their weight loss and frenetic activity represent an attempt to free themselves of their passive (and, to their mind, feminine) longings by becoming lean, masculine, and self-sufficient (Sours, 1980). At the same time, however, diminished gonadotropin and testosterone levels (brought on by starvation) may result in impotence and decreased libido (Wheeler et al., 1983). Persistent anorexia may cause delayed puberty and diminished growth with the risk of short stature as an adult (Pugliese et al., 1983).

ETIOLOGY

In attempting to understand eating disorders, we are gradually assembling the pieces of a complex etiological puzzle (Yates, 1989, 1990). Individual and family psychodynamics, cultural influences, genetic factors, and neurobiological mechanisms all play a part in the genesis and course of anorexia nervosa and bulimia. How these pieces fit together is as yet unclear. This discussion thus far has focused primarily on the individual psychodynamics of the anorectic or bulimic patient and has alluded only in passing to the family and cultural setting in which these illnesses occur. A more detailed examination of the various proposed causal factors follows.

Cultural Factors

The recent wave of popular and scientific interest first in anorexia nervosa and then in bulimia coincides with an apparent increase in their incidence. They were the "in" diseases of the 1970s and 1980s. Twenty years ago, the typical anorectic girl not only regarded herself as special by virtue of her asceticism, but also as unique. In contrast, an anorectic or bulimic subculture now exists within many populations of school-age girls, and miniepidemics of at least transient eating disorders are common at various schools. Powerful cultural pressures toward thinness that resonate with characteristic adolescent concerns about identity, the body, and instinctual life help recruit many girls to experiment with bulimic and anorectic symptoms; most, however, do not develop full-blown, fixed eating disorders (Schotte & Stunkard, 1987). Researchers are only beginning to learn which vulnerabilities characterize those girls whose flirtation with bulimia and anorexia becomes a more serious engagement.

As the sustainer of life, food has always been endowed with near magical powers, both good and ill. In almost all cultures, people have intimately linked the customs surrounding food, its preparation, and ingestion to the central values of the culture (Levi-Strauss, 1969). American society is no exception. As noted in the introduction to this chapter, some observers have considered anorexia to be emblematic of a prevalent *culture of narcissism* (Lasch, 1978). Within that framework, self-sufficient perfection and transformation of the body through diet and exercise are regarded as a means of achieving individual perfection (Sours, 1980). The devotees of this contemporary secular form of asceticism often rationalize their regimen in terms of physical or psychological health. Viewed historically, however, it is but the latest manifestation of a long tradition of ascetic attitudes toward food and the instinctual life in general. During the Middle Ages, for example, many accounts were recorded of "fasting saints," young women who defied their families and the church authorities by starving themselves in a quest for spiritual perfection (Bell, 1985; Brumberg, 1988).

Western culture currently emphasizes slimness as an important physical ideal, especially for women (Boskind-White & White, 1983; Garner et al., 1983a; Garner & Garfinkel, 1980; Schwartz et al., 1982). Surveying the measurements of Miss America contestants and *Playboy* centerfold models for the past 20 years, Garner et al. (1980) found a significant trend toward slimness. Yet, these authors observed, this emphasis on slimness was occurring in a society where the average weight of women in all height categories had actually *increased* over the same 20 years. It is, therefore, no surprise that they also found a substantial increase in the number of diet articles in women's magazines during this same period. The simultaneous turn toward gourmet cooking by an affluent society, on the one hand, and the interest in natural foods and "lean cuisine," on the other, represent the same cultural ambivalence toward food (as well as more rational concerns over health).

Women are generally more preoccupied than men with dieting and are more likely to be dissatisfied with their body image. These attitudes begin early, with children as young as 6 years rating pictures of endomorphs more negatively than those of ectomorphs (Yates, 1989). In surveys of high school populations about 42% to 50% of girls classified themselves as fat, although only 10% to 25% of them were actually overweight (Hsu et al., 1982; Hueneman et al., 1966); in contrast, only a small percentage of boys showed such a discrepancy. Correspondingly, Hsu and colleagues (1982) found that 29% of girls reported dieting "often" to "always," compared with only 8% of boys. Data from a recent large survey in this country identified more people who were dissatisfied with their body dimensions than had been the case in a similar survey 13 years earlier; save in the area of height, more women than men were dissatisfied with their body dimensions and weight (Cash et al., 1986). Studies comparing nonclinical subjects' perceived and actual body dimensions found that a more substantial proportion of women than men overestimate their body size (Thompson & Thompson, 1986). To what extent these distortions are culturally determined is unclear.

Although historically the prevalence of cases among the poor, the black, and the working class has been said to be low (Jones et al., 1980), reports of anorexia nervosa and bulimia in nonwhite and low-income populations have recently increased (Lacey & Dolan, 1988; Pope et al., 1987; Pumariega et al., 1984; Yates, 1989). In Hispanic adolescents, attitudes typical of patients with an eating disorder show a weak but positive correlation with socioeconomic class status and a strong correlation with acculturation to the predominant Anglo culture (Pumariega, 1986). Kenyan and Egyptian women living in Great Britain have a higher rate of eating disorders and dissatisfaction with their bodies than do their compatriots in their native lands, where different ideals of the female physique prevail. How the dynamics of eating disorders differs with cultural context has not yet been systematically studied.

Upward mobility or acculturation to contemporary Western norms entails more than changing notions of feminine beauty. It also involves complex issues of women's attitudes about achievement, competition, and autonomy, as well as broader issues of women's relationship to their bodies and the instinctual life (Brumberg, 1988).

Family Factors

The families of eating disorder patients compel attention. In such cases the clinician must deal with a patient and family who are locked in a life-and-death struggle about food that often appears to express wider conflicts. Furthermore, the family members of patients with eating disorders themselves have a higher-than-expected incidence of eating difficulties, depression, and alcoholism.

Various research groups have approached these facts in diverse fashion, according to their own theoretical predisposition. An extensive family-systems literature has studied anorexia and bulimia from the perspective of maladaptive family processes and structure (Humphrey, 1987; Ravenscroft, 1988; Sargent et al., 1985; Schwartz et al., 1985; Yager & Strober, 1985). Clinicians as diverse as Minuchin and colleagues (1978), Bruch (1978), Sours (1980), and Selvini-Palazzoli (1978) believe these families' disordered relationships, communication patterns, and modes of dealing with stress play an important role in shaping and maintaining the child's symptoms. Approaching the problem within a biological framework, other researchers have suggested that the patient and family may share presumed genetically transmitted biological vulnerabilities, with individual or environmental factors accounting for family members' diverse symptomatic patterns. As yet, the data from both the family systems and biological perspectives are merely suggestive rather than conclusive. It seems likely that the pathogenesis of the eating disorders will prove to involve a complex interplay of psychological factors (individual, familial, and cultural) affecting a particular biological predisposition.

Family Dynamic Factors

Families of Anorectics.   In the United States, most anorectics who come to clinical attention are from the white middle- and upper-middle-class strata. However, more than affluence characterizes the families of these anorectics; they are typically perfectionistic, striving, and, despite their apparent successes, ever envious. (As the Duchess of Windsor allegedly put it, "No girl can be too rich or too thin.") The education of these anorectics is a long apprenticeship in the control of impulses and the limiting of gratification; the illness flourishes largely in the soil of family values that encourage perfectionistic striving and emphasize external appearances.

Minuchin and colleagues (1978) have stressed the importance of examining the total family structure of the anorectic patient, whose milieu they call a *psychosomatic family.* Minuchin identified four aspects of overall family functioning that he felt encouraged somatization and somatic solutions to psychological problems: enmeshment, overprotectiveness, rigidity, and lack of conflict resolution. *Enmeshment* is defined as an "extreme form of proximity and intensity in family interaction." Such families display poor differentiation among family members with extreme togetherness and intrusion into each other's thoughts and feelings. Boundaries between the generations are poor, with the parents' spousal relationship being subordinated to their parental roles. In such families, *overprotectiveness* predates the anorectic's illness, with family members showing high levels of concern for and sensitivity to each other's welfare. As a child, the anorectic is highly attuned to what will upset her family. Through the years, the *rigidity* of such families makes it difficult for parents to deal flexibly with the changes in their children's developmental needs. Often culturally accomplished, such families may be highly perfectionistic, stressing the externals of achievement rather than the development of the child's own sense of pleasure and growth. These families often need to see and to present themselves as unmitigatedly happy or normal, save for the anorectic child's symptoms. Because they deny or diffuse disagreement, they neither negotiate nor resolve their differences. In Minuchin's view, the anorectic's symptoms are not simply the end product of these family characteristics; to understand these disturbances, the clinician must regard them as both a regulatory and a responsive part of a resonating family transactional system.

Anorectics often have a history of not having shown much negativism or opposition as toddlers. Within the framework of their families, compliance and good behavior are rewarded rather than separation and individuation. The rewards of control outweigh the pleasures of drive gratification; the high achievement of such children is thus often joyless (Sours, 1980). As a child, the anorectic dreads displeasing her mother for fear of losing her love; instead, the youngster attempts to anticipate her parents' wishes. She does not permit herself to have imperfections, nor can she openly acknowledge or discuss the parents' imperfections. Both the child herself and the family deny aggression rather than cope with it. Bruch (1975, 1978) hypothesized that although the parents of the anorectic emphasize their child's previous happiness and seeming normality, they are poorly attuned to the child's autonomous strivings. They thus respond inappropriately to behavior initiated by the child (as opposed to the child's responses to their cues). As a result, the anorectic fails to develop a sense of ownership of her own body. In their interactions with the child the parents' continual labeling of her feelings and bodily sensations tells the child how she *must* be feeling, regardless of how she does feel; the child thus comes to doubt the legitimacy of her own feelings. Under the developmental demands of adolescence, however, the facade of compliance gives way to a relentless negativism in the form of dieting and weight loss—being a good girl literally with a vengeance.

The proposed family dynamics described above, however, also characterize many nonanorectic families and appear in the background of many adolescents with serious narcissistic, borderline, or psychosomatic pathology. Similarly, the cultural influences that overemphasize thinness, physical self-mastery, and perfectionism are also widespread in contemporary middle class society. Further research and clinical studies are needed to delineate how these general determinants interact with individual developmental and constitutional factors to produce the symptomatic features of anorexia or bulimia in specific cases.

Families of Bulimics.   In comparison with anorectics, bulimics describe their families as more rejecting, negligent, and blameful (Humphrey, 1988). The families of bulimics appear to be less cohesive and organized and to express greater conflict and negative emotions than those of anorectics.

Genetic Factors

Anorexia occurs with increased frequency in the siblings of anorectics, especially in their younger sisters with whom there may be intense rivalry. Concordant and discordant sets of identical twins have been described (Holland et al., 1984; Wiener, 1976). Among female twin pairs, monozygotic twins are more likely than dizygotic pairs to be concordant for anorexia (Holland et al., 1984). Although such findings suggest a genetic predisposition, they do not rule out environmental factors, because parents may treat identical twins in a more similar way than they do fraternal ones.

The Relationship between Eating Disorders and Affective Disorders

Considerable recent research has focused on the relationship between anorexia and bulimia on the one hand and affective disorders on the other. Researchers have suggested that these disorders may be variant expressions of a primary affective disorder; this theory is based on several observations: the apparent high incidence of affective disorders in patients with eating disorders and in their families; altered biological markers associated with primary affective disorders; and the improvement of many cases of bulimia with antidepressant medication (Eckert & Mitchell, 1986; Swift et al., 1986).

Given family patterns of perfectionism, rigid morality, and difficulties with separation, it comes as no surprise that depression is common both in anorectics and bulimics and in their families. Because of the absence of adoption studies, investigators have not yet determined the extent to which this high prevalence reflects genetic as opposed to sociofamilial transmission. Cantwell and colleagues (1977) noted a particularly high incidence of affective disorder in the mothers of anorectics and of frequent depression in the anorectics themselves, both in the premorbid and postmorbid state and at 5-year follow-up. Other family studies have also shown an increased prevalence of affective disorders in the families of both anorectics (Gershon et al., 1983; Winokur et al., 1980) and bulimics (Hudson et al., 1982). In some studies, the morbid risk for affective disorder in relatives of anorectic probands is as high as that found in families of probands with affective disorders. In addition, the families of normal-weight bulimics and bulimic anorectics show a higher prevalence of depression, alcoholism, and drug abuse than do those of fasting anorectics (Eckert & Mitchell, 1986; Strober et al., 1982). Other studies, however, suggest that vulnerability to eating disorders and affective disorders is independently transmitted and that the two conditions are not genetically related (Yates, 1989). Thus, although depressed eating-disordered patients may have an increased family prevalence of depression, nondepressed eating-disordered patients do not (Wilson & Lindholm, 1987).

Empirically, certain antidepressants have proven to be useful in treating bulimia; however, this observation lends only equivocal support to the notion of bulimia as a *forme fruste,* or variant of depression. The far-reaching effects of antidepressant drugs extend well beyond relieving depression; they have proven useful in treating enuresis, panic disorder, obsessive-compulsive disorder, and attention deficit disorder. Furthermore, their antibingeing efficacy in individual patients bears no simple relationship to the patient's degree of depression or to its improvement (Swift et al., 1986).

Neurobiological Factors

The basic mechanisms regulating food intake and body weight appear to be located in specific hypothalamic nuclei (Morley & Levine, 1983), giving rise to the hypothesis that anorexia and bulimia reflect a primary hypothalamic dysfunction (Hsu, 1987). Starvation simultaneously produces far-reaching metabolic and hormonal changes of its own. Consequently, it is difficult to distinguish those abnormalities that might be etiologically specific to anorexia nervosa from those caused by the self-imposed weight loss (Fichter et al., 1984).

Although the evidence remains controversial, certain abnormalities in hypothalamically regulated hormonal functions may not be solely attributable to starvation (Herzog, 1987). Even before losing substantial weight, a significant number of anorectics develop amenorrhea and revert to a prepubertal pattern of gonadotropin secretion and estrogen deficiency (Hsu, 1980; Miles & Wright, 1984; Yates, 1989). On subsequent recovery, ovulatory and gonadotropin abnormalities may persist well beyond the restoration of normal weight. Similarly, for months after weight restoration, abnormalities can be detected in the levels of vasopressin and certain central nervous system metabolites of norepinephrine; these irregularities raise the possibility of underlying disturbances in neurotransmitter regulation (Gold et al., 1983; Kaye et al., 1984). In cases of both anorexia nervosa and normal-weight bulimia, alterations have been found in the regulation of cortisol, thyrotropin, and gonadotropin secretion, suggesting that these neuroendocrine abnormalities may not be solely artifacts of low weight (Devlin et al., 1990; Hudson & Pope, 1987).

The intense, addictive pattern of bingeing and purging developed by many bulimics has also prompted speculation about possible underlying neurobiological mechanisms. Feelings of tension, loneliness, boredom, or depression often precipitate binges (Abraham & Beaumont, 1982). Given the association of bulimia with mood disorders, bulimics may be particularly prone to such dysphoria. In many bulimics, bingeing and vomiting transiently relieve these dysphoric mood states (Kaye et al., 1986, 1988; Kaye & Gwirtsman, 1985). Kaye and colleagues have proposed that some bulimics, much like drug addicts or alcoholics, may come to depend on a frequent "fix," especially when under stress.

Thus, bulimia may involve disorders in both mood regulation and satiety. The same monoamine neurotransmitter systems (i.e., norepinephrine and serotonin (5-HT)) implicated in mood disorders are also believed to play a role in hypothalamic regulation of appetite and neuroendocrine functions (Herzog & Copeland, 1988; Morley & Levine, 1983). This has led to the hypothesis that shared neurochemical mechanisms modulate appetite, mood, and certain neuroendocrine systems (Kaye & Gwirtsman, 1985). Dietary intake in turn may have complex effects on brain chemistry. Because the body synthesizes monoamine neurotransmitters from simple amino acid precursors, the dietary balance of various food constituents such as proteins and carbohydrates may influence neurotransmitter synthesis and hence also appetite, mood, and arousal (Kaye et al., 1988; Wurtman, 1987).

Activation of serotonergic pathways appears to reduce appetite, especially carbohydrate craving (Herzog & Copeland, 1988). Reciprocally, carbohydrate ingestion boosts serotonin synthesis. Kaye et al. (1988) have suggested that bulimics' carbohydrate binges may constitute an attempt to compensate for a central serotonin deficiency in order to improve mood and reduce hunger. Thus, the characterological, mood, and appetive differences between bulimic and fasting anorectics may be reflected in differences in serotonin metabolism. Even after regaining their normal weight, the bulimic anorectics show lower levels of the serotonin metabolite 5-HIAA in their cerebrospinal fluid than do the fasting anorectics.

In addition to serotonin, other neurotransmitter systems may play a role in these disorders. In animals, adrenergic stimulation of the medial hypothalamus increases appetite, whereas adrenergic stimulation of the lateral hypothalamus induces satiety (Morley & Levine, 1983). Endorphins also appear to be involved in the regulation of appetite and separation distress (Hudson & Pope, 1987).

Various drugs that alter neurotransmitter systems show some potential for relieving bulimia and provide another tantalizing clue about possible underlying neuromechanisms.

Bulimia often makes its appearance during weight-reduction dieting. Following the termination of a World War II semistarvation experiment, many volunteer subjects reported uncontrollable eating binges (Keys et al., 1950). These observations have led researchers to suggest that certain patterns of overstringent dieting may distort appetite and satiety mechanisms, predisposing vulnerable dieters to bingeing (Yates, 1989).

TREATMENT

Anorexia Nervosa

The treatment of anorexia nervosa involves (1) restoring normal weight, nutrition, and eating attitudes and (2) resolving the anorectic patient's conflicts and fostering alternative coping mechanisms so that she need not cling to anorexia as the only solution to her developmental quandary. Integrating these tasks is difficult (Bruch, 1973, 1975, 1978). On the one hand, reflective psychotherapy is virtually impossible when the patient is in a state of starvation because her physiological condition distorts her mental content and psychological processes. On the other hand, it is hard to foster the anorectic's autonomy while employing the coercive measures that refeeding often entails. Chronicity is a serious danger, particularly if the focus remains simply on refeeding; many a pseudocompliant patient has regained her normal weight to get out of the hospital and has returned home only furtively to resume her symptoms. At the same time, anorexia is a potentially life-threatening illness; if weight loss continues, it is important to confront the patient and her family's denial of the seriousness of her condition, and to hospitalize her. Hospitalization is indicated if starvation is severe, persistent, and progressive; if severe metabolic disturbance is present; if ongoing direct confrontations between patient and parents seem to exacerbate the symptoms; or if psychotic or suicidal decompensation is likely (Sours, 1980). Many pediatricians hospitalize when loss amounts to 25% of the usual body weight. Hospitalization is often advocated either to provide a therapeutic parentectomy or to protect the child from malignant family interactions; nonetheless, psychological work with both family and child during the hospital stay is essential to ensure cooperation with treatment. Other indications for hospitalization are serious bingeing and vomiting that threaten dangerous electrolyte imbalance. It is important to emphasize to the patient, repeatedly if necessary, that hospitalization is not a punishment but is necessary to protect her life and health (Herzog, 1987).

After a careful evaluation, the clinician devises an integrated treatment plan involving the collaboration of the pediatrician and psychiatrist (Anyan & Schowalter, 1983). Usually a degree of "judicious coercion" (Sours, 1980) is required to get the patient to maintain and gradually to increase her weight. If the patient does not maintain a steady weight gain in an outpatient setting, confronting her with the imminence of hospitalization may be necessary.

Inpatient Treatment.
Many inpatient units employ a highly structured treatment protocol similar to the following one. The physician makes clear to the patient that (among other criteria) discharge depends on her achieving and maintaining a specified body weight, that is, 90% of her normal

body weight. The patient is free to order in advance from the hospital menu for each meal, provided that each meal includes enough calories to achieve a weight gain of about 200 grams per day. (One kilogram of weight gain requires an excess caloric balance of 7500 calories.) Weekly consultations with the ward dietician concerning preferences and overall balance are permitted and encouraged. The patient is required to finish the meal within a specified time limit. If the meal is not finished within that time, the remaining calories are given to the patient in the form of a liquid high-calorie supplement; if that is refused by mouth, it is given by nasogastric tube. Nasogastric feeding, however, is to be avoided whenever possible, as it can perpetuate a coercive sadomasochistic struggle between the staff and patient (Garner, 1985). The patient is carefully observed during the meal and for an hour afterward to guard against her secreting food or self-inducing vomiting. Exercise is not controlled directly. However, the patient is weighed daily or every other day, with appropriate precautions against large fluid intake. If she fails to gain the requisite amount of weight (i.e., 200–300 grams per day) or if she loses weight, she is placed on complete bedrest for a prespecified number of hours that day. Because anorectics tend to be motorically hyperactive, this restriction is usually quite unpleasant. It is not surprising that for such ambivalent and reclusive girls, restriction from visitors or from social activities is often less effective.

Treatment of anorectics is frequently arduous for ward staff because the patient seeks to draw them into the struggle for control that she re-creates in the hospital (Garner, 1985). It requires much thoughtfulness and planning by staff to encourage the patient to learn to feed herself properly, rather than allowing staff to take over and thus deprive her of that function. An additional aspect of milieu treatment is encouraging the patient to learn to choose pleasurable activities based on her own preferences, rather than on either pseudocompliance or prescription (Galdston, 1974).

Psychotherapy. If the change in the patient's attitude and eating habits is to be more than transient, it is necessary to initiate both individual and family work coincident with refeeding. Establishing a treatment alliance is difficult because the patient is frequently wary that the therapist will seek intrusively to control her. Bruch (1970, 1973, 1978) had several important caveats about the psychotherapy of anorectic patients. These children were previously overly compliant with parents who often told them how they ought to feel, so it is important for the therapist not to "interpret at" the patient as though telling her what she really thinks. Bruch (1973) recommended instead a fact-finding approach (which she called "the constructive use of ignorance"), whereby the therapist emphasizes that he or she can understand the situation only with the help of the patient. The treatment should focus on the previously stunted process of individuation. The therapist gives careful attention to the patient's sense of what she feels and thinks.

Increasing the patient's awareness of her own (as opposed to others') feelings, needs, and impulses and exploring her difficulty in organizing and expressing these needs and feelings are key aspects of the treatment. The anorectic's perfectionistic starving wards off both her own harshly critical views of herself and those that she attributes to others; her self-starvation thus props her shaky self-esteem, a support which she is reluctant to relinquish. Bruch saw the main goal of the individual psychotherapy as helping the anorectic to understand that she has worth in her own right and does "not need the strained and stressful superstructure of artificial perfection." The therapist must actively help the anorectic to recognize that her need to be in control wards off intolerable feelings of helplessness and loneliness; in particular, the therapist needs to help the patient see how this struggle leads her to mistrust the therapist. Only late in the poststarvation phase, after establishing a good treatment alliance is it possible to work through the patient's moral masochism and age-appropriate individuation from her parents.

Family Therapy. Family therapy is important, not only to support the rest of the treatment plan, but to help untie the knot that binds the patient and her family; this will tend to prevent relapse on return home. Minuchin and co-workers (Liebman et al., 1974a, 1974b; Minuchin et al., 1978) have utilized structural family therapy, together with an operant reinforcement paradigm of privileges geared to weight gain, as the principal treatment of anorexia. Although not all clinicians accept Minuchin's extravagant claims for the exclusive efficacy of family therapy or the adynamic, adiagnostic, and adevelopmental bias of his systems theory, there is a general consensus that family treatment is an important ingredient of an overall treatment plan. The family format exposes and addresses the family members' enmeshment; the parents' narcissistic use of the anorectic child; the anorectic's attempt in turn to manipulate and control her parents; and the family's mutual difficulties in coping with conflict. An English study found that patients less than 19 years old did better with family therapy, whereas those 19 and older profited more from individual psychotherapy (Russell et al., 1987).

Medication. Medication has been used adjunctively, especially in the hospital treatment of anorectics (Mitchell, 1988). The ancillary use of medication should not obscure the need to elucidate and resolve the sources of the anorectic's anxiety and low self-esteem. Chlorpromazine has been used to allay agitation and anxiety about regaining weight; it may be particularly helpful in patients with evidence of psychotic thinking in areas other than food and body image. In the presence of depressive symptoms, tricyclic antidepressants (such as amitriptyline) have improved both weight gain and depressed mood. However, it remains unclear whether subgroups of patients respond differentially to various antidepressants (Biederman et al., 1985). Caution is needed in using the tricyclics in physiologically unstable patients (Riddle et al., 1991). Experimental animal evidence indicating a role for serotonergic mechanisms in the regulation of hunger and satiety has prompted interest in the use of antiserotonergic drugs such as cyproheptadine. In some short-term studies with nonbulimic anorectics cyproheptadine produced weight gains superior to placebo (Halmi et al., 1986). The effect of all of these agents on the long-term course of the illness is unknown.

Bulimia Nervosa

Therapeutic Approaches. With the recent increase in clinical interest in bulimia, clinicians have employed a wide variety of treatment methods (Yager & Edelstein, 1985; Yates, 1990) including individual psychodynamic psychotherapy (Schwartz, 1988), cognitive-behavioral therapy (Fairburn, 1985), family therapy (Ravenscroft, 1988), group therapy (Mitchell et al., 1990; Pyle & Mitchell, 1985), and pharmacotherapy (Herzog, 1987). Outcome studies of these different modalities are just beginning (Herzog et al., 1988a, 1988b; Mitchell et al., 1990). Given the many personality types and social contexts in which bulimia occurs, it seems probable that no one treatment will be suitable for all bulimics.

Appropriate treatment requires a comprehensive assessment of the patient's overall interpersonal and psychological functioning, as well as a detailed examination of her eating symptoms (Swift, 1985). From a psychological perspective, bingeing and purging may serve several functions: They may represent attempts to reduce tension or relieve a depressed mood; they may take on the form of an ingrained habit or addiction; or they may become a form of masochistic gratification (Schwartz, 1988; Yager & Edelstein, 1985). From an object relations viewpoint, the bulimic's bingeing may represent an attempt to evoke the internal image and soothing presence of a nurturing other; alternately it may represent a regressive use of the bulimic's own body as an object of rage and desire in a defensive attempt at narcissistic self-sufficiency (Ritvo, 1984; Schwartz, 1988). These symptom dynamics may occur in persons of diverse character and biological makeup.

Assessment must address the bulimic's pattern of bingeing and purging, including antecedents and consequences. The degree to which these symptoms are ego-alien or acceptable to the patient has important prognostic implications. Careful evaluation of the patient's overall character organization and psychosocial functioning sheds light on the role that the eating symptoms play in her life and the painful affects that the bingeing may transiently relieve.

The therapist must also assess the extent of depressive symptoms. If depression is present, to what extent is it secondary to the bulimia and to what extent does it appear primary, reflecting perhaps current life stresses or developmental struggles? A careful family history for eating and affective disorders may add useful information about this dimension.

Regardless of the treatment modality and the focus of the issues, the therapist needs to attend actively to the eating disorder symptoms themselves. It is a mistake to believe the symptoms will simply remit spontaneously with the resolution of underlying issues (Yager & Edelstein, 1985).

Medication. In both open trials and double-blind controlled studies, certain antidepressants have proven useful in reducing bulimics' binge eating and vomiting (Mitchell, 1988; Yates, 1990). These include the tricyclic antidepressants imipramine (Mitchell et al., 1990; Pope et al., 1983a, 1985) and desipramine (Hughes et al., 1986), the monoamine oxidase inhibitor phenelzine (Walsh et al., 1988), and the specific serotonergic antidepressant, fluoxetine. There appears to be no simple relationship between the binge-reducing effect of these drugs and either the patient's preexisting level of depression or concomitant degree of improvement in depression.

Outcome. Even with vigorous psychotherapy and pharmacotherapy, bulimia may remain a tenacious symptom. Various follow-up studies have found a 2 to 5 year improvement rate that ranges from 13% to 71% (Herzog et al., 1988a, 1988b). The course of bulimia appears to fluctuate with remissions and relapses. Thus, a recent carefully controlled prospective study found that only 66% of bulimics showed improvement during 18 months of treatment; however, 50% of those who showed improvement relapsed by the end of the study. The coexistence of an affective disorder had no effect on the treatment outcome (Herzog, 1988b).

Chapter 20

Gender Identity Disorders

INTRODUCTION

Nothing about our bodies is taken so much for granted as the fact of gender; conceptually, however, it remains in many ways profoundly uncertain. Although a number of different definitions are available in the literature, it has turned out to be inordinately difficult merely to describe the essential nature of gender. For example, Freud's (1953b) theory asserted that the awareness of the presence or absence of the penis during certain vulnerable periods of development was the critical variable determining the sense of gender, whereas Stoller (1964) spoke of an innate sense of masculinity and femininity. However, the supporting evidence for these theories stems chiefly from psychoanalytically oriented clinical practice, and the empirical investigators have found it difficult to confirm either hypothesis.

During a recent review, Fagot and Leinbach (1985) described several dimensions of gender and summarized a number of applicable theories. Thus, there is the cognitive-developmental theory (Kohlberg, 1966), social learning theory (Mischel, 1966), information-processing models (Constantinople, 1979; Martin & Halverson, 1981), a multidimensional matrix approach (Huston, 1983), and straight developmental theory. Some of the terms used are *sex*, which refers to the anatomical dimension of gender; *gender identity*, which usually means the subjective sense of being male or female (regardless of anatomical sex); *sex-role behavior*, which pertains to how a person speaks, walks, gestures, moves, or otherwise communicates a sense of gender in behavioral ways; and *sexual preference*, which describes whether the individual seeks same-sex or opposite-sex partners, or both, as well as whether the person's own body, things, animals, or some other target is the necessary vehicle for full sexual gratification. Earlier investigators gave great weight to the question of which orifice or other body part was the primary source of sexual discharge or which particular practice was preferentially sought for by the subject of the assessment. Today, researchers no longer emphasize these issues and concern themselves instead with how the sense of gender identity is formed and how it finds expression. In keeping with this developmental interest, investigators have devoted a good deal of attention to when accurate *self-labeling* as boy or girl appears. They have also studied the emergence of *gender stability*, that is, the awareness that boys become men and girls, women; *constancy*, the sense of the stability and unchanging character of gender; and *motive*, the recognition that a person cannot change gender by wishing to do so.

In contrast to the developmental view, clinical studies of gender disorder in childhood have come to focus on rather a different set of concerns. These include:

1. *Effeminacy* in boys and excessive *tomboyishness* in girls.
2. *Cross-dressing* of a kind and to a degree that suggests early transvestitism.

3. *Homosexuality,* in essence, seeking sexual engagements with same-sex partners.
4. *Transsexuality,* as manifested by a person's expressed distaste for his or her anatomical sex; a declared preference for being a member of the opposite sex; and a pattern of behavior in keeping with that declared gender preference.

HISTORY

In Freud's original conceptualizations, the critical factor that dominated childhood sexual concerns was, as noted earlier, the presence or the absence of the penis. As a visible, palpable, sensuously alive part of the male child's body, this organ thrust itself on the youngster's attention in an absorbing way and led to boys' feeling at once gratified that they had something extra and worried that it could be taken away. As for the girls, Freud stated that awareness of the penis led them to feel envious of the boys' special "gift" and hence insecure about the worth of their own bodies and about their femininity. Freud believed that children elaborated theories of castration. The boy with such thoughts would begin to feel concerned that his penis could be taken away and that he could be made into a girl (a condition Freud called *castration anxiety*); the girl would be jealous of what the boy had apparently been given and would be inclined to sustain feelings of longing and inadequacy thereafter (a state of affairs Freud called *penis-envy*).

In terms of Freud's theory, the essential drive that made for sexual engagement was the product of a kind of sexual energy, the *libido.* This libido was the source of sexual yearning; it sought a particular kind of partner (male, female, older, younger, family member, nonfamily member, self, animal, cadaver, thing, etc.); it sought to engage the significant other via a particular body zone (the mouth, the anus, or the penis, clitoris, or vagina), and it sought to do so by playing an active or a passive role (i.e., it sought entrance into the other's body, or it offered to receive the thrust of penetration by the other). Other conditions for gratification might also prevail. For example, excrement might be needed to attain maximum satisfaction, or a dimension of suffering, engendered or experienced, might be necessary for fulfillment. Hence, the description of sexual behavior was complex, with numerous developmental, behavioral, and attitudinal components. In addition, Freud attempted to give a developmental account of the instinctual vicissitudes that shaped the ultimate form of the individual's sexuality (Nagera, 1966).

Alfred Adler (1929), a prominent contemporary of Freud, saw the social position of men as being far more highly regarded than that of women and assumed that the little girl perceived that the role of women involved inferiority, weakness, and lowered status. Hence, little girls would have doubts about the desirability of being feminine and would sometimes demonstrate an assertiveness and competitiveness with men that Adler called "masculine protest."

However, even in those early days, the psychoanalysts did not have the field all to themselves. The biological underpinnings of sexuality were attracting attention as well.

C. A. Pfeiffer, in 1936, and Vera Dantchakoff, in 1938, performed the first crucial experiments on sexual differentiation of the brain. Baraclough and Gorski demonstrated that testosterone was the mediator of sex-specific differentiation of the brain (Dorner, 1981). In 1938 Dantchakoff reported that prenatally androgenized female guinea pigs showed increased male behavior in adulthood. Dorner later found sexual *dimorphism* (i.e., within a given context, males displayed a fixed tendency to act one way, females another) in rats that was dependent on prenatal testosterone levels. Ultimately his laboratory was able to develop an androgenized female who displayed mounting behavior toward a castrated male who invited in a female fashion.

The indefatigable Lauretta Bender, one of the first modern authors to attempt a careful documentation of the syndromes of childhood, described her observations of homosexual behavior in children (Bender & Paster, 1941). However, it was the 1947 Kinsey Report that ushered in a new era in addressing the issues of sexuality on all levels; it was not long before the work with children showed the effect of these studies. The first study that reflected, at least in part, the influence of this new outlook was the Bakwins' (1953) work, *Homosexual Behavior in Children*. In a paper addressed to pediatricians, the Bakwins quoted Kinsey as saying that 50% or more of preadolescent boys engaged in homosexual play "without erotic arousal." In addition to Bender's work, they also cited Greco and Wright who had, in 1944, described a group of 10 youths in an institution; during a time of need each youngster had been befriended by an older man and had been seduced into homosexuality. There was the suggestion that the boys may have abandoned the pattern after losing the friend.

During this same interval, Kallman began publishing his seminal twin studies that reported concordance rates for many varieties of mental disorders. In one paper (1944) he described 40 pairs of monozygotic twins; in each pair one twin was homosexual. After he had contacted the homosexual twin, he was able to locate 37 of the cotwins, all of whom turned out to be homosexual as well. As controls, he studied a contrasting group of 45 dizygotic twin pairs in which one twin was homosexual. In these instances he found that only three of the cotwins were homosexual. Of the remainder, 23 were heterosexual and 19 could not be reached for investigation. The clinician should, perhaps, be cautious in interpreting such findings because the environment of identical twins can be unique. Some of this uncertainty is evident in the Bakwins' conclusion that environmental factors play a minor role in the genesis of homosexuality even though, at the same time, they suggest that the dominating mother needs curbing, the passive father needs encouragement, and the youngster needs help in learning to behave appropriately.

In 1956 Brown observed that although studies on sex-role differentiation had been carried out with adults, practically no work had been done in this area with children. He devised a projective study of 5- and 6-year-olds in which the youngsters made choices for a cutout figure of a child designated as an *it*. In a game format the children examined pictures of toys, clothes, and activities that they could choose or reject for the It child. Brown found that boys showed a strikingly higher and more consistent preference for assigning the It a masculine role than girls did for assigning the feminine role. However, he cautioned that a cross-sex role preference did not indicate a problem with sex role identification.

The modern approach to the issues of incongruous gender role behavior has been in large measure the outcome of the seminal work of three different practitioners: the psychoanalyst, Robert Stoller; the psychologist, John Money; and the child psychiatrist, Richard Green. A number of other serious investigators in this realm such as Zucker, Zuger, Mayer, Person, and Mayer-Bahlberg, have also done excellent work.

Money's research began in the mid 1950s with a number of studies that were directed toward children born with ambiguous genitalia. Money et al. (1955) studied the consequences of sex assignment of babies whose sexual anatomy was not explicit. From the time of birth, these children's hermaphroditic bodies had rendered their sex an uncertain quantity. As a result, early on, the babies received an arbitrary assignment to one sex or the other, and they were then reared according to that sexual identity. In some instances, this was, in fact, contrary to the child's chromosomal gender (as later determined). When the correct gender was finally ascertained, Money observed that severe psychological consequences followed efforts to alter the established state of affairs. On the basis of these findings, gender determination appeared to be primarily a product of upbringing rather than genetics. The authors concluded that once such an anatomically uncertain child had been set on a particular course and had continued to live that way through the first two years of life, it was wiser not to attempt to change that pattern. This was true even if, from a chromosomal view, the original decision had been in error. This "sensitive period" phenomenon strengthened Money's impression that the assignment of gender identity took place by means of a form of imprinting (as that term was employed by Lorenz).

In 1964 Stoller introduced the term *gender identity*, which he defined as a person's sense of knowing to which sex he or she belongs. Stoller thus carved out a single clear signpost that was of inestimable value in the subsequent delineation of the transsexual. He ascribed gender first to sexual anatomy, second to the attitudes of family and peers, and third to a hidden but powerful biological force that drives the sense of gender. He illustrated this with the case of a child with ambiguous genitalia who had been reared as a girl until age 14—with disastrous psychological consequences. Once the child learned that he was a boy, however, and assumed his genetically correct sexual identity, he appeared to recover from his pronounced psychological difficulties and was subsequently found to be free of significant emotional disturbance. In the face of such findings, Stoller introduced the concept of the *core gender identity,* an unalterable sense of gender that becomes established by age 3 years and remains unchanged throughout life.

Stoller believed that core gender identity is largely determined by the strength of the silent biological drive; where this is strong (as in the above case of the 14-year-old), then no amount of social influence, or even the evidence of the individual's own anatomy, can overcome it. Where it is weak, however, and the child is exposed to noxious environmental factors that tend to subvert the youngster's commitment to one gender or the other, then states of gender confusion (such as transvestism) will ensue.

Historically, at just this time attention came to be directed toward a newly defined syndrome called *transsexualism.* In 1966 Benjamin described individuals who were, anatomically, of one sex, but whose sense of gender was totally committed to the opposite sex. The patients would say, for example, "I am a man trapped in a woman's body"—or the reverse, as the case might be. So novel and so striking was this syndrome, that once encountered, it caught the professional imagination. Indeed, the identification of this group and its study did much to increase the interest in the field and to attract a good many investigators.

Richard Green, the third major contributor, worked for a time in Baltimore, Maryland, with Money and subsequently moved to California, where he worked with Stoller. In the interim, around 1970, a new journal *Archives of Sexual Behavior,* was initiated and became one of the rallying points for researchers who were entering the field.

An early study carried out by Green and Stoller attempted to highlight the role of postnatal environmental factors in influencing the formation of gender disturbance. They reported (1971) on two pairs of monozygotic twins who differed radically in gender behavior. The first pair were boys, one of whom was described as being effeminate to the point of prissiness, and the other as being markedly masculine. The other pair were 24-year-old women: one wanted to get married and have 5 children, and the other wanted a sex-change operation. In both instances it was possible to discern important differences in rearing style that could account for the divergence in gender behavior. The authors drew attention to the role of environmental factors in the formation of gender identity but warned against drawing hasty conclusions from insufficient data.

The distinction between nature and nurture continues to be a central issue in the field.

In 1968 Green began a long-range study of 60 feminine boys matched with 50 normal controls. It was the first prospective study of its kind, and it continues at present. A series of papers have appeared presenting the clinical picture of the subjects (Green, 1974, 1987) and their demographic characteristics, compared with the controls (Green, 1976). Some of the results will be referred to later.

Meanwhile, the results of a study on adult homosexuality that appeared in 1973 (Saghir & Robins, 1973) were destined to influence greatly all further work in the field. The investigators interviewed a sizable population of homosexual men and women and inquired carefully into their childhood histories. It turned out that more than two-thirds (67%) of the men had been considered sissies or described themselves as effeminate during childhood, whereas only a tiny proportion of the controls (3%) reported this as a factor in their backgrounds. Among the females, 70% of the subjects spoke of being arrant tomboys in their grade-school years, whereas 16% of the controls reported behavior of comparable character. Later, in their teens, 35% of the future homosexual women were still so characterized, whereas this was true for none of the controls. These data suggest strongly that adult gender deviance is not a late arrival on the scene, but rather the outcome of a lifelong process.

In the 1970s the structuring of research underwent a good deal of change. Biological studies made a great leap forward. For example, in 1977 Ward demonstrated that stress during gestation could lower the testosterone levels in maternal (and hence fetal) rat blood and thus affect the degree of brain masculinization. If the lowered levels occurred during gestational days 14 to 21 (the critical period for brain masculinization in the rat), it predisposed the animal to bisexual or even homosexual behavior.

A new diagnostic manual for psychiatric disorders, the DSM-III, ushered in the 1980s. In particular, the approach utilized in this manual sought to establish specific descriptive criteria for measuring a patient's behavior. Only if the patient's clinical picture was consonant with those criteria could the patient be assigned a given diagnosis. The subsequent influence of this work has been particularly powerful in shaping both the research into and the overall clinical approach to gender disturbances in childhood.

DIAGNOSIS

Symptom Lists and Criteria

In a relatively early paper, Bakwin (1968) used the term *gender role* to describe behavior characteristic of a particular sex. He provided one of the early symptom lists to depict the clinical picture of both the effeminate boys and the masculine girls. For the boy he listed:

1. Dress repeatedly in women's clothes.
2. Experiment with cosmetics.
3. Have posture and gestures like those of females.
4. Avoid boys' toys, games and rough sports.
5. Prefer to play with dolls.
6. Prefer girls to boys as playmates.
7. Tend to be "loners."
8. Ingratiating and clinging attitude toward adults.
9. Tend to be gentle.
10. Helpful around the house.
11. Tend to be unusually neat.
12. Are generally obedient.
13. Show a marked preference for mother.
14. Admire mother's clothes and general appearance.
15. Display a precocious interest in art.
16. Love beautiful materials.
17. Enjoy dancing.
18. Express a desire to be dancers and/or actors.
19. Are often noted to be bossy (bossy and parental toward dolls).
20. As apt to draw a female as a male figure when asked to draw a person.
21. Show precocious and exaggerated feminine behavior. (In particular, their exhibitionism, precocious esthetic development, excessive dependency on mother, and unwillingness to make friends are not typical of little girls.)

For masculine-behaving girls Bakwin listed the following characteristics:
1. Show deviant behavior dating back to earliest childhood.
2. Prefer boys' clothes.
3. Prefer boys' haircuts.
4. Actively object to wearing girls' clothes.
5. Refuse to play with dolls.
6. Choose to play with guns and boys' games.
7. Resent feminine activities such as housework and sewing.
8. Want to play with boys and not with girls.
9. Want to be called by boys' names.
10. Display a masculine carriage and mannerisms.
11. Like to play with other children.
12. Later, may resent menstruation.

A somewhat similar list had been arrived at independently by Zuger and Taylor (1969). These authors noted many of the same symptoms of boyhood effeminacy that Bakwin had mentioned. In addition, they observed that such boys stated a desire to be a girl; role-played as a girl in games; and tended to dress up and fantasy feminine roles in order to allay anxiety. These boys were preoccupied with how women looked, especially their mothers. They had difficulty playing with other boys, who considered them bossy; on the other hand, they were popular with girls because they liked dancing and music (a pattern noted especially in high school). Later follow-up was difficult because as adults they were furtive about their effeminacy or homosexual orientation.

More recently, Meyer and Dupkin (1985) summarized the standard descriptive criteria for documenting childhood gender disturbance:

- Early onset of cross-dressing.
- Consistency of cross-dressing.
- The wish to be of the opposite sex.
- Reversed sex-roles in pretend play.
- Preference for games of opposite sex.
- Favorite playmates of opposite sex.

These criteria discriminate significantly between typical and atypical boys and girls (Green, 1976).

Zucker (1982) reviewed the three major diagnostic schemata proposed for childhood gender disturbances. In all of these approaches, the salient finding (as Zucker saw it) was the child's persistent negative feeling about his or her gender.

DSM-III Criteria

The first schema is DSM-III-R (1987), which employs the term *Gender Identity Disorder of Childhood* both for boys and for girls. The DSM-III-R criteria are based on observable phenomena. For each gender, there are two classes of criteria, designated respectively as *Group A* criteria and *Group B* criteria. The A group comprises views expressed by the child; such statements must be at odds with the child's anatomic gender. Thus, in the case of the prepubertal boy, in order to make the diagnosis, a boy may state that he *is* a girl or persistently insist that he wishes to be one. In line with this, he may attempt to hide his penis, he may pretend to have a vagina, or he may prefer to sit while urinating. However, this criterion does not require that he be unaware of his actual sex. In fact, by latency, all boys know what sex they are—although they may not be happy about it.

With respect to the B group of criteria, there must be *anatomic dysphoria* and/or *feminine behaviors*. The anatomic dysphoria means that the boy is unhappy or disgusted with his genitals or thinks he will outgrow them. Examples of feminine behaviors include:

- Cross dressing.
- A preference for the games and pastimes of girls.
- Female mannerisms.
- Preference for female playmates.
- Rejection of or little interest in masculine activities.

For girls, the criteria differ: The A group is the same, that is, the girl expresses her distress about being a girl and her desire to be a boy. The B criteria include persistent *anatomic dysphoria* or aversion to feminine clothing and insistence on wearing masculine clothing.

The anatomic dysphoria may include:

- Wanting a penis (It is rare for the girl child to claim she already has a penis).
- Standing to urinate.
- Being critical of female sexual anatomy.

In the case of the girl, the reason for omitting any reference to masculine behavior is to protect the normal tomboys from false diagnosis. However, Green et al. (1982) report that most tomboys are content to be girls and would therefore not meet the group A criteria. Hence, a behavioral criterion could be included because, in fact, most adult female homosexuals and transsexuals demonstrate extreme and persistent cross-gender behavior in childhood.

Both reliability and validity studies have supported the DSM-III-R diagnostic criteria. However, several authors have felt that DSM-III-R is not "fine-grained" enough and have sought to distinguish further clinical subgroups that the manual lumps together.

Cross-Gender and Gender Behavior Disorders

The second diagnostic schema was developed by Rosen et al. (1977) and represents the work of "splitters" rather than "joiners." This group sought to distinguish between two different categories of gender disturbance: a *cross-gender identification* syndrome and a *gender behavior disturbance*. Of the two, investigators considered the cross-gender identification syndrome to be the more severe condition, whereas they regarded gender behavior disturbance as a less deviant configuration. The two proposed diagnostic categories differed along three parameters. First, in these authors' view, not all youngsters with such a problem will make statements to the effect that they want to be of the opposite sex. For boys, only the cross-gender identity cases assert such a preference; the gender-behavior-disturbance children do not. Second, the degree of cross-dressing is far more severe in the cases of cross-gender identification. And third, the cross-gender boy has a much closer and more dependent relationship with his mother than does the boy with gender behavior disorder. In sum, the cardinal differences lie in the following areas: Does the boy state he wants to be or should have been a girl (or that someday he will be a woman), or does he play and behave in a feminine manner without making such assertions? In DSM-III-R both behaviors are required for the diagnosis; Rosen et al. (1977) would distinguish between the two in terms of diagnostic significance. However, within the current literature, this distinction has not been widely accepted, and the DSM-III-R criteria remain the most widely used standard.

Stoller's Transsexual Theory

A third and final diagnostic formulation is that of Stoller (1968), who felt that the diagnosis of *male transsexualism* was a distinct syndrome with specific dynamics and well-delineated etiology. The transsexual boy was different from other effeminate boys in two respects. First, he manifested a fixed belief that he was a member of the opposite sex and would grow up to be a woman. Here was no simple *wish* to be a girl; these youngsters insisted that they *were*, in fact, girls.

The second element in the diagnosis was the presence of the necessary and characteristic family dynamics. Stoller considered these to be essential components of the syndrome; without the specific conditions being present the label cannot be applied. The particular familial configuration that Stoller thus required (and that will be described shortly) has not been confirmed by most other investigators, and the validity of this formulation remains uncertain. In contrast to Stoller, the DSM-III-R criteria are purely descriptive; they make no etiologic hypothesis.

Diagnostic Instruments

Zucker (1982) emphasizes that during childhood the condition, by whatever name it is called, will typically undergo meaningful change. The symptoms will usually appear in boldest relief during the earlier (usually preschool) years and then will exhibit a lessening of intensity as childhood progresses. As they grow older, some youngsters display an attenuation of the more severe aspects of the syndrome (presumably in an attempt to avoid teasing and gain social acceptance), although others do not. Thus the diagnosis may be affected by the point in childhood at which the child is observed. By and large, however, it is a stable condition, and, although its intensity may become muted, there is usually much to indicate that the underlying disturbance persists.

Investigators have proposed a number of specific diagnostic instruments to distinguish those children who display signs of gender identity disorder. One of the oldest instruments is the Draw-a-Person test (Zucker et al., 1983). In this test the diagnostician simply asks the child to draw anyone he or she likes. Most children will draw a person of their own gender first; in contrast, the child who is vulnerable to gender disorder will draw an opposite-sexed individual.

More recent instruments are the Child Game Participation Questionnaire (Bates & Bentler, 1973) and the Child Behavior and Attitude Questionnaire (Bates et al., 1973). The Child Game Participation Questionnaire essentially evaluates the games that children play and that they prefer. With slight modifications this instrument can also be given to the parents. The Child Behavior and Attitude Questionnaire is a much wider ranging review of behaviors and attitudes that researchers have found to be relevant in the diagnostic study of gender-disordered youngsters. Investigators recently evaluated these instruments (Meyer-Bahlberg et al., 1985) and found them to be dependable measures for assessment purposes. Although relatively new emergents, both of these questionnaires seem likely to contribute to the specificity and accuracy of psychiatric evaluation. As such, they indicate the direction of future diagnostic efforts in this area, that is, toward greater emphasis on reliable structured instruments for assessment.

A major diagnostic issue that has recently surfaced is the question of comorbidity or specificity of the diagnosis. Is it an isolated condition that occurs in the occasional boy or girl, or is it usually associated with other significant disturbances so that it is best regarded as part of some larger personality configuration?

Coates and Person (1985) make the point that Stoller saw gender disturbance as a unique condition coming from a distinctive family pattern and having no associated personality involvements. In contrast, however, Coates and Person have concluded that "boyhood femininity occurs in the context of behavioral disturbance" (p. 703). They also note that such youngsters are not well related to peers and display poor social skills. In support of this view they cite the work of Bates and colleagues (1973, 1974, 1975a, 1975b), which suggests the presence of associated diagnoses reflecting such symptoms as defiance, tantrums, hyperactivity, readiness to cry, inhibition, and fearfulness. Coates and Person (1985) themselves studied a group of 25 boys, all of whom met the DSM-III criteria for Childhood Gender Disturbance. Of these, on the Child Behavior Checklist, 21 scored in the clinical range for total behavior problem, and about two-thirds did poorly on the Social Competence scale. In particular, in a great many of their cases these authors documented the co-occurrence of separation anxiety and effeminacy. Indeed, out of their population of 25 children, 15 (60%) met the criteria for separation anxiety disorder; this included many with school-avoidant behavior. Behaviorally, these boys had great difficulties leaving their mothers and could not even tolerate having their mothers talk to anyone on the phone. In their therapy sessions, the boys found it difficult to leave at the end of the hour; some of them would fight against departure or would suddenly become very effeminate. In some instances the children had to be treated with the mother present in the room. Moreover, 5 of the 25 youngsters had histories of chronic asthma.

In addition, these children had severe problems with peer relationships. They did not relate well to other boys; girls tolerated them as playmates without developing lasting friendships. Many of the boys were very lonely. They were often teased and hated gym class; these stresses may have contributed to their school avoidance. A significant depressive factor was present in at least half the patients, with many expressed feelings of self-hatred. By and large they were not psychotic (although two of the 25 had transient delusional episodes). On the Rorschach test, however, the majority tended to display poor personality integration.

In sum, Coates and Person concluded that boys with gender identity disorder suffer significantly from pervasive psychological difficulties manifested by social incompetence, behavioral disturbance, and separation problems. The extent to which these additional symptoms are caused by the child's gender disorder and the degree to which they reflect common etiologic factors will be discussed later in this chapter.

PREVALENCE AND EPIDEMIOLOGY

From the outset, there has been a considerable degree of interest in determining the percentage of children referred to mental health clinics that show any evidence of gender disturbance. For example, Zuger and Taylor (1969) studied a group of boys referred for psychiatric evaluation. Of these, one in every 20 was found to be effeminate. They compared this to the findings for schoolchildren in general, where not more than 15% (and usually less than 10%) showed any one symptom of effeminacy. Thus, doll play was reported in 15% and cross-dressing in 10%. Other estimates of these symptoms in the general population are 5% or less.

Among the 26 effeminate boys, the incidence of such cross-gender behavior was 65% to 100%. Symptoms tended to be multiple rather than singular, and enduring rather than transient (Zuger & Taylor, 1969, p. 380).

Estimates of prevalence of gender identity disorder in the general child population are more difficult to ascertain. Achenbach and Edelbrock (1981) carried out a survey on a nonclinical population of children ages 4 to 11 using a research questionnaire called the DIS. According to their parents' report, 3% to 6% of boys and 10% to 12% of girls acted as though they belonged to the opposite sex. However, when the parents asked the child whether he or she wanted to *be* a member of the opposite sex, only 0% to 2% of the boys and 2% to 5% of the girls gave affirmative responses. (When such a survey was made of children attending a psychiatric clinic, the percentages were much higher in each category.) As for the prevalence of adult transsexualism, figures from Sweden (Walinder, 1967), England and Wales (Hoenig & Kenna, 1974), and Australia (Ross et al., 1981), indicate that one man in 24,000 to 34,000 is transsexual, whereas this is true only for one woman in 103,000 to 150,000.

There is a high prevalence of gender disorder among children referred for other serious psychiatric conditions. Conversely, children with gender identity disorder often meet the criteria for other psychiatric disorders, suggesting that gender identity disorder is not an isolated finding but part of a more pervasive psychological disturbance (Coates & Person, 1985). These findings suggest that children with gender identity disorders "are a heterogeneous group, and that the etiology of Gender Identity Disorder is multifactorial" (Meyer-Bahlburg, 1985, p. 682).

To predict the possibility of future gender disorders, investigators assayed the frequency of such problems within the population attending a children's psychiatric clinic at a pediatric general hospital (Sreenivasan, 1985). They evaluated the first 100 boys to come through during a given interval. When all the data were in, the first 50 of these admissions were studied to determine which ones met the criteria for effeminate behavior. Once the researchers had selected this subgroup, they sifted the results of their evaluation to ascertain the background findings associated with the effeminacy. With the correlations established, the workers then used these factors to predict which of the next 50 boys would also rank high on effeminacy scores.

The main finding of the project was that evidence of effeminacy was not uncommon among the child psychiatric patients. Fifteen out of the 100 patients had high scores for effeminacy—although, in fact, not one had been referred for this reason. (None of the 15 had symptoms that were sufficiently severe to merit the DSM-III diagnosis of Gender Identity Disorder.) In addition, a number of background factors could successfully predict the appearance of this trait. In brief, the boy fated to become effeminate was perceived by his mother from birth on as being soft or pretty rather than manly. More often than not there was no father in the home; when there was a father present, the mother appeared nonetheless to be the more powerful parent. She encouraged cuddliness and clinging and devalued autonomy; the child tended to sleep in the same bed with the mother till late in childhood. In time, the boy who emerged from these child-rearing practices was hypersensitive and insecure, and showed strong effeminate tendencies.

In terms of nonpredictive factors, the largest prospective demographic study (Green, 1976) of gender-discordant children reported that gender was not related to the religion of either parent or to their ethnic background or educational level. Nor did the mother's age at the time she delivered or the number of years between siblings influence the outcome.

CLINICAL DESCRIPTION

The Childhood Syndromes

As already noted, in Freud's original conceptualization of the nature of the psychological differences between the sexes, the primary emphasis fell on the presence or absence of the penis (Freud, 1953b/1905). Freud believed this factor achieved a special importance in the life of the child during the phallic phase of psychosexual development (at approximately age 3 years or thereabouts). Subsequent direct observations of children (Galenson, 1974) have made it plain that the awareness of sexual differences comes into being somewhere during the first half of the 2nd year of life, roughly between the 12th and the 18th month, and that a sense of gender can be identified as early as age 2 years, and sometimes even earlier. Erotic feelings appear early in childhood (Bakwin, 1968); young children who masturbate speak of it "feeling good." In short, it is likely that gender and genital sensations are established as presences in a child's awareness and sense of self well before the phallic phase commences.

In the case of effeminate boys, the onset is often as far back as they can remember. Observers report that symptoms have been noted "almost as soon as motor and speech development allowed their manifestation" (Zuger, 1969, p. 1099). In most instances, the father was initially affectionate but the boy withdrew; the effeminate boy had no interest in his father as a person. For their part, the fathers tried to get their sons interested in boyish things and ended up feeling frustrated. In time the fathers became alienated, and the gap between father and son widened progressively. Most of the mothers took a strong stand against the effeminate behavior. The sex of the nearest siblings appeared not to fit any characteristic pattern.

Green has begun an extensive study of tomboys as a developmental phenomenon (Williams et al., 1985; R. Green et al., 1982). In a preliminary report, Green (1974) had described four girls who had shown cross-gender tendencies. They insisted on donning boys' clothes, on avoiding doll play, on engaging in boys' sports, and on associating with boys as their primary peers. These girls stated explicitly that they wished they were boys. The degree of their tomboyism seemed greater than usual, even for tomboyish girls. Follow-up data as these subjects moved into young adulthood showed that they varied all the way from conventional femininity to one who was living as a man.

In their latency years, the boy's tendencies toward effeminate behavior can be very powerful. Because of the social opprobrium entailed, these boys very often strive to suppress at least the more overt aspects of these behavioral inclinations, and to some extent the symptoms tend to fade. Much depends on the attitude of the parents; this can range from gross denial of any problem to the most intense concern about the child's lack of manliness. Parents typically seek help during this period, and active involvement with the father as well as positive support can go far toward altering the child's behavior (although the basic tendencies may remain untouched).

In general, the tomboy girl faces far less social pressure than her male equivalent. Because the large majority of these girls do not become homosexual later in life, parents express far less concern. Behaviorally these girls are inclined to active outdoor interests that may vary from conventional team sports to more generally rugged preoccupations, such as tree climbing, wilderness activities, or exploring. A characteristic finding is a disinclination to don the more obviously feminine garb; this varies a great deal with the cultural milieu, but the tendency to prefer pants (especially jeans) to skirts, and sneakers or boots to obviously girlish shoes is ubiquitous. Where there are sexually grouped clusters, these youngsters sometimes insist on entering into the all-boy games and frequently win acceptance in such contexts. Such girls may disparage their more feminine same-sex peers, calling them sissies and prissies. On the other hand, many tomboy girls are well related to other girls as well as to boys.

Typically this pattern begins to attenuate after puberty. The interest in boys that comes with early adolescence evokes an active desire in these youngsters to achieve within the boy–girl arena, and they address these issues as actively as they formerly tackled sports and tree climbing. The tomboy orientation does not disappear however, and in a variety of ways this element in their makeup finds expression in their adaptive patterns. It often conditions career choice, style of garb, and quality of interpersonal address. These youngsters are more likely to be drawn toward professional careers and are less likely to become hairdressers or to work in the garment industry. They prefer tailored clothes, and they are inclined to be very direct and sometimes confronting in their interpersonal style. On the whole, their orientation is unequivocally heterosexual both in fantasy as well as in the way they choose to live. On the other hand, although the superficial boyishness of the latency years tends to disappear and these women lead conventional lives, the tomboy element persists and must somehow be integrated into the final personality organization.

For the effeminate boys, however, the transition into adolescence often marks the beginning of a homosexual career. During the teen years the pressure of sexual fantasy and erotic yearning begins to make itself felt on a new and intense level; a given boy may find that his arousal is confined strictly to male objects, his fantasies are strongly homosexual, and his desires for love and closeness are directed only toward other boys. Perhaps more commonly the youngster is torn between the attraction toward boys and an interest in girls. This arouses the utmost confusion; a true identity crisis ensues, and the youngster may suffer from great gusts of anxiety and depression. Suicidal preoccupation may color this era of floundering.

It is difficult to generalize about the sequences that follow, and much depends on the social surround. Sometimes the boy's recognition of his homosexual orientation engenders the most profound depression and personal devaluation. The teenager may become isolated and ascetic in his efforts to curb what he regards as unwholesome tendencies. In other instances, the boy's acceptance of the homosexual identity as a reality provides a sense of relief; at least he is no longer in doubt.

If the young person falls in love, it introduces an urgent and powerful variable. He may experience a particular relationship as an ecstatic release. It sweeps away all other considerations; he is in love and that is all that matters. Another powerful element that may be present is the encounter with a society of homosexual peers. Once the youngster discovers the homosexual community, many forces come into play. In general, they reenforce the homosexual identity, and many compensatory gratifications become available in terms of social and companionable supports as well as sexual and love relationships. At the same time, this sort of identification has caused youngsters to distance themselves from the society of their "straight" peers.

The psychiatrist tends to see young people who are in doubt about their sexual proclivities, who are at once drawn to the more conventional aspects of social integration and to gay relationships. In recent years the fear of acquired immune deficiency syndrome (AIDS) has added additional stress and insecurity to the engagement in homosexual practices. Families who might once have made their peace with a youngster's sexual difference now press all the more fervently for the boy to reconsider. To say the least, AIDS has vastly complicated an already difficult situation.

Potential Adult Gender Disorders: Transsexualism, Transvestism, and Homosexuality

There is a curious disjunction between the gender identity syndromes of adulthood, and their childhood precursors. Currently only one condition is diagnosable in childhood—gender identity disorder. In adulthood, however, at least three major syndromes are the focus of recent investigations: *transsexualism, transvestism,* and *homosexuality.* In pure form they are reasonably distinct entities although, clinically, a great deal of crossover exists among them. Nonetheless, enough distinctions are present to make them the subjects of much current research.

All three syndromes tend to have their onset early in life; at this point, it is difficult to divine the likely outcome of a particular case of childhood gender identity disorder. In any case, the *transsexual* is defined by a global sense of belonging to the other sex. These are the people who lay siege to the centers that perform sex-change surgery, and who seek by every possible means to convince the surgeons that they are the proper candidates for such an operation. They speak of being trapped in a body of the wrong anatomy and plead for surgery to right this wrong. Meyer (1982) observes that transsexuals do not deny the realities of their bodies; what they challenge is the significance of that anatomy for their identity. (The frequent presence of deviant character structure and perversions leads Meyer to regard the transsexual state as an expression of the borderline syndrome.)

The *transvestite* has no such illusion about his gender and does not challenge it. He does, however, need to don the garments of the other sex from time to time in order to feel good. This urge may be primarily a compulsive need to act in a way that relieves anxiety; in effect, the tension mounts and mounts and will not allow the person to be at peace until he performs the garbing ritual. Alternatively (or additionally), the behavior may become erotically charged so that the dressing up provides sexual discharge as well as tension relief. In its pure form, the condition is defined exclusively by the wearing of cross-sex clothing; the affected individual does not have to be homosexual. On the other hand, a sizable percentage of homosexuals do engage in cross-dressing.

Finally, the *homosexual* is defined by his or her preference for a sexual partner who is a member of the same sex. As a rule, there is no question of gender identity; indeed, certain homosexual men are very proud of and concerned about maintaining their feeling of masculinity. Nor is there any inherent disposition on the part of many homosexuals to don the garments or simulate the appearance of the other sex. To be sure, some homosexuals do cross-dress, but the majority probably do not. In any case, in all these instances, the clinician is probably dealing with a spectrum of conditions (e.g., borderline, neurotic, or personality disorder), one of whose manifestations is some disturbance in gender-related behavior.

Transvestism (Bakwin, 1968) can be distinguished from transsexualism in several ways. The onset of transvestism is later, the cross-dressing is accompanied by sensual pleasure in childhood, and, in the teens, by masturbation, erection, and fantasies. Transsexual behavior starts very early, and the individual does not cross-dress so much as assume what seems to be the correct garb for the felt state of gender. Normal boys may cross-dress occasionally, but not with the same excitement and pleasure, and not as consistently.

Person and Ovesey (1984) have studied the relationship of homosexuality to transsexuality in considerable depth. They classify two forms of transsexualism: *primary* and *secondary*. Those with the primary form are essentially asexual; they seek out neither transvestitic nor homosexual avenues of discharge, but they do feel transsexual urges (i.e., the wish to be transformed into a member of the opposite sex). The secondary types are either homosexual or transvestite (or combined) transsexuals. They started out as cross-dressing homosexuals, or as transvestites, and eventually shifted to the transsexual level. Person and Ovesey note that, in the pure transvestite or the secondary transsexual, the impulse to cross-dress is compulsive and difficult to control. In the cross-dressing homosexual, however, this is not the case.

DYNAMICS AND ETIOLOGY

Three classes of theory attempt to account for gender disorder: biological, identificatory, and conflict/defense theories (Meyer & Dupkin, 1985).

Biological Hypotheses

This group of theories asserts that the key variables are neurobiological. According to this view, during fetal growth critical brain structures can either remain feminine in development (their basic state), or, subject to the proper biochemical influences, they can be masculinized. This is the essential determinant; all the rest is a matter of shaping influences on an already predisposed individual. Gender problems emerge, as Meyer and Dupkin put it, when the ". . . concentration or activity of fetal hormones is modified during the critical period of their influence upon the brain, leading to an aberrant brain set that governs subsequent gender orientation, masculine or feminine role preference, and sexual object choice" (p. 237).

Clinical Studies. By using various clinical evaluations, a number of researchers have sought to establish the presence of biological determinants of gender. For example, in a study of effeminate and noneffeminate boys, Zuger (1974) attempted to compare genetic and environmental influences. To do this, he weighed such factors as developmental delays as well as other biological elements for their possible etiologic force. Zuger found no difference between the groups in parental age, birth weights, birth order, number of miscarriages, or perinatal deaths of siblings. On the other hand, effeminate boys suffered more frequently from certain maturational or developmental difficulties. They had a higher incidence of inguinal hernia and undescended testicles and were more likely to have had herniorrhaphies before age 4 years than were controls. Enuresis and speech delay were also more common in the effeminate group. Overall, 27 of the 43 effeminate boys had one or more *developmental delays;* 16 had none. In summing up, the authors concluded that the co-occurrence of effeminacy and developmental delays was compatible with a hypothesis of genetic disposition, although acknowledging that there was no direct evidence to support it.

In cases that resist the gender lessons of the rearing adults, the youngsters may insist on changing their sex of rearing at puberty (Diamond, 1965). Even when sex-role deviance is present, the boys tend to tone down their behavior after they enter school because of the social reaction they encounter. The gender-discordant girls endure less social criticism, and their behavior does not change. This can be construed as arguing for a genetic pattern that responds to social pressure. (It is obviously capable of other interpretations as well.)

Genetics. Bakwin (1968) speaks for evidence of genetic influence on gender role. He notes that from birth on, there are many biological differences between boys and girls besides their genital distinctions; for example, ossification of girls is more advanced, and boys are taller and weigh more. In addition, many more boys than girls die in the first days of life (ratio 1:32).

Another suggestive proof of genetic influence is the presence of gender deviance in the near relatives of some of these boys (Holeman & Winokur, 1965).

The Role of Endocrines. A more direct demonstration that biology establishes gender requires tracing out the specific mechanisms that structure the way a sense of gender is formed. Animal studies with both guinea pigs and rhesus monkeys offer evidence of the androgenizing effects on the brain of prenatal administration of male hormones (Young et al., 1964). In one study with rats, castration carried out during the first 10 days after birth had a feminizing effect; if it was carried out later than the 10th day, however, it did not. In another (Harris & Levine, 1962), the critical period for most animals was the second day; animals castrated after the third postnatal day remained masculine. It could be demonstrated that the hypothalamus mediated the effect, that is, the presence or absence of testosterone during the critical postnatal period permanently fixed the hypothalamic regulation of gonadotropic secretion in either a masculine or feminine pattern.

An area of great interest has been the effect on children of their mothers' receiving sex hormones during pregnancy. Hormones with virilizing properties (such as diethylstilbesterol (DES)) have been administered to many women in an effort to prevent spontaneous abortion. In addition to suffering many serious gynecological malformations, daughters born of such pregnancies are known to be more tomboyish than average. In other instances, women have been administered female hormones during pregnancy; in particular, estrogens and progesterones have been given to diabetic mothers, whose pregnancies are always at risk. In 1973, Yalom et al. studied a group of boys, some of whom were 16 years old and some, 6 years old, whose diabetic mothers had all received feminizing hormones to help them through gestation; the estrogen level that reached the fetus was calculated to be particularly high. On measurement, the 16-year-olds were significantly less masculine than controls. They displayed more feminine movements, were less aggressive and assertive, less competitive and success oriented, and showed less determination to achieve. They did less well on an embedded figure task. The 6-year-olds differed from controls only on teachers' ratings, but, here again, at school the experimental subjects were poorer athletically and less assertive than were the controls. Yalom and colleagues speculated:

> There may be more than one developmental route to "femininity." That which is largely a product of psychological identification with a woman and with female peers would be more likely to include cross-dressing, taking the role of a girl in games, and playing with girls' toys. That which is largely a product of a neuroendocrine factor may be more nonspecific and primordial such as general level of aggressivity. (p. 560)

Perhaps the most striking work in this realm has been carried out by Dorner (1981). He observed that among rats, estrogens function specifically to activate female behavior in a female-differentiated brain, and, paradoxically enough, male behavior in a male-differentiated brain. In contrast to this, among primates, only androgens activate male behavior in a male-differentiated brain and female behavior in a female-differentiated brain. From an etiologic view Dorner considers this to be important because if a mother is stressed during gestation, her male fetus may become brain-feminized. Then, after birth, the normal endogenous levels of testosterone will have the effect of enhancing female tendencies, which makes for effeminate behavior during childhood and homosexual behavior during adolescence.

Consistent with this belief, a survey of 800 homosexual men in East Germany revealed that the large majority were born during the stressful war years. Specific inquiry among 100 homosexual men, compared with 100 controls, revealed that the mothers of the homosexuals had experienced a much higher incidence of stressful happenings (bereavement, rape, abandonment by partner, or severe anxiety) during their gestations with these sons. Hence, prenatal maternal stress is regarded by Dorner as a risk factor for gender disorder later in life. It is noteworthy that such sexual differentiation of the brain takes place roughly between weeks 16 and 28 of gestation. To be sure, other interpretations of these data are possible because such life events might also have had nonbiologically mediated effects on the subsequent mother–son relationship, for example, the mother may have become depressed or might have developed a hatred of men, or there may have been a lack of available masculine role models. In view of these considerations, Dorner's work is at best controversial.

The Role of Neurotransmitters. One plausible hypothesis is that sex hormones exert their organizing impact on brain function by influencing the various neurotransmitter systems. Evidence to support this view has arisen in other contexts. Thus, researchers have found female rats to be higher in brain serotonin content and lower in monoamine oxidase than males. If male rats are castrated, however, they too develop higher levels of brain serotonin, whereas if females are androgenized, their serotonin level falls. Moreover, if males are treated at birth with a monoamine oxidase inhibitor (pargyline), it permanently decreases their male sexual activity.

Current research suggests that neurotransmitters can be regarded as environment-dependent organizers of the brain; influences on this system can stem either from endogenous (perhaps genetic) causes or from exogenous (environmentally induced) factors. Neurotransmitters may thus play a role in mediating the impact of various environmental influences such as stress or disturbances in attachment.

Nonconflictual Identity Hypotheses

In essence, the most prominent theory of this kind regarding the origins of male transsexuality is that of Stoller (1964). He describes an extended blissful symbiosis between the boy and a mother of somewhat mixed gender affinities, in the context of an uninvolved or distant father. Given such a family setting, Stoller predicates an intense, virtually perfect fixation that heads off separation–individuation or oedipal conflicts, but only if the boy remains psychologically fused with his mother, even on the level of gender identity. Based on his work with transsexuals seeking sex-change operations, Volkan drew similar conclusions, noting the intense separation anxiety and overattachment these patients manifested toward their mothers (although Volkan perceived this as defensive behavior rather than as nonconflictual fixation).

Imprinting Theory. Curiously, Money et al. (1957) appear to have elaborated a conflict-free theory as well. The author most prominently associated with the imprinting concept is Money. He had observed the effect of early sex assignment in children with ambiguous genitalia, and the powerful role such assignment seemed to play in determining how the child constructed his own gender identity. For Money, such early sex assignment had the effect of imprinting. He suggested that the critical period for gender role imprinting in the human was the first $2\frac{1}{2}$ to 3 years. Puberty, according to this thinking, is a second critical time that allows for limited imprinting. Sears, too, believes that such socially induced sex-typing trains the child in gender qualities as do Kagan et al. and Handrich (all quoted in Bakwin, 1968, p. 624). Aberrations are the result of *misprinting,* in which the response is associated with the wrong stimulus at a critical period. In an early and influential article, Green and Money (1960) reviewed a number of possible etiologic factors: the status of the parental relationship, the sexual preferences of the parents, the child's physique, IQ, ordinal position and gender of siblings, family attitudes (especially taboos) toward sex, desire by parents for opposite-sexed child, tendency toward mother identification, play patterns, awareness of sex differences, and overall mental health. No consistent patterns emerged other than the lack of paternal forcefulness within these households and the mother's tendency to be more concerned about the child's effeminate behavior than was the father. The authors proposed that a genetic factor might be at work but turned to the imprinting concept as a causal paradigm.

Lorenz's (1970) original ethological account of imprinting described a type of biological survival mechanism developed by many animals to ensure the immediate attachment of the offspring to their caretaker: During the early critical moments of their existence, the babies simply and automatically became profoundly attached to whatever large moving presence came into their ken. Lorenz demonstrated that it could be a large red balloon, or it could be the investigator himself; at one point he had a gaggle of little goslings following him about wherever he went. Apparently, a perceptual image printed itself on their awareness and thereafter they followed it and accepted it as their guide for that early part of their lives. Thus newly hatched goslings did not need to be watched or to be taught to follow the mother goose; once they had imprinted upon her, they followed her automatically. This obviously had enormous survival value.

In seeking to apply this kind of thinking to the establishment of gender identity (as Money et al., 1957, construed it), human beings are also assumed to imprint (although in the human instance the mechanism is less obvious). Where a gender disorder appears, a sort of misprinting is then assumed to have taken place. During a critical period, the child inappropriately takes the parent of the opposite sex as the focus of identification and accepts the incorrect gender as his own. But the impact of imprinting is not uniform, although not all of the variables are well understood. Some individual animals appear genetically better or worse at achieving a solid imprinting. In similar fashion, some humans may be especially likely to be shaped by their particular environment. In any case, these authors conclude, having good gender role models is likely to be an important aspect of child rearing.

Temperament.   By the end of the 1960s, Green was speculating independently about *temperament,* a constitutional factor (reflecting perhaps a particular neuroendocrine organization) that makes a child more vulnerable to certain aspects of his postnatal experience. Such constitutional factors could be expressed in levels of cuddliness or aggressivity that would affect the mother–child interaction and presently find expression in particular varieties of gender patterning.

Familial Influences.   Many investigators have sought to determine whether any recognizable family patterns accompany the appearance of gender identity disorder in childhood.

In 1968, Bakwin studied 14 effeminate boys and 3 masculine girls and their families in an effort to sort out possible etiologic factors. He found that:

1. Of the families, 13 were intact.
2. None of the boys' fathers were effeminate.
3. One of the girls' mothers had acted similarly as a girl.
4. One of the boys' mothers had wanted a girl.

Zuger (1970) compared two groups, the parents of effeminate boys and the parents of routine psychiatric admissions. As he summed it up, the marital relationship was not different for the two groups. In the homes of the effeminate boys, there was a tendency for the mothers to be dominant, but not to the point of significance. Nor was there any significant increase in the expressed desire of the parents for girls as against boys. The patterns of parental affection were not significantly different. With respect to parental attitudes toward effeminacy, of the 25 parents in the study, 19 were unaware, confused, or tolerant. Twenty-one of the 22 effeminate boys felt closer to the mother than to the father, but the quality of the closeness was also different. Those noneffeminate boys who were attached to their mothers expressed this by wanting her attention; in contrast to this, the effeminate boys expressed their attachment by aligning themselves with mother in many aspects of her personality and functioning. It is, of course, difficult to ascertain whether such a pattern of family dynamics represents a cause or an effect of the boys' femininity.

Social Learning Theory.   Another nonconflictual group of formulations are those proposed by the social learning theorists (Mischel, 1966). In particular, these theories assume that two mechanisms underlie the formation of personality traits: *direct operant conditioning* and *vicarious learning.* The conditioning occurs when parents selectively reward certain kinds of behavior so that the child tends to repeat them until the patterns become habitual. There are also several types of vicarious learning. One kind takes place when the child attempts to model his behavior after that of one of the parents. Another type of social learning occurs when the parents direct the child to act in certain ways and, in seeking to comply, he makes the sequence part of his own persona (overt prescriptive behavior).

The tendency to imitate can be enhanced when:

1. There is a nurturant relationship between the model and the observing child.
2. When the child perceives the model to have power and to control things that are important to him.
3. When the child perceives that the model's behavior brings rewards.
4. When the model gives direct rewards for the imitative behavior (the parents think that the little boy who dresses up like Mommy or the little girl who acts boyish is cute).

In other cases, the reinforcement of deviant gender role behavior by the parents may be more subtle and less conscious. The combined processes of differential reinforcement and imitation are thus thought to determine gender behavioral choice.

The results of a research project into the tomboy phenomenon (Williams et al., 1985) exemplified this approach. This study compared 50 tomboys and their parents with 49 nontomboy girls and their parents by means of a questionnaire, psychological tests, and semistructured interview. The tomboys preferred rough-and-tumble play and eschewed dolls, in marked contrast to the controls. The tomboys were well socialized for the most part, took the male role in fantasy play, and often (41%) expressed a wish to be boys.

In discussions with the family, there were no differences between the tomboys and the controls on most family variables. When differences did appear, however, they suggested that the tomboys had less contact with their mothers during their early years of life than did the controls. There were no significant differences in father–daughter interaction. Asked about modeling behavior, the parents reported that the tomboys were less likely than the nontomboys to model themselves after the mother or to state a wish to grow up to be like her. Instead, they modeled themselves after the father and expressed a desire someday to be like him. Both the parents and the children perceived the tomboys as preferring the father to the mother.

In respect to their own gender affinities, mothers of the tomboys were rated as less feminine than mothers of the nontomboys and were more likely to have been tomboys themselves in childhood. More than that, as adults, these women were more likely to be in charge of disciplining their children than were the mothers of the nontomboys.

In summary, these data do not seem to present a very strong argument in favor of social learning theory.

Conflict/Defense Hypothesis

In a general sense, this approach involves the concept of trauma in early childhood with severe psychological consequences including:

- Disturbance in object relations.
- Conflicts from an early developmental level.
- The subsequent institution of defensive measures involving regression and symptom formation.

There are several varieties of theory within this framework. The first theory involves arrest of development. This approach assumes that, at a certain stage of personality, cross-gender behavior is a normal presence and that the child ordinarily lives through it and puts it behind him as he continues to grow (Lampl-De Groot, 1946; Stoller, 1964). As a phase-specific state of affairs, the boy identifies with his mother and needs a certain amount of parental support to grow past this developmental moment. If he lacks this support, or receives messages that encourage him to remain at that level, he fails to proceed along his normal growth trajectory, and the gender identity disorder appears (Greenson, 1966).

In particular, where this takes place, a characteristic familial pattern is often present. The mother is resentful toward men, is jealous of them, scorns masculinity, and either encourages the boy to be feminine or accepts effeminate acts and gestures as perfectly desirable forms of behavior. For example, she might call such behavioral patterns cute or funny. The clinician could view this as well as a form of operant conditioning, with the mother responding selectively to effeminate behaviors and thus fostering their persistence, while disregarding the child's more masculine efforts, which are thus extinguished. The fathers are usually the less powerful presences in the home; they may deny that any problem exists or, at any rate, are unable to counteract the mother's influence.

A second variety of conflict/defense theory has to do with the dynamic sequence that ensues in the wake of object loss. If a boy loses the presence of his maternal caretaker or feels that he has (e.g., she becomes pregnant and preoccupied or depressed and withdrawn), he might then seek to compensate by becoming like the lost person and thus retaining her (Gilpin et al., 1979; Fischoff, 1964; Stone & Bernstein, 1980). In effect, his way of mourning is to assume a feminine identity and thus, in a primitive sense, to undo the painful loss.

A third explanatory concept is that of defense against castration anxiety. This hypothesis invokes the classic psychoanalytic formulation—that at a certain moment in development, there is a normal rise in the child's fear of losing his genitalia. In a panicky anticipatory attempt to defend against such an occurrence, the youngster symbolically (and preemptively) "castrates" himself; he takes on a girlish manner and says in effect: "There is no need to turn me into a girl: I already am a girl so do not hurt me" (Friend et al., 1954; Sperling, 1964). In the resulting paradoxical pattern, the boy clings to effeminacy to preserve and protect his masculinity. This pattern often occurs in the context of a boy who sees normal masculine assertiveness as a dangerously aggressive act that threatens either to injure his parent or to invite frightening retaliation against himself. Thus, Meyer and Dupkin (1985) document a case in which "the longing to be a female appeared to compensate for traumatic object relationships and to serve as a regressive defense against the dangers of masculine assertiveness" (p. 257).

Yet another formulation is that of the child's self-defense against the mother as aggressor. The boy feels threatened and powerless in the face of his mother's overwhelming behavior; he gains some small access to power by becoming like the one he fears. The basic mechanism at work is "identification with the aggressor," and the child is trying literally (as he perceives things) to protect himself against being killed or totally destroyed. In response to the boy's maladaptive pattern, some parents attempt to extinguish the effeminate behaviors, whereas others overtly or covertly support them.

The chances are that in most instances, many of these mechanisms are present simultaneously and are acting in concert. Thus, all the children in Meyer and Dupkin's study were involved with dyadic preoedipal concerns (they had problems with their earliest relationships during the oral and anal periods of development). Where the boys disavowed castration fears and the associated phallic concerns (by giving up on attempts to assert their masculinity), these anxieties tended to return disguised as fetishes, scopophilia, and hostile effeminate exhibitionism (dressing in women's clothes, female impersonation, etc.). These boys repudiated the phallus to bring about the reappearance of the lost object or to win the mother's favor. There was a failure of object constancy in the sense of trust in a stable attachment to a parent; this lack was expressed in object hunger (a constant seeking for attachments followed by clinging, smothering, controlling behavior), narcissistic vulnerability (a hypersensitivity to criticism, constant demand for attention, plus an insistent sense of entitlement), separation anxiety (a pressing fear of losing attachments, which causes inordinate pain at even brief separations), and a yearning for material things—presumably as a substitute for persons. General ego impairment was apparent in preoccupation with part objects (which gives rise to the fetishistic behavior), aggression, regressive behavior (infantile posturing and emotionality), and drive regression (preoccupation with oral and anal interests, or with primitive phallic concerns such as inappropriate showing off, pornography, or peeping). In psychoanalytic terms, the boys seemed fixated at a phallic-narcissistic phase. Edgcumbe and Burgner (1975) analyzed a number of such patients and commented that gender disturbance emerges piecemeal from compromised object relations, developmental interferences, drive regression, and ego impairment.

Stoller subsequently narrowed the scope of the nonconflictual cases he had originally described to a few rare patients (Stoller, 1978; Person & Ovesey, 1974). Now called *primary transsexuals*, these cases are thought to involve trauma, developmental interference, and ego impairment. There has been little corroboration of the dynamics Stoller originally suggested, with their retrospectively reconstructed account of prolonged symbiotic attachment. Person and Ovesey (1974a; 1974b) suggest that the reported blissful symbiosis never really happened. Instead, it was a reparative retrospective fantasy constructed by those patients who gave this history in an unconscious effort to avoid the early pain and loss.

Many authors have noted the onset of fetishistic (erotic attachment to objects such as shoes or undergarments that have been used in childhood masturbatory rituals and which become necessary for adult sexual interactions), transvestitic (cross-dressing), and gender-disturbed behavior in children less than 2 years of age (Meyer & Dupkin, 1985, p. 266). Galenson and Roiphe (1974) postulate that the rapprochement period (roughly the second half of the second year of life) is a time of integration among sex drive, self-image and object images; in effect, it is a preoedipal phase of body–genital schematization (i.e., a time when the sense of having a male or a female body becomes established). As a result, at the time of gender formation, children are coping with heightened sexual drives, incomplete discrimination between self and object, recurrent waves of separation anxiety, and intensified aggression. Anxieties about anatomical differences tend therefore to be indistinguishable from anxieties about object loss and global annihilation.

In a 1985 paper, Coates and Person describe their work with 25 effeminate boys. They note that several of the youngsters first began to cross-dress when they suffered a sudden loss of their mother. During therapy the youngsters played out "being Mommy" as a way of "having Mommy" and used the effeminacy to cope with separation fears. The conclusions of these investigators thus emerge at polar opposites from those of Stoller; for Coates and Person, the effeminacy results not from blissful symbiosis but from object loss.

However, Coates and Person note as well that 40% of their group did not display separation difficulties, and this may well indicate that there are alternate routes to arriving at this symptomatology.

Again, these authors challenge the theoretical position that some of the boys' peer difficulties are the product of peer disapproval. In fact, Coates and Person note that the youngsters often arrived at their condition by dint of excessive family approval of the effeminate behavior, with the peer behavior and reactions serving as secondary phenomena.

Cultural Factors

Beyond the three groups of explanatory theories listed by Meyer and Dupkin, the clinician should consider the etiologic force of cultural factors (Bakwin, 1968). There are periods in the history of given cultures when effeminate behaviors seem to be more acceptable, present in greater degree, or encountered with greater frequency than in other epochs. This acceptance also varies with locale, even within a given culture. Religious beliefs, legal realities, basic social acceptability and the availability of social groups, all bear on the frequency of occurrence and the form of this syndrome.

PROGNOSIS

Retrospective studies support the conclusion that early effeminate behavior may be the commonest form of onset of later homosexuality. Thus, Saghir and Robins (1973) found that two-thirds of their nonhospitalized homosexuals gave a history that suggested early effeminate behavior. Zuger (1978) saw a random group of 20 adult male homosexuals and more than three-fourths of them gave such a history.

Psychoanalytically Based Outcome Studies

Turning to more specific symptomatic behaviors, Person and Ovesey (1984) have studied the dynamics of cross-dressing in adults whose gender aberrations were very severe. The investigators concluded that the meanings of such cross-dressing behavior are different among homosexuals, transsexuals, and transvestites. That is to say, although repeated cross-dressing can occur as part of any one of these conditions, in each instance its origins and dynamics will vary. In particular, the homosexuals who cross-dress are acting out fluctuating identifications with a variety of idealized women, whereas the transsexuals and transvestites who engage in this practice are seeking thus to identify with—and in this way to retain—a lost object, presumably the mother. The "loss" referred to here is the psychological experience of failing to achieve an adequate caring and nurturant relationship during an early and vulnerable developmental period. Sometimes this loss is part of a syndrome following the death of the mother or her abandonment of the home; typically, however, the issue is one of psychological loss. This identification paradigm is designed to undo or to compensate for that loss; it extends to fantasy life, sense of self, object-relations, and affect.

Adequate prospective longitudinal data to predict which childhood symptom patterns characteristically evolve into each of the adult gender-disorder syndromes are not yet available. Despite the hazards of retrospective reconstruction, Ovesey and Person attempted to trace the pathological developmental sequences that presage the various forms of adult gender identity disorder. Based on data garnered in the course of adult psychoanalyses, they concluded that the fixations leading to each of the several disorders come at different moments in the sequence of personality unfolding.

At the earliest fixation level stands the transsexual, who fantasies symbiotic fusion with the mother as a means of allaying separation anxiety (Person & Ovesey, 1984). The ultimate expression of this defensive stance is to seek genital change by means of surgery and thus to achieve the dreamed-of fusion by literally becoming the mother.

The transvestite addresses a similar problem but the loss and the ensuing fixation come later in development, and the compensatory effort can therefore employ different means. The transvestite attempts to relieve the anxiety of object loss by incorporating transitional objects—female clothing—into his inner sense of self. A part of his mother (her clothes) becomes a part of him; he thus possesses her and has not lost her. In the oedipal period, the final transition to transvestism takes place; the garments change from instruments of identification to fetishes. If this happens, the use of these garments is associated not merely with avoiding anxiety but with attaining direct sexual pleasure.

Finally, the homosexual cross-dresser is reworking a still later stage in development. Accordingly, he is less concerned with the kinds of merger experiences that so preoccupy the transsexual or pure transvestite and that characterize the first and second years of life. Instead he is coping with trauma by means of the kinds of role-play typical of the third and fourth years. He relieves anxiety by shifting identifications. Rather than becoming one with his mother, the goal of the child's efforts is assuming the mother's power. In effect, he has emerged from the work of separation–individuation with a distinct, albeit fragile, identity. His sense of gender, however, remains in jeopardy, and it is there that he must expend enormous efforts. The investigators believe that these efforts represent a form of borderline pathology.

According to Person and Ovesey, these male homosexual cross-dressers can be further subdivided into two major personality types: passive-effeminate homosexuals with hysterical personalities and hyperaggressive effeminate homosexuals with narcissistic personalities (drag queens). During development, they both show a marked preference for girls as playmates and for girlish things as play objects. The little boy shadows his mother and shares in her activities; as a result, these youngsters are consistently teased by other children. Feminine mannerisms and interest in feminine dress-up may appear as early as age 2 years, and in each case is present well before puberty. Although the dress-up behavior is sometimes said to be merely relaxing, more typically fantasies of impersonating women such as the mother, a sister, or a baby-sitter accompany the behavior. The child shows much interest in the mother's clothes and makeup and is noted to have good taste. The interest extends beyond mere clothing to hairdo, makeup, nail polish, and so on.

In a dynamic sense, the effeminate prehomosexual boy wishes to do to himself, or to a woman, what the transvestite wishes done to him. The transvestite fantasizes that a woman will make him beautiful; the homosexual who cross-dresses wishes to make the woman, and himself, beautiful. By latency, the homosexual boy is thinking of various actresses and identifying with them. In general, these youngsters take great pleasure in imitating, and they display a "mimetic hunger." Deep down they dislike themselves. In particular, they do not like who they are, and they accordingly spend time posing and role-playing as someone else. Their families support the theatrics and, to a lesser extent, the cross-dressing. Role-playing is central to the lives of these children, and they may become very skillful performers. The roles the youngsters assume may be grandiose, for example, royalty, and they often involve pregnancy (with a fluctuating impersonation between the roles of mother and child). The closeness to the mother is not so much tinged with seduction as with imitation. The child ignores his father as well as the usual boyish games and activities of latency. Although some emotional lability may be noted, the child's chief interest is his fantasy play.

In adolescence, the troubles accelerate. Ostracized by peers, such teenagers are often solitary. Typically, they respond to pubertal changes in one of two ways: They may resent the masculinization of their bodies, and in those instances, cross-dressing becomes even more pervasive. Or they may resent the lack of masculinity in themselves and seek and imitate macho models. Cross-dressing is less characteristic in such cases, and later on, their preferred sex partners turn out to be "tough" men.

During the teens, the style later associated with the drag queen appears—typically an arch, sarcastic bitchiness. Person and Ovesey remark that this is a defensive pattern, is common within the gay community, and is designed to elicit admiration. With this show of bravado, these cross-dressers, at once, plead for recognition and declare their independence of it.

As adults, some homosexuals will become the incurable feminine ultraromantics who adore refinement and abhor masculine crudeness, whereas others will be flamboyant, vulgar, and aggressive, and will make a fine art of shocking their associates. Both groups are severely narcissistic and suffer from many identity problems. Miming and imitating are second nature, to the point that some individuals may no longer be sure who they are. The cross-dressing is not erotic (fetishistic) so much as it serves the playing out of fantasies. However, fetishistic behavior (involving an attachment to uniforms, buttocks, etc.) to heighten sexual excitement is not uncommon within this part of the gay community.

The passive hysterical effeminate types caricature feminine norms. They take particular pleasure in having a male companion for whom they act the role of the woman. Through the very excess of their solicitude, ultimately they come to dominate, and they may thus lose their lovers who eventually begin to feel smothered. By way of contrast, the drag queen builds a life around the endless series of balls and parties that demand continuous involvement in elaborate makeup and dressing rituals. Grandiose and psychopathic trends are common.

Within both contexts, a characteristic type of fantasy emerges—the *transformation fantasy* (Person & Ovesey, 1984, p. 178). In their dreams, members of the drag queen group become female celebrities who already enjoy wide acclaim and who dominate with their sexuality and charisma. In particular these objects of imitation can then dominate powerful men. Individuals in the passive hysterical group dream of being the glamorous, passionate, helpless child-waif, who experiences masochistic, dependent need-gratification. In both instances the cross-dressing, the transformation fantasies, and the impersonations give life to the sense of inner deadness and lack of identity that characterize these individuals. During the role play they experience a sense of actually being someone. The drag can thus become addictive.

Because the male transsexual, does not establish a male core gender identity, the merger fantasy is predominant, and the man feels himself to *be* a woman. In the transvestite, on the other hand, there is a *vertical split* (Kohut, 1977), and the self-representation simultaneously maintains male and female identities. There is, however, a general lack of depth and richness to such an individual's personality; the female identity is confined to garments and appearance and lacks all complexity and nuance. To the extent that it continues to be present, however, this female identity does represent an abiding identification with the mother.

In contrast to both these types, homosexual cross-dressers show truly feminine identifications along with intense dramatizations and, not infrequently, emotional storms and lability. Therefore, identity and role often shift and change, but the roles are genuinely feminine. This group of individuals is identifying with mature and deeply admired women; the transvestite and the transsexual identify with a pregenital child's version of mother. The cross-dressing homosexual is so preoccupied with role play and the living out of fantasy that it gives him a quality of being creative; this stands in marked contrast to the obsessive quality of the transvestite. Even the cross-dressing homosexual, however, must devote so much energy to ego consolidation that many of his behaviors, albeit colorful, are in reality a kind of pseudocreativity.

Within these several conditions, object relations vary in keeping with the basic psychodynamics. Thus, the transsexual is committed to merging with the female and wants nothing so much as his surgery. The transvestite is devoted to his female self-object and spends his time and energy enacting that merger fantasy. His world consists of his body in its feminine garb. He thinks of it obsessively, and this infantile symbolic dyad forms the center of his life.

The cross-dressing homosexual, on the other hand, obsesses about romantic themes or magical sexuality. He dreams of being admired, dominating through sex, seducing and controlling. He wants two forms of object attachment: the connection with other "queens," or with women who he views as powerful; and the tie to an erotic other, in whose admiration he confirms his sense of self. He is thus forced into object seeking within the outside world, although his frequent outbursts of emotion tend to make his relationships and the connections he forms inherently stormy and unstable. It is difficult for the transvestite and the cross-dressing homosexual to accept the separateness of their partners, and their relationships are a welter of introjected and projected partial identifications.

Longitudinal Studies

This area of childhood gender disorders is fortunate in having a number of carefully executed and faithfully reported longitudinal studies. They allow for a measure of predictability that is often lacking in the study of childhood disorders. Thus, Bakwin (1968) reported on a follow-up in adulthood of 10 (out of an original population of 14) effeminate boys. Only 3 of the subjects no longer showed signs of effeminacy. Bakwin found that two had become effeminate homosexuals. One had died of alcoholism and cirrhosis; he too had been homosexual with some traces of effeminacy. Another boy had become more generally social but had retained feminine interests and was at odds with his father. Yet another was still effeminate but was no longer cross-dressing. Two others had displayed no further effeminacy, and of the ninth, the mother said that the effeminate behavior had largely disappeared and he now had male friends. Two cross-gender girls were followed into adulthood as well. One still retained some masculine posturing but had married and had six children, and the other, also married, was a contented wife and mother.

One of the earliest and most extended longitudinal studies (Zuger, 1966, 1969, 1978) indicated clearly that early cross-gender behavior predisposes to adult disturbances in the areas of eroticism, object choice, and gender identity. As they grew toward adulthood, 75% of effeminate boys became either homosexual, transvestite, or transsexual. Although the initial symptoms were remarkably similar for all the boys, the outcome was not obviously related to the character of these symptoms. At the 10-year follow-up, 12 of the 16 youngsters demonstrated evidently deviant development; 2 of the remaining 4 were uncertain, and 2 were heterosexual. Most of the 12 were simply homosexual. Of that group, 9 members did not have markedly effeminate mannerisms; 3 did. Preference was generally for the passive sex role, although this particular aspect of outcome was rather variable. One case became transsexual and another transvestite; what distinguished both of these cases was the persistence of their childhood cross-dressing into later life. This stood in contrast to the sporadic resort to this practice by the other boys in the series.

Among other observations, the author noted the youngsters' eventual choice of occupation; these choices included attending art school, studying music, or acting (one of those who chose acting had considered architecture and interior decorating), hairdressing, social work, and grocery clerking.

Perhaps the most ominous finding was that, of the 16 boys, 4 had attempted suicide, and 1 had succeeded.

Green and Money (1961) and then Green (1974) saw five effeminate boys at 5 to 10 years of age, and followed them up 12 to 15 years later. By the time they were approaching or had reached adulthood, three were homosexual, one was probably homosexual, and one was uncertain. Combining these and other studies (Bakwin, 1968; Lebovitz, 1972), at least half of such boys end up with deviant gender adjustment.

Green also carried out a follow-up on the group of boys he had originally studied with Stoller. These youngsters had been observed as children, and a prospective study was initiated. With the boys now in adolescence, Green (1979) concluded that "feminine boyhood behavior as defined by clothing, toy, peer group, activity, and role-playing preferences, does not consistently predict later homosexual orientation. However, from preliminary data, it does appear to load in favor of such an outcome in some persons" (p. 107). Nonetheless, in a later publication, Green (1987) emphasized again the variability of outcome, both for boys and girls, among youngsters who show cross-gender tendencies in childhood.

Money and Russo (1979) followed up a series of 11 effeminate youngsters who had been diagnosed before puberty. Several years later 5 of these former patients could be located. All 5, now in their 20s, reported that they were fully or predominantly homosexual.

In his definitive review of all the available studies, Zucker (1985) concluded that if the investigator excludes the uncertain cases, then in terms of outcome, "70% of the cases are either transsexual, homosexual or bisexual, or transvestitic, and 30% are heterosexual" (p. 150).

Similarly, Coates and Person (1985) concluded that over the long term, some form of atypical outcome is reported in 37% to 75% of such youngsters.

Some interesting observations have been made concerning the individual symptoms. In the boys, the high level of effeminacy is most striking from about age 3 years to 6 or 7 years. Thereafter, perhaps because of social disapproval, it diminishes but usually does not disappear. By the time the youngster gets into the teens, as a rule, only minor residua are seen. Nonetheless, the vulnerability to less overt gender disorder remains. In girls, the masculinelike behavior tends to persist until adolescence and then attenuates, although again, residua persist. Where social sanctions are likely, the teenager tends to establish a more furtive pattern of behavior.

Where youngsters begin to display sexually discordant behavior, the attitudes of the parents are crucial in supporting or inhibiting this tendency. Green (1975) hazards the suggestion that the natural course of boyhood effeminacy, if not addressed by parents, may be transsexualism or transvestism. Zuger (1978) makes much the same observation. Where adult intervention interrupts this natural course, the outcome may be homosexuality.

In Green's experience, a key (and perhaps somewhat paradoxical) variable appears to be the nature of the child's preferred peer group. Where the childhood peer group is heterosocial (i.e., where the little boy plays with both boys and girls), the youngster is the more likely to become homosexual as an adult. Where, however, the peer group is homosocial (the boy plays only with other boys), the adult outcome is more likely to be heterosexuality.

As a rule, the symptoms seen in early childhood do not persist (Zuger, 1978):

> What seems to be happening as one follows these children, is a kind of "decay" or burning out of these symptoms, completely in some, partially in others, and not at all in a few. This gives rise to the spectrum of cases actually seen. (p. 368)

In fact, Zucker et al. (1985) recently explored this pattern by taking a careful observational cross-section of a number of such boys, paying special attention to their symptoms (effeminate mannerisms, gait, play patterns, etc.) and then repeating the studies one year later. The siblings of these youngsters served as controls and received the same evaluative tests. It turned out that evaluators could reliably discriminate the sex-atypical children from the controls. More than that, one year later, the gender-atypical group continued to display its distinguishing features; however, some members showed a decrease in the cross-gender behavior whereas others maintained it at the same level. The authors speculate that there might be at least two different populations here, and that "such within-group variations may be related to long-term differences in both psychosocial and psychosexual behavior" (p. 718).

One interesting observation is the relatively low rate of transsexuality among those effeminate boys followed up in the various studies. This rate may occur because among the families who do come to professional attention, either the family attitudes are already changing, or the mental health efforts that are then invoked may, separately or together, redirect the potential transsexual away from that particular outcome. It is also possible that transsexualism is a very rare phenomenon, which would make it hard to trace statistically within the framework of a prospective study. In any case, Green (1974) observed that most adult transsexuals were never brought to medical attention as children.

On the other hand, the likelihood of a homosexual outcome is very well documented indeed.

THERAPY

One issue that must be addressed is whether cross-gender–identified children should be treated at all. If homosexuality is not to be construed as a pejorative term, or, more to the point, to be diagnosed as a psychiatric disorder, then why treat a child who manifests tendencies to develop in that direction? Indeed, many parents who are initially upset by recognizing homosexual tendencies in their child eventually come to accept this outcome reasonably well (Zucker, 1985, p. 116). At best, the physician does have the obligation to inform the parents of this finding. However, two reasons for active intervention have been advanced (Zucker, 1985): The affected child is at risk for transsexualism and transvestism, as well as for homosexuality, and these have serious consequences for the life course; during childhood, especially late childhood, peer ostracism can weigh heavily on a child's development. Zucker remarks that he is "not convinced that this rationale is a compelling one." He states further that a more reasonable treatment goal is to make children feel more comfortable about their sex.

In any case, numerous investigators employing a number of different modalities have attempted to treat such children. Thus, Meyer and Dupkin (1985) treated 12 children with signs of gender disturbance. Because the children were so young, the therapists could not limit their work to the usual tactics of the psychotherapist, that is, encouraging the elaboration of material, clarification, and interpretation. However, the therapists sought as best they could to maintain a psychodynamic posture; that is, they avoided resorting to explanation, education, and suggestion as much as possible and maintained therapeutic neutrality. Their major strategy was to seek the recovery, expression, and discussion of the underlying conflict.

Other therapists maintain that nonconflictual processes are responsible for such symptoms. Accordingly, in their therapeutic efforts these clinicians employ explanation, suggestion, and modeling as primary instruments for change.

Bakwin (1968) advocates that the therapist indicate approval of appropriate gender-role behavior and disapproval of deviance—but not too vigorous disapproval, lest it engender feelings of failure, loss of self-esteem, guilt, and futility. Fathers should be encouraged to become more involved in the boy's everyday activities, or, father lacking, some other male presence should take an active role in the boy's life. There is no place for nagging, teasing, or ridiculing t child or punishing him for effeminate behavior.
He should not be allowed to associate with homosexuals who may act seductively toward him. (Those homosexuals who have been studied as adults have reported that their first sexual experiences occurred at very early ages.) Placement in coeducational schools is preferable. If the boy shows any tendencies to be a loner, parents and therapist should address this pattern and encourage socialization. The clinician needs to explore and review the parental attitudes toward sex and provide adequate information to the child. The gender-disordered child is often a lonely social outsider. His peers will not talk with him, he fails to get the corrective experience of social exchange, and he is likely to harbor distorted ideas.

In a series of papers, Green, in collaboration with various colleagues, set out the principles for managing cases of gender incongruence in boys. The initial statement (Green & Money, 1961) offered 13 principles:

1. Identify the extent to which such a gender problem really exists.
2. Interview each parent separately. Sometimes one or the other (usually the father) plays ostrich to the existence of the difficulty.
3. Interview the child alone to ascertain whether he knows the reason for his referral. It is wise for the doctor to initiate discussion if necessary.
4. Where it is evident that the problem is present, convey to the parents that the child has a chronic handicap and needs support rather than criticism.
5. Get the parents to see that these are not physiological but psychological problems, although that does not make treating them any easier. Emphasize the advantages of early intervention.
6. Respect the fact that the child cannot change himself by will power. There are limitations to what the therapist can do, it takes time, and there may be regressions.
7. As therapist, do not veto any particular effeminate behavior. The child needs to feel the therapist's acceptance.
8. Encourage the father, or other male family member, to involve himself with the child as actively as possible.
9. Explore the amount of time spent by the child with same-sex peers, and gently encourage him to increase such contacts. Some individual tutoring in game-playing skills may help.

10. Observe parental patterns that might support girlishness and that might interfere with attempts at more masculine behavior.

11. Study the sexual patterns of the parents and their ways of relating to one another.

12. Explore the details of the child's sexual education and the extent of his knowledge. In particular, how aware is the child of the fixed character of sexual anatomy?

13. In the earliest formulation, the 13th principle was a suggestion to arrange for follow-up at 6-month intervals. Subsequently the authors recognized that more extended courses of therapy were indicated along with appropriate follow-up.

The later papers (Green, 1969; Green et al., 1972) further developed these ideas with the addition of special attention to the sex of the therapist. Green and his colleagues emphasized the importance, for two reasons, of having a male therapist treat such a boy: the therapist provides an important role model, and the therapist makes up for the (relatively) absent father (although the therapist avoids competitive play or activities that the child might find threatening). The tendencies of the families in these studies to support the feminine posturing was evident in their readiness to photograph the child in dress-up and to gush over his effeminacy as cute. The therapist must interrupt these behaviors and consistently disapprove of this family attitude. The parents' ability to tolerate the child's reaction to frustration is crucial. Moreover, the parents, especially the fathers, have to learn to reinforce more masculine behavior; often they need special support to do so. This may require reorienting the balance of power within the family so that the existing male role no longer emerges as passive, denigrated, and second best.

As for the boy's environment, some regulation of peer exposure can be essayed. Parents can discourage play with girls and attempt to find some less boisterous and less aggressive boys to be the child's playmates. On an individual level, the therapist can sensitize the child to his own gait and gestures and teach him to behave differently. The child can be coached and assisted to learn many acceptably masculine games and play activities that are not excessively rough or frightening. Work with a therapist whom the child comes to trust can help him address his fantasies and inner preoccupations and give him insight into his motivations. Identification with a therapist who is comfortable in his maleness is, in Green's opinion, of considerable value.

Finally, this work addresses effeminacy as such; its effects on the possible later emergence of homosexuality are unknown.

In a recent project aimed at evaluating the stability of gender-discordant behavior during childhood, Zucker et al. (1985) also studied the effects of therapy on the expression of such behavior. The findings suggested both a *dosage* and a *therapy-characteristic* effect, that is, the number of sessions (dosage) for both children and parents was a significant factor, and the amount of time in therapy specifically devoted to work on gender issues (therapy-characteristic) made an important difference as well. It was particularly noteworthy that the authors could trace a highly significant influence to the amount of work with parents, more so, in fact, than they could account for by the child work. However, the efforts on the part of the child therapists to work out the underlying dynamics of the condition during the play sessions with the individual children were also determined to be of considerable significance.

Overall, researchers have found therapeutic intervention to be helpful; indeed, even boys who have merely been evaluated for gender difficulties without receiving subsequent formal therapy of any kind have shown improvement (Green, 1975, p. 342).

Behavior modification, in the form of positive and negative reinforcement within the laboratory (Rekers & Lovaas, 1974) and within the home (Bates et al., 1975b), has been tried both by itself and in conjunction with group work, all with some evident benefit. The goal of Rekers' work in particular was to extinguish feminine behavior and to develop masculine behavior in boys with evidence of cross-gender identity. Eight children were treated (summarized in table form in Zucker, 1985, pp. 118–122). The following techniques were used: (1) social attention and differential social reinforcement by an adult for the sex-appropriate play along with verbal prompting by the mother for the avoidance of cross-sexed toys, (2) having the mother engage in such gender-inappropriate play as a means of telling him not to do so. Although these approaches did lessen the amount of cross-sex play, they did not generalize well to situations other than the play therapy. However, the addition of self-monitoring and self-reinforcing procedures had an equivocal impact.

Using similar techniques, the same investigators have attempted to modify nine specific effeminate mannerisms (flexed elbow, limping-the-wrist, feminine running, etc.). They utilized such behavioral tactics as maternal prompts, response costs, training the child before a TV monitor, modeling, and reinforcement of successive approximations.

Other investigators (Hay et al., 1981) have used covert modeling procedures to teach an effeminate boy to imagine how the 6-Million-Dollar Man would carry out one of the target behaviors, and then do it that way. The authors felt that the method showed promise.

The long-range follow-up with the behaviorally treated children has characteristically indicated the disappearance of much of the cross-gender behavior; indeed, investigators could no longer distinguish these patients behaviorally from the other children in their immediate environment. Group therapy has been essayed (Green & Fuller, 1973; Bates et al., 1975a) with ambiguous results. A male therapist saw a group of effeminate boys together, and their parents in a parallel but separate group process. The focus was on encouraging father–son interaction. In particular, it is uncertain whether the group work with the youngsters or with the parents is more influential. In any case, formal behavioral and group approaches seem worth pursuing as part of a broad spectrum approach to the treatment of gender identity disorders. The physician should always keep in mind the same caveat noted for individual therapy: It is unclear whether these approaches reduce the child's vulnerability to the later development of gender difficulties in adulthood.

PART VI

Impact of Traumatic Environments

Chapter 21

Child Physical Abuse

INTRODUCTION

The past two decades have seen an explosion in public and medical awareness of the alarming magnitude of physical and emotional child abuse, neglect, and sexual exploitation. Since the passage of state laws based on the Children's Bureau's 1963 Model Child Abuse Reporting Statute, the number of abuse cases reported has risen dramatically; for example, reports of child abuse in the state of Florida jumped from 10 cases in 1968 to more than 30,000 in 1972 (Kempe & Kempe, 1978). Yet most evidence indicates that it is not so much the actual incidence of child abuse that has suddenly increased; rather, our awareness of it has grown.

Throughout most of human history, the mistreatment and even the death of children have been matters of relative social indifference (Radbill, 1980; Robin, 1982; for a dissenting view, see Demos, 1986; Kroll & Bachrach, 1986). High infant mortality rates, widespread poverty, and a culturally sanctioned view of children as chattels in need of punitive discipline made the lives of many children (to invoke the spirit of Hobbes) nasty, mean, brutish, and short. Even societies whose cultural achievements were otherwise impressive have frequently treated their children badly. For example, the worldly Roman historian Tacitus, in his history of the Judean campaign, regarded the Jews' abhorrence of child sacrifice as a quaint and unusual scruple. During the Industrial Revolution, the pauper apprentice system subjected thousands of children, many as young as five years of age, to long hours of brutal and dangerous factory labor. Even the passage of the first Factory Act in 1802 protected only pauper and orphan children; it did nothing for those still under their parents' supervision. Today, in many countries such as China, infanticide, especially of female infants, remains a widespread (if not an officially tolerated) practice (Burke, 1984); throughout history this practice has probably served as the most commonly employed means of population control.

The 18th and 19th centuries saw a gradual change in European societies' attitudes toward children. Under the influence of the Enlightenment and writers such as Rousseau, concern for children as cherished beings requiring special protection and treatment became more widespread (Aries, 1962; Robin, 1982).

In this country, the first half of the 19th century saw the establishment of houses of refuge in several of the states. Although intended primarily for wayward children, these shelters also admitted children who were neglected and abused. During the same period, state courts first established the principle that in extreme cases children could be removed from the care of their parents and placed in the hands of an institution that would act *in loco parentis*. Such actions, however, appear to have been rare exceptions. The case of Mary Ellen, a young girl who was regularly beaten and starved by her adoptive parents inspired the founding of the Society for the Prevention of Cruelty to Children in 1871. Because of the absence of child protection laws, initially people could do little to help Mary Ellen. According to several accounts, concerned church workers were finally able to obtain help from the authorities only by involving key members of the Society for the Prevention of Cruelty to Animals.

Although 17th-century physicians described autopsy findings of children who had died of trauma, the first systematic medicolegal study of child abuse was Ambroise Tardieu's *Étude médico-légale sur l'infanticide* (1868). Tardieu summarized the autopsies of 32 children who had met violent deaths. He noted that the perpetrators were usually the parents and that they often gave suspicious accounts of the injuries. Although the X ray had not yet been invented, Tardieu noted that these children displayed multiple traumatic lesions of bone, skin, and brain.

Widespread medical recognition of child abuse did not come until a century later, with the publication of Kempe and colleagues' (1962) now-classic paper, "The Battered Child Syndrome." These authors described a pattern of serious physical abuse, generally inflicted by a parent or foster parent. They urged that the clinician seriously consider the syndrome in any child exhibiting unexplained fractures, subdural hematoma, failure to thrive, bruises, or sudden death, especially when the extent of the injury is at variance with the history given. In their opinion, ongoing abuse is especially likely when X rays reveal multiple fractures in different stages of healing. Kempe and his colleagues also commented on the extent to which physicians miss abuse because of an emotional unwillingness to consider the diagnosis.

The publication of this paper galvanized medical, legislative, and media attention on the problem of child abuse and neglect. A crescendo of activity at the local, state, and federal levels culminated in the establishment of protective service agencies and mandatory reporting laws in all of the states. It also led to the creation of the National Center on Child Abuse and Neglect for the purpose of funding research and demonstration projects and coordinating and assisting states and communities in program implementation. As the federal agency charged with collecting, analyzing, and disseminating information on child abuse, the Center is also the source of many useful publications and documents (e.g., National Center on Child Abuse and Neglect, 1984).

As a result of the increased awareness and study, researchers have learned a great deal about *overt* physical abuse in childhood. As professionals became more aware, their attention began to extend to the less obvious forms of child abuse: the nonorganic *failure-to-thrive syndrome,* chronic neglect, and, most recently, sexual abuse. Here too, as health care professionals became sensitized to the signs of these conditions, the reported incidences rocketed.

This chapter and the next examine child abuse, child neglect, and sexual abuse; nonorganic failure to thrive is discussed in Chapter 1.

DEFINITION

Many definitions have been proposed for child abuse and neglect; none is universally accepted. Different purposes such as research, legislation, or advocacy may well require different criteria, in some cases narrower, in some cases more broadly drawn.

The Federal Child Abuse Prevention and Treatment Act of 1974 (P.L. 93-247) defines child abuse and neglect as the

> . . . physical or mental injury, sexual abuse, negligent treatment or maltreatment of a child under the age of eighteen by a person who is responsible for the child's welfare under circumstances which indicate that the child's health or welfare is harmed or threatened thereby. . . .

Polansky et al. (1975) (quoted in Mrazek & Mrazek, 1985) have proposed the following operational definition of *child neglect:*

> Child neglect may be defined as a condition in which a caretaker responsible for the child either deliberately or by extraordinary inattentiveness permits the child to experience avoidable present suffering and/or fails to provide one or more of the ingredients generally deemed essential for developing a person's physical, intellectual, and emotional capacities. (p. 682)

Five subtypes of child neglect are defined by Schmitt (1981): medical care neglect, safety neglect, emotional deprivation, educational neglect, and physical neglect.

Kempe and Helfer's (1972) definition of the "battered child" sums up the notion of physical child abuse succinctly: "Any child who receive[s] nonaccidental physical injury or injuries as a result of acts (or omissions) on the part of his parents or guardians."

EPIDEMIOLOGY

In 1982, 929,310 cases of child abuse and neglect were reported nationwide; of these, 26% involved abuse, 43% neglect, and 19% a combination of both (American Humane Association, cited in Heins, 1984). A Department of Health and Human Services study estimated that 1,025,900 children suffered "demonstrable harm" from abuse or neglect in 1986, and abusive or neglectful treatment endangered the health of an additional half-million (*Washington Post,* June 30, 1988, p. A26). These figures almost certainly understate the full magnitude of the problem. The true incidence of child abuse and neglect is difficult to estimate precisely because of the many cases that go unreported and the lack of uniformity in definition. Prevalence estimates range from 340 cases to 570 cases per 100,000 children per year (Mrazek & Mrazek, 1985; Heins, 1984). Up to 10% of all injuries seen in hospital emergency wards in children under 5 years are attributable to abuse and an additional 10% to gross neglect (Holter & Friedman, 1968). Between 2000 and 5000 children are killed by their parents each year, with many more reported as having succumbed to "accidents" rather than homicide (Gelles, 1982). Abuse is the commonest single cause of death in infants between 6 and 12 months of age (Heins, 1984).

Straus and colleagues (1980; summarized in Gelles, 1982) conducted an intensive investigation of the incidence of child abuse and family violence in a nationally representative sample of intact families. Mild forms of violence were very common; 82% of children 3 to 9 years old and 66% of children 10 to 14 years old had been hit during the survey year. More extreme violence was less common but still astonishingly frequent. Three percent of children had been kicked, bitten, or punched by their parents in the survey year, and as many as 8% had received such treatment in the course of their lifetime. Parents had threatened nearly 3% of children with a gun or knife at some point during childhood. Violence was rarely limited to a single episode or type. Thus, children who had objects thrown at them were also hit an average of 4.5 times during the survey year. "Single incident" cases made up only 6% of the reported cases of abuse in this survey; the median number of serious assaults per year experienced by children whose parents reported at least one abusive act was 4.5.

Furthermore, violence toward children frequently occurs in the context of other types of family violence. Thus, in families with child abuse, investigators also often find sexual abuse, wife beating, and spousal rape.

CLINICAL FEATURES

Presentation

Children old enough to speak may report that a physical injury has been inflicted. Investigators should take such reports seriously and carefully examine the facts. In the absence of a direct report or witnesses, certain features of the history may strongly suggest that an injury is an inflicted one (Green, 1985; Mrazek & Mrazek, 1985). An implausible or contradictory account of how the injury occurred should alert the physician to the possibility of abuse, as should a history of repeated suspicious injuries. Some abusing parents "shop" from one hospital emergency ward to another with each new injury to avoid arousing suspicion. In order to circumvent these furtive attempts, hospitals in many areas maintain a central citywide registry of suspicious pediatric trauma cases. Attributing the injury to an abusive sibling is a common evasion. Even when substantiated, sibling abuse usually requires protective and/or therapeutic intervention, because it often indicates laxness of parental supervision and serious problems with resentment or impulse control in the sibling (Rosenthal & Doherty, 1984); in many cases, the abusive sibling has himself been a victim of abuse (Green, 1985). When present, all these factors leave the index patient at continued risk. Unexplained delays in bringing the child for treatment are also a common indicator of a deliberately inflicted injury.

Certain patterns of physical injuries characterize abuse (Bittner & Newberger, 1982; Snyder et al., 1983). Multiple bruises on the buttocks and lower back; bruises or scars at different stages of healing; and rope burns, choke marks, hand marks, or strap marks are all symptoms of serious abuse, often administered under the pretext of discipline. In young non-Caucasian children, it is important not to mistake for a bruise the common bluish nontender areas of skin pigmentation known as the *mongolian spot* (Oates, 1984). Deliberately inflicted burns are also a common form of abuse; these include scalds on the feet and buttocks and multiple cigarette burns or other branding marks. Abdominal trauma may produce rupture of the liver or spleen, whereas head trauma may result in skull fracture, ruptured eardrum, subdural hematoma, retinal detachment, or intraocular hemorrhage. Severely shaken infants may show characteristic joint avulsions and intracranial hemorrhage (Caffey, 1972). Radiological examination may reveal old fractures in different stages of healing, indicating repeated trauma. Abused children may also show evidence of physical neglect such as poor nutrition, filthy clothes or diapers, chronic diaper rash, and a lack of well-baby care.

Newberger and colleagues (1977, 1986) have used the concept of *pediatric social illness* to include a range of conditions strongly influenced by family environment and social conditions; these include inflicted trauma, accidental trauma, failure to thrive, and poisoning. On the whole, the families of preschool children with these conditions appeared to be experiencing more stress and greater isolation in their lives than were control families. The findings also suggested that the parents' difficulties in protecting children from environmental hazards may have stemmed from excessive expectations of the child. The authors speculated that these preschoolers' propensity for accidents partially reflected their inability to "internalize self-protection," even as their parents failed to protect them. (For a review of psychosocial factors in ingestions and accidents, see Cohen, 1983; Graham, 1983).

Effects of Abuse on Child Development

Abused children show a wide gamut of symptoms and developmental delays and deviations (Green, 1978b). It may be difficult in any given case to distinguish clearly among the preexisting developmental difficulties that might have predisposed the child to abuse, the effects of the more general parental deficits and the accompanying deprived environment that originally gave rise to abuse, and the impact of the long-standing abuse and neglect. In reviewing the symptoms of abused children, it is important not to conceptualize them merely as deficits and psychopathology; they also represent the coping patterns of children at different levels of development and skill as these youngsters attempt to deal with stressful family conditions and destructive parental behavior (Cicchetti & Aber, 1980; Crittenden, 1985).

In infancy, the earliest sign of neglect or abuse may be failure to thrive. Abused infants show frequent irritable crying, feeding difficulties, and delays in motor and social development. During the second 6 months of life, deficits in social responsiveness become more obvious as the infants display a tendency toward affective withdrawal, a lack of pleasure in social interactions, and a predominately irritable or unhappy mood (Gaensbauer & Sands, 1979). Failure of these children to attach adequately to their mothers is apparent in their relative lack of stranger and separation anxiety. Such youngsters have failed to develop Erikson's (1950) sense of "basic trust." (See the section Child Factors for a description of the cycle that results as the infant's negative and maladaptive social responses tax the abusive mother's inadequate parenting skills and self-esteem, leading to further abuse and rejection by the mother and increased negativity by the infant.)

Abused toddlers and preschoolers continue to show delays in language, motor, and social development. Socially, they are anxious, fearful, and hypervigilant, scanning the environment with "frozen watchfulness" (Kempe & Kempe, 1978). Along with a general emotional blunting and lack of spontaneity, their ability to play may be impaired and they are often unable to use toys imaginatively (Galdston, 1965). When they do play, punitive themes of "identification with the aggressor" may be apparent in their attacks on and harsh punishment of play figures. Although many abused preschoolers (especially girls) are passive and overcompliant, not all are so submissive. As many as 25% are negativistic, aggressive to peers and adults, and hyperactive (Kempe & Kempe, 1978). Some children alternate between submissive withdrawal and aggressive oppositionality.

During the school years, abused children are lonely, withdrawn, mistrustful, and joyless (Kempe & Kempe, 1978; Martin & Beezley, 1977). Many are overcompliant, pseudomature, and compulsive; others continue to have difficulty with poor impulse control, oppositionality, and aggressive and destructive behavior. The self-esteem of these children is low, and they seem to regard themselves "with the same displeasure and contempt that their parents directed toward them" (Green, 1985, p. 324). This incorporation of the parents' punitive attitudes into the child's own harsh superego is apparent both in the abused child's self-deprecatory attitude and in his readiness to see others as critical and attacking; it is also apparent in these children's high incidence of masochistic and self-destructive behaviors. Such behaviors include actual suicide attempts or gestures, self-mutilation, and accident proneness. Green (1978c) found a record of such assaults on the self in 40% of a sample of abused children. He noted that the self-destructive behavior was most often precipitated by parental physical abuse or actual or threatened separation from parents. These effects may be long-lasting; a study of psychiatric inpatients with major depressions (Yesavage & Widrow, 1985) found that the severity of self-destructive behavior during hospitalization correlated significantly with a childhood history of extremely severe physical discipline.

School-age children who have been abused often retain contradictory, irreconcilable images of their parents. Fear is not the only reason that many children fail to report the abuse they suffer. (More baffling, some children even defend their parents' motives.) Maintaining an internal image of a "good parent" may be so important to the child that he prefers to see himself as evil, and his parent's punitiveness as justified. The child's preference for seeing himself rather than his abusing parent as the bad one has several roots (Wasserman & Rosenfeld, 1985). First, to paraphrase Fairbairn (1952), it is better to see oneself as a sinner in a world ruled by the good Lord, than as a saint in a world ruled by the Devil. This view is congruent with what the child's parents have already told him—that he is to blame. Secondly, it also fits with the child's inherent egocentrism, the notion that he is the cause of whatever happens, both good and bad. Finally, and perhaps most important, by preserving an internal image of a good parent (never mind how inaccurate a representation of his real parent it may be), the child maintains hope. The typical unpredictability of abusive parents leaves some abused children "anxiously attached" (Bowlby, 1973). Despite, or perhaps because of the abuse, the parents' presence and approval become all the more desperately important. The isolated and mistrustful attitudes of such families further discourage the child from turning to potentially ameliorating relationships outside the home.

Many abused children show signs of mental retardation and central nervous system impairment (Martin, 1981). In one uncontrolled sample of abused children, 33% were mentally retarded and 43% showed signs of neurological damage (Martin et al., 1974). In most cases, these deficits do not appear to be due to major head trauma. Comparing matched groups of abused, neglected, and normal controls, Green and colleagues (1981) found only insignificant differences in the incidence of neurological impairment between the abused children and those in the neglected group, who had not suffered physical abuse. Green and colleagues proposed that alternative causes for this neurological impairment might include poor prenatal and infant care, malnutrition, and other abnormal child-rearing factors, including relative maternal deprivation and inadequate (or excessive) sensory and cognitive stimulation.

Not surprisingly, the school adjustment of most abused children is poor. Their attentional, neurological, and cognitive deficits place them at an intellectual disadvantage; and their aggressiveness, poor impulse control, and difficulty in establishing cooperative relations with teachers and peers compound these problems. Industrious application to schoolwork, hobbies, and activities requires attaining a certain developmental readiness. In many cases, the necessary competencies never emerge because the constant inner and outer emotional turmoil that preoccupies these children interferes with consolidating latency-age defenses and ego skills.

All of these difficulties persist into adolescence. Aggressive and self-destructive behavior may become more ominous, and serious delinquency, violent behavior, and suicide attempts are common. As might be expected, in populations of adolescent psychiatric inpatients (Monane et al., 1984; Rogeness et al., 1986) and juvenile delinquents, histories of abuse are all too common. In particular, juvenile delinquents who have been physically abused as children are more likely than nonabused delinquents to commit violent offenses and to have had parents who were criminals or alcoholics (Tarter et al., 1984). Such abused adolescents frequently abuse drugs and alcohol in an effort both to identify with an addicted or alcoholic parent and to cope with low self-esteem and overwhelming problems with their family, school, and peers. Repeated episodes of running away are also common. In some instances, as the child enters puberty, the trauma of sexual abuse may be heaped on the already existing burden of physical abuse.

Goodwin (1987) has argued cogently that many children's reactions to sexual abuse can best be understood as a form of posttraumatic stress syndrome, analogous to that described in survivors of war, crime, or disaster. The analogy might profitably be extended to the physically abused child. The cardinal features of the posttraumatic syndrome include anxiety, guilt, sleep disturbance, and disturbances of mood, concentration, and memory. The victim may reexperience the trauma suddenly and intrusively, either as a recollection or as an abrupt feeling of reliving the event.

CASE EXAMPLE

Derek, a 13-year-old boy, was hospitalized for unmanageable aggressive behavior. For many years, Derek's mother and stepfather had regularly subjected him to physical abuse. Because of an intense identification with the aggressor, Derek attempted to frighten those about him in his social interactions. He cultivated an intimidating swagger and glare that were highly effective. His favorite motto was a Marine slogan from Vietnam: "Yea, though I walk through the Valley of the Shadow of Death, I will fear no evil, for I am the meanest mother-fucker in the valley." Although he could recall the many times since early childhood that he had been viciously beaten by his parents, he denied feeling afraid or helpless and acknowledged only defiance. Similarly, in discussing his fights with peers (which he was quick to excuse as justifiable self-defense) he usually showed little discomfort.

Despite his sufferings at his parents' hands, Derek was quick to side with his parents in their suspicious stance toward and numerous grievances against the hospital. Indeed, when his first-grade teacher had filed an abuse complaint after finding numerous whip marks on his back, Derek had fearfully refused to corroborate her suspicions. During his hospitalization, Derek's mother would frequently simply fail to show up for his home passes. At such times, Derek would feign indifference, make alibis for his mother, or lash out at sympathetic staff whom he perceived as being upset with his mother for having disappointed him.

During his first year as an inpatient, as Derek began to feel more secure at the hospital and in therapy, he gradually became more in touch with the extreme helplessness and humiliation he had felt during his parents' whippings. One day, following a fight in which he beat up his roommate, he appeared uncharacteristically distressed. He anxiously volunteered that his assaultive response had been all out of proportion to the provocation. "It's funny," he added, "when Jim [his roommate] started calling me names, I had a picture in my mind of my mother with a two-by-four. . . . You know, it's like I wasn't really fighting with Jim; I was fighting with a flashback of my mother."

ETIOLOGY

From one viewpoint, the cause of child abuse is simple—namely, an abusing parent. Indeed, serious psychopathology is common in parents who injure their offspring. Nonetheless, a narrow focus on parent personality factors alone omits other crucial variables such as dysfunctional family interactions, social stressors, violence-promoting cultural values, and characteristics of the child that elicit abuse (Gelles, 1973, 1978). Belsky (1980), Garbarino (1977a, 1982), and Bronfenbrenner (1977) have emphasized the necessity of what they term an *ecological model* of child abuse. This model attempts to integrate two sets of factors: on the one hand there is the impact of parental developmental histories and cultural values that predispose to abuse, and on the other the influence of stressful forces within and about the family that increase the likelihood of conflict. The abusive act is the final outcome of interacting family disturbances produced by social-situational stressors (e.g., poverty, isolation, marital tensions), child-mediated stressors (e.g., temperamental difficulties, stepchild status), and parent-mediated stressors (e.g., alcoholism, history of abuse as a child) (Bittner & Newberger, 1982). Parents respond to such conflicts and stressors by becoming violent not only because of psychological factors, but also because of cultural norms concerning corporal punishment and other child-rearing practices.

In an article pessimistically entitled "Controlling Child Abuse in America: An Effort Doomed to Failure," Zigler (1979) observed, "Undoubtedly the single most important determinant of child abuse is the willingness of adults to inflict corporal punishment upon children in the name of discipline" (p. 198). The Supreme Court (*Ingraham v. Wright*, 1977) has recently affirmed the legality of corporal punishment in schools, a practice that is permitted in all but nine states; it is estimated that there are 2 to 3 million incidents of corporal punishment in public schools each year (Hyman & Wise, 1979).

Social-Situational Factors

In many cases of child abuse, economic and social stresses are undoubtedly important contributing factors (Garbarino, 1976). Poor families are greatly overrepresented in reports to child protection agencies. Gil (1970) found that 60% of families involved in reported abuse incidents were or had been on welfare; more than half of the reported abusing families had incomes below $5000, placing them in the bottom quartile of all American families. The same study found that during the year prior to the reported abuse episode almost half of the fathers in the sample of reported families were unemployed. Pending better controlled studies, however, it is unclear to what extent these figures are skewed by the fact that abuse occurring in poor families is far more likely to be reported than similar episodes occurring in more affluent families. Snyder et al. (1983) noted that in white or upper-middle-class families childhood physical trauma stands a much better chance of being misdiagnosed as accidental injury.

Socioeconomic status (SES) bears a strong relationship to child-rearing style. Low-SES parenting attitudes and values generally stress greater punitiveness and restrictiveness, with a correspondingly greater reliance on authoritarian disciplinary practices (see Kohn, 1969; Susman et al., 1985). Herrenkohl and colleagues (1984) found that income was significantly correlated with broad aspects of parental style, with more child-centered and supportive behavior at upper income levels and more parent-centered and child-rejecting behavior at lower income levels. At the same income level, however, physically abusive parents were more likely to show hostile behavior toward their children than were nonabusive parents.

Low SES is associated with a host of frustrating and stressful life circumstances—unemployment, illness, poor housing, limited education, and lack of access to supportive services—all of which increase the strain of family life. Abusing parents have also been described as socially isolated (Garbarino, 1977b), a condition Kempe (1973) referred to as lacking a "lifeline." Some social historians, such as Demos (1986), see the isolation of family life from the broader life of the community as a modern phenomenon that also encourages a narcissistic overinvestment in children. When children do not meet the ensuing excessive expectations, this overinvestment then results in violence. Similarly, Galdston (1981) sees abusive parents as victims of "disenculturation." Taking issue with those who see brutalization of children in earlier times as ubiquitous, Demos contends that the socially integrated pattern of preindustrial American family life encouraged the humane treatment of children. Prospective studies (Altemeier et al., 1982) however, have not found social isolation to be an *antecedent* of abuse, suggesting that once abuse has begun, furtiveness and withdrawal from the broader community may represent an attempt to hide the family's shameful secret. Abuse is more common in nonnuclear and single-parent families, especially those that are the result of divorce rather than death (Gil, 1970; Sack et al., 1985). A variety of studies (Eiduson, 1983; Straus et al., 1980) attest to the greater stressfulness of life in single-parent households, although these findings no doubt reflect in part the greater poverty of such households.

The importance of socioeconomic factors to the genesis of child abuse involves many hotly debated issues, both methodological and ideological. Social psychologists and policy planners have emphasized these factors for pragmatic as well as conceptual reasons. Gil (1970) goes so far as to assert that the primary prevention of child abuse is essentially a political issue, rather than a purely technical or clinical one.

In certain predisposed parents, socioenvironmental stresses can serve as the catalyst for abuse. Furthermore, the culture of poverty often provides the context for the intergenerational transmission of an abuse-prone personality. But socioenvironmental difficulties alone do not adequately explain or predict abuse. Despite deprivation and difficult life circumstances, most poor parents do *not* abuse their children. More than that, abuse also occurs in affluent, well-educated families.

Parental Factors

Early impressionistic clinical studies of abusive parents described them variously as immature, rigid, suspicious, suffering from low self-esteem, dependent on their children, and freely expressive of aggressive impulses (e.g., Steele & Pollock, 1968). In recent years, more systematic, better controlled studies have shown that speaking of a specific "abusive" personality is a drastic oversimplification. Using a lifetime psychopathology scale, Green et al. (1980) found that abusive mothers obtained high scores on the Anger-Excitability and Disorganized subscales. Kaplan et al. (1983) employed a structured interview and found a high incidence of psychopathology among abusive mothers; depressive disorders and alcoholism were especially common.

The data thus suggest a rather more complex formulation. As A. H. Green (1980) observed:

> Individuals with a certain psychological makeup operating in combination with the burden of a painfully perceived childhood and immediate environ-

> mental stress might be likely to abuse the offspring who most readily elicits the unhappy childhood imagery of the past. (p. 38)

Indeed, it is a near-ubiquitous finding of one study after another that abusive parents, in their own childhoods, frequently experienced emotional privation, rejection, harsh criticism, inordinate demands, and overt abuse at the hands of *their* parents. Such traumatic childhood experiences have severely deleterious effects on later adult functioning, especially in the realm of parenting. The abusive parent has strong identifications with his or her own harsh, rejecting parent. Even when he or she struggles consciously against the image, this identification with a wrathful, violently punitive other exerts a powerful influence. Linked to the internalized image of the parent's own angry parent is the equally insidious and powerful image of the "bad" child of the past, which the abused (and now potentially abusive) parent felt herself to be when criticized and rejected as a child. This "bad" self-image of childhood makes for fragile self-esteem and pervasive feelings of worthlessness. These painful feelings of self-devaluation are often defended against with a brittle positive facade of conscientiousness and affection. More fatefully for their offspring however, such parents project their own "bad" self-image onto their child, while at the same time making him the target of the hatred felt toward their own abusive parent. The child singled out for abuse may have temperamental or other features that make him an easy vehicle for such scapegoating.

Even when such features are missing, however, another powerful dynamic can make a child the focus of rage and reproach from his abuse-prone parent. Such a parent typically has strong unmet (and often unacknowledged) dependency needs. These painful longings result from profound emotional deprivation in childhood and are often exacerbated by characteristically unsatisfactory marriages that frequently reflect the same unhappy repetition of traumatic early relationships. The unfulfilled parent frequently turns toward her own child for the gratifications her spouse or family of origin have failed to meet (A. H. Green, 1980). This role reversal, whereby the parent seeks sustenance from the child, places impossible demands on such a "parentified" child. Inevitably, the child fails to gratify the parent adequately, whereupon the parent comes to perceive the child not only as the "bad" child out of his or her own past, who should be punished, but also unconsciously as his or her own rejecting, depriving mother, the focus of childhood hurt and rage. As A. H. Green (1980) pointed out, the tragedy of abusive parents is that "they cannot envision any parent–child relationship as a mutually gratifying experience, since the task of parenting mobilizes identifications with the parent–aggressor, child–victim dyad of the past" (p. 41).

Although fathers abuse children as frequently do mothers, the fathers have been far less studied. In one of the few such studies, A. H. Green (1979) found that abusing fathers share many of the personality features and socioeconomic background factors that had been previously reported in abusing mothers. Alcoholism was common and fathers were often intoxicated when they attacked their children. Limited vocational skills, low job satisfaction, and the frequent actual or threatened loss of a job all undermined these fathers' self-esteem and sense of masculinity while simultaneously exacerbating marital tensions. Deprived in their own childhood, male abusers are often intensely jealous of the attention the child receives from the mother, especially during infancy. Often, such jealous rage is even more intense when the abusing man is not the child's father, but rather a stepfather or paramour. The mother's sudden unavailability may precipitate paternal abuse by placing the father in reluctant charge of the child, while increasing his own sense of deprivation.

In cases of child abuse by the father, the mother's role varies. In Green and colleagues' (1974) sample, 14% of abused children were abused jointly by their mothers and fathers. Although mothers may sometimes instigate or passively collude with fathers beating their children, both mother and child are often the victims of a father's brutality. Child abuse frequently occurs against a background of domestic violence (often exacerbated by alcohol) that includes wife beating and sexual abuse. Contributing factors may include a cultural tradition of physical intimidation of women and rage at feeling excluded from the mother and child's close relationship. Battered wives often have a history of having been physically abused during their own childhood; they later choose a violence-prone mate who resembles their own abusive parent (A. H. Green, 1980). Yet Gayford (1975) noted that in a significant number of cases, the battered women (at least 37% in one sample) in turn abused their children. Child abuse is thus frequently but one facet of a complex, often multigenerational, pattern of family violence. Not only are the children of such families traumatized by being victims, they are exposed to an atmosphere of pervasive violence that they identify with and come to expect as an inevitable feature of all relationships.

At the same time, not all abused children inexorably end up abusing their own children (Cicchetti & Aber, 1980). Kaufman and Zigler (1987) estimate that about one-third of all individuals who have been abused or severely neglected as children will abuse or neglect their own offspring. This rate is about six times higher than the base rate for abuse in the general population. Despite an abusive, stressful upbringing, some children not only develop adequate coping skills but also deliberately "disidentify from the aggressor" and, as a self-reparative act, attempt to provide a better home for their children than they themselves ever knew. Other protective factors that help break the cycle of abuse include the availability of a supportive spouse or boyfriend, a lower level of current stress, and the presence during childhood of a supportive parent or foster parent.

Child Factors

Given abuse-prone parents, some children are more likely to be abused than are others. In general, certain characteristics of children render parent–child interactions more difficult and frustrating, or less gratifying, and thus increase the risk of abuse. As might be expected, younger children (Straus et al., 1980), step- and foster children (Bittner & Newberger, 1982), and handicapped children (White et al., 1986) are all especially vulnerable to abuse.

Children who get off to a difficult start in any of several ways are particularly likely to be targets. Illegitimacy, unwanted pregnancy, and young maternal age are all associated with increased abuse (Altemeier et al., 1982; Herrenkohl & Herrenkohl, 1979). Children born prematurely seem to be at greater risk for subsequent abuse than are full-term infants. It is unclear to what extent this association, if valid, is due to the increased fussiness and temperamental difficulties of premature infants; in addition, if the infant must be kept in an incubator away from the mother in the first days of life, this may disrupt the early attachment ("bonding") between the mother and the premature infant (Egeland & Sroufe, 1981).

When abused or neglected children and their nonabused siblings were compared by Herrenkohl and Herrenkohl (1979), the abused children were more likely to have been premature. The same comparison showed that children described by their mothers as having had developmental difficulties such as slow weight gain, fussiness, or poor coordination were more likely than their normal siblings to have been the targets of gross, life-threatening neglect. In some studies, mental retardation and physical handicaps in the child have also been associated with increased risk of abuse or neglect (Wasserman et al., 1983).

In about 50% of abusive families, one child is singled out for abuse; in the remainder, more than one (and often several) children are the targets (Herrenkohl & Herrenkohl, 1979). Friedrich and Boriskin (1976) observed that abuse is commonly associated with parental perception of a child as "difficult" or "different." This conclusion was confirmed by the findings of Herrenkohl and Herrenkohl (1979) and Estroff et al. (1984) who compared maltreating parents' perceptions of their abused children versus their nonabused children. Of course, the extent to which the abusive parents' perceptions of the child are objectively valid remains open to question. Also unanswered is the question of how to determine which aberrant child behaviors may have provoked the abuse and which behaviors were the result of it. Estroff et al. (1984) found that the maltreating mothers' degree of psychopathology was strongly associated with how disturbed they perceived their abused child to be. It is noteworthy that mothers regarded the nonabused siblings as markedly less deviant than the abused child.

Abusive parents often speak of their abused child as being "just like" some hated person in their own life, such as a detested parent, sibling, or (ex)-spouse. Clinically, such a global, negative identification of the child's appearance, behavior, or gender with a malign figure from the parent's past is an ominous sign that deserves further exploration. Maltreating parents have often had an unhappy childhood and experience low self-esteem. In many cases, what the abusive parent cannot bear is some perceived characteristic in the child that resembles a despised part of the parent's self.

As should be clear from this discussion, goodness of fit between the personality and temperament of the parent and child plays a major role in the vulnerability to abuse. The social resources, coping skills, and expectations with which the parent approaches a given child will vary, as will the temperamental difficulty and responsiveness of the child; what resonances the child strikes in the parent will be as fateful as the effectiveness of the parent's responses to the child's demands, capacities, and expectations.

Several observational studies have attempted to give an interactional account of the abused child and parent (Burgess & Conger, 1977, 1978; Crittenden, 1985; Gaensbauer & Sands, 1979; George & Main, 1979; Herrenkohl et al., 1983, 1984; Martin & Beezley, 1977; Wasserman et al., 1983). Overt abuse cannot be understood simply in terms of child factors or parent factors taken in isolation. The clinician must look not only at the overt acts of abuse, but also at the complex, often reciprocal pattern of negative interactions between parent and child that reinforce the parent's deficient coping skills and transmit them to the child (Herrenkohl et al., 1984). The deficiencies in the parent and child's coping skills are thus mutually reinforced in a spiral of ever-increasing frustration.

For example, Gaensbauer and Sands (1979) found that abused (or neglected) infants showed a variety of distortions in their affective communication with their caretakers. These aberrant patterns interfered with mutual engagement and elicited negative caretaker responses. These maltreated infants rarely made positive overtures toward others, tended to withdraw affectively from interpersonal interactions, and in the interactions that did take place, seemed joyless and apathetic. Their mothers often saw this withdrawal as a rebuff, an especially devastating (and enraging) experience for the narcissistically vulnerable mother. Characteristically, these infants' emotional responses were also labile, shallow, and frequently ambivalent to the point of ambiguity. Such infants often appeared forlorn and dejected, cried readily, and were prone to lash out angrily with little provocation. The mothers perceived their children as demanding and implacable and felt inadequate to satisfy their needs. The intensity and inconsolability of these easily upset infants exacerbated the difficulties and further alienated these mothers.

Because these infants' affects are so frequently negative, unpredictable, or hard to read, at best they are difficult to engage in a positive and sustained interaction, even by patient, well-intentioned adults. Not surprisingly, abused children's maladaptive interactions are not confined to their parents (Wasserman et al., 1987). In a day-care setting, when compared with matched, nonabused controls, the abused toddlers tended to harass staff both verbally and nonverbally and were more frequently assaultive toward their peers (George & Main, 1979). Indeed, they were the only children who assaulted or threatened to assault staff caregivers. Even when adults or peers made friendly overtures, abused toddlers were far warier than controls; they were more likely to withdraw and, if they did approach, they did so anxiously, guardedly, and ambivalently. Interestingly, a similar behavior pattern of ambivalence and avoidance toward caregivers has been observed in maternally rejected but apparently nonabused infants (George & Main, 1979).

Milowe and Lourie (1964) were the first to report on some children who were abused in more than one home, and the investigators speculated on the child's role in provoking abuse. As noted earlier, children who are the victims of abuse often develop patterns that may enrage their caregivers. Without "blaming the victim," it is fair to say that the infant characteristics described above will at the least exacerbate an already tense, dysynchronous, and mutually ungratifying relationship with the parents.

In turn, parents prone to abuse show complementary difficulties in relating to their infants, and often enough, to other children and adults as well. For example, Burgess and Conger (1977, 1978) found that abusive parents initiated fewer contacts with their child. Of those exchanges that did occur, more were negative and fewer were positive than with nonabusive controls. Similarly, abusive mothers often show an impoverished repertoire of responses to their infants and react to them with either passivity or withdrawal (Dietrich, 1977, cited in Herrenkohl et al., 1984). Abusive mothers are not only more hostile and inconsistent than normal mothers; they are more likely to use anxiety and guilt-inducing methods to control their children in conjunction with harsh authoritarian practices (Susman et al., 1985). The inconsistency of these parents' interactions is evident in the high degree of both permissiveness *and* punitiveness found by Wasserman and colleagues (1983). Significantly, in their classic study of child-rearing patterns, Sears and colleagues (1957) found this parenting style to be associated with the most frequent expressions of serious aggression. Herrenkohl and colleagues (1983) found maltreating parents to be generally more rejecting toward their children; the investigators noted that abusive episodes frequently involved parental overreaction to irritating child behavior that was still within the normal range, such as ignoring a parental request.

Retrospectively, it is often difficult to distinguish which temperamental and personality features of abused children are *antecedent*, rendering abuse more likely, and which are the *result* of abusive, negligent, or otherwise pathological parenting. Yet another possibility is that both the apparently predisposing child factor (e.g., prematurity, difficult temperament) and the parent's abuse potential might each be independently associated with a third causal factor (e.g., maternal alcoholism or low SES).

Although dramatic (and traumatic) acts of violence usually bring such troubled parent–child dyads to clinical or legal attention, the research cited indicates that these sporadic eruptions of violence occur against an ongoing pattern of destructive and maladaptive affective interactions. Whether these patterns begin with constitutional factors in the child or defects in parenting, once they become established, they develop a persistent life of their own and take a heavy toll on both parent and child (Gaensbauer & Sands, 1979; Greenspan, 1981). It is therefore essential that any assessment and intervention with the abusive family take into account the potential for such a destructive cycle of interaction that conditions the interpersonal reality of each of its members.

As the ecological model alluded to earlier implies, environmental and personality variables do not operate in isolation from each other. An ambitious prospective study by Egeland and colleagues (1980) explored their complex interactions. As elaborated in the discussion of psychosomatic processes (Chapter 15), a wide variety of psychological factors mediate the subjective impact of stressful life events. For example, the investigators found that maltreating mothers experienced more chaotic, traumatic, and disruptive life events during the first year after giving birth than mothers who gave adequate care. In another study, maltreating and adequate mothers had had an equal number of stressful life events, but those involving family alcoholism, marital discord, and separation events were particularly likely to be associated with maltreatment (Salzinger et al., 1986). Yet many adequate mothers also experienced high levels of disruptive life events without mistreating their children. What made the difference? First, Egeland and colleagues found that, compared with adequate mothers, the inadequate mothers were quicker to respond to their frustrations with hostility. They were more anxious, suspicious, defensive, and rigid; in addition, they were less likely to seek help from others, thereby cutting themselves off from potentially supportive relationships (Egeland et al., 1980). Maltreating mothers also perceive fewer events in their lives as positive than do adequate mothers (Salzinger et al., 1986), perhaps because such mothers have an increased incidence of depression (Kaplan et al., 1983). Egeland found the maltreating mothers were less able to cope with the ambivalent feelings that accompany healthy mothering, were less sensitive and responsive to their infants, and had less ability to perceive accurately the child's aggressive impulses or to help the child modulate them. Thus, whether changing life events were related to later abuse or neglect seemed to depend on various personality characteristics and parenting capacities of the mother.

Ethological Factors

Infanticide and abuse of offspring are found in nonhuman primates (Burke, 1984; Goodall, 1986; Reite & Caine, 1983; Troisi & D'Amato, 1984). Predisposing factors seem to include overcrowding, social disruption, and selective breeding pressures. In addition, separation experiences in young female monkeys may be deleterious to their later maternal behavior. Some monkey mothers have adequate mothering skills but show intense ambivalence toward their offspring, alternating intense attachment behavior with abuse (Troisi & D'Amato, 1984). Such maternal behavior appears to fit Bowlby's (1973) model of "anxious attachment."

INTERVENTION AND TREATMENT

Primary Prevention

We already know a good deal about what is needed to diminish the incidence of child maltreatment. As Gil (1970) noted, many crucial questions in primary prevention of child abuse are political rather than professional ones. Reducing the level of poverty, unemployment, and poor housing would go far toward mitigating environmental stresses on family life. The associations between child maltreatment and unwanted pregnancy, prematurity, and teenage parenthood are reasonably clear. Improving potential teenage mothers' access to sex education, family planning resources, incentives to remain in school, and alternative means of economic emancipation (other than motherhood) would all tend to lower the incidence not only of teenage pregnancy and associated prematurity but also of child abuse. Other measures include family-life education and counseling programs for adolescents in preparation for parenthood, better access to and utilization of perinatal and well-baby care, wider availability of quality day care and other child-care resources, and neighbor-based social services geared to reducing stresses on family life (Cicchetti & Aber, 1980).

Treatment

Under the impetus of the Federal Child Abuse Prevention and Treatment Act of 1974, state and local jurisdictions have implemented procedures to encourage reporting of suspected child abuse and neglect and to ensure timely, effective investigative and treatment services (Besharov, 1981). These procedures include requirements mandating certain professionals to report suspected cases, with penalties for failure to report. In most states, medical professionals, school personnel, and law enforcement officers are required to report such cases; some states' reporting mandates cover all citizens. Mandated reporters are granted immunity from liability in any suits arising out of good faith reports. Because of some ambivalence on the part of legislators regarding whether to treat child abuse as a criminal or rehabilitative matter, states vary in designating social service agencies or the police as the agency to receive abuse reports. Ultimately, most reports are referred to a child protective agency. Such agencies, in responding to a report, have the obligation to take the following steps (Besharov, 1981):

1. Investigating the validity of the report and determining the degree of danger to the child.
2. Ensuring the immediate safety of the child, either through crisis intervention in the home or, when necessary, by placing the child in protective custody.
3. Assessing the family and child's service needs.
4. Providing (or arranging for) appropriate protective and treatment services.
4. When necessary, seeking court action to remove the child from the home or to require family involvement in treatment.

Optimally, the specific approach to a given family should be designed on the basis of a careful evaluation. All too often, however, the evaluation and treatment resources available to abusing families are limited in availability and scope. Although all states mandate local child protective services, the quality, staffing, and funding of such programs vary considerably. Excessive case loads and the emotional wear and tear of such work lead to premature burnout and frequent staff turnover, so that many public agencies experience difficulty in retaining trained staff. A review of 3300 county child-protection departments nationwide revealed an annual staff turnover rate among primary caseworkers of 50% to 100% (Kempe & Kempe, 1978).

The multidisciplinary child protection team, first pioneered in Denver by Kempe and colleagues, has proved its usefulness in a number of ways: providing better integrated services, avoiding fragmentation of responsibility and follow-up, and combating staff burnout (Green, 1983; Kempe & Helfer, 1972; Kempe & Kempe, 1978; Schmitt, 1981). Such teams may operate either within the setting of a local protective service agency or in a hospital. Demonstration hospital-based programs, such as those found at many children's hospitals, have proven effective in centralizing and preventing duplication of services and initiating early intervention with families. Optimally, such teams would include pediatricians, psychiatrists, psychologists, legal counsel, nurses, social workers, and representatives from the local protective services agency, public schools, and visiting nurses agency.

One of the most difficult decisions the community faces is whether to place a child in protective custody outside the home. Where there has been life-threatening trauma or neglect, repeated abuse, obvious parental rejection, or active parental psychosis involving the child, the decision may seem relatively straightforward. The caseworker, and ultimately the judge, must weigh the immediate safety of the child, the positive and the traumatic aspects of the separation process, and the long-term benefits and hazards of removal (Wasserman & Rosenfeld, 1985). Even with a clear picture of the facts and careful evaluation of the parent–child relationship, the judgment often would challenge Solomon. The ability of professionals to predict which families are likely to repeat abuse (other than those who are already recidivists) is poor. On the one hand, a good foster home may seem like an attractive alternative to returning the child home and trusting to the vagaries of treatment and monitoring to ensure his safety. On the other hand, for many children, short-term foster placement becomes long-term foster placement, frequently for the remainder of their childhood years (Holman, 1983). All too often, this means a disruptive series of foster homes that may themselves engender enormous stress. Such multiple placements are especially likely when the child has not received adequate psychotherapy so that his own aggressive behaviors and interpersonal difficulties threaten the stability of his placement. Even when parental rights have been permanently terminated, such personality problems often limit the possibilities for adoption or stable long-term foster placement.

Another complication arises because the courts are reluctant to interfere with the sanctity of families. As required by the Federal Child Abuse Act, states must provide a guardian *ad litem,* often an attorney, to represent the child in child protective judicial proceedings. (For a discussion of the legal complexities, see Besharov, 1981.) Some child advocates have argued that the outcome of long-term foster placement is so dismal that state agencies must make every effort to work with the child in the context of his family (Cicchetti & Aber, 1980). Without adequate treatment programs, however, changes in child welfare policy that preclude long-term placement may merely expose children to repeated abuse (Holman, 1983). (For a further discussion of the issues involved in involuntary placement and the notion of "the least detrimental alternative," see Gerbner et al., 1980, and the two influential works by Goldstein, Freud, & Solnit, *Beyond the Best Interests of the Child,* 1973, and *Before the Best Interests of the Child,* 1979.)

The treatment of abusing families is still an evolving art. The causal factors in child abuse are multiple and complexly related. Correspondingly, the treatment and prevention of child abuse require intervention on many fronts. Green (1985) and Cohn (1979) have summarized the goals of intervention with abusing parents as follows:

1. Providing crisis intervention to reduce stress from family conflict and the environment.

2. Decreasing parents' social isolation by fostering supportive relationships with members of the treatment team and other adults.

3. Helping parents enhance their chronically low self-esteem.

4. Providing parents with positive child-rearing models for identification.

5. Helping parents develop more effective child-rearing techniques, with special emphasis on nonabusive disciplinary methods.

6. Providing parents with a greater awareness of child development in general and specific counseling regarding physical or developmental difficulties the child may be encountering.

7. Correcting parental misperceptions of the child.

8. Helping parents understand the relationship between their own painful childhood experiences and their misperceptions and inappropriate handling of the child.

9. Helping parents derive pleasure from the child.

10. Fostering an ability to talk out problems and to substitute more appropriate expressions of anger in place of action.

Effective treatment thus requires not only dealing with the individual parents and family's coping skill and dynamics, but also the overall social context of the family. In his article, "Healing the Wounds of Social Isolation," Garbarino (1982) offers the exhortation: "Treat the social network." Pioneering programs such as the demonstration projects of the National Center for the Prevention and Treatment of Child Abuse and Neglect in Denver, Colorado, have developed innovative interventions in addition to traditional modes of individual psychotherapy and parent casework. These include crisis telephone assistance (hot lines), crisis and therapeutic nurseries, residential family treatment, lay therapists and foster grandparents, social service homemakers, and self-help groups such as Parents Anonymous (for a detailed description of such programs, see Kempe & Kempe, 1978). Work with abusive families requires flexible treatment planning with strong outreach and crisis intervention services.

The efficacy of such intervention programs is difficult to assess. Because of problems with ascertainment and the moral unacceptability of untreated control groups, the prognosis and natural history of untreated child abuse is unclear, although undoubtedly poor. Kempe and Kempe (1978) estimate that without intervention about 5% of abused children are ultimately killed, and about 35% are subjected to repeated nonlethal abuse. It is against this untreated baseline that the effectiveness of treatment programs must be measured.

In their experience at the National Center in Denver, Kempe and Kempe (1978) found that about 10% of abusive parents were too seriously disturbed for successful treatment. Included in this group were actively psychotic parents whose child was the object of paranoid delusions or hallucinations; impulsive "aggressive sociopaths" whose addiction to drugs or alcohol may also have exacerbated hair-trigger tempers; deliberately sadistic parents who premeditatedly tortured their children, often in the self-righteous guise of "discipline"; and parents who physically abused their children as part of a fanatic religious or ideological belief.

With an additional 10% of families, clinicians attempted treatment but were not successful. The remaining 80% were judged treatment successes, with half requiring "only short-term" help (1 to 3 years) and half requiring long-term support. Although the criterion for success was no serious reinjury, in only about half the families did clinicians judge there to be a change in the parents' basic feeling for their child, "their capacity to be truly loving."

Whether as a result of less extensive resources or different client populations, other programs appear to have had less promising results than those cited for the Denver project. For a period of almost $3\frac{1}{2}$ years the First National Child Abuse Program Evaluation evaluated 11 different child abuse and neglect demonstration projects (Cohn 1979, 1982); these included programs organized on the public protective service agency model, the hospital-based model, the private family service agency model, and the volunteer model. Of the 1724 cases served, 30% of the parents were said to have severely reabused or neglected their children while receiving treatment services. By the end of treatment investigators judged that only 42% of the parents were less likely to reabuse or neglect their children; and no more than 28% were judged to have accomplished any of the treatment goals listed earlier (see pp. 34–35). Reviewing the efficacy of various treatment components, Cohn found that parents who participated in a self-help organization (such as Parents Anonymous), irrespective of whatever other services they received, did significantly better than parents who did not. It is not clear whether this finding indicates that self-help groups are especially efficacious; abusive parents who join and maintain participation in such groups may represent a self-selected sample high in motivation and readiness to examine and accept responsibility for their behavior. Finally, the survey found that only 100 children (fewer than 6%) received direct therapeutic services.

The data on the psychological and developmental sequelae of abuse reviewed above suggest that abused children require a good deal of direct therapeutic and special educational help. In addition to possible emergency, interim, and long-term placement, many such children profit from services such as individual or group psychotherapy, therapeutic nursery or day-care services, and special educational resource help (Green, 1985; Kempe & Kempe, 1978). The treatment of such children often requires much skill both in handling the technical aspects of the work and in managing the difficult countertransference issues activated in the therapy (Green, 1978a).

Chapter 22

Child Sexual Abuse

INTRODUCTION

Beginning in the 1960s, the belated recognition of child abuse as a social and medical problem of immense magnitude led to a burgeoning of professional and public concern. Despite this dramatic increase in awareness, the sexual abuse of children continued to be a curiously and woefully unattended problem, frequently undiagnosed and untreated in clinical practice and almost universally ignored as a social phenomenon (Herman, 1981). In the words of Suzanne Sgroi (1975), it remained "the last frontier in child abuse."

There appear to be many reasons for this relative neglect. The sexual molestation of children, especially when it involves incest, is a topic that arouses profound discomfort in most adults. In this sense, the taboo against sexual abuse is more highly charged than that against physical mistreatment. Although repelled by actual physical abuse, most parents, if candid, can recall having occasionally entertained conscious violent, even murderous, feelings toward their children. Yet far fewer parents can contemplate without extreme discomfort the notion of explicit sexual longings toward their offspring. Some feminist writers (Herman, 1981) have also discerned a sexist bias in the historical reluctance of male investigators to acknowledge the full extent of child sexual abuse, a form of abuse perpetrated almost exclusively by males (Finkelhor, 1984). These feminist writers regard this disinclination as part of a larger reluctance to confront the deleterious consequences of a patriarchal tradition that they contend provides the impetus for sexually exploiting women and children. They believe that, as a result, the widespread prevalence of child molestation was largely ignored until recently; moreover, when it was finally acknowledged, society shifted the blame to the victim.

In contrast, the past decade has seen a greatly heightened awareness of sexual abuse, in large part reflecting the combined impact of both the child advocacy and women's movements. Sexual abuse has become an "in" topic, with articles, TV documentaries, dramatic court cases, and painful personal testimonies appearing frequently in the mass media. Recent years have seen several highly controversial legal cases involving allegations of sex abuse in child custody suits between divorced parents or against day-care workers (the latter cases sometimes involving scores of plaintiffs). As Green (1988) observed, these cases have generated intense emotions, pitting partisans of alleged victims against those of the alleged perpetrator, expert against expert, and, at times, the wrongfully accused against the legal system. Some experts believe that the field of child sexual abuse is now moving from underreporting and neglect of the problem to "hypervigilance and frequent overreporting" (Schetky, 1986).

Ironically, heightened public awareness and concern have been paralleled by a small but strident group of proincest apologists who purport to find positive values in incest, such as the alleged liberation of the child from repressive sexual taboos (Herman, 1981). Like many self-exculpatory molesters, these advocates rationalize away the exploitative element of incest and minimize its serious, adverse impact on the child.

The intense passions aroused by the topic of childhood sexual abuse are not new. For example, widespread hostility greeted Freud's (1896/1957a) contention that child sexual abuse, often incestuous, was far more widespread than generally supposed and his initial hypothesis (later revised) that it lay behind most cases of adult neurosis (see below). His icy reception, Freud (1914/1957d) remarked ruefully, was the sort reserved for "those who had 'disturbed the sleep of the world'" (p. 21).

Whether the actual incidence of childhood sexual abuse has increased during this century is unclear. There are some indications that the overall rate of sexual victimization of children has remained relatively stable for the past several decades (Finkelhor, 1984); on the other hand, compared to Alfred Kinsey's survey data from the 1940s, recent surveys suggest an increase in both the prevalence and seriousness of child sexual abuse (Leventhal, 1988). Better discovery and improved reporting procedures undoubtedly account for much of the increased incidence of *reported* sexual abuse. Parents, teachers, and physicians have become more highly attuned to the menace of sexual abuse and are less likely to dismiss children's hints or allegations regarding its occurrence.

Some authorities are alarmed by what they perceive as a pervasive loosening of societal prohibitions concerning sexual matters. This permissive trend has been apparent in many ways, such as in the increased availability and semilegitimization of pornography (including child pornography) and in the prevalence of explicit sexual and violent themes in the popular media. Unfortunately, few reliable data exist to help determine whether this barrage of sexual stimulation actually encourages sexual abuse (Finkelhor, 1979).

DEFINITION

The term *sexual abuse* (or *sexual exploitation*) covers a wide variety of sins against children. The actual sexual behaviors that victimize children include exhibitionism, genital fondling (molestation), intercourse (oral, anal, or genital), and rape. Less than 50% of the reported cases of abuse involve actual or attempted coitus (Conte & Berliner, 1981); in some studies the figure is less than 5% (Finkelhor, 1979). Victims may range from infants or toddlers too young to comprehend the sexual nature of what is being done to them, through physically mature adolescents close to the legal age of consent. The abuse may occur only once or be repeated for a period of months and years. Overt coercion or violence often accompanies such acts.

In yet other cases, children may compliantly cooperate, either out of deference to adult authority or from a profound (albeit misdirected) hunger for adult affection at any cost. It is important to emphasize that neither the child's apparent consent nor the absence of coercion renders the sexual encounter between an adult and a child nonabusive. The immense differences in power and status between the two make any sexual relationship between them inherently exploitative. In this sense, an abuser need not be an adult but could be an older child or sibling who is in a position of power or control.

Variations in Definitions

The legal definitions of sexual abuse embodied in state sexual assault statutes are often narrowly drawn in anatomical terms and degree of relationship between the victim and perpetrator. From the psychological viewpoint the salient formulation is Schecter and Roberge's (1976) definition of sexual abuse as "the involvement of dependent, developmentally immature children and adolescents in sexual activities that they do not fully comprehend, to which they are unable to give informed consent, or that violate the social taboos of family roles" (cited in Mrazek & Kempe, 1981, p. 11). The essential characteristics of an abusive sexual interaction thus include (1) the exploitation of a child for an elder's sexual gratification; (2) the exposure of that child to sexual activities inappropriate to his developmental level or to his role in the family; and (3) the inability of the child to give true informed consent because of an inherent disadvantage in terms of age, power, or status relative to the other person (Snyder et al., 1983).

As is true of physical abuse, the definition of sexual abuse is not culture-free. Societies have differed as to the age at which sexual activity is deemed appropriate for young people, the types of sexual activity permitted, and the degrees of consanguinity within which sexual relations are permitted or forbidden (Fox, 1967).

Clinical Varieties

In order to understand fully the psychological impact of a sexual experience for a child, the professional must comprehend several crucial dimensions (Mrazek & Mrazek, 1985):

1. What was the nature and frequency of the sexual act or acts—who did what with whom and on what occasion(s)?
2. Did the act(s) involve violence, threats, or blandishments; and if so, what were they?

3. What was the chronological, emotional, and mental maturity of the persons involved?
4. What was the quality of the relationship between the abuser and the child; that is, how did they know each other prior to the event, what were their respective motives for and attitudes about the sexual interaction, and how did they perceive what happened?
5. What were the attitudes of other family members before and after the event?
6. What were the prevailing cultural norms concerning such sexual practices?

Several of these distinctions carry very important clinical implications. One major distinction is between incestuous (or intrafamilial) abuse, where the sexual interaction takes place with a family member, and nonincestuous (or extrafamilial) abuse. A second important distinction is whether the abusive act was a single isolated episode or was repeated for a period of time. In general, a child who is molested on a single occasion by a stranger and has a supportive family to which to turn is likely to experience a less profound trauma and fewer long-term sequelae than the child who is abused repeatedly by a family member while feeling that there is no one to look to for help (Finkelhor, 1987).

EPIDEMIOLOGY AND PREVALENCE

The incidence of sexual abuse varies depending on the definition and the means of verification. However, state statistics of reported cases, which serve as one yardstick, totaled 123,000 cases in 1985, up from an estimate of only 7,559 in 1976 (Finkelhor, 1987). About 58% of these remain unsubstantiated (Schetky, 1986). Despite the methodological difficulties in obtaining precise figures, it is obvious that the prevalence of sexual abuse is shockingly high. Rape is the most serious form of sexual abuse; each year in this country it is estimated to involve about 18,000 children under age 13 years (Khan, 1979). In Brooklyn, based on actual reports to the police during the years 1962 to 1967, the annual incidence of sexual crimes against children involving physical contact was 149.2 per 100,000 children (ages 7–14) (De Francis, 1969). If one includes the full gamut of sexual abuse from exhibitionism to rape, retrospective studies of nonclinical populations suggest that even 40 years ago prevalence rates were very high. Reanalysis of Kinsey's data from the 1950s indicated that, prior to age 13 years, 28% of adult women had had at least one such sexual experience with an adult (Gagnon, 1965). More recently, in a study of 796 college students, 20% of the women and 9% of the men claimed to have experienced some sort of sexual abuse as children (Finkelhor, 1979). Of these experiences 80% to 85% involved physical contact, of which genital fondling was the most common; the remainder involved such experiences as seeing an exhibitionist. Of the women, 50% reported that the perpetrator was a family member; of the men, 17% stated that a family member was involved. Similarly, using a random sample of adult women, Russell (1983, 1986) found that 12% reported having had at least one experience of intrafamilial sexual abuse prior to age 14; 20% reported having experienced extrafamilial sexual abuse prior to the same age.

These retrospective studies also confirm the widespread suspicion that the events reported to social agencies and police represent only a small fraction of the actual incidence of sexual abuse. For example, 25% to 33% of child victims queried as adults stated that as children they had never told anyone of their experience (Finkelhor, 1979). Even when revealed to the family, cases of sexual abuse are rarely reported to the authorities, especially when they involve relatives. In one study, only 2% of sexual abuse cases involving family members were ever brought to police attention versus 6% of cases of extrafamilial abuse (Russell, 1983, 1986).

By a ratio of anywhere from 2 to 1 (Finkelhor, 1979) to 12 to 1 (De Francis, 1969), girls are much more likely than boys to be the victims of sexual abuse. Boys are more likely than girls to be abused by nonfamily members, and in their case, the abuse appears even less likely to be reported to authorities (Finkelhor, 1979).

The early teen years seem to be the most likely age for rape victimization, for both boys and girls (Khan, 1979). In recent years, reports of abuse involving boys and young children under 5 years have increased dramatically (Kempe & Kempe, 1984; Mrazek et al., 1981). As noted earlier, it is difficult to determine whether this reflects an actual increase in incidence or merely improved reporting.

CLINICAL FEATURES

In most instances, the abuser is someone the child already knows either as a family member or as an acquaintance, a neighbor, or a babysitter. Despite the myth of the dangerous stranger, less than 25% of the perpetrators of sexual abuse are truly unknown to the child or his family (De Francis, 1969); indeed, family members are as likely to be the offender as are other acquaintances of the child (Mrazek et al., 1981; Conte & Berliner, 1981). In one English study, natural fathers were responsible in 20% of the cases coming to official attention, stepparents in 12%, natural mothers in 2%, and other relatives in 9% (Mrazek et al., 1981). In both intrafamilial and extrafamilial abuse, 85% to 95% of the perpetrators are male. In those instances where the sexual experiences are repeated for a long period of time, family members are more likely to be involved than are nonfamily members (Greenberg, 1979).

A common notion prevails that child molestation is usually a nonviolent affair, perpetrated by passive introverts who rely more on blandishments and seduction than force. Although coercion may not be involved in many cases of exhibitionism, in sexual crimes involving physical contact with the child, physical violence and threats do appear to be very common (Becker & Skinner, 1985; Finkelhor, 1980).

Perpetrators

A detailed review of pedophilia is beyond the scope of this discussion (see Howells, 1981; Langevin, 1985). As noted above, the overwhelming majority of sexual abusers are male. Behaviorally, these offenders show wide variation in their predilections concerning the sex and age of their preferred victim (e.g., exclusively male, exclusively female, or both); their relationship to their victims; the degree of violence employed; and the nature of the perverse act. Equally diverse character pathologies may be found. Our knowledge of pedophilia is limited because, in general, only apprehended offenders have been studied in clinical detail; the members of the apprehended cohort may be more likely to be persons who commit aggravated assaults or repeat their crime recklessly many times. Most nonincestuous sex abusers probably molest a large number of children before being apprehended. The statistics suggest that large numbers of child molesters are never discovered or reported; of them we know little.

Even when overt violence is absent, child molestation combines both sexual and aggressive motives. An erotic component is certainly present; by exploiting a child, the pedophile can obtain the sexual gratification that he frequently is incapable of achieving by means of adult heterosexual relations. The molester realizes and enjoys the enactment of primitive fantasies involving triumph over fears of castration and loss of bodily integrity. Pedophiles' sexual responses to various stimuli have been studied experimentally using physiological indices, such as penile tumescence. Many of these molesters show unusual levels of sexual arousal in response to pictures of children, preferring them to those of adult women (Finkelhor, 1984). How child molesters come to develop such deviant patterns of arousal is the object of much speculation from both the psychoanalytic and operant conditioning perspectives (Howells, 1981).

In addition to the erotic element, however, part of the molester's gratification appears to come from controlling and triumphantly dominating a submissive child, thereby compensating for his own sense of powerlessness. For some molesters, many of whom have a childhood history of having, themselves, been sexually exploited, this symbolic mastery may involve undoing a traumatic past via an explicit identification with the aggressor.

Many theories of pedophilia emphasize the ways in which the pedophile is thwarted in his adult sexual relationships by both external and internal factors. Several observers have described the child molester as inhibited and even inadequate with adult women (Langevin, 1985); in the case of the incestuous father, marital relations have usually deteriorated profoundly so that husband and wife have become sexually alienated.

An important dichotomy lies between child sexual abusers who are termed *fixated* offenders and those who are termed *regressed* offenders (Groth, 1982). The fixated offenders are those men who from adolescence on show a primary or exclusive sexual interest in children, usually male. Their pedophiliac interests are persistent, often compulsive, and their offenses are frequently premeditated. As many as 80% of such offenders have been sexually victimized themselves as children (Groth, 1985 cited in Lourie & Blick, 1987a). In contrast, the regressed offender has a more conventional peer-oriented sexual development. Among this latter group, the sexual interest in children is likely to be episodic, impulsive, and in response to stress. Their involvement with a child (usually female) provides a regressive substitute for a conflictual adult relationship.

Victims

As might be expected from the great prevalence of sexual abuse, its victims include children of all social classes and backgrounds. Certain social and family factors, however, appear to increase children's risk of sexual exploitation. Retrospective questionnaire studies, such as Finkelhor's (1979), avoid some of the sampling biases involved in studying only reported cases of abuse. Finkelhor identified eight characteristics that placed girls at high risk of abuse: having a stepfather, having not received physical affection from father, having lived away from the natural mother, having an emotionally unavailable or sexually punitive mother, having a mother who had not finished high school, having an annual family income under $10,000, and having had less than three friends in childhood. The sort of correlational multiple-regression analysis that identifies these factors does not explain *why* they predispose children to sexual abuse. Investigators can only speculate about the various mechanisms that might be at work. For example, the most powerful predictor that Finkelhor found—having a stepfather—correctly identified many girls who had been molested; in a number of cases, however, the molestation had occurred even prior to meeting the stepfather. It is possible to speculate that these girls' single mothers were more preoccupied, emotionally less available, less vigilant about their daughter's safety, or more likely to bring sexually opportunistic men into the house in the course of their own dating (Finkelhor, 1984); on the other hand, these girls, whose natural fathers were less available to them, might also, in dealing with men, have had a diminished ability to discriminate between exploitative interest and genuine concern (Finkelhor, 1980). Finally, as Finkelhor noted, it is important not to use these predictors to blame the victim. All but a tiny fraction of episodes of abuse are initiated by the older person. Thus, some of these risk indicators, such as lacking an involved, protective parent, might in fact represent selection criteria by which perpetrators identify children who will be "easy marks." Furthermore, to the extent that perpetrators and victims share the same social (and even family) environment, some of the socioeconomic factors (i.e., low-income status) may prove to be more usefully conceptualized as perpetrator characteristics. As noted earlier, it is not possible to study directly representative samples of unapprehended abusers.

In light of the ongoing debate concerning the effects of sexual permissiveness, it is interesting to note Finkelhor's (1979) finding that victimized girls were much more likely than nonvictimized girls to report that their mothers were punitive about sexual matters. Even when other variables were controlled for, this remained one of the most striking correlates of victimization.

Clinical Presentation

As retrospective studies indicate, during their childhood many victims of sexual abuse never tell anyone about their experiences (Finkelhor, 1979; Russell, 1986). Many toddlers, of course, may be too young to communicate verbally what has happened to them. The commonest motives for concealment are probably shame and the fear of retaliation by the perpetrator or punishment by parents. The perpetrator may threaten to hurt or kill the child or other family members should the incident be revealed. For example, in one recent widely publicized case of ongoing sexual abuse at a daycare center, the defendants allegedly slaughtered classroom pets in front of the children as an intimidating warning. Children are quite likely to reveal abuse at the hands of a stranger, whereas incestuous abuse may well remain a secret, even for years. In cases of incestuous abuse, the perpetrator may play upon the child's loyalty or intimidate his victim by warning that the family will break up if the abuse is disclosed. Much depends on the child's perception of whether adults are open to hearing about what has happened and whether they are more likely to react with punishment or protection. In many cases of incest, the mother's powerful, implicit message to the child is "I don't want to know!" Not surprisingly, many incest victims may first reveal their secret to a best friend or trusted teacher, rather than to their mother.

Symptoms and Behavioral Sequelae of Sexual Abuse

Even when the child has kept silent about the abuse or is too young to tell anyone, various physical symptoms and nonspecific behavioral signs may suggest the truth.

When violence has been used against the child, bruises or lacerations may be present. In the postpubertal girl, pregnancy is, of course, a conclusive sign of sexual activity. In children of all ages genital irritation, discharge, or bleeding; venereal disease; urinary tract infections; or proctitis may provide the first clues. The incidence of diagnosed gonorrhea in children under 10 years has increased dramatically in the past several years. Compulsive masturbation may reflect sexual overstimulation with or without urogenital inflammation. The majority of victims, however, have no physical signs of sexual abuse.

Children who have been sexually abused may also show abrupt changes in behavior (Rosenfeld, 1979a). Fearfulness, withdrawal, school phobia, or night terrors of acute onset require careful investigation. Sudden fearfulness in the presence of unfamiliar adults, especially males, should arouse suspicions. Previously well-behaved children may develop school difficulties, peer problems, or moodiness. Other behavioral symptoms may include signs of developmental regression such as enuresis, encopresis, clinginess, or temper tantrums. And, as Freud (1896/1957a, 1896/1962a) noted long ago, conversion disorder is frequently associated with sexual abuse in children. Because most occurrences of the above long list of nonspecific symptoms are *not* caused by sexual abuse, only careful questioning and a high index of suspicion will make an accurate diagnosis possible (Rosenfeld, 1979a).

Goodwin (1987) has argued cogently that many children's reactions to sexual abuse can be best understood as a form of posttraumatic stress syndrome, analogous to that described in adult and child survivors of war, crime, or disaster (Terr, 1987). The cardinal features of the posttraumatic stress syndrome include symptoms such as anxiety, guilt, sleep disturbance, and flattened or labile mood. In addition, victims are prone to reexperiencing the trauma either in sudden intrusive recollections or through abruptly acting or feeling as though the original event were recurring. Difficulties with concentration and memory as well as a general ego constriction are also common. How these features manifest themselves in a given child victim will depend on individual and developmentally determined factors.

Goodwin (1987) traced the manner in which the characteristic concerns of each developmental period shape the child's symptomatic response to the abuse experience. The preschool victim may regress in areas of speech, toilet training, and ability to function independently of mother, becoming clingy and withdrawn. The child may reenact fragments of the traumatic experience in the form of inappropriate sexual behavior or driven, stereo-typed play involving annihilation and primitive retaliation.

In contrast, the oedipal child of 4 to 6 years is more troubled with issues of guilt, badness, and self-blame. Especially in cases of incest, these children are concerned about retribution and are fearful of being responsible for the breakup of the family. As the child seeks external punishment to relieve internal guilt, masochistic character features may appear including compulsively repeated themes of punishment and reparation during play. At this age, regression may take more subtle forms than it does in the younger child. Girls may simply become passive, overly docile, and lack the curiosity and initiative essential for moving into latency and the school years.

In the school-age child, Goodwin noted, identification with the aggressor may take the form of inappropriate sexual or aggressive behaviors with peers and younger children. In school, ego constriction may be limited to difficulty with specific school subjects, such as biology, that impinge on the child's areas of anxiety; or the constriction may take more global forms, such as pseudostupidity, elective mutism, or conversion symptoms.

The adolescent's efforts to individuate from the family are complicated by the incest victim's premature precipitous deidealization of both parents as well as by what is often an intense, ambivalent enmeshment with the abusing father. For girls who have been the victim of sexual abuse, the move into age-appropriate involvement with boys may be complicated by anxiety in the presence of males and intrusive recollections of the abuse experience. Acting-out behaviors, such as running away, promiscuity, substance abuse, and suicide attempts, are frequent concomitants of incestuous abuse. Sexual abuse, especially incest, is thus an important and often overlooked part of the differential diagnosis of adolescent behavior problems. However, as Rosenfeld (1979a) pointed out, incestuous families often suffer from pervasive defects in impulse control, limit setting, and interpersonal boundaries, so the link may not be one of simple cause and effect.

Heightened eroticization is frequently apparent in children subjected to ongoing molestation. Yates (1987b) found that such children view "the world through libidinous glass: seeking, expecting, and yearning for further sexual experience" (p. 258). She noted several other characteristics of the eroticized child. Their anatomical knowledge is precociously advanced. They are readily aroused by casual interaction; indeed, they may have difficulty differentiating sexual from nonsexual touching. Sexual activity may become their primary means of tension release and principal mode of trying to form relationships with others. Increased eroticization may also be seen to a lesser degree in nonmolested children reared in sexually permissive or overly stimulating homes; however, Yates believes that in the absence of actual sexual experiences, such children are unlikely to act-out sexually.

Incest

Narrowly defined, the term *incest* (from the Latin *incestus,* meaning "not chaste") refers to sexual intercourse between family members too closely related to marry legally. In this chapter incest (or incestuous abuse) refers more broadly to sexual activity between a child and any family member, including steprelatives.

Although the most extensively studied form of incest has been that between father and daughter, there is evidence that incest between siblings or stepsiblings is the commonest form of this behavior (Finkelhor, 1979; Laredo, 1982; Nakashima & Zakus, 1977). Finkelhor (1979) found that homosexual incest between brothers was almost as common as heterosexual incest involving a brother and sister. A casual attitude toward sibling incest and a tacitly condoning view of rape appear to be prevalent in some isolated rural subcultures; such a cynically permissive view is reflected in the old country saw that "a virgin is a girl who can run faster than her brothers."

Participants. Homosexual father–son incest occurs less commonly and appears to involve dynamics that differ from father–daughter incest. Mother–son sexual engagement appears to be the rarest form of incest. In general, women are rarely the perpetrators of sexual abuse toward children. As previously noted, natural mothers are involved in only 2% of all sexual abuse cases.

Many cases of incest involve relatives outside the nuclear family, such as uncles, cousins, and grandfathers. Increasing numbers of children now live at close quarters with stepparents and stepsiblings of the opposite sex. In cases where a divorced mother has not remarried, children may have extended contact with their mother's boyfriends. The apparent recent increase in incestuous abuse may partially reflect the attenuation of the incest taboo in such nontraditional family arrangements. As many as 17% of women who grow up with a stepfather for a significant part of childhood recall having suffered some form of sexual abuse at his hands; in comparison, only 2% of women report having been abused by their biological fathers (Russell, 1986). Hence, the broad definition of incest cited above includes sexual activity with family members who are not blood relatives.

Types and Dynamics. Weinberg's (1955) classic study of incest distinguished two different types of incestuous fathers: the *promiscuous* and the *endogamic.* The first type, the indiscriminately *promiscuous* incestuous father, is characteristically found in chaotic, disorganized, multiproblem families. In such contexts, incest is but one facet of a complex pattern of family difficulties, often of overwhelming character, that may include alcoholism, violence, and antisocial behavior.

CASE EXAMPLE

Sammy S. was a 12-year-old boy in fourth grade who was admitted to an inpatient child psychiatry unit after a suicide attempt in a foster home. He had been placed there after running away from home, a desperate gesture precipitated by a severe beating at the hands of his father. Sammy soon revealed to his doctor that he had frequently been abused both sexually and physically by his violent, alcoholic father. Through the years, the Department of Protective Services had become well-acquainted with the family; three elder siblings had been removed from the home during the previous decade. Sammy's mother was an alcoholic and a suspected prostitute; she had long ago abandoned the family. The father's current common-law wife was herself a teenager and could offer little protection from the physical abuse to which she was also victim. Terrified phone calls from Sammy's younger sisters soon made it apparent that they too were being sexually abused. In addition to attacking the girls himself, Mr. S. would, for a nominal fee, often permit male acquaintances to molest the children as well.

Incest in such multiproblem families is often associated with poverty, poor education, isolation, and other socioeconomic stressors. Rural children and low-income children appear to be at increased risk for sexual abuse of all types (Finkelhor, 1980). Nonetheless, incest is not confined to economically disadvantaged or geographically isolated families. The statistics cited earlier make it clear that incest is common in urban middle-class families as well (Giaretto, 1981; Russell, 1986).

Incest in middle-class, seemingly respectable families is often of the type Weinberg (1955) termed *endogamic*. The endogamic incestuous father, Weinberg felt, concentrated most of his social and sexual interests within the family and turned to his daughter(s) to gratify dependent longings unmet by the adult women in his life, notably his wife (and, earlier, his mother).

Endogamic father–daughter incest has been the most thoroughly studied type, and much has been written about its dynamics (see reviews by Mrazek, 1981a; Mrazek & Bentovim, 1981; Rosenfeld, 1979b; Swanson & Biaggio, 1985). Two differing perspectives on it can be discerned in the literature (Lourie, 1984; Rosenfeld, 1979b), each with important implications for treatment. The first perspective, which has been characterized as the *victim/perpetrator* model, draws heavily on the paradigms of rape and child battering; by extension, this model sees the daughter as the helpless victim of a disturbed, often tyrannical father who uses her to meet his sexual and narcissistic needs. The second, *family dynamic* perspective, rather than viewing endogamic incest simply as deviant behavior on the part of a disturbed father, sees it as the product of familywide pathology (Lourie & Blick, 1987a). This second perspective does not seek to exculpate the offending father or to blame the daughter, who is indeed an exploited minor. It does, however, emphasize various fundamental defects in family organization. For example, such families blur generational boundaries so that a kind of role reversal exists between mother and daughter. By a sort of mutual consent, the incest victim (who is often the eldest daughter) assumes many of the other maternal functions in the family in addition to the sexual one. The fathers, who are often sexually estranged from their wives and, indeed, generally unable to deal with grown women, turn toward their daughters for gratification of strong unmet dependency needs. These men fear sexual intimacy with adult women, which prevents them from turning to adulterous gratifications; indeed, strangely enough, many of these men have a paradoxically puritanical attitude regarding sex.

To be sure, in many families extreme seductiveness may occur between father and daughter without actual incest taking place. In general, the mother plays a key role. Incest is most likely to occur in those families where illness, alcoholism, chronic depression, repeated childbearing, or other difficulties have rendered the mother psychologically or physically unavailable (Herman & Hirschman, 1981). The mother's abdication (voluntary or involuntary) of her parental and spousal roles seems to set the stage for her daughter to take over the mother's maternal and sexual functions in the family. Within such families, the mother often implicitly encourages the father's turning sexually toward the daughter; at the least, many of these mothers manage to look the other way. In incestuous families the adults seem unable to provide the basic parental functions of psychological protection for their children.

According to some authors, incestuous families have a rigidly patriarchal structure. The father not only perceives the females in the family as his possessions but also in many cases resorts to violence and intimidation in order to maintain his dominance (Herman & Hirschman, 1981). Wife beating is common in such families, although the daughter singled out for the father's sexual attentions may enjoy a protected status. Contradicting the common view that incest is usually a nonviolent crime, Becker and Skinner's study concludes that physical aggression is involved in almost two-thirds of incest cases (Becker & Skinner, 1985). Girls whose mothers have little power in their marriages appear more vulnerable to both incestuous and nonincestuous sexual abuse, perhaps because they more readily fall into the victim role themselves (Finkelhor, 1984). Finkelhor (1984) examined parental educational level as an indirect measure of the relative power distribution between mother and father. Although the risk of sexual abuse was increased in families where both parents had failed to complete a high school education, it was even higher in families where the father was well educated and the mother was not.

As children, many parents of incestuous families themselves suffered from emotional deprivation (sometimes including physical or sexual abuse), which deprived them of adequate role models for their subsequent parenting. Diagnostically, these parents present a heterogeneous pattern of psychopathology. Incestuous fathers represent a mixed group with respect to personality type, degree of violence, and degree of pedophilic interest in children other than their own (Groth, 1982; Langevin, 1985). Although many incest offenders are shy, inhibited, and ineffectual in family relationships, others are violent and tyrannical. Some have deviant sexual interest only toward their own pubescent daughters, whereas others are also attracted to other children. Some of these fathers are bisexual in their incestuous interests, and those fathers who molest a son are more likely than not to be involved in molesting a daughter as well (Finkelhor, 1984). In a minority of cases, alcoholism plays an important contributing role.

Clinical Course.　Incestuous sexual activity usually begins insidiously in preadolescence; initially it takes the form of genital fondling and often progresses to intercourse when the girl reaches puberty (Swanson & Biaggio, 1985). Such incestuous abuse characteristically continues for several years. Most often the victim is the eldest daughter of the family. As she grows older, however, and becomes less compliant or leaves home, the father may victimize each younger daughter in turn. Incestuous fathers are often jealous and sexually possessive of their daughters. They may resent and resist the daughter's attempts to establish relationships with boys her own age. Some girls remain socially isolated, sexually inhibited, and avoid age-appropriate relationships with boys, whereas others plunge into sexual acting-out. Many resort to marrying at an early age in what seems to be the only way to escape from their father's (and family's) clutches.

Coercion in Cases of Incest.　Many incest victims are forced to participate unwillingly by dint of coercion or fear of physical violence. Others may feel they have no other recourse. Girls often fear that, if they tell, they will not be believed, they will be blamed and punished, or their revelations will result in their father's imprisonment and destruction of the family. The intense insecurity and deprivation that characterizes so many incestuous families may lead the girl to cling all the more intensely to the incestuous relationship, albeit with great guilt and ambivalence. Some incest victims see their fathers as the only source of nurturance in the family; these deprived and exploited girls may view sexual submission as the only way to obtain care and affection. For them, sexualized love may seem preferable to no love at all. Girls in this group suffer great pangs of guilt and conflict; unlike victims who can more unambivalently hate a brutal father, these girls remain strongly attached to and protective of their fathers. The affectionate facade, however, does not diminish the exploitation of these girls. As Herman (1981) pointedly observed, "The father, in effect, forces the daughter to pay with her body for affection and care which should be freely given. . . . This is the reality of incest from the point of view of the victim" (p. 4).

The Incestuous Family.   Despite strenuous efforts to maintain a facade of respectability, normality, and competency, many incestuous families suffer from a pervasive fear of separation and family disintegration. The incestuous bonding between father and daughters in such families may serve a *tension-reducing* function in a desperate attempt to hold the family together (Lustig et al., 1966). There is an omnipresent fear (or threat) that the family will disintegrate if the child refuses or incriminates the father; it is because of this fear—which may be well founded—that children often continue to participate in an incestuous relationship.

Thus for a period of months or years, the entire family may collude in permitting unchecked incestuous activity. When this occurs, the victim, in turn, is caught up in what Summit (1982) has described as the *sexual abuse accommodation syndrome*. The child is entrapped and coerced into keeping the secret, frequent / at the cost of a high level of inner stress. Such children often feel helpless, guilty, isolated, and burdened. The overt and covert pressures exerted on them to deny what is happening compel them to sacrifice their own sense of reality and foster dissociation and primitive denial mechanisms. These children are thus deprived of what they desperately need—the firm support of a protective adult to help counter the inner feelings of badness, helplessness, and denied reality (Goodwin, 1987).

In a study of the nonabused siblings of incest victims, Lourie (1984) concluded that the disturbed dynamics of incestuous families were often as damaging as the sexual abuse itself. Within these families, the parents are unable to view their children's needs as separate from their own. Whether such parents' demands are sexual or nonsexual, their children's emotional growth is devastated because they are used as objects for gratifying the parents' narcissistic and infantile needs.

Effects of Sexual Abuse

Questions concerning the pathogenic impact of childhood sexual abuse have played a crucial and controversial role in the historical evolution of dynamic psychiatry (Garcia, 1987; Jones, 1953; Malcolm, 1984; Masson, 1984). On the basis of his early analytic work, Freud (1896/1957a, 1896/1962a) initially concluded that childhood sexual abuse, frequently of an incestuous nature, laid the groundwork for most, if not all, cases of neurosis, both hysterical and obsessional. It was Freud's public assertion of this belief that initially aroused scandalized hostility from his colleagues. Anticipating such incredulity, Freud (1896/1957a) noted:

It seems to me certain that our children are far more often exposed to sexual assaults than the few precautions taken by parents in this connection would lead us to expect. . . . It is to be expected that increased attention to the subject will very soon confirm the great frequency of sexual experiences and sexual activity in childhood. (p. 207)

However, by the next year Freud himself had growing doubts that actual sexual abuse had really occurred in all cases of neurosis, although he continued to believe, even late in life, that "seduction retains a certain aetiological importance" (Freud, 1896/1962a, p. 168). For one thing, Freud had come to believe increasingly that in the course of childhood development, sexual impulses and conflicts occurred normally even in the absence of externally inflicted trauma (Freud, 1905/1953b; 1985, p. 272). Thus, from a theoretical view, Freud no longer required actual abuse as an explanatory and essential noxious factor in the genesis of sexual conflict. Furthermore, for complex reasons, Freud also came to believe that in the case of some (but not all) of his patients, the apparent memories of incest recovered during analysis represented fantasies rather than real events (Freud, 1985, p. 264–267; Garcia, 1987; Jones, 1953). Masson (1984) has argued, unjustly and, in our view, unconvincingly, that Freud had self-serving motives for this shift, which allegedly predisposed Freud and subsequent generations of psychoanalytic psychotherapists to dismiss accusations of incest out of hand (see also Malcolm, 1984). It is fair to say, however, that Freud's heightened appreciation of the importance of inner fantasy and psychic reality implies that the clinician cannot understand the pathogenic impact of an externally inflicted sexual trauma without reference to how the child interprets the experience in terms of her inner life (A. Freud, 1981a).

During the century that has elapsed since Freud's first speculations, the effects of sexual abuse on the child's ongoing development continue to be debated. Investigators have attributed almost every conceivable disturbance to childhood sexual trauma. Much of the literature on the topic comes from anecdotal clinical material. Because of the lack of adequate controls for comparison, however, the significance of these data is equivocal. More recently, systematic studies of various troubled groups (e.g., prostitutes, runaways, drug abusers, psychiatric hospital inpatients, and patients with conversion disorder or multiple personality (Putnam et al., 1986)) indicate an increased incidence of childhood sexual abuse relative to controls. Even these cases, however, prove little about cause and effect. Because certain types of sexual abuse are correlated with disturbed or stressful family dynamics, later difficulties may reflect the pathogenic force of these family factors, rather than of the sexual abuse itself (Finkelhor, 1984).

Despite the methodological limitations of most studies, various opinions repeatedly appear in the literature concerning the long-term effects of childhood sexual abuse (see reviews by Mrazek & Mrazek, 1981, 1985).

These include difficulties in sexual adjustment (such as sexual inhibition, preoccupation with sexual matters, promiscuity, unwanted pregnancy, prostitution, or homosexuality); interpersonal problems; damaged self-concept; behavior problems; and vulnerability to becoming a child molester. Lowered sexual self-esteem appears to be one of the best documented sequelae (Finkelhor, 1984).

It is generally assumed that children who have experienced only a single, unrepeated episode of sexual abuse by a stranger and receive support from their families suffer fewer long-term sequelae than do victims of repeated incest (Synder et al., 1983). In contrast, incest with a parent is the most traumatic form of abuse (Finkelhor, 1979). The degree of force and aggression used to exact compliance from the child seems to be the single most important additional determinant of how traumatically a child experiences an episode of sexual abuse. Finkelhor (1979) also found that the age of the participants was a major predictor of psychological trauma. The older the child and the greater the disparity of age between victim and perpetrator, the more negative the experience.

Family factors, especially the mother's response, have a powerful influence on the aftermath of sexual abuse. Children from multirisk, multiproblem families enter the traumatic situation already burdened by a higher level of psychopathology. Clinically, children appear to fare worse when the mother is either punitive or trivializes the event, is unable to comfort the child, or makes the child feel unprotected (Gomes-Schwartz et al., 1985).

If the current high prevalence estimates are correct, more children are now exposed to incest than to tonsillectomy (Rush, 1980). Professionals cannot conceptualize sexual abuse as a unitary, pathogenic factor with uniform sequelae. Instead, many factors shape, mitigate, or exacerbate the ultimate meaning of the abuse experience; these include the child's developmental status, family context, parental reaction, and cultural mores. There is still much to learn about the elements that distinguish the children who cope relatively effectively with sexual abuse, showing perhaps only subtle impairments in adult life, from those who go on to develop severe, disabling pathology.

EVALUATION

The management of sexual abuse cases is complex and demanding, frequently involving multifaceted legal and clinical decisions. For this reason, such cases should usually be handled by a well-coordinated and experienced multidisciplinary team; such teams are now common at major pediatric treatment centers and are increasingly recognized as an essential component of effective child protective services (Seidl & Paradise, 1984). Close liaison among the caseworkers of the public child protection agency, pediatricians, mental health clinicians, prosecutors, and police is essential. The elements of effective evaluation and management are detailed in several comprehensive works addressing the treatment of childhood sexual abuse (Mrazek & Kempe, 1981; Sgroi, 1982). Unfortunately, outside the setting of demonstration projects and university-affiliated centers, services to sexually abused children are frequently poorly coordinated, fragmentary, and inadequate. All too often cases are inadequately investigated, are prematurely closed, or do not get referred for needed psychiatric evaluation and treatment Adams-Tucker, 1984; Kaplan & Zitrin, 1983).

Clinical evaluation of the sexually abused child involves several key elements, distinct from the legal issues concerning credibility, validation, and confirmation (Lourie & Blick, 1987b; Mrazek, 1981a, 1981b; for a discussion of these important evidentiary considerations, see Sgroi et al., 1982). These clinical essentials include assessment of the following factors:

1. What has been the impact of the abuse on the child and family? How are they coping? How has the trauma of abuse interacted with preexisting vulnerabilities and difficulties?
2. What immediate steps are necessary to prevent future abuse and to provide emotional security for the child?
3. What crisis management is necessary to help the family deal with the immediate emotional and legal sequelae of the trauma?
4. What long-term interventions are indicated for the child and/or family to minimize recurrences of abuse and long-term sequelae?

TREATMENT OF INTRAFAMILIAL ABUSE

Disclosure of incest triggers a family crisis with many reverberations, disrupting a precarious balance that has been established about the incest secret (Swanson & Biaggio, 1985). The father may face the possibility of incarceration, and the entire family may be threatened with humiliation, loss of income, and disintegration. In a family organized around a long-standing secret (maintained at the expense of the child, but basic to the family's homeostasis), the first reaction is often denial; the family may attempt, sometimes with intense pressure, to coerce the child into retracting the charges. Hence, following the revelation of incest, the clinician's first task is to assure the child's safety both from the ongoing sexual abuse and from parental retaliation. There is a critical decision to be faced: When does the situation require removal of either the father or the child from the family home? Resolving this issue is difficult, but necessary. In addition to physical or psychological reprisals against the child, other immediate hazards include suicidal ideation or actual attempts at self-destruction on the part of the mother, father, or the victim.

Assessing the Accuracy of Allegations of Incest

One of the most difficult tasks that faces the clinician is assessing the veracity of a child's allegation of incest when there is no corroborative physical evidence and the parents deny the charge (Terr, 1986). The child often further compounds the problem by retracting the accusation, either because of guilt feelings or fears of parental reprisal, family dissolution, or incarceration of the father. As noted earlier, the term "child sexual abuse accommodation syndrome" was coined by Summit (1982) to describe those sexually abused children who sense that the adults want them to remain silent or to "take back" the accusation, recanting it as fantasy or a lie.

Freud's difficulty in distinguishing between incestuous fantasies and actual occurrences had fateful consequences, and the same problem increasingly vexes the contemporary clinician. (For perceptive discussions of this troublesome clinical task, see Benedek and Schetky, 1987a, 1987b; A. H. Green, 1986, 1988; Hanson, 1988; Rosenfeld et al., 1979; Terr, 1986, 1988a, 1988b; Yates, 1988a, 1988b.) Very young children may have trouble separating fantasy from reality or may attribute actual abuse to the wrong person. On the other hand, young children are likely to confuse, distort, or repudiate their memories of actual incestuous events in order to maintain a good internal image of a parent or to protect against the overwhelming feelings of helplessness that the experience of abuse produces (Rosenfeld et al., 1979). Despite these caveats, a report of incest coming from a school-age child whose thinking is not disordered and whose account remains relatively precise and consistent over time is usually accurate and deserves credence. The conclusion that the child has mistaken a fantasy for reality should be grounded in actual evidence, rather than mere theoretical predilection.

Exaggerated or maliciously false accusations *do* occur and in themselves are prima facie evidence of serious family problems (Schuman, 1987). Such false accusations are most likely to arise in certain situations (A. H. Green, 1986): The first involves acrimonious custody cases in which a vindictive parent, usually the mother, brainwashes the child into accusing the other parent of sexual abuse. The accusation is then used as grounds to justify terminating visitation rights. Unfortunately, this destructive tactic appears to be increasingly common (Benedek & Schetky, 1985, 1987b; Bresee et al., 1986; Schetky, 1986). Indeed, some lawyers have labeled it the "nuclear weapon" of custody litigation. In three series of sexual abuse allegations occurring in the context of custody and/or visitation disputes, the accusations could not be clinically confirmed in 36% to 75% of the cases (A. H. Green, 1986).

A second, somewhat similar circumstance arises when a delusional or paranoid mother misperceives the relationship between the child and father and then influences the child into acquiescence or *folie à deux* acceptance of the allegations (A. H. Green, 1986). The vindictive or delusional mother often resents any positive ties between the father and child and may subject the child to great pressure.

A third type of false accusation of sex abuse is that made by a vengeful child seeking to retaliate against the father for some other grievance. Even when deliberately fabricated, such accusations may reflect a sexually overstimulating family atmosphere or serious sexual conflicts and concerns on the child's part.

There are, unfortunately, no hard and fast criteria for distinguishing between true and false accusations of sex abuse (Benedek and Schetky, 1987a, 1987b; Hanson, 1988). In the absence of clear-cut guidelines, the courts must often make an agonizing choice between two terrible possibilities: (1) condemning an innocent parent or adult to public stigma, criminal penalties, and the loss of custody or visitation or (2) leaving a child unsupported and unprotected in the face of ongoing trauma. These are terrifying alternatives indeed. Such cases have aroused intense passions and near hysteria with accused adults often being assumed guilty unless proven innocent.

In a controversial article, A. H. Green (1986, 1988) tentatively suggested several characteristics to help differentiate true allegations of sexual abuse from vindictively false ones. True disclosures are often delayed and conflicted, are made with considerable hesitancy, and are usually accompanied by painful or depressed affect. Unless the molestation was gentle and nonthreatening, the molested child is usually fearful in the father's presence and is unwilling to confront him with the accusation, even in the mother's presence. Such children also usually demonstrate the characteristic signs or symptoms of sexual abuse noted earlier: anxiety, regression, sexual preoccupation, depression, or full-blown posttraumatic stress disorder.

In contrast, Green contends, false accusations of sexual abuse are usually made easily and apparently spontaneously, with little painful affect. Despite the accusations, the child appears at ease with the father when the mother is not present. When she *is* present, the child willingly confronts the father with the alleged abuse but keeps a careful eye on the mother as though checking for approval or cues about how to proceed. In addition, the child often does not exhibit the characteristic symptoms of sexual abuse (other than perhaps sexual preoccupation). However, Green's observations have recently been sharply challenged by Hanson (1988), and further research is clearly needed.

A related controversy concerns the increasingly widespread use of anatomically correct dolls (Realmuto et al., 1990; Terr, 1988a, 1988b; Yates,

1988a, 1988b). The admissibility in court of sex abuse assessments using such dolls has been questioned in recent appeals court decisions. Defenders of the dolls' use maintain that such dolls give young children both tacit permission and the means to reveal their sexual traumas (Leventhal et al., 1989; Yates, 1988a, 1988b). They point to controlled studies showing that significantly more victims of suspected sex abuse engage in sexual play with such dolls than do control children. The differences, however, are not absolute (Glaser & Collins, 1989; Everson & Boat, 1990). Critics of the dolls, however, charge that the dolls are overly suggestive and implicitly urge sexual play from the child. Especially in the hands of unskilled examiners and when coupled with persistent direct leading questions, interviews using the dolls may elicit totally erroneous "evidence" from impressionable pre-schoolers (Renshaw, 1987; Terr, 1988a, 1988b). Great caution and more systematic research are necessary.

In the absence of corroborating testimony or physical evidence, it may remain impossible to validate the young child's testimony (in terms of the standard required for criminal proceedings), especially in the face of adversarial cross-examination of the child. Courts continue to struggle with the knotty questions of how old children must be to give reliable, admissible testimony, and how legal authorities can conduct interrogations that will protect both the children and the rights of the accused (Claman et al., 1986; Nurcombe, 1986; Terr, 1986).

Treatment Models

Coordination of clinical assessment and treatment with the legal and protective management of the case is often complicated. The threat of legal proceedings inclines some families to an adversarial stance that impedes adequate evaluation and treatment. Generally speaking, families who bend all their energies to contesting or repudiating the charges are the most difficult to engage therapeutically.

Two conceptual models for incest—the *victim/perpetrator* model and the *family-dynamic* model (Rosenfeld, 1979b)—have important implications for treatment. The victim/perpetrator model emphasizes the necessity of protecting the incest victim and the importance of sanctions against the perpetrator. The family-dynamic model emphasizes the importance of treating the family dysfunction that is expressed by the incestuous behavior; this model implies that each member of the family, including the perpetrator, needs and deserves compassionate, therapeutic intervention. To a large extent these two models parallel the dichotomy that Rosenfeld and Newberger (1977) have labeled *compassion versus control*, a familiar dialectic at the interface between psychiatry and the law. Effective intervention programs for incestuous families must include elements of both compassion and control. Thus, incarceration of an incestuous father protects the child, satisfies the impulse for punishment, and may even prevent recidivism upon release (Mrazek & Mrazek, 1985). Yet, incarceration exacts a high cost in terms of family disintegration and loss of economic status; further, by itself, incarceration leaves untouched the individual and family psychopathology that facilitated the abuse and that renders the child vulnerable to repeated victimization and other sequelae. At the same time, it must also be emphasized that without the force of the courts and protective services, many families will not accept treatment or continue it, and ongoing supervision of the child's safety is impossible. As in the treatment of physical abuse, court-ordered and supervised treatment is far more efficacious than treatment that is offered on a purely voluntary basis (Mrazek, 1981b).

Giarretto (1981) has developed an innovative treatment program for incest that combines intensive family treatment with deferred prosecution or probation. This multidisciplinary team approach combines court-supervised counseling (including individual, marital, and family modalities) with self-help peer support groups of parents and victims (such as Parents United and Daughters and Sons United). The program counselor and the juvenile probation officer responsible for the legal supervision of the case jointly devise the treatment plan. The counseling emphasizes first the individual level and then the mother–daughter dyad, with the dual goals of reestablishing a sound mother–daughter relationship and, if possible, rebuilding the family about that core. If the family wishes to be reunited, marital and family counseling can follow.

Giarretto (1981) claims a very high rate of success in reuniting those families who completed the program, with no recurrence of incest and a marked improvement in several measures of family functioning; however, his data are not clear about the drop-out rate. Other intensive treatment programs present a less sanguine picture. For example, Sgroi and colleagues' (1982) multiple-impact treatment project was effective in providing ongoing protective services; nonetheless, at the end of treatment, less than half the perpetrators had admitted guilt, one-third of the parents had separated or divorced, and barely a third of the victims and perpetrators were still living in the same household.

Therapeutic Considerations

In working with incestuous families, most therapists and caseworkers experience a considerable degree of discomfort; many authors have remarked on this reaction (Herman, 1981; Krieger et al., 1980). The clinician must struggle hard with the intense feelings of erotic excitement, anxiety, rage, and repugnance that these cases may stir up. Sexual titillation by or anxious avoidance of investigating the sexual details are common hazards for the therapist, as are the pitfalls of overidentification with either the victim or the parent.

The sense of shame, along with the intense mistrust of adults, that characterizes many victims of incest requires careful handling. On the other hand, many such children have learned to use sexual seductiveness as a means of obtaining love and affection (Yates, 1987b); the therapist must therefore be prepared to deal with sexualized behavior in the treatment situation. As a transference repetition, such behavior may have a variety of meanings: competitiveness with the mother, identification with the adult sexual aggressor, an attempt to obtain nurturance from the therapist, a need to control the level of intimacy, and/or a test of the therapist's reliability and nonexploitiveness (Krieger et al., 1980). At the same time, these children have an extreme need for feeling safe in the therapeutic setting. Their sexualized behavior requires a steadfast, nonjudgmental, and nonpunitive stance on the part of the therapist. The complex feelings that the child's behavior evokes in the therapist (e.g., flattered pleasure, harsh disapproval, guilty excitement) make treating sexually abused children an exacting and difficult task.

Diagnostic Appendix
Child Psychiatric Diagnosis

OVERVIEW

In initiating a psychiatric assessment, the mental health professional is likely to take for granted that he or she is examining not only a child or an adolescent, but is, in fact, exploring the child's family and larger milieu. In effect, the clinician assumes that a dynamic interplay of forces between the child and his environment has brought the existing problems into being and is maintaining them in place. The work of evaluation then has two facets; how to assess the factors at work within the child, and how to discern those that reflect the interplay between child and environment.

Underlying this approach is another assumption: both the child as a unit and the family as a system seek to maintain a steady state of homeostatic equilibrium. Tensions rise and fall; interactions provoke and soothe; but the tendency is always to return to some optimal level of adjustment. The final configuration need not be in any sense normative or conventional. To an outside observer, the homeostatic balance maintained by a given individual and family may seem wildly askew; nonetheless, however pathological its form, this dynamic equilibrium persists.

The homeostatic model implies as well that the therapist must consider ongoing factors of growth and change in the child himself, in the people around the child (for the adults also grow and develop), and in the subcultural surround (albeit somewhat slower paced, communities are as dynamic and fluid as are the people who compose them). For better or for worse, growth and change are forever disturbing the equilibria, bringing about some degree of transformation, and creating imbalances. Hence, the child repeatedly must accommodate and adapt to these changes. Good health (whether in the individual or the family) implies the ability to adapt readily, an ease and a comfort in so doing, and a usual state of inner and outer harmony. On the other hand, the youngster who is hindered in coping and whose adaptive capacities are limited by genetic (constitutional) disadvantages or by excessive environmental stress becomes increasingly troubled— and the environment immediately senses, echoes, resonates with, and responds to the child's distress. This, in turn, affects the youngster, creating a feedback loop that is thus constantly in play. It is the diagnostician's task to discern the nature of this system. The professional must identify the inner and outer disabilities, seek their source, find the factors that tend to perpetuate them, and consider ways to unravel this disturbing situation.

DIAGNOSTIC TECHNIQUES: TACTICS AND METHOD

The Initial Contact

In concrete terms, the clinician may first encounter the diagnostic situation in any one of many different ways. For the private practitioner, the most common channel is a phone call or a letter from a variety of sources. The commonest first contact is a family member, but the alert will often come from a physician (usually a pediatrician or child psychiatrist) or some other mental health professional. Alternatively, the call may come from a staff member of a hospital, a clinic, or a school; from a lawyer or a clergyman; or from some kind of social agency (welfare, child protection, family service, etc.). Occasionally, a teenager may make the call himself or may just walk into an office or clinic (grade school children seldom call on their own, and preschoolers, never).

Whatever the source, as a rule, the initial information involves some account of a problem, most often in the form of a concrete question such as these: Why is this intellectually competent child performing so poorly at school? With which of two litigating parents should the child live? Would it damage the child to be held back at school for a year? What can be done about the child's unwillingness to go to school? The informant will often mention the source of the referral, for example, "We got your name from our family doctor [or a friend, or from some other source]," and this is often a significant factor in the subsequent work. In any case, an appointment is set up, and the study is under way.

As noted, the first encounter may arise because a doctor or agency has made the referral. Sometimes a report is forwarded, such as a school psychological evaluation, a hospital case summary, or some other datum that tells a great deal about the youngster; for the most part, however, even when available, such documents are often late in coming. Regardless of the initial contact, it is important for the family to call the clinician directly to set up the appointment. Making such an appointment will mobilize a great deal of concerned anticipatory internal work in the people who initiate the call. Contemplating a mental health interview is no minor matter. It implies that the person stands ready to reveal highly personal details about himself and/ or his family and faces the need to "explain" himself, or his motives or actions, to a stranger—well-reputed, perhaps, or vouched for by credentials—but yet a stranger. The interview may open the floodgates on a world of emotion that the person has rigorously repressed to get through each day. And all of these fears jostle side by side with hopes for a magical cure and instant relief from the pain of the existing problem.

The sensitive clinician will be alive to all these nuances, and will respond to them from the first phone exchange. The essential qualities the clinician seeks to convey are interest, empathy, and reality. He or she can express awareness of how distressing or how challenging the situation sounds, and readiness to look at it with the caller. Sometimes, with very anxious communicants, the clinician can offer minimal reassurance: "Yes, I have worked with such situations before, and there is often something that can be done, but we have to look at it together and talk it over before I can tell you anything about your particular circumstance." In this connection questions may arise about seeing people at unusual times or places; the patient or the family would rather arrange an evening or weekend appointment, or they ask if the doctor could come to their homes or if they could go to the doctor's residence. In the face of such requests, it is important for the clinician to clarify the structure of the office appointment schedule, including any evening or weekend hours, if such are available. The physician must emphasize that he or she does not depart from the established schedule.

The therapist may address the matter of fee but usually omits it from this initial exchange. It is often quite helpful to say to prospective patients something to this effect: "There are expenses associated with such consultations; do you know whether your current health insurance program will help you with that aspect of things?" If the patient knows this information, then no further discussion is necessary at that point. Where the answer is negative, however, it is wise to ask callers to contact the insurance company representative and to ascertain the status of their coverage. It can save some very unpleasant and uncomfortable complications later on. Inevitably, a subset of callers will regard so early a reference to fee as proof of a predatory attitude on the part of the clinician. ("All they are really interested in is your money.") In the long run, however, introducing realistic considerations early is more likely to prevent problems than augment them.

There is another essential issue to address in initiating any sort of clinical arrangement: whom to see first. With preteen children, the rule of thumb is to see the parents first without the child being present. In the case of teenagers, a different set of considerations prevail. Where the young person is, in fact, the one who initiates the call, he should always be seen first. Where a troubled youth is involved but the parent calls (the usual case), it is often wise nonetheless to see the teenager before seeing his family (however, regardless of the youngster's age, sooner or later the clinician should always see the parents). If the parents of the adolescent seem very troubled and under great pressure, they might then need immediate contact with the examiner. On the other hand, where the caller says, "We have a family problem," the professional might suggest that they all come as a family for the first interview and let the quality of the response to that offer guide the structuring of subsequent meetings.

In the situation of a preteen child, the parents, during the initial phone call, are asked to come to the first interview without the child. When the time for the appointment arrives, however, the doctor may open the reception room door only to find the youngster sitting with the parents, and, when the interviewer appears, they all stand up. Under such circumstances, it is best, at first, to see the whole family together. Later, the therapist may ask the older child, if appropriate, to sit in the waiting room for a while. Where the child is too young or it is clinically inadvisable for the boy or girl to sit outside alone, the clinician can arrange subsequent appointments.

The Initial Interview

The initial interview must accomplish a number of missions. To begin with, people who are meeting for the first time need to "size each other up," to get a sense of how each communicates, how each relates, and whether there is enough sense of a feeling of engagement to allow for constructive work. This holds true for both parties, and parents are well advised not to continue to work with someone whom they do not feel able to trust or to exchange with in a reasonably comfortable fashion. A certain subjective component to such work, no doubt derived from residual transferences from the past, bears meaningfully on the outcome of the therapeutic process. In a similar way experienced clinicians learn that they should refer some situations to a colleague rather than attempt to handle them. Perhaps the examiner does not do well with teenagers or very depressed people or very aggressive patients or individuals who appear to be very seductive, or whatever. If the clinician encounters such a clinical situation, he or she should not undertake the case if there is any alternative. This should be a guiding principle in determining with whom the clinician contracts a working relationship.

A second mission of the first contact is to develop a picture of the expectations that have brought the clinician and the family (or patient) together. The therapist's clarity or vagueness in addressing this issue is of signal importance in the outcome of the study. Often, the attempt to clarify what the parents want, what they hope might emerge from the evaluation, and what role they expect the interviewer to play reveal immediately whether it is a "workable" situation. Sometimes the expectations are so unreal that no possible action, no matter how skillfully or zealously undertaken, could provide the desired response. People under great stress often have magical expectations, and confronting this kind of yearning with a frank admission that it is impossible to fulfill such wishes might be a critical factor in setting the work on a realistic course. Not infrequently a parent implies that the clinician's task is to get the other parent to understand the problem, or to persuade the youngster to behave, for example, by making a mute child talk or an oppositional child comply. Again and again, the clinician's response must be: "I cannot do the things you wish me to do, but if we work together and get a better understanding of what has happened, and is perhaps continuing to happen, then, out of such a mutual effort, we have a chance of doing something that could help." Some parents will not be satisfied with such an answer; they will presently abandon the evaluation and shop for someone who will promise more. But it is better to have that outcome at this early point than to become more deeply involved in a situation that is doomed to failure.

Where the sought-for solution is within the reach of a reasonable effort, the work of evaluation can then get under way. The third mission of the first interview is to begin data collection. Several kinds of data are needed. At best, any division of the information into categories is arbitrary. The web of human interaction is so continuous that past and present overlap, internal factors and environmental factors are in a state of constant dynamic flux, and the relative weight of individual components and family vectors is always the resultant of a mutually interacting system. Still, for purposes of study, it is necessary to channel the initial wash of material into orderly conduits, to develop data streams of different ranks of primacy, and to conduct the inquiry in a systematic way (or in as organized a fashion as that particular situation will allow).

A fourth mission of the first interview is to convey to the parents the nature of the evaluation process and to give some picture of what is entailed. For example, the clinician can spell out what a developmental history involves, can underline the importance of getting a picture of family tensions and family coping strategies, and can describe the roles of the various family members in the evaluation. The therapist should mention the possibility of additional studies, depending on what emerges. It is important for the clinician thoroughly to inform the family about the details of the process into which he or she is inviting them; their readiness to engage and their ability to cooperate are critical.

Realms of Inquiry: The Chief Complaint

The first area to cover is the *chief (or presenting) complaint*. In essence, this is the trigger that occasioned the visit. Sometimes it is a specific event, for example, a position taken by the school or by a neighbor that threatens the current family equilibrium. Sometimes it is the last in a series of recurrent events that have cumulatively raised the stress level in the family to an intolerable pitch. Sometimes a child surprises parents by announcing that he wants to talk to someone about troubles or is contemplating self-destruction. Sometimes it is part of a larger therapeutic effort: the child has been in a psychiatric setting and is now coming out with a recommendation for continued outpatient care. Whatever form it takes, it is the point from which the study departs. The statement of this chief complaint invites exploration into the nature of the child's and the family's current problem. The clinician probes gently to find out how long the situation has existed, whether it has changed over time, how the different family members are involved, what theories various family members have as to the cause, what attempts have been made heretofore to deal with the problem, and what the family (and/or the child) are doing about it now. Of particular importance is the question: Why is the difficulty coming to attention at this point?

The responses to these queries can take the family members far afield from the area of initial exploration. Sometimes it is best to allow such freely associative expression; in other instances, it is important to curb the tendency to move off into adjacent realms and to seek instead to keep the material centered on the current problem. A certain amount of clinical judgment will be necessary to determine how much the family talks, for example, about the origins of the problem, or the previous attempts at intervention. The therapist can say, truthfully, "We will come back to that presently and pick up all those items, but for the moment I see the general picture, and could we talk about another component of the problem"—and move on to the next area. In sum, the key point is to find out what has transpired that is being experienced as a problem, and why it is coming to attention now.

Realms of Inquiry: Family Background

A second area for early exploration is the nature of both the larger family background and the human context within which the child now lives. In particular, the clinician should identify any major mental or neurological illness in the family's lineage so that he or she can incorporate at least a preliminary sense of the genetic loading of the situation. Next it is important to ascertain a sense of the significant presences in the child's life: Who else lives at home and what is their relationship with the child? Are grandparents active participants in the youngster's relationship world? Are there siblings in or out of the household? Are there other close relatives who are not living at home, such as a divorced parent, an older sibling, an uncle, or a cousin who are key figures in the child's network of attachments? Has a housekeeper or other caretaker played (or is currently playing) an important role in the child's life?

Overall, this kind of review will illumine both the character of the difficulty and the people involved. In particular it will show their natural approach to problem-solving and their style of interpersonal relationship and child management. These data will play a significant role in determining the later formulation of dynamics and eventual treatment planning.

Finances. The discussion of the areas noted above may well take up much of the first hour. Before the end of the hour is reached, however, the examiner should initiate an exploration into the financial implications of the study. The therapist should clarify the amount of the fee and the method and time of payment, and should offer some estimate of the number of hours needed for the study. The parents should also receive some account of additional studies that may be necessary including endocrinological study, neurological examination, EEG, CAT scan, MRI, psychological and/or neuropsychological testing, genetic screening where that may be indicated, or any other specialized study that the available data suggest. To the extent that it is feasible, the therapist should discuss the implications of the fee with the family. Within the private practice, insurance issues are of primary importance; where possible, the mental health professional should ask the parents to pay him or her directly and then to seek reimbursement from the insurance company. The direct exchange of money for service is an important psychological as well as material presence in the outcome of the evaluation.

It is advisable to ask for at least a partial payment at the time of the first hour. People who have made a financial investment at the outset will often be more inclined to move past the normal initial ambivalence and to make at least the necessary psychological commitment to see the evaluation through. Some clinics and some practitioners ask for payment with each session. That is probably a sound approach, but it may be technically difficult for certain patients.

Medical Studies.   No mental health evaluation is complete unless the practitioner has considered the child's overall health and physical status as integral parts of the emerging profile. The necessity for contact with and (if the child has not been seen recently) a clinical examination by the pediatrician are emphasized, and the name and address of the pediatrician (or family physician) are noted. The evaluator should plan to talk to the pediatrician by phone and should ask the parents to sign a release permitting the necessary exchange of information.

Closing the First Interview.   Where possible, the time for the next appointment should now be established. Many parents will need some help in how to prepare the child for his first appointment. The clinician can set this appointment up or can schedule another interview with the parents to take a more detailed history of child and family, and to address the preparation issues. The discussion of how to go about this should be deferred until the clinician has reviewed the details of history taking.

Finally, the parents should fill out one (or several) of the standard instruments (such as the Child Behavioral Checklist (Achenbach, 1983) or, where relevant, the Conner's Hyperactivity Rating Scale, 1973). These are gaining acceptance as important sources of basic information; they have the special virtue of covering a great deal of terrain (which builds in a measure of protection against possible errors of omission), and, in certain instances, they can help materially with making a diagnostic formulation (see Checklists and Rating Scales, later in this Appendix).

Developmental History

The evaluator devotes the next hour with the parents to a review of the child's developmental history, again subdividing it into areas of exploration. To best accomplish this component of the work, the therapist should pursue such material systematically and in some detail.

In conducting the developmental study, the physician encourages the parent to speak freely about the child's development and to mention any areas that seem to merit special concern and exploration. This will usually generate a number of recollections and associations that are often of rather helter-skelter character but that nonetheless offer some valuable leads. The examiner should then begin to review the history of the child thoroughly and in detail. This is a laborious and time-consuming process, but only such a careful and systematic survey will reveal the essential information.

Pregnancy. It is best to begin with a general history of the mother's encounter with pregnancy: Were there previous pregnancies and what was their quality and outcome? Were there some lingering states of feeling because of prior stressful experiences? That clarified, the clinician then investigates three areas concerning the beginning of this child's life: circumstances of conception, gestation, and delivery. Thus, the questions range from whether the child was a wanted baby and what the family circumstances were at the time of conception through a review of the mother's physical and emotional status during pregnancy. These factors include her use of drugs, tobacco, or alcohol during the months of gestation, any illnesses she may have had (especially viral infections, such as rubella), any threats of miscarriage and the occurrence of any external traumatic events in her life (marital difficulties, financial reversals, illnesses or deaths in her family of origin, disasters that might have overtaken a close friend, etc.) between conception and delivery. It is important as well to explore the mother's fantasies and hopes during pregnancy. Did she want, expect, or dream of a child of a given gender? What age child did the mother tend to picture to herself? Did the pregnancy evoke any special fears or anxieties? Did the mother picture the kind of person this child would someday be, or the kind of relationship she would have with the baby?

The therapist should review the paternal involvement in the pregnancy, touching on any childbirth courses the parents may have taken together, and the father's activities, feelings, and responses during this time. Where relevant, the involvement of other family members should also be explored.

Finally the questions turn to the delivery itself, its nearness to term, its duration, its level of difficulty, the character of the mother's experience, whether anesthesia was employed (and, if so, what kind), the degree of the father's presence and support, any complications that might have been present, and the baby's condition at the time of birth. Many mothers are aware of Apgar scores, and many mothers and fathers can describe their first encounter with the newborn in the delivery or the recovery room. If a Caesarean section was performed, what were the indications, and how did the mother feel about that?

A different but parallel set of considerations pertain when a baby is adopted shortly after birth. Obviously the issues of pregnancy and delivery are not applicable, but the meaning of the new arrival, the parents' fantasies, aspirations as to gender, and various aspects of anticipation are all important.

The Newborn.   Often the parents have quite specific recollections of the quality of the baby's interactive pattern shortly after birth. Such observations are particularly likely concerning untoward incidents, for example, the baby did not like to be held, or had a milk allergy, or cried all the time, or turned day into night and night into day. Many mothers can describe the kind of person their baby was literally from the outset. The clinician can ask about temperamental characteristics, such as mood, intensity, regularity, consolability, threshold, adaptability, activity level, and reactivity to new experiences, and the mother will often offer vivid memories. The clinician can thus begin to build an image of this child's welcome into the world and his equipment on arrival.

Where the baby was premature or had severe congenital problems, the evaluator should survey such circumstances carefully, with special emphasis on the parents' reactions. Where obtainable, the associated hospital records should be reviewed. Where no pertinent neonatal observations can be reported, however, and patient questioning fails to reveal any further details, the examination proceeds to the first year of life.

Beginning with the history of the newborn period and throughout the child's subsequent development, it is important to explore how this particular child fits into this particular family pattern. Every family has its own complex system of aspirations, values, identifications, expectations, and mutual projections. Where does the newborn (and growing child) stand in this rich web? Was the child conceived in an attempt to save a failing marriage or to replace a lost sibling or grandparent? If the child is adopted, what did that choice mean to the parents? What fantasies (and facts) concern the child's origins?

The child has been the recipient of what identifications or projections, and how do these color the parents' perceptions of the child's temperament? Did the fussy infant offer a hateful presence "just like" the mother's memories of her own ungratifying mother? Or did the child's handicaps or difficulties become emblematic to a parent of his or her own sense of defectiveness or badness? Did the baby's feeding pattern raise doubts about or affirm the mother's sense of her own nurturant capacities? Did the baby's voracity stir uneasy reminders in the father of his own neediness? How did the baby's siblings greet and perceive the baby's arrival?

What aspirations attend a new boy or girl in their family? To go to an Ivy League college, to be a football player, a concert artist, a debutante? What perceived dangers must be guarded against in this particular family? Being too aggressive, too timid, too sexual, too compliant, or too defiant?

Thus, although the infant has his own unique personality and constitutional endowment, each family "invents" their infant, just as the infant will, in the course of development, construct and invent his own representation of his family (Scharff & Scharff, 1987). It is crucial for the diagnostician to learn the unique and special meanings that the family embraces concerning the child and his behavior. All this may not be open to exploration at the outset, but some of it will, and in any case there will be many hints and references that the clinician should note for subsequent study.

The First Year. For many parents inquiry into details about events in the first 12 months becomes a particularly difficult part of the study. They simply do not recall much of what happened, and they often cannot even tell about landmarks (such as when the baby first started to smile, or when he could sit up by himself). Where the family has reared several children, it is not unusual for a parent to have difficulty differentiating one child's developmental story from another's, and things get mixed up. Such failure to recall may indicate some early barrier in the establishment of the parent–infant relationship; the inability of parents to give much of a picture of early development should be weighed as an evaluative factor.

Throughout, it is important to keep in mind that parental experience was continuing alongside the childhood events; as the evaluation goes along, the clinician needs to incorporate questions that will illuminate the parents' lives and that will shed light as well on the child's reactions to family events and stresses. The inquiry turns to anything that would have been distracting or upsetting to parents, for example, a move, an illness, the loss of a grandparent, a difficult episode in the marriage, a business reverse (such as job loss, bankruptcy, or failure of promotion), or any other source of stress that might have impinged significantly on the baby's emotional growth. The fate of nonfamily members can also be important. The infant is specially vulnerable to separations in the first year of life, and the loss of a housekeeper or maid to whom the child had become attached is usually of considerable significance.

The examiner may explore how the previously noted temperamental traits matured, and when major developmental landmarks were reached. These include the infant's capacity to be soothed, social smiling (how early and how readily), cuddlesomeness, alertness, responsiveness (especially to invitations to play), mood, activity level, regularity of behavior, and length of time the child could concentrate on a particular item. How distractible was the baby? How did he respond to new situations such as a new maid or babysitter; how did the baby react to strangers in general; and how happy was the baby overall? How readily did the child make eye contact and was there anything unusual about that? Was the baby particularly tense or unusually floppy? Was the baby surprisingly vulnerable to touch, sound, or light—or otherwise hypersensitive? Or was the opposite true, with a logy unresponsiveness present at the outset?

Starting from birth onward, how did the newborn take nourishment? Was the child breast-fed, and what went into the decisions around that? Were there any problems with feeding, then or later? Was a pacifier important, and for what interval? During the first year was there any problem with food refusal, excessive pickiness, or other aspects of nurturance? Was the child very selective in whom he would allow to feed him, or did he fall asleep during most feedings?

It is important to know who cared for the child, how many caretakers were involved, and how consistently any one person was in charge. Finally, in the latter part of the first year, the mastery of motor behavior, speech, walking, and preferred patterns of play are all significant. At this point stranger reactions tend to appear, and the child's way of coping with new people and novel situations should be surveyed. Separation too should receive special emphasis. The parents' responses to the first-year-of-life events, the character of their handling of the infant, plus an account of the parental emotional state are interwoven with this exploration.

One to Three Years. Evaluation of the next developmental stage—ages 1 to 3 years—includes reviewing the baby's responses as he learned to walk, talk, climb, and manipulate the world. The clinician examines patterns of self-protection and self-preservation as opposed to a readiness to court disaster through excessive "fearlessness," along with any tendency to have accidents or to be hurt a great deal. Note should be taken of any history of ingestion of toxic substances. If, on the other hand, the child was unduly fearful and always ready for tearful panic, that too is important.

The patterning of relationship is a key factor. Did the child run away early on; was he very attached to caretakers so that he seldom left their side? What, in fact, was the youngster's reaction if left for a short time? Activity level should be explored: Was the child always in motion? Poorly coordinated? Was the youngster destructive so that toys never endured very long no matter how much they seemed to be valued, and were other household items always in danger? In terms of preferences, did the child have a favorite toy or some particular object that he carried about everywhere, and if so, when did this pattern begin and end? What about weaning: Did the child stop the bottle or breast spontaneously, or was it withdrawn by the caretakers—and if this did happen, how did the child react? Did the child take a nighttime bottle for some extended period? Until when?

What about *eating patterns?* In general, was this a greedy child who devoured everything that he could get? Or was the child excessively abstemious and hard to feed? Did he beg for food, hide food, or eat inedible items, such as paint, rust, and dirt? Did he bite adults or other children?

Conative behaviors need review: Was the child willful and insistent and obstinate, or overly compliant and unwilling (or unable) to assert his own interests? Were there ever moments when the child seemed to want to be provocative and acted deliberately to disobey? Did the child ever seem to turn against himself and slap his own face or otherwise seem to seek injury? If corrected, how did he respond? Was he concerned by the caretaker's anger? What was the usual manner of correcting the child? Was there ever any question of abuse at anyone's hands? What went on and how long did it last?

Did the child go through a stage of "terrible twos," with negativism, tantrums, protest, oppositional behavior, refusal to obey instructions, deliberate misbehavior, overt provocativeness, destructiveness, repeated upsets about trivia, demandingness, insatiability, and other evidences of attempting to pit himself against the adults? Did this take the form of a genuine *power struggle,* and if so, how was it handled and how long did it last? Did some elements of this pattern never resolve, so that they continue to persist at present?

How was the child's *health*—were there any serious illnesses or hospitalizations? Were there any allergies? Was surgery necessary at any time, and did it involve a separation? How did the youngster handle it? How did the family deal with it?

What about *speech*—when did the child say his first words, and has there been any problem with the clarity of speech? Was there any difficulty with using pronouns, making use of "I" in referring to himself, or with saying "yes" or "no?" When did the child first use sentences? Are there any ambiguities or odd usages in the child's speech, and does the quality of communication pose any kind of problem? Did the child go through a period of stuttering? Did he tend to remain mute a good deal of the time, speaking only to a very few, select people?

When and how did the caretaker initiate toilet training, and what was the outcome of these efforts? Did the child fight being changed; were there episodes of smearing behavior; did the child characteristically hide when defecating? Was training successfully achieved; and, if so, has it been adequately maintained, or have there since been "accidents?" To what extent are the parents currently involved in supervising or assisting the child's toileting?

Three to Five Years. As the child grew older, were there any *sleep disturbances* such as difficulty falling asleep, nightmares, sleepwalking, or night terrors? Did the child try to get into the parents' bed a great deal?

How was this managed? Does this continue; if not, when and how did it stop?

What about *sexual patterns*—did the child manipulate his genitals a great deal? Was there some tendency to exhibit the genitals? Was the child ever concerned about the size, the form, or the safety of his genitals? Did he express envy of anyone else's body? And in each instance, what were the parental reactions to this behavior? During development, did the child display a preference for the playthings of or the companionship of children of the opposite sex? Did the child like to play with the clothing or personal ornaments of the opposite-sexed parent? Did the child have a tendency to cross-dress? Was there ever any interest expressed in changing to the opposite sex?

Most children will have attended some kind of *nursery school* or play school during these preschool years; did this youngster have such an experience and what was its character? In particular, what observations did the teachers report about peer relationships and the child's general sociability? Do the parents have any comments about the way the youngster got on with other children at this time? Was there anything special about the materials the child chose as playthings, and the way these were used? Were there problems in separation from the parent when the child was dropped off? How long did this last and how was it handled?

Were there any *fears* present, for example, did the youngster have a pronounced reaction to fire, thunder, animals, insects, storms, noise, or darkness? Did the child ever behave oddly, or in a way that caused the parents worry? Did the child have an imaginary companion or live in a world of make-believe? Did the child go through an epoch of complaining that something frightening was present, which other people could not see?

Some children display odd habits, for example, they constantly twirl a lock of hair, pull out strands of hair, rub their heads, pull at an ear, or twirl objects for extended periods of time. Were any such habits present? Was the child fascinated by fire, or did he tend to play with fire (light matches one after another or set small fires)?

Was the general behavior of this child essentially compliant or did some oppositional behavior appear now and then? Was this an impulsive child who constantly had to be kept under observation? Did the youngster tend to wander off or to run away outright? Did adults find the child provocative, always "pushing someone's button" and forever getting people upset? Was this a destructive child? Did the parents note a malicious quality that might be expressed by destroying or acquiring other children's possessions? Did the child treat pets nicely, or was he ever cruel or mean to them? Was this an open child, or did he show a certain slyness, craftiness, or dissimulation in dealing with adults? For example, did the child steal? Tell lots of lies? Sometimes beg from neighbors or even from strangers?

Latency—School-Related Behavior.   From age 5, when most children start kindergarten, the school-related behavior reports are of primary importance in composing the database for the evaluation. They are by no means the only essential areas, but they are nonetheless significant. These school-related behaviors have three basic dimensions: the child's relationship to his teachers, the child's relationship to peers, and the child's relationship to academics. Each is of considerable diagnostic and prognostic weight and must be evaluated with great care.

THE CHILD'S RELATIONSHIP TO TEACHERS.   Any problems with authority and obedience that have transpired at home can make themselves dramatically evident within the school context. To be sure, some children discriminate sharply between the home and the school settings; they display little at school to cause concern, whereas at home their behavior may continue to be problematic to the point that it is insufferable. Or, contrariwise, a child may be regarded as a major problem within the school context; yet the parents may perceive him as being essentially conforming and unremarkable. A common pattern, however, arises when there is a lack of adequate controls at home; all too often, this is accompanied by a general disinhibition of behavior, so that the children are likely to be quite problematic everywhere they go. At school they may disrupt the class or confront and challenge the teacher, or they may simply refuse to comply with instructions and rules. Hence, investigating this aspect of their lives requires a careful review of school adjustment within the framework of obedience, conformity, adaptability to social structures, acceptance of rules, and maintenance of elementary respect for authority. In particular, the examiner seeks to ascertain whether the child's troublemaking is devious or covert, whether it involves an element of willfulness, or whether the child gives the impression of being unable to control himself because of some difficulty in mastering impulse. For example, the child's state of uncontrollable restlessness and constant driven activity might result in frequent clashes with his teacher but could still convey the sense of difficulty in inner control rather than intentional disruptiveness. Even so, anyone whose behavior regularly interferes with the smooth running of a sizable group poses a very real classroom problem.

Quite a different variety of school-based difficulty arises with the inhibited and anxious child. Here the youngster is, if anything, too dependent on the positive regard of teacher and lives in dread of a frown or a cross word. The child greets any reproof or any less-than-perfect grade with a kind of despair and a feeling of impending disaster. Many teachers are astute in perceiving their students' nuances of neediness, and the instructors compensate automatically for these vulnerabilities. Other teachers are less perceptive and unwittingly wreak havoc in the lives of such anxious and dependent children. The relationships with teachers, as described both by child and instructors, are of critical importance.

ACCEPTANCE OF AND ACCEPTANCE BY PEERS.   This is a vital area of adjustment during the grade-school years; indeed, the mastery of the social skills necessary for adequate peer relationships is a major criterion for successful—or failed—development. The inquiry here reviews the question of relationships with friends, a realm with many dimensions. These include:

- Having same-age friends (as against seeking out or associating only with adults, older children, or younger children).
- Having same-gender friends (as against primarily preferring opposite-gender children).
- Being an accepted member of a peer group.
- Defining the child's role within that group and whether it expresses conventional or unconventional social attitudes toward peers:
  Would the child tattle on peers?
  Does the child worry if peers are in trouble?
  Is there trust in peers?
  Does the child feel liked by peers?
  Does the child feel excluded by others?
  Is the child able to make new friends?
  Is the child able to keep friends?
  Is the child invited to parties or to overnights?
  Does the child fight occasionally, or often?
  Is the child regarded as a bully, a target, or a scapegoat by his peers?
- Does the child have close friends or only acquaintances? Is there a current best friend? Are there youngsters with whom the child habitually associates, for example, youngsters with whom he sits on the school bus or with whom he walks to school?
- Does the child belong to any sort of team, club, or gang?

The events aboard the school bus (where this is a factor in the child's life) are usually suggestive. This is a transitional moment in the child's experience: It exposes the vulnerable youngster to a relatively high level of stress, and symptomatic behavior frequently appears. Again, observations taken during recess are often diagnostic. The schoolyard is a site of maximal peer pressure, and supervision is often relatively minimal; as a result, latent interpersonal difficulties will appear with particular intensity in this context.

An important datum is the diagnosis that peers may chance to make. If they regard the child as a queer duck, an oddball, or a weirdo, or as crazy or peculiar in some way, this suggestive finding may well indicate an important pattern of aberrant behavior.

THE CHILD'S RELATIONSHIP TO ACADEMICS. Many children have problems that interfere with their learning, and sorting out the various causes of this interference is one of the commonest issues posed to the mental health professional. It is therefore important to obtain as much detail as possible about the youngster's approach to each specific area of learning, and about whatever impedes or influences the learning process in any way. Where a problem is present, a series of questions arise. When, how, and to whom did the difficulty first become manifest, and what were the circumstances in the child's life at the time? The extent of the problem needs to be determined; if the child seems to have a learning difficulty, is this pervasive and affecting all subjects, or is it discrete and operating only in specific areas (with no obvious impediment in other aspects of learning)? In particular, which areas are affected? The following are suggested areas of possible difficulties: reading, calculation, handwriting, spelling, learning through hearing, learning through seeing, remembering certain kinds of material, getting the gist of a paragraph, being able to grasp or to apply grammatical rules, organizing work, understanding verbal instructions, responding when questioned, reasoning from a given datum using a set of rules, classifying, putting things in series, sorting out among similarities, and abstracting a general principle from a series of instances. The various kinds of learning dysfunction can come about in many ways, and they all need exploration. The commonest cause of learning problems is some disturbance in attention (such as that associated, at least in theory, with attention-deficit hyperactivity disorder), but it is by no means the only cause. Even in that instance the problem may have different origins. Thus, there can be a diffuse inability to concentrate along with a ready distractibility that makes it virtually impossible for the child consistently to keep his mind on his work. The difficulty here lies not so much in the ability to use or to absorb information as in the capacity to concentrate. Alternatively, there may be an additional (perhaps genetically transmitted) lack of ability to function in just one area, because the child's brain is different in a delimited and specific fashion. In effect, the trouble could lie with a specific learning difficulty that accompanies the attentiveness problem but is actually a separate and parallel condition. As a result, if the child were able to concentrate, he might conceivably do as well as any student, except for that area of specific deficit (numbers, letters, diagrams, reading, writing, or whatever the problem may happen to be).

There are also emotional reasons why a child might not learn. Chronic anxiety can interfere radically with the ability to attend to and to take in information. Depression, too, can inhibit such functioning; the youngster is then too preoccupied with thoughts of wrongdoing, worthlessness, family difficulties, or concern about some form of abuse to be able to learn. Or the child simply lacks the energy; the pervasive sadness puts a damper on all effort. Some children are so caught up in feelings of guilt and worthlessness that they see little point in trying to succeed at anything.

On a different level of pathology, any of the major mental illnesses (with their clouding of consciousness, intrusion of primitive ideation, perceptual disturbances, confusion between reality and fantasy perceptions, and general sense of illness and stress) may form a major block to learning. The borderline child may be so preoccupied with fantasies that he does not hear what is being said and has to be poked by someone when the teacher calls on him. The child who dissociates or who is in the throes of a posttraumatic stress disorder may go through periods of blankness or selectively forget what he has just mastered. It takes careful questioning to sort out these possibilities and to discern the nature of the learning problem. Not infrequently, a number of factors coexist, that is, a child may have ADHD alongside a considerable burden of depression or may have a specific learning deficit accompanied by a high level of anxiety. The inquiry must be particularly precise to help sort out such complexity.

Finally, where the child refuses to learn as an expression of defiance, learning problems can arise from chronic anger. Many conduct-disordered children present severe learning problems on this basis. Sometimes, the youngster's attempts to keep anger at bay fill his head with fantasies of revenge or torture. Staying on task is difficult, not so much because the child cannot control these fantasies (as is the case with the borderline), as because the child, rather than doing necessary tasks, is trying to control his behavior by imagining what he would like to do.

Substance abuse can be a very real problem in connection with learning difficulties. The young adolescent who comes to class "stoned" on marijuana or under the influence of alcohol (let alone phencyclidine [or "angel dust"], heroin, or cocaine) is physically as well as emotionally in no condition to learn. As a youngster gets ever deeper into a pattern of substance use, one of the first victims will be attention to academics. Ultimately, nothing in the youngster's life will be important except the substance and its effects.

The Grade-School Years—Nonschool Areas.   In addition to the issues arising in connection with school, this age group requires exploring and evaluating two other major fields of study: the home-related behavioral pattern, including the youngster's adjustment within the neighborhood; and the inner world of the grade-school child.

THE HOME-RELATED BEHAVIORAL PATTERN.   The great world of parent–child and sibling interactions is dominant in human adjustment, but the study must extend to the child's relationship to the home, to the things within the home, and to the care of and regulation of that environment. And it must go still further—to the family's immediate neighbors and broader community.

● *The Nature of Home.* It is important for the diagnostician to have an accurate definition of "home," because for certain children, this is a highly uncertain aspect of their lives. Some youngsters live half the time in their father's home and half in their mother's. Where parent(s) move(s) every few months, the child has no (or, at best, a dim) sense of having a particular geographic locus. Some youngsters grow up in trailers or work with the family as migrant agricultural labor and follow the crops for a good part of every year. Other youngsters, during these formative years, are shunted from foster home to foster home, or from relative to relative. They may respond by becoming more and more unruly and are thus more and more quickly expelled from one environment after another in an ever-increasing spiral of misfortune and maladjustment. And, finally, there are the off-spring of the homeless parents whose dwelling is the street or a series of shelters. Hence, a first dimension of concern is the nature of home.

● *Who Lives at Home?* First, the diagnostician seeks the child's definition of home, as best the youngster can offer it. Accepting for the moment that a recognizable home does exist, the next consideration is, Who lives within it, and what kinds of interactions take place between the youngster and those people? The population of a household is often quite different from a catalog of family members. Brothers and sisters or fathers or mothers may be out-of-house dwellers, whereas cousins, grandparents, stepparents, parental companions, or boarders may be ubiquitous and prominent presences for the child. It is important to explore thoroughly the relationships with each and, to the extent possible, the role that particular people play in the child's life.

Special emphases emerge that are contingent on the chief complaint. For example, if the problem is one of misbehavior, defiance of authority, and oppositional attitudes, then the issues of behavioral management (by whom, and in what manner) become the foci of special study. On the other hand, where depression and withdrawal are the reasons for coming to evaluation, then it is far more useful to direct the limited study time to attachment issues, the management of separations, and responses to the child's expressed concerns than to the specifics of behavioral control.

● *Siblings.* The role of siblings should never be underestimated as the begetter and conditioner of behavioral disturbance. A boy whose sibling has an accident or illness may blame himself for what happened. He may then act up to get punished for his "wrongdoing" without ever communicating these feelings to the parents (except through his misbehavior). Only the careful analysis of the time when the sibling's problem occurred and determining the time of onset of the behavioral difficulties may give the clue to the cause of the problem. In this connection the clinician must keep in mind siblings whom the patient may never have known; an idealized first baby lost to the mother before the birth of the present child can lead to a mythical presence in the lives of both that mother and her current offspring.

OTHER RELATIONSHIPS.   Within peer relationships, both dominance–submission and gender issues are often lived out with great intensity and in remarkable detail. Queries about intimacy, attachment, teasing, abuse, rejection, support, and cooperation will highlight some of the issues, whereas attachment paradigms with parents will throw light on others.

The school years are the age at which earlier attachment problems can blossom into major symptom pictures, so that such conditions as school avoidance, or school phobia, emerge as relatively common difficulties. Again, a careful history of the attachment paradigm within that family must be elicited as part of the study of this condition.

Within the neighborhood context, the same considerations that were present in evaluating school peer behavior determine the line of exploration for neighborhood friendships and relationships. As noted earlier, the age group and sex of preferred playmates are both significant. There are boys who prefer to play with girls and girls who would much rather consort with boys than with the members of their own sex. Some children consistently avoid their same-age playmates—a pattern of behavior that is all too likely to be associated with developmental difficulties. Such youngsters may play only with younger peers, whereas others seek primarily older children or adults. Again, group roles and the inclusion/exclusion paradigm are significant and should be carefully reviewed.

The relationships with the adults in a neighborhood are often important. Some children steal from neighbors, tell outlandish lies, or beg from door to door; other youngsters set fires to or vandalize nearby dwellings; in short, a host of problematic behaviors enacted with those on the periphery of the child's life serve as displacements from and thus as protection from disturbing interactions with immediate caretakers. The diagnostician may also discover areas of strength; some children are helpful to neighbors and are highly valued members of the local community.

The Grade-School Years—The Child's Inner Life.   Two dimensions to a child's inner life require review: the way the child structures his cognitive world, and the inner universe of personal fantasy.

The rules for cognitive organization, especially as outlined by Piaget, have been reviewed in the Developmental History section. The clinician can evaluate the levels of preoperational, concrete operational, and formal operational thinking in relation to the child's chronological age and can estimate the child's level of attainment. A mental status examination will consider the child's ability to read, write, and express himself verbally in coherent and communicative fashion. The child's reality orientation and awareness of general information in keeping with his age and cultural background can be readily estimated by asking him questions about what date it is, where he is, the distance he is from home, and the names of significant persons in his life. Memory can be evaluated by asking the child to recall three objects and by having the child repeat back numbers; intellectual functioning, by asking the child to do appropriate calculations. Judgment can be estimated by posing questions about simple ethical dilemmas (What would you do if you found a stamped unopened letter or if you saw a fire starting in a movie theater?). In short, the evaluator can and should readily explore a host of cognitive capacities.

In addition, it is important to inquire about the presence of specific symptoms. Does the child ever have a feeling that someone is saying something to him when there is no one there? Does the child sometimes see things moving, out of the corner of his eye, or maybe even when gazing full on, that no one else can see? Does the child ever feel that something terrible is about to happen without knowing exactly what it is, or even why this feeling should come up? Does the child find himself compelled to perform odd rituals, such as counting common objects in the environment, or cleaning something, or washing his hands? A variety of cognitive issues of this sort sooner or later must be addressed, and for the most part, the child will offer the pertinent information only if the evaluator asks the proper questions.

The other aspect of the inner world that requires study is the realm of wish and fantasy.

It is a curious reality that among the fields open to science, so little has been done with the rich universe of human fantasy. Freud was the great pioneer in studying this remarkable area, and psychoanalysis continues to be the site of major research for elaborating such knowledge, but there are still vast gaps in our understanding. Aside from the relatively small group of psychoanalytically oriented psychiatrists, medicine in general has neglected this realm, although fantasies about the body and about health matters in general have a great deal to do with both illness and wellness.

For any meaningful study of childhood, some knowledge of the child's inner imaginings is critically important. It does not take the place of detailed knowledge about the youngster's behavior, but it opens another domain for study and insight. It gives the investigator a grasp on important emotional motivations, such as guilt or rage or fear, that can be profound determinants of the child's actions. To obtain access to this normally obscure terrain, the clinician can ask the parents a number of questions such as these: Did the child ever describe a dream, or make up a story, or tell of wishes, or draw a picture that communicated something of his inner life? Many parents have such material that they have kept from earlier times, and sometimes these data can be remarkably illuminating. Often, repeated reports of the same nightmare reveal a central concern: A robber will come and take me away; someone is in the house and will stab me in my sleep; there is a monster under the bed who will get me; and so forth. Occasionally the dream is transparently oedipal, is evidently concerned with separation, or is an obvious expression of some other problem; at other times work in therapy must continue for a long time before the meaning becomes clear. In any case, data of this kind are important components of the study.

Areas of strength need to be explored as well. The therapist should inquire into competences, interests, and hobbies related to both academic realms and extracurricular activities. Sometimes these abilities reflect important family traditions, such as sports participation, a military career, and musical performance, that become vital issues in acceptance of or conformity with family values. In this connection it is important to make some estimate of the ideals and models that the family, implicitly or overtly, offers to—or thrusts upon—a given child.

Prepuberty and Puberty. At about 10 or 11 years old, the child enters the epoch of prepuberty and puberty, which involves an additional array of issues. These, in a sense, complement the material that has been discussed thus far. Home interactions, neighborhood experiences, inner life, and school adjustment in its several realms are as relevant to puberty as they were to latency. Indeed, many such matters retain their importance throughout the life span, so the material to be gathered next supplements these several fields of data collection.

The area of growth and the youngster's feelings about growing up lead to the next areas of inquiry, which are concerned with sexuality, body changes, and the increased potential for aggression. A major component of pubertal work is the child's beginning address to the issues related to independence and autonomy. And the final realm for inquiry is identity formation.

GROWTH AND GROWING UP. Youngsters are bombarded with advance notice regarding the meaning of puberty. Often enough they are learning the music and the dances of puberty well before the biological changes are in evidence. But a catalog of their interests at the end of the grade-school years will reveal a picture that is essentially different from the one created by the subsequent developmental advance.

Late latency is a time for sex education, preparation for menstruation, early steps toward autonomy, and the anticipation of change. Accordingly, the therapist poses questions, such as the following, that involve the parents' and child's views of growth and change: Do you like the idea of your son or daughter growing up? What are you doing to prepare him for change? What does he think about changing and developing—does he express any attitudes about independence, romance, or sexuality? Are his attitudes different from yours? Are there difficulties about this? Does the youngster seem to desire change or does he prefer to defer it? Is he content to remain where he is or is he eager for the next step?

Does the youngster say or do anything that suggests he is being exposed to drugs? Has he hinted at some experience in taking or trying drugs? Does he talk about other children who are using or experimenting with such agents? Have the parents had reason to suspect or have they ever accused the youngster of such behavior? The usual age of onset for drug usage is typically somewhat later, but the problem does appear frequently during these late latency years and should be kept in mind in conducting the evaluation.

Is independence recognized by allowing the youngster to use money? Does he do some of the shopping for himself or for the family? Does he get an allowance and the freedom to spend it on his own? Does he earn money, either for work done at home or by babysitting or running errands or having a paper route? Does he have a say in selecting his own clothes? Does he take some forms of public transportation on his own?

As the pubertal process gets underway, youngsters must master many aspects of coping and learning. In particular, the issues of sexuality can be challenging to many families, and the diagnostician needs to explore this area, with tact and sensitivity to be sure, but to explore it. Among the many questions that can come up, some of the important ones are, Is there much concern with modesty at home? With nakedness? Has the youngster chanced to see parental nudity and/or sexuality? Has he expressed any feelings about these topics? Has he shown much curiosity; has he asked questions? If so, of whom and concerning what?

To what extent has the child been formally prepared for pubertal development (has the girl been told about menstruation and the boy about erections and nocturnal emissions)? Has he been informed about human reproduction? Has the child attended sex-ed classes at school? Did the parents have any particular feelings about that? Did they feel it necessary to supplement that material with teaching at home?

What about family attitudes toward sexuality—are many sexual jokes told at home? What sort of language does the youngster hear? What is the level of explicit language in his own conversation? Does the child have access to *Playboy*, X-rated videos, or other suggestive material? If so, how does he get to see them, and what does he do with the experience? Do the parents keep pornographic materials about, or do they find that the youngster has brought them into the house? When rape, abortion, or child molestation come up on TV or arise within the context of the family or the neighborhood, does the family discuss such topics? Is the youngster concerned about any of these?

PUBERTY. Where puberty is already in process, then the meaning of the ensuing changes to the parents becomes singularly important. How did it make mother and father feel to learn of their daughter's menarche? What happened, and how did the parents respond? If the youngster was troubled in any way, how did the family help her? Has the boy begun to have wet dreams? Is there any family response—and, if so, what is it? Does the youngster express concern or curiosity about parental sexuality? Is there any hint of sex play between the siblings, or is there any such behavior with other children? Is the child beginning to worry the parents in terms of dress, language, hair style, or makeup? Is there reason to suspect that the youngster is engaging in sexual activity of some kind with peers, or with someone older than the peer group? How long have the parents suspected this, and how have they addressed the issue? Or does the child express a sense of fear and inhibition where heterosexual interactions are concerned, and if so, what have the parents done about that?

How about the larger community—have the school or the neighbors ever complained about the youngster's sexual behavior? How was it handled? Have the parents worried that the youngster is growing in a homosexual direction or is confused about sexuality? Where do the parental concerns arise—have there been specific incidents, things the youngster has said, or worries that have been expressed? How did the parents respond? Where are things now?

Is masturbation ever mentioned at home, and is there reason to believe the youngster is concerned about this? Was it ever a subject of discussion between parents and child? Is it the subject of much humor or teasing at home? Are the parents concerned about it?

Can the youngster talk about any of this? Whom does he confide in most readily? Does he try to deny any of the developmental happenings and act as though nothing has changed? What could have led him to assume such an attitude?

AGGRESSION.   What about the aggressive component of development: Is the teenager quarrelsome, provocative, confronting? Are there house rules for everyone and has the youngster previously obeyed them? Does the youth now invite power struggles and seek to defy these house rules? What is the authority structure of the home: Who sets the limits, who decides on and who carries out disciplinary action, and what happens if the youngster does not comply? Have there been major confrontations? Has there been a gradual—or an abrupt—transition in freedoms and responsibilities as the youngster has grown older?

Have there been changes in the way the youth interacts with siblings? Have things taken a turn for the worse—what has happened? Are there evidences of trouble and dismay in other realms, among friend relationships, or at school? Does the youngster seem more angry than before, or more depressed? Moody or unpredictable? Does the teenager lash out suddenly for what seems insufficient reason, and, if this should happen, is there a subsequent apology? Is there an emphasis on revenge behavior, and is there any reason to suspect that, in fact, the youth has covertly caused someone injury or has injured someone's possessions? Is there a quality of the youngster trying deliberately to be provocative and seeming to need limits and even a measure of punishment? Has the youth become difficult, irascible, explosive, and impossible to reason with? Does he accept responsibility for his own acts, or is it always someone else's fault? Does the youth tend to accuse others of being "against me"—how unrealistic do the accusations become? What triggers a reaction? Do particular people serve as the target for the youth's rage? Or does the aggression take the form of sly and covert acts, such as maliciously spreading false gossip, stealing others' precious possessions, teasing others sadistically, telling secrets that will obviously hurt someone's feelings, or covertly destroying highly valued property—an airplane model, a letter, a photograph, a valued garment, or a treasured record?

AUTONOMY AND INDEPENDENCE.   A major dimension of the work of puberty is the beginning *struggle for independence* (the separation component) and for *genuine autonomy* (the individuation component). All too often it begins by the youngster making all sorts of unreasonable demands or insisting on impossible rights, and it may take considerable empathic tolerance (not to mention adroit management) to bring the situation into line. How does this struggle manifest itself in this home—is the youngster insisting on more entitlements than before? Does the teenager assert that he is no longer a child and hence may do things that were previously, and are perhaps currently, forbidden? How do the parents deal with such issues, and what is the outcome of these exchanges?

Do some of these assertions of greater autonomy take the form of smoking, drinking, or drug usage, with all sorts of rationalizations to defend this behavior? Do the parents believe that substance abuse is occurring, but is not being admitted at home? Does the child demand sexual freedoms that seem, in some measure, to reflect the struggles for a greater sense of independence? Or does the youngster seem immature and dependent, resisting parental suggestions to go out more with friends or to go to parties and mingle with mixed groups? Does the youngster prefer instead to stay home and watch TV, play games with parents, or consort with younger children? How much withdrawal has been noted? For example, to what extent does the young person remain alone in a room or refuse to accept invitations to parties and other social events? Has the behavior changed in this respect?

IDENTITY.   Finally, do the youngsters talk at all about the person they would like to be, or would like to resemble? Do the youngsters have a sense of the future and talk about possible courses of study or interests that would take them forward in their lives? Are they ambitious, and what do they dream of? Do they have heroes or heroines, people to whom they look up or whom they admire? Does this translate into specific behavior—do they follow some singer or a name band, or study a particular subject? Does some area of athletics or art capture their interest, and what do they do about it? What do the parents think of these interests: Do they support the youngsters' interests, oppose them, or stay out of it?

Is reading important? For example, has a novel taken possession of the teenager for a while, so that he dreams of living in the same way as one of the characters? Or a TV show he follows because it chimes with some sense of his own interests or future? Is there a movie or fictional character he idolizes? Does he point to the great success someone has achieved and does he dream of imitating or outdoing that person? To what extent are the young person's choices consonant or dissonant with parental values? Does he change heroes or idols rapidly, or does he follow a steady course leading the observer to think that this is indeed an important choice and one that the child is likely to pursue in the future?

How about the sense of self—does the youngster seem to change rapidly and radically from time to time? Are there up periods and down periods? Are there odd episodes of forgetfulness that the youth has trouble explaining? Are there odd posturings or rituals the youth apparently has to carry out? The later era of adolescence brings with it an increase in the frequency of manic-depressive disorder, multiple personality disorder, and changes in a preexisting obsessive-compulsive disorder. The patient may not speak about any of these conditions spontaneously, and they are likely to be detected only if the evaluator maintains a high index of suspicion and asks the appropriate questions.

OBJECT RELATIONS.   Yet another important realm concerns the emerging shape of the adolescent's interpersonal relations: How does the youth regard and treat the significant people about himself? Is he capable of empathy and concern for others, or are friends and parents seen as objects for manipulation and exploitation? Is the teenager capable of maintaining a balanced view of others even in the face of frustration (i.e., sees others as a mixture of good and bad), or does the youngster's perspective allow for only two polar extremes: idealization and devaluation? Similarly, how balanced is the young person's view of the self? Does he see himself as having a blend of strengths and weaknesses, or does he unrealistically see himself as being filled with grandiosity or with self-loathing? What is the quality of the youngster's friendships with peers of both sexes? Is the youth popular or close to one or two good friends? Does he have a lover? Can the adolescent see the world from another's perspective even when disagreeing? The work of object attachment undergoes profound alterations during the teenage interval, and the diagnostician must be endlessly alert to its many nuances.

Middle and Late Adolescence. The earlier themes continue, but with a greater accent on patterns of overall mental health and mental illness. The issues include idealism, sexuality, delinquency, identity consolidation, career choice and preparation, and capacity for independent functioning and self-regulation. Such major issues as driving, pregnancy, abortion, arrest and imprisonment, venereal disease, AIDS, sexual orientation, suicide, breakdowns of various kinds, as well as creative achievements, talents, awards, and other forms of recognition must all be explored. Family relationships continue to be central in the youngsters' lives and merit careful and extended inquiry. At this point in the unfolding of personality the quality of these interactions differs greatly from that at earlier ages, and the character of inquiry must shift accordingly.

A major difference in conducting such a study in adolescence relates to the new emergents in the subject's developmental level. Midadolescent youngsters have acquired considerable independence; they may have many negative feelings about meeting the examiner with their parents present and, indeed, about having the parents share the study in any way. Yet, the diagnostician cannot successfully conclude such an exploration without parental participation. As a rule, the youngsters still live at home; no matter where they live, they are likely still to be financially dependent on their parents; and they are even more likely to be emotionally dependent on the parents—even if they deny this vociferously. Moreover, the parents can often provide critical developmental information. In most instances the parents are also deeply invested in and concerned about their offspring and need to be able to share, at least to some extent, in what is happening. Nonetheless, the study is still more the youth's to influence in form and content than is the case with the younger adolescent. Thus, when younger children assert they do not wish to come for their interview, the parents can often make them do so, whereas the decisions of the older teenagers are often critical. On the other hand, the teen years see great changes with each passing month, and both the scope and the depth of an interview with older adolescents can far surpass the limitations on topics and tactics necessary with prepubertal children. In particular, the levels of ethical development, cognitive maturity, emotional attainment, empathic concern, social ripeness, sublimatory potential, self-direction, and overall identification with adulthood are at quite a different order of magnitude for this midadolescent cohort, compared with the pubertal youngsters. Accordingly, the therapist's work with these young people has far less about it of play (as it often must in the treatment of younger children) than it does of serious and focused exchange.

ADDITIONAL ELEMENTS IN THE EVALUATIVE PROCESS

Once the examiner has obtained the data and has shaped a preliminary sketch of the problem, he or she must decide whether it makes sense to go ahead, and, if so, in what way. There is the question of whether there is a problem present at all, or whether the child is going through a normal variation of development about which the parents need only to receive reassurance. If there is enough suggestion of disordered function to require further exploration, is it primarily a psychiatric problem? Should it rather be referred first to a neurologist? Is there a hint here of a genetic component? Should the pediatrician be the logical professional to orchestrate this study? In brief, a plan must be established for the next step.

The ensuing task implies that the evaluator has a thorough knowledge of both normal development and the syndromes of childhood and adolescence. The kinds of decisions that have to be made and the plans that must be formulated will be direct applications of this basic information. If, at this point, the examiner has reviewed the alternatives and the problem sounds as if it lies primarily within the psychiatric realm, he or she must then arrange for the interview with the child.

As noted, to a certain extent, how the clinician approaches this interview relates directly to the child's developmental level, that is, initially, the therapist sometimes sees the preschool child with his parents present, whereas the adolescent is usually alone. In the grade-school years the arrangement may go either way depending on the nature of the case. The site of interview may also vary. Preschool and grade-school children are best seen in a playroom, and adolescents are interviewed in a conventional office setting. Then there is the matter of how to prepare the youngster for the interview. Many parents ask rather anxiously how to explain to children that they will be seeing a psychiatrist or a psychologist. In response, the interviewer should communicate to the parents a sense of realistic and sensible action. The parents need to sit down with the child and talk about the existence of the problem and their concerns regarding it. It is best to caution the parents about the need to avoid accusation or condemnation; it is quite important that the child or teenager should not confuse the consultation with a punishment or threat. It is not the long-heralded final crackdown on bad behavior or the first step in getting rid of the child. It is a serious attempt to seek help for a problem that the parents, on their own, do not know how to resolve; and that idea needs to be put into words in direct form. The notion that the child is going to see a healer should be in the forefront, and the need to work cooperatively with the examiner should be emphasized from the outset.

The clinician should urge the parents to be as empathic as possible, to focus on how everyone in the situation feels, to speak directly about their worries for the child, and to talk about their own and the child's discomfort. In effect the parents should tell their child the truth in as supportive, sympathetic, and understanding a way as possible, but, in any case, the truth. As far as what the doctor will do, the parents can say simply that the doctor talks and plays with children and tries to understand their problems and worries, and that the doctor will talk with the parents and try to help them too.

At this point the parents should hear about confidentiality, and the therapist should encourage them to introduce that concept to the child. The clinician should make clear that what goes on between the child and the doctor will not automatically be passed on to the parents; if the youngster wants the doctor to keep things private, and if the information is not about something dangerous, the doctor will certainly do so. The parents should encourage the child to question the doctor if he has any doubts or worries about the confidentiality of the interview.

The clinician then asks the parents to make another appointment, and next time to bring the child. Not infrequently, at this point one or both parents may indicate a need to think over what has been said; if so, the professional should encourage the parents not to make the appointment immediately but rather to take the time and think it through, and then to call back if they decide to go ahead. If, however, the parents are sure that they wish to begin the evaluation, the therapist should set up separate appointments for both the child and the parents. It is important to see the child early in the process, so that as the developmental history unfolds, the physician can relate the account to a concrete person.

Child Interview

For purposes of exposition, assume that the child is a preschooler 3 or 4 years of age and that the interview takes place in a public clinic. The examiner receives a call that the patient has arrived and accordingly proceeds to the waiting room. The receptionist indicates that a particular woman is Mrs. Jones, who has arrived with her son Johnny. Once they are identified, the examiner begins the process of evaluation, for the first important observation deals with the nature of the interaction between caretaker and child. The mother (to be sure, it is not always the mother—it might be the father, grandmother, big sister, foster parent, or even the maid—but the commonest combination is for the young child to arrive with the mother) might be reading or watching TV (if that is available), while the child is on the floor playing either by himself or with other children who happen to be present. Or the youngster might be on his mother's lap while she shows him pictures in a magazine. Any one of many sequences might occur, but whichever it is, it is relevant to the data the clinician seeks to collect at this point.

First Encounter.   The examiner introduces him- or herself to the mother and turns to Johnny saying something to this effect: "Johnny, I am Dr. Brown, and you and I are going to spend the next little while together in the playroom back there. We will talk together and play and get to know one another. Afterward you and I will come back here to Mother, and then you will go home." It is rather important to spell all this out for such a little boy because he may already have had some painful experiences with doctors; he may have been left in a hospital at some point for a medical emergency or for elective surgery, such as a tonsillectomy; or his caretakers may have threatened him with being given away or taken away by someone because he was not a good boy. The therapist may not know this information at the outset, so it is best to be quite explicit.

In the large majority of cases the child will interrupt whatever he is doing and look over at the caretaker, who will usually say something such as: "Now go along with the nice doctor Johnny, just like I told you." Whereupon Johnny will pick himself up and, indeed, do just that. Without further fuss, he will go along with the doctor, often reaching up automatically to take his or her hand. Nor does the physician refuse such an invitation from a preschooler; he or she takes the child's hand and the two march off to the playroom.

THE RESISTANT CHILD.   When the doctor makes the introductory speech to the child, a number of alternative sequences may ensue. The youngster may simply ignore the doctor, continue playing (or whatever he is doing), and act as though he had not been addressed. Or, alternatively, the child might rush to his mother's side, begin to cling to her, and set up a dolorous clamor—"I don't want to go, I don't like that doctor, don't leave me, I'm scared"—and other such declarations of negation and refusal, strongly tinged with piteous or angry overtones.

The usual course is for the doctor, first, to specially note how the mother handles this contretemps, what she does, what she says, and what she conveys. The range of responses varies widely, extending on the one hand from the mother who returns the child's agonizing clutching with interest and seizes him in a death grip, holding him tightly to her bosom and reassuring him, while asking why won't he go (at this point he could not get away if he wanted to). Or, the mother might hold up her hands helplessly as the child clings to her, turn to the examiner with a certain sense of vindication, and say: "You see, it's always like this, I can't do a thing with him."

On the other hand, there are also quite mature responses, such as the mother who says: "It's always a little hard for Johnny with new situations; once he is more familiar with things he won't have this trouble—come on young man, you can manage it, let's try now, come on, upsy daisy, just go along with the doctor and you will be all right." Or, an occasional mother will say: "Johnny feels better if I start out with him; why not let me help him get back there until he gets over the first minute or two and he'll do fine."

For the most part, the tactics the clinician pursues at this point should emerge to some extent from reading the clinical situation. The usual thing is to talk to the child for a moment or two essentially repeating the initial message in somewhat different language. Where that proves ineffectual (as usually it does), the therapist invites the mother to accompany the child to the playroom.

When the three arrive at the open playroom door, the doctor goes into the room and says to the child: "See, it is really a room just for talking and playing, and that's where we will meet for the next little while, while your mother waits [or sees a social worker—or whatever the plan may be]". After seeing the playroom and noting the absence of examining tables and glass cabinets filled with shiny instruments, many a child can take the plunge. He will relinquish his hold on mother and enter the room. The mother can then be excused and the interview can proceed. But, to assume the worst, if the child still refuses, saying to mother "I want you to come in with me," the doctor can then suggest: "Why doesn't Mother come in for about 5 minutes until Johnny gets used to the office, and then she can leave and meet him again when we are through."

Once in, the mother is asked to sit on a chair, and the doctor begins actively to invite the child to play. Most youngsters of this age are readily engaged by asking them to look at the toys in the room and to pick out something they would like to play with. Where a child accepts this gambit, and some sort of interactive play gets under way, the doctor can wait a few minutes and then suggest that Johnny is doing fine now and would mother go outside and wait, or see her worker in the other office? Again, for many children this will work out well, and they can accept the separation at this point. However, where this suggestion still precipitates a major reaction on the child's part, the interview might have to be conducted with the mother and child both in the room for the rest of the hour. If mother is indeed scheduled to see another professional, that colleague might now be called in to conduct at least a modified interview with mother, while the child's examiner continues with the youngster.

Either because of an oppositional orientation or great panic, the occasional child will continue to be obdurate, even with mother present for the entire hour. This can reach such proportions that, despite the examiner's best efforts, the child will not join in any kind of joint play and will instead continue to avoid all interaction. Under such circumstances, the doctor can try talking to him for a bit to see what comes of gentle interpretative efforts; if no communicative exchange is possible, the doctor can spend the rest of the hour drawing the child. Such an effort can go on indefinitely, and numerous observations can be made about the child's appearance and deportment while this is proceeding. The doctor can ask the child to help with the drawing by holding still for a moment and take up the fact that the child is being so actively uncooperative (if that is the case) in an interested and exploratory way. Then, if the child's avoidant stance persists, the doctor can speculate out loud (as the drawing continues) about the child's motivations; maybe the child is trying to control the situation, frustrate the examiner, or keep possession of Mommy—or whatever seems to be the case within that context. There are many opportunities to make observations and to register responses that emerge naturally from such an engagement, and the ensuing reactions may shed some light on the child's problems.

THE COOPERATIVE CHILD.   Where the child and the doctor leave the waiting room together without any problem, the average child is a little hesitant when he reaches the door of the playroom and must be invited in. There are, however, some children, not very often met with but by no means rare, who come to the doorway of a room with playthings, give an enthusiastic whoop—"Hey, toys!"—and plunge in actively. They need no prompting but instead take over immediately and structure the play: "I'm the teacher and you are the student and you don't know how to do the problem, and I show you how," and so on—and things proceed from there. Or it might be a war game with the child playing the good guys and the examiner assigned the role of the bad guys; planes proceed to fly, bombs to fall, and all sorts of hectic activity to follow, with the examiner having no chance to get a word in edgewise. This is a perfectly workable situation, and the examiner has no need to act other than as directed, while trying to remember the details of the play sequences as they unroll. The examiner can afford to be passive and to learn just by letting the child find his own level of expression.

The more usual situation, however, is for the child to enter the room at the doctor's invitation and to stand uncertainly until invited to sit on a designated chair. It is quite striking that many 4-year-old children are capable of sitting through an entire interview and talking seriously with the doctor. As a rule, however, most of the younger children become restless after a while and begin to look over at the toys and to ask arch questions such as "What's that in the box there?" When this happens, it is a cue for the examiner to invite the child to go to the toys and pick out what he would like to play with. Indeed, it is almost an ethical question whether a mental health professional should invite a young child into a room with toys and not let him at them at some point.

On the other hand, the goal of the interview is not to play but rather to conduct a psychiatric exploration, to work together in addressing some of the child's problems, and to seek to understand the child's inner experience and relationship world. Hence, it is essential to seek ways of talking with the child about personal and touchy subjects, and to do this without being invasive or heavy-handed. This goal implies working close to the bone, but in a way that is tactful and responsive to the child's feelings. Throughout the entire evaluation, the essence of what the examiner does can best be described as sensitive clinical exploration. The word *sensitive* here refers specifically to a heightened aliveness to and awareness of the patient's emotional state. The physician achieves this through a process of attunement, in part conscious and to a large extent unconscious, by opening him- or herself up to feel with the child, to sense the pain, anxiety, reactivity, and concern with shaming and humiliation. The examiner sends messages in the form of certain tones of voice or particular kinds of inquiry (direct questions, very gentle attempts at humor, empathic reflections, tentative challenges, overt expressions of sympathy, etc.) and watches carefully to judge the effects of each gambit. The examiner's basic principle must always be the same: Protect the patient; do not frighten, humiliate, or wound the patient in any way. Children are considerably more vulnerable than adults and require special care. Much of the skill and basic competence of the able clinician lies precisely in being able to address and to explore delicate issues with children in nonhurtful ways, or at least to keep the level of hurt tolerable for the child.

The word *clinical* implies a pattern of continuous correction that begins with such an exploration. The examiner rapidly formulates possible positions that the patient might be maintaining: The youngster is unusually self-conscious and ever on the verge of embarrassment; the youngster is seething with anger and barely containing the impulse to lash out; the youngster is grandiose and is watching to see if the doctor is sufficiently appreciative; the youngster is terrified to losing control and is afraid to refer to that lest it pitch him over the edge; the youngster is subtly demeaning the doctor and is acting provocatively to prove that the doctor cannot help. At the same time the clinician is ready to discard or alter these views as soon as the next shift in the patient's posture, eye movement, facial expression, or verbal response suggests that the previous assumptions were wrong. The process resembles constructing an image out of clay; the therapist may add too much in one area and find an unfilled space somewhere else. The image is forever changing, but the goal is to approach ever more closely to a suitable representation.

Sometimes an initial construction of this kind must be rejected in toto as a new basic concept arises. Thus, in speaking with an adolescent who is talking about hallucinations, the doctor gradually gets the impression that this is all make-believe and that the youngster is faking it. Dealing with a state of hallucinosis and formulating the youngster's problem in those terms then give way to considering the youngster in terms of deceitful manipulative behavior with the attendant characteriologic problems. *Dealing with* and *considering* refer to the doctor's inner processes—the internal image of the patient that has thus far been constructed and that the professional will seek to refine and to extend.

The Interview Proper.   As with chess, the child psychiatric interview has a variety of opening moves, each with its own strengths and weaknesses, and each clinician must develop a style with which he or she feels comfortable. What follows is a composite of a number of clinicians' approaches to this task; in no sense is it definitive. At this moment in the formation of the field, there is no single, universally accepted model.

One way of beginning the interview is to talk about names. A person's name is at once the handle extended toward society that anyone may grasp, and yet at the same time it is a deeply and peculiarly personal area. So the clinician says to the child: "I know your name is Johnny, but I don't know your whole name. Do you have a middle name?" Depending on his response, the doctor carefully and gingerly, launches a series of questions, posing each after the previous one has been answered and adapting each in terms of the preceding response. Taken out of context, the questions sound something like this: "Do you have a nickname? Is there a name you're called at home which no one else uses? What do you like best to be called?"

The doctor then repeats his or her own name and asks whether the child knows what kind of doctor he is seeing. Again, it is surprising how many quite little children are capable of answering, "psychiatrist." Where even an approximation is forthcoming, the doctor says something complimentary and gives the child some recognition for knowing a difficult word and saying it correctly. An important principle of interviewing is that, wherever an appropriate way can be found, the clinician supports the youngster's narcissism. The interview context, by nature, causes the patient to doubt whether he is doing well and to wonder what the doctor thinks of him; being praised within such a situation carries great weight.

"What does a psychiatrist do?" asks the doctor. Many small children can say something to the effect that that kind of doctor helps you with your worries, or treats your problems, or you tell them your troubles. And, again, the clinician remarks on how well the youngster has said it. Then it is generally a good idea to repeat the thought in some such terms as:

> There are special doctors you go to if your eye hurts, and there are special doctors if you have a pain in your arm or leg. Then there are doctors who help with tummy aches. In the same way, there are doctors whom you see if there are hurting places in your feelings, if you feel unhappy, or if there is some trouble in your life, maybe in the way you get along with other people. Now, here we are meeting together—Johnny and the psychiatrist. It sounds as if something in your life must be troubling you, something that brings us together. Could you tell me something about that?

THE CHIEF COMPLAINT.   This is a critical point in the work. In a few instances, the response is a clear and accurate account of the chief complaint that the doctor can then follow up and explore in some detail: When did it all begin, how did it feel while it was happening, what do you think was on your mind when it happened, what did the people at home say or do, what happened at school, and so on. With most youngsters, however, things take a different tack. As a rule, in the child's home, the question of whether or not to see a professional has been hanging in the air for weeks. There has been much telephoning about it to friends, relatives, or schoolteachers, and perhaps there have even been several direct discussions between the parents and the child. When the parents have reached a decision to take the child to a therapist, the parents will often sit down with the child and describe the doctor and instruct the youngster to tell the doctor all about the trouble and answer all the questions. (Sometimes they also warn the child *not* to tell about something, to preserve some family secret.)

On the way out to the clinic, the parents may repeat the instructions: "Now be sure to tell the doctor all about what that person did to you [or—how you set the fires, hurt your little sister, started to mess in your pants—whatever the basis of the referral might be]." But at the point in the clinical interview when the doctor asks the child: "What brings you to see the psychiatrist?" in about four cases out of five the child's answer is "I don't know."

This is not difficult to understand. It is hard for children to tell about many things that they feel ashamed of, or that they fear will make people laugh, be angry, or disbelieve them. Worst of all, they may feel that disclosure will cause people to dislike them—and they defend themselves accordingly. They avoid self-incrimination by saying "I don't know." If that is the answer, the doctor then responds: "Well my understanding of what it is all about is . . . " The doctor tells whatever the chief complaint is reported to have been and adds: "Do you think we can talk about it?" In response the youngster may say, "I don't want to," may merely fall silent, or may breathe a sigh of relief and say, in effect, "Yes, this is what happened." Where the child can talk about it, the examiner proceeds as before, and they explore the area as best the child is able. However, where the youngster does not respond or refuses to discuss it, then the interviewer says: "OK, tell you what, let's talk about something else, and maybe later on if you feel like it, we can come back to this and see how we can do."

REVIEW OF CURRENT STATUS. With that, the doctor turns to other aspects of the child's life and tries gently to explore one of them. It might be useful to ask "Who lives at home?" As noted earlier, it is better to query this than to ask who is in the child's family. Family membership is often complex and sometimes uncertain, whereas who lives at home is usually concrete and specific, as well as being very important. If the child names some people, then the clinician can begin to inquire into these relationships: Whom does the child feel closest to? With whom does the child spend time? Who disciplines the youngster? What kinds of things does the child do with others he has named? Is anyone at home sick a lot? Does the child worry about that? Is anyone very mean to the child? Does the person sometimes hurt the child or leave marks? Does anyone play with the child or touch the child in ways that make the youngster feel upset or that he would not like his mother to know about. Does anyone scare the child? Is anyone the youngster's best friend? Is there anyone who is not home whom the child misses and wishes were there?

Not all these questions will be appropriate in all situations, and, as always, the therapist must exercise clinical judgment about what to ask, and when to interrupt and change the subject. Still, these are important areas, and sooner or later the clinician must get to them and see what the child does with them.

As noted earlier, there are three main loci for exploration of the child's life: home, school, and inner life. The *school,* the second locus, affects most youngsters because even very little children are likely to be spending at least a few hours a week in nursery school or play school. This then becomes a site for review, with questions directed first toward how hard is it to leave home to go to school, and then toward interactions with other children and group adjustment, as well as teacher and authority issues. The clinician may explore the child's feeling about naps and various activities: How do you feel about going to school? How did you feel the first day? How was it when you saw Mommy leaving? How is it now when you are left? What do you like best to do there? What do you think you are best at doing? Could you show me an example of what you do? These are among the topics that can be covered.

An area in the child's life associated with home is the *neighborhood.* In the case of the preschooler, this includes the other children who live nearby and who might be brought over by an adult occasionally, or whom the child might visit: How does the youngster get on with these friends? Do they ever fight? Who is the most fun to be with and what do they like best to do together? Is there a favorite game they like to play and how does it go? Are there secret games that no one is supposed to know about? If there are, do children take off their clothes to play those games? Who likes those games best? Who wants to play them a lot?

THE EXPLORATION OF COGNITION.   It is often possible to study the child's thought processes without the need for formal exploration. However it is accomplished, it is important for the therapist to try to estimate the child's intelligence and general store of information. For school-age children, the examiner can review some of the child's class work; for younger children an elementary knowledge of colors, the ability to name common objects, the level at which the child draws a human figure, and the level of sentence structure employed can all provide ready hints to the youngster's intellectual level.

The following areas all inform the examiner about the quality of the child's cognition: the present level of thought (preoperational, concrete operations, etc.), the ability to concentrate (the length of time during which the child can keep his attention fixed on a game or activity), the level of distractibility, the presence of intrusive fantasy as a distracting inner aspect of the child's thinking, the coherence with which the child can follow an idea, any evidence of incoherence or confusion in the ordering of thoughts, any hint of bizarre elements in the child's ideation or play, hints of hallucinatory experiences during the interaction (and affirmative answers to questions about any previous encounter with such phenomena). The ability to distinguish between reality and fantasy, between play roles and actual identity, between make-believe and the quiddity of things should be solidly in place by the third year. For example, such a young child can have a phobia and be able to say, in effect: "I know there is no reason to be as scared as I am, but I'm still afraid." The clinician can sense all these factors during play or can inquire about them directly. Memory may be tested by any of the time-honored devices (repeating numbers or recalling three words, etc., although this might also be a measure of concentration). The examiner should note language usage; sometimes aphasic children or youngsters with speech disorders may offer confusing diagnostic profiles that then require the assistance of a speech and language pathologist. The doctor can observe mood directly and can ask the child about feelings of excitement, elation, unhappiness, sadness, or shifting, changing emotional states. The examiner must, in fact, perform a brief mental status evaluation while interacting with the child.

THE EXPLORATION OF FANTASY.   The last area of study is the child's *inner life*. Doctors are trained to inquire into every aspect of a person's adaptation with no restrictions and no taboos; as long as it is part of the health profile, the doctor feels that it is necessary to thoroughly explore the area. With the adult patient, for example, this includes relationships with the patient's children, spouse, and employer, with sexuality, with living conditions, with money—there are literally no holds barred. If it touches on health to any degree, it is the doctor's right and duty to look into it.

The one exception is the realm of fantasy; it would be most unusual for the average physician to inquire into a patient's dreams, daydreams, or inner life. And this for very good reason; if the information were forthcoming, the doctor would not be able to use it. Physicians in general, are not trained to interpret such data, and it would not help their work. For the mental health practitioner, however, exploring fantasy and inner processes is of central importance, and he or she must gain access to this area to accomplish an adequate examination. With the preschool child the problem is rather special.

In a sense, the youngster's developmental level makes it easier to access this aspect of his life. The preschooler is at the Piagetian stage of preoperational thinking, so that fantasy-tinged material is a normal part of the child's thoughts. At this lifestage, the preferred mode of self-expression is play, which offers an automatic window on the child's inner life; by its very nature, play is a form of fantasy expression. That is why the examiner can afford to take the passively observant stance when the child plays so actively; in effect, the data are pouring in.

In addition to play, however, a number of other evocative tactics are useful in exploring fantasy life. It is important for the examiner to have such techniques available to address the various patterns of relationship and interaction offered by different children. There is, first of all, the direct method: Simply ask the child to tell the doctor a dream. Many children will say that they don't remember their dreams, to which the examiner may respond: "Well, we certainly do forget most dreams, but maybe you can remember a bad dream, did you ever have a nightmare?" Many children who have no recollection of a dream do, indeed, remember a bad dream and can say at least something about it. This is especially true for recurrent nightmares.

The same approach serves often for daydreams; the clinician has but to ask and the child offers a remembered daydream, which is sometimes unhappy as well. Frequently, external triggers for some of these inner events—a movie or a TV show, especially the frightening variety—may trouble the youngster's thinking for a while. Such information, in turn, can open the way to a discussion of fears, nighttime fears, and specific fears in the child's life: darkness, animals, insects, snakes, storms, monsters, masks, heights, and the like.

Drawings are a common form for expressing fantasy. Many children, even nonverbal youngsters, will agree to make a picture for the doctor, and they will draw spontaneously as well as what the examiner requests. One possibility is to ask the child to draw a picture of his family. (Many children will say they cannot draw people; in such instances, resorting to stick figures will often overcome that hurdle.) The ensuing portraits are powerful images of the child's feelings within the hierarchies of valuation and devaluation, dominance–submission, inclusion–rejection, and other such polarities that may obtain within the family context. Drawings of a genderless person or of a boy or girl will give vital information about the child's gender organization. Both the gender that the child draws first and the details depicting each gender provide valuable hints to his perspective.

Then the doctor can ask a child the obvious question: What do you want to be when you grow up? Albeit obvious, it is not a simple query; it is actually a rather penetrating probe that touches on deep reservoirs of identification (and, sometimes, self-doubt) as well as grandiosity. Nor should the examiner be led astray by apparently obvious answers; whatever the child offers has many roots. Thus, to be a fireman has the superficial image of riding an interesting truck through the streets while making a loud noise; but firemen also put out fires and rescue people, and to what extent is the youngster concerned with the need for emotional containment, or rescue?

Most children have encountered the idea of a fairy godmother, or a genie. Hence, the therapist may couch the next question in terms such as "Let's make believe that a fairy godmother suddenly appeared and said to you: I hereby grant you three wishes. You may only have three, and you cannot wish for any others (there is always the bright youngster whose first wish will be for lots more wishes), but those you do make may be for anything in the world that you would like to have, for things to be any way you want, or for *you* to be any way you want. Now what would you wish for?" Or the question may be couched in terms of finding a lamp and rubbing it, and the genie appears who makes a similar offer. This is a powerful means for glimpsing a child's inner yearnings and hidden desires, and the answers will often be quite revealing. Sometimes, however, children are so concrete or so defended that they say they don't know what their wishes are, or that they can't think of any wishes. The doctor may then try an alternative means of viewing this aspect of the child's inner life by saying: "Well, let's imagine that one day you are in your backyard, with your shovel and pail, and you are digging in the ground. You dig deeper and deeper, and suddenly— clunk!—you hit something hard. So you clear out all the dirt on top of it and dig around it—and wow!—it turns out to be a great big bag of money. And it's all yours. Now, what would you want to buy with that money—what's the first thing you would buy and what's the second, and the third? Would you want to buy something for Mommy—what do you think she would want most? How about daddy, and brother, or sister?"

Thus the examiner can try to create a question that is sufficiently concrete to free up a response from even a limited or constricted youngster. With luck, it will then be possible to extend the query into some of the family relationships as well.

Yet another device is to begin a story and then to interrupt it and ask the youngster to finish it any way he wants to. This tactic was introduced by Dr. Louise Despert of New York City, with a series of 19 stories that she translated from the French and presented to the American literature. These stories subsequently came to be known as the Despert Fables (much to the dismay of Dr. Despert who was at pains to say that she did not write them, she merely translated them. But her caution was of no avail; they remain the Despert Fables to this day).

Only one of the stories has actually become incorporated into the general practice of the field; it is called the *Baby Bird Story,* and it goes something like this (there are many variations):

Once upon a time in a big forest, there was a very tall tree. And high in the tree there was a nest with three birds in it; one was a mama bird, one a papa bird, and one a baby bird. It was quite a little baby bird, so little, indeed, that it had not yet learned to fly. One fine morning, they woke up, and the mamma bird said: "Goodness, there is nothing to eat in the nest; I will have to fly off over that way and bring something back." So off she flew and the papa bird and baby bird waited in the nest. Time passed and they were getting pretty hungry so the papa bird said: "Maybe there isn't anything off that way where she is looking; I will fly off the other way and see what I can find." So off he flew in the opposite direction, and there was baby bird all alone in the nest. Well, after a while baby bird began to get kind of bored, so it started to look around, first on one side of the nest and then the other, and then it decided to look down at the forest floor and see what it could see. But it was too little to see much over the edge of the nest, so it hopped up on the edge and it leaned over, only it still couldn't see, so it leaned over a little farther, and then a little farther, and then, uh oh, it leaned over a little too far and down it went! As I told you, it was still quite young and had not yet learned how to fly, so it just tumbled and dropped, fluttering and falling, and down and down—and now you finish the story, what happens to the baby bird?

Younger children tend to get quite caught up in stories of this sort, and from their responses the clinician gets a revealing glimpse of the youngster's feelings about separation, his sense of security, and the quality of his attachment to his parents. The more secure children will think of some way to achieve a happy outcome; the more troubled youngsters will weave in themes of injury, loss, and revenge. One school-age boy told one of the authors that the baby bird fell to the forest floor where some predators seized it and devoured it. When the father and mother bird returned and found out what had happened, they flew down and killed the predators. In brief, this child voiced his concerns with the absence of support, the lack of anyone in his environment whom he could trust, and the dominance of the themes of revenge and aggression in his life. In contrast to this, another child described mama and papa birds both coming back with worms and finding baby bird on the forest floor. They fed it, taught it to fly, and they all flew back to the nest.

These, then, are some of the devices that are commonly used to elicit fantasy material from the child; these data, along with the rest of the study, are an invaluable addition to the profile of personality organization.

Much of what a child communicates by means of play can be thought of as metaphor. The various play figures, be they stuffed animals, dolls, puppets, or toy soldiers, are ultimately the significant figures in the child's life and the child's history—including the child himself. The actions in the play drama are some version of the child's memories of significant events, traumatic or gratifying as the case may be, or some wish for a revision of his reality, past and present. Sometimes the images thus created include the examiner. Thus, a child who during a first diagnostic contact plays out rescue by an ambulance is probably hoping the examiner will indeed act to rescue him from his current straits. The child who, during the first hour, plays out a war in which all the participants are killed is telling something of his depressed state of mind and his feelings of rage, hopelessness, and helplessness. The grandiose child who begins from the outset to lord it over the examiner and to show how successful he is and how deplorable is the examiner's performance or behavior (Let's play that I'm the best student in the class and you're the dumbest student and you did something bad and you have to be punished) is likely to be expressing his narcissistic orientation, his grandiosity, and his need to be dominant at all costs. Play is, in effect, the child's own language, and the therapist must learn it gradually by working with the youngster. The rules and logic of play are acquired as the product of much supervision and experience. It is a language whose message is often crucial in unraveling the hidden component of a child's disturbance.

Other Developmental Levels. The tactics for evaluating a preschooler are, in some respects, similar to the techniques employed with older age groups, but certain striking differences necessarily emerge. A major theme that clinicians do not try to explore extensively with younger children but that older children can address involves the past, especially previous experiences with trauma. The usual approach is to ask the child to recall his earliest memory and then to build up recollections from there about the preschool years. Gradually the therapist uses this information to reconstruct those events that may have contributed in some measure to the current problems: divorce, accidents, fires, moves, illnesses, school changes, separations from parents, bouts of physical abuse or seduction, and the like. The goal of the work is to assess what any of these experiences may have meant to the child, and whether he is still experiencing the effects.

Beyond those topics, the substance of the examination is very much as described earlier; the clinician seeks to assess the child's ability to discuss the chief complaint and follows that with an exploration of the home, the school, and the neighborhood dimensions of the child's life. The therapist does a brief mental status survey and encourages the expression of fantasy, using as many of the aforementioned methods as possible. The examiner stays particularly alert to the way the child relates in the sessions, tries to put into words any problematic aspects of the child's relationship behavior, and raises any such perceived difficulties as areas for study. The need to do this in a nonthreatening and noncritical way is often a confronting test of the examiner's sensitivity and ingenuity. In general, if the examiner thinks that a given line of inquiry will be too much for a youngster, it is better not to press the question.

The same holds true for teenagers. Once again, the topics are essentially those listed. The emergents that development brings, however, require certain additions to the questions, and the style and language are necessarily quite different. The therapist should not use street talk or adolescent jargon; neither should he or she speak in an excessively sophisticated or academic fashion. Straight, simple, declarative, and essentially adult language is best, with an approach that conveys a basic quality of dealing with issues directly and expecting the youngster to do the same. The areas to address are those listed for the latency child, but with the addition, now, of some references to sexuality, growing up, body changes, sex education, sexual experience, and erotic fantasy. In addition, the doctor seeks to ascertain the youngster's ideal formations and visions of the future, the career choices he is contemplating, and the sort of family life the youth wishes for in his dreams.

Again, great tact and sensitivity are necessary to determine how far to carry such an inquiry. It is usually better to approach these areas gingerly until learning where a given youngster stands in terms of facing these aspects of life. In general, direct questions about sexual activity and masturbation are not advisable in the first hour unless the discussion suggests that the youngster is prepared to talk about these areas. It is appropriate to broach the subject in a tactful way, but it is not wise to press it. The clinician can ask, "Have you ever felt that you were in love?" or "Is romance an important part of your life?" as an opening gambit. If there is real doubt after a few general queries, the examiner could speak of the problem: "You know, sexuality is a part of teenage life, but not all young people can talk about it very comfortably. It seems to me I've raised the topic but I get the feeling you edge away. Where are you with all this?" Sometimes this kind of statement can help lead in and allow the youngster to say at least something about the sexual aspect of his experience. In general, it is more important to convey empathy and understanding than it is to pin down the youth to hard answers during the opening hours. But the therapist should mention that things are not being said or that some topics are hard to talk about. He or she should identify the topics and give the failure to talk about them the quality of an understandable problem.

Talking about ideals and religious attitudes, especially as these involve concepts of an afterlife, can be of considerable importance. Sometimes these are very touchy areas, especially where this has caused contention within the family, but the subject needs at least to be identified as important, even if the physician does not press it.

In some instances it is crucial to take a firm position in conducting the evaluation. There are situations where the doctor simply cannot ethically proceed with the usual pattern of interviewing; it becomes essential for the therapist to tell the youth that as a professional he or she must take some action to interfere. Sometimes it comes down to a decision: either the youngster addresses the problem and shares it with the parents, or the doctor will. This comes up when the youngster tells of possessing a lethal weapon, using hazardous drugs, having a venereal disease, planning suicide, or being involved in active criminality—or a host of similar dangerous or potentially dangerous situations. The injunction "First do no harm" applies to diagnostic as well as to therapeutic contacts; in the case of younger teenagers (and most older teenagers as well), serious or threatening matters must be shared with parents. The only degree of freedom is who tells them. From a mental health view it is better if the youngster tells them directly; optimally this can be done in the doctor's office, and the doctor can then back it up with support, explanation, suggestions, and further discussion.

Neurological Observations. While the interview is progressing, the doctor is noting the child's neurological patterns as well. If a neurological deficiency is present, many of the child's behaviors may suggest a possible diagnosis, including the following: coordination, concentration, distractibility, hearing, vision, the presence of petit mal seizures or "absences," weakness of some part of the body, hints of memory difficulties or capacities, unusual strengths or weaknesses in short-term memory, ability to do sequential actions, fine motor and gross motor skills, restlessness, hyperactivity, or constriction of activity, competencies at reading, writing, and drawing, ability to understand and obey verbal commands, ability to respond to limits, flightiness, fragmentation of play patterns, impulsivity, suggestibility, word-finding difficulties, articulation difficulties, stuttering and other disturbances of speech and languge usage, nystagmus, unusual patterns of eye contact, odd patterns of motor behavior (such as automatisms, blindisms, hand fluttering, toe walking, or other peculiarities of posture or gait), and tics (including random twitching of any muscle group, sniffing, throat clearing, or making odd sounds). Clinicians vary in the degree to which they themselves conduct various neurological tests or refer the child to a neurologist; in any case, the normal course of interaction and play offers many opportunities for observations.

Enrichment and Review of Data. The next step in the evaluation may involve additional interviews with one or both parents and more visits with the child. The parent contacts are intended to clarify the current status of the home, to obtain a more detailed picture of the parent–child interactive pattern, to achieve further developmental clarification, and to attempt constructing a model of the family pattern that would help explain the current state of affairs. With the child the effort is, on the one hand, to build a firm relationship within whose context the data can be developed in greater detail, and, on the other, to test out the limits of the child's relationship potential. Thus, if the youngster has been rather reserved, is it possible to achieve a more open state? Or if the child has been rather winning and confiding, does that persist or does it mask a manipulative orientation? For many relationship questions, only a certain amount of time and work can give adequate answers; where doubt exists, it is necessary to extend the evaluation and to give the process the time it needs. This can also be true where certain questions about organicity arise. Weighing the effect of a given biological problem against the contribution of emotional factors to a particular structural pattern of symptomatology can be a complex diagnostic challenge that cannot always be satisfactorily resolved. It might take a rather extended exposure to the youngster's pattern of behavior along with an in-depth study of school behavior and teachers' observations to sort out the relevant information. In addition, formal neurological and neuropsychological testing may be necessary.

Meanwhile, the diagnostician should write letters, make calls, and invite information from the appropriate pediatrician, neurologist, psychologist, educator, and/or social worker who has seen the child and family. In addition, hospital records (both psychiatric and medical/surgical) and laboratory studies should be reviewed. In more complex cases, it is wise to hold a multidisciplinary conference with the other professionals who have participated in the evaluation to clarify obscure areas and to ascertain the need for additional studies. Where other agencies are involved (such as welfare or child protection), it is important for the evaluator to meet with representatives of these organizations in order to get a sense of their position in the case, and, in particular, the services they can offer the child and family.

Interpretative Conference. Finally, armed with all these data, the examiner does some quiet thinking and perhaps some additional reading as well. Diagnosis is often an extended and painstaking process; the diagnostician is considering a large volume of data and trying to build a model of the child's functioning that will account for his condition within the context of his human and physical environment. Once such an initial schema emerges, then the therapist can devise a plan that seeks to meet the needs of the situation by helping the child, the family, and the school, as well as providing counsel to the other involved professionals.

A major product of an evaluation is the establishment of a definitive diagnosis. This is important for a variety of reasons: it allows for collecting meaningful demographic data; it permits researchers to know they are dealing with conditions that their protocols either include or exclude; it communicates necessary information to funding sources such as government programs or insurance companies; it offers justification (for either medicolegal or peer review) for pursuing suitable diagnostic measures and initiating particular therapies; and, of special importance, it causes the diagnostician to think through the case carefully and to formulate a picture appropriate to existing classifications. The criteria for specific diagnostic labels are delineated in the chapters of the present volume that deal with particular syndromes. Where appropriate, the clinician should use more than one diagnostic label in the evaluation.

In addition to diagnosis, the evaluation should provide some sense of how to proceed with future work on the problem. Formulating recommendations is no simple matter. It implies an in-depth understanding of the child and family, as well as a thorough knowledge of the community and its facilities. The diagnostician needs a grasp on the full array of both the supportive and the therapeutic modalities in the field, and this comprehension must range over the biopsychosocial sphere in a valid and realistic way. Most troubled youngsters who are properly evaluated will require multiple modalities of intervention at the same time, and the examiner must have a good command of the ways of bringing these several techniques to bear. This will be true whether or not that particular practitioner is personally qualified to carry them out. Thus, a psychologist may turn to a psychiatrist to administer the medication for a case being seen in individual psychotherapy; and the same psychiatrist may send a family to that psychologist for parent training while the psychiatrist him- or herself continues to work with the child. The key point here is that each professional can diagnose a need and get the child to an appropriate treatment modality, even if it is not one that the particular professional is trained to administer.

The next step in the process is to meet with the family and to explain the plan. As the work has gone on, it is likely that enough of the elements being recommended have already been touched upon so they do not come as a shock or a surprise to the people involved. Thus, if a youngster with anorexia is being evaluated, the final recommendation might be for immediate pediatric hospitalization and the initiation of family and individual therapy. During the study, however, these options should have been mentioned as among the possible outcomes of the study, the health issues should have been spelled out, the dangers underlined, and the potential need for hospitalization foreshadowed. Much of this will probably already have been done by the pediatrician or the specialist in adolescent medicine. Again, where the character of the case suggests the possibility of childhood depression, then, as part of an overall treatment plan, the clinician should have spoken early of antidepressant medication as among the interventions that he or she would consider. All in all, the interpretative conference should sum up the findings and communicate the recommendations, but optimally, it should not spring surprises. Instead, it should be a calculated drawing together of the several threads of explanation and anticipation that the preceding hours of study brought to the fore and clarified, and that have now been woven together into a coherent pattern. In a properly managed conference, the conclusions and recommendations would be experienced as a logical outcome of the hints, the possibilities, and the data the clinician has communicated thus far.

As the diagnostic process unfolds, the professional's impressions and recommendations are likely to stir many questions and concerns in the parents' minds, and a vital function of the integrative session is to air and discuss these reactions. If the parents are to follow through effectively with proffered recommendations, it is essential for them to be able to ask questions, to understand the logic of the proposed formulation, and to be able adequately to express their concerns.

It is important to keep in mind that one of the possible outcomes of a study is the decision to postpone a final formulation until obtaining more data, and a family must be prepared for this possibility as well. This is often one of the hardest recommendations for people to accept, because it flies in the face of both the practical need systems that have brought the family to the assessment situation and their magical expectations with regard to the study's outcome. It is common for parents to look to the final hour of evaluation as the moment of closure, the point at which they will receive the magical solution to all the problems that have beset them so grievously. An inconclusive result will fall far short of their expectations. Nonetheless the decision to extend the assessment process is often the best position to assume, and the family has to be told what else needs to be done, and why (e.g., a trial of treatment or a change in caretakers followed by a waiting period and then a reevaluation).

The child must also hear about the findings and recommendations. There is no cut-and-dried way to do this, and optimally it should vary with the case. The approach will reflect the relationship that the examiner has been able to establish with the youngster as well as the quality of the child's communication pattern with the family. Many professionals prefer to have the child present with the parents for the review and the conveyance of interpretative information. Others see the child separately, either before or after seeing the parents. Some do both; they have the child in when explaining the recommendations, and they then see the child separately to allow the youngster to express any feelings or reactions that may have arisen in response to the review. In many instances this is the optimal plan; but no one procedure covers all contingencies, diagnoses, and developmental levels.

Teenagers who are seeking actively to distance themselves from what they experience as the domination of the parents may present special problems. Some of these cases will require considerable tact and firmness on the examiner's part. Sometimes the best way to handle necessary but difficult communication is to have the youngster convey the news; in the presence of the doctor the youth can tell the parents what the situation is and what the doctor has said needs to be done. This is particularly true where issues such as pregnancy or drug use have not previously been revealed to the parents. This then opens the door for the doctor to discuss these matters with the parents in a constructive way.

CHECKLISTS AND RATING SCALES

There are several reasons for using checklists and rating scales (Edelbrock, 1987):

- Certain childhood disorders represent a disturbance in the *degree* of some behavior pattern that is normally present during development (the very structure of such terms as *undersocialized* or *hyperactive* betrays this quality). Rating scales are a way of quantifying the degree of this disturbance. Such scales establish both whether or not a deviation is present and the extent of its salience. In particular, the scales allow for evaluating behavior within a developmental context.

- Certain scales allow untrained observers to report data in specific and quantitative terms rather than in a vague, global, and approximate fashion.

- Such devices also permit the observer to follow behavioral changes. When combined with developmental norms, these scales approach a way of stating quantitatively whether, and to what extent, a condition is worsening or improving, or whether it is remaining at a plateau.

- The scales allow for objective reporting under conditions where inter-rater reliability can be measured and validity issues addressed. As a result, they are basic to research efforts into the nature and extent of childhood disorders.

Most professionals who employ these measures refer to the individual rating scales or questionnaires as *instruments*. Some instruments are designed for use by adults (parents, teachers, ward personnel, therapists, etc.) to describe what they see in children; others are intended for self-ratings by the children themselves. All in all, these various instruments have been remarkably useful (e.g., under proper conditions a teenager's self-rating about the number or seriousness of his delinquent acts or about the level of his sexual activity might be quite different from—and far more revealing than—the reports of the significant adults in that youngster's life). To obtain the most clinically useful information, a number of ratings, made by different adults as well as by the youngster, should be assembled and considered side by side. This gives a sense of the behavior in different contexts, as seen from various perspectives, and allows the richest clinical profile to emerge.

The Scales

Introduction. Perhaps the two most common instruments currently in use are the Conner's Rating Scale for Parents (along with the accompanying

Conner's Rating Scale for Teachers) (Conners, 1969,1973), and the Child Behavioral Checklist and Profile (developed by Achenbach and Edelbrock and commonly referred to as the CBCL).

CONNERS RATING SCALE.   The original Conner's Parent Scale offered the parents 73 items for responses, whereas the Conner's Scale for Teachers presented 39 items for the teacher to rate. Over time, it was possible to select out particularly sensitive and consistent items from each scale, and currently an abbreviated form has been developed that contains only 10 items and is quick, easy to use, valid, and reliable. The more expanded forms were also shortened (the parents taking a full Conner's are now asked to respond to 48 items; the teachers, to 28).

CHILD BEHAVIOR CHECKLIST.   The Child Behavior Checklist (CBCL) is a more complex instrument. (There are actually two separate devices involved: The Child Behavioral Checklist and the Child Behavioral Profile.) It has many versions, depending on whether a parent, teacher, researcher, or the child is doing the rating, and depending as well on the age and sex of the child being rated. It is a far more searching instrument than the Conner's checklist. Thus, parents must fill out 138 items, and teachers face a similar list. An advantage of this scale is that it rather effectively groups children into one of two large categories, *internalizers* and *externalizers*. Properly used, it can also approximate more specific diagnostic categories, for example, schizoid, depressed, hyperactive, delinquent. One of the strengths of the instrument is that it teases out *patterns* of behavior rather than emphasizing the *frequency* of a given behavior.

BEHAVIOR PROBLEM CHECKLIST.   Quite a different approach was taken by Quay and Peterson in their research studies, and their efforts gave rise to an alternative instrument, The Behavior Problem Checklist (BPC). The first manual was formally available in 1967; in time, it was expanded to offer an overall means for identifying and quantifying childhood psychopathology. Again it provides two broad factors, called respectively: *Personality* and *Conduct Problems* (roughly equivalent to the internalizing/externalizing dimensions of the CBCL). In addition, however, it provides for several more specific categories that approach individual diagnoses, such as, psychotic behavior and conduct disorder. During its rather long history it has been revised repeatedly and has had varying numbers of items (55 to 150). Currently there are 89 scorable lines, 12 of which are designed specifically for very young children. This checklist has a relatively strong record of validity and reliability.

OTHER INSTRUMENTS.   Although these three checklists are the most frequently employed, numerous additional instruments have been designed to measure and evaluate a specific form of behavior, for example, gender disorder, hyperkinesis, anxiety, and depression. Only a few will be mentioned; literally dozens are available.

1. The Child Behavior Inventory (CBI, Eyberg, 1980) allows parents to recount both the *frequency* and the *degree* of problem associated with a particular behavior. Thus, talking back may occur repeatedly (behavior with high-level frequency but low-level seriousness) yet never have the impact of threatening or attacking a sibling with a knife once (low-frequency behavior, but with high-level seriousness).
2. The Louisville Fear Survey assists in estimating the kinds and qualities of childhood fears.
3. The Werry-Weiss-Peters Activity Scale, the Hyperkinesis Index, and the Hyperactivity Rating Scale are each designed to help evaluate activity level and to sort out hyperactive youngsters from normals.

In addition to the many scales that assess specific psychopathology, some instruments have been designed to evaluate children at different developmental levels. Thus, the Preschool Behavior Questionnaire and the Symptom Checklist and Social Competence Scale are both designed to identify deviant conditions in preschool populations. The School Behavior Checklist is targeted for the grade-school child and seeks, as its name indicates, to throw light on school adjustment problems. There is a Teacher Referral Form for those working with children in a school-based mental health program, and Walker's Checklist addresses behavior problems in the classroom.

In addition to these parent- or teacher-report scales, there is now a strong movement afoot to develop self-report instruments for children and adolescents. Experience has shown that these are valid and informative, yielding sensitive information that can be obtained in no other fashion. Thus, anxiety can be measured with the Children's Manifest Anxiety Scale and the State-Trait Anxiety Inventory for Children. Depression is addressed (in adolescents) via the Beck Depression Inventory. There is also a Child Depression Inventory and a derivative short form, the Short Child Depression Inventory.

Other factors for which specific self-report instruments have been created are children's social behavior and their capacity for self-control. The Children's Action Tendency Scale offers the subject choices of response in conflicted situations. (If someone tries to bully you, would you do *a*, or *b*, or *c*?) The Children's Assertive Behavior Scale also confronts the child with a choice among social behaviors and is useful in assessing social skills.

The Children's Perceived Self-Control Scale offers a series of *yes–no* choices to test how well the child can restrain impulse, resist temptation, and anticipate consequences. Such instruments may someday be important in designing preventive programs.

STRUCTURED (AND SEMISTRUCTURED) INTERVIEWS

With the introduction of DSM-III and DSM-III-R, the emphasis has fallen on how to elicit the kinds of information that would allow for the application of this diagnostic system. The traditional clinical interview has been notoriously inexact in this respect. Checklists and rating scales provided one means of compensating for this deficiency; it is inherent in their structure, however, that they cannot clarify the ambiguous or pursue what is only hinted at. Hence, in addition to the instruments already described, a number of structured and semistructured interviews have also emerged. These devices seek to address diagnostic issues in a more open, more exploratory, and less constricted fashion than is true for checklists.

One surprising aspect of the attempt to develop these interview instruments was the discovery that when questioned directly (in an appropriate and tactful fashion), children will reveal many hitherto unsuspected and highly troubled emotions. This has been found true for suicidal ideation as well as for concerns about separation. In many instances, the parents were essentially unaware of these feelings.

Nonstructured Interviews

There are many sources of variation in formulating diagnoses. Different clinicians, using the conventional unstructured interview as their diagnostic tool, approach data collection in highly diverse fashion, making for profound degrees of uncertainty. It is this aspect of the process that the structured interview seeks to correct.

The structured interview implies a standard set of queries to put to the patient in a predetermined order. The array of questions is printed out, and, for reasons of comparability, the interviewer is usually instructed to read the exact language of each question to the patient. By and large, those who construct such instruments put together what they think of as a *schedule* of questions. Hence, the word schedule tends to appear in the title, for example, the NIMH Diagnostic Interview Schedule for Children or the Child Assessment Schedule.

Criteria

To serve well, such an interview must meet several criteria:

- Raters must record answers reliably.
- Different raters should rate symptoms in similar fashion.

- The rules by which diagnoses are made should give good results.
- The instrument should be reasonably sensitive and specific. That is to say, it should identify most of the cases where pathology exists, and it should not find pathology in most of the normals.

In addition, on the face of it, the questions asked and the nature of the diagnostic category being explored should fit together in a way that makes sense (face validity).

Currently, several instruments have emerged that approach these criteria, and they are finding ever-increasing application.

1. *Behavior Screening Questionnaire (BSQ).* This 60-question schedule is designed to identify problems in preschool children. The questions are read to the parents and are scored as "behavior absent," "sometimes present," or "frequently present." Although it does not give rise to diagnostic labels, it will pick up a large majority of the children who clinically are recorded as disturbed. It thus lends itself to epidemiological survey work (although it is best administered by a trained professional).

2. *Diagnostic Interview for Children and Adolescents (DICA).* This instrument was designed to fit itself to the child's areas of interest. Created in counterpoint to the Kiddie-SADS (Schedule for Affective Disorders and Schizophrenia), it sought to make less burdensome demands on the respondent and to be easier to use. There is no parent form for this schedule; it is best used with 7- to 12-year-olds. One part includes direct questions for the child to answer, a second part involves ratings by the examiner, and the third part covers details in the child's life history. As a rule, it requires 45 to 60 minutes to complete.

3. *Interview Schedule for Children (ISC).* This is a research instrument intended specifically for repeated administration thus permitting sequential follow-up studies. It is a lengthy procedure that entails in-depth questioning of both parent and child and requires trained clinicians for its adminsitration.

4. *Diagnostic Interview Schedule for Children (DISC-II).* A highly structured interview, this recently revised instrument is intended for use by laypersons doing epidemiological surveys. It will produce DSM-III-R diagnoses for children between ages 6 and 17 years. There is both a child interview and a parent form; together they take about 2 hours to administer.

These then are a sampling of the kinds of instruments currently employed as screening, survey, and diagnostic assists. At this point, they are not widely used in clinical practice. This is gradually changing, however, and individual practitioners and clinics are beginning to "find" these instruments and to use them routinely.

PSYCHOLOGICAL TESTING

Introduction

Broadly speaking, three main categories of psychological testing are currently in use. The first involves the *assessment of intelligence* and is pointed generally toward measuring cognitive and perceptual functioning. The second is called *neuropsychological testing* and is designed to identify and perhaps localize specific functional deficits. The third category consists of a rather diverse group of instruments collectively called *projective tests*. These are intended to explore different aspects of personality functioning ranging from impulse control, through affect regulation and reality testing, to patterns of attachment—along with many points in between.

In addition to these principal groups, many kinds of specific instruments seek to illuminate the patient's status in respect to some particular aspect of functioning such as anxiety, hyperactivity, depression, and gender identity. We cannot here do more than mention a few of the principal or most commonly used instruments within each category.

Intelligence Testing

Binet-Simon and Stanford-Binet.   This was initiated in France in the early 1900s when a psychologist, Binet, and a psychiatrist, Simon, sought to devise a means for estimating the competence of children to be educated (Binet & Simon, 1916; Terman & Merrill, 1973). One of their goals was to do this in a way that would avoid the subjective and the impressionistic and would allow for a valid and reliable measurement. That is to say, they sought to develop a test that would offer a true measurement of what it undertook to assess, and that would give similar results no matter who used it or how often it was given. To achieve these goals, the investigators put together a series of tasks that they posed to sizable cohorts of children of different ages. They winnowed out only those tasks where children showed a steady improvement with increasing age, that is, the investigators culled out those tasks that most 8-year-olds both did well and did better than 6-year-olds, that most 10-year-olds did well and did better than most 8-year-olds, and so on. Because the goal of the undertaking was to study school performance, the emphasis fell on tasks that did not depend on reading or writing. Once the authors identified a task that met such developmental criteria, the ability to perform that task was assumed to represent the mental age of that child. In other words, because the majority of the children within a given age cohort were able to perform that task successfully whereas most younger children could not, success at its performance represented the attainment of a given mental age.

This was the breakthrough. Later, this conception was further elaborated (at Stanford) by seeking a quotient, that is, mental age divided by chronological age (times 100 to eliminate decimal points); this was the original Intelligence Quotient (as measured on the Stanford-Binet). Ultimately the reckoning was accomplished by using standard deviations to determine the intellectual status of the individual; the final score was a measure of how many standard deviations above, at, or below the mean each given subtest attained. (See Chapter 2 for further discussion of intelligence tests).

Wechsler-Bellevue. This notion of employing standard deviations came from the work of David Wechsler in New York. Working with adults, he had developed a somewhat similar set of tasks that became the popular and widely used Wechsler-Bellevue. Scoring was based on deviations from the mean, and the test consisted of a series of structured subtests (rather than a cluster of age-graded items). There were a group of verbal subtests and a group of performance subtests; two separate scores were thus arrived at that the examiner could then combine by formula to offer a full-scale IQ. Eventually the Wechsler was adapted for children in two forms: the WISC–R (the Wechsler Intelligence Scale for Children–Revised), and the WIPPSI [pronounced *wip-see*] (the Wechsler Pre-School and Primary Scale for Intelligence).

The scoring of the Wechsler tests is in itself informative, because different patterns of response can suggest important differential diagnostic possibilities. Thus a spread of 7 points between the lowest and the highest point reached on any of these subtests can be considered within the average range; greater differences imply the possible presence of some deviation of function. Unless the difference amounts to 22 points, however, it is not statistically significant.

Unusually high or low scores on given subtests should always be pursued for their possible implications. Similarly, wide discrepancies between performance and verbal scores might suggest anything from organicity to specific learning deficits.

Nonverbal Tests. Raven's Progressive Matrices offers the patient a series of designs where some element is lacking. The patient is then shown a number of alternative forms (any one of which might be used to fill in the pattern) and is asked to select the one that best occupies the missing space. The abilities involved in this kind of task allow for a rapid estimate of IQ. Because it is essentially nonverbal, the test is used in cross-cultural studies.

Other tests also minimize demands for language competence. In the

Goodenough Draw-A-Person test, for example, the child is instructed to draw a picture of a person, and the test is then scored according to a set of established norms. Sometimes psychologists prefer to start with this as a way of inviting cooperation, while simultaneously getting a rough idea of the level at which the child is functioning.

Verbal Tests. A widely used instrument is the Peabody Picture Vocabulary Test. The examiner shows the child a chart with pictures and then pronounces a word. The child is asked to point to the picture corresponding to that word.

Another, and a particularly sensitive test of this type, is the Illinois Test of Psycholinguistic Abilities. This involves a series of evaluations of the child's comprehension and ability to use language; it is commonly employed to measure the progress of children in remedial programs.

Cognitive Processes. The Visual-Aural Digit Span Test, although simple in format, is intended to examine not so much *what* a child can do as *how* the child goes about doing it. To this end, the examiner reads aloud a sequence of numbers to the child and then shows the child the numbers on printed cards. In each instance, the child is asked to remember the numbers and to repeat them—on some occasions by saying them and on others by writing them. Thus, four kinds of results can be evaluated, and the examiner is able to assess the child's ability to transfer information between sight and sound, along with the child's ability to maintain and recall an inner sequence. This is a sensitive instrument and can tap into learning difficulties that the usual IQ tests will miss.

Achievement Tests

A number of tests measure the child's level of academic accomplishment. This is a matter of considerable moment to the educator because anything that interferes with academic progress, or that sets the child apart from his peers, is profoundly significant to that child's adjustment. Best known among these instruments are the Wide Range Achievement Test, the Peabody Individual Achievement Test, and the Woodcock-Johnson Psychoeducational Battery. Any of these will give a good estimate of a child's educational attainment at a given point in time.

Personality Assessment—The Projective Hypothesis

Among clinicians, the use of nonstructured materials (such as a drawing the patient creates, a story the patient makes up, or the meanings the patient attributes to an amorphous form (such as an inkblot)) has achieved a considerable level of acceptance. Research psychologists, on the other hand, have raised many questions concerning whether such an approach can offer a valid kind of test. All of these techniques derive from an essential concept, namely, that the response to such nonstructured stimuli captures an *externalization* of the patient's personality in whole or in part. In other words, the patient who is offered a very general or an ambiguous framework for response will project onto this evocative prompting something of what he is, on many levels. Therefore, by properly analyzing the obtained response, the tester can view the inner workings of the patient's mind.

Rorschach Test. The most famous of such projective devices is the Rorschach Test. This involves a series of 10 standard inkblots (some black and white, and some with different colored inks, against a white background) that possess no inherent or predetermined meaning. The patient is given the cards one at a time in a prescribed sequence; the instructions are for the child to say whatever the inkblots look like, whatever he sees, and whatever they make him think of. The examiner notes the time it takes to obtain a response, the number of responses, the way the card is handled, and, in particular, the nature of the response. This last dimension involves the forms that are seen, the responses to the different colors, the relationship of percept and background, whether bizarre or unrelated percepts are reported, the specificity of the responses, the clarity or the vagueness of the images, and so on. Once completed, the patient is asked to review the cards and to indicate the perceived elements that led to formulating the particular images (these are scored on miniature reproductions of each blot).

As noted, the test is much criticized for its lack of precision and low reliability; its powerful and suggestive qualities, however, foster its continued use.

Thematic Apperception Test (TAT). The test includes 30 cards, each bearing a black and white picture (plus one blank card), from among which the examiner can select appropriate items; as a rule, the average test protocol involves only about 10 of the cards. The subject is handed the cards one at a time, and instructed to create a story based on the card and to say something about each character in the story. The stories are formally scored in terms of the motives, the concerns, and the avoidances depicted in the ensuing accounts. On a clinical level, the stories are often used as indices both of the patient's ongoing personality conflicts and of the primary attempts being made to solve those difficulties. Paradoxically, delinquents (presumably those with a strong inclination to engage in covert antisocial behavior) will often recount blander stories than will normal youngsters).

Children's Apperception Test (CAT). This was designed for children aged 3 to 10. It consists of 10 cards with pictures of animals engaged in meaningful (presumably evocative) behavior—getting married, getting punished, fighting, and so on. It is scored very much like the TAT. A similar but more objectively scored instrument is the Blackie Test. Blackie is a dog who is pictured in a number of emotionally charged interactions (about to lose its tail, etc.). In responding to these images, however, the child is asked to select among a group of multiple-choice possibilities about how and why Blackie feels. The test thus seeks to capture projected feelings in objective fashion.

Drawing Techniques

DRAW-A-PERSON TEST. In recent years this once widely used projective test has become far less commonly employed. It consists of asking the child to draw a person and to follow that with a second drawing of someone of the opposite sex. The examiner can then pose a battery of 33 questions about the drawings. The essential data, however, are contained in the drawings themselves, and the strength of the test resides in their interpretation. This is also its greatest weakness, because the findings from this test have not correlated well with the results obtained by other means. Nonetheless, some *emotional indicators* (continuous vs. broken lines, shading, the angle of placement of the drawing, and omission of important details, to name a few) are strongly suggestive.

HOUSE-TREE-PERSON TEST. Four drawings are required for this test: a house, a tree, a person, and a person of the opposite sex. The house is interpreted as the locus for portraying family life; the tree as the vehicle for deeper unconscious feelings about the self; and the person as the means of expressing more conscious and conventional concerns about the self.

PEN AND PENCIL TESTS

- *Sentence Completion Test.* Unlike most of the projective tests, this instrument is essentially verbal. Here the child is offered a series of incomplete statements, each in the form of a few words that begin a sentence but stop in the middle, and the child must complete the sentence (e.g., I am most worried about . . .). Several versions of this test now exist, and it is sometimes used to screen children who betray evidence of significant psychopathology.
- *Minnesota Multiphasic Personality Inventory (MMPI).* This test has achieved a great deal of recognition and stands in a class by itself in terms of widespread use and general acceptance. It offers 556 items (posed in the form of statements about oneself) in respect to which the respondent has three choices: "true," "false," and "cannot say." One of the strengths of the test lies in its scoring. A number of individual scales emerge that offer a

profile made up of categories such as mania, depression, schizophrenia, and hysteria. The configuration of the scores on the several scales shows high correlations with diagnoses. Although designed for adults, the test can be used successfully with teenagers. A version for parents of young children, the Personality Inventory for Children (PIC), has been developed; it is, however, not geared to diagnostic categories in the same way as the MMPI.

Tests for Organic Dysfunction: Neuropsychological Testing

These tests seek to identify children with organic brain damage. A number of such instruments have been developed including a wide variety of subtests that seek to pinpoint specific kinds of brain dysfunction. In a statistical sense, it is not difficult to demonstrate evidence of brain damage. Thus, even on the Wechsler (where one group of subtests offers a verbal IQ and another, a performance IQ), the brain-injured child will tend to achieve lower performance levels than verbal scores, often by a considerable margin. This, however, is far too nonspecific to use as a diagnostic measure.

Bender Visual-Gestalt Test (usually referred to as the Bender or the Bender-Gestalt). This is probably the most widely used test of its kind and forms part of the typical test battery ordinarily administered by clinical psychologists. It is essentially a test of visual–motor function and requires children to copy various complex line drawings. The children are shown the drawings one at a time and asked to reproduce them. After completing the copy, they are allowed to scrutinize the model again and then to repeat the drawings to see if they perceive and/or can correct any errors. Scoring correlates well with development (younger children normally make more errors) and with cognitive status. The number of errors, the quality of errors, and the ability to recognize and correct errors together make for significant identification of organic damage.

Halstead-Reitan Test Battery. This complex text involves many subtests and is intended to assess perceptual–motor functioning. It was designed for adults, but simplified versions are now available for children (one for 5- to 8-year olds, and another for 9- to 14-year-olds). The battery includes a test of abstract concept formation; a modification of the Seguin Formboard designed to measure speed, memory, and tactile competence; the Seashore rhythm test; a trail-making test; an assessment of hand-grip strength; an aphasia screening instrument; procedures to evaluate sensory perception; plus the WISC and the Wide Range Achievement Test as allied procedures. Another test that conveys much the same information is the Luria-Nebraska Neuropsychological Test Battery.

Goldstein-Scherer Color-Form Sorting Test.   This is supposed to measure the degree of facility with which the patient forms abstract concepts (tested by asking the patient to cluster a variety of different objects).

Frostig Developmental Test of Visual Perception.   Here a series of drawing tasks assess functioning in a number of predetermined areas. Spatial, figure–ground, and coordination functions are evaluated to arrive at a perceptual score. A number of remedial methods are designed to flow from these findings, but the long-range benefit of this approach remains to be demonstrated.

Graham-Kendall Memory for Designs Test.   This is much like the Bender but has an additional demand. The child is shown a design for 5 seconds but is then asked to reproduce it from memory. The test is easy to score and discriminates between brain-injured and normal youngsters.

There are many tests for specific functions. The Continuous Performance Test, for example, measures attention and concentration. The child is shown a series of stimuli (letters or numbers that pop into view on a video screen) with instructions to press a button when a particular item appears or when a given sequence occurs. The omission of correct answers is thought to indicate that attention is not being maintained; a pattern of frequent incorrect responses indicates impulsivity.

Bibliography

Aarkrog, T., & Mortensen, K. V. (1985). Schizophrenia in early adolescence. *Acta Psychiatrica Scandinavica, 72,* 422–429.

Abe, K. (1972). Phobias and nervous symptoms in childhood and maturity: Persistence and associations. *British Journal of Psychiatry, 120,* 275–283.

Abikoff, H., & Gittelman, R. (1984). Does behavior therapy normalize the classroom behavior of hyperactive children? *Archives of General Psychiatry, 41,* 449–454.

Abikoff, H., & Gittelman, R. (1985a). Hyperactive children treated with stimulants. Is cognitive training a useful adjunct? *Archives of General Psychiatry, 42,* 953–961.

Abikoff, H., & Gittelman, R. (1985b). The normalizing effects of methylphenidate on the classroom behavior of ADDH children. *Journal of Abnormal Child Psychology, 13,* 33–44.

Abikoff, H., Gittelman, R., & Klein, D. F. (1980). Classroom observation code for hyperactive children: A replication of validity. *Journal of Consulting and Clinical Psychology, 48,* 555–565.

Abraham, K. (1916). The first pregenital stage of the libido. In *Selected papers on psycho-analysis.* London: Hogarth Press, 1927.

Abraham, S. F., & Beumont, P. J. V. (1982). How patients describe bulimia or binge eating. *Psychological Medicine, 12,* 625–635.

Abramson, L. Y., Seligman, M. E. P., & Teasdale, J. D. (1978). Learned helplessness in humans: Critique and reformulation. *Journal of Abnormal Psychology, 87,* 49–74.

Achenbach, T. M. (1966). The classification of children's psychiatric symptoms: A factor analytic study. *Psychological Monographs, 80*(7) No. 615.

Achenbach, T. M. (1980). DSM-III in light of empirical research on classification of child psychopathology. *Journal of the American Academy of Child Psychiatry, 19,* 395–412.

Achenbach, T. M. (1982). *Developmental psychopathology* (2nd ed.). New York: Wiley.

Achenbach, T. M., & Edelbrock, C. S. (1978). The classification of child psychopathology: A review and analysis of empirical efforts, *Psychological Bulletin, 85,* 1275–1301.

Achenbach, T. M., & Edelbrock, C. S. (1979). The child behavior profile: II. Boys aged 12–16 and girls aged 6–11 and 12–16. *Journal of Consulting and Clinical Psychology, 47,* 223–233.

Achenbach, T. M., & Lewis, M. (1971). A proposed model for clinical research and its application to encopresis and enuresis. *Journal of the American Academy of Child Psychiatry, 10,* 535–554.

Ackerman, P. T., Anhalt, J. M., Holcomb, P. J., & Dykman, R. A. (1986). Presumably innate and acquired automatic processes in children with attention and/or reading disorders. *Journal of Child Psychology and Psychiatry, 27,* 513–529.

Ackerman, S. H., Manaker, S., & Cohen, M. I. (1981). Recent separation and the onset of peptic ulcer disease in older children and adolescents. *Psychosomatic Medicine, 43,* 305–310.

Adams, P. L. (1973). *Obsessive children.* New York: Brunner/Mazel.

Adams, P. L. (1985, October). *Childhood obsessive compulsive disorder: Spectrum or single disorder?* Paper presented at the American Academy of Child Psychiatry Annual Meeting, San Antonio, TX.

Adams-Tucker, C. (1984). The unmet psychiatric needs of sexually abused youths: Referrals from a child protection agency and clinical evaluations. *Journal of the American Academy of Child Psychiatry, 23,* 659–667.

Adelman, H. S., & Taylor, L. (1986). The problems of definition and differentiation and the need for a classification schema. *Journal of Learning Disabilities, 19,* 514–520.

Ader, R. (1983). Developmental psychoneuroimmunology. *Developmental Psychobiology, 16,* 251–267.

Ader, R., & Cohen, N. (1985). High time for psychoimmunology. *Nature, 315,* 103–104.

Ader, R., Grota, L. J., & Cohen, N. (1987). Conditioning phenomena and immune function. *Annals of New York Academy of Sciences, 496,* 532–544.

Adler, A. (1929). *Individual psychology* (2nd ed.). London: Kegan Paul, Trench, Trübner.

Adler, R., Bongar, B., & Katz, E. R. (1982). Psychogenic abdominal pain and parental pressure in childhood athletics. *Psychosomatics, 23,* 1185–1186.

Agras, S. (1959). The relationship of school phobia to childhood depression. *American Journal of Psychiatry, 116,* 533–539.

Agras, S., Sylvester, D., & Oliveau, D. C. (1969). The epidemiology of common fears and phobia. *Comprehensive Psychiatry, 10,* 151–156.

Agras, W. S., Chapin, H. N., & Oliveau, D. C. (1972). The natural history of phobia: Course and prognosis. *Archives of General Psychiatry, 26,* 315–317.

Aichorn, A. (1935). *Wayward youth.* New York: Viking.

Ainsworth, M. D. S. (1982). Attachment: Retrospect and prospect. In C. M. Parkes & J. Stevenson-Hinde (Eds.), *The place of attachment in human behavior* (pp. 3–30). New York: Basic Books.

Ainsworth, M. D. S., Blehar, M. C., Waters, E., & Wall, S. (1978). *Patterns of attachment: A psychological study of the strange situation.* Hillsdale, NJ: Erlbaum.

Akesson, H. O. (1986). The biological origin of mild mental retardation: A critical review. *Acta Psychiatrica Scandinavica, 74,* 3–7.

Akiskal, H. S., Downs, J., Jordan, P., Watson, S., Daugherty, D., & Pruitt, D. B. (1985). Affective disorders in referred children and younger siblings of manic-depressives. *Archives of General Psychiatry, 42,* 996–1003.

Akiskal, H. S., Hirschfeld, R. M. A., & Yerevanian, B. I. (1983). The relationship of personality to affective disorders. *Archives of General Psychiatry, 40,* 801–810.

Akiskal, H. S., Rosenthal, R. H., Rosenthal, T. L., Kashgarian, M., Khani, M. K., & Puzantian, V. R. (1979). Differentiation of primary affective illness from situational, symptomatic and secondary depressions. *Archives of General Psychiatry, 36,* 635–644.

Albert, N., & Beck, A. T. (1975). Incidence of depression in early adolescence: A preliminary study. *Journal of Youth and Adolescence, 4,* 301–307.

Alberts-Corush, J., Firestone, P., & Goodman, J. T. (1986). Attention and impulsivity characteristics of the biological and adoptive parents of hyperactive and normal control children. *American Journal of Orthopsychiatry, 56,* 413–423.

Albin, R. L., Young, A. B., Penney, J. B. (1989). The functional anatomy of basal ganglia disorders. *Trends in Neuroscience, 12,* 366–375.

Alexander, A. B. (1972). Systematic relaxation and flow rates in asthmatic children: Relationship to emotional precipitants and anxiety. *Journal of Psychosomatic Research, 16,* 405–410.

Alexander, A. B., Cropp, G. J. A., & Chai, H. (1979). Effects of relaxation training on pulmonary mechanics in children with asthma. *Journal of Applied Behavioral Analysis, 12,* 27–35.

Alexander, F. (1950). *Psychosomatic medicine.* New York: Norton.

Alpert, J. E., Cohen, D. J., Shaywitz, B. A., & Piccirillo, M. (1981). Neurochemical and behavioral organization: Disorders of attention, activity, and aggression. In D. O. Lewis (Ed.), *Vulnerabilities to delinquency* (pp. 109–186). New York: SP Medical & Scientific Books.

Altemeier, W. A., III, O'Connor, S. M., Sherrod, K. B., & Vietze, P. M. (1985). Prospective study of antecedents for nonorganic failure to thrive. *Journal of Pediatrics, 106,* 360–365.

Altemeier, W. A., III, O'Connor, S. M., Vietze, P. M., Sandler, H. M., & Sherrod, K. B. (1982). Antecedents of child abuse. *The Journal of Pediatrics, 100,* 823–829.

Aman, M. G., & Kern, R. A. (1989). Review of fenfluramine in the treatment of the developmental disabilities. *Journal of the American Academy of Child and Adolescent Psychiatry, 28,* 549–565.

American Psychiatric Association. (1980). *Diagnostic and statistical manual of mental disorders* (DSM-III) (3rd ed.). Washington, DC: American Psychiatric Association.

American Psychiatric Association. (1987). *Diagnostic and statistical manual of mental disorders* (DSM-III-R) (3rd ed.–revised). Washington, DC: American Psychiatric Association.

Anderson, C. D. (1981). Expression of affect and physiological response in psychosomatic patients. *Journal of Psychosomatic Research, 25,* 143–149.

Anderson, D. J., Noyes, R., & Crowe, R. R. (1984). A comparison of panic disorder and generalized anxiety disorder. *American Journal of Psychiatry, 141,* 572–575.

Anderson, G. M., & Hoshino, Y. (1987). Neurochemical studies of autism. In D. J. Cohen & A. M. Donnellan (Eds.), *Handbook of autism and pervasive developmental disorders* (pp. 166–191). New York: Wiley.

Anderson, J. C., Williams, S., McGee, R., & Silva, P. A. (1987). DSM-III disorders in preadolescent children: Prevalence in a large sample from the general population. *Archives of General Psychiatry, 44,* 69–76.

Anderson, L. T., Campbell, M., Grega, D. M., Perry, R., Small, A. M., & Green, W. H. (1984). Haloperidol in the treatment of infantile autism: Effects on learning and behavioral symptoms. *American Journal of Psychiatry, 141,* 1195–1202.

Andreasen, N. C. (Ed.) (1986). *Can schizophrenia be localized in the brain?* Washington, DC: American Psychiatric Press.

Andreasen, N. C. (1987). The diagnosis of schizophrenia. *Schizophrenia Bulletin, 13,* 9–22.

Andreasen, N. C., Nasrallah, H. A., Dunn, V., Olson, S. C., Grove, W. M., Ehrhardt, J. C., Coffman, J. A., & Crossett, J. H. W. (1986). Structural abnormalities in the frontal system in schizophrenia: A magnetic resonance imaging study. *Archives of General Psychiatry, 43,* 136–144.

Angold, A. (1988). Childhood and adolescent depression. I. Epidemiological and aetiological aspects. *British Journal of Psychiatry, 152,* 601–617.

Annett, M., & Manning, M. (1989). Reading and a balanced polymorphism for laterality and ability. *Journal of Child Psychology and Psychiatry, 31,* 511–529.

Anthony, E. J. (1957). An experimental approach to the psychopathology of childhood: encopresis. *British Journal of Medical Psychology, 30,* 146–175.

Anthony, E. J. (1975a). Childhood depression. In E. J. Anthony & T. Bencdek (Eds.), *Depression and human existence* (pp. 231–277). Boston: Little, Brown.

Anthony, E. J. (1975b). The influence of a manic-depressive environment on the developing child. In E. J. Anthony & T. Benedek (Eds.), *Depression and human existence* (pp. 279–315). Boston: Little, Brown.

Anthony, E. J. (1975c). Neurotic disorders. In A. M. Freedman, H. I. Kaplan, & B. J. Sadock (Eds.), *Comprehensive textbook of psychiatry* (Vol. 2, pp. 2143–2160). Baltimore: Williams & Wilkins.

Anthony, E. J. (1975d). Two contrasting types of adolescent depression and their treatment. In E. J. Anthony & T. Benedek (Eds.), *Depression and human existence* (pp. 445–460). Boston: Little, Brown.

Anthony, E. J. (1976). How children cope in families with a psychotic parent. In E. N. Rexford, L. W. Sander, & T. Shapiro (Eds.), *Infant psychiatry: A new synthesis* (pp. 239–247). New Haven, CT: Yale University Press.

Anthony, E. J. (1981). The phenomenon of anxiousness. In E. J. Anthony & D. C. Gilpin (Eds.), *Three further clinical faces of childhood* (pp. 127–133). New York: Spectrum.

Anthony, E. J. (1983a). An overview of the effects of maternal depression on the infant and child. In H. L. Morrison (Ed.), *Children of depressed parents: Risk, identification, and intervention* (pp. 1–16). New York: Grune & Stratton.

Anthony, E. J. (1983b). Foreword. In J. D. Call, E. Galenson, & R. L. Tyson (Eds.), *Frontiers of infant psychiatry* (Vol. 1, pp. xvi–xxiv). New York: Basic Books.

Anthony, E. J. (1983c). Prologue. In K. S. Robson (Ed.), *The borderline child: Approaches to etiology, diagnosis, and treatment* (pp. 1–9). New York: McGraw-Hill.

Anthony, E. J. (1984). The influence babies bring to bear on their upbringing. In J. D. Call, E. Galenson, & R. L. Tyson (Eds.), *Frontiers of infant psychiatry* (Vol. II, pp. 259–266). New York: Basic Books.

Anthony, E. J. (1987). Children at high risk for psychosis growing up successfully. In E. J. Anthony & B. J. Cohler (Eds.), *The invulnerable child* (pp. 147–184). New York: Guilford.

Anthony, E. J., & Cohler, B. J. (Eds.). (1987). *The invulnerable child.* New York: Guilford.

Anthony, E. J., & Scott, P. D. (1960). Manic-depressive psychosis in childhood. *Journal of Child Psychology and Psychiatry, 1,* 53–72.

Anyan, W. R., & Showalter, J. E. (1983). A comprehensive approach to anorexia nervosa. *Journal of the American Academy of Child and Adolescent Psychiatry, 22,* 122–127.

Apley, J., & Hale, B. (1973). Children with recurrent abdominal pain: How do they grow up? *British Medical Journal, 3,* 7–9.

Apley, J., MacKeith, R., & Meadow, R. (1978). *The child and his symptoms: A comprehensive approach* (3rd ed.). Oxford: Blackwell.

Apter, A., Borengasser, M. A., Hamovit, J., Bartko, J. J., Cytryn, L., & McKnew, D. H. (1982). A four-year follow-up of depressed children. *Journal of Preventive Psychiatry, 1*, 331–335.

Arboleda, C., & Holzman, P. S. (1985). Thought disorder in children at risk for psychosis. *Archives of General Psychiatry, 42*, 1004–1013.

Aries, P. (1962). *Centuries of childhood.* New York: Alfred A. Knopf.

Arson: How to defend against the most destructive school crime. (1976, December). *School Security 1*, pp. 1–8.

Arthur, B., & Kemme, M. L. (1964). Bereavement in children. *Journal of Child Psychology and Psychiatry, 5*, 37–49.

Asarnow, J. R. (1988). Children at risk for schizophrenia: Converging lines of evidence. *Schizophrenia Bulletin, 14*, 613–631.

Asarnow, J. R., & Ben-Meir, S. (1989). Children with schizophrenia spectrum and depressive disorders: A comparative study of premorbid adjustment, onset pattern, and severity of impairment. *Journal of Child Psychology and Psychiatry, 29*, 477–488.

Asarnow, J. R., Goldstein, M. J., & Ben-Meir, S. (1988). Parental communication deviance in childhood onset schizophrenia spectrum and depressive disorders. *Journal of Child Psychology and Psychiatry, 29*, 825–838.

Asarnow, R., Sherman, T., & Strandburg, R. (1986). The search for the psychobiological substrate of childhood onset schizophrenia. *Journal of the American Academy of Child Psychiatry, 25*, 601–604.

Asberg, M. (1989). Neurotransmitter monoamine metabolites in the cerebrospinal fluid as risk factors for suicidal behavior. In Alcohol, Drug Abuse, and Mental Health Administration (Ed.), *Report of the Secretary's Task Force on Youth Suicide: Vol. 2. Risk factors for youth suicide* (DHHS Publication No. ADM 89-1622, pp. 193–212). Washington, DC: U.S. Government Printing Office.

Ashkenazi, Z. (1975). The treatment of encopresis using a discriminative stimulus and positive reinforcement. *Journal of Behavior Therapy and Experimental Psychiatry, 6*, 155–157.

Aston-Jones, G., Ennis, M., Pieribone, V. A., Nickell, W. T., & Shipley, M. T. (1986). The brain nucleus locus coeruleus: Restricted afferent control of a broad efferent network. *Science, 234*, 734–737.

Aston-Jones, G., Foote, S. L., & Bloom, F. E. (1984). Anatomy and physiology of locus coeruleus neurons: Functional implications. In M. G. Ziegler & C. R. Lake (Eds.), *Norepinephrine* (Vol. 2, pp. 92–116). Baltimore: Williams & Wilkins.

Atkinson, L., Quarrington, B., & Cyr, J. J. (1985). School refusal: The heterogeneity of a concept. *American Journal of Orthopsychiatry, 55*, 83–101.

August, G. J., Raz, N., & Baird, T. D. (1987). Fenfluramine response in high and low functioning autistic children. *Journal of the American Academy of Child and Adolescent Psychiatry, 26*, 342–346.

August, G. J., & Stewart, M. A. (1982). Is there a syndrome of pure hyperactivity? *British Journal of Psychiatry, 140*, 305–311.

August, G. J., Stewart, M. A., & Tsai, L. (1981). The incidence of cognitive disabilities in the siblings of autistic children. *British Journal of Psychiatry, 138,* 416–422.

Ayllon, T., Simon, S. J., & Wildman, R. W. (1975). Instructions and reinforcement in the elimination of encopresis: A case study. *Journal of Behavior Therapy and Experimental Psychiatry, 6,* 235–238.

Ayoub, C., Pfeifer, D., & Leichtman, L. (1979). Treatment of infants with non-organic failure to thrive. *Child Abuse and Neglect, 3,* 937–941.

Azrin, N. H., & Foxx, R. M. (1974). *Toilet training in less than a day.* New York: Simon & Schuster.

Azrin, N. H., & Nunn, R. G. (1973). Habit-reversal: A method of eliminating nervous habits and tics. *Behavior Research and Therapy, 11,* 619–628.

Azrin, N. H., & Thienes, P. M. (1978). Rapid elimination of enuresis by intensive learning without a conditioning apparatus. *Behavior Therapy, 9,* 342–354.

Bach-y-Rita, G., Lion, J. R., Climent, C. E., & Ervin, F. R. (1971). Episodic dyscontrol: A study of 130 violent patients. *American Journal of Psychiatry, 127,* 1473–1478.

Baker, H., & Wills, U. (1978). School phobia: Classification and treatment. *British Journal of Psychiatry, 132,* 492–499.

Baker, L., & Cantwell, D. (1985). Developmental arithmetic disorder. In H. Kaplan & B. Sadock (Eds.), *Comprehensive textbook of psychiatry* (Vol. 2, pp. 1697–1700). Baltimore: Williams & Wilkins.

Bakwin, H. (1961). Enuresis in children. *Journal of Pediatrics, 58,* 806–819.

Bakwin, H. (1968). Deviant gender-role behavior in children: Relation to homosexuality. *Pediatrics, 41,* 620–629.

Bakwin, H. (1973). The genetics of enuresis. In I. Kolvin, R. MacKeith, & S. R. Meadow (Eds.), *Bladder control and enuresis* (pp. 73–77). (Clinics in Developmental Medicine, Nos. 48/49). London: Heinemann.

Bakwin, H., & Bakwin, R. (1953). Homosexual behavior in children. *Journal of Pediatrics, 43,* 108–111.

Balint, M. (1955). Friendly expanses—Horrid empty spaces. *International Journal of Psycho-Analysis, 36,* 225–241.

Balla, D., & Zigler, E. (1979). Personality development in retarded persons. In N. R. Ellis (Ed.), *Handbook of mental deficiency: Psychological theory and research* (pp. 143–168). Hillsdale, NJ: Erlbaum.

Ballenger, J. C., Gibson, R., Peterson, G. A., & Laraia, M. T. (1986, May). *"Functional" MVP in agoraphobia/panic disorder.* Paper presented at American Psychiatric Association Annual Meeting, Washington, DC.

Ballenger, J. C., Reus, V. I., & Post, R. M. (1982). The "atypical" clinical picture of adolescent mania. *American Journal of Psychiatry, 139,* 602–606.

Balson, P. M. (1973). Case study: encopresis. A case with symptom substitution? *Behavior Therapy, 4,* 134–136.

Bandura, A. (1977). *Social learning theory.* Englewood Cliffs, NJ: Prentice-Hall.

Bandura, A., & Walters, R. H. (1963). *Social learning and personality development.* New York: Holt, Rinehart & Winston.

Bareggi, S. R., Becker, R. E., Ginsburg, B. E., & Genovese, E. (1979). Neurochemical investigation of an endogenous model of the "hyperkinetic syndrome" in a hybrid dog. *Life Sciences, 24,* 481–488.

Barkley, R. A. (1977). A review of stimulant drug research with hyperactive children. *Journal of Child Psychology and Psychiatry, 18,* 137–165.

Barkley, R. A. (1981). *Hyperactive children: A handbook for diagnosis and treatment.* New York: Guilford.

Barkley, R. A. (1982). Specific guidelines for defining hyperactivity in children (Attention Deficit Disorder). In B. Lahey & A. Kazdin (Eds.), *Advance in Child Clinical Psychology* (Vol. 5, pp. 137–180). New York: Plenum.

Barkley, R. A. (1985). The parent–child interaction patterns of hyperactive children: Precursors to aggressive behavior? *Advances in Developmental and Behavioral Pediatrics, 6,* 117–150.

Barkley, R. A., & Cunningham, C. E. (1978). Do stimulant drugs improve the academic performance of hyperkinetic children? A review of outcome studies. *Clinical Pediatrics, 17,* 85–92.

Barkley, R. A., Karlsson, J., Pollard, S., & Murphy, J. V. (1985). Developmental changes in the mother–child interactions of hyperactive boys: Effects of two dose levels of Ritalin. *Journal of Child Psychology and Psychiatry, 26,* 705–715.

Barlett, D., Hurley, W., & Brand, C. (1968). Chromosomes of male patients in a security hospital, *Nature, 219,* 351–354.

Barnes, D. M. (1987). Biological issues in schizophrenia. *Science, 235,* 430–433.

Barnes, D. M. (1988). Meeting on the mind: Need for mother's touch is brain-based. *Science, 239,* 142–144.

Baron, M., Gruen, R., Rainer, J. D., Kane, J., Asnis, L., & Lord, S. (1985). A family study of schizophrenic and normal control probands. *American Journal of Psychiatry, 142,* 447–455.

Barr, R. G., Levine, M. D., & Watkins, J. B. (1979a). Recurrent abdominal pain of childhood due to lactose intolerance. *New England Journal of Medicine, 300,* 1149–1452.

Barr, R. G., Levine, M. D., & Wilkinson, R. H. (1979b). Chronic and occult stool retention: A clinical tool for its evaluation in school-aged children. *Clinical Pediatrics, 18,* 674–686.

Barraclough, C. A., & Gorski, R. A. (1961). Evidence that the hypothalamus is responsible for androgen-induced sterility in the female rat. *Endocrinology, 68,* 68–70.

Barrios, B., Hartmann, D., & Shigetomi, C. (1981). Fears and anxieties in children. In E. J. Mash & L. X. Terdal (Eds.), *Behavioral assessment of childhood disorders.* New York: Guilford.

Barton, R. (1976). Diabetes insipidus and obsessional neurosis. *American Journal of Psychiatry, 133,* 235–236.

Bates, J. M., & Bentler, P. M. (1973). Play activities of normal and effeminate boys. *Developmental Psychology, 9,* 20–27.

Bates, J. M., Bentler, P. M., & Thompson, S. K. (1973). Measurement of deviant gender development in boys. *Child Development, 44,* 591–598.

Bates, J. M., Bentler, P. M., & Thompson, S. K. (1975a). Gender deviant boys compared with clinical control boys. *Journal of Abnormal Child Psychology, 7,* 243–259.

Bates, J. M., Skilbeck, W. M., Smith, K. V. R., & Bentler, P. M. (1974). Gender role abnormalities in boys: An analysis of clinical ratings. *Journal of Abnormal Child Psychology, 2,* 1–16.

Bates, J. M., Skilbeck, W. M., Smith, K. V. R., & Bentler, P. M. (1975b). Intervention with families of gender-disturbed boys. *American Journal of Orthopsychiatry, 45,* 150–157.

Battle, E. S., & Lacey, B. (1972). A context for hyperactivity in children over time. *Child Development, 43,* 757–773.

Bauer, D. H. (1976). An exploratory study of developmental changes in children's fears. *Journal of Child Psychology and Psychiatry, 17,* 69–74.

Baxter, L. R., Schwartz, J. M., Mazziotta, J. C., Phelps, M. E., Pahl, J. J., Guze, B. H., & Fairbanks, L. (1988). Cerebral glucose metabolic rates in nondepressed patients with obsessive-compulsive disorder. *American Journal of Psychiatry, 145,* 1560–1563.

Beardslee, W. R. (1986). The need for the study of adaptation in the children of parents with affective disorders. In M. Rutter, C. E. Izard, & P. B. Read (Eds.), *Depression in young people: Developmental and clinical perspectives* (pp. 189–204). New York: Guilford.

Beardslee, W. R., Bemporad, J., Keller, M. B., & Klerman, G. L. (1983). Children of parents with major affective disorder: A review. *American Journal of Psychiatry, 140,* 825–832.

Beck, A. T. (1976). *Cognitive therapy and the emotional disorders.* New York: International Universities Press.

Beck, A. T., & Emery, G. (1985). *Anxiety disorders and phobias: A cognitive perspective.* New York: Basic Books.

Beck, A. T., Rush, A. J., Shaw, B. F., & Emery, G. (1979). *Cognitive therapy of depression.* New York: Guilford.

Becker, J. V., & Skinner, L. J. (1985). Sexual abuse in childhood and adolescence. In D. Shaffer, A. A. Ehrhardt, & L. L. Greenhill (Eds.), *The clinical guide to child psychiatry* (pp. 336–352). New York: Free Press.

Beech, H. R. (Ed.). (1974). *Obsessional states.* London: Methuen.

Behar, D., Rapoport, J. L., Adams, A. J., Berg, C. J., & Cornblath, M. (1984a). Sugar challenge testing with children considered behaviorally "sugar reactive." *Nutrition and Behavior, 1,* 277–288.

Behar, D., Rapoport, J. L., Berg, C. J., Denckla, M. B., Mann, L., Cox, C., Fedio, P., Zahn, T., & Wolfman, M. G. (1984b). Computerized tomography and neuropsychological test measures in adolescents with obsessive-compulsive disorder. *American Journal of Psychiatry, 141,* 363–369.

Bell, R. Q. (1974). Contributions of human infants to caregiving and social interaction. In M. Lewis & L. Rosenblum (Eds.), *The effect of the infant on its caregiver.* New York: Wiley.

Bellak, L. (Ed.). (1979). *Psychiatric aspects of minimal brain dysfunction in adults.* New York: Grune & Stratton.

Bellak, L. (1985). ADD psychosis as a separate entity. *Schizophrenia Bulletin, 11*, 523–527.

Bellman, M. (1966). Studies on encopresis. *Acta Paediatrica Scandinavica (Supplement), 170.*

Belsky, J. (1980). Child maltreatment: An ecological integration. *American Psychologist, 35*, 320–335.

Belson, W. A. (1978). *Television violence and the adolescent boy.* Farnborough, England: Teakfield.

Bemporad, J. R. (1978). Encopresis. In B. Wolman, J. Egan, & A. Ross (Eds.), *Handbook of treatment of mental disorders in childhood and adolescence* (pp. 161–178). Englewood Cliffs, NJ: Prentice-Hall.

Bemporad, J. R., Pfeifer, C. M., Gibbs, L., Cortner, R. H., & Bloom, W. (1971). Characteristics of encopretic patients and their families. *Journal of the American Academy of Child Psychiatry, 10*, 272–292.

Bemporad, J. R., Ratey, J. J., O'Driscoll, G., & Daehler, M. L. (1988). Hysteria, anorexia and the culture of self-denial. *Psychiatry, 51*, 96–103.

Bemporad, J. R., Smith, H. F., & Hanson, G. (1987a). The borderline child. In J. D. Noshpitz (Ed.), *Basic handbook of child psychiatry* (vol. 5, pp. 305–312). New York: Basic Books.

Bemporad, J. R., Smith, H. F., & Hanson, G. (1987b). Treatment of the borderline child. In J. D. Noshpitz (Ed.), *Basic handbook of child psychiatry* (vol. 5, pp. 450–457). New York: Basic Books.

Bemporad, J. R., Smith, H. F., Hanson, G., & Cicchetti, D. (1982). Borderline syndromes in children: Criteria for diagnosis. *American Journal of Psychiatry, 139*, 596–602.

Bemporad, J. R., & Wilson, A. (1978). A developmental approach to depression in childhood and adolescence. *Journal of the American Academy of Psychoanalysis, 6*, 325–352.

Benbow, C. P., & Stanley, J. C. (1980). Sex differences in mathematical ability: Fact or artifact? *Science, 210*, 1262–1264.

Bender, B. G., Lerner, J. A., & Kollasch, E. (1988). Mood and memory changes in asthmatic children receiving corticosteroids. *Journal of the American Academy of Child and Adolescent Psychiatry, 27*, 720–725.

Bender, L. (1947). Childhood schizophrenia. *American Journal of Orthopsychiatry, 17*, 40–56.

Bender, L. (1954). *A dynamic psychopathology of childhood.* Springfield: Charles C. Thomas.

Bender, L. (1971). The nature of childhood psychosis. In J. G. Howells (Ed.), *Modern perspectives in international child psychiatry* (pp. 649–684). New York: Brunner/Mazel.

Bender, L., & Paster, S. (1941). Homosexual trends in children. *American Journal of Orthopsychiatry, 11*, 730.

Benedek, E. P., & Schetky, D. H. (1985). Allegations of sexual abuse in child custody and visitation disputes. In D. H. Schetky & E. P. Benedek (Eds.), *Emerging issues in child psychiatry and the law* (pp. 145–156). New York: Brunner/Mazel.

Benedek, E. P., & Schetky, D. H. (1987). Problems in validating allegations of sexual abuse. Part I: Factors affecting perception and recall of events. *Journal of the American Academy of Child and Adolescent Psychiatry, 26*, 912–915.

Benedek, E. P., & Schetky, D. H. (1987). Problems in validating allegations of sexual abuse. Part II: Clinical evaluation. *Journal of the American Academy of Child and Adolescent Psychiatry, 26*, 916–921.

Benjamin, H. (1966). *The transsexual phenomenon.* New York: Julian.

Bentivegna, S. W., Ward, L. B., & Bentivegna, N. P. (1985). Study of a diagnostic profile of the borderline syndrome in childhood and trends in treatment outcome. *Child Psychiatry and Human Development, 15*, 198–205.

Berg, C. Z., Rapoport, J., & Behar, D. (1986). Childhood obsessive-compulsive disorder: An anxiety disorder? In R. Gittelman (Ed.), *Anxiety syndromes in children* (pp. 126–135). New York: Guilford.

Berg, C. Z., Rapoport, J., Whitaker, A., Davies, M., Leonard, H., Swedo, S., Braiman, S., & Lenane, M. (1989). Childhood obsessive-compulsive disorder: A two-year prospective follow-up of a community sample. *Journal of the American Academy of Child and Adolescent Psychiatry, 28*, 528–533.

Berg, C. Z., Whitaker, A., Davies, M., Flament, M. F., & Rapoport, J. L. (1988). The survey form of the Leyton Obsessional Inventory—Child version: Norms from an epidemiological study. *Journal of the American Academy of Child and Adolescent Psychiatry, 27*, 759–763.

Berg, I. (1976). School phobia in the children of agoraphobic women. *British Journal of Psychiatry, 128*, 86–89.

Berg, I., Butler, A., & Hall, G. (1976). The outcome of adolescent school phobia. *British Journal of Psychiatry, 128*, 80–85.

Berg, I., & Jackson, A. (1985). Teenage school refusers grow up: A follow-up study of 168 subjects, ten years on average after in-patient treatment. *British Journal of Psychiatry, 147*, 366–370.

Berg, I., Marks, I., McGuire, R., & Lipsedge, M. (1974). School phobia and agoraphobia. *Psychological Medicine, 4*, 428–434.

Berger, H. G., Honig, P. J., & Liebman, R. (1977). Recurrent abdominal pain: Gaining control of the symptom. *American Journal of Diseases of Children, 131*, 1340–1344.

Berger, M., Yule, W., & Rutter, M. (1975). Attainment and adjustment in two geographic areas: II. The prevalence of specific reading retardation. *British Journal of Psychiatry, 126*, 510–519.

Bergman, P., & Escalona, S. K. (1949). Unusual sensitivities in very young children. *Psychoanalytic Study of the Child, 3–4*, 333–352.

Berlin, F. S., Bergey, G. K., & Money, J. (1982). Periodic psychosis of puberty: A case report. *American Journal of Psychiatry, 139*, 119–120.

Berman, K. F., Illowsky, B. P., & Weinberger, D. R. (1988). Physiological dysfunction of dorsolateral prefrontal cortex in schizophrenia: IV. Further evidence for regional and behavioral specificity. *Archives of General Psychiatry, 45*, 616–622.

Bernstein, G. A., & Garfinkel, B. D. (1986). School phobia: The overlap of affective and anxiety disorders. *Journal of the American Academy of Child Psychiatry, 25,* 235–241.

Bernstein, G. A., & Garfinkel, B. D. (1988). Pedigrees, functioning, and psychopathology in families of school phobic children. *American Journal of Psychiatry, 145,* 70–74.

Bernstein, G. A., Svingen, P. H., & Garfinkel, B. D. (1990). School phobia: Patterns of family functioning. *Journal of the American Academy of Child and Adolescent Psychiatry, 29,* 24–30.

Besharov, D. J. (1981). What physicians should know about child abuse reporting laws. In N. S. Ellerstein (Ed.), *Child abuse and neglect: A medical reference* (pp. 21–49). New York: Wiley.

Bettelheim, B. (1959). Joey: A "mechanical boy." *Scientific American, 200,* 116–127.

Bettelheim, B. (1967). *The empty fortress.* New York: Free Press.

Bettelheim, B. (1974). *A home for the heart.* New York: Alfred A. Knopf.

Bettes, B. A., & Walker, E. (1987). Positive and negative symptoms in psychotic and other psychiatrically disturbed children. *Journal of Child Psychology and Psychiatry, 28,* 555–568.

Bibring, E. (1953). The mechanism of depression. In P. Greenacre (Ed.), *Affective disorders* (pp. 13–48). New York: International Universities Press.

Biederman, J., Baldessarini, R. J., Wright, V., Knee, D., Harmatz, J. S. (1989a). A double-blind placebo-controlled study of desipramine in the treatment of ADD: I. Efficacy. *Journal of the American Academy of Child and Adolescent Psychiatry, 28,* 777–784.

Biederman, J., Baldessarini, R. J., Wright, V., Knee, D., Harmatz, J. S., Goldblatt, A. (1989b). A double-blind placebo-controlled study of desipramine in the treatment of ADD: II. Serum drug levels and cardiovascular findings. *Journal of the American Academy of Child and Adolescent Psychiatry, 28,* 903–911.

Biederman, J., Herzog, D. B., Rivinus, T. M., Harper, G. P., Ferber, R. A., Rosenbaum, J. F., Harmatz, J. S., Tondorf, R., Orsulak, P. J., & Schildkraut, J. J. (1985). Amitriptyline in the treatment of anorexia nervosa: A double-blind, placebo-controlled study. *Journal of Clinical Psychopharmacology, 5,* 10–16.

Binet, A., & Simon, T. (1916). *The development of intelligence in children* (E.S. Kite, Trans.). Baltimore: William & Wilkins.

Birch, H. G., Richardson, S. A., Baird, D., Horobin, G., & Illsley, R. (1970). *Mental subnormality in the community: A clinical and epidemiologic study.* Baltimore: Williams & Wilkins.

Bittner, S., & Newberger, E. H. (1982). Pediatric understanding of child abuse and neglect. In E. H. Newberger (Ed.), *Child abuse* (pp. 137–157). Boston: Little, Brown.

Black, A. (1974). The natural history of obsessional neurosis. In H. R. Beech (Ed.), *Obsessional states* (pp. 19–54). London: Methuen.

Black, B., & Robbins, D. R. (1990). Panic disorder in children and adolescents. *Journal of the American Academy of Child and Adolescent Psychiatry, 29,* 36–44.

Black, D. W., Yates, W. R., Noyes, R., Pfohl, B., & Kelley, M. (1989). DSM-III personality disorder in obsessive-compulsive study volunteers: A controlled study. *Journal of Personality Disorders, 3*, 58–62.

Bleiberg, E. (1984). Narcissistic disorders in children: A developmental approach to diagnosis. *Bulletin of the Menninger Clinic, 48*, 501–517.

Bleuler, E. (1950). *Dementia praecox or the group of schizophrenias* (J. Zinkin, Trans.). New York: International Universities Press. (Original work published 1911)

Bliss, J. (1980). Sensory experiences of Gilles de la Tourette syndrome. *Archives of General Psychiatry, 37*, 1343–1347.

Bloch, H. A., & Niederhoffer, A. (1958). *The gang*. New York: Philosophical Library.

Block, J. (1968). Further considerations of psychosomatic predisposing factors in allergy. *Psychosomatic Medicine, 30*, 202–208.

Block, J., Jennings, P. H., Harvey, E., & Simpson, E. (1964). Interaction between allergic potential and psychopathology in childhood. *Psychosomatic Medicine, 26*, 307–320.

Blos, P. (1962). *On adolescence*. New York: Free Press.

Bolton, D., Collins, S., & Steinberg, D. (1983). The treatment of obsessive-compulsive disorder in adolescence: A report of fifteen cases. *British Journal of Psychiatry, 142*, 456–464.

Bolton, D., & Turner, T. (1984). Obsessive-compulsive neurosis with conduct disorder in adolescence: A report of two cases. *Journal of Child Psychology and Psychiatry, 25*, 133–139.

Borcherding, B. G., Keysor, C. S., Rapoport, J. L., Elia, J., & Amass, J. (1990). Motor/vocal tics and compulsive behaviors on stimulant drugs: Is there a common vulnerability. *Psychiatric Research, 33*, 83–94.

Borland, B. L., & Heckman, H. K. (1976). Hyperactive boys and their brothers: A 25-year follow-up study. *Archives of General Psychiatry, 33*, 669–675.

Boskind-White, M., & White, W. C., Jr. (1983). *Bulimarexia: The binge/purge cycle*. New York: Norton.

Bouchard, T. J., & McGue, M. (1981). Familial studies of intelligence: A review. *Science, 212*, 1055–1059.

Bowlby, J. (1944). Forty-four juvenile thieves: Their characters and home life. *International Journal of Psychoanalysis, 25*, 19–52, 107–127.

Bowlby, J. (1969). *Attachment*. New York: Basic Books.

Bowlby, J. (1973). *Attachment and loss: Vol. II. Separation anxiety and anger*. New York: Basic Books.

Bowlby, J. (1980). *Attachment and loss: Vol. III. Loss, sadness and depression*. New York: Basic Books.

Bowlby, J. (1982). *Attachment* (2nd ed.). New York: Basic Books.

Bowlby, J. (1988). Developmental psychiatry comes of age. *American Journal of Psychiatry, 145*, 1–10.

Boyd, M. M. (1960). The depth of sleep in enuretic school children and in non-enuretic controls. *Journal of Psychosomatic Research, 4*, 274–281.

Bradley, C. (1937). The behavior of children receiving Benzedrine. *American Journal of Psychiatry, 94*, 577–585.

Brady, N. P., & Lind, D. L. (1961). Experimental analysis of hysterical blindness. *Archives of General Psychiatry, 4,* 331–339.

Brand, C. (1987). A touch of (social) class [Book review]. *Nature, 325,* 767–768.

Brazelton, T. B. (1962a). A child-oriented approach to toilet training. *Pediatrics, 29,* 121–128.

Brazelton, T. B. (1962b). Crying in infancy. *Pediatrics, 29,* 579–588.

Brazelton, T. B. (1973). Is enuresis preventable? In I. Kolvin, R. C. MacKeith, & S. R. Meadow (Eds.), *Bladder control and enuresis* (pp. 281–284). Clinics in Developmental Medicine, Nos. 48/49. London: Heinemann.

Brazelton, T. B. (1974). Coping with a colicky baby. *Redbook Magazine,* 70–72.

Brazelton, T. B., Koslowski, B., & Main, B. (1974). The origins of reciprocity: The early mother–infant interaction. In M. Lewis & L. Rosenblum (Eds.), *The effect of the infant on its caregiver.* New York: Wiley-Interscience.

Bregman, J. D., Dykens, E., Watson, M., Ort, S. I., & Leckman, J. F. (1987). Fragile-X syndrome: Variability of phenotypic expression. *Journal of the American Academy of Child and Adolescent Psychiatry, 26,* 463–471.

Bregman, J. D., Leckman, J. F., & Ort, S. I. (1988). Fragile-X syndrome: Genetic predisposition to psychopathology. *Journal of Autism and Developmental Disorders, 18,* 343–354.

Breier, A., Charney, D. S., & Heninger, G. R. (1985). The diagnostic validity of anxiety disorders and their relationship to depressive illness. *American Journal of Psychiatry, 142,* 787–797.

Brenner, C. (1955). *An elementary textbook of psychoanalysis.* New York: International Universities Press.

Brent, D. A. (1987). Correlates of the medical lethality of suicide attempts in children and adolescents. *Journal of the American Academy of Child and Adolescent Psychiatry, 26,* 87–89.

Brent, D. A., Kalas, R., Edelbrock, C., Costello, A. J., Dulcan, M. K., & Conover, N. (1986). Psychopathology and its relationship to suicidal ideation in childhood and adolescence. *Journal of the American Academy of Child Psychiatry, 25,* 666–673.

Brent, D. A., Kerr, M. M., Goldstein, C., Bozigar, J., Wartella, M., & Allan, M. J. (1989). An outbreak of suicide and suicidal behavior in a high school. *Journal of the American Academy of Child and Adolescent Psychiatry, 28,* 918–924.

Brent, D. A., Perper, J. A., & Allman, C. J. (1987). Alcohol, firearms, and suicide among youth: Temporal trends in Allegheny County, Pennsylvania. *Journal of the American Medical Association, 257,* 3369–3372.

Bresse, P., Stearns, G. B., Bess, B. H., & Packer, L. S. (1986). Allegations of child sexual abuse in child custody disputes: A therapeutic assessment model. *American Journal of Orthopsychiatry, 56,* 560–569.

Breslau, N., Davis, G. C., & Prabucki, K. (1987). Searching for evidence on the validity of generalized anxiety disorder: Psychopathology in children of anxious mothers. *Psychiatry Research, 20,* 285–297.

Breuer, J., & Freud, S. (1955). Studies on hysteria. In J. Strachey (Ed.), *The standard edition of the complete psychological works of Sigmund Freud* (Vol. 2). London: Hogarth. (Original work published 1893–1895).

Breznitz, Z., & Friedman, S. L. (1988). Toddlers' concentration: Does maternal depression make a difference? *Journal of Child Psychology and Psychiatry, 29,* 267–279.

Briar, S., & Piliavin, I. (1965, summer). Delinquency, situational inducements, and committment to conformity. *Social Problems, 13,* 35–45.

Broadhurst, P. H. (1981). The making and unmaking of behaviour. In R. Lynn (Ed.), *Dimensions of personality.* New York: Pergamon.

Bronfenbrenner, U. (1977). Toward an experimental ecology of human development. *American Psychologist, 32,* 513–531.

Brown, D. G. (1956). Sex-role preference in young children. *Psychological Monographs: General and Applied, 70*(14), 1–19.

Brown, G. L., & Goodwin, F. K. (1984). Aggression, adolescence and psychobiology. In Keith, C. R. (Ed.), *The aggressive adolescent* (pp. 63–69). New York: Free Press.

Brown, G. L., Hunt, R. D., Ebert, M. H., Bunney, Jr., W. E., & Kopin, I. J. (1979). Plasma levels of *d*-amphetamine in hyperactive children. *Psychopharmacology, 62,* 133–140.

Brown, G. W., Harris, T. O., & Bifulco, A. (1986). Long-term effects of early loss of parent. In M. Rutter, C. E. Izard, & S. B. Read (Eds.), *Depression in young people: Developmental and clinical perspectives* (pp. 251–296). New York: Guilford.

Bruch, H. (1970). Psychotherapy in primary anorexia nervosa. *Journal of Nervous and Mental Disease, 150,* 51–67.

Bruch, H. (1971a). Anorexia nervosa in the male. *Psychosomatic Medicine, 33,* 31–47.

Bruch, H. (1971b). Death in anorexia nervosa. *Psychosomatic Medicine, 33,* 135–144.

Bruch, H. (1973). *Eating disorders: Obesity, anorexia nervosa and the person within.* New York: Basic Books.

Bruch, H. (1975). Anorexia nervosa. In M. Reiser (Ed.), *American handbook of psychiatry* (Vol. 4, pp. 787–809). New York: Basic Books.

Bruch, H. (1978). *The golden cage: The enigma of anorexia nervosa.* Cambridge: Harvard University Press.

Bruininks, R. H., Hauber, F. A., & Kudla, M. J. (1980). National survey of community residential facilities: A profile of facilities and residents in 1977. *American Journal of Mental Deficiency, 84,* 470–478.

Brumback, R. A., & Weinberg, W. A. (1977). Mania in childhood. II. Therapeutic trial of lithium carbonate and further description of manic-depressive illness in children. *American Journal of Diseases of Children, 131,* 1122–1126.

Brumberg, J. J. (1988). *Fasting girls: The history of anorexia nervosa.* Cambridge, MA: Harvard University Press.

Brunn, R. D. (1988). The natural history of Tourette's syndrome. In D. J. Cohen, R. D. Brunn, & J. F. Leckman (Eds.), *Tourette's syndrome and tic disorders: Clinical understanding and treatment* (pp. 21–39). New York: Wiley.

Buchsbaum, M. S., & Haier, R. J. (1978). Biological homogeneity, symptom heterogeneity, and the diagnosis of schizophrenia. *Schizophrenia Bulletin, 4,* 473–475.

Buchsbaum, M. S., & Haier, R. J. (1987). Functional and anatomical brain imaging: Impact on schizophrenia research. *Schizophrenia Bulletin, 13,* 115–132.

Bullard, D. M., Jr., Glaser, H. H., Heagarty, M. C., & Pivchik, E. C. (1967). Failure to thrive in the "neglected" child. *American Journal of Orthopsychiatry, 37,* 680–690.

Bunney, W. E., Jr. (moderator). (1977). The switch process in manic-depressive psychosis. *Annals of Internal Medicine, 87,* 319–335.

Burbeck, T. W. (1979). An empirical investigation of the psychosomatogenic family model. *Journal of Psychosomatic Research, 23,* 327–337.

Burd, L., Fisher, W., Knowlton, D., & Kerbeshian, J. (1987). Hyperlexia: A marker for improvement in children with pervasive developmental disorder? *Journal of the American Academy of Child and Adolescent Psychiatry, 26,* 407–412.

Burd, L., & Kerbeshian, J. (1987). A North Dakota prevalence study of schizophrenia presenting in childhood. *Journal of the American Academy of Child and Adolescent Psychiatry, 26,* 347–350.

Burd, L., Kerbeshian, J., Wikenheiser, M., & Fisher, W. (1986). Prevalence of Gilles de la Tourette's syndrome in North Dakota adults. *American Journal of Psychiatry, 143,* 787–788.

Burg, C., Rapoport, J. L., Bartley, L. S., Quinn, P. O., & Timmins, P. (1980). Newborn minor physical anomalies and problem behavior at age three. *American Journal of Psychiatry, 137,* 791–796.

Burgess, R. L., & Conger, R. D. (1977). Family interaction patterns related to child abuse and neglect: Some preliminary findings. *Child Abuse and Neglect, 1,* 269–277.

Burgess, R. L., & Conger, R. (1978). Family interaction in abusive, neglectful, and normal families. *Child Development, 49,* 1163–1173.

Burke, B. (1984). Infanticide: Why does it happen in monkeys, mice, and men? *Science 84, 5,* 26–31.

Burnham, D. L., Gladstone, A. I., & Gibson, R. W. (1969). *Schizophrenia and the need-fear dilemma.* New York: International Universities Press.

Burrows, B., Martinez, F. D., Halonen, M., Barbee, R. A., & Cline, M. G. (1989). Association of asthma with serum IgE levels and skin-test reactivity to allergens. *New England Journal of Medicine, 320,* 271–277.

Byers, R., & Lord, E. (1943). Late effects of lead poisoning in young children. *Journal of Pediatrics, 93,* 709–720.

Caffey, J. (1972). On the theory and practice of shaking infants: Its potential residual effects of permanent brain damage and mental retardation. *American Journal of Diseases of Children, 124,* 161–169.

Cain, A. C. (1969). Special "isolated" abilities in severely psychotic young children. *Psychiatry, 32,* 137–149.

Calabrese, J. R., Kling, M. A., & Gold, P. W. (1987). Alterations in immunocompetence during stress, bereavement, and depression: Focus on neuroendocrine regulation. *American Journal of Psychiatry, 144,* 1123–1134.

Caldwell, B. M. (1964). The effects of infant care. In M. L. Hoffman & L. W. Hoffman (Eds.), *Review of child development research* (Vol. 1, pp. 9–87). New York: Russell Sage Foundation.

Callaway, E., Halliday, R., & Naylor, H. (1983). Hyperactive children's event-related potentials fail to support underarousal and maturational-lag theories. *Archives of General Psychiatry, 40,* 1243–1248.

Campbell, L. M. (1973). A variation of thought stopping in a twelve year old boy: A case report. *Journal of Behavior Therapy and Experimental Psychiatry, 4,* 69–70.

Campbell, M. (1985). Schizophrenic disorders and pervasive developmental disorders/infantile autism. In J. M. Wiener (Ed.), *Diagnosis and psychopharmacology of childhood and adolescent disorders* (pp. 113–150). New York: Wiley.

Campbell, M., Adams, P., Small, A. M., Curren, E. L., Overall, J. E., Anderson, L. T., Lynch, N., & Perry, R. (1988). Efficacy and safety of fenfluramine in autistic children. *Journal of the American Academy of Child and Adolescent Psychiatry, 27,* 434–439.

Campbell, M., Anderson, L. T., Green, W. H., & Deutsch, S. I. (1987). Psychopharmacology. In D. J. Cohen & A. M. Donnellan (Eds.), *Handbook of autism and pervasive developmental disorders* (pp. 545–565). New York: Wiley.

Campbell, M., Green, W. H., & Deutsch, S. I. (1985). *Child and adolescent psychopharmacology.* Beverly Hills: Sage Publications.

Campbell, M., Perry, R., & Green, W. H. (1984). Use of lithium in children and adolescents. *Psychosomatics, 25,* 95–106.

Campbell, M., Perry, R., Polonsky, B. B., Deutsch, S. I., Palij, M., & Lukashok, D. (1986). Brief report: An open study of fenfluramine in hospitalized young autistic children. *Journal of Autism and Developmental Disorders, 16,* 495–506.

Campbell, M., Schulman, D., & Rapaport, J. L. (1978). The current status of lithium therapy in child and adolescent psychiatry: A report of the Committee on Biological Aspects of Child Psychiatry, December 1977. *Journal of the American Academy of Child Psychiatry, 17,* 717–780.

Campbell, S. B. (1979). Mother–infant interaction as a function of maternal ratings of temperament. *Child Psychiatry and Human Development, 10,* 67–76.

Campbell, S. B. (1986). Developmental issues in childhood anxiety. In R. Gittelman (Ed.), *Anxiety disorders of childhood* (pp. 24–57). New York: Guilford.

Campbell, S. B., Breaux, A. M., Ewing, L. J., & Szumowski, E. K. (1984). A one-year follow-up study of parent-referred hyperactive preschool children. *Journal of the American Academy of Child Psychiatry, 23,* 243–249.

Campbell, S. B., Endman, M. W., & Bernfeld, G. (1977). A three-year follow-up of hyperactive preschoolers into elementary school. *Journal of Child Psychology and Psychiatry, 18,* 239–249.

Campbell, S. B., & Paulauskas, S. (1979). Peer relations in hyperactive children. *Journal of Child Psychology and Psychiatry, 20,* 233–246.

Campbell, S. B., Schleifer, M., & Weiss, G. (1978). Continuities in maternal reports and child behaviors over time in hyperactive and comparison groups. *Journal of Abnormal Child Psychology, 6,* 33–45.

Campbell, S. B., & Werry, J. S. (1986). Attention deficit disorder (hyperactivity). In H. C. Quay & J. S. Werry (Eds.), *Psychopathological disorders of childhood* (pp. 111–155). New York: Wiley.

Cannon, T. D., Mednick, S. A., & Parnas, J. (1989). Genetic and perinatal determinants of structural brain deficits in schizophrenia. *Archives of General Psychiatry, 46,* 883–889.

Cannon, W. B. (1929). *Bodily changes in pain, hunger, fear and rage: An account of recent researches into the function of emotional excitement* (2nd ed.). New York: Appleton-Century-Crofts.

Cannon, W. B. (1932). *The wisdom of the body.* New York: Norton.

Cantor, S. (1988). *Childhood schizophrenia.* New York: Guilford.

Cantor, S., Evans, J., Pearce, J., & Pezzot-Pearce, T. (1982). Childhood schizophrenia: Present but not accounted for. *American Journal of Psychiatry, 139,* 758–762.

Cantor, S., & Kestenbaum, C. (1986). Psychotherapy with schizophrenic children. *Journal of the American Academy of Child Psychiatry, 25,* 623–630.

Cantwell, D. P. (1972). Psychiatric illness in the families of hyperactive children. *Archives of General Psychiatry, 27,* 414–417.

Cantwell, D. P. (1975). Genetic studies of hyperactive children. In R. R. Fieve, D. Rosenthal, & H. Brill (Eds.), *Genetic research in psychiatry.* Baltimore: Johns Hopkins University Press.

Cantwell, D. P. (1981). Hyperactivity and antisocial behavior revisited: A critical review of the literature. In D. O. Lewis (Ed.), *Vulnerabilities to delinquency* (pp. 21–38). New York: SP Medical and Scientific Books.

Cantwell, D. P. (1983). Depression in childhood: Clinical picture and diagnostic criteria. In D. P. Cantwell & G. A. Carlson (Eds.), *Affective disorders in childhood and adolescence: An update* (pp. 3–18). New York: Spectrum.

Cantwell, D. P. (1985). Hyperactive children have grown up: What have we learned about what happens to them? *Archives of General Psychiatry, 42,* 1026–1028.

Cantwell, D. P., Baker, L., & Rutter, M. (1978). Family factors. In M. Rutter & E. Schopler (Eds.), *Autism: A reappraisal of concepts and treatment* (pp. 269–296). New York: Plenum.

Cantwell, D. P., Russell, A. T., Mattison, R., & Will, L. (1979). A comparison of DSM-II and DSM-III in the diagnosis of childhood psychiatric disorders: I. Agreement with expected diagnosis. *Archives of General Psychiatry, 36,* 1208–1213.

Cantwell, D. P., Sturzenberger, S., Burroughs, J., Salkin, B., & Green, J. K. (1977). Anorexia nervosa: An affective disorder? *Archives of General Psychiatry, 34,* 1087–1093.

Caparulo, B. K., & Cohen, D. J. (1977). Cognitive structures, language, and emerging social competence in autistic and aphasic children. *Journal of the American Academy of Child Psychiatry, 16,* 620–645.

Caparulo, B. K., Cohen, D. J., Rothman, S. L., Young, J. G., Katz, J. D., Shaywitz, S. E., & Shaywitz, B. A. (1981). Computed tomographic brain scanning in children with developmental neuropsychiatric disorders. *Journal of the American Academy of Child Psychiatry, 20,* 338–357.

Capitanio, J. P., Rasmussen, K. L. R., Snyder, D. S., Laudenslager, M., & Reite, M. (1986). Long-term follow-up of previously separated pigtail macaques: Group and individual differences in response to novel situations. *Journal of Child Psychology and Psychiatry, 27,* 531–538.

Caplan, R., Guthrie, D., Fish, B., Tanguay, P. E., & David-Lando, G. (1989). The Kiddie Formal Thought Disorder Rating Scale: Clinical assessment, reliability, and validity. *Journal of the American Academy of Child and Adolescent Psychiatry, 28,* 408–416.

Capron, C., & Duyme, M. (1989). Assessment of effects of socioeconomic status on IQ in a full cross-fostering study. *Nature, 340,* 552–554.

Capstick, N., & Seldrup, U. (1977). Obsessional states: A study in the relationship between abnormalities occurring at birth and the subsequent development of obsessional symptoms. *Acta Psychiatrica Scandinavica, 56,* 427–439.

Carey, G. (1987). Big genes, little genes, affective disorder, and anxiety. *Archives of General Psychiatry, 44,* 486–491.

Carey, G., & Gottesman, I. (1981). Twin and family studies of anxiety, phobic, and obsessive disorders. In D. F. Klein & J. Rabkin (Eds.), *Anxiety: New research and changing concepts* (pp. 117–136). New York: Raven.

Carlson, G. A. (1985). Bipolar disorder in adolescence. *Psychiatric Annals, 15,* 379–386.

Carlson, G. A., & Cantwell, D. P. (1980). Unmasking masked depression in children and adolescents. *American Journal of Psychiatry, 137,* 445–449.

Carlson, G. A., & Cantwell, D. P. (1982). Suicidal behavior and depression in children and adolescents. *Journal of the American Academy of Child Psychiatry, 21,* 361–368.

Carlson, G. A., & Garber, J. (1986). Developmental issues in the classification of depression in children. In M. Rutter, C. E. Izard, & P. B. Read (Eds.), *Depression in young people: Developmental and clinical perspectives* (pp. 399–434). New York: Guilford.

Carlson, G. A., & Kashani, J. H. (1988). Phenomenology of major depression from childhood through adulthood: Analysis of three studies. *American Journal of Psychiatry, 145,* 1222–1225.

Carpenter, W. T., Jr. (1987). Approaches to knowledge and understanding of schizophrenia. *Schizophrenia Bulletin, 13,* 1–8.

Carpenter, W. T., Jr., McGlashan, T. H., & Strauss, J. S. (1977). The treatment of acute schizophrenia without drugs: An investigation of some current assumptions. *American Journal of Psychiatry, 134,* 14–20.

Cash, T. F., Winstead, B. A., & Janda, L. H. (1986, April). The great American shape-up. *Psychology Today,* pp. 30–37.

Casper, R. C., & Davis, J. M. (1977). On the course of anorexia nervosa. *American Journal of Psychiatry, 134,* 974–978.

Casper, R. C., Eckert, E. D., Halmi, K. A., Goldberg, S. C., & Davis, J. M. (1980). Bulimia: Its incidence and clinical importance in patients with anorexia nervosa. *Archives of General Psychiatry, 37,* 1030–1035.

Caspi, A., Elder, G. H., & Bem, D. J. (1988). Moving away from the world: Life-course patterns of shy children. *Developmental Psychology, 24,* 824–831.

Centers for Disease Control. (1986). *Youth Suicide Surveillance Summary: 1970–1980.* Atlanta: U.S. Department of Health and Human Services.

Centers for Disease Control. (1988). CDC recommendations for a community plan for the prevention and containment of suicide clusters. *Morbidity and Mortality Weekly Report, 37* (Supp. S-6), 1–12.

Cernkovich, S. A., & Giordano, P. C. (1979). A comparative analysis of male and female delinquency. *Sociological Quarterly, 20,* 131–145.

Chambers, W. J., Puig-Antich, J., Hirsch, M., Paez, P., Ambrosini, P. J., Tabrizi, M. A., & Davies, M. (1985). The assessment of affective disorders in children and adolescents by semistructured interview. Test-retest reliability of the Schedule for Affective Disorders and Schizophrenia for school-age children, present episode version. *Archives of General Psychiatry, 42,* 696–702.

Chambers, W. J., Puig-Antich, J., Tabrizi, M. A., & Davies, M. (1982). Psychotic symptoms in prepubertal major depressive disorder. *Archives of General Psychiatry, 39,* 921–927.

Chapin, H. D. (1908). A plan of dealing with atrophic infants and children. *Archives of Pediatrics, 25,* 491–496.

Chapin, H. D. (1915). A plea for accurate statistics in infants' institutions. *Archives of Pediatrics, 32,* 724–726.

Chappell, P. B., Leckman, J. F., Pauls, D., & Cohen, D. J. (1990). Biochemical and genetic studies of Tourette's syndrome: Implications for treatment and future research. In S. I. Deutsch (Ed.), *Application of basic neuroscience to child psychiatry.* New York: Plenum.

Charles, L., Schain, R., & Zelniker, T. (1981). Optimal dosages of methylphenidate for improving the learning and behavior of hyperactive children. *Developmental and Behavioral Pediatrics, 2,* 78–81.

Charney, D. S., Heninger, G. R., & Breier, A. (1984). Noradrenergic function in panic anxiety. *Archives of General Psychiatry, 41,* 751–763.

Chase, T. M., Foster, N. L., Fedro, P., Brooks, R., Mansi, L., Kessier, R., & DiChiro, G. (1984). Gilles de la Tourette syndrome: Studies with the fluorine-18-labeled fluorodeoxyglucose positron emission topographic method. *Annals of Neurology, 15,* S175.

Chatoor, I., Dickson, L., & Einhorn, A. (1984). Rumination: Etiology and treatment. *Pediatrics Annals, 13,* 924–929.

Chatoor, I., & Egan, J. (1983). Nonorganic failure to thrive and dwarfism due to food refusal: A separation disorder. *Journal of the American Academy of Child Psychiatry, 22,* 294–301.

Chatoor, I., & Egan, J. (1987a). Etiology and diagnosis of failure to thrive and growth disorders in infants and children. In J. D. Noshpitz (Ed.), *Basic handbook of child psychiatry* (Vol. 5, pp. 272–279). New York: Basic Books.

Chatoor, I., & Egan, J. (1987b). Treatment of failure to thrive and growth disorders in infants and children. In J. D. Noshpitz (Ed.), *Basic handbook of child psychiatry* (Vol. 5, pp. 421–425). New York: Basic Books.

Chatoor, I., Schaefer, S., Dickson, L., & Egan, J. (1984). Non-organic failure to thrive: A developmental perspective. *Pediatrics Annals, 13,* 829–842.

Chatoor, I., Wells, K. C., Conners, C. K., Seidel, W. T., & Shaw, D. (1983). The effects of nocturnally administered stimulant medication on EEG sleep and behavior in hyperactive children. *Journal of the American Academy of Child Psychiatry, 22,* 337–342.

Chelune, G. J., Ferguson, W., Koon, R., & Dickey, T. O. (1986). Frontal lobe disinhibition in attention deficit disorder. *Child Psychiatry and Human Development, 16,* 221–232.

Chess, S. (1973). Marked anxiety in children. *American Journal of Psychotherapy, 17,* 390–395.

Chess, S. (1977). Follow-up report on autism in congenital rubella. *Journal of Autism and Childhood Schizophrenia, 7,* 69–81.

Chess, S., & Hassibi, M. (1978). *Principles and practice of child psychiatry.* New York: Plenum.

Chess, S., & Korn, S. (1970). Temperament and behavior disorders in mentally retarded children. *Archives of General Psychiatry, 23,* 122–130.

Chess, S., Korn, S. J., & Fernandez, P. B. (1971). *Psychiatric disorders of children with congenital rubella.* New York: Brunner/Mazel.

Chess, S., & Thomas, A. (1984). *Origins and evolution of behavior disorders: From infancy to early adult life.* New York: Brunner/Mazel.

Chethik, M. (1969). The therapy of an obsessive-compulsive boy. *Journal of the American Academy of Child Psychiatry, 8,* 465–484.

Chethik, M. (1979). The borderline child. In J. D. Noshpitz (Ed.), *Basic handbook of child psychiatry* (Vol. 2, pp. 304–321). New York: Basic Books.

Chodoff, P. (1954). A re-examination of some aspects of conversion hysteria. *Psychiatry, 17,* 75–81.

Chodoff, P. (1974). The diagnosis of hysteria: An overview. *American Journal of Psychiatry, 131,* 1073–1078.

Chodoff, P., and Lyons, H. (1958). Hysteria, the hysterical personality, and "hysterical" conversion. *American Journal of Psychiatry, 114,* 734–740.

Cicchetti, D., & Aber, L. (1980). Abused children—abusive parents: An overstated case? *Harvard Educational Review, 50,* 244–255.

Cicchetti, D., & Rizley, R. (1981). Developmental perspectives on the etiology, intergenerational transmission, and sequelae of child maltreatment. In R. Rizley & D. Cicchetti (Eds.), *New directions for child development* (pp. 31–55). San Francisco: Jossey-Bass.

Cicchetti, D., & Schneider-Rosen, K. (1986). An organizational approach to childhood depression. In M. Rutter, C. E. Izard, & P. B. Read (Eds.), *Depression in young people: Developmental and clinical perspectives* (pp. 71–134). New York: Guilford.

Claman, L., Harris, J. C., Bernstein, B. E., & Lovitt, R. (1986). The adolescent as a witness in a case of incest: Assessment and outcome. *Journal of the American Academy of Child Psychiatry, 25,* 457–461.

Clark, N. M., Feldman, C. H., Evans, D., Millman, E. J., Wailewski, Y., & Valle, I. (1981). The effectiveness of education for family management of asthma in children: A preliminary report. *Health Education Quarterly, 8,* 166–174.

Cleckly, H. (1964). *The mask of sanity* (4th ed.). St. Louis: Mosby.

Clemens, J. A., & Fuller, R. W. (1979). Differences in the effects of amphetamine and methylphenidate on brain dopamine turnover and serum prolactin concentration in reserpine-treated rats. *Life Sciences, 24,* 2077–2081.

Clements, S. D. (1966). Task force one: Minimal brain dysfunction in children. *National Institute of Neurological Disease and Blindness, Monograph No. 3.* Washington, DC: U.S. Department of Health, Education and Welfare.

Clements, S. D., & Peters, J. E. (1962). Minimal brain dysfunctions in the school-age child. *Archives of General Psychiatry, 6,* 185–197.

Clerget-Darpoux, F., Goldin, L. R., & Gershon, E. S. (1986). Clinical methods in psychiatric genetics. *Acta Psychiatrica Scandinavica, 74,* 305–311.

Cloninger, C. R. (1987). A systematic method for clinical description and classification of personality variants. *Archives of General Psychiatry, 44,* 573–588.

Cloninger, C. R., Christiansen, K. O., Reich, T., & Gottesman, I. I. (1978). Implications of sex differences in the prevalence of antisocial personality, alcoholism, and criminality for familial transmission. *Archives of General Psychiatry, 35,* 941–951.

Cloward, R. A., & Ohlin, L. E. (1960). *Delinquency and opportunity.* New York: Free Press.

Coates, S., & Person, E. S. (1985). Extreme boyhood femininity: Isolated behavior or pervasive disorder? *Journal of the American Academy of Child Psychiatry, 24,* 702–709.

Cobb, S. (1976). Social support as a moderator of life stress. *Psychosomatic Medicine, 38,* 300–314.

Cohen, A. K. (1955). *Delinquent boys: The culture of the gang.* Glencoe, IL: Free Press.

Cohen, D. J., (1975). Psychosomatic models of development. In E. J. Anthony (Ed.), *Explorations in child psychiatry* (pp. 197–212). New York: Plenum.

Cohen, D. J. (1980a). Constructive and reconstructive activities in the analysis of a depressed child. *Psychoanalytic Study of the Child, 35,* 237–266.

Cohen, D. J. (1980b). The pathology of the self in primary childhood autism and Gilles de la Tourette syndrome. *Psychiatric Clinics of North America, 3,* 383–402.

Cohen, D. J., Caparulo, B., & Shaywitz, B. (1976). Primary childhood aphasia and childhood autism: Clinical, biological and conceptual observations. *Journal of the American Academy of Child Psychiatry, 15,* 604–645.

Cohen, D. J., Caparulo, B. K., & Shaywitz, B. A. (1978). Neurochemical and developmental models of childhood autism. In G. Serban (Ed.), *Cognitive defects in the development of mental illness* (pp. 66–100). New York: Brunner/Mazel.

Cohen, D. J., Detlor, J., Young, J. G., & Shaywitz, B. A. (1980). Clonidine ameliorates Gilles de la Tourette syndrome. *Archives of General Psychiatry, 37,* 1350–1357.

Cohen, D. J., & Donnellan, A. M. (Eds.). (1987). *Handbook of autism and pervasive developmental disorders.* New York: Wiley.

Cohen, D. J., Leckman, J. F., & Shaywitz, B. A. (1985). The Tourette syndrome and other tics. In D. Shaffer, A. A. Ehrhardt, & L. L. Greenhill (Eds.), *The clinical guide to child psychiatry* (pp. 3–28). New York: Free Press.

Cohen, D. J., & Nadelson, T. (1971). The impact of skin disease on the person. In T. Fitzpatrick (Ed.), *Dermatology in general medicine.* New York: McGraw-Hill.

Cohen, D. J., Ort, S. I., Leckman, J. F., Riddle, M. A., & Hardin, M. T. (1988). Family functioning and Tourette's syndrome. In D. J. Cohen, R. D. Brunn, & J. F. Leckman (Eds.), *Tourette's syndrome and tic disorders: Clinical understanding and treatment* (pp. 179–196). New York: Wiley.

Cohen, D. J., Paul, R., & Volkmar, F. R. (1986a). Issues in the classification of pervasive and other developmental disorders: Toward DSM-IV. *Journal of the American Academy of Child Psychiatry, 25,* 213–220.

Cohen, D. J., Paul, R., & Volkmar, F. R. (1987a). Issues in the classification of pervasive developmental disorders and associated conditions. In D. J. Cohen & A. M. Donnellan (Eds.), *Handbook of autism and pervasive developmental disorders* (pp. 20–40). New York: Wiley.

Cohen, D. J., Riddle, M. A., & Leckman, J. F. (1987b). Tourette syndrome: Clinical features, etiology, and pathogenesis. In J. D. Noshpitz (Ed.), *Basic handbook of child psychiatry* (Vol. 5, pp. 319–327). New York: Basic Books.

Cohen, D. J., Shaywitz, B. A., Young, J. G., Carbonari, C. M., Nathanson, J. A., Lieberman, D., Bowers, M. B., Jr., & Maas, J. W. (1979). Central biogenic amine metabolism in children with the syndrome of chronic multiple tics of Gilles de la Tourette. *Journal of the American Academy of Child Psychiatry, 18,* 320–341.

Cohen, D. J., Shaywitz, S. E., Young, J. G., & Shaywitz, B. A. (1983). Borderline syndromes and attention deficit disorders of childhood: Clinical and neuro-chemical perspectives. In K. S. Robson (Ed.), *The borderline child: Approaches to etiology, diagnosis and treatment* (pp. 197–221). New York: McGraw-Hill.

Cohen, D. J., Volkmar, F. R., & Paul, R. (1986b). Issues in the classification of pervasive developmental disorders: History and current status of nosology. *Journal of the American Academy of Child Psychiatry, 25,* 158–161.

Cohen, G. J. (1983). The accident-prone child. *Clinical Proceedings Children's Hospital National Medical Center, 39,* 5–10.

Cohen, R. (1979a). The approach to assessment. In J. D. Noshpitz, (Ed.), *Basic handbook of child psychiatry* (Vol. 1, pp. 485–505). New York: Basic Books.

Cohen, R. (1979b). Direct examination of the child. In J. D. Noshpitz, (Ed.), *Basic handbook of child psychiatry* (Vol. 1, pp. 505–529, 547–551), New York: Basic Books.

Cohen-Sandler, R., & Berman, A. L. (1982). Training suicidal children to problem-solve in nonsuicidal ways. In C. Pfeffer & J. Richman (Eds.), *Suicide and the Life Cycle: Proceedings of the 15th Annual Meeting of the American Association of Suicidology,* New York.

Cohen-Sandler, R., Berman, A. L., & King, R. A. (1982a). A follow-up study of hospitalized suicidal children. *Journal of the American Academy of Child Psychiatry, 21,* 398–403.

Cohen-Sandler, R., Berman, A. L., & King, R. A. (1982b). Life stress and symp-tomatology: Determinants of suicidal behavior in children. *Journal of the American Academy of Child Psychiatry, 21,* 178–186.

Cohler, B. J. (1987). Adversity, resilience, and the study of lives. In E. J. Anthony & B. J. Cohler (Eds.), *The invulnerable child* (pp. 363–424). New York: Guilford.

Cohn, A. H. (1979). Essential elements of successful child abuse and neglect treatment. *Child Abuse and Neglect, 3,* 491–496.

Cohn, A. H. (1982). Organization and administration of programs to treat child abuse and neglect. In E. H. Newberger (Ed.), *Child abuse* (pp. 89–101). Boston: Little, Brown.

Coll, C. G., Kagan, J., & Reznick, J. S. (1981). Behavioral inhibition in young children. *Child Development, 55,* 1005–1019.

Compton, A. (1972a). A study of the psychoanalytic theory of anxiety: I. The development of Freud's theory of anxiety. *Journal of the American Psychoanalytic Association, 20,* 3–44.

Compton, A. (1972b). A study of the psychoanalytic theory of anxiety: II. Developments in the theory of anxiety since 1926. *Journal of the American Psychoanalytic Association, 20,* 311–394.

Conners, C. K. (1969). A teacher rating scale for use in drug studies with children. *American Journal of Psychiatry, 126,* 884.

Conners, C. K. (1973). Rating scales for use in drug studies with children. *Psychopharmacology Bulletin* [Special issue, *Pharmacotherapy of Children*], 24–84.

Conners, C. K. (1975). Controlled trial of methylphenidate in preschool children with minimal brain dysfunction. In R. Gittelman-Klein (Ed.), *Recent advances in child psychopharmacology* (pp. 64–78). New York: Human Sciences Press.

Conners, C. K. (1980). *Food additives and hyperactive children.* New York: Plenum.

Conners, C. K. (1981). *Food additives and hyperactive children: Controlled experiments.* Unpublished lecture.

Conners, C. K. (1983). Psychological management of the asthmatic child. *Clinical Reviews in Allergy, 1,* 163–177.

Conners, C. K. (1984). Nutritional therapy in children. In J. R. Galler (Ed.), *Nutrition and Behavior* (pp. 159–192). New York: Plenum.

Conners, C. K. (1985). Methodological and assessment issues in pediatric psychopharmacology. In J. M. Wiener (Ed.), *Diagnosis and psychopharmacology of childhood and adolescent disorders* (pp. 69–110). New York: Wiley.

Conners, C. K. (1987). Event-related potentials and quantitative EEG brain-mapping in dyslexia. *Child Health and Development, 5,* 9–21.

Conners, C. K., & Barkley, R. A. (1985). Rating scales and checklists for child psychopharmacology. *Psychopharmacology Bulletin, 21,* 809–851.

Conners, C. K., & Blouin, A. G. (1983). Nutritional effects on behavior of children. *Journal of Psychiatric Research, 17,* 193–201.

Conners, C. K., Caldwell, J., Caldwell, L., Schwab, E., Kronsberg, S., Wells, K. C., Leong, N., & Blouin, A. G. (1986, October). Experimental studies of sugar and aspartame on autonomic, cortical, and behavioral responses of children. *Proceedings of Interfaces in Psychology.* Lubbock, TX: Texas Tech Press.

Conners, C. K., Glasgow, A., Raiten, D., Caldwell, J., Caldwell, L., & Clymer, R. (1987, August). Hyperactives differ from normals in blood sugar and hormonal response to sucrose. Presented at the Annual Meeting of the American Psychological Association, New York.

Conners, C. K., Goyette, C. H., Southwick, D. A., Lees, J. M., & Andrulonis, P. A. (1976). Food additives and hyperkinesis. *Pediatrics, 58,* 154–166.

Conners, C. K., & Reader, M. J. (1987). The effects of piracetam on reading achievement and visual event-related potentials in dyslexic children. *Child Health and Development, 5,* 75–90.

Conners, C. K., & Solanto, M. V. (1984). The psychophysiology of stimulant drug response in hyperkinetic children. In L. M. Bloomingdale (Ed.), *Attention deficit disorder: Diagnostic, cognitive, and therapeutic understanding* (pp. 191–204). New York: SP Medical and Scientific Books.

Conners, C. K., & Taylor, E. (1980). Pemoline, methylphenidate, and placebo in children with minimal brain dysfunction. *Archives of General Psychiatry, 37,* 922–930.

Conners, C. K., & Wells, K. C. (1986). *Hyperkinetic children: A neuropsychosocial approach.* Beverly Hills: Sage Publications.

Consensus Development Conference (NIH). (1982). Defined diets and childhood hyperactivity. *Journal of the American Medical Association, 248,* 290–292.

Constantinople, A. (1979). *Sex-role acquisition: In search of the elephant. Sex Roles, 2,* 121–133.

Conte, J. R., & Berliner, L. (1981). Sexual abuse of children: Implications for practice. *Social Casework, 62,* 601–606.

Cookson, W. O. C. M., & Hopkin, J. M. (1988, January 16). Dominant inheritance of atopic immunoglobulin-E responsiveness. *Lancet,* pp. 86–88.

Coolidge, J. C., Brodie, R. D., & Feeney, B. (1964). A ten-year follow-up study of sixty-six school-phobic children. *American Journal of Orthopsychiatry, 34,* 675–684.

Coolidge, J. C., Hahn, P. B., & Peck, A. L. (1957). School phobia: Neurotic crisis or way of life. *American Journal of Orthopsychiatry, 27,* 296–306.

Coolidge, J. C., Willer, M. L., Tessman, E., & Waldfogel, S. (1960). School phobia in adolescence: A manifestation of severe character disturbance. *American Journal of Orthopsychiatry, 30,* 599–608.

Coons, H. W., Klorman, R., & Borgstedt, A. D. (1987). Effects of methylphenidate on adolescents with a childhood history of attention deficit disorder: II. Information processing. *Journal of the American Academy of Child and Adolescent Psychiatry, 26,* 368–374.

Cooper, C. E. (1973). Cross-cultural aspects of bedwetting. In I. Kolvin, R. C. MacKeith, & S. R. Meadow (Eds.), *Bladder control and enuresis* (pp. 53–57). (Clinics in Developmental Medicine, Nos. 48/49). London: Heinemann.

Corbett, J. A. (1985). Mental retardation: psychiatric aspects. In M. Rutter & L. Hersov (Eds.), *Child and adolescent psychiatry, modern approaches* (pp. 661–678). Oxford: Blackwell.

Cornblatt, B. A., & Erlenmeyer-Kimling, L. (1985). Global attentional deviance as a marker of risk for schizophrenia: Specificity and predictive validity. *Journal of Abnormal Psychology, 94,* 470–486.

Coryell, W., & Tsuang, M. T. (1986). Outcome after 40 years in DSM-III Schizophreniform Disorder. *Archives of General Psychiatry, 43,* 324–328.

Costello, A. J. (1986). Assessment and diagnosis of affective disorders in children. *Journal of Child Psychology and Psychiatry, 27,* 565–574.

Costello, A. J. (1987). Structured interviewing for the assessment of child psychopathology. In J. D. Noshpitz (Ed.), *Basic handbook of child psychiatry* (Vol. 5, pp. 143–153). New York: Basic Books.

Costello, E. J., & Angold, A. (1988). Scales to assess child and adolescent depression: Checklists, screens, and nets. *Journal of the American Academy of Child and Adolescent Psychiatry, 27,* 726–737.

Courchesne, E., Yeung-Courchesne, R., Press, G. A., Hesselink, J. R., & Jernigan, T. L. (1988). Hypoplasia of cerebellar vermal lobules VI and VII in autism. *New England Journal of Medicine, 318,* 1349–1354.

Cowdry, R. W. (1987). Psychopharmacology of borderline personality disorder: A review. *Journal of Clinical Psychiatry, 48*(8, Suppl.), 15–22.

Cowdry, R. W., & Gardner, D. L. (1988). Pharmacotherapy of borderline personality disorder. *Archives of General Psychiatry, 45,* 111–119.

Creak, M. (1938). Hysteria in childhood. *British Journal of Children's Diseases, 35,* 85–95.

Creak, M. (1961). Schizophrenic syndrome in childhood: Report of a working party. *British Medical Journal, 2,* 889–890.

Creer, T. L. (1970). The use of a timeout from positive reinforcement procedure with asthmatic children. *Journal of Psychosomatic Research, 14,* 117–120.

Crisp, A. H. (1979). Early recognition and prevention of anorexia nervosa. *Developmental Medicine and Child Neurology, 21,* 393–395.

Crisp, A. H., Burns, T., & Bhat, A. V. (1986). Primary anorexia nervosa in the male and female: A comparison of clinical features and prognosis. *British Journal of Medical Psychology, 59,* 123–132.

Crisp, A. H., Palmer, R. L., & Kalucy, R. S. (1976). How common is anorexia nervosa? A prevalence study. *British Journal of Psychiatry, 128,* 549–554.

Crittenden, P. M. (1985). Maltreated infants: Vulnerability and resilience. *Journal of Child Psychology and Psychiatry, 26,* 85–96.

Crocker, A. C., & Nelson, R. P. (1983). Mental retardation. In M. D. Levine, W. B. Carey, A. C. Crocker, & R. T. Gross (Eds.), *Developmental-behavioral pediatrics* (pp. 756–770). Philadelphia: Saunders.

Crow, T. J. (1985). The two-syndrome concept: Origins and current status. *Schizophrenia Bulletin, 11,* 471–486.

Crowe, R. R., Noyes, R., Pauls, D. L., & Slymen, D. (1983). A family study of panic disorder. *Archives of General Psychiatry, 40,* 1065–1069.

Crowe, R. R., Noyes, R., Jr., Wilson, A. F., Elston, R. C., & Ward, L. J. (1987). A linkage study of panic disorder. *Archives of General Psychiatry, 44,* 933–937.

Cunningham, C. E., & Barkley, R. A. (1979). The interactions of normal and hyperactive children with their mothers in free play and structured tasks. *Child Development, 50,* 217–224.

Cytryn, L., & Lourie, R. S. (1980). Mental retardation. In H. I. Kaplan, A. M. Freedman, & B. J. Sadock, *Comprehensive textbook of psychiatry* (Vol. 3, pp. 2484–2526). Baltimore: Williams & Wilkins.

Cytryn, L., & McKnew, D. H., Jr. (1972). Proposed classification of childhood depression. *American Journal of Psychiatry, 129,* 149–155.

Cytryn, L., & McKnew, D. H., Jr. (1974). Factors influencing the changing clinical expression of the depressive process in children. *American Journal of Psychiatry, 131,* 879–881.

Cytryn, L., & McKnew, D. H., Jr. (1979). Affective disorders. In J. D. Noshpitz (Ed.), *Basic handbook of child psychiatry* (Vol. 2, pp. 321–340). New York: Basic Books.

Cytryn, L., & McKnew, D. H., Jr. (1980). Affective disorders. In H. I. Kaplan, A. M. Freedman, & B. J. Sadock (Eds.), *Comprehensive textbook of psychiatry* (Vol. 3, 3rd ed., pp. 2798–2809). Baltimore: Williams & Wilkins.

Cytryn, L., & McKnew, D. H., Jr. (1987). Childhood depression: An update. In J. D. Noshpitz (Ed.), *Basic handbook of child psychiatry* (Vol. 5, pp. 286–293). New York: Basic Books.

Cytryn, L., McKnew, D. H., Jr., Bartko, J. J., Lamour, M., & Hamovitt, J. (1982). Offspring of patients with affective disorders: II. *Journal of the American Academy of Child Psychiatry, 21,* 389–391.

Cytryn, L., McKnew, D. H., Zahn-Waxler, C., & Gershon, E. S. (1986). Developmental issues in risk research: The offspring of affectively ill parents. In M. Rutter, C. E. Izard, & P. B. Read (Eds.), *Depression in young people: Developmental and clinical perspectives* (pp. 163–188). New York: Guilford.

Cytryn, L., McKnew, D. H., Zahn-Waxler, C., Radke-Yarrow, M., Gaensbauer, T. J., Harmon, R. J., & Lamour, M. (1984). A developmental view of affective disturbances in the children of affectively ill patients. *American Journal of Psychiatry, 141,* 219–222.

Dahl, E. K., Cohen, D. J., & Provence, S. (1986). Clinical and multivariate approaches to the nosology of pervasive developmental disorders. *Journal of the American Academy of Child Psychiatry, 25,* 170–180.

Dally, P., & Gomez, J. (1979). *Anorexia nervosa.* London: Heinemann.

Daniels, D., & Plomin, R. (1985). Origins of individual differences in shyness. *Developmental Psychology, 21,* 118–121.

Dantchakoff, V. (1938). Roles des Hormones dans les Manifestations des Instincts Sexuels. *C. R. Academie de Science, Paris, 206,* 945–947.

Davidson, L., & Gould, M. (1989). Contagion as a risk factor in youth suicide. In Alcohol, Drug Abuse, and Mental Health Administration (Ed.), *Report of the Secretary's Task Force on Youth Suicide: Vol. 2. Risk factors for youth suicide* (DHHS Publication No. ADM 89-1622, pp. 88–106). Washington, DC: U.S. Government Printing Office.

Davidson, M., Kugler, M., & Bauer, C. (1963). Diagnosis and management in children with severe and protracted constipation and obstipation. *Journal of Pediatrics, 62,* 261–275.

Davidson, S. (1960). School phobia as a manifestation of family disturbance: Its structure and treatment. *Journal of Child Psychology and Psychiatry, 1,* 270–287.

Davison, I. S., Faull, C., & Nicol, A. R. (1986). Temperament and behaviour in six-year-olds with recurrent abdominal pain: A follow-up [Research Note]. *Journal of Child Psychology and Psychiatry, 27,* 539–544.

Davison, K., & Bagley, C. R. (1969). Schizophrenia-like psychoses associated with organic disorders of the central nervous system: A review of the literature. In R. N. Herrington (Ed.), *Current problems in neuropsychiatry* (pp. 113–184). Ashford, Kent: Headley Bros.

Decarie, T. G. (1965). *Intelligence and affectivity in early childhood.* New York: International Universities Press.

Decina, P., Kestenbaum, C. J., Farber, S., Kron, L., Gargan, M., Sackeim, H. A., & Fieve, R. R. (1983). Clinical and psychological assessment of children of bipolar probands. *American Journal of Psychiatry, 140,* 548–553.

Delamater, A. M., Rosenbloom, N., Conners, C. K., & Hertweck, L. (1983). The behavioral treatment of hysterical paralysis in a ten-year-old boy: A case study. *Journal of the American Academy of Child Psychiatry, 22,* 73–79.

Del Beccaro, M. A., Burke, P., & McCauley, E. (1988). Hallucinations in children: A follow-up study. *Journal of the American Academy of Child and Adolescent Psychiatry, 27,* 462–465.

De Francis, V. (1969). *Protecting the child victim of sex crimes committed by adults.* Denver: American Humane Association.

DeFries, J. C., Singer, S. M., Foch, T. T., & Lewitter, F. I. (1978). Familial nature of reading disability. *British Journal of Psychiatry, 132,* 361–367.

De Leon, G., & Mandell, W. (1966). A comparison of conditioning and psychotherapy in the treatment of functional enuresis. *Journal of Clinical Psychology, 22,* 326–330.

DeLisi, L. E. (1986). Neuroimmunology: Clinical studies of schizophrenia and other psychiatric disorders. In H. A. Nasrallah & D. R. Weinberger (Eds.), *The neurology of schizophrenia* (Vol. 1, pp. 377–396). Amsterdam: Elsevier.

Delong, G. R., & Aldershof, A. L. (1987). Long-term experience with lithium treatment in childhood: Correlation with clinical diagnosis. *Journal of the American Academy of Child and Adolescent Psychiatry, 26,* 389–394.

Delprato, D. J. (1980). Hereditary determinants of fears and phobias: A critical review. *Behavior Therapy, 11,* 79–103.

Demos, J. (1986). *Past, present, and personal: The family and the life course in American history.* New York: Oxford University Press.

DeMyer, M. K. (1987). Treatment of psychotic children. In J. D. Noshpitz (Ed.), *Basic handbook of child psychiatry* (Vol. 5, pp. 502–511). New York: Basic Books.

Denckla, M. B. (1972). Clinical syndromes in learning disabilities: The case for "splitting" vs. "lumping." *Journal of Learning Disabilities, 5,* 401–406.

Denckla, M. B. (1978). Minimal brain dysfunction. In J. S. Chall & A. F. Mirsky (Eds.), *Seventy-seventh yearbook of the National Society for the Study of Education* (pp. 223–268). Chicago: University of Chicago Press.

Denckla, M. B. (1983). The neuropsychology of social-emotional learning disabilities. *Archives of Neurology, 40,* 461–462.

Denckla, M. B. (1985). Revised neurological examination for subtle signs. *Psychopharmacology Bulletin, 21,* 773–800.

Denckla, M. B. (1986). New diagnostic criteria for autism and related behavioral disorders: Guidelines for research protocols. *Journal of the American Academy of Child Psychiatry, 25,* 221–224.

Denckla, M. B. (1989). Neurological examination. In J. L. Rapoport (Ed.), *Obsessive-compulsive disorder in children and adolescents* (pp. 107–115). Washington, DC: American Psychiatric Press.

Denckla, M. B., LeMay, M., & Chapman, C. A. (1985). Few CT scan abnormalities found even in neurologically impaired learning disabled children. *Journal of Learning Disabilities, 18,* 132–135.

Denckla, M. B., & Rudel, R. G. (1976). Rapid "automatized" naming (R.A.N.): Dyslexia differentiated from other learning disabilities. *Neuropsychologia, 14,* 471–479.

DeSanctis, S. (1971). On some varieties of dementia praecox. Translated by Maria-Livia Osborn in J. G. Howells (Ed.), *Modern perspectives in international child psychiatry* (pp. 590–609). New York: Brunner/Mazel. (Original work published 1906)

Des Lauriers, A. (1967). The schizophrenic child. *Archives of General Psychiatry, 16,* 194–201.

Detera-Wadleigh, S. D., Berrettini, W. H., Goldin, L. R., Boorman, D., Anderson, S., & Gershon, E. S. (1987). Close linkage of c-Harvey-ras-1 and the insulin gene to affective disorder is ruled out in three North American pedigrees. *Nature, 325,* 806–808.

Deutsch, C. K., Matthysse, S., Swanson, J. M., & Farkas, L. G. (1990). Genetic latent structure analysis of dysmorphology in attention deficit disorder. *Journal of the American Academy of Child and Adolescent Psychiatry, 29,* 189–194.

Deutsch, C. K., Swanson, J. M., Bruell, J. H., Cantwell, D. P., Weinberg, F., & Baren, M. (1982). Overrepresentation of adoptees in children with the attention deficit disorder. *Behavior Genetics, 12,* 231–238.

Deutsch, F. (Ed.). (1959). *On the mysterious leap from the mind to the body.* New York: International Universities Press.

Deutsch, H. (1942). Some forms of emotional disturbance and their relationship to schizophrenia. *Psychoanalytic Quarterly, 11,* 301–321.

Devlin, M. J., Walsh, B. T., Kral, J. G., Heymsfield, S. B., Pi-Sunyer, F. X., & Dantzic, S. (1990). Metabolic abnormalities in bulimia nervosa. *Archives of General Psychiatry, 47,* 144–148.

Di Nardo, P. A., O'Brien, G. T., Barlow, D. H., Waddell, M. T., & Blanchard, E. B. (1983). Reliability of DSM-III anxiety disorder categories using a new structured interview. *Archives of General Psychiatry, 40,* 1070–1074.

Diamond, M. (1965). A critical evaluation of the ontogeny of human sexual behavior. *Quarterly Review of Biology, 40,* 147–175.

Dirks, J. F., Robinson, S. K., & Dirks, D. L. (1981). Alexithymia and the psycho-maintenance of bronchial asthma. *Psychotherapy and Psychosomatics, 36,* 63–71.

Dirks, J. F., Jones, N. F., & Kinsman, R. A. (1977). Panic-fear: A personality dimension related to intractability in asthma. *Psychosomatic Medicine, 39,* 120–126.

Dirks, J. F., Schraa, J. C., Brown, E. L., & Kinsman, R. A. (1980). Psycho-maintenance in asthma: Hospitalization rates and financial impact. *British Journal of Medicine and Psychology, 53,* 349–354.

Dische, S. (1973). Treatment of enuresis with an enuresis alarm. In I. Kolvin, R. C. MacKeith, & S. R. Meadow (Eds.), *Bladder control and enuresis* (pp. 211–230). (Clinics in Developmental Medicine, Nos. 48/49). London: Heinemann.

Doctors, S. (1981). The symptom of delicate self-cutting in adolescent females: A developmental view. *Adolescent Psychiatry, 9,* 443–460.

Dodge, W. F., West, E. F., Bridgforth, E. B., & Travis, L. B. (1970). Nocturnal enuresis in 6- to 10-year-old children. *American Journal of Diseases of Children, 120,* 32–35.

Doherty, M. B., Madansky, D., Kraft, J., Carter-Ake, L. L., Rosenthal, P. A., & Coughlin, B. F. (1986). Cortisol dynamics and test performance of the dexamethasone suppression test in 97 psychiatrically hospitalized children aged 3–16 years. *Journal of the American Academy of Child Psychiatry, 25,* 400–408.

Doleys, D. M. (1977). Behavioral treatment for nocturnal enuresis in children: A review of the recent literature. *Psychological Bulletin, 84,* 30–54.

Doleys, D. M. (1983). Enuresis and encopresis. In T. H. Ollendick & M. Hersen (Eds.), *Handbook of child psychopathology* (pp. 201–226). New York: Plenum.

Doleys, D. M., & Arnold, S. (1975). Treatment of childhood encopresis: full cleanliness training. *Mental Retardation, 13,* 14–16.

Donnelly, M., Zametkin, A. J., Rapoport, J. L., Ismond, D. R., Weingartner, H., Lane, E., Oliver, J., Linnoila, M., & Potter, W. Z. (1986). Treatment of childhood hyperactivity with desipramine: plasma drug concentration, cardiovascular effects, plasma and urinary catecholamine levels, and clinical response. *Clinical Pharmacology and Therapeutics, 39,* 72–81.

Dorner, G. (1981). Sex hormones and neurotransmitters as mediators for sexual differentiation of the brain. *Endokronologie, 78* (2/3), 129–138.

Dorow, R., Horowski, R., Paschelke, G., Amin, M., & Braestrup, C. (1983). Severe anxiety induced by FG 7142, a Betacarboline ligand for benzodiazepine receptors. *Lancet, 8341,* 98–99.

Douglas, J. W. B. (1973). Early disturbing events and later enuresis. In I. Kolvin, R. C. MacKeith, & S. R. Meadow (Eds.), *Bladder control and enuresis* (pp. 109–117). (Clinics in Developmental Medicine, Nos. 48/49). London: Heinemann.

Douglas, M. (1970). *Purity and danger: An analysis of concepts of pollution and taboo.* Hammondsworth, England: Penguin.

Douglas, V. I. (1983). Attentional and cognitive problems. In M. Rutter (Ed.), *Developmental neuropsychiatry* (pp. 280–329). New York: Guilford.

Douglas, V. I. (1984). The psychological processes implicated in ADD. In L. M. Bloomingdale (Ed.), *Attention deficit disorder: Diagnostic, cognitive, and therapeutic understanding* (pp. 147–162). New York: SP Medical and Scientific Books.

Douglas, V. I., Barr, R. G., O'Neill, M. E., & Britton, B. G. (1986). Short term effects of methylphenidate on the cognitive, learning and academic performance of children with attention deficit disorder in the laboratory and the classroom. *Journal of Child Psychology and Psychiatry, 27,* 191–211.

Draeger, S., Prior, M., & Sanson, A. (1986). Visual and auditory attention performance in hyperactive children: Competence or compliance. *Journal of Abnormal Child Psychology, 14,* 411–424.

Drotar, D., Malone, C. A., Negray, J., & Dennstedt, M. (1981). Psychosocial assessment and care for infants hospitalized for non-organic failure to thrive. *Journal of Clinical Child Psychology, 10,* 63–66.

Duane, D. D. (1989). Neurobiological correlates of learning disorders. *Journal of the American Academy of Child and Adolescent Psychiatry, 28,* 314–318.

Dubo, S., McLean, J. A., Ching, A. Y. T., Wright, H. L., Kauffman, P. E., Sheldon, J. M. (1961). A study of relationships between family situation, bronchial asthma, and personal adjustment in children. *The Journal of Pediatrics, 59,* 402–414.

Dubowitz, V., & Hersov, L. (1976). Management of children with non-organic (hysterical) disorders of motor function. *Developmental Medicine and Child Neurology, 18,* 358–368.

Duffy, F. H., Denckla, M. B., Bartels, P. H., & Sandini, G. (1980). Dyslexia: Regional differences in brain electrical activity by topographic mapping. *Annals of Neurology, 7,* 412–420.

Dunbar, H. F. (1943). *Psychosomatic diagnosis.* New York: Harper & Row (Hoeber).

Dwyer, J. T., & Delong, G. R. (1987). A family history study of twenty probands with childhood manic-depressive illness. *Journal of the American Academy of Child and Adolescent Psychiatry, 26,* 176–180.

Dykman, R. A., Murphree, O. D., & Peters, J. E. (1969). Like begets like: Behavioral tests, classical autonomic and motor conditioning, and operant conditioning in two strains of pointer dogs. *Annals of the New York Academy of Sciences, 159,* 976–1007.

Eaton, L. F., & Menolascino, F. J. (1982). Psychiatric disorders in the mentally retarded: Types, problems and challenges. *American Journal of Psychiatry, 139,* 1297–1303.

Ebaugh, F. G. (1923). Neuropsychiatric sequelae of acute epidemic encephalitis in children. *American Journal of Diseases of Children, 25,* 89–97.

Eckert, E. D., & Mitchell, J. E. (1986). Anorexia nervosa and bulimia. In G. Winokur & P. Clayton (Eds.), *The medical basis of psychiatry* (pp. 171–182). Philadelphia: Saunders.

Edelbrock, C. (1987). Behavioral checklists and rating scales. In J. D. Noshpitz (Ed.), *Basic handbook of child psychiatry* (Vol. 5, pp. 153–164). New York: Basic Books.

Edfors-Lubs, M. L. (1971). Allergy in 7000 twin pairs. *Acta-Allergologica, 26,* 249–285.

Edgcumbe, R., & Burgner, M. (1975). The phallic-narcissistic phase: A differentiation between preoedipal and oedipal aspects of phallic development. *Psychoanalytic Study of the Child, 30,* 161–180.

Education for All Handicapped Children Act. (1975). Public Law No. 94–142. S. 6, 94th Congress, 1st Sess. Report No. 94–168.

Egan, J., & Kernberg, P. (1984). Pathological narcissism in childhood. *Journal of the American Psychoanalytic Association, 32,* 39–62.

Egeland, B., Breitenbucher, M., & Rosenberg, D. (1980). Prospective study of the significance of life stress in the etiology of child abuse. *Journal of Consulting and Clinical Psychology, 48,* 195–205.

Egeland, B., & Sroufe, L. A. (1981). Attachment and early maltreatment. *Child Development, 52,* 44–52.

Egeland, J. A., Gerhard, D. S., Pauls, D. L., Sussex, J. N., Kidd, K. K., Allen, C. R., Hostetter, A. M., & Housman, D. E. (1987). Bipolar affective disorders linked to DNA markers on chromosome 11. *Nature, 325,* 783–787.

Eggers, C. (1978). Course and prognosis of childhood schizophrenia. *Journal of Autism and Childhood Schizophrenia, 8,* 21–26.

Eggers, C. (1989). Schizo-affective psychoses in childhood: A follow-up study. *Journal of Autism and Developmental Disorders, 19,* 327–342.

Eiduson, B. (1983). Conflict and stress in nontraditional families: Impact on children. *American Journal of Orthopsychiatry, 53,* 426–435.

Eisenberg, L. (1958a). School phobia: Diagnosis, genesis and clinical management. *Pediatric Clinics of North America, 5,* 645–666.

Eisenberg, L. (1958b). School phobia: A study of communication of anxiety. *American Journal of Psychiatry, 114,* 712–718.

Eisenberg, L. (1959). The pediatric management of school phobia. *Journal of Pediatrics, 55,* 758–766.

Eisenberg, L. (1978). Definitions of dyslexia: Their consequences for research and policy. In A. L. Benton & D. Pearl (Eds.), *Dyslexia: An appraisal of current knowledge* (pp. 29–42). New York: Oxford University Press.

Eisenberg, L. (1986). Editorial: Does bad news about suicide beget bad news? *New England Journal of Medicine, 315,* 705–707.

Eissler, K. R. (Ed.) (1949). *Searchlights on delinquency.* New York: International Universities Press.

Ekman, P., Levenson, R. W., & Friesen, W. V. (1983). Autonomic nervous system activity distinguishes among emotions. *Science, 221,* 1208–1210.

Ekstein, R. (1966). *Children of time and space, of action and impulse: Clinical studies on the psychoanalytic treatment of severely disturbed children.* New York: Appleton-Century-Crofts.

Ekstein, R., & Wallerstein, J. (1954). Observations on the psychology of borderline and psychotic children. *Psychoanalytic Study of the Child, 9,* 344–369.

Elkins, R. N., Rapoport, J. L., & Lipsky, A. (1980). Obsessive-compulsive disorder of childhood and adolescence. *Journal of the American Academy of Child Psychiatry, 19,* 511–524.

Elkins, R. N., Rapoport, J. L., Zahn, T. P., Buchsbaum, M. S., Weingartner, H., Kopin, I. J., Langer, D., & Johnson, C. (1981). Acute effects of caffeine in normal prepubertal boys. *American Journal of Psychiatry, 138,* 178–183.

Elledge, S. (1984). *E. B. White: A Biography.* New York: Norton.

Ellis, E. F. (1983). Allergic disorders. In R. E. Behrman & V. C. Vaughan, III (Eds.), *Nelson textbook of pediatrics* (pp. 524–561). Philadelphia: Saunders.

Elmer, E., Gregg, G. S., & Ellison, P. (1969). Late results of the "failure to thrive" syndrome. *Clinical Pediatrics, 8,* 584–589.

Emde, R. N., Harmon, R. J., & Good, W. V. (1986). Depressive feelings in children: A transactional model for research. In M. Rutter, C. E. Izard, & P. B. Read (Eds.), *Depression in young people: Developmental and clinical perspectives* (pp. 135–160). New York: Guilford.

Engel, G. L. (1967). A psychological setting of somatic disease: The 'giving up–given up' complex. *Proceedings of the Royal Society of Medicine, 60,* 533–555.

Engel, G. L. (1977). The need for a new medical model: A challenge for biomedicine. *Science, 196,* 129–136.

English, P. C. (1978). Failure to thrive without organic reason. *Pediatric Annals, 7,* 774–781.

Erikson, E. H. (1950). *Childhood and society.* New York: Norton.

Erikson, E. H. (1963). *Childhood and society* (2nd ed.). New York: Norton.

Erlenmeyer-Kimling, L., & Cornblatt, B. (1984). Biobehavioral risk factors in children of schizophrenic parents. *Journal of Autism and Developmental Disorders, 14,* 357–374.

Erlenmeyer-Kimling, L., & Cornblatt, B. (1987a). High-risk research in schizophrenia: A summary of what has been learned. *Journal of Psychiatric Research, 21,* 401–411.

Erlenmeyer-Kimling, L., & Cornblatt, B. (1987b). The New York high-risk project: A follow-up report. *Schizophrenia Bulletin, 13,* 451–461.

Erlenmeyer-Kimling, L., Kestenbaum, C., Bird, H., & Hilldoff, U. (1984). Assessment of the New York high-risk project subjects in sample A who are now clinically deviant. In N. F. Watt, E. J. Anthony, L. C. Wynne, & J. E. Rolf (Eds.), *Children at risk for schizophrenia: A longitudinal perspective* (pp. 227–239). Cambridge: Cambridge University Press.

Eron, L. D. (1980). Prescription for reduction of aggression. *American Psychologist, 35,* 244–252.

Escalona, S. (1953). Emotional development in the first year of life. In M. Senn (Ed.), *Transactions of the Sixth Conference on Problems of Infancy and Childhood.* New York: Josiah Macy Foundation.

Escalona, S. (1964). Some considerations regarding psychotherapy with psychotic children. In M. R. Haworth (Ed.), *Child Psychotherapy* (pp. 50–58). New York: Basic Books.

Estes, H. R., Haylett, C. H., & Johnson, A. M. (1956). Separation anxiety. *American Journal of Psychotherapy, 10,* 682–695.

Estroff, T. W., Herrera, C., Gaines, R., Shaffer, D., Gould, M., & Green, A. H. (1984). Maternal psychopathology and perception of child behavior in psychiatrically referred and child maltreatment families. *Journal of the American Academy of Child Psychiatry, 23,* 649–652.

Eth, S., & Pynoos, R. S. (1985). *Post-traumatic stress disorder in children.* Washington, DC: American Psychiatric Press.

Evans, S. L., Reinhart, J. B., & Succop, R. A. (1972). Failure to thrive. *Journal of the American Academy of Child Psychiatry, 11,* 440–457.

Evans-Jones, L. G., & Rosenbloom, L. (1978). Disintegrative psychosis in childhood. *Developmental Medicine and Child Neurology, 20,* 462–470.

Everson, M. D., & Boat, B. W. (1990). Sexualized doll play among young children: Implications for the use of anatomical dolls in sexual abuse evaluations. *Journal of the American Academy of Child and Adolescent Psychiatry, 29,* 736–742.

Eysenck, H. J., & Rachman, S. J. (1965). The application of learning theory to child psychiatry. In J. G. Howells (Ed.), *Modern perspectives in child psychiatry.* Edinburgh: Oliver & Boyd.

Fagot, B., & Leinbach, M. D. (1985). Gender identity: Some thoughts on an old concept. *Journal of the American Academy of Child Psychiatry, 24,* 684–688.

Fairbairn, W. R. D. (1952). *Psychoanalytic studies of the personality.* London: Routledge & Kegan Paul.

Fairburn, C. G. (1985). Cognitive-behavioral treatment for bulimia. In D. M. Garner & P. E. Garfinkel, *Handbook of psychotherapy for anorexia nervosa and bulimia.* New York: Guilford.

Fairburn, C. G., & Cooper, P. J. (1984). The clinical features of bulimia nervosa. *British Journal of Psychiatry, 144,* 238–246.

Faraone, S. V., & Tsuang, M. T. (1985). Quantitative models of the genetic transmission of schizophrenia. *Psychological Bulletin, 98,* 41–66.

Farran, C. (1983). *Infant Colic: What it is and what you can do about it.* New York: Scribner's.

Faull, C., & Nicol, A. R. (1986). Abdominal pain in six-year-olds: An epidemiological study in a new town. *Journal of Child Psychology and Psychiatry, 27,* 251–260.

Federn, P. (1952). *Ego psychology and the psychoses.* New York: Basic Books.

Fein, D., Pennington, B., Markowitz, P., Braverman, M., & Waterhouse, L. (1986). Toward a neuropsychological model of infantile autism: Are the social deficits primary? *Journal of the American Academy of Child Psychiatry, 25,* 198–212.

Feingold, A. (1988). Cognitive gender differences are disappearing. *American Psychologist, 43,* 95–103.

Feingold, B. F. (1975). *Why your child is hyperactive.* New York: Random House.

Feinstein, S. C., & Miller, D. (1979). Psychoses of adolescence. In J. D. Noshpitz (Ed.), *Basic handbook of child psychiatry* (Vol. 2, 708–722). New York: Basic Books.

Feinstein, S. C., & Wolpert, E. A. (1973). Juvenile manic-depressive illness. *Journal of the American Academy of Child Psychiatry, 12,* 123–136.

Feldman, G. (1976). The effect of biofeedback training on respiratory resistance of asthmatic children. *Psychosomatic Medicine, 38,* 27–34.

Fenton, G. W. (1986). Epilepsy and hysteria. *British Journal of Psychiatry, 149,* 28–37.

Fenton, W. S., & McGlashan, T. H. (1986). The prognostic significance of obsessive-compulsive symptoms in schizophrenia. *American Journal of Psychiatry, 143,* 437–441.

Ferenczi, S. (1926). *Further contributions to the theory and technique of psychoanalysis.* London: Hogarth Press.

Ferguson, H. B., & Pappas, B. A. (1979). Evaluation of psychophysiological, neurochemical, and animal models of hyperactivity. In R. L. Trites (Ed.), *Hyperactivity in children* (pp. 61–92). Baltimore: University Park Press.

Ferguson, H. B., & Rapoport, J. L. (1983). Nosological issues and biological validation. In M. Rutter (Ed.), *Developmental Neuropsychiatry* (pp. 369–384). New York: Guilford.

Fichter, M. M., Pirke, K-M., & Holsboer, F. (1984). Weight loss causes neuroendocrine disturbances: Experimental study in healthy starving subjects. *Psychiatry Research, 17,* 61–72.

Field, T. (1984). Separation stress of young children transferring to new schools. *Developmental Psychology, 20,* 786–792.

Fine, S. (1973). Family therapy and a behavioral approach to childhood obsessive-compulsive neurosis. *Archives of General Psychiatry, 28,* 695–697.

Fineman, K. R. (1980). Firesetting in childhood and adolescence. *Psychiatric Clinics of North America, 3,* 483–500.

Finkelhor, D. (1979). *Sexually victimized children.* New York: Free Press.

Finkelhor, D. (1980). Risk factors in the sexual victimization of children. *Child Abuse and Neglect, 4,* 265–273.

Finkelhor, D. (1984). *Child sexual abuse: New theory and research.* New York: Free Press.

Finkelhor, D. (1987). The sexual abuse of children: Current research reviewed. *Psychiatric Annals, 17,* 233–241.

Finlay-Jones, R. A. (1981). Showing that life events are a cause of depression: A review. *Australian and New Zealand Journal of Psychiatry, 15,* 229–238.

Fischoff, J. (1964). Preoedipal influences in a boy's determination to be "feminine" during the oedipal period. *Journal of the American Academy of Child Psychiatry, 3,* 273–286.

Fish, B. (1977). Neurobiologic antecedents of schizophrenia in children: Evidence for an inherited, congenital neurointegrative defect. *Archives of General Psychiatry, 34,* 1297–1313.

Fish, B. (1986). Antecedents of an acute schizophrenic break. *Journal of the American Academy of Child Psychiatry, 25,* 595–600.

Fish, B. (1987). Infant predictors of the longitudinal course of schizophrenic development. *Schizophrenia Bulletin, 13,* 395–409.

Fish, B., & Ritvo, E. R. (1979). Psychoses of childhood. In J. D. Noshpitz (Ed.), *Basic handbook of child psychiatry* (Vol. 2, pp. 249–304). New York: Basic Books.

Fish, B., Shapiro, T., & Campbell, M. (1966). Long-term prognosis and the response of schizophrenic children to drug therapy: A controlled study of trifluoperazine. *American Journal of Psychiatry, 123,* 32–39.

Fisher, L., Harder, D. W., & Kokes, R. F. (1980). Child competence and psychiatric risk: III. Comparisons based on diagnosis of hospitalized parent. *Journal of Nervous and Mental Disorder, 168,* 338–342.

Flament, M. F., & Rapoport, J. L. (1984). Childhood obsessive-compulsive disorder. In T. R. Insel (Ed.), *Obsessive-compulsive disorder* (pp. 24–43). Washington, DC: American Psychiatric Press.

Flament, M. F., Rapoport, J. L., Berg, C. J., Sceery, W., Kilts, C., Mellstrom, B., & Linnoila, M. (1985). Clomipramine treatment of childhood obsessive-compulsive disorder. *Archives of General Psychiatry, 42,* 977–983.

Flament, M. F., Rapoport, J. L., Murphy, D. L., Berg, C. J., & Lake, C. R. (1987). Biochemical changes during clomipramine treatment of childhood obsessive-compulsive disorder. *Archives of General Psychiatry, 44,* 219–225.

Flament, M. F., Whitaker, A., Rapoport, J. L., Davies, M., Berg, C. Z., Kalikow, K., Sceery, W., & Shaffer, D. (1988). Obsessive-compulsive disorder in adolescence: An epidemiological study. *Journal of the American Academy of Child and Adolescent Psychiatry, 27,* 764–771.

Fleming, J. E., & Offord, D. R. (1990). Epidemiology of childhood depressive disorders. A critical review. *Journal of the American Academy of Child and Adolescent Psychiatry, 29,* 571–580.

Foa, E. B., & Goldstein, A. (1978). Continuous exposure and complete response prevention in the treatment of obsessive-compulsive neurosis. *Behavior Therapy, 9,* 821–829.

Foa, E. B., & Steketee, G. (1984). Behavioral treatment of obsessive-compulsive ritualizers. In T. R. Insel (Ed.), *Obsessive-compulsive disorder* (pp. 46–69). Washington, DC: American Psychiatric Press.

Folkman, W., & Siegelmam, E. (1972). *Youthful firesetters: An exploratory study in personality and background.* Washington, DC: Department of Agriculture, Forest Service.

Folstein, S., & Rutter, M. (1978). A twin study of individuals with infantile autism. In M. Rutter & E. Schopler (Eds.), *Autism: A reappraisal of concepts and treatment* (pp. 219–242). New York: Plcnum.

Fontaine, R., & Chouinard, G. (1986). An open clinical trial of fluoxetine in the treatent of obsessive-compulsive disorder. *Journal of Clinical Psychopharmacology, 6,* 98–101.

Foote, S. L., Aston-Jones, G., & Bloom, F. E. (1980). Impulse activity of locus coeruleus neurons in awake rats and monkeys is a function of sensory stimulation and arousal. *Proceedings of the National Academy of Science, 77,* 3033–3037.

Foote, S. L., Bloom, F. E., & Aston-Jones, G. (1983). Nucleus locus ceruleus: New evidence of anatomical and physiological specificity. *Physiological Reviews, 63,* 844–914.

Forbis, O. L., & Jones, R. H. (1965). Hysteria in childhood. *Southern Medical Journal, 58,* 1221–1225.

Forsythe, W. I., & Redmond, A. (1974). Enuresis and spontaneous cure rate. Study of 1129 enuretics. *Archives of Disease in Childhood, 49,* 259–263.

Fournier, J. P., Garfinkel, B. D., Bond, A., Beauchesne, H., & Shapiro, S. K. (1987). Pharmacological and behavioral management of enuresis. *Journal of the American Academy of Child and Adolescent Psychiatry, 26,* 849–853.

Fox, R. (1967). *Kinship and marriage: An anthropological perspective.* Harmondsworth, England: Penguin.

Fraiberg, S. (1969). Libidinal object constancy and mental representation. *Psychoanalytic Study of the Child, 24,* 9–47.

Fraiberg, S. (Ed.) (1980). *Clinical studies in infant mental health: The first year of life.* New York: Basic Books.

Fraiberg, S., Adelson, E., & Shapiro, V. (1975). Ghosts in the nursery. *Journal of the American Academy of Child Psychiatry, 14,* 387–421.

Fraiberg, S., Shapiro, V., & Cherniss, D. (1983). Treatment modalities. In J. D. Call, E. Galenson, & R. L. Tyson (Eds.), *Frontiers of infant psychiatry* (pp. 56–73). New York: Basic Books.

Frances, A. (1985). Validating schizotypal personality disorders: Problems with the schizophrenia connection. *Schizophrenia Bulletin, 11,* 595–597.

Frances, A., & Blumenthal, S. J. (1989). Personality as a predictor of youthful suicide. In Alcohol, Drug Abuse, and Mental Health Administration (Ed.), *Report of the Secretary's Task Force for Youth Suicide: Vol. 2. Risk factors for youth suicide* (DHHS Publication No. ADM 89-1622, pp. 160–171). Washington, DC: U.S. Government Printing Office.

Francis, J. J. (1965). Passivity and homosexual predisposition in latency boys. *Bulletin of the Philadelphia Association of Psychoanalysis, 15,* 160–174.

Frankel, R. M., Leary, M., & Kilman, B. (1987). Building social skills through pragmatic analysis: Assessment and treatment implications for children with autism. In D. J. Cohen & A. M. Donnellan (Eds.), *Handbook of autism and pervasive developmental disorders* (pp. 333–359). New York: Wiley.

Freedman, D. X. (1984). Overview of panic disorders. *Psychosomatics, 25*(Suppl. 10), 37–39.

Freeman, B. J., Ritvo, E. R., Needleman, R., & Yokota, A. (1985). The stability of cognitive and linguistic parameters in autism: A five-year prospective study. *Journal of the American Academy of Child Psychiatry, 24,* 459–464.

Freeman, B. J., Ritvo, E. R., Schroth, P. E., Tonick, I., Guthrie, D., Wake, L. (1981). Behavioral characteristics of high- & low-IQ autistic children. *American Journal of Psychiatry, 138,* 25–29.

French, T. M., & Alexander, F. (1941). *Psychogenic factors in bronchial asthma.* Washington, DC: National Research Council.

Freud, A. (1926). A hysterical symptom in a child of two years and three months. *International Journal of Psychoanalysis, 7,* 227–229.

Freud, A. (1937). *The ego and the mechanisms of defense.* New York: International Universities Press.

Freud, A. (1946). *The ego and the mechanisms of defense.* New York: International Universities Press. (Original work published 1936)

Freud, A. (1965). *Normality and pathology in childhood: Assessments of development.* New York: International Universities Press.

Freud, A. (1966). Obsessional neurosis: A summary of psychoanalytic views as presented at the congress. *International Journal of Psycho-Analysis, 47,* 116–122.

Freud, A. (1981a). A psychoanalyst's view of sexual abuse by parents. In P. B. Mrazek & C. H. Kempe (Eds.), *Sexually abused children and their families* (pp. 33–34). Oxford: Pergamon.

Freud, A. (1981b). A study guide to Freud's writings. In *Psychoanalytic psychology of normal development* (pp. 209–276). New York: International Universities Press.

Freud, A. (1981c). *Psychoanalytic psychology of normal development, 1970–1980.* New York: International Universities Press.

Freud, S. (1946). *New introductory lectures on psychoanalysis.* London: Hogarth Press.

Freud, S. (1953a). Inhibitions, symptoms and anxiety. In J. Strachey (Ed. and Trans.), *The standard edition of the complete psychological works of Sigmund Freud* (Vol. 20, pp. 87–172). London: Hogarth Press. (Original work published 1926)

Freud, S. (1953b). Three essays on the theory of sexuality. In J. Strachey (Ed. and Trans.), *The standard edition of the complete psychological works of Sigmund Freud* (Vol. 7, pp. 125–245). London: Hogarth Press. (Original work published 1905)

Freud, S. (1953c). Totem and taboo. In J. Strachey (Ed. and Trans.), *The standard edition of the complete psychological works of Sigmund Freud* (Vol. 13, pp. 1–162). London: Hogarth Press. (Original work published 1912)

Freud, S. (1955a). The acquisition of power over fire. In J. Strachey (Ed. and Trans.), *The standard edition of the complete psychological works of Sigmund Freud* (Vol. 22, pp. 185–193). London: Hogarth Press. (Original work published 1932)

Freud, S. (1955b). Notes upon a case of obsessional neurosis. In J. Strachey (Ed. and Trans.), *The standard edition of the complete psychological works of Sigmund Freud* (Vol. 10, pp. 153–326). London: Hogarth Press. (Original work published 1909)

Freud, S. (1957a). The aetiology of hysteria. In J. Strachey (Ed. and Trans.), *The standard edition of the complete psychological works of Sigmund Freud* (Vol. 14, pp. 189–221). London: Hogarth Press. (Original work published 1896)

Freud, S. (1957b). On the history of the psychoanalytic movement. In J. Strachey (Ed. and Trans.), *The standard edition of the complete psychological works of Sigmund Freud* (Vol. 14, pp. 1–66). London: Hogarth Press. (Original work published 1914)

Freud, S. (1957c). Mourning and melancholia. In J. Strachey (Ed. and Trans.), *The standard edition of the complete psychological works of Sigmund Freud* (Vol. 14, pp. 243–258). London: Hogarth Press. (Original work published 1917)

Freud, S. (1957d). On narcissism. In J. Strachey (Ed. and Trans.), *The standard edition of the complete psychological works of Sigmund Freud* (Vol. 14, pp. 69–102). London: Hogarth Press. (Original work published 1914)

Freud, S. (1957e). Some character types met with in psychoanalytic practice. In J. Strachey (Ed. and Trans.), *The standard edition of the complete psychological works of Sigmund Freud* (Vol. 14, pp. 309–333). London: Hogarth Press. (Original work published 1916)

Freud, S. (1958). The disposition to obsessional neurosis. In J. Strachey (Ed. and Trans.), *The standard edition of the complete psychological works of Sigmund Freud* (Vol. 12, pp. 317–326). London: Hogarth Press. (Original work published 1913)

Freud, S. (1959). Character and anal eroticism. In J. Strachey (Ed. and Trans.), *The standard edition of the complete psychological works of Sigmund Freud,* (Vol. 9, pp. 167–175). London: Hogarth Press. (Original work published 1908)

Freud, S. (1961). The ego and the id. In J. Strachey (Ed. and Trans.), *The standard edition of the complete psychological works of Sigmund Freud* (Vol. 19, pp. 12–59). London: Hogarth Press. (Original work published 1923)

Freud, S. (1962b). Further remarks on the neuro-psychoses of defence. In J. Strachey (Ed. and Trans.), *The standard edition of the complete psychological works of Sigmund Freud* (Vol. 3, pp. 162–185). London: Hogarth Press. (Original work published 1896)

Freud, S. (1962c). The neuro-psychoses of defence. In J. Strachey (Ed. and Trans.), *The standard edition of the complete psychological works of Sigmund Freud* (Vol. 3, pp. 45–61). London: Hogarth Press. (Original work published 1894)

Freud, S. (1985). *The complete letters of Sigmund Freud to Wilhelm Fliess (1887–1904)* (J. M. Masson, Ed. & Trans.). Cambridge, MA: Harvard University Press.

Friedman, S. B. (1973). Conversion symptoms in adolescents. *Pediatric Clinics of North America, 20,* 873–882.

Friedmann, C. T., & Silvers, F. M. (1977). A multimodality approach to in-patient treatment of obsessive-compulsive disorder. *American Journal of Psychotherapy, 31,* 456–465.

Friedrich, W. N., & Boriskin, J. A. (1976). The role of the child in abuse: A review of the literature. *American Journal of Orthopsychiatry, 46,* 580–589.

Friend, M. R., Schiddel, L., Klein, B., & Dunaeff, D. (1954). Observations on the development of transvestism in boys. *American Journal of Orthopsychiatry, 24,* 563–575.

Frijling-Schreuder, E. C. M. (1969). Borderline states in children. *Psychoanalytic Study of the Child, 24,* 307–327.

Frith, U. (1983). The similarities and differences between reading and spelling problems. In M. Rutter (Ed.), *Developmental neuropsychiatry* (pp. 453–472). New York: Guilford.

Frith, U., & Baron-Cohen, S. (1987). Perception in autistic children. In D. J. Cohen & A. M. Donnellan (Eds.), *Handbook of autism and pervasive developmental disorders* (pp. 85–102). New York: Wiley.

Fromm-Reichmann, F. (1948). Notes on the development of treatment of schizophrenics by psychoanalytic psychotherapy. *Psychiatry, 11*, 263–273.

Fromm-Reichmann, F. (1950). *Principles of intensive psychotherapy.* Chicago: University of Chicago Press.

Fyer, A. J., Mannuzza, S., Gallops, M. S., Martin, L. Y., Aaronson, C., Gorman, J. M., Liebowitz, M. R., Klein, D. F. (1990). Familial transmission of simple phobias and fears. *Archives of General Psychiatry, 47*, 252–256.

Gaensbauer, T. J., Harmon, R. J., Cytryn, L., & McKnew, D. H. (1984). Social and affective development in infants with a manic-depressive parent. *American Journal of Psychiatry, 141*, 223–229.

Gaensbauer, T. J., & Sands, K. (1979). Distorted affective communications in abused/neglected infants and their potential impact on caretakers. *Journal of the American Academy of Child Psychiatry, 18*, 236–250.

Gaffney, G. R., Kuperman, S., Tsai, L. Y., Minchin, S. (1989). Forebrain structure in infantile autism. *Journal of the American Academy of Child and Adolescent Psychiatry, 28*, 534–537.

Gaffney, G. R., & Tsai, L. Y. (1987). Brief report: Magnetic resonance imaging of high level autism. *Journal of Autism and Developmental Disorders, 17*, 433–438.

Gagnon, J. H. (1965). Female child victims of sex offenses. *Social Problems, 13*, 176–192.

Galaburda, A. M., Sherman, G. F., Rosen, G. D., Aboitiz, F., & Geschwind, N. (1985). Developmental dyslexia: Four consecutive patients with cortical anomalies. *Annals of Neurology, 18*, 222–233.

Galdston, R. (1965). Observations on children who have been physically abused and their parents. *American Journal of Psychiatry, 122*, 440–443.

Galdston, R. (1974). Mind over matter: Observations on fifty patients hospitalized with anorexia nervosa. *Journal of the American Academy of Child Psychiatry, 13*, 246–263.

Galdston, R. (1981). The domestic dimensions of violence: Child abuse. *Psychoanalytic Study of the Child, 36*, 391–414.

Galenson, E., & Roiphe, H. (1974). The emergence of genital awareness during the second year of life. In R. C. Friedman, R. M. Richert, & R. L. Van de Wiele (Eds.), *Sex differences in behavior* (pp. 223–231). New York: Wiley.

Galenson, E., (1979). Psychological development during the second year. In J. Noshpitz, R. Cohen, S. Morrison, J. Call, I. Behin, & L. Stone (Eds.), *Handbook of child psychiatry* (vol. 1, pp. 144–156). New York: Basic Books.

Galler, J. R., Neustein, S., & Walker, W. A. (1980). Clinical aspects of recurrent abdominal pain in children. *Advances in Pediatrics, 27*, 31–53.

Gallico, R. P., Burns, T. J., & Grob, C. S. (1987). *Emotional and behavioral problems in children with learning disabilities.* Boston: Little, Brown.

Gammon, G. D., John, K., Rothblum, E. D., Mullen, K., Tischler, G. L., & Weissman, M. M. (1983). Use of a structured diagnostic interview to identify bipolar disorder in adolescent inpatients: Frequency and manifestation of the disorder. *American Journal of Psychiatry, 140,* 543–547.

Gans, H. J. (1962). *The urban villagers.* New York: Free Press.

Garbarino, J. (1976). A preliminary study of some ecological correlates of child abuse: The impact of socioeconomic stress on mothers. *Child Development, 47,* 178–185.

Garbarino, J. (1977a). The human ecology of child maltreatment: A conceptual model for research. *Journal of Marriage and the Family, 39,* 721–735.

Garbarino, J. (1977b). The price of privacy in the social dynamics of child abuse. *Child Welfare, 56,* 565–575.

Garbarino, J. (1982). Healing the social wounds of isolation. In E. H. Newberger (Ed.), *Child abuse* (pp. 43–55). Boston: Little, Brown.

Garber, H., & Heber, F. R. (1977). The Milwaukee Project: Indications of the effectiveness of early intervention in preventing mental retardation. In P. Mittler (Ed.), *Research to practice in mental retardation* (Vol. 1, pp. 119–127). Baltimore: University Park Press.

Garber, J., Zeman, J., & Walker, L. (1988, October). *Recurrent abdominal pain in children: "Masked" anxiety?* Paper presented at the Annual Meeting of American Academy of Child and Adolescent Psychiatry, Seattle, WA.

Garber, J., Zeman, J., & Walker, L. S. (1990). Recurrent abdominal pain in children: Psychiatric diagnoses and parental psychopathology. *Journal of the American Academy of Child and Adolescent Psychiatry, 29,* 648–656.

Garcia, E. E. (1987). Freud's seduction theory. *Psychoanalytic Study of the Child, 42,* 443–468.

Gardner, R. A. (1973). *MBD: The family book about minimal brain dysfunction.* New York: Jason Aronson.

Garfinkel, B. D., Wender, P. H., Sloman, L., & O'Neil, I. (1983). Tricyclic antidepressant and methylphenidate treatment of attention deficit disorder in children. *Journal of the American Academy of Child Psychiatry, 22,* 343–348.

Garfinkel, P. E., Moldofsky, H., & Garner, D. M. (1980). The heterogeneity of anorexia nervosa: Bulimia as a distinct subgroup. *Archives of General Psychiatry, 37,* 1036–1040.

Garmezy, N. (1986). Developmental aspects of children's responses to the stress of separation and loss. In M. Rutter, C. E. Izard, & P. B. Read (Eds.), *Depression in young people* (pp. 297–323). New York: Guilford.

Garmezy, N. (1987). Stress, competence, and development: Continuities in the study of schizophrenic adults, children vulnerable to psychopathology, and the search for stress-resistant children. *American Journal of Orthopsychiatry, 57,* 159–174.

Garmezy, N., & Rutter, M., (Eds.) (1983). *Stress, coping, and development in children.* New York: McGraw-Hill.

Garner, D. M. (1985). Iatrogenesis in anorexia nervosa and bulimia nervosa. *International Journal of Eating Disorders, 4,* 701–726.

Garner, D. M., & Garfinkel, P. E. (1980). Socio-cultural factors in the development of anorexia nervosa. *Psychological Medicine, 10,* 647–656.

Garner, D. M., Garfinkel, P. E., & Olmsted, M. P. (1983a). An overview of the sociocultural factors in the development of anorexia nervosa. In P. L. Darby, P. E. Garfinkel, & D. M. Garner (Eds.), *Anorexia nervosa: Recent developments in research* (pp. 65–82). New York: Alan R. Liss.

Garner, D. M., Garfinkel, P. E., Schwartz, D., & Thompson, M. (1980). Cultural expectations of thinness in women. *Psychological Reports, 47,* 483–491.

Garner, D. M., Olmsted, M. P., & Polivy, J. (1983b). Development and validation of a multidimensional eating disorder inventory for anorexia nervosa and bulimia. *International Journal of Eating Disorders, 2,* 15–33.

Garner, D. M., Olmsted, M. P., Polivy, J., & Garfinkel, P. E. (1984). Comparison between weight-preoccupied women and anorexia nervosa. *Psychosomatic Medicine, 46,* 255–266.

Gauthier, Y., Fortin, C., Drapeau, P., Breton, J.-J., Gosselin, J., Quintal, L., Weisnagel, J., & Lamarre, A. (1978). Follow-up study of 35 asthmatic preschool children. *Journal of the American Academy of Child Psychiatry, 17,* 679–694.

Gauthier, Y., Fortin, C., Drapeau, P., Breton, J.-J., Gosselin, J., Quintal, L., Weisnagel, J., Tetreault, L., & Pinard, G. (1977). The mother–child relationship and the development of autonomy and self-assertion in young (14–30 months) asthmatic children. *Journal of the American Academy of Child Psychiatry, 16,* 109–131.

Gayford, J. J. (1975). Wife battering: A preliminary survey of 100 cases. *British Medical Journal, 1,* 194–197.

Geleerd, E. R. (1958). Borderline states in childhood and adolescence. *The Psychoanalytic Study of the Child, 13,* 279–295.

Geller, B., Chestnut, E. C., Miller, M. D., Price, D. T., & Yates, E. (1985). Preliminary data on DSM-III associated features of major depressive disorder in children and adolescents. *American Journal of Psychiatry, 142,* 643–644.

Gelles, R. J. (1973). Child abuse as psychopathology: A sociological critique and reformulation. *American Journal of Orthopsychiatry, 43,* 611–621.

Gelles, R. J. (1978). Violence toward children in the United States. *American Journal of Orthopsychiatry, 48,* 580–592.

Gelles, R. J. (1982). Child abuse and family violence: Implications for medical professionals. In E. H. Newberger (Ed.), *Child abuse* (pp. 25–41). Boston: Little, Brown.

George, C., & Main, M. (1979). Social interactions of young abused children: Approach, avoidance, and aggression. *Child Development, 50,* 306–318.

George, D. T., Weiss, S. R., & Jimerson, D. C. (1985). Clinical characteristics of normal weight bulimia. In W. H. Kaye & H. E. Gwirtsman (Eds.), *The treatment of normal weight bulimia* (pp. 1–18). Washington, DC: American Psychiatric Press.

Gerald, P. S., & Meryash, D. L. (1983). Chromosomal disorders other than Down syndrome. In M. D. Levine, W. B. Carey, A. C. Crocker, & R. T. Gross (Eds.), *Developmental-behavioral pediatrics* (pp. 346–353). Philadelphia: Saunders.

Gerbner, G., Ross, C., & Zigler, E. (1980). *Child abuse: An agenda for action.* New York: Oxford University Press.

Gershon, E. S., Hamovit, J., Guroff, J. J., Dibble, E., Leckman, J. F., Sceery, W., Targum, S. D., Nurnberger, J. I., Jr., Goldin, L. R., & Bunney, W. E., Jr. (1982). A family study of schizoaffective, bipolar I, bipolar II, unipolar, and normal control probands. *Archives of General Psychiatry, 39,* 1157–1167.

Gershon, E. S., Hamovit, J. R., Schreiber, J. L., Dibble, E. D., Kaye, W., Nurnberger, J. I., Andersen, A., & Ebert, M. (1983). Anorexia and major affective disorders associated in families: A preliminary report. In S. B. Guze, F. J. Earls, & J. E. Barrett (Eds.), *Childhood psychopathology and development* (pp. 279–286). New York: Raven Press.

Geschwind, N., & Galaburda, A. M. (1985). Cerebral lateralization. Biological mechanisms, associations, and pathology: I. A hypothesis and a program for research. *Archives of Neurology, 42,* 428–459.

Gesell, A., & Amatruda, C. S. (1941). *Developmental diagnosis.* New York: Paul B. Hoeber.

Giarretto, H. (1981). A comprehensive child sexual abuse treatment program. In P. B. Mrazek & C. H. Kempe (Eds.), *Sexually abused children and their families* (pp. 179–198). Oxford: Pergamon.

Gil, D. G. (1970). *Violence against children.* Cambridge, MA: Harvard University Press.

Gillberg, C., Persson, E., Grufman, M., & Themner, U. (1986). Psychiatric disorders in mildly and severely mentally retarded urban children and adolescents: epidemiological aspects. *British Journal of Psychiatry, 149,* 68–74.

Gillberg, C., & Svennerholm, L. (1987). CSF monoamines in autistic syndromes and other pervasive developmental disorders of early childhood. *British Journal of Psychiatry, 151,* 89–94.

Gillberg, C., Svennerholm, L., & Hamilton-Hellberg, C. (1983). Childhood psychosis and monoamine metabolites in spinal fluid. *Journal of Autism and Developmental Disorders, 13,* 383–396.

Gillberg, C., Wahlstrom, J., Forsman, A., Hellgren, L., & Gillberg, I. C. (1986). Teenage psychoses: epidemiology, classification and reduced optimality in the pre-, peri- and neonatal periods. *Journal of Child Psychology and Psychiatry, 27,* 87–98.

Gilles de la Tourette, G. (1982). Study of a neurologic condition characterized by motor incoordination accompanied by echolalia and coprolalia (C. G. Goetz & H. L. Klawans, Trans.). In A. J. Friedhoff & T. N. Chase (Eds.), *Gilles de la Tourette syndrome.* New York: Raven Press. (Original work published 1885)

Gilpin, D. C., Raza, S., & Gilpin, D. (1979). Transsexual symptoms in a male child treated by a female therapist. *American Journal of Psychotherapy, 33,* 453–463.

Gittelman, R. (1983a). Hyperkinetic syndrome: Treatment issues and principles. In M. Rutter (Ed.), *Developmental neuropsychiatry* (pp. 437–449). New York: Guilford.

Gittelman, R. (1983b). Treatment of reading disorders. In M. Rutter (Ed.), *Developmental neuropsychiatry* (pp. 520–541). New York: Guilford.

Gittelman, R. (1985). Controlled trials of remedial approaches to reading disability. *Journal of Child Psychology and Psychiatry, 26,* 843–846.

Gittelman, R. (1986). Childhood anxiety disorders: Correlates and outcome. In R. Gittelman (Ed.), *Anxiety disorders of childhood* (pp. 101–125). New York: Guilford.

Gittelman, R., & Klein, D. F. (1984). Relationship between separation anxiety and panic and agoraphobic disorders. *Psychopathology, 17*(Suppl.), 56–65.

Gittelman, R., & Mannuzza, S. (1985). Diagnosing ADD-H in adolescents. *Psychopharmacology Bulletin, 21,* 237–242.

Gittelman, R., Mannuzza, S., Shenker, R., & Bonagura, N. (1985). Hyperactive boys almost grown up: I. Psychiatric status. *Archives of General Psychiatry, 42,* 937–947.

Gittleman-Klein, R. (1977). Definitional and methodological issues concerning depressive illness in children. In J. G. Schulterbrandt & A. Raskin (Eds.), *Depression in childhood: diagnosis, treatment, and conceptual models* (pp. 69–81). New York: Raven Press.

Gittleman-Klein, R. (1988). Childhood anxiety disorders. In C. J. Kestenbaum & D. T. Williams (Eds.), *Handbook of clinical assessment of children and adolescents* (Vol. 2, pp. 722–742). New York: New York University Press.

Gittelman-Klein, R., & Klein, D. F. (1973). School phobia: Diagnostic considerations in the light of imipramine effects. *Journal of Nervous and Mental Disease, 156,* 199–215.

Gittelman-Klein, R., & Klein, D. F. (1976). Methylphenidate effects in learning disabilities. Psychometric changes. *Archives of General Psychiatry, 33,* 655–664.

Gittelman-Klein, R., & Klein, D. F. (1980). Separation anxiety in school refusal and its treatment with drugs. In L. Hersov & I. Berg (Eds.), *Out of school: Modern perspectives in school refusal and truancy* (pp. 321–341). Chichester: Wiley.

Gittelman-Klein, R., Klein, D. F., Katz, S., Saraf, K., & Pollack, E. (1976). Comparative effects of methylphenidate and thioridazine in hyperkinetic children: I. Clinical results. *Archives of General Psychiatry, 33,* 1217–1231.

Glasberg, R., & Aboud, F. E. (1982). Keeping one's distance from sadness: Children's self-reports of emotional experience. *Developmental Psychology, 18,* 287–293.

Glaser, D., & Collins, C. (1989). The response of young, nonsexually abused children to anatomically correct dolls. *Journal of Child Psychology and Psychiatry, 30,* 547–560.

Glaser, H. H., Heagarty, M. C., Bullard, D. M., Jr., & Pivchik, E. C. (1968). Physical and psychological development of children with early failure to thrive. *Journal of Pediatrics, 73,* 690–698.

Gleuck, S., & Gleuck, E. (1950). *Unravelling juvenile delinquency.* Cambridge, MA: Harvard University Press.

Gloor, P., Olivier, A., Quesney, L. F., Andermann, F., & Horowitz, S. (1982). The role of the limbic system in experiential phenomena of temporal lobe epilepsy. *Annals of Neurology, 12,* 129–144.

Glosser, G., & Koppell, S. (1987). Emotional-behavioral patterns in children with learning disabilities: Lateralized hemispheric differences. *Journal of Learning Disabilities, 20,* 365–368.

Glow, R. A. (n.d.). *Children's behavior problems.* Unpublished monograph.

Goetz, C. G., Tanner, C. M., Wilson, R. S., Carroll, V. S., Como, P. G., & Shannon, K. M. (1987). Clonidine and Gilles de la Tourette syndrome: Double-blind study using objective rating methods. *Annals of Neurology, 21,* 307–310.

Goetz, P. L., Succop, R. A., Reinhart, J. B., & Miller, A. (1977). Anorexia nervosa in children: A follow-up study. *American Journal of Orthopsychiatry, 47,* 597–603.

Gold, P. W., Goodwin, F. K., & Chrousos, G. P. (1988). Clinical and biochemical manifestations of depression: Relation to the neurobiology of stress (Part Two). *New England Journal of Medicine, 319,* 413–420.

Gold, P. W., Kaye, W., Robertson, G. L., & Ebert, M. (1983). Abnormalities in plasma and cerebrospinal-fluid arginine vasopressin in patients with anorexia nervosa. *New England Journal of Medicine, 308,* 1117–1123.

Goldberg, T. E., Weinberger, D. R., Berman, K. F., Pliskin, N. H., & Podd, M. H. (1987). Further evidence for dementia of the prefrontal type in schizophrenia? *Archives of General Psychiatry, 44,* 1008–1014.

Golden, G. S. (1977). The effect of central nervous system stimulants on Tourette syndrome. *Annals of Neurology, 2,* 69–70.

Golden, G. S. (1984). Psychologic and neuropsychologic aspects of Tourette's syndrome. *Neurology Clinics of North America, 2,* 91–102.

Golden, G. S. (1987). Neurological functioning. In D. J. Cohen & A. M. Donnellan (Eds.), *Handbook of autism and pervasive developmental disorders,* 133–147. New York: Wiley.

Golden, G. S. (1988). The use of stimulants in the treatment of Tourette's syndrome. In D. J. Cohen, R. D. Brunn, & J. F. Leckman (Eds.), *Tourette's syndrome and tic disorders: Clinical understanding and treatment* (pp. 317–325). New York: Wiley.

Goldfarb, W. (1970). Childhood psychosis. In P. H. Mussen (Ed.), *Carmichael's manual of child psychology* (Vol. 2, pp. 765–830). New York: Wiley.

Goldfarb, W. (1974). *Growth and change of schizophrenic children: A longitudinal study.* New York: Wiley.

Goldfarb, W., Meyers, D., Florsheim, J., & Goldfarb, N. (1978). *Psychotic children grown up: A prospective follow-up study in adolescence and adulthood.* New York: Human Sciences Press.

Goldsmith, H. H., & Gottesman, I. I. (1981). Origins of variation in behavioral style: A longitudinal study of temperament in young twins. *Child Development, 52,* 91–103.

Goldstein, J., Freud, A., & Solnit, A. J. (1973). *Beyond the best interests of the child.* New York: Free Press.

Goldstein, J., Freud, A., & Solnit, A. J. (1979). *Before the best interests of the child.* New York: Free Press.

Goldstein, K. (1942). *After-effects of brain injuries in war.* New York: Grune & Stratton.

Goldstein, M. J. (1987a). Psychosocial issues. *Schizophrenia Bulletin, 13,* 157–171.

Goldstein, M. J. (1987b). The UCLA high-risk project. *Schizophrenia Bulletin, 13,* 505–514.

Gomes-Schwartz, B., Horowitz, J. M., & Sauzier, M. (1985). Severity of emotional distress among sexually abused preschool, school-age, and adolescent children. *Hospital Community Psychiatry, 36,* 503–508.

Goodall, J. (1986). *The chimpanzees of Gombe.* Cambridge, MA: Harvard University Press.

Goodman, W. K., Price, L. H., Delgado, P. L., Palumbo, J., Krystal, J. H., Nagy, L. M., Rasmussen, S. A., Heninger, G. R., & Charney, D. S. (1990). Specificity of serotonin reuptake inhibitors in the treatment of obsessive-compulsive disorder: Comparison of fluvoxamine and desipramine. *Archives of General Psychiatry, 47,* 577–585.

Goodman, W. K., Price, L. H., Rasmussen, S. A., Mazure, C., Fleischman, R. L., Hill, C. L., Heninger, G. R., & Charney, D. S. (1989). The Yale-Brown Obsessive Compulsive Scale: I. Development, use, and reliability. *Archives of General Psychiatry, 46,* 1006–1011.

Goodwin, D. W., Guze, S. B., & Robins, E. (1969). Follow-up studies in obsessional neurosis. *Archives of General Psychiatry, 20,* 182–187.

Goodwin, J. (1985). Post-traumatic symptoms in incest victims. In S. Eth & R. S. Pynoos (Eds.), *Post-traumatic stress disorder in children* (pp. 155–168). Washington, DC: American Psychiatric Press.

Goodwin, J. (1987). Developmental impacts of incest. In J. D. Noshpitz (Ed.), *Basic handbook of child psychiatry* (Vol. 5, pp. 103–111). New York: Basic Books.

Goodwin, J., Simms, M., & Bergman, R. (1979). Hysterical seizures: A sequel to incest. *American Journal of Orthopsychiatry, 49,* 698–703.

Goodyer, I. (1981). Hysterical conversion reactions in childhood. *Journal of Child Psychology and Psychiatry, 22,* 179–188.

Gordon, D. A., & Young, R. D. (1976). School phobia: A discussion of etiology, treatment, and evaluation. *Psychological Reports, 39,* 783–804.

Gorenstein, E. E., & Newman, J. P. (1980). Disinhibitory psychopathology: A new perspective and a model for research. *Psychological Review, 87,* 301–315.

Gorman, J. M. (1984). The biology of anxiety. In L. Grinspoon (Ed.), *Psychiatry update* (Vol. 3, pp. 467–482). Washington, DC: American Psychiatric Press.

Gorman, J. M. (1986, May). *Panic disorder: Focus on cardiovascular status.* Paper read at the American Psychiatric Association Annual Meeting, Washington, DC.

Gorman, J. M., Liebowitz, M. R., Fyer, A. J., & Stein, J. (1989). A neuroanatomical hypothesis for panic disorder. *American Journal of Psychiatry, 146,* 148–161.

Gottesman, I. I., & Bertelsen, A. (1989). Confirming unexpressed genotypes for schizophrenia: Risks in the offspring of Fischer's Danish identical and fraternal discordant twins. *Archives of General Psychiatry, 46,* 867–872.

Gottesman, I. I., McGuffin, P., & Farmer, A. E. (1987). Clinical genetics as clues to the "real" genetics of schizophrenia: A decade of modest gains while playing for time. *Schizophrenia Bulletin, 13,* 23–47.

Gottesman, I. I., & Shields, J. (1972). *Schizophrenia and genetics: A twin study vantage point.* New York: Academic.

Gould, M. S., & Shaffer, D. (1986). The impact of suicide in television movies: Evidence of imitation. *New England Journal of Medicine, 315,* 690–694.

Gould, M.S., Wallenstein, S., & Kleinman, M. (1990). Time-space clustering of teenage suicide. *American Journal of Epidemiology, 131,* 71–78.

Gould, R., Miller, B. L., Goldberg, M. A., & Benson, D. F. (1986). The validity of hysterical signs and symptoms. *Journal of Nervous and Mental Disease, 174,* 593–597.

Gould, S. J. (1981). *The mismeasure of man.* New York: Norton.

Goyer, P. F., Davis, G. C., & Rapoport, J. L. (1979). Abuse of prescribed stimulant medication by a 13-year-old hyperactive boy. *Journal of the American Academy of Child Psychiatry, 18,* 170–175.

Goyette, C. H., Conners, C. K., & Ulrich, R. F. (1978). Normative data on revised Conners parent and teacher rating scales. *Journal of Abnormal Child Psychology, 6,* 221–236.

Grad, L. R., Pelcovitz, D., Olson, M., Matthews, M., & Grad, G. J. (1987). Obsessive-compulsive symptomatology in children with Tourette's syndrome. *Journal of the American Academy of Child and Adolescent Psychiatry, 26,* 69–73.

Graham, P. J. (1979). Epidemiologic studies. In H. C. Quay and J. S. Werry, *Psychopathological disorders of childhood* (pp. 185–209). New York: Wiley.

Graham, P. J. (1983). Poisoning in childhood. In M. Rutter (Ed.), *Developmental neuropsychiatry* (pp. 52–67). New York: Guilford.

Graham, P. J., Rutter, M. L., Yule, W., & Pless, I. B. (1967). Childhood asthma: A psychosomatic disorder? Some epidemiological considerations. *British Journal of Preventive and Social Medicine, 21,* 78–85.

Graham, P. J., & Stevenson, J. (1985). A twin study of genetic influences on behavioral deviance. *Journal of the American Academy of Child Psychiatry, 24*(1), 33–41.

Granell de Aldaz, E., Feldman, L., Vivas, E., & Gelfand, D. M. (1987). Characteristics of Venezuelan school refusers: Toward the development of a high-risk profile. *Journal of Nervous and Mental Disease, 175,* 402–407.

Granell de Aldaz, E., Vivas, E., Gelfand, D. M., & Feldman, L. (1984). Estimating the prevalence of school refusal and school-related fears: A Venezuelan sample. *Journal of Nervous and Mental Disease, 172,* 722–729.

Gray, J. A. (1979). Anxiety and the brain: Not by neurochemistry alone. *Psychological Medicine, 9,* 605–609.

Graziano, A. M., DeGiovanni, I. S., & Garcia, K. A. (1979). Behavioral treatment of children's fears: A review. *Psychological Bulletin, 86,* 804–830.

Greco, M. C., & Wright, J. C. (1944). The correctional institution in the etiology of chronic homosexuality. *American Journal of Orthopsychiatry, 14,* 295.

Green, A. H. (1978a). Psychiatric treatment of abused children. *Journal of American Academy of Child Psychiatry, 17,* 356–371.

Green, A. H. (1978b). Psychopathology of abused children. *Journal of American Academy of Child Psychiatry, 17,* 92–103.

Green, A. H. (1978c). Self-destructive behavior in battered children. *American Journal of Psychiatry, 135,* 579–582.

Green, A. H. (1979). Child-abusing fathers. *Journal of American Academy of Child Psychiatry, 18,* 270–282.

Green, A. H. (1980). *Child maltreatment: A handbook for mental health and child care professional.* New York: Jason Aronson.

Green, A. H. (1983). Hospital-based intervention in child abuse. *Resident and Staff Physician, 29,* 76–88.

Green, A. H. (1985). Child abuse and neglect. In D. Shaffer, A. A. Ehrhardt, & L. L. Greenhill (Eds.), *The clinical guide to child psychiatry* (pp. 315–335). New York: Free Press.

Green, A. H. (1986). True and false allegations of sexual abuse in child custody disputes. *Journal of the American Academy of Child Psychiatry, 25,* 449–456.

Green, A. H. (1988). The sex abuse controversy [Letter]. *Journal of the American Academy of Child and Adolescent Psychiatry, 27,* 259.

Green, A. H., Gaines, R. W., & Sandgrund, A. (1974). Child abuse: Pathological syndrome of family interaction. *American Journal of Psychiatry, 131,* 882–886.

Green, A. H., Liang, V., Gaines, R., & Sultan, S. (1980). Psychopathological assessment of child-abusing, neglecting, and normal mothers. *Journal of Nervous and Mental Disease, 168,* 356–360.

Green, A. H., Voeller, K., Gaines, R., & Kubie, J. (1981). Neurological impairment in maltreated children. *Child Abuse and Neglect, 5,* 129–134.

Green, D. (1980). A behavioural approach to the treatment of obsessional rituals: An adolescent case study. *Journal of Adolescence, 3,* 297–306.

Green, M. (1967). Diagnosis and treatment: Psychogenic, recurrent abdominal pain. *Pediatrics, 40,* 84–89.

Green, R. (1969). Childhood cross-gender identification. In R. Green & J. Money (Eds.), *Transsexualism and sex reassignment.* Baltimore: Johns Hopkins Press.

Green, R. (1971). Diagnosis and treatment of gender identity disorders during childhood. *Archives of Sexual Behavior, 1,* 167–173.

Green, R. (1974). *Sexual identity conflict in children and adults.* Baltimore: Penguin.

Green, R. (1975). The significance of feminine behavior in boys [Annotation]. *Journal of Child Psychology and Psychiatry, 16,* 341–344.

Green, R. (1976). One-hundred ten feminine and masculine boys: Behavioral contrasts and demographic similarities. *Archives of Sexual Behavior, 5,* 425–446.

Green, R. (1979). Childhood cross-gender behavior and subsequent sexual preference. *American Journal of Psychiatry, 136,* 106–108.

Green, R. (1987). *The "sissy boy syndrome" and the development of homosexuality.* New Haven: Yale University Press.

Green, R., & Fuller, M. (1973). Group therapy with feminine boys and their parents. *International Journal of Group Psychotherapy, 23,* 54–68.

Green, R., & Money, J. (1960). Incongruous gender role: Nongenital manifestations in prepubertal boys. *Journal of Nervous and Mental Diseases, 130,* 160–168.

Green, R., & Money, J. (1961, February). Effeminacy in prepubertal boys: Summary of eleven cases and recommendations for case management. *Pediatrics,* pp. 286–290.

Green, R., Newman, L., & Stoller, R. (1972). Treatment of boyhood "transsexualism:" An interim report of four years' experience. *Archives of General Psychiatry, 26,* 213–217.

Green, R., & Stoller, R. (1971). Two monozygotic (identical) twin pairs discordant for gender identity. *Archives of Sexual Behavior, 1,* 321–327.

Green, R., Williams, K., & Goodman, K. (1982). Ninety-nine "tomboys" and "nontomboys:" Behavioral contrasts and demographic similarities. *Archives of Sexual Behavior, 11,* 247–266.

Green, W. H. (1986). Psychosocial dwarfism: Psychological and etiological considerations. In B. B. Lahey & A. E. Kazdin (Eds.), *Advances in clinical child psychology* (Vol. 9, pp. 245–278). New York: Plenum.

Green, W. H., Campbell, M., Hardesty, A. S., Grega, D. M., Padron-Gayol, M., Shell, J., & Erlenmeyer-Kimling, L. (1984). A comparison of schizophrenic and autistic children. *Journal of the American Academy of Child and Adolescent Psychiatry, 23,* 399–409.

Green, W. H., & Deutsch, S. I. (1990). Biological studies of schizophrenia with childhood onset. In S. I. Deutsch (Ed.), *Application of basic neuroscience to child psychiatry* (pp. 217–229). New York: Plenum Medical.

Greenbaum, R. S. (1964). Treatment of school phobias: Theory and practice. *American Journal of Psychotherapy, 18,* 616–634.

Greenberg, D., Witztum, E., & Pisante, J. (1987). Scrupulosity: Religious attitudes and clinical presentations. *British Journal of Medical Psychology, 60,* 29–37.

Greenberg, J. R., & Mitchell, S. A. (1983). *Object relations in psychoanalytic theory.* Cambridge, MA: Harvard University Press.

Greenberg, N. H. (1979). The epidemiology of childhood sexual abuse. *Pediatric Annals, 8,* 289–299.

Greenhill, L. L. (1984). Stimulant related growth inhibition in children: A review. In L. L. Greenhill & B. Shopsin (Eds.), *The Psychobiology of Childhood* (pp. 135–157). New York: Spectrum.

Greenman, D. A., Gunderson, J. G., Cane, M., & Saltzman, P. R. (1986). An examination of the borderline diagnosis in children. *American Journal of Psychiatry, 143,* 998–1003.

Greenson, R. (1966). A transvestite boy and a hypothesis. *International Journal of Psychoanalysis, 47,* 396–403.

Greenspan, S. I. (1981). *Psychopathology and adaptation in infancy and early childhood.* New York: International Universities Press.

Greenspan, S. I., & Lourie, R. S. (1981). Developmental structuralist approach to classification of adaptive and pathologic personality organizations: Infancy and early childhood. *American Journal of Psychiatry, 138,* 725–735.

Gross, M. (1979). Pseudoepilepsy: A study in adolescent hysteria. *American Journal of Psychiatry, 136,* 210–213.

Gross, R. T., & Dornbusch, S. M. (1983). Enuresis. In M. D. Levine, W. B. Carey, A. C. Crocker, & R. T. Gross (Eds.), *Developmental-Behavioral Pediatrics* (pp. 573–586). Philadelphia: Saunders.

Grossman, H. J. (Ed.) (1983). *Classification in mental retardation.* Washington, DC: American Association on Mental Deficiency.

Groth, A. N. (1982). The incest offender. In S. M. Sgroi (Ed.), *Handbook of clinical intervention in child sexual abuse* (pp. 215–239). Lexington, MA: Lexington Books.

Group for the Advancement of Psychiatry, Committee on Child Psychiatry. (1966). *Psychopathological disorders of childhood: Theoretical considerations and a proposed classification* (Vol. 6, Report No. 62). New York: GAP.

Groves, J. E. (1981). Current concepts in psychiatry: Borderline personality disorder. *New England Journal of Medicine, 305,* 259–262.

Gualtieri, C. T., & Hicks, R. E. (1985). Neuropharmacology of methylphenidate and a neural substrate for childhood hyperactivity. *The Psychiatric Clinics of North America, 8,* 875–892.

Gualtieri, C. T., Quade, D., Hicks, R. E., Mayo, J. P., and Schroeder, S. R. (1984). Tardive dyskinesia and other clinical consequences of neuroleptic treatment in children and adolescents. *American Journal of Psychiatry, 141*, 20–23.

Gualtieri, C. T., & Van Bourgondien, M. E. (1987). So-called borderline children [Letter]. *American Journal of Psychiatry, 144*, 832.

Gualtieri, C. T., Wargin, W., Kanoy, R., Patrick, K., Shen, C. D., Youngblood, W., Mueller, R. A., & Breese, G. R. (1982). Clinical studies of methylphenidate serum levels in children and adults. *Journal of the American Academy of Child Psychiatry, 21*, 19–26.

Gunderson, J. G. (1984). *Borderline personality disorder.* Washington, DC: American Psychiatric Press.

Gunderson, J. G., & Elliott, G. R. (1985). The interface between borderline personality disorder and affective disorder. *American Journal of Psychiatry, 142*, 277–288.

Gunderson, J. G., Kerr, J., & Englund, D. W. (1980). The families of borderlines. *Archives of General Psychiatry, 37*, 27–33.

Gunderson, J. G., & Siever, L. J. (1985). Relatedness of schizotypal to schizophrenic disorders. *Schizophrenia Bulletin, 11*, 532–537.

Gunderson, J. G., & Singer, M. T. (1975). Defining borderline patients: An overview. *American Journal of Psychiatry, 132*, 1–10.

Gunderson, J. G., & Zanarini, M. C. (1987). Current overview of the borderline diagnosis. *Journal of Clinical Psychiatry, 48*(8, Suppl.), 5–11.

Gunn, P., Berry, P., & Andrews, R. J. (1981). The temperament of Down's syndrome infants: A research note. *Journal of Child Psychology and Psychiatry, 22*, 189–194.

Guth, D. L. (Ed.). (1976). *Letters of E. B. White.* New York: Harper & Row.

Gwirtsman, H. E., Roy-Byrne, P., Yager, J., & Gerner, R. H. (1983). Neuroendocrine abnormalities in bulimia. *American Journal of Psychiatry, 140*, 559–563.

Haber, S. N., Kowall, N. W., Vonsattel, J. P., Bird, E. D., & Richardson, E. P. (1986). Gilles de la Tourette's syndrome: A postmortem and neurohistochemical study. *Journal of Neurological Sciences, 75*, 225–241.

Haggerty, R. J. (1980). Life stress, illness and social supports. *Developmental Medicine and Child Neurology, 22*, 391–400.

Hagin, R. A., & Kugler, J. (1988). School problems associated with Tourette's syndrome. In D. J. Cohen, R. D. Brunn, & J. F. Leckman (Eds.), *Tourette's syndrome and tic disorders: Clinical understanding and treatment* (pp. 223–236). New York: Wiley.

Hahn, W. (1966). Autonomic responses of asthmatic children. *Psychosomatic Medicine, 28*, 323–332.

Hallgren, B. (1956). Enuresis. A study with references to certain physical, mental, and social factors possibly associated with enuresis. *Acta Psychiatrica et Neurologica Scandinavica, 31*, 405–436.

Halmi, K. A. (1974). Anorexia nervosa: Demographic and clinical features in 94 cases. *Psychosomatic Medicine, 36*, 18–26.

Halmi, K. A. (1985a). The diagnosis and treatment of anorexia nervosa. In D. Shaffer, A. A. Ehrhardt, & L. L. Greenhill (Eds.), *The clinical guide to child psychiatry* (pp. 218–228). New York: Free Press.

Halmi, K. A. (1985b). Medical aberrations in bulimia nervosa. In W. H. Kaye & H. E. Gwirtsman (Eds.), *The treatment of normal weight bulimia* (pp. 37–46). Washington, DC: American Psychiatric Press.

Halmi, K. A., Eckert, E., LaDu, T. J., & Cohen, J. (1986). Anorexia nervosa: Treatment efficacy of cyproheptadine and amitriptyline. *Archives of General Psychiatry, 43,* 177–181.

Halmi, K. A., Falk, J. R., & Schwartz, E. (1981). Binge eating and vomiting: A survey of a college population. *Psychological Medicine, 11,* 697–706.

Halperin, J. M., Gittelman, R., Katz, S., & Struve, F. A. (1986). Relationship between stimulant effect, electroencephalogram, and clinical neurological findings in hyperactive children. *Journal of the American Academy of Child Psychiatry, 25,* 820–825.

Halperin, J. M., Gittelman, R., Klein, D. F., & Rudel, R. G. (1984). Reading disabled hyperactive children: A distinct subgroup of attention deficit disorder with hyperactivity? *Journal of Abnormal Child Psychology, 12,* 1–14.

Halverson, C. F., & Waldrop, M. F. (1976). Relations between preschool activity and aspects of intellectual and social behavior at age 7+. *Developmental Psychology, 12,* 107–112.

Hammer, H. M. (1967). Astasia-Abasia: A report of two cases at West Point. *American Journal of Psychiatry, 124,* 671–674.

Handford, H. A., Mattison, R., Humphrey, II, F. J., & McLaughlin, R. E. (1986). Depressive syndrome in children entering a residential school subsequent to parent death, divorce, or separation. *Journal of the American Academy of Child Psychiatry, 25,* 409–414.

Hannaway, P. (1970). Failure to thrive: A study of 100 infants and children. *Clinical Pediatrics, 9,* 96–99.

Hansen, C. R., & Cohen, D. J. (1984). Multimodality approaches in the treatment of attention deficit disorders. *Pediatric Clinics of North America, 31,* 499–513.

Hanson, D. R., & Gottesman, I. I. (1976). The genetics, if any, of infantile autism and childhood schizophrenia. *Journal of Autism and Childhood Schizophrenia, 6,* 209–234.

Hanson, G. (1988). The sex abuse controversy [Letter]. *Journal of the American Academy of Child and Adolescent Psychiatry, 27,* 258.

Harder, D. W., Kokes, R. F., Fisher, L., & Strauss, J. S. (1980). Child competence and psychiatric risk. IV. Relationship of parent diagnostic classification and parent psychopathology severity to child functioning. *Journal of Nervous and Mental Disorders, 168,* 343–347.

Harkavy Friedman, J. M., Asnis, G. M., Boeck, M., DiFiore, J. (1987). Prevalence of specific suicidal behaviors in a high school sample. *American Journal of Psychiatry, 144,* 1203–1212.

Harley, J. P., Matthews, C. G., & Eichman, P. (1978). Synthetic food colors and hyperactivity in children: A double-blind challenge experiment. *Pediatrics, 62,* 975–983.

Harlow, H. F. (1961). The development of affectional patterns in infant monkeys. In B. M. Foss (Ed.), *Determinants of infant behavior* (pp. 75–88). New York: Wiley.

Harmon, R. J., Wagonfeld, S., & Emde, R. N. (1982). Anaclitic depression: A follow-up from infancy to puberty. *Psychoanalytic Study of the Child, 37,* 67–94.

Harris, E. L., Noyes, R., Jr., Crowe, R. R., & Chaudhry, S. R. (1983). Family study of agoraphobia. *Archives of General Psychiatry, 40,* 1061–1064.

Harris, G., & Levine, S. (1962). Sexual differentiation of the brain and its experimental control. *Journal of Physiology, 163,* 42P–43P.

Hartnell, L. (1987). Post-viral fatigue syndrome: A canker in my brain. *Lancet, 1,* 910.

Havens, L. (1973). *Approaches to the mind.* Boston: Little, Brown.

Havighurst, R. J., & Davis, A. (1955). A comparison of the Chicago and Harvard studies of social class differences in child rearing. *American Sociological Review, 20,* 438–442.

Hay, G. G., & Leonard, J. C. (1979). Anorexia nervosa in males. *Lancet, 2,* 574–575.

Hay, W. M., Barlow, D. H., & Hay, L. R. (1981). Treatment of stereotypic cross-gender motor behavior using covert modeling in a boy with gender identity confusion. *Journal of Consulting and Clinical Psychology, 49,* 388–394.

Haynes, C. F., Cutler, C., Gray, J., & Kempe, R. S. (1984). Hospitalized cases of nonorganic failure to thrive: The scope of the problem and short-term lay health visitor intervention. *Child Abuse and Neglect, 8,* 229–242.

Haynes, C. F., Cutler, C., Gray, J., O'Keefe, K., & Kempe, R. S. (1983). Non-organic failure to thrive: Decision for placement and videotaped evaluations. *Child Abuse and Neglect, 7,* 309–319.

Hayward, C., Killen, J. D., & Taylor, C. B. (1989). Panic attacks in young adolescents. *American Journal of Psychiatry, 146,* 1061–1062.

Heal, L. W., Sigelman, C. K., & Switzky, H. N. (1978). Research on community residential alternatives for the mentally retarded. In N. R. Ellis (Ed.), *International review of research in mental retardation* (Vol. 9, pp. 209–249). New York: Academic.

Hechtman, L., Weiss, G., Perlman, T., & Amsel, R. (1984). Hyperactives as young adults: Initial predictors of adult outcome. *Journal of the American Academy of Child Psychiatry, 23,* 250–260.

Hechtman, L., Weiss, G., Perlman, T., & Tuck, D. (1981). Hyperactives as young adults: Various clinical outcomes. *Adolescent Psychiatry, 9,* 295–306.

Heimlich, E. P. (1972). Paraverbal techniques in the therapy of childhood communication disorders. *International Journal of Child Psychotherapy, 1,* 65–83.

Heins, M. (1984). The "battered child" revisited. *Journal of the American Medical Association, 251,* 3295–3300.

Heisel, J. S., Ream, S., Raitz, R., Rappaport, M., & Coddington, R. D. (1973). The significance of life events as contributing factors in the diseases of children. *Journal of Pediatrics, 83,* 119–123.

Hellgren, L., Gillberg, C., & Enerskog, I. (1987). Antecedents of adolescent psychoses: A population-based study of school health problems in children who develop psychosis in adolescence. *Journal of the American Academy of Child and Adolescent Psychiatry, 26,* 351–355.

Hellman, D., & Blackman, N. (1966). Enuresis, firesetting, and cruelty to animals: A triad predictive of adult crime. *American Journal of Psychiatry, 122,* 1431–1435.

Hendren, R. L., Barber, J. K., & Sigafoos, A. (1986). Eating-disordered symptoms in a nonclinical population: A study of female adolescents in two private schools. *Journal of the American Academy of Child Psychiatry, 25,* 836–840.

Herman, B. H., Hammock, M. K., Arthur-Smith, A., Egan, J., Chatoor, I., Zelnik, N., Corradine, M., Appelgate, K., Boeckx, R. L., & Sharp, S. D. (1986). Role of opioid peptides in autism: Effects of acute administration of naltrexone. *Society for Neuroscience Abstracts, 12,* 468.

Herman, B. H., & Panksepp, J. (1981). Ascending endorphin inhibition of distress vocalization. *Science, 211,* 1060–1062.

Herman, J. L. (1981). *Father–daughter incest.* Cambridge: Harvard University Press.

Herman, J., & Hirschman, L. (1981). Families at risk for father–daughter incest. *American Journal of Psychiatry, 138,* 967–970.

Herman, S. P., Stickler, G. B., & Lucas, A. R. (1981). Hyperventilation syndrome in children and adolescents: Long-term follow-up. *Pediatrics, 67,* 183–187.

Herrenkohl, E. C., & Herrenkohl, R. C. (1979). A comparison of abused children and their nonabused siblings. *Journal of the American Academy of Child Psychiatry, 18,* 260–269.

Herrenkohl, E. C., Herrenkohl, R. C., Toedter, L., & Yanushefski, A. M. (1984). Parent–child interactions in abusive and nonabusive families. *Journal of the American Academy of Child Psychiatry, 23,* 641–648.

Herrenkohl, R. C., Herrenkohl, E. C., & Egolf, B. P. (1983). Circumstances surrounding the occurrence of child maltreatment. *Journal of Consulting and Clinical Psychology, 51,* 424–431.

Hersen, M. (1971). The behavioral treatment of school phobia: Current techniques. *Journal of Nervous and Mental Disease, 153,* 99–107.

Hersov, L. A. (1960a). Persistent non-attendance at school. *Journal of Child Psychology and Psychiatry, 1,* 130–136.

Hersov, L. A. (1960b). Refusal to go to school. *Journal of Child Psychology and Psychiatry, 1,* 137–145.

Hersov, L. A. (1980). Hospital in-patient and day-patient treatment of school refusal. In L. Hersov & I. Berg (Eds.), *Out of school: Modern perspectives in school refusal and truancy* (pp. 303–320). Chichester: Wiley.

Hersov, L. A. (1985a). Faecal soiling. In M. Rutter & L. Hersov (Eds.), *Child and adolescent psychiatry: Modern approaches* (2nd ed.). Oxford: Blackwell.

Hersov, L. A. (1985b). School refusal. In M. Rutter & L. Hersov (Eds.), *Child and adolescent psychiatry* (2nd ed., pp. 382–399). Oxford: Blackwell.

Hersov, L. A., & Berg, I. (1980). *Out of school: Modern perspectives in school refusal and truancy.* Chichester: Wiley.

Herzog, D. B. (1987). *Advances in psychiatry: Focus on eating disorders.* New York: Park Row (Wiley).

Herzog, D. B., & Copeland, P. M. (1988). Bulimia nervosa: psyche and satiety. *The New England Journal of Medicine, 319,* 716–718.

Herzog, D. B., Keller, M. B., & Lavori, P. W. (1988a). Outcome in anorexia nervosa and bulimia nervosa: A review of the literature. *The Journal of Nervous and Mental Disease, 176,* 131–143.

Herzog, D. B., Keller, M. B., Lavori, P. W., & Ott, I. L. (1988b). Short-term prospective study of recovery in bulimia nervosa. *Psychiatry Research, 23,* 45–55.

Hetherington, E. M., & Brackbill, Y. (1963). Etiology and covariation of obstinacy, orderliness, and parsimony in young children. *Child Development, 34,* 919–943.

Hibbert, G. A. (1984). Ideational components of anxiety: Their origin and content. *British Journal of Psychiatry, 144,* 618–624.

Higgins, J. (1976). Effects of child rearing by schizophrenic mothers: A follow-up. *Journal of Psychiatric Research, 13,* 1–9.

Hinde, R. A. (1970). *Animal behavior: A synthesis of ethology and comparative psychology* (2nd ed.). New York: McGraw-Hill.

Hiscock, M., & Kinsbourne, M. (1987). Specialization of the cerebral hemispheres: Implications for learning. *Journal of Learning Disabilities, 20,* 130–143.

Hoag, J. M., Norriss, N. G., Himeno, E. T., & Jacobs, J. (1971). The encopretic child and his family. *Journal of the American Academy of Child Psychiatry, 10,* 242–256.

Hoberman, H. M., & Garfinkel, B. D. (1988). Completed suicide in children and adolescents. *Journal of the American Academy of Child and Adolescent Psychiatry, 27,* 689–695.

Hobson, R. P. (1986a). The autistic child's appraisal of expressions of emotion. *Journal of Child Psychology and Psychiatry, 27,* 321–342.

Hobson, R. P. (1986b). The autistic child's appraisal of expressions of emotion: A further study. *Journal of Child Psychology and Psychiatry, 27,* 671–680.

Hobson, R. P. (1989). On sharing experiences. *Development and Psychopathology, 1,* 197–203.

Hoch, P. H., & Cattell, J. P. (1959). The diagnosis of pseudoneurotic schizophrenia. *Psychiatric Quarterly, 33,* 17–43.

Hodges, K., Kline, J. J., Barbero, G., & Flanery, R. (1985). Depressive symptoms in children with recurrent abdominal pain and in their families. *Journal of Pediatrics, 107,* 622–626.

Hodgkinson, S., Sherrington, R., Gurling, H., Marchbanks, R., Reeders, S., Mallet, J., McInnis, M., Petursson, H., & Brynjolfsson, J. (1987). Molecular genetic evidence for heterogeneity in manic depression. *Nature, 325,* 805–806.

Hoehn-Saric, R. (1982). Neurotransmitters in anxiety. *Archives of General Psychiatry, 39,* 735–742.

Hoehn-Saric, R., & Barksdale, V. C. (1983). Impulsiveness in obsessive-compulsive patients. *British Journal of Psychiatry, 143,* 177–182.

Hoenig, J., & Kenna, J. C. (1974). The prevalence of transsexualism in England and Wales. *British Journal of Psychiatry, 124,* 181–190.

Hofer, M. A., Wolff, C. T., Friedman, S. B., & Mason, J. W. (1972a). A psychoendocrine study of bereavement: Part I. *Psychosomatic Medicine, 34,* 481–491.

Hofer, M. A., Wolff, C. T., Friedman, S. B., and Mason, J. W. (1972b). A psychoendocrine study of bereavement: Part II. *Psychosomatic Medicine, 34,* 492–504.

Hoffman, H. (1845). *Struwwelpeter*. London: Routledge & Kegan Paul. (undated English translation)

Hohman, L. B. (1922). Post-encephalitic behavior disorders in children. *Johns Hopkins Hospital Bulletin, 33*, 372–375.

Holden, C., Head Start enters adulthood. *Science, 247*, 1400–1402.

Holemon, R. E., & Winokur, G. (1965). Effeminate homosexuality: A disease of childhood. *American Journal of Orthopsychiatry, 35*, 48–56.

Holinger, P. C., Offer, D., & Ostrov, E. (1987). Suicide and homicide in the United States: An epidemiologic study of violent death, population changes, and the potential for prediction. *American Journal of Psychiatry, 144*, 215–219.

Holland, A. J., Hall, A., Murray, R., Russell, G. F. M., & Crisp, A. H. (1984). Anorexia nervosa: A study of 34 twin pairs and one set of triplets. *British Journal of Psychiatry, 145*, 414–419.

Hollender, M. H. (1972). Conversion hysteria. A post-Freudian reinterpretation of 19th century psychosocial data. *Archives of General Psychiatry, 26*, 311–314.

Hollingsworth, C. E., Tanguay, P. E., Grossman, L., & Pabst, P. (1980). Long-term outcome of obsessive-compulsive disorder in children. *Journal of American Academy of Child Psychiatry, 19*, 134–144.

Holman, M. L. (1983). A study of recidivism in child abuse and neglect. *Clinical Proceedings Children's Hospital National Medical Center, 39*, 100–107.

Holmes, G. L., Sackellares, J. C., McKiernan, J., Ragland, M., & Dreifuss, F. E. (1980). Evaluation of childhood pseudoseizures using EEG telemetry and video tape monitoring. *Journal of Pediatrics, 97*, 554–558.

Holmes, T. H., & Masuda, M. (1974). Life change and illness susceptibility. In B. S. Dohrenwend & B. P. Dohrenwend (Eds.), *Stressful life events: Their nature and effects* (pp. 45–72). New York: Wiley.

Holstrom, D. (1983, November 2). Firemen's companionship keeps boys from becoming fire-setters. *The Christian Science Monitor*, p. 7.

Holter, J. C., & Friedman, S. B. (1968). Child abuse: Early case finding in the emergency department. *Pediatrics, 42*, 128–138.

Holzman, P. S. (1986). Thought disorder in schizophrenia: Editor's introduction. *Schizophrenia Bulletin, 12*, 342–346.

Holzman, P. S., & Grinker, R. R., Sr. (1977). Schizophrenia in adolescence. *Adolescent Psychiatry, 5*, 276–290.

Hoover, C. F., & Insel, T. R. (1984). Families of origin in obsessive-compulsive disorder. *Journal of Nervous and Mental Disease, 172*, 207–215.

Horn, J. M., Loehlin, J. C., & Willerman, L. (1979). Intellectual resemblance among adoptive and biological relatives: The Texas adoption project. *Behavior Genetics, 9*, 177–207.

Horn, W. F., Chatoor, I., & Conners, C. K. (1983). Additive effects of dexedrine and self-control training: A multiple assessment. *Behavior Modification, 7*, 383–402.

Horowitz, M. J., Wilner, N., Marmar, C., & Krupnick, J. (1980). Pathological grief and the activation of latent self-images. *American Journal of Psychiatry, 137*, 1157–1162.

Horwood, L. J., Fergusson, D. M., Hons, B. A., & Shannon, F. T. (1985). Social and familial factors in the development of early childhood asthma. *Pediatrics, 75,* 859–868.

Howells, J. G., & Guirguis, W. R. (1984). Childhood schizophrenia 20 years later. *Archives of General Psychiatry, 41,* 123–128.

Howells, K. (1981). Adult sexual interest in children: Considerations relevant to theories of aetiology. In M. Cook & K. Howells (Eds.), *Adult Sexual Interest in Children* (pp. 55–94). New York: Academic.

Hsu, L. K. G. (1980). Outcome of anorexia nervosa: A review of the literature (1954 to 1978). *Archives of General Psychiatry, 37,* 1041–1046.

Hsu, L. K. G. (1987). An overview of the eating disorders. In J. D. Noshpitz (Ed.), *Basic handbook of child psychiatry* (Vol. 5, pp. 374–388). New York: Basic Books.

Hsu, L. K. G., Crisp, A. H., & Harding, B. (1979). Outcome of anorexia nervosa. *Lancet, 1,* 61–65.

Hsu, L. K. G., Milliones, J., Friedman, L., Holder, D., & Klepper, T. (1982, October). *A survey of eating attitudes and behavior in adolescents.* Paper presented at the 25th annual meeting of the American Academy of Child Psychiatry, Washington, DC.

Hudson, J. I., Laffer, P. S., & Pope, H. G., Jr. (1982). Bulimia related to affective disorder by family history and response to dexamethasone suppression test. *American Journal of Psychiatry, 139,* 685–687.

Hudson, J. I., & Pope, H. G., Jr. (1987). *The psychobiology of bulimia.* Washington, DC: American Psychiatric Press.

Hudson, J. I., Pope, H. G., Jr., Jonas, J. M., & Yurgelun-Todd, D. (1983). Phenomenologic relationship of eating disorders to major affective disorder. *Psychiatry Research, 9,* 345–354.

Huenemann, R. L., Shapiro, L. R., Hampton, M. C., & Mitchell, B. W. (1966). A longitudinal study of gross body composition and body conformation and their association with food and activity in a teenage population. *American Journal of Clinical Nutrition, 18,* 325–338.

Huessy, H. R. (1984). Remarks on the epidemiology of MBD/ADD. In L. M. Bloomingdale (Ed.), *Attention deficit disorder: Diagnostic, cognitive, and therapeutic understanding* (pp. 1–9). New York: SP Medical and Scientific Books.

Hufton, I. W., & Oates, R. K. (1977). Nonorganic failure to thrive: A long-term follow-up. *Pediatrics, 59,* 73–77.

Hughes, M. C. (1984). Recurrent abdominal pain and childhood depression: Clinical observations of 23 children and their families. *American Journal of Orthopsychiatry, 54,* 146–155.

Hughes, P. L., Wells, L. A., Cunningham, C. J., & Ilstrup, D. M. (1986). Treating bulimia with desipramine. *Archives of General Psychiatry, 43,* 182–186.

Humphrey, L. L. (1987). Comparison of bulimic-anorexic and nondistressed families using structural analysis of social behavior. *Journal of the American Academy of Child and Adolescent Psychiatry, 26,* 248–255.

Humphrey, L. L. (1988). Relationships within subtypes of anorexics, bulimics, and normal families. *Journal of the American Academy of Child and Adolescent Psychiatry, 27,* 544–551.

Hunt, R. D., Minderaa, R., & Cohen, D. J. (1985). Clonidine benefits children with attention deficit disorder and hyperactivity: Report of a double-blind placebo crossover therapeutic trial. *Journal of the American Academy of Child Psychiatry, 24,* 617–629.

Hurst, M. W., Jenkins, C. D., & Rose, R. M. (1978). The assessment of life change stress: A comparative and methodological inquiry. *Psychosomatic Medicine, 40,* 126–141.

Huschka, M. (1942). The child's response to coercive bowel training. *Psychosomatic Medicine, 4,* 301–308.

Huston, A. C. (1983). Sex-typing. In P. H. Mussen (Ed.), *Handbook of child psychology* (Vol. 4, pp. 387–467). New York: Wiley.

Hutchings, B., & Mednick, S. (1974). Registered criminality in the adoptive and biologic parents of registered male adoptees. In S. A. Mednick, S. Schulsinger, & F. Higgins (Eds.), *Genetics, environment and psychopathology.* Amsterdam: North Holland.

Hyman, I. A., & Wise, J. H. (1979). *Corporal punishment in American education: Readings in history, practice, and alternatives.* Philadelphia: Temple Press.

Imperato-McGinley, J., Peterson, R. E., Gautier, T., & Sturla, E. (1979). Male pseudohermaphroditism secondary to 5α-reductase deficiency: A model for the role of androgens in both the development of the male phenotype and the evolution of a male gender identity. *Journal of Steroid Biochemistry, 11,* 637–645.

Ingraham v. Wright. 430 U.S. 651 (1977).

Insel, T. R. (1984). Obsessive-compulsive disorder: The clinical picture. In T. R. Insel (Ed.), *Obsessive-compulsive disorder* (pp. 1–22). Washington, DC: American Psychiatric Press.

Insel, T. R., Hoover, C., & Murphy, D. L. (1983a). Parents of patients with obsessive-compulsive disorder. *Psychological Medicine, 13,* 807–811.

Insel, T. R., & Mueller, E. A. (1984). The psychopharmacologic treatment of obsessive-compulsive disorder. In T. R. Insel (Ed.), *Obsessive-compulsive disorder* (pp. 72–88). Washington, DC: American Psychiatric Press.

Insel, T. R., Murphy, D. L., Cohen, R. M., Alterman, I., Kilts, C., & Linnoila, M. (1983b). Obsessive-compulsive disorder: A double-blind trial of clomipramine and clorgyline. *Archives of General Psychiatry, 40,* 605–612.

Insel, T. R., Ninan, P. T., Aloi, J., Jimerson, D. C., Skolnick, P., & Paul, S. M. (1984). A benzodiazepine receptor-mediated model of anxiety. *Archives of General Psychiatry, 41,* 741–750.

Interagency Committee on Learning Disabilities. (1987). *Learning disabilities: A report to the U.S. Congress* (pp. 107–118). Washington, DC: Department of Health and Human Services.

Izard, C. E., & Schwartz, G. M. (1986). Patterns of emotion in depression. In M. Rutter, C. E. Izard, & P. B. Read (Eds.), *Depression in young people: Developmental and clinical perspectives* (pp. 33–70). New York: Guilford.

Jacobs, S., & Ostfeld, A. (1977). An epidemiological review of the mortality of bereavement. *Psychosomatic Medicine, 39,* 344–357.

Jacobs, T. J., & Charles, E. (1980). Life events and the occurrence of cancer of children. *Psychosomatic Medicine, 42,* 11–24.

Jacobson, A. M., & Leibovich, J. B. (1984). Psychological issues in diabetes mellitus. *Psychosomatics, 25,* 7–15.

Jacobziner, H. (1965). Attempted suicides in adolescence. *Journal of the American Medical Association, 191,* 7–11.

Jacques, E. (1965). Death and the mid-life crisis. *International Journal of Psycho-Analysis, 46,* 502–514.

Jagger, J., Prusoff, B., Cohen, D. J., Kidd, K. K., Carbonari, C., & John, K. (1982). The epidemiology of Tourette's syndrome: A pilot study. *Schizophrenia Bulletin, 8,* 267–278.

James, W. (1890). *Principles of psychology.* New York: Holt.

Jansky, J. J. (1988). Assessment of learning disabilities. In C. J. Kestenbaum & D. T. Williams (Eds.), *Handbook of clinical assessment of children and adolescents* (pp. 296–311). New York: New York University Press.

Jenike, M. A., Baer, I., Minichiello, W. E., Schwartz, C. E., & Carey, R. J., Jr. (1986). Concomitant obsessive-compulsive disorder in schizotypal personality disorder. *American Journal of Psychiatry, 143,* 530–532.

Jenkins, R. L. (1973). *Behavior disorders of childhood and adolescence.* Springfield, IL: Charles C Thomas.

Jensen, A. R. (1980). *Bias in mental testing.* New York: Free Press.

Jensen, J. B., & Garfinkel, B. D. (1990). Growth hormone dysregulation in children with major depressive disorder. *Journal of the American Academy of Child and Adolescent Psychiatry, 29,* 295–301.

Jersild, A. T., & Holmes, B. G. (1935). Children's fears. *Child Development Monographs, No. 20.*

Jersild, A. T., Telford, C. W., & Sawrey, J. M. (1975). *Child psychology* (7th ed.). Englewood Cliffs, NJ: Prentice-Hall.

Jessner, L., Lamont, J., Long, R., Rollins, N., Whipple, B., & Prentice, N. (1955). Emotional impact of nearness and separation for the asthmatic child and his mother. *Psychoanalytic Study of the Child, 10,* 353–375.

Johnson, A. M., Falstein, E. I., Szurek, S. A., & Svendsen, M. (1941). School phobia. *American Journal of Orthopsychiatry, 11,* 702–711.

Johnson, A. M., & Szurek, S. A. (1952). The genesis of antisocial acting out in children and adults. *Psychoanalytic Quarterly, 21,* 323–343.

Johnson, C., & Larson, R. (1982). Bulimia: An analysis of moods and behavior. *Psychosomatic Medicine, 44,* 341–351.

Johnson, C. L., Lewis, C., & Hagman, J. (1984). The syndrome of bulimia: Review and synthesis. *Psychiatric Clinics of North America, 7,* 247–273.

Johnson, C. L., Stuckey, M. K., Lewis, L. D., & Schwartz, J. M. (1982). Bulimia: A descriptive survey of 316 cases. *International Journal of Eating Disorders, 2,* 3–16.

Johnson, R. E. (1979). *Juvenile delinquency and its origins: An integrated theoretical approach.* Cambridge: Cambridge University Press.

Jones, D. J., Fox, M. M., Barbigian, H. M., & Hutton, H. E. (1980). Epidemiology of anorexia nervosa in Monroe County, New York: 1960–1976. *Psychosomatic Medicine, 42,* 551–558.

Jones, E. (1953). *The life and work of Sigmund Freud* (Vol. 1). New York: Basic Books.

Jorgensen, O. S., Lober, M., Christiansen, J., & Gram, L. F. (1980). Plasma concentration and clinical effect in imipramine treatment of childhood enuresis. *Clinical Pharmacokinetics, 5,* 386–393.

Judd, L. L. (1965). Obsessive compulsive neurosis in children. *Archives of General Psychiatry, 12,* 136–143.

Kaffman, M., & Elizur, E. (1977). Infants who become enuretics. A longitudinal study of 161 kibbutz children. *Monographs of the Society for Research in Child Development, 42*(2), 170.

Kafka, J. S. (1969). The body as transitional object: A psychoanalytic study of a self-mutilating patient. *British Journal of Medical Psychology, 42,* 207–212.

Kafry, D. (1978). *Fire survival skills: Who plays with matches?* (Technical Report for Pacific Southwest Range and Forest Stations). Washington, DC: U.S. Department of Agriculture.

Kagan, J. (1966). Psychological development of the child. In F. Faulkner (Ed.), *Human development* (p. 341). Philadelphia: Saunders.

Kagan, J. (1983). Stress and coping in early development. In N. Garmezy & M. Rutter (Eds.), *Stress, coping, and development in children* (pp. 191–216). New York: McGraw-Hill.

Kagan, J. (1987). Perspectives on infancy. In J. Osofsky (Ed.), *Handbook of infant development* (2nd ed., pp. 1150–1198). New York: Wiley.

Kagan, J., Reznick, J. S., & Snidman, N. (1988). Biological bases of childhood shyness. *Science, 240,* 167–171.

Kahn, E., & Cohen, L. H. (1934). Organic drivenness: A brain-stem syndrome and an experience. *New England Journal of Medicine, 210,* 748–756.

Kaliner, M. (Moderator) (1982). Autonomic nervous system abnormalities and allergy. *Annals of Internal Medicine, 96,* 349–357.

Kaliner, M., Eggleston, P. A., & Mathews, K. P. (1987). Rhinitis and asthma. *Journal of the American Medical Association, 258,* 2851–2873.

Kallman, F. J. (1944). Twin and sibship study of overt male homosexuality. *American Journal of Human Genetics, 4,* 136.

Kallman, F. J., & Roth, B. (1956). Genetic aspects of preadolescent schizophrenia. *The American Journal of Psychiatry, 112,* 599–606.

Kandel, D. B., & Davies, M. (1986). Adult sequelae of adolescent depressive symptoms. *Archives of General Psychiatry, 43,* 255–262.

Kandel, E. R. (1983). From metapsychology to molecular biology: Explorations into the nature of anxiety. *American Journal of Psychiatry, 140,* 1277–1293.

Kandt, R. S. (1984). Neurologic examination of children with learning disorders. *Pediatric Clinics of North America, 31,* 297–315.

Kanner, L. (1943). Autistic disturbances of affective contact. *Nervous Child, 2,* 217–250.

Kanner, L. (1957). *Child psychiatry* (3rd ed.). Springfield: Charles C Thomas.

Kanner, L. (1971). Follow-up study of eleven autistic children originally reported in 1943. *Journal of Autism and Child Schizophrenia, 1,* 119–145.

Kanner, L., Rodriguez, A., & Ashenden, B. (1972). How far can autistic children go in matters of social adaptation? *Journal of Autism and Child Schizophrenia, 2,* 9–33.

Kaplan, A. P., Buckley, R. H., & Mathews, K. P. (1987). Allergic skin disorders. *Journal of the American Medical Association, 258,* 2900–2909.

Kaplan, H. I. (1980). History of psychosomatic medicine. In H. I. Kaplan, A. M. Freedman, & B. J. Sadock (Eds.), *Comprehensive textbook of psychiatry* (Vol. 2, pp. 1843–1853). Baltimore: Williams & Wilkins.

Kaplan, S. J., Pelcovitz, D., Salzinger, S., & Ganeles, D. (1983). Psychopathology of parents of abused and neglected children and adolescents. *Journal of the American Academy of Child Psychiatry, 22,* 238–244.

Kaplan, S. J., & Zitrin, A. (1983). Psychiatrists and child abuse: I. Case assessment by child protective services. *Journal of the American Academy of Child Psychiatry, 22,* 253–256.

Kaplan, S. L., Hong, G. K., & Weinhold, C. (1984). Epidemiology of depressive symptomatology in adolescents. *Journal of the American Academy of Child and Adolescent Psychiatry, 23,* 91–98.

Karno, M., Golding, J. M., Sorenson, S. B., & Burnam, M. A. (1988). The epidemiology of obsessive-compulsive disorder in five U.S. communities. *Archives of General Psychiatry, 45,* 1094–1099.

Kashani, J. H., Barbero, G. J., & Bolander, F. D. (1981a). Depression in hospitalized pediatric patients. *Journal of the American Academy of Child Psychiatry, 20,* 123–134.

Kashani, J. H., Beck, N. C., Hoeper, E. W., Fallahi, C., Corcoran, C. M., McAllister, J. A., Rosenberg, T. K., & Reid, J. C. (1987). Psychiatric disorders in a community sample of adolescents. *American Journal of Psychiatry, 144,* 584–589.

Kashani, J. H., & Carlson, G. A. (1985). Major depressive disorder in a preschooler. *Journal of the American Academy of Child Psychiatry, 24,* 490–494.

Kashani, J. H., & Carlson, G. A. (1987). Seriously depressed preschoolers. *American Journal of Psychiatry, 144,* 348–350.

Kashani, J. H., Holcomb, W. R., & Orvaschel, H. (1986). Depression and depressive symptoms in preschool children from the general population. *American Journal of Psychiatry, 143,* 1138–1143.

Kashani, J. H., Husain, A., Shekim, W. O., Hodges, K. K., Crytryn, L., & McKnew, D. H. (1981b). Current perspectives on childhood depression: An overview. *American Journal of Psychiatry, 138,* 143–153.

Kashani, J. H., McGee, R. O., Clarkson, S. E., Anderson, J. C., Walton, L. A., Williams, S., Silva, P. A., Robins, A. J., Cytryn, L., & McKnew, D. H. (1983). Depression in a sample of nine-year-old children: Prevalence and associated characteristics. *Archives of General Psychiatry, 40,* 1217–1223.

Kashani, J. H., & Orvaschel, H. (1988). Anxiety disorders in mid-adolescence: A community sample. *American Journal of Psychiatry, 145,* 960–964.

Kashani, J. H., Ray, J. S., & Carlson, G. A. (1984). Depression and depressive-like states in preschool-age children in a child development unit. *American Journal of Psychiatry, 141,* 1397–1402.

Kashani, J. H., & Simonds, J. F. (1979). The incidence of depression in children. *American Journal of Psychiatry, 136,* 1203–1205.

Kasl, S. V. (1983). Pursuing the link between stressful life experiences and disease: A time for reappraisal. In C. L. Cooper (Ed.), *Stress research.* New York: Wiley.

Kauffman, C., Grunebaum, H., Cohler, B., & Gamer, E. (1979). Superkids: Competent children of psychotic mothers. *American Journal of Psychiatry, 136,* 1398–1402.

Kaufman, I., Heims, L., & Reiser, D. (1967). A reevaluation of the psychodynamics of firesetting. *American Journal of Orthopsychiatry, 31,* 123–137.

Kaufman, J., & Zigler, E. (1987). Do abused children become abusive parents? *American Journal of Orthopsychiatry, 57,* 186–192.

Kaye, W. H., Ebert, M. H., Raleigh, M., & Lake, C. R. (1984). Abnormalities in CNS monoamine metabolism in anorexia nervosa. *Archives of General Psychiatry, 41,* 350–355.

Kaye, W. H., & Gwirtsman, H. E. (1985). Mood changes and patterns of food consumption during bingeing and purging: Are there underlying neurobiologic relationships? In W. H. Kaye & H. E. Gwirtsman (Eds.), *The treatment of normal weight bulimia* (pp. 19–36). Washington, DC: American Psychiatric Press.

Kaye, W. H., Gwirtsman, H. E., Brewerton, T. D., George, D. T., & Wurtman, R. J. (1988). Bingeing behavior and plasma amino acids: A possible involvement of brain serotonin in bulimia nervosa. *Psychiatry Research, 23,* 31–43.

Kaye, W. H., Gwirtsman, H. E., George, D. T., Weiss, S. R., & Jimerson, D. C. (1986). Relationship of mood alterations to bingeing behaviour in bulimia. *British Journal of Psychiatry, 149,* 479–485.

Kazdin, A. E., Esveldt-Dawson, K., French, N. H., & Unis, A. S. (1987). Effects of parent-management training and problem-solving skills training combined in the treatment of antisocial child behavior. *Journal of the American Academy of Child and Adolescent Psychiatry 26,* 416–424.

Keith, C. (1987). The violent youth. In J. D. Noshpitz (Ed.), *Basic handbook of child psychiatry* (Vol. 5, pp. 111–122). New York: Basic Books.

Keller, M. B., Beardslee, W. R., Dorer, D. J., Lavori, P. W., Samuelson, H., & Klerman, G. L. (1986). Impact of severity and chronicity of parental affective illness on adaptive functioning and psychopathology in children. *Archives of General Psychiatry, 43,* 930–937.

Kelsoe, J. R., Ginns, E. I., Egeland, J. A., Gerhard, D. S., Goldstein, A. M., Bale, S. J., Pauls, D. L., Long, R. T., Kidd, K. K., Conte, G., Housman, D. E., & Paul, S. M. (1989). Reevaluation of the linkage relationship between chromosome lip loci and the gene for bipolar affective disorder in the Old Order Amish. *Nature, 342,* 238–243.

Kempe, C. H. (1973). A practical approach to the protection of the abused child and rehabilitation of the abusing parent. *Pediatrics, 51,* 804–812.

Kempe, C. H., & Helfer, R. E. (Eds.) (1972). *Helping the battered child and his family.* Philadelphia: Lippincott.

Kempe, R. S., Cutler, C., & Dean, J. (1980). The infant with failure to thrive. In C. H. Kempe & R. E. Helfer (Eds.), *The battered child* (3rd ed.). Chicago: University of Chicago Press.

Kempe, R. S., & Kempe, C. H. (1978). *Child abuse.* Cambridge, MA: Harvard University Press.

Kempe, R. S., & Kempe, C. H. (1984). *The common secret: Sexual abuse of children and adolescents.* New York: Freeman.

Kempe, ꞌC. H., Silverman, F. N., Steele, B. F., Droegemueller, W., & Silver, H. (1962). The battered child syndrome. *Journal of the American Medical Association, 181,* 17–24.

Kemph, J. P. (1987). Hallucinations in psychotic children. *Journal of the American Academy of Child and Adolescent Psychiatry, 26,* 556–559.

Kendell, R. E., Hall, D. J., Hailey, A., & Babigian, H. M. (1973). The epidemiology of anorexia nervosa. *Psychological Medicine, 3,* 200–203.

Kendler, K. S. (1985). Diagnostic approaches to schizotypal personality disorder: A historical perspective. *Schizophrenia Bulletin, 11,* 538–553.

Kendler, K. S. (1986). Genetics of schizophrenia. In R. E. Hales & A. J. Frances (Eds.), *Psychiatry update: American Psychiatric Association Annual Review* (Vol. 5, pp. 25–41). Washington, DC: American Psychiatric Association Press.

Kendler, K. S., Heath, A. C., Martin, N. G., & Eaves, L. J. (1986). Symptoms of anxiety and depression in a volunteer twin population. *Archives of General Psychiatry, 43,* 213–221.

Kendler, K. S., Heath, A. C., Martin, N. G., & Eaves, L. J. (1987). Symptoms of anxiety and symptoms of depression. Same genes, different environments? *Archives of General Psychiatry, 44,* 451–457.

Kendler, K. S., & Robinette, C. D. (1983). Schizophrenia in the National Academy of Sciences–National Research Council twin registry: A 16-year update. *American Journal of Psychiatry, 140,* 1551–1563.

Kendler, K. S., & Tsuang, M. T. (1988). Outcome and familial psychopathology in schizophrenia. *Archives of General Psychiatry, 45,* 338–346.

Kennedy, J. L., Giuffra, L. A., Moises, H. W., Cavalli-Sforza, L. L., Pakstis, A. J., Kidd, J. R., Castiglione, C. M., Sjogren, B., Wetterberg, L., & Kidd, K. K. (1988). Evidence against linkage of schizophrenia to markers on chromosome 5 in a northern Swedish pedigree. *Nature, 336,* 167–170.

Keogh, B. K. (1986). Future of the LD field: Research and practice. *Journal of Learning Disabilities, 19,* 455–460.

Kernberg, O. F. (1975). *Borderline conditions and pathological narcissism.* New York: Jason Aronson.

Kernberg, O. F. (1976). *Object-relations theory and clinical psychoanalysis.* New York: Jason Aronson.

Kernberg, O. F. (1977). The structural diagnosis of borderline personality organization. In P. Hartocollis (Ed.), *Borderline personality disorders: The concept, the syndrome, the patient* (pp. 87–121). New York: International Universities Press.

Kernberg, O. F. (1984). *Severe personality disorders: Psychotherapeutic strategies.* New Haven: Yale University Press.

Kernberg, P. F. (1978, October). *Minimal brain dysfunction and borderline personality disorder in adolescence.* Paper read at the Annual Meeting of the Academy of Child Psychiatry, San Diego, California.

Kernberg, P. F. (1979). Childhood schizophrenia and autism: A selective review. In L. Bellak (Ed.), *Disorders of the schizophrenic syndrome* (pp. 509–559). New York: Basic Books.

Kernberg, P. F. (1983a). Borderline conditions: Childhood and adolescent aspects. In K. S. Robson (Ed.), *The borderline child: Approaches to etiology, diagnosis, and treatment* (pp. 101–119). New York: McGraw-Hill.

Kernberg, P. F. (1983b). Issues in the psychotherapy of borderline conditions in children. In K. S. Robson (Ed.), *The borderline child: Approaches to etiology, diagnosis, and treatment* (pp. 223–234). New York: McGraw-Hill.

Kernberg, P. F. (1984, October). *Treatment of narcissistic personality disorder in children.* Paper presented at the Annual Meeting of the American Academy of Child Psychiatry, Toronto, Canada.

Kernberg, P. F. (1990). Resolved: Borderline personality exists in children under twelve. *Journal of the American Academy of Child and Adolescent Psychiatry, 29,* 478–482.

Kessler, J. W. (1980). History of minimal brain dysfunctions. In H. E. Rie & E. D. Rie (Eds.), *Handbook of minimal brain dysfunctions: A critical view.* New York: Wiley.

Kessler, R. C., Downey, G., Milavsky, J. R., & Stipp, H. (1988). Clustering of teenage suicides after television news stories about suicides: A reconsideration. *American Journal of Psychiatry, 145,* 1379–1383.

Kestenbaum, C. J. (1978). Childhood psychosis: Psychotherapy. In B. B. Wolman, J. Egan, & A. O. Ross (Eds.), *Handbook of treatment of mental disorders in childhood and adolescence* (pp. 354–384). Englewood Cliffs, NJ: Prentice-Hall.

Kestenbaum, C. J. (1983). The borderline child at risk for major psychiatric disorder in adult life. In K. S. Robson (Ed.), *The borderline child: Approaches to etiology, diagnosis, and treatment* (pp. 49–81). New York: McGraw-Hill.

Kestenbaum, C. J. (1985). Putting it all together: A multidimensional assessment of psychotic potential in adolescence. *Adolescent Psychiatry, 12,* 5–16.

Kestenbaum, C. J. (1986). Thoughts on the precursors of affective and cognitive disturbance in schizophrenia. In D. B. Feinsilver (Ed.), *Towards a comprehensive model for schizophrenic disorders* (pp. 211–233). Hillsdale, NJ: Analytic Press.

Kety, S. S. (1985). Schizotypal personality disorder: An operational definition of Bleuler's latent schizophrenia? *Schizophrenia Bulletin, 11,* 590–597.

Keyes, A., Brozek, J., Henschel, A., Mikelsen, O., & Taylor, H. L. (1950). *The biology of human starvation.* Minneapolis: University of Minnesota Press.

Khan, A. U. (1979). *Psychiatric emergencies in pediatrics.* Chicago: Year Book Medical Publishers.

Khan, A. U. (1987a). Biochemical profile of depressed adolescents. *Journal of the American Academy of Child and Adolescent Psychiatry, 26,* 873–878.

Khan, A. U. (1987b). Heterogeneity of suicidal adolescents. *Journal of the American Academy of Child and Adolescent Psychiatry, 26,* 92–96.

Khantzian, E. J., Dalsimer, J. S., & Semrad, E. V. (1969). The use of interpretation in the psychotherapy of schizophrenia. *American Journal of Psychotherapy, 23,* 182–197.

Kidd, K. K., Egeland, J. A., Molthan, L., Pauls, D. L., Kruger, S. D., & Messner, K. H. (1984). Amish study: IV. Genetic linkage study of pedigrees of bipolar probands. *American Journal of Psychiatry, 141,* 1042–1048.

Kiernan, C. (1983). The use of nonvocal communication techniques with autistic individuals. *Journal of Child Psychology and Psychiatry, 24,* 339–375.

King, A. (1963). Primary and secondary anorexia nervosa syndromes. *British Journal of Psychiatry, 109*, 470–479.

King, R. A. (1988). Pre-pubertal schizophrenia [Letter]. *Archives of General Psychiatry, 45*, 1051.

King, R. A., Pfeffer, C., Gammon, G. D., & Cohen, D. J. (1991). Suicidality of childhood and adolescence: Review of the literature and proposal for establishments of a DSM-IV category. In B. B. Lahey & A. E. Kazdin (Eds.), *Advances in Clinical Child Psychology* (Vol. 14). New York: Plenum.

Kinsbourne, M. (1984). Beyond attention deficit: Search for the disorder in ADD. In L. M. Bloomingdale (Ed.), *Attention deficit disorder: Diagnostic, cognitive, and therapeutic understanding* (pp. 133–145). New York: SP Medical and Scientific Books.

Kinsey, A., Pomeroy, W. B., & Martin, C. E. (1947). *Sexual behavior in the human male.* Philadelphia: Saunders.

Kinsman, R. A., Dahlem, N. W., Spector, S., & Staudenmayer, H. (1977). Observations on subjective symptomatology, coping behavior, and medical decisions in asthma. *Psychosomatic Medicine, 39*, 102–119.

Kirch, D. G., & Weinberger, D. R. (1986). Anatomical neuropathology in schizophrenia: Post-mortem findings. In H. A. Nasrallah & D. R. Weinberger (Eds.), *The neurology of schizophrenia* (pp. 325–348). Amsterdam: Elsevier.

Klaus, M., & Kennell, M. H. (1982). *Parent–infant bonding.* St. Louis: Mosby.

Klein, D. F. (1964). Delineation of two drug-responsive anxiety syndromes. *Psychopharmacologia, 5*, 397–408.

Klein, D. F. (1981). Anxiety reconceptualized. In D. F. Klein & J. G. Rabkin (Eds.), *Anxiety: New research and changing concepts* (pp. 235–263). New York: Raven Press.

Klein, D. F., Gittelman, R., Quitkin, F., & Rifkin, A. (1980). *Diagnosis and drug treatment of psychiatric disorders: Adults and children* (2nd ed.). Baltimore: Williams & Wilkins.

Klein, D. F., & Gorman, J. M. (1987). A model of panic and agoraphobic development. *Acta Psychiatrica Scandinavica, 76*(Suppl.), 87–95.

Klein, M. (1932). *The psychoanalysis of children.* London: Hogarth Press.

Klein, M. (1948). *Contributions to psycho-analysis, 1921–1945.* London: Hogarth Press.

Klein, M. (1952a). On observing the behaviour of young infants. In J. Riviere & E. Jones (Eds.), *Developments in psycho-analysis* (pp. 237–270). London: Hogarth Press.

Klein, M. (1952b). On the theory of anxiety and guilt. In J. Riviere & E. Jones (Eds.), *Developments in psycho-analysis* (pp. 271–291). London: Hogarth Press.

Klerman, G. L. (1986). Current trends in clinical research on panic attacks, agoraphobia, and related anxiety disorders. *Journal of Clinical Psychiatry, 47*(Suppl.), 37–39.

Klerman, G. L. (1988). The current age of youthful melancholia. Evidence for increase in depression among adolescents and young adults. *British Journal of Psychiatry, 152*, 4–14.

Klorman, R., Coons, H. W., & Borgstedt, A. D. (1987). Effects of methylphenidate on adolescents with a childhood history of attention deficit disorder: I. Clinical findings. *Journal of the American Academy of Child and Adolescent Psychiatry, 26,* 363–367.

Knapp, P. H. (1963). The asthmatic child and the psychosomatic problem of asthma: Towards a general theory. In H. I. Schneer (Ed.), *The asthmatic child* (pp. 234–255). New York: Harper & Row.

Knapp, P. H. (1975). Psychosomatic aspects of bronchial asthma. In S. Arieti & M. F. Reiser (Eds.), *American handbook of psychiatry* (Vol. 4, pp. 693–708). New York: Basic Books.

Knapp, P. H. (1980). Current theoretical concepts in psychosomatic medicine. In H. I. Kaplan, A. M. Freedman, & B. J. Sadock (Eds.), *Comprehensive textbook of psychiatry* (Vol. 2, pp. 1853–1862). Baltimore: Williams & Wilkins.

Knapp, P. H., & Mathe, A. A. (1985). Psychophysiologic aspects of bronchial asthma. In E. B. Weiss, M. S. Segal, & M. Stein (Eds.), *Bronchial asthma mechanisms and therapeutics* (2nd ed., pp. 914–931). Boston: Little, Brown.

Knight, R. B., Atkins, A., Eagle, C. J., Evans, N., Finkelstein, J. W., Fukushima, D., Katz, J., & Weiner, H. (1979). Psychological stress, ego defenses, and cortisol production in children hospitalized for elective surgery. *Psychosomatic Medicine, 41,* 40–49.

Knight, R. P. (1953). Borderline states. *Bulletin of the Menninger Clinic, 17,* 1–12.

Knobloch, H., & Pasamanick, B. (1975). Some etiologic and prognostic factors in early infantile autism and psychosis. *Pediatrics, 55,* 182–191.

Koegel, R. L., & Mentis, M. (1985). Motivation in childhood autism: Can they or won't they? *Journal of Child Psychology and Psychiatry, 26,* 185–191.

Kog, E., Vertommen, H., & Vandereycken, W. (1987). Minuchin's psychosomatic family model revised: A concept-validation study using a multitrait-multimethod approach. *Family Process, 26,* 235–253.

Kohlberg, L. (1966). A cognitive-developmental analysis of children's sex-role concepts and attitudes. In E. E. Maccoby (Ed.), *The development of sex differences.* Stanford, CA: Stanford University Press.

Kohn, M. L. (1969). *Class and conformity: A study in values.* Homewood, IL: Dorsey Press.

Kohut, H. (1971). *The analysis of the self: A systematic approach to the psychoanalytic treatment of narcissistic character disorders.* New York: International Universities Press.

Kohut, H. (1977). *The restoration of the self.* New York: International Universities Press.

Kohut, H. (1972). Thoughts on narcissism and narcissistic rage. *The Psychoanalytic Study of the Child, (27,* 360–440).

Kokes, R. F., Harder, D. W., Fisher, L., & Strauss, J. S. (1980). Child competence and psychiatric risk: V. Sex of patient parent and dimensions of psychopathology. *Journal of Nervous and Mental Disorders, 168,* 348–352.

Kolvin, I. (1971). Studies in the childhood psychoses: I. Diagnostic criteria and classification. *British Journal of Psychiatry, 118,* 381–384.

Kolvin, I., Berney, T. P., & Bhate, S. R. (1984). Classification and diagnosis of depression in school phobia. *British Journal of Psychiatry, 145,* 347–357.

Kolvin, I., Ounsted, C., Humphrey, M., & McNay, A. (1971). Studies in the childhood psychoses: II. The phenomenology of childhood psychoses. *British Journal of Psychiatry, 118,* 385–395.

Kolvin, I., Taunch, J., Currah, J., Garside, R. F., Nolan, J., & Shaw, W. B. (1972). Enuresis: A descriptive analysis and a controlled trial. *Developmental Medicine and Child Neurology, 14,* 715–726.

Koon, R. E. (1983). Conversion dysphagia in children. *Psychosomatics, 24,* 182–184.

Korenblum, M., Marton, P., Kutcher, S., Stein, B., Kennedy, B., & Pakes, J. (1988, October). *Personality dysfunction in depressed adolescents: State or trait?* Poster presented at the American Academy of Child and Adolescent Psychiatry Annual Meeting, Seattle, WA.

Korner, A. F. (1983). Individual differences in neonatal activity: Implications for the origins of different coping styles. In J. D. Call, E. Galenson, & R. L. Tyson (Eds.), *Frontiers of infant psychiatry* (pp. 379–387). New York: Basic Books.

Kosslyn, S. M. (1988). Aspects of cognitive neuroscience of mental imagery. *Science, 240,* 1621–1626.

Kotelchuck, M. (1980). Nonorganic failure to thrive: The status of interactional and environmental etiologic theories. *Advances in Behavioral Pediatrics, 1,* 29–51.

Kotses, H., & Glaus, K. D. (1981). Applications of biofeedback to the treatment of asthma: A critical review. *Biofeedback Self Regulation, 6,* 573–593.

Kotsopoulos, S., Kanigsberg, J., Cote, A., & Fiedorowicz, C. (1987). Hallucinatory experiences in nonpsychotic children. *Journal of the American Academy of Child and Adolescent Psychiatry, 26,* 375–380.

Kovacs, M. (1985a). The Children's Depression Inventory (CDI). *Psychopharmacology Bulletin, 21,* 995–998.

Kovacs, M. (1985b). The natural history and course of depressive disorders in childhood. *Psychiatric Annals, 15,* 387–389.

Kovacs, M., & Beck, A. T. (1977). An empirical-clinical approach toward a definition of childhood depression. In J. G. Schulterbrandt & A. Raskin (Eds.), *Depression in childhood: Diagnosis, treatment and conceptual models* (pp. 1–25). New York: Raven Press.

Kovacs, M., Feinberg, T. L., Crouse-Novak, M. A., Paulauskas, S. L., & Finkelstein, R. (1984a). Depressive disorders in childhood. *Archives of General Psychiatry, 41,* 229–237.

Kovacs, M., Feinberg, T. L., Crouse-Novak, M., Paulauskas, S. L., Pollock, M., & Finkelstein, R. (1984b). Depressive disorders in childhood: II. A longitudinal study of the risk of a subsequent major depression. *Archives of General Psychiatry, 41,* 643–649.

Kovacs, M., & Puig-Antich, J. (1989). Major psychiatric disorders and risk factors in youth suicide. In Alcohol, Drug Abuse, and Mental Health Administration (Ed.), *Report of the Secretary's Task Force for Youth Suicide: Vol. 2. Risk factors for youth suicide* (DHHS Publication No. ADM 89-1622, pp. 143–159). Washington, DC: U.S. Government Printing Office.

Krauthammer, C., & Klerman, G. L. (1978). Secondary mania. *Archives of General Psychiatry, 35,* 1333–1339.

Krieger, I. (1982). *Pediatric disorders of feeding, nutrition, and metabolism.* New York: Wiley.

Krieger, M. J., Rosenfeld, A. A., Gordon, A., & Bennett, M. (1980). Problems in the psychotherapy of children with histories of incest. *American Journal of Psychotherapy, 34,* 81–88.

Kringlen, E. (1965). Obsessional neurotics: A long-term follow-up. *British Journal of Psychiatry, 111,* 709–722.

Kroll, J., & Bachrach, B. (1986). Child care and child abuse in early medieval Europe. *Journal of the American Academy of Child Psychiatry, 25,* 562–568.

Kron, L., & Kestenbaum, C. J. (1988). Children at risk for psychotic disorder in adult life. In C. J. Kestenbaum & D. T. Williams (Eds.), *Handbook of clinical assessment of children and adolescents* (Vol. 2, pp. 650–672). New York: New York University Press.

Krupnick, J. L. (1984). Bereavement during childhood and adolescence. In M. Osterweis, F. Solomon, & M. Green (Eds.), *Bereavement: Reactions, consequences, and care* (pp. 99–141). Washington, DC: National Academy Press.

Krupski, A. (1986). Attention problems in youngsters with learning handicaps. In J. K. Torgesen & B. Y. L. Wong (Eds.), *Psychological and educational perspectives on learning disabilities* (pp. 161–192). New York: Academic.

Kuczenski, R. (1983). Biochemical actions of amphetamines and other stimulants. In I. Crease (Ed.), *Stimulants: Neurochemical, behavior and clinical perspectives* (pp. 31–63). New York: Raven Press.

Kupietz, S., Winsberg, B. G., & Sverd, J. (1982). Learning ability and methylphenidate (Ritalin) plasma concentration in hyperkinetic children: A preliminary investigation. *Journal of the American Academy of Child Psychiatry, 21,* 27–30.

Kurlan, R., Behr, J., Medved, L., & Como, P. (1988). Transient tic disorder and the spectrum of Tourette's syndrome. *Archives of Neurology, 45,* 1200–1201.

Kydd, R. R., & Werry, J. S. (1982). Schizophrenia in children under 16 years. *Journal of Autism and Developmental Disorders, 12,* 343–357.

Kysar, J. E. (1968). The two camps in child psychiatry: A report from a psychiatrist-father of an autistic and retarded child. *American Journal of Psychiatry, 125,* 141–147.

LaBarbera, J. D., & Dozier, J. E. (1980). Hysterical seizures: The role of sexual exploitation. *Psychosomatics, 21,* 897–903.

LaBuda, M. C., & DeFries, J. C. (1990). Genetic etiology of reading disability: Evidence from a twin study. In G. T. Pavlidis (Ed.), *Perspectives on dyslexia* (Vol. 1, pp. 47–76). Chichester: Wiley.

Lacey, J. H., & Dolan, B. M. (1988). Bulimia in British blacks and Asians: A catchment area study. *British Journal of Psychiatry, 152,* 73–79.

Lacey, J. H., & Smith, G. (1987). Bulimia nervosa: The impact of pregnancy on mother and baby. *British Journal of Psychiatry, 150,* 777–781.

Lacey, J. I., & Lacey, B. C. (1958). Verification and extension of the principle of autonomic response-stereotypy. *American Journal of Psychology, 71,* 50–73.

Lacey, J. I., & VanLehn, R. (1952). Differential emphasis in somatic response to stress. *Psychosomatic Medicine, 14,* 71–81.

Lader, M. H. (1967). Palmar skin conductance measures in anxiety and phobic states. *Journal of Psychosomatic Research, 11,* 271–281.

Lader, M. H. (1980). The psychophysiology of anxiety. In H. M. Van Praag, M. H. Lader, O. J. Rafaelsen, & E. J. Sachar (Eds.), *Handbook of Biological Psychiatry. Part II: Brain Mechanisms and Abnormal Behavior: Psychophysiology.* New York: Marcel Dekker.

Lader, M. H. (1972). The nature of anxiety. *British Journal of Psychiatry, 121,* 481–491.

La Greca, A., & Quay, H. (1984). Behavioral disorders of children. In N. S. Endler & J. M. Hunt (Eds.), *Personality and the Behavioral Disorders* (pp. 711–713). New York: Wiley.

Lahey, B. B., Green, K. D., & Forehand, R. (1980). On the independence of ratings of hyperactivity, conduct problems, and attention deficits in children: A multiple regression analysis. *Journal of Consulting and Clinical Psychology, 48,* 566–574.

Lahey, B. B., Schaughency, E. A., Hynd, G. W., Carlson, C. L., & Nieves, N. (1987). Attention deficit disorder with and without hyperactivity: Comparison of behavioral characteristics of clinic-referred children. *Journal of the American Academy of Child and Adolescent Psychiatry, 26,* 718–723.

Lambert, N. M., Sandoval, J., & Sassone, D. (1978). Prevalence of hyperactivity in elementary school children as a function of social system definers. *American Journal of Orthopsychiatry, 48,* 446–463.

Lampl-de Groot, J. (1946). The pre-oedipal phase in the development of the male child. *Psychoanalytic Study of the Child, 2,* 75–83.

Lander, E. S. (1988). Splitting schizophrenia. *Nature, 336,* 105–106.

Lancet (1982, May 29). Autonomic abnormalities in asthma [Editorial]. *Lancet,* pp. 1224–1225.

Langevin, R. (Ed.) (1985). *Erotic preference, gender identity, and aggression in men: New research studies.* Hillsdale, NJ: Erlbaum.

Langhorne, J. E., Loney, J., Paternite, C. E., & Bechtoldt, H. P. (1976). Childhood hyperkinesis: A return to the source. *Journal of Abnormal Psychology, 85,* 201–209.

Lapouse, R., & Monk, M. A. (1958). An epidemiologic study of behavior characteristics in children. *American Journal of Public Health, 48,* 1134–1144.

Lapouse, R., & Monk, M. A. (1959). Fears and worries of a representation sample of children. *American Journal of Orthopsychiatry, 29,* 803–818.

Laprade, K., & Trites, R. L. (1985). Is there an independent syndrome of hyperactivity? A reply to our critics. *Journal of Child Psychology and Psychiatry, 26,* 491–493.

Laredo, C. M. (1982). Sibling incest. In S. M. Sgroi (Ed.), *Handbook of clinical intervention in child sexual abuse* (pp. 177–189). Lexington, MA: Lexington Books.

Lasch, C. (1978). *The culture of narcissism:* American life in an age of diminishing expectations. New York: Norton.

Lask, B., & Matthew, D. (1979). Childhood asthma. A controlled trial of family psychotherapy. *Archives of Disease in Childhood, 54,* 116–119.

Last, C. G., & Francis, G. (1988). School phobia. In B. B. Lahey & A. A. Kazdin (Eds.), *Advances in Clinical Child Psychology* (Vol. 11). New York: Plenum.

Last, C. G., Francis, G., Hersen, M., Kazdin, A. E., & Strauss, C. C. (1987a). Separation anxiety and school phobia: A comparison using DSM-III criteria. *American Journal of Psychiatry, 144,* 653–657.

Last, C. G., Phillips, J. E., & Statfeld, A. (1987b). Childhood anxiety disorders in mothers and their children. *Child Psychiatry and Human Development, 18,* 103–110.

Last, C. G., & Strauss, C. C. (1990). School refusal in anxiety-disordered children and adolescents. *Journal of the American Academy of Child and Adolescent Psychiatry, 29,* 31–35.

Laufer, M. W., & Denhoff, E. (1957). Hyperkinetic behavior syndrome in children. *Journal of Pediatrics, 50,* 463–474.

Laufer, M. W., Denhoff, E., & Solomons, G. (1957). Hyperkinetic impulse disorder in children's behavior problems. *Psychosomatic Medicine, 19,* 39–49.

LaVigna, G. W. (1987). Non-aversive strategies for managing behavior problems. In D. J. Cohen & A. M. Donnellan (Eds.), *Handbook of autism and pervasive developmental disorders* (pp. 418–429). New York: Wiley.

Laybourne, P. C., & Churchill, S. W. (1972). Symptom discouragement in treating hysterical reactions of childhood. *International Journal of Child Psychotherapy, 1,* 111–123.

Lazare, A. (1981). Conversion symptoms. *New England Journal of Medicine, 305,* 745–748.

Lazarus, R. S. (1979). Positive denial: The case for not facing reality. *Psychology Today, 13*(6), 44–60.

Lebenthal, E., Rossi, T. M., Nord, K. S., & Branski, D. (1981). Recurrent abdominal pain and lactose absorption in children. *Pediatrics, 67,* 828–832.

Lebovitz, P. S. (1972). Feminine behavior in boys: Aspects of its outcome. *American Journal of Psychiatry, 128,* 1283–1289.

Leckman, J. F. (1983). The dexamethasone suppression test. *Journal of American Academy of Child Psychiatry, 22,* 477–479.

Leckman, J. F., Detlor, J., Harcherik, D. F., Ort, S., Shaywitz, B. A., & Cohen, D. J. (1985). Short- and long-term treatment of Tourette's disorder with clonidine: A clinical perspective. *Neurology, 35,* 343–351.

Leckman, J. F., Dolansky, E. S., Hardin, M. T., Clubb, M., Walkup, J. T., Stevenson, J., & Pauls, D. L. (1990). Perinatal factors in the expression of Tourette's syndrome: An exploratory study. *Journal of the American Academy of Child and Adolescent Psychiatry, 29,* 220–226.

Leckman, J. F., Price, R. A., Walkup, J. T., Ort, S. I., Pauls, D. L., & Cohen, D. J. (1987a). Nongenetic factors in Gilles de la Tourette's syndrome [Letter to the editor]. *Archives of General Psychiatry, 44,* 100.

Leckman, J. F., Riddle, M. A., Berrettini, W. H., Anderson, G. M., Hardin, M., Chappell, P., Bissette, G., Nemeroff, C. B., Goodman, W. K., & Cohen, D. J. (1988a). Elevated CSF dynorphin A [1–8] in Tourette's syndrome. *Life Sciences, 43,* 2015–2023.

Leckman, J. F., Riddle, M. A., & Cohen, D. J. (1988b). Pathobiology of Tourette's syndrome. In D. J. Cohen, R. D. Brunn, & J. F. Leckman (Eds.), *Tourette's syndrome and tic disorders: Clinical understanding and treatment* (pp. 103–116).

Leckman, J. F., Towbin, K. E., Ort, S. I., & Cohen, D. J. (1988c). Clinical assessment of tic disorder severity. In D. J. Cohen, R. D. Brunn, & J. F. Leckman (Eds.), *Tourette's syndrome and tic disorders: Clinical understanding and treatment* (pp. 55–78). New York: Wiley.

Leckman, J. F., Walkup, J. T., & Cohen, D. J. (1988d). Clonidine treatment of Tourette's syndrome. In D. J. Cohen, R. D. Brunn, & J. F. Leckman (Eds.), *Tourette's syndrome and tic disorders: Clinical understanding and treatment* (pp. 103–116). New York: Wiley.

Leckman, J. F., Walkup, J. T., Riddle, M. A., Towbin, K. E., & Cohen, D. J. (1987b). Tic disorders. In H. Y. Meltzer, W. Bunney, J. Coyle, J. Davis, I. Kopin, C. Schuster, R. Shader, & G. Simpson (Eds.), *Psychopharmacology: The third generation of progress* (pp. 1239–1246). New York: Raven Press.

Leckman, J. F., Weissman, M. M., Merikangas, K. R., Pauls, D. L., & Prusoff, B. A. (1983). Panic disorder and major depression. *Archives of General Psychiatry, 40,* 1055–1060.

Leckman, J. F., Weissman, M. M., Pauls, D. L., & Kidd, K. K. (1987c). Family-genetic studies and identification of valid diagnostic categories in adult and child psychiatry. *British Journal of Psychiatry, 151,* 39–44.

Leckman, J. F., Weissman, M. M., Prusoff, B. A., Caruso, K. A., Merikangas, K. R., Pauls, D. L., & Kidd, K. K. (1984). Subtypes of depression: Family study perspective. *Archives of General Psychiatry, 41,* 833–838.

Leff, J., & Vaughn, C. (1985). *Expressed emotion in families.* New York: Guilford.

Lenane, M. C., Swedo, S. E., Leonard, H., Pauls, D. L., Sceery, W., & Rapoport, J. L. (1990). Psychiatric disorders in first degree relatives of children and adolescents with obsessive-compulsive disorder. *Journal of the American Academy of Child and Adolescent Psychiatry, 29,* 407–412.

Leichtman, M., & Shapiro, S. (1983). A clinical approach to the psychological testing of borderline children. In K. S. Robson (Ed.), *The borderline child: Approaches to etiology, diagnosis, and treatment* (pp. 121–170). New York: McGraw-Hill.

Lentz, K. A. (1985). The expressed fears of young children. *Child Psychiatry and Human Development, 16,* 3–13.

Leonard, H. L. (1989a). Childhood rituals and superstitions: Developmental and cultural perspective. In J. L. Rapoport (Ed.), *Obsessive-compulsive disorder in children and adolescents* (pp. 289–309). Washington, DC: American Psychiatric Press.

Leonard, H. L. (1989b). Drug treatment of obsessive-compulsive disorder. In J. L. Rapoport (Ed.), *Obsessive-compulsive disorder in children and adolescents* (pp. 217–236). Washington, DC: American Psychiatric Press.

Leonard, H. L., Goldberger, E. L., Rapoport, J. L., Cheslow, D. L., Swedo, S. E. (1990). Childhood rituals: Normal development or obsessive compulsive symptoms? *Journal of the American Academy of Child and Adolescent Psychiatry, 29,* 17–23.

Leonard, H. L., Swedo, S. E., Rapoport, J. L., Coffey, M., & Cheslow, D. (1988). Treatment of childhood obsessive-compulsive disorder with clomipramine and desmethylimipramine: A double-blind crossover comparison. *Psychopharmacology Bulletin, 24,* 93–95.

Leonard, H. L., Swedo, S. E., Rapoport, J. L., Koby, E. V., Lenane, M. C., Cheslow, D. L., Hamburger, S. D. (1989). Treatment of obsessive-compulsive disorder with clomipramine and desipramine in children and adolescents: A double-blind crossover comparison. *Archives of General Psychiatry, 46,* 1088–1092.

Leonard, M. F., Rhymes, J. P., & Solnit, A. J. (1966). Failure to thrive in infants. *American Journal of Diseases of Children, 111,* 600–612.

Lerner, J. W. (1989). Educational interventions in learning disabilities. *Journal of the American Academy of Child and Adolescent Psychiatry, 28,* 326–331.

Leroy, J. G. (1983). Heredity, development, and behavior. In M. D. Levine, W. B. Carey, A. C. Crocker, & R. T. Gross (Eds.), *Developmental-behavioral pediatrics* (pp. 315–345). Philadelphia: Saunders.

Lesser, I. M., & Lesser, B. Z. (1983). Alexithymia: Examining the development of a psychological concept. *American Journal of Psychiatry, 140,* 1305–1308.

Lesser, I. M., & Rubin, R. T. (1986). Diagnostic considerations in panic disorders. *Journal of Clinical Psychiatry, 47*(Suppl. 6), 4–10.

Leventhal, J. M. (1988). Have there been changes in the epidemiology of sexual abuse of children during the 20th century? *Pediatrics, 82,* 766–773.

Leventhal, T., Weinberger, G., Stander, R. J., & Stearns, R. P. (1967). Therapeutic strategies with school phobics. *American Journal of Orthopsychiatry, 37,* 64–70.

Levi-Strauss, C. (1969). *The raw and the cooked: Introduction to a science of mythology.* Chicago: University of Chicago Press.

Levine, M. D. (1975). Children with encopresis: a descriptive analysis. *Paediatrics, 56,* 412–416.

Levine, M. D. (1982). Encopresis: Its potentiation, evaluation and alleviation. *Pediatric Clinics of North America, 29,* 315–330.

Levine, M. D., & Bakow, H. (1976). Children with encopresis: A study of treatment outcome. *Paediatrics, 58,* 845–852.

Levine, M. D., Mazonson, P., & Bakow, H. (1980). Behavioral symptom substitution in children cured of encopresis. *American Journal of Diseases of Children, 134,* 663–667.

Levine, M. D., & Zallen, B. G. (1984). The learning disorders of adolescence: Organic and nonorganic failure to strive. *Pediatric Clinics of North America, 31,* 345–369.

Levy, D. (1955). Oppositional syndrome and oppositional behavior. In R. H. Hoch & J. Zubin (Eds.), *Psychopathology of childhood* (pp. 204–226). New York: Grune & Stratten.

Lewinsohn, P., Hops, H., Williams, J. A., Clarke, G., & Andrews, J. (1987, October). *Cognitive-behavioral treatment for depressed adolescents.* New Research Poster presented at the annual meeting of the American Academy of Child and Adolescent Psychiatry, Washington, DC.

Lewis, D. O. (1981a). Delinquency and psychotic disorders. In D. O. Lewis (Ed.), *Vulnerabilities to delinquency* (p. 16). Jamaica, NY: Spectrum.

Lewis, D. O. (1981b). Treatment programs for delinquent children: Implications of the psychobiological vulnerabilities to delinquency. In D. O. Lewis, (Ed.) *Vulnerabilities to delinquency* (pp. 313–320). Jamaica, NY: Spectrum.

Lewis, D. O. (1987). New perspectives on juvenile delinquency. In J. D. Noshpitz, (Ed.), *Basic handbook of child psychiatry* (Vol. 5, pp. 581–590). New York: Basic Books.

Lewis, D. O., Lewis, M., Unger, L., & Goldman, G. (1984). Conduct disorder and its synonyms: Diagnoses of dubious validity and usefulness. *American Journal of Psychiatry, 141,* 514–519.

Lewis, D. O., Shanok, S. S., & Balla, D. A. (1979). Perinatal difficulties, head and face trauma, and child abuse in the medical histories of seriously delinquent children. *American Journal of Psychiatry, 136,* 419–423.

Lewis, D. O., Shanok, S. S., Balla, D. A., & Bard, B. (1980). Psychiatric correlates of severe reading disabilities in an incarcerated delinquent population. *Journal of the American Academy of Child Psychiatry, 19,* 611–622.

Lewis, M., & Michalson, L. (1983). *Children's emotions and moods.* New York: Plenum.

Lewis, N., & Yarnell, H. (1951). Pathological firesetting (Pyromania): *Nervous and Mental Disease Monographs, 82.*

Lewiston, N. J., & Rubinstein, S. (1986). Sudden death in adolescent asthma. *New England and Regional Allergy Proceedings, 7,* 448–453.

Lewitter, F. I., DeFries, J. C., & Elston, R. C. (1980). Genetic models of reading disability. *Behavior Genetics, 10,* 9–30.

Lidz, T., Cornelison, A., Terry, D., & Fleck, S. (1958). Intrafamilial environment of the schizophrenic patient: VI. The transmission of irrationality. *Archives of Neurology and Psychiatry, 79,* 305–316.

Liebman, R., Honig, P., & Berger, H. (1976a). An integrated treatment program for psychogenic pain. *Family Process, 15,* 397–405.

Liebman, R., Minuchin, S., & Baker, L. (1974a). An integrated treatment program for anorexia nervosa. *American Journal of Psychiatry, 131,* 432–436.

Liebman, R., Minuchin, S., & Baker, L. (1974b). The role of the family in the treatment of anorexia nervosa. *Journal of Child Psychiatry, 13,* 264–274.

Liebman, R., Minuchin, S., & Baker, L. (1974c). The use of structural family therapy in the treatment of intractable asthma. *American Journal of Psychiatry, 131,* 535–540.

Liebman, R., Minuchin, S., Baker, L., & Rosman, B. (1976b). The role of the family in the treatment of chronic asthma. In P. Guerin (Ed.), *Family therapy* (pp. 309–324). New York: Gardner Press.

Liebman, W. M. (1978). Recurrent abdominal pain in children. *Clinical Pediatrics, 17,* 149–153.

Liebman, W. M. (1979). Recurrent abdominal pain in children: Lactose and sucrose intolerance: A prospective study. *Pediatrics, 64,* 43–45.

Liebowitz, M. R., Gorman, J. M., Fyer, A. J., & Klein, D. F. (1985). Social phobia: Review of a neglected anxiety disorder. *Archives of General Psychiatry, 42,* 729–736.

Liem, J. H. (1980). Family studies of schizophrenia: An update and commentary. *Schizophrenia Bulletin, 6,* 429–455.

Linet, L. S. (1985). Tourette syndrome, pimozide, and school phobia: The neuroleptic separation anxiety syndrome. *American Journal of Psychiatry, 142,* 613–615.

Linn, M. W., Linn, B. S., & Jensen, J. (1984). Stressful events, dysphoric mood, and immune responsiveness. *Psychological Reports, 54,* 219–222.

Lipowski, Z. J. (1977). Psychosomatic medicine in the seventies: An overview. *American Journal of Psychiatry, 134,* 233–244.

Loeber, R., & Schmaling, K. B. (1985). Empirical evidence for overt and covert patterns of antisocial conduct problems: A metaanalysis. *Journal of Abnormal Child Psychology, 13,* 337–352.

Loening-Baucke, V. A., & Cruikshank, B. M. (1986). Abnormal defecation dynamics in chronically constipated children with encopresis. *Journal of Pediatrics, 108,* 562–566.

Loewald, H. W. (1980). *Papers on psychoanalysis.* New Haven: Yale University Press.

Lombroso, C. (1911). *Crime: Its causes and remedies.* (Horton, Trans.) Boston: Little, Brown.

Loney, J., Kramer, J., & Milich, R. (1981). The hyperactive child grows up: Prediction of symptoms, delinquency, and achievement and follow-up. In K. Gadow & J. Loney (Eds.), *Psychosocial aspects of drug treatment for hyperactivity.* Boulder, CO: Westview Press.

Long, R. T., Lamont, J. H., Whipple, B., Bandler, L., Blom, G. E., Burgin, L., & Jessner, L. (1958). A psychosomatic study of allergic and emotional factors in children with asthma. *American Journal of Psychiatry, 114,* 890–899.

Loranger, A. W., & Levine, P. M. (1978). Age at onset of bipolar affective illness. *Archives of General Psychiatry, 35,* 1345–1348.

Loranger, A. W., Oldham, J. M., & Tulis, E. H. (1982). Familial transmission of DSM-III borderline personality disorder. *Archives of General Psychiatry, 39,* 795–799.

Lorenz, K. (1970). *Studies in animal and human behavior.* London: Methuen.

Lorenz, K. (1981). *The foundations of ethology.* New York: Springer-Verlag.

Lotter, V. (1978). Follow-up studies. In M. Rutter & E. Schopler (Eds.), *Autism: A reappraisal of concepts and treatment* (pp. 475–496). New York: Plenum.

Lou, H. C., Henriksen, L., & Bruhn, P. (1984). Focal cerebral hypoperfusion in children with dysphasia and/or attention deficit disorder. *Archives of Neurology, 41,* 825–829.

Lou, H. C., Henricksen, L., & Bruhn, P. (1990). Focal cerebral dysfunction in developmental learning disabilities. *Lancet, 335,* 8–11.

Lourie, I. S. (1984). The locus of emotional harm in incest: The study of "non-victims" of incestuous families. *Clinical Proceedings: Children's Hospital National Medical Center, 40,* 46–54.

Lourie, I. S., & Blick, L. C. (1987a). Child sexual abuse. In J. D. Noshpitz (Ed.), *Basic handbook of child psychiatry* (Vol. 5, pp. 280–286). New York: Basic Books.

Lourie, I. S., & Blick, L. C. (1987b). Intervention in cases of child sexual abuse. In J. D. Noshpitz (Ed.), *Basic handbook of child psychiatry* (Vol. 5, pp. 431–439). New York: Basic Books.

Lourie, R. S. (1955). Treatment of psychosomatic problems in infants. *Clinical Proceedings of Children's Hospital of DC, 11,* 142–152.

Lovaas, O. I. (1978). Parents as therapists. In M. Rutter & E. Schopler (Eds.), *Autism: A reappraisal of concepts and treatments* (pp. 369–378). New York: Plenum.

Lowe, T. L., & Cohen, D. J. (1980). Mania in childhood and adolescence. In R. H. Belmaker & H. M. van Praag (Eds.), *Mania: An evolving concept* (pp. 111–117). New York: Spectrum.

Lowe, T. L., Cohen, D. J., Detlor, J., Kremenitzer, M. W., & Shaywitz, B. A. (1982). Stimulant medications precipitate Tourette's syndrome. *Journal of the American Medical Association, 247,* 1729–1731.

Lowing, P. A., Mirsky, A. F., & Pereira, R. (1983). The inheritance of schizophrenic spectrum disorders: A reanalysis of the Danish adoptee study data. *American Journal of Psychiatry, 140,* 1167–1171.

Lukeman, D. (1975). Conditioning methods of treating childhood asthma. *Journal of Child Psychology and Psychiatry, 16,* 165–168.

Luparello, T. J., Leist, N., Lourie, C. N., & Sweet, P. (1970). The interaction of psychological stimuli and pharmacologic agents on airway reactivity in asthmatic subjects. *Psychosomatic Medicine, 32,* 509–513.

Luparello, T. J., Lyons, H. A., Bleecker, E. R., & McFadden, E. R., Jr. (1968). Influences of suggestion on airway reactivity in asthmatic subjects. *Psychosomatic Medicine, 30,* 819–825.

Luria, A. R. (1963). *The mentally retarded child.* New York: Macmillan.

Lustig, N., Dresser, J. W., Spellman, S. W., & Murray, T. B. (1966). Incest. *Archives of General Psychiatry, 14,* 31–40.

Luxenberg, J. S., Swedo, S. E., Flament, M. F., Friedland, R. P., Rapoport, J., & Rapoport, S. I. (1988). Neuroanatomical abnormalities in obsessive-compulsive disorder detected with quantitative x-ray computed tomography. *American Journal of Psychiatry, 145,* 1089–1093.

Lykken, D. T. (1957). A study of anxiety in the sociopathic personality. *Journal of Abnormal and Social Psychology, 55,* 6–10.

Maas, J. W. (1975). Biogenic amines and depression: Biochemical and pharmacological separation of two types of depression. *Archives of General Psychiatry, 32,* 1357–1361.

Maccoby, E. E., & Jacklin, C. N. (1974). *The psychology of sex differences.* Stanford, CA: Stanford University Press.

Mack, J. E., & Hickler, H. (1981). *Vivienne: The life and suicide of an adolescent girl.* Boston: Little, Brown.

Mackay, A. V. (1980). Positive and negative schizophrenic symptoms and the role of dopamine. *British Journal of Psychiatry, 137,* 379–386.

MacKay, M. C., Beck, L., & Taylor, R. (1973). Methylphenidate for adolescents with minimal brain dysfunction. *New York State Journal of Medicine, 73,* 550–554.

Mackay, R. I. (1982). The causes of severe mental handicap. *Developmental Medicine and Child Neurology, 24,* 386–388.

MacKeith, R., Meadow, R., & Turner, R. K. (1973). How children become dry. In I. Kolvin, R. C. MacKeith, & S. R. Meadow (Eds.), *Bladder control and enuresis* (pp. 3–21) (Clinics in Developmental Medicine, Nos. 48/49). London: Heinemann.

MacKenzie, J. N. (1886). The production of "rose asthma" by an artificial rose. *American Journal of Medical Science, 91,* 45–57.

MacQueen, G., Marshall, J., Perdue, M., Siegel, S., & Bienenstock, J. (1989). Pavlovian conditioning of rat mucosal mast cells to secrete rat mast cell protease II. *Science, 243,* 83–85.

Mahler, M. S. (1949). A psychoanalytic evaluation of tic in psychopathology of children: Symptomatic and tic syndrome. *The Psychoanalytic Study of the Child, 3/4,* 279–310.

Mahler, M. S. (1952). On child psychosis and schizophrenia: Autistic and symbiotic infantile psychoses. *Psychoanalytic Study of the Child, 7,* 286–305.

Mahler, M. S. (1966). Notes on the development of basic moods: The depressive affect in psychoanalysis. In R. Loewenstein (Ed.), *Psychoanalysis: A general psychology.* New York: International Universities Press.

Mahler, M. S. (1968). *On human symbiosis and the vicissitudes of individuation: Vol. 1. Infantile psychosis.* New York: International Universities Press.

Mahler, M. S., Pine, F., & Bergman, A. (1975). *The psychological birth of the human infant.* New York: Basic Books.

Malatesta, C. Z., Jonas, R., & Izard, C. E. (1987). The relation between low facial expressivity during emotional arousal and somatic symptoms. *British Journal of Medical Psychology, 60,* 169–180.

Malcolm, J. (1984). *In the Freud archives.* New York: Knopf.

Malmquist, C. P. (1965). School phobia: A problem in family neurosis. *Journal of Child Psychiatry, 4,* 293–319.

Malone, C., & Drotar, D. (1983, October). *A prospective study of failure to thrive: Outcome data for the children up to the age of two.* Paper presented at the 30th annual meeting of the American Academy of Child Psychiatry, San Francisco.

Maloney, M. J. (1980). Diagnosing hysterical conversion reactions in children. *Journal of Pediatrics, 97,* 1016–1020.

Mann, H. B., & Greenspan, S. I. (1976). The identification and treatment of adult brain dysfunction. *American Journal of Psychiatry, 133,* 1013–1017.

Mann, V. A. (1986). Why some children encounter reading problems: The contribution of difficulties with language processing and phonological sophistication to early reading disability. In J. K. Torgesen & B. Y. L. Wong (Eds.), *Psychological and educational perspectives on learning disabilities* (pp. 133–160). New York: Academic.

Mannuzza, S., Klein, R. G., Konig, P. H., & Giampino, T. L. (1989). Hyperactive boys almost grown up: IV. Criminality and its relationship to psychiatric status. *Archives of General Psychiatry, 46,* 1073–1079.

Marchi, M., & Cohen, P. (1990). Early childhood eating behaviors and adolescent eating disorders. *Journal of the American Academy of Child and Adolescent Psychiatry, 29,* 112–117.

Marcus, J., Hans, S. L., Lewow, E., Wilkinson, L., & Burack, C. M. (1985a). Neurological findings in high-risk children: Childhood assessment and 5-year followup. *Schizophrenia Bulletin, 11,* 85–100.

Marcus, J., Hans, S. L., Mednick, S. A., Schulsinger, F., & Michelsen, N. (1985b). Neurological dysfunctioning in offspring of schizophrenics in Israel and Denmark: A replication analysis. *Archives of General Psychiatry, 42,* 753–761.

Marcus, J., Hans, S. L., Nagler, S., Auerbach, J. G., Mirsky, A. F., & Aubrey, A. (1987). Review of the NIMH Israeli Kibbutz-City Study and the Jerusalem Infant Development Study. *Schizophrenia Bulletin, 13*, 425–438.

Margraf, J., Ehlers, A., & Roth, W. T. (1986). Sodium lactate infusions and panic attacks: A review and critique. *Psychosomatic Medicine, 48*, 23–51.

Marks, I. (1983). Are there anticompulsive or antiphobic drugs? Review of the evidence. *British Journal of Psychiatry, 143*, 338–347.

Marks, I. M. (1986). Genetics of fear and anxiety disorders. *British Journal of Psychiatry, 149*, 406–418.

Marks, I. M. (1987). *Fears, phobias, and rituals: Panic, anxiety, and their disorders.* New York: Oxford University Press.

Marohn, R., Dalle-Molle, D., McCarter E., & Linn, D. (1980). *Juvenile delinquents: Psychodynamic assessment and hospital treatment.* New York: Brunner/Mazel.

Martin, C., & Halversod, C. F. (1981). A schematic-processing model of sex typing and stereotyping in children. *Child Development, 52*, 1119–1134.

Martin, H. P. (1981). The neuro-psycho-developmental aspects of child abuse and neglect. In N. S. Ellerstein (Ed.), *Child abuse and neglect: A medical reference* (pp. 95–119). New York: Wiley.

Martin, H. P., & Beezley, P. (1977). Behavioral observations of abused children. *Developmental Medicine and Child Neurology, 19*, 373–387.

Martin, H. P., Beezley, P., Conway, E. F., & Kempe, C. H. (1974). The development of abused children. *Advances in Pediatrics, 21*, 25–72.

Martin, J. M., & Fitzpatrick, J. P. (1965). *Delinquent behavior.* New York: Random House.

Mason-Brothers, A., Ritvo, E. R., Guze, B., Mo, A., Freeman, B. J., Funderburk, S. J., & Schroth, P. C. (1987). Pre-, peri-, and postnatal factors in 181 autistic patients from single and multiple incidence families. *Journal of the American Academy of Child and Adolescent Psychiatry, 26*, 39–42.

Masson, J. M. (1984). *Freud, the assault on truth: Freud's suppression of the seduction theory.* New York: Farrar, Straus, & Giroux.

Masterson, J. (1985). Family assessment of the child with intractable asthma. *Developmental and Behavioral Pediatrics, 6*, 244–251.

Masterson, J. F. (1967). *The psychiatric dilemma of adolescence.* Boston: Little, Brown.

Masterson, J. F. (1972). *Treatment of the borderline adolescent: A developmental approach.* New York: Wiley.

Masterson, J. F. (1981). *The narcissistic and borderline disorders: An integrated developmental approach.* New York: Brunner/Mazel.

Masterson, J. F., & Costello, J. (1980). *From borderline adolescent to functioning adult: The test of time.* New York: Brunner/Mazel.

Mattes, J. A. (1980). The role of frontal lobe dysfunction in childhood hyperkinesis. *Comprehensive Psychiatry, 21*, 358–369.

Mattes, J. A., Boswell, L., & Oliver, H. (1984). Methylphenidate effects on symptoms of attention deficit disorder in adults. *Archives of General Psychiatry, 41*, 1059–1063.

Mattes, J. A., & Gittelman, R. (1981). Effects of artificial food colorings in children with hyperactive symptoms. *Archives of General Psychiatry, 38*, 714–718.

Mattes, J. A., & Gittelman, R. (1983). Growth of hyperactive children on maintenance regimen of methylphenidate. *Archives of General Psychiatry, 40,* 317–321.

Matthysse, S. (1987). Schizophrenic thought disorder: A model theoretic perspective. *Schizophrenia Bulletin, 13,* 173–184.

Mattis, S. (1978). Dyslexia syndromes: A working hypothesis that works. In A. L. Benton & D. Pearl (Eds.), *Dyslexia: An appraisal of current knowledge* (pp. 43–60). New York: Oxford University Press.

Mattison, R., Cantwell, D. P., Russell, A. T., & Will, L. (1979). A comparison of DSM-II and DSM-III in the diagnosis of childhood psychiatric disorders: II. Interrater agreement. *Archives of General Psychiatry, 36,* 1217–1222.

Matza, D., & Sykes, G. M. (1961). Juvenile delinquency and subterranean values. *American Sociological Review, 26,* 712–719.

May, J. G. (1979). Nosology and diagnosis. In J. D. Noshpitz (Ed.), *Basic handbook of child psychiatry* (Vol. 2, pp. 111–144). New York: Basic Books.

Mayes, L. C., & Carter, A. S. (1990). Emerging social regulatory capacities as seen in the still-face situation. *Child Development, 61,* 754–763.

Mayes, S. D., Humphrey, F. J., II., Handford, H. A., & Mitchell, J. F. (1988). Rumination disorder: Differential diagnosis. *Journal of the American Academy of Child and Adolescent Psychiatry, 27,* 300–302.

McConville, B. J., Boag, L. C., & Purohit, A. P. (1973). Three types of childhood depression. *Canadian Psychiatric Association Journal, 18,* 133–138.

McCord, W., McCord, J., & Zola, I. K. (1959). *Origins of crime.* New York: Columbia University Press.

McDermott, J. F., Jr. (1985). Anxiety disorder in children and adults: Coincidence or consequence? *Integrative Psychiatry, 3,* 158–167.

McFadden, E. R., Jr., Luparello, T., Lyons, H. A., Bleeker, E. (1969). The mechanism of action of suggestion in the induction of acute asthma attacks. *Psychosomatic Medicine, 31,* 134–143.

McGee, R., & Share, D. L. (1988). Attention deficit disorder-hyperactivity and academic failure: Which comes first and what should be treated? *Journal of the American Academy of Child and Adolescent Psychiatry, 27,* 318–325.

McGee, R., Williams, S., Share, D. L., Anderson, J., & Silva, P. A. (1986). The relationship between specific reading retardation, general reading backwardness and behavioural problems in a large sample of Dunedin boys: A longitudinal study from five to eleven years. *Journal of Child Psychology and Psychiatry, 27,* 597–610.

McGee, R., Williams, S., & Silva, P. A. (1984a). Background characteristics of aggressive, hyperactive, and aggressive-hyperactive boys. *Journal of the American Academy of Child Psychiatry, 23,* 280–284.

McGee, R., Williams, S., & Silva, P. A. (1984b). Behavioral and developmental characteristics of aggressive, hyperactive, and aggressive-hyperactive boys. *Journal of the American Academy of Child Psychiatry, 23,* 270–279.

McGee, R., Williams, S., & Silva, P. A. (1987). A comparison of girls and boys with teacher-identified problems of attention. *Journal of the American Academy of Child and Adolescent Psychiatry, 26,* 711–717.

McGlashan, T. H. (1982). Aphanisis: The syndrome of pseudo-depression in chronic schizophrenia. *Schizophrenia Bulletin, 8,* 118–134.

McGlashan, T. H. (1983a). The borderline syndrome: I. Testing three diagnostic systems. *Archives of General Psychiatry, 40,* 1311–1318.

McGlashan, T. H. (1983b). The borderline syndrome: II. Is it a variant of schizophrenia or affective disorder? *Archives of General Psychiatry, 40,* 1319–1323.

McGlashan, T. H. (1983c). Intensive individual psychotherapy of schizophrenia: A review of techniques. *Archives of General Psychiatry, 40,* 909–920.

McGlashan, T. H. (1986a). Predictors of shorter-, medium-, and longer-term outcome in schizophrenia. *American Journal of Psychiatry, 143,* 50–55.

McGlashan, T. H. (1986b). Schizotypal personality disorder. Chestnut Lodge Follow-Up Study: VI. Long-term follow-up perspectives. *Archives of General Psychiatry, 43,* 329–334.

McGlashan, T. H. (1986c) Schizophrenia: Psychosocial treatments and the role of psychosocial factors in its etiology and pathogenesis. In A. J. Frances & R. E. Hales (Eds.), *Psychiatry Update Annual Review* (Vol. 5, pp. 96–111). Washington, DC: American Psychiatric Association.

McGlashan, T. H. (1987). Testing DSM-III symptom criteria for schizotypal and borderline personality disorders. *Archives of General Psychiatry, 44,* 143–148.

McGlashan, T. H. (1988). Adolescent versus adult onset of mania. *American Journal of Psychiatry, 145,* 221–223.

McGue, M. (1989). Nature-nurture and intelligence. *Nature, 340,* 507–508.

McGuffin, P., Farmer, A., & Gottesman, I. I. (1987). Is there really a split in schizophrenia? The genetic evidence. *British Journal of Psychiatry, 150,* 581–592.

McKenna, P. J. (1987). Pathology, phenomenology and the dopamine hypothesis of schizophrenia. *British Journal of Psychiatry, 151,* 288–301.

McKeon, P., & Murray, R. (1987). Familial aspects of obsessive-compulsive neurosis. *British Journal of Psychiatry, 151,* 528–534.

McKinney, J. D. (1984). The search for subtypes of specific learning disability. *Journal of Learning Disabilities, 17,* 41–50.

McKinney, W. T., Jr. (1977). Animal behavioral/biological models relevant to depressive and affective disorders in humans. In J. G. Schulterbrandt & A. Raskin (Eds.), *Depression in childhood: Diagnosis, treatment, and conceptual models* (pp. 107–122). New York: Raven Press.

McKnew, D. H., Jr., Cytryn, L., Efron, A. M., Gershon, E. S., & Bunney, W. E., Jr. (1979). Offspring of manic-depressive patients. *British Journal of Psychiatry, 134,* 148–152.

McLean, J. A., & Ching, A. Y. T. (1973). Follow-up study of relationships between family situation and bronchial asthma in children. *Journal of American Academy of Child Psychiatry, 12,* 142–161.

McMahon, R. C. (1980). Genetic etiology in the hyperactive child syndrome: A critical review. *American Journal of Orthopsychiatry, 50,* 145–150.

McNichol, K. N., & Williams, H. E. (1973a). Spectrum of asthma in children: I. Clinical and physiological components. *British Medical Journal, 4,* 7–11.

McNichol, K. N., & Williams, H. E. (1973b). Spectrum of asthma in children: II. Allergic components. *British Medical Journal, 4,* 12–16.

Mechanic, D. (1962). The concept of illness behavior. *Journal of Chronic Diseases, 15,* 189–194.

Mednick, S., Gabrielli, W., & Hutchings, B. (1984). Genetic influences in criminal convictions: Evidence from an adoptive cohort. *Science, 224,* 891–894.

Mednick, S. A., Machon, R. A., Huttunen, M. O., & Bonett, D. (1988). Adult schizophrenia following prenatal exposure to an influenza epidemic. *Archives of General Psychiatry, 45,* 189–192.

Mednick, S. A., Parnas, J., & Schulsinger, F. (1987). The Copenhagen High-Risk Project, 1962–1986. *Schizophrenia Bulletin, 13,* 485–495.

Meehl, P. E. (1962). Schizotaxia, schizotypy, schizophrenia. *American Psychologist, 17,* 827–838.

Meehl, P. E. (1989). Schizotaxia revisited. *Archives of General Psychiatry, 46,* 935–944.

Meers, D. (1970). Contribution of a ghetto culture to symptom formation: Psychoanalytic studies of ego anomalies in childhood. *Psychoanalytic Study of the Child, 25,* 209–230.

Meijer, A. (1978). Sources of dependency in asthmatic children. *Psychosomatics, 19,* 351–355.

Meltzer, H. Y. (1987). Biological studies in schizophrenia. *Schizophrenia Bulletin, 13,* 77–111.

Mendlewicz, J., Linkowski, P., Guroff, J. J., & Van Praag, H. M. (1979). Color blindness linkage to bipolar manic-depressive illness: New evidence. *Archives of General Psychiatry, 36,* 1442–1447.

Menkes, M., Rowe, J., & Menkes, J. (1967). A twenty-five year follow-up study on the hyperkinetic child with minimal brain dysfunction. *Pediatrics, 39,* 393–399.

Mercer, J. R. (1975). Sociocultural factors in educational labeling. In M. J. Begab & S. A. Richardson (Eds.), *The mentally retarded and society* (pp. 141–157). Baltimore: University Park Press.

Merton, R. K. (1935). Social structure and anomie. *American Sociological Review, 3,* 672–682.

Merton, R. K. (1957). *Social theory and social structure.* Glencoe, IL: Free Press.

Merz, B. (1988). Tourette's syndrome hypothesis creates controversy among geneticists. *Journal of the American Medical Association, 260,* 2619.

Meyer, J. K. (1982). The theory of gender identity disorders. *Journal of the American Psychoanalytic Association, 30,* 381–418.

Meyer, J. K., & Dupkin, C. (1985). Gender disturbance in children: An interim clinical report. *Bulletin of the Menninger Clinic, 49,* 236–269.

Meyer, R. J., & Haggerty, R. (1962). Streptococcal infections in families: Factors altering individual susceptibility. *Pediatrics, 29,* 539–549.

Meyer, V., Levy, R., & Schnurer, A. (1974). The behavioural treatment of obsessive-compulsive disorders. In H. R. Beech (Ed.), *Obsessional states* (pp. 233–258). London: Methuen.

Meyer-Bahlburg, H. F., Feldman, J. & Ehrhardt, A. A. (1985). Questionnaire for the assessment of atypical gender role behavior: A methodological study. *Journal of the American Academy of Child Psychiatry, 24,* 695–701.

Michaels, J. J. (1938). Incidence of enuresis and age of cessation in 100 delinquents and 100 sibling controls. *American Journal of Orthopsychiatry, 8,* 460–465.

Mikkelsen, E. J., Detlor, J., & Cohen, D. J. (1981). School avoidance and social phobia triggered by haloperidol in patients with Tourette's disorder. *American Journal of Psychiatry, 138,* 1572–1576.

Mikkelsen, E. J., Rapoport, J. L., Nee, L., Gruenau, C., Mendelson, W., & Gillin, J. C. (1980). Childhood enuresis: I. Sleep patterns and psychopathology. *Archives of General Psychiatry, 37,* 1139–1144.

Miklich, D. R., Rewey, H. H., Weiss, J. H., & Kolton, S. (1973). A preliminary investigation of psychophysiological responses to stress among different subgroups of asthmatic children. *Journal of Psychosomatic Research, 17,* 1–8.

Miles, S. W., & Wright, J. J. (1984). Psychoendocrine interaction in anorexia nervosa, and the retreat from puberty: A study of attitudes to adolescent conflict, and luteinizing hormone response to luteinizing hormone releasing factor, in refed anorexia nervosa subjects. *British Journal of Medical Psychology, 57,* 49–56.

Milich, R. S., & Loney, J. (1979). The factor composition of the WISC for hyperkinetic/MBD males. *Journal of Learning Disabilities, 12,* 491–495.

Milich, R. S., Loney, J., & Landau, S. (1982). Independent dimensions of hyperactivity and aggression: A validation with playroom observation data. *Journal of Abnormal Psychology, 91,* 183–198.

Miller, A. (1981). *Prisoners of childhood.* New York: Basic Books.

Miller, D., & Looney, J. (1974). The prediction of adolescent homicide: Episodic dyscontrol and dehumanization. *The American Journal of Psychoanalysis, 34,* 187–198.

Miller, L. C., Barrett, C. L., Hampe, E., & Noble, H. (1972a). Comparison of reciprocal inhibition, psychotherapy, and waiting list control for phobic children. *Journal of Abnormal Psychology, 79,* 269–279.

Miller, L. C., Barrett, C. L., Hampe, E., & Noble, H. (1972b). Factor structure of childhood fears. *Journal of Consulting and Clinical Psychology, 39,* 264–268.

Miller, T. W. (Ed.) (1989). *Stressful life events.* Madison, CT: International Universities Press.

Miller, W. (1958). Lower class culture as a generating milieu of gang delinquency. *Journal of Social Issues, 14,* 15–19.

Millon, T. (1986a). Personality prototypes and their diagnostic criteria. In T. Millon & G. L. Klerman (Eds.), *Contemporary directions in psychopathology: Toward the DSM-IV* (pp. 671–712). New York: Guilford.

Millon, T. (1986b). A theoretical derivation of pathological personalities. In T. Millon & G. L. Klerman (Eds.), *Contemporary directions in psychopathology: Toward the DSM-IV* (pp. 639–669). New York: Guilford.

Milowe, I. D., & Lourie, R. S. (1964). The child's role in the battered child syndrome. *Journal of Pediatrics, 65,* 1079–1081.

Minuchin, S., Baker, L., Rosman, B. L., Liebman, R., Milman, L., & Todd, T. C. (1975). A conceptual model of psychosomatic illness in children: Family organization and family therapy. *Archives of General Psychiatry, 32,* 1031–1038.

Minuchin, S., Rosman, B., & Baker, L. (1978). *Psychosomatic families: Anorexia nervosa in context.* Cambridge: Harvard University Press.

Mirksy, A. F., Silberman, E. K., Latz, A., & Nagler, S. (1985). Adult outcomes of high-risk children: Differential effects of town and kibbutz rearing. *Schizophrenia Bulletin, 11,* 150–154.

Mischel, W. (1966). A social learning view of sex differences in behavior. In E. E. Maccoby, (Ed.), *The development of sex differences.* Stanford, CA: Stanford University Press.

Mitchell, J. E. (1988). The pharmacologic management of bulimia nervosa: A critical review. *International Journal of Eating Disorders, 7,* 29–41.

Mitchell, J. E., & Bantle, J. P. (1983). Metabolic and endocrine investigations in women of normal weight with the bulimia syndrome. *Biological Psychiatry, 18,* 355–365.

Mitchell, J. E., Pyle, R. L., & Eckert, E. D. (1981). Frequency and duration of binge-eating episodes in patients with bulimia. *American Journal of Psychiatry, 138,* 835–836.

Mitchell, J. E., Pyle, R. L., Eckert, E. D., Hatsukami, D., Pomeroy, C., & Zimmerman, R. (1990). A comparison study of antidepressants and structured intensive group psychotherapy in the treatment of bulimia nervosa. *Archives of General Psychiatry, 47,* 149–157.

Mitchell, W. G., Gorrell, R. W., & Greenberg, R. A. (1980). Failure-to-thrive: A study in a primary care setting: Epidemiology and follow-up. *Pediatrics, 65,* 971–977.

Modell, J. G., Mountz, J. M., Curtis, G. C., & Greden, J. F. (1989). Neurophysiological dysfunction in basal ganglia/limbic striatal and thalamocortical circuits as a pathogenetic mechanism of obsessive-compulsive disorder. *Journal of Neuropsychiatry, 1,* 27–36.

Moffatt, M. E. K., Kato, C., & Pless, I. B. (1987). Improvements in self-concept after treatment of nocturnal enuresis: Randomized controlled trial. *Journal of Pediatrics, 110,* 647–652.

Mogul, S. L. (1980). Asceticism in adolescence and anorexia nervosa. *Psychoanalytic Study of the Child, 35,* 155–175.

Moldofsky, H., & Sandor, P. (1988). Pimozide in the treatment of Tourette's syndrome. In D. J. Cohen, R. D. Brunn, & J. F. Leckman (Eds.), *Tourette's syndrome and tic disorders: Clinical understanding and treatment* (pp. 281–289). New York: Wiley.

Monahan, J. (1984). The prediction of violent behavior: Toward a second generation of theory and policy. *American Journal of Psychiatry, 141,* 10–15.

Monane, M., Leichter, D., & Lewis, D. O. (1984). Physical abuse in psychiatrically hospitalized children and adolescents. *Journal of the American Academy of Child Psychiatry, 23,* 653–658.

Money, J., Hampson, J. G., & Hampson, J. L. (1955). Hermaphroditism: Recommendations concerning assignment of sex, change of sex and psychologic management. *Bulletin of Johns Hopkins Hospital, 97,* 284–300.

Money, J., Hampson, J. G., & Hampson, J. L. (1957). Imprinting and the establishment of gender role. *Archives of Neurology and Psychiatry, 77,* 333–336.

Money, J., & Russo, A. J. (1979). Homosexual outcome of discordant gender identity role: Longitudinal follow-up. *Journal of Pediatric Psychology, 4,* 29–41.

Moreau, D. L., Weissman, M., & Warner, V. (1989). Panic disorder in children at high risk for depression. *American Journal of Psychiatry, 146,* 1059–1060.

Morillo, E., & Gardner, L. I. (1979). Bereavement as an antecedent factor in thyrotoxicosis of childhood: Four case studies with survey of possible metabolic pathways. *Psychosomatic Medicine, 41,* 545–555.

Morley, J. E., & Levine, A. S. (1983). The central control of appetite. *Lancet, 1,* 398–401.

Morris, A. H., Escoll, M. D., & Wexler, R. (1956). Aggressive behavior disorders of childhood. *American Journal of Psychiatry, 112,* 991–997.

Morris, R. J., & Kratochwill, T. R. (1983). *Treating children's fears and phobias: A behavioral approach.* New York: Pergamon.

Morrison, J. R. (1980). Adult psychiatric disorders in parents of hyperactive children. *American Journal of Psychiatry, 137,* 825–827.

Morrison, J. R., & Stewart, M. A. (1971). A family study of the hyperactive child syndrome. *Biological Psychiatry, 3,* 189–195.

Morrison, J. R., & Stewart, M. A. (1973). The psychiatric status of the legal families of adopted hyperactive children. *Archives of General Psychiatry, 28,* 888–891.

Mrazek, D. A. (1981). The child psychiatric examination of the sexually abused child. In P. B. Mrazek & C. H. Kempe (Eds.), *Sexually abused children and their families* (pp. 143–153). Oxford: Pergamon.

Mrazek, D. A. (1986). Childhood asthma: Two central questions for child psychiatry. *Journal of Child Psychiatry, 27,* 1–5.

Mrazek, D. A., Casey, B., & Anderson, I. (1987). Insecure attachment in severely asthmatic preschool children: Is it a risk factor? *Journal of the American Academy of Child and Adolescent Psychiatry, 26,* 516–520.

Mrazek, D., & Mrazek, P. (1985). Child maltreatment. In M. Rutter & L. Hersov (Eds.), *Child and adolescent psychiatry: Modern approaches* (pp. 679–697). Oxford: Blackwell.

Mrazek, D. A., & Strunk, R. (1984). Psychological adjustment of severely asthmatic preschool children: Allergic considerations. *Psychosomatic Medicine, 46,* 85.

Mrazek, P. B. (1981a). The nature of incest: A review of contributing factors. In P. B. Mrazek & C. H. Kempe (Eds.), *Sexually abused children and their families* (pp. 97–108). Oxford: Pergamon.

Mrazek, P. B. (1981b). Special problems in the treatment of child sexual abuse. In P. B. Mrazek & C. H. Kempe (Eds.), *Sexually abused children and their families* (pp. 159–166). Oxford: Pergamon.

Mrazek, P. B., & Bentovim, A. (1981). Incest and the dysfunctional family system. In P. B. Mrazek & C. H. Kempe (Eds.), *Sexually abused children and their families* (pp. 167–178). Oxford: Pergamon.

Mrazek, P. B., Lynch, M., & Bentovim, A. (1981). Recognition of child sexual abuse in the United Kingdom. In P. B. Mrazek & C. H. Kempe (Eds.), *Sexually abused children and their families* (pp. 35–50). Oxford: Pergamon.

Mrazek, P. B., & Mrazek, D. A. (1981). The effects of child sexual abuse: Methodological considerations. In P. B. Mrazek & C. H. Kempe (Eds.), *Sexually abused children and their families* (pp. 235–245). Oxford: Pergamon.

Mundy, P., Sigman, M., Ungerer, J., & Sherman, T. (1986). Defining the social deficits of autism: The contribution of non-verbal communication measures. *Journal of Child Psychology and Psychiatry, 27*, 657–669.

Nadi, N. S., Nurnberger, J. I., & Gershon, E. S. (1984). Muscarinic cholinergic receptors on skin fibroblasts in familial affective disorder. *New England Journal of Medicine, 311*, 225–230.

Nagera, H. (1976). *Obsessional neuroses: Developmental psychopathology.* New York: Jason Aronson.

Nagera, U. (1966). *Early childhood disturbances, the infantile neurosis, and the adult disturbances.* New York: International Universities Press.

Nakashima, I. I., & Zakus, G. E. (1977). Incest: Review and clinical experience. *Pediatrics, 60*, 696–701.

Nasrallah, H. A., Loney, J., Olson, S. C., McCalley-Whitters, M., Kramer, J., & Jacoby, C. G. (1986). Cortical atrophy in young adults with a history of hyperactivity in childhood. *Psychiatry Research, 17*, 241–246.

National Center for Health Statistics. (1989). Monthly vital statistics report. *Advance Report of Final Mortality Statistics, 1987, 38*(Suppl. 5), 19.

National Center on Child Abuse and Neglect (1984). *Perspectives on child maltreatment in the mid '80s.* Washington, DC: U.S. Department of Health and Human Services.

National Institute of Mental Health (NIMH). (1985). *Psychopharmacology Bulletin, 21*(4), 951–988.

Needleman, H. L. (1981). *Studies in children exposed to low levels of lead.* EPA-600/1-81-066, North Carolina 27711. Washington, DC: Environmental Protection Agency.

Needleman, H. L., Gunnoe, C., Leviton, A., Reed, R., Peresie, H., Maher, C., & Barrett, P. (1979). Deficits in psychologic and classroom performance of children with elevated dentine lead levels. *New England Journal of Medicine, 300*, 689–695.

Neill, J. R., & Sandifer, M. G. (1982). The clinical approach to alexithymia: A review. *Psychosomatics, 23*, 1223–1231.

Nelson, J. C., Bowers, M. B., & Sweeney, D. R. (1979). Exacerbation of psychosis by tricyclic antidepressants in delusional depression. *American Journal of Psychiatry, 136*, 574–576.

Nelson, S. H., & Grunebaum, H. (1971). A follow-up study of wrist slashers. *American Journal of Psychiatry, 127*, 1345–1349.

Nemiah, J. C. (1984). Foreword. In T. R. Insel (Ed.), *Obsessive-compulsive disorder* (pp. ix-xi). Washington, DC: American Psychiatric Press.

Neuhaus, E. (1958). A personality study of asthmatic and cardiac children. *Psychosomatic Medicine, 20*, 181–186.

Newberger, E. H., Hampton, R. L., Marx, T. J., & White, K. M. (1986). Child abuse and pediatric social illness: An epidemiological analysis and ecological reformulation. *American Journal of Orthopsychiatry, 56*, 589–601.

Newberger, E. H., Reed, R. B., Daniel, J. H., Hyde, J. N., & Kotelchuck, M. (1977). Pediatric social illness: Toward an etiologic classification. *Pediatrics, 60*, 178–185.

Newcorn, J., Halperin, J. M., Healey, J., O'Brien, J., Morganstein, A., Sharma, V., & Young, J. G. (1987, October). *Are ADDH and ADHD children the same or different?* Paper read at the American Academy of Child and Adolescent Psychiatry Convention, Washington, DC.

Nichols, K. A. (1974). Severe social anxiety. *British Journal of Medical Psychology, 47,* 301–306.

Nichols, P. L., & Chen, T.-C. (1981). Minimal brain dysfunction: A prospective study. Hillsdale, NJ: Erlbaum.

Nieman, G. W., & Delong, R. (1987). Use of the Personality Inventory for Children as an aid in differentiating children with mania from children with attention deficit disorder with hyperactivity. *Journal of the American Academy of Child and Adolescent Psychiatry, 26,* 381–388.

Nixon, H. (1975). The diagnosis and management of faecal incontinence in children. *Archivum Chirurgicum Neerlandicum, 27,* 171–177.

Nordahl, T. E., Benkelfat, C., Semple, W. E., Gross, M., King, A. C., & Cohen, R. M. (1989). Cerebral glucose metabolic rates in obsessive-compulsive disorder. *Neuropsychopharmacology, 2,* 23–28.

Noshpitz, J. D. (1960). On the etiology of adolescent delinquency. *Pediatric Clinics of North America, 7,* 97–114.

Noshpitz, J. D. (1962). Notes on the theory of residential treatment. *Journal of the American Academy of Child Psychiatry, 1,* 284–296.

Noshpitz, J. D. (1980). Disturbances in early adolescent development. In S. I. Greenspan & G. H. Pollock (Eds.), *The course of life: Psychoanalytic contributions toward understanding personality development* (Vol. 2, pp. 309–356). Washington, DC: NIMH.

Noshpitz, J. D. (1984). Narcissism and aggression. *American Journal of Psychotherapy, 38,* 17–34.

Nuechterlein, K. H. (1986). Childhood precursors of adult schizophrenia. *Journal of Child Psychology and Psychiatry, 27,* 133–144.

Nunn, K. P. (1986). Annotation: The episodic dyscontrol syndrome in childhood. *Journal of Child Psychology and Psychiatry, 27,* 439–446.

Nunn, K. P., Lask, B., & Cohen, M. (1986). Viruses, neurodevelopmental disorder and childhood psychosis. *Journal of Child Psychology and Psychiatry, 27,* 55–64.

Nurcombe, B. (1964). Children who set fires. *Medical Journal of Australia, 1*(16), 579–584.

Nurcombe, B. (1986). The child as witness: Competency and credibility. *Journal of the American Academy of Child Psychiatry, 25,* 473–480.

Nurnberger, J. I., Jr., & Gershon, E. S. (1982). Genetics. In E. S. Paykel (Ed.), *Handbook of affective disorders.* Edinburgh and London: Churchill-Livingstone.

Nyhan, W. L. (1978). The Lesch-Nyhan syndrome. *Developmental Medicine and Child Neurology, 20,* 376–380.

Oates, K. (1986). *Child abuse and neglect: What happens eventually?* New York: Brunner/Mazel.

Oates, R. K. (1984). Overturning the diagnosis of child abuse. *Archives of Disease in Childhood, 59,* 665–677.

Oates, R. K., & Hufton, I. W. (1977). The spectrum of failure to thrive and child abuse: A follow-up study. *Child Abuse and Neglect, 1,* 119–124.

O'Carroll, P. W., Mercy, J. A., & Steward, J. A. (1988). CDC recommendations for a community plan for the prevention and containment of suicide clusters. *Morbidity and Mortality Weekly Report, 37*(Suppl. 6), 1–12.

O'Connor, J. (1983). Why can't I get hives: Brief strategic therapy with an obsessional child. *Family Process, 22,* 201–209.

Offer, D. (1969). *The psychological world of the teen-ager.* New York: Basic Books.

Offer, D., Marohn, R. C., & Ostrov, E. (1979). *The psychological world of the juvenile delinquent.* New York: Basic Books.

Offer, D., Ostrov, E., & Howard, K. I. (Eds.). (1984). Patterns of adolescent self-image. *New Directions for Mental Health Services* (p. 22). San Francisco: Jossey-Bass.

Offer, D., Ostrov, E., & Howard, K. I. (1987). Epidemiology of mental health and mental illness among adolescents. In J. D. Noshpitz (Ed.), *Basic handbook of child psychiatry* (Vol. 5, pp. 82–88). New York: Basic Books.

Office of Education (1976). Assistance to states for education of handicapped children: notice of proposed rulemaking. *Federal Register, 41,* 52404–52407.

Olatawura, M. (1973). Encopresis: A review of thirty-two cases. *Acta Paediatrica Scandanavica, 62,* 358–364.

Ollendick, T. H., & Mayer, J. A. (1984). School phobia. In S. M. Turner (Ed.), *Behavioral theories and treatment of anxiety* (pp. 367–411). New York: Plenum.

Olweus, D. (1979). Stability of aggressive reaction patterns in males: A review. *Psychological Bulletin, 86,* 852–875.

Olweus, D. (1980). Familial and temperamental determinants of aggressive behavior in adolescent boys: A causal analysis. *Developmental Psychology, 16,* 644–660.

Olweus, D., Mattson, A., Schalling, D., & Low, H. (1980). Testosterone, aggression, physical and personality dimensions in normal adolescent males. *Psychosomatic Medicine, 42,* 253–269.

Onnis, L., Tortolani, D., & Cancrini, L. (1986). Systemic research on chronicity factors in infantile asthma. *Family Process, 25,* 107–122.

Oppel, W. C., Harper, P. A., & Rider, R. (1968a). The age of attaining bladder control. *Journal of Pediatrics, 42,* 614–626.

Oppel, W. C., Harper, P. A., & Rider, R. V. (1968b). Social, psychological, and neurological factors associated with nocturnal enuresis. *Pediatrics, 42,* 627–641.

Ornitz, E. M. (1974). The modulation of sensory input and motor output in autistic children. *Journal of Autism and Childhood Schizophrenia, 4,* 197–215.

Ornitz, E. M. (1985). Neurophysiology of infantile autism. *Journal of the American Academy of Child Psychiatry, 24,* 251–262.

Ornitz, E. M. (1987). Neurophysiologic studies of infantile autism. In D. J. Cohen & A. M. Donnellan (Eds.), *Handbook of autism and pervasive developmental disorders* (pp. 148–165). New York: Wiley.

Ornitz, E. M., & Ritvo, E. R. (1968). Perceptual inconstancy in early infantile autism. *Archives of General Psychiatry, 18,* 76–98.

Ornstein, A. (1981). Self pathology in childhood: Developmental and clinical considerations. In K. Robson (Ed.), *The psychiatric clinics of North America: Development and pathology of the self* (Vol. 4, pp. 435–453). Philadelphia: Saunders.

Ornstein, A. (1984, October) *The treatment of the "Narcissistic Child."* Unpublished manuscript presented at the Annual Meeting of the American Academy of Child Psychiatry, Toronto, Ontario.

Orvaschel, H., & Weissman, M. M. (1986). Epidemiology of anxiety disorders in children: A review. In R. Gittelman (Ed.), *Anxiety disorders of childhood* (pp. 58–72). New York: Guilford.

Oster, J. (1972). Recurrent abdominal pain, headache and limb pains in children and adolescents. *Pediatrics, 50,* 429–436.

Owen, F. (1963). Patterns of respiratory disturbance in asthmatic children evoked by the stimulus of the mother's voice. *Acta Psychotherapeutica and Psychosomatica, 11,* 228–241.

Oxman, T. E., Rosenberg, S. D., Schnurr, P. P., & Tucker, G. J. (1985). Linguistic dimensions of affect and thought in somatization disorder. *American Journal of Psychiatry, 142,* 1150–1155.

Panksepp, J., Herman, B. H., Vilberg, T., Bishop, P., & DeEskinazi, F. G. (1980). Endogenous opioids and social behavior. *Neuroscience and Biobehavioral Review, 4,* 473–487.

Pao, P.-N. (1969). The syndrome of delicate self-cutting. *British Journal of Medical Psychology, 42,* 195–206.

Pao, P.-N. (1979). *Schizophrenic disorders: Theory and treatment from a psychodynamic point of view.* New York: International Universities Press.

Paradise, J. L. (1966). Maternal and other factors in the etiology of infantile colic. *Journal of the American Medical Association, 197,* 123–131.

Pardes, H., Kaufmann, C. A., & West, A. (1987). Update on research in schizophrenia: Report on the Tarrytown Conference, April 13–15, 1986. *Schizophrenia Bulletin, 13,* 185–198.

Parkes, C. M., & Brown, R. J. (1972). Health after bereavement: A controlled study of young Boston widows and widowers. *Psychosomatic Medicine, 34,* 449–461.

Parkes, C. M., & Stevenson-Hinde, J. (1982). *The place of attachment in human behavior.* New York: Basic Books.

Pasamanick, B., & Kawi, A. (1956). A study of the association of prenatal and paranatal factors in the development of tics in children. *Pediatrics, 48,* 596–601.

Pasamanick, B., Rogers, M. E., & Lilienfeld, A. M. (1956). Pregnancy experience and the development of behavior disorder in children. *American Journal of Psychiatry, 112,* 613–618.

Paternite, C. E., & Loney, J. (1980). Childhood hyperkinesis: Relationships between symptomatology and home environment. In C. K. Whalen & B. Henker (Eds.), *Hyperactive children: The social ecology of identification and treatment.* New York: Academic.

Paternite, C. E., Loney, J., & Langhorne, J. E. (1976). Relationships between symptomatology and SES-related factors in hyperkinetic/MBD boys. *American Journal of Orthopsychiatry, 46,* 291–301.

Pato, M. T., Zohar-Kadouch, R., Zohar, J., & Murphy, D. L. (1988). Return of symptoms after discontinuation of clomipramine in patients with obsessive-compulsive disorder. *American Journal of Psychiatry, 145,* 1521–1525.

Patterson, G. R. (1965). A learning theory approach to the problem of the school phobic child. In L. P. Ullman & L. Krasner (Eds.), *Case studies in behavior modification* (pp. 279–285). New York: Holt, Rinehart & Winston.

Patterson, G. R. (1976). The aggressive child: Victim and architect of a coercive system. In E. J. Mash, L. J. Hamerlynk, & L. C. Handy (Eds.), *Behavioral modification and families*. New York: Brunner/Mazel.

Patterson, G. R. (1982). *Coercive family process*. Eugene, OR: Castalia.

Patterson, T. (1986). Electrophysiological studies of schizophrenia. *Bulletin of the Menninger Clinic, 50,* 238–256.

Paul, R. (1987). Communication. In D. J. Cohen & A. M. Donnellan (Eds.), *Handbook of autism and pervasive developmental disorders* (pp. 61–84). New York: Wiley.

Paul, S. M., & Skolnick, P. (1984). The biochemistry of anxiety: From pharmacotherapy to pathophysiology. In L. Grinspoon (Ed.), *Psychiatry update* (Vol. 3, pp. 482–490). Washington, DC: American Psychiatric Press.

Pauls, D. L. (1987). The familiality of autism and related disorders: A review of the evidence. In D. J. Cohen & A. M. Donnellan (Eds.), *Handbook of autism and pervasive developmental disorders* (pp. 192–198). New York: Wiley.

Pauls, D. L., Bucher, K. D., Crowe, R. R., & Noyes, R. (1980). A genetic study of panic disorder pedigrees. *American Journal of Human Genetics, 32,* 639–644.

Pauls, D. L., Hurst, C. R., Kruger, S. D., Leckman, J. F., Kidd, K. K., & Cohen, D. J. (1986a). Gilles de la Tourette's syndrome and attention deficit disorder with hyperactivity: Evidence against a genetic relationship. *Archives of General Psychiatry, 43,* 1177–1179.

Pauls, D. L., Hurst, C. R., Leckman, J. F., Cohen, D. J., Kruger, S. D., and Kidd, K. K. (1987). Tourette's syndrome and attention deficit disorder with hyperactivity [Reply to letter]. *Archives of General Psychiatry, 44,* 1025–1026.

Pauls, D. L., Kruger, S. D., Leckman, J. F., Cohen, D. J., & Kidd, K. K. (1984). The risk of Tourette's syndrome and chronic multiple tics among relatives of Tourette's syndrome patients obtained by direct interview. *Journal of the American Academy of Child Psychiatry, 23,* 134–137.

Pauls, D. L., & Leckman, J. F. (1986). The inheritance of Gilles de la Tourette's syndrome and associated behaviors. *New England Journal of Medicine, 315,* 993–997.

Pauls, D. L., & Leckman, J. F. (1988). The genetics of Tourette's syndrome. In D. J. Cohen, R. D. Brunn, & J. F. Leckman (Eds.), *Tourette's syndrome and tic disorders: Clinical understanding and treatment* (pp. 91–101). New York: Wiley.

Pauls, D. L., Pakstis, A. J., Kurlan, R., Kidd, K. K., Leckman, J. F., Cohen, D. J., Kidd, J. R., Como, P., Sparkes, R. (1990). Segregation and linkage analyses of Tourette's syndrome and related disorders. *Journal of the American Academy of Child and Adolescent Psychiatry, 29,* 195–203.

Pauls, D. L., Towbin, K. E., Leckman, J. F., Zahner, G. E. P., & Cohen, D. J. (1986b). Gilles de la Tourette's syndrome and obsessive-compulsive disorder. *Archives of General Psychiatry, 43,* 1180–1182.

Paykel, E. S., & Rassaby, E. (1978). Classification of suicide attempters by cluster-analysis. *British Journal of Psychiatry, 133,* 45–52.

Payton, J. B., Steele, M. W., Wenger, S. L., Minshew, N. J. (1989). The fragile X marker and autism in perspective. *Journal of the American Academy of Child and Adolescent Psychiatry, 28,* 417–421.

Pearl, R., Donahue, M., & Bryan, T. (1986). Social relationships of learning-disabled children. In J. K. Torgesen & B. Y. L. Wong (Eds.), *Psychological and educational perspectives on learning disabilities* (pp. 193–224). New York: Academic.

Pelham, W. E. (1982). Childhood hyperactivity: Diagnosis, etiology, nature and treatment. In R. Gatchel, A. Baum, & J. Singer (Eds.), *Clinical psychology and behavioral medicine: Overlapping disciplines*. Hillsdale, NJ: Erlbaum.

Pelham, W. E., & Bender, M. E. (1982). Peer relationships in hyperactive children: Description and treatment. In K. D. Gadow & I. Bialer (Eds.), *Advances in learning and behavioral disabilities, Vol. 1*. Greenwich, CT: JAI.

Pelham, W. E., & Milich, R. (1984). Peer relations in children with hyperactivity/attention deficit disorder. *Journal of Learning Disabilities, 17*, 560–567.

Pennington, B. F. (1990). Annotation: The genetics of dyslexia. *Journal of Child Psychology and Psychiatry, 31*, 193–201.

Perry, R., Campbell, M., Adams, P., Lynch, N., Spencer, E. K., Curren, E. L., & Overall, J. E. (1989). Long-term efficacy of haloperidol in autistic children: Continuous versus discontinuous drug administration. *Journal of the American Academy of Child and Adolescent Psychiatry, 28*, 87–92.

Person, E. S., & Ovesey, L. (1974a). The transsexual syndrome in males: I. Primary transsexualism. *American Journal of Psychotherapy, 28*, 4–20.

Person, E. S., & Ovesey, L. (1974b). The transsexual syndrome in males: II. Secondary transsexualism. *American Journal of Psychotherapy, 28*, 174–193.

Person, E. S., & Ovesey, L. (1984). Homosexual cross-dressers. *Journal of the American Academy of Psychoanalysis, 12*, 167–186.

Petti, T. A. (1983). Psychopharmacologic treatment of borderline children. In K. S. Robson (Ed.), *The borderline child: Approaches to etiology, diagnosis, and treatment* (pp. 235–256). New York: McGraw-Hill.

Petti, T. A., Bornstein, M., Delamater, A., & Conners, C. K. (1980). Evaluation and multimodality treatment of a depressed prepubertal girl. *Journal of the American Academy of Child Psychiatry, 19*, 690–702.

Petti, T. A., & Law, W., III. (1982). Borderline psychotic behavior in hospitalized children: Approaches to assessment and treatment. *Journal of the American Academy of Child Psychiatry, 21*, 197–202.

Petti, T. A., & Unis, A. (1981). Imipramine treatment of borderline children: Case reports with a controlled study. *American Journal of Psychiatry, 138*, 515–518.

Petti, T. A., & Vela, R. M. (1990). Borderline disorders of childhood: An overview. *Journal of the American Academy of Child and Adolescent Psychiatry, 29*, 327–337.

Petty, L. K., Ornitz, E. M., Michelman, J. D., & Zimmerman, E. G. (1984). Autistic children who become schizophrenic. *Archives of General Psychiatry, 41*, 129–135.

Pfeffer, C. R. (1986). *The suicidal child*. New York: Guilford.

Pfeffer, C. R. (1988). Suicidal behavior among children and adolescents: Risk identification and intervention. In A. J. Frances & R. E. Hales (Eds.), *Review of psychiatry* (pp. 386–402). Washington, DC: American Psychiatric Press.

Pfeffer, C. R. (1989). Family characteristics and support systems as risk factors for youth suicide. In Alcohol, Drug Abuse, and Mental Health Administration (Ed.), *Report of the Secretary's Task Force for Youth Suicide: Vol. 2. Risk factors for youth suicide*

(DHHS Publication No. ADM 89-1622, pp. 71–87). Washington, DC: U.S. Government Printing Office.

Pfeffer, C. R., Adams, D. A., Weimer, A., & Rosenberg, J. (1987, October). *Parental stresses of suicidal child and young adolescent psychiatric inpatients.* New research poster at the Annual Meeting of the American Academy of Child and Adolescent Psychiatry, Washington, DC.

Pfeffer, C. R., Conte, H. R., Plutchik, R., & Jerret, I. (1979). Suicidal behavior in latency-age children: An empirical study. *Journal of the American Academy of Child and Adolescent Psychiatry, 18,* 679–692.

Pfeffer, C. R., Lipkins, R., Plutchik, R., & Mizruchi, M. (1988). Normal children at risk for suicidal behavior: A two-year follow-up study. *Journal of the American Academy of Child and Adolescent Psychiatry, 27,* 34–41.

Pfeffer, C. R., Solomon, G., Plutchik, R., Mizruchi, M. S., & Weiner, A. (1982). Suicidal behavior in latency-age psychiatric inpatients: A replication and cross-validation. *Journal of the American Academy of Child and Adolescent Psychiatry, 21,* 564–569.

Pfeffer, C. R., Zuckerman, S., Plutchik, R., & Mizruchi, M. S. (1984). Suicidal behavior in normal school children: A comparison with child psychiatric inpatients. *Journal of the American Academy of Child and Adolescent Psychiatry, 23,* 416–423.

Pfeiffer, C. A. (1936). Sexual differences of the hypophyses and their determination by the gonads. *American Journal of Anatomy, 58,* 195–225.

Phillips, D. P., & Carstensen, L. L. (1986). Clustering of teenage suicides after television news stories about suicide. *New England Journal of Medicine, 315,* 685–689.

Phillips, D. P., & Paight, D. J. (1987). The impact of televised movies about suicide: A replicative study. *New England Journal of Medicine, 317,* 809–811.

Piaget, J. (1954). *The construction of reality in the child.* New York: Basic Books.

Piaget, J. (1965). *The moral judgement of the child.* New York: Free Press.

Pickar, D. B. (1986). Psychosocial aspects of learning disabilities. *Bulletin of the Menninger Clinic, 50,* 22–32.

Pine, F. (1974). On the concept "borderline" in children. *Psychoanalytic Study of the Child, 29,* 341–368.

Pine, F. (1983). A working nosology of borderline syndromes in children. In K. S. Robson (Ed.), *The borderline child: Approaches to etiology, diagnosis, and treatment* (pp. 83–99). New York: McGraw-Hill.

Pine, F. (1986). On the development of the "borderline-child-to-be." *American Journal of Orthopsychiatry, 56,* 450–457.

Pinkerton, P. (1958). Psychogenic megacolon in children: The implications of bowel negativism. *Archives of Disease in Childhood, 33,* 371–380.

Pipp, S. & Harmon, R. J. (1987). Attachment as Regulation: A Commentary. *Child Development, 58,* 648–652.

Pitman, R. K., & Jenike, M. A. (1988). Coprolalia in obsessive-compulsive disorder: A missing link. *Journal of Nervous and Mental Disease, 176,* 311–313.

Piven, J., Berthier, M. L., Starkstein, S. E., Nehme, E., Pearlson, G., & Folstein, S. (1990). Magnetic resonance imaging evidence for a defect of cerebral cortical development in autism. *American Journal of Psychiatry, 147*, 734–739.

Plachetta, K. E. (1976). Encopresis: A case study utilizing contracting, scheduling and self-charting. *Journal of Behavior Therapy and Experimental Psychiatry, 7*, 195–196.

Plato (1889). *The Dialogues of Plato: Vol. II. Timaeus* (B. Jowett, Trans.). New York: Scribner.

Pliszka, S. R. (1987). Tricyclic antidepressants in the treatment of children with attention deficit disorder. *Journal of the American Academy of Child and Adolescent Psychiatry, 26*, 127–132.

Plomin, R. (1983). Developmental behavioral genetics. *Child Development, 54*, 253–259.

Plomin, R., & DeFries, J. C. (1980). Genetics and intelligence: Recent data. *Intelligence, 4*, 15–24.

Polansky, N., Hally, D., & Polansky, N. F. (1975). *Profile of neglect: A survey of the state of knowledge of child neglect.* Department of Health, Education, and Welfare: Community Services Administration, Social and Rehabilitation Services.

Pollitt, E., Eichler, A. W., & Chan, C-K. (1975). Psychosocial development and behavior of mothers of failure-to-thrive children. *American Journal of Orthopsychiatry, 45*, 525–537.

Pope, H. G., Champoux, R. F., & Hudson, J. I. (1987). Eating disorder and socioeconomic class: Anorexia nervosa and bulimia in nine communities. *The Journal of Nervous and Mental Disease, 175*, 620–623.

Pope, H. G., Jonas, J. M., Hudson, J. I., Cohen, B. M., & Gunderson, J. B. (1983b). The validity of DSM-III borderline personality disorder. *Archives of General Psychiatry, 40*, 23–30.

Pope, H. G., Jr., Hudson, J. I., Jonas, J. M., & Yurgelun-Todd, D. (1983a). Bulimia treated with imipramine: A placebo-controlled, double-blind study. *American Journal of Psychiatry, 140*, 554–558.

Pope, H. G., Jr., Hudson, J. I., Jonas, J. M., & Yurgelun-Todd, D. (1985). Antidepressant treatment of bulimia: A two-year follow-up study. *Journal of Clinical Psychopharmacology, 5*, 320–327.

Pope, H. G., Jr., Hudson, J. I., & Yurgelun-Todd, D. (1984). Anorexia nervosa and bulimia among 300 suburban women shoppers. *American Journal of Psychiatry, 141*, 292–293.

Popper, K. R., & Eccles, J. C. (1977). *The self and its brain.* London: Routledge & Kegan Paul.

Porges, S. W. (1984). Physiologic correlates of attention: A core process underlying learning disorders. *Pediatric Clinics of North America, 31*, 371–385.

Porrino, L. J., Rapoport, J. L., Behar, D., Ismond, D. R., & Bunney, W. E. (1983a). A naturalistic assessment of the motor activity of hyperactive boys: II. Stimulant drug effects. *Archives of General Psychiatry, 40*, 688–693.

Porrino, L. J., Rapoport, J. L., Behar, D., Sceery, W., Ismond, D. R., & Bunney, W. E. (1983b). A naturalistic assessment of the motor activity of hyperactive boys: I. Comparison with normal controls. *Archives of General Psychiatry, 40*, 681–687.

Posner, M. I., Petersen, S. E., Fox, P. T., & Raichle, M. E. (1988). Localization of cognitive operations in the human brain. *Science, 240,* 1627–1631.

Powell, G. F., Brasel, J. A., & Blizzard, R. M. (1967a). Emotional deprivation and growth retardation simulating idiopathic hypopituitarism: I. Clinical evaluation of the syndrome. *New England Journal of Medicine, 276,* 1271–1278.

Powell, G. F., Brasel, J. A., Raiti, S., & Blizzard, R. M. (1967b). Emotional deprivation and growth retardation simulating idiopathic hypopituitarism: II. Endocrinological evaluation of the syndrome. *New England Journal of Medicine, 276,* 1279–1283.

Poznanski, E. O., Krahenbuhl, V., & Zrull, J. P. (1976). Childhood depression: A longitudinal perspective. *Journal of the American Academy of Child Psychiatry, 15,* 491–501.

Prendergast, M., Taylor, E., Rapoport, J. L., Bartko, J., Donnelly, M., Zametkin, A., Ahearn, M. B., Dunn, G., & Wieselberg, H. M. (1988). The diagnosis of childhood hyperactivity: A U.S.-U.K. cross-national study of DSM-III and ICD-9. *Journal of Child Psychology and Psychiatry, 29,* 289–300.

President's Panel on Mental Retardation (1963). *Chart book: Mental retardation, a national plan for a national problem.* Washington, DC: U.S. Department of Health, Education, and Welfare.

Price, R. A., Kidd, K. K., Cohen, D. J., Pauls, D. L., & Leckman, J. F. (1985). A twin study of Tourette syndrome. *Archives of General Psychiatry, 42,* 815–820.

Price, R. A., Leckman, J. F., Pauls, D. L., Cohen, D. J., & Kidd, K. K. (1986). Gilles de la Tourette's syndrome: Tics and central nervous system stimulants in twins and nontwins. *Neurology, 36,* 232–237.

Prior, M., & Sanson, A. (1986). Attention deficit disorder with hyperactivity: A critique. *Journal of Child Psychology and Psychiatry, 27,* 307–319.

Prizant, B. M., & Schuler, A. L. (1987a). Facilitating communication: Language approaches. In D. J. Cohen & A. M. Donnellan (Eds.), *Handbook of autism and pervasive developmental disorders* (pp. 316–332). New York: Wiley.

Prizant, B. M., & Schuler, A. L. (1987b). Facilitating communication: Theoretical foundations. In D. J. Cohen & A. M. Donnellan (Eds.), *Handbook of autism and pervasive developmental disorders* (pp. 289–300). New York: Wiley.

Prizant, B. M., & Wetherby, A. M. (1987). Communicative intent: A framework for understanding social-communicative behavior in autism. *Journal of the American Academy of Child and Adolescent Psychiatry, 26,* 472–479.

Propping, P. (1983). Genetic disorders presenting as "schizophrenia." *Human Genetics, 65,* 1–10.

Provence, S. A. (1985). On the efficacy of early intervention programs. *Developmental and Behavioral Pediatrics, 6,* 363–366.

Provence, S. A., & Lipton, R. C. (1963). *Infants in institutions.* New York: International Universities Press.

Prugh, D. G. (1954). Childhood experience and colonic disorder. *Annals of New York Academy of Science, 58,* 355–376.

Prugh, D. G. (1983). *The psychosocial aspects of pediatrics.* Philadelphia: Lea & Febiger.

Pueschel, S. M. (1983). The child with Down syndrome. In M. D. Levine, W. B. Carey, A. C. Crocker, & R. T. Gross (Eds.), *Developmental-behavioral pediatrics* (pp. 353–362). Philadelphia: Saunders.

Pugliese, M. T., Lifshitz, F., Grad, G., Fort, P., & Marks-Katz, M. (1983). Fear of obesity: A cause of short stature and delayed puberty. *New England Journal of Medicine, 309,* 513–518.

Puig-Antich, J. (1982). Major depression and conduct disorder in prepuberty. *Journal of the American Academy of Child Psychiatry, 21,* 118–128.

Puig-Antich, J. (1986). Psychobiological markers: Effects of age and puberty. In M. Rutter, C. E. Izard, P. B. Read (Eds.), *Depression in young people* (pp. 341–381). New York: Guilford.

Puig-Antich, J. (1987). Biological tests in the diagnosis of affective disorders in children and adolescents. In J. D. Noshpitz (Ed.), *Basic handbook of child psychiatry* (pp. 177–184). New York: Basic Books.

Puig-Antich, J., Blau, S., Marx, N., Greenhill, L. L., & Chambers, W. (1978). Prepubertal major depressive disorder: A pilot study. *Journal of the American Academy of Child Psychiatry, 17,* 695–707.

Puig-Antich, J., Goetz, D., Davies, M., Kaplan, T., Davies, S., Ostrow, L., Asnis, L., Twomey, J., Iyengar, S., & Ryan, N. (1989). A controlled family history study of prepubertal major depressive disorder. *Archives of General Psychiatry, 46,* 406–418.

Puig-Antich, J., Goetz, R., Davies, M., Tabrizi, M. A., Novacenko, H., Hanlon, C., Sachar, E. J., & Weitzman, E. D. (1984b). Growth hormone secretion in prepubertal children with major depression: IV. Sleep-related plasma concentrations in a drug-free, fully recovered clinical state. *Archives of General Psychiatry, 41,* 479–483.

Puig-Antich, J., Lukens, E., Davies, M., Goetz, D., Brennan-Quattrock, J., & Todak, G. (1985a). Psychosocial functioning in prepubertal major depressive disorders: I. Interpersonal relationships during the depressive episode. *Archives of General Psychiatry, 42,* 500–507.

Puig-Antich, J., Lukens, E., Davies, M., Goetz, D., Brennan-Quattrock, J., & Todak, G. (1985b). Psychosocial functioning in prepubertal major depressive disorders: II. Interpersonal relationships after sustained recovery from affective episode. *Archives of General Psychiatry, 42,* 511–517.

Puig-Antich, J., Novacenko, H., Davies, M., Tabrizi, M. A., Ambrosini, P., Goetz, R., Bianca, J., Goetz, D., & Sachar, E. J. (1984a). Growth hormone secretion in prepubertal children with major depression: III. Response to insulin-induced hypoglycemia after recovery from a depressive episode and in a drug-free state. *Archives of General Psychiatry, 41,* 471–475.

Puig-Antich, J., Perel, J. M., Lupatkin, W., Chambers, W. J., Tabrizi, M. A., King, J., Goetz, R., Davies, M., & Stiller, R. L. (1987). Imipramine in prepubertal major depressive disorders. *Archives of General Psychiatry, 44,* 81–89.

Puig-Antich, J., & Rabinovich, H. (1986). Relationship between affective and anxiety disorders in childhood. In R. Gittelman (Ed.), *Anxiety disorders of childhood* (pp. 136–156). New York: Guilford.

Pumariega, A. J. (1986). Acculturation and eating attitudes in adolescent girls: A comparative and correlational study. *Journal of the American Academy of Child Psychiatry, 25,* 276–279.

Pumariega, A. J., Edwards, P., & Mitchell, C. B. (1984). Anorexia nervosa in black adolents. *Journal of the American Academy of Child Psychiatry, 23,* 111–114.

Purcell, K. (1963). Distinctions between subgroups of asthmatic children: Children's perceptions of events associated with asthma. *Pediatrics, 31,* 486–494.

Purcell, K., Bernstein, L., & Bukantz, S. C. (1961). A preliminary comparison of rapidly remitting and persistently "steroid dependent" asthmatic children. *Psychosomatic Medicine, 23,* 305–310.

Purcell, K., Brady, K., Chai, H., Muser, J., Molk, L., Gordon, N., & Means, J. (1969a). The effect on asthma in children of experimental separation from the family. *Psychosomatic Medicine, 31,* 144–164.

Purcell, K., & Metz, J. (1962). Distinctions between subgroups of asthmatic children: Some parent attitude variables related to age on onset of asthma. *Journal of Psychosomatic Research, 6,* 251–258.

Purcell, K., Muser, J., Miklich, D., & Dietiker, K. E. (1969b). A comparison of psychologic findings in variously defined asthmatic subgroups. *Journal of Psychosomatic Research, 13,* 67–75.

Purcell, K., Turnbull, J., & Bernstein, L. (1962). Distinctions between subgroups of asthmatic children: Psychological test and behavior rating comparisons. *Journal of Psychosomatic Research, 6,* 283–291.

Purcell, K., & Weiss, J. H. (1970). Asthma. In C. Costello (Ed.), *Symptoms of psychopathology* (pp. 597–623). New York: Wiley.

Purcell, K., Weiss, J., & Hahn, W. (1972). Certain psychosomatic disorders. In B. B. Wolman (Ed.), *Manual of child psychopathology* (pp. 706–740). New York: McGraw-Hill.

Putnam, F. W., Guroff, J. J., Silberman, E. K., Barban, L., & Post, R. M. (1986). The clinical phenomenology of multiple personality disorder: Review of 100 recent cases. *Journal of Clinical Psychiatry, 47,* 285–293.

Pyle, R. L., & Mitchell, J. E. (1985). Psychotherapy of bulimia: The role of groups. In W. H. Kaye & H. E. Gwirtsman (Eds.), *The treatment of normal weight bulimia* (pp. 77–100). Washington, DC: American Psychiatric Press.

Pyle, R. L., Mitchell, J. E., & Eckert, E. D. (1981). Bulimia: A report of 34 cases. *Journal of Clinical Psychiatry, 42,* 60–64.

Pyle, R. L., Mitchell, J. E., Eckert, E. D., Halvorson, P. A., Neuman, P. A., & Goff, G. M. (1983). The incidence of bulimia in freshman college students. *International Journal of Eating Disorders, 2,* 75–85.

Quay, H. C. (1964). Personality dimensions in delinquent males as inferred from the factor analysis of behavior ratings. *Journal of Research in Crime and Delinquency, 1,* 33–36.

Quay, H. C. (1965). Psychopathic personality as pathological stimulation seeking. *American Journal of Psychiatry, 122,* 180–183.

Quay, H. C., & LaGreca, A. M. (1986). Disorders of anxiety, withdrawal, and dysphoria. In H. C. Quay & J. S. Werry (Eds.), *Psychopathological disorders of childhood* (3rd ed.). New York: Wiley.

Quay, H. C., & Peterson, D. (1967). *Manual for the Behavior Problem Checklist.* Champaign, IL: Author.

Quay, H. C., & Werry, J. S. (1979). *Psychopathologic disorders of childhood* (2nd ed.) New York: Wiley.

Quay, H. C., & Werry, J. S. (1986). *Psychopathologic disorders of childhood* (3rd ed.) New York: Wiley.

Rabkin, J. G., & Streuning, E. L. (1976). Life events, stress, and illness. *Science, 194,* 1013–1020.

Rabkin, R. (1964). Conversion hysteria as social maladaption. *Psychiatry, 27,* 349–363.

Rachman, S. J., & Hodgson, R. J. (1980). *Obsessions and compulsions.* Englewood Cliffs, NJ: Prentice Hall.

Rachman, S. J., & de Silva, P. (1978). Abnormal and normal obsessions. *Behavior Research and Therapy, 16,* 233–248.

Rada, R. T., Krill, A. E., Meyer, G. G., & Armstrong, D. (1973). Visual conversion reaction in children: II. Follow-up. *Psychosomatics, 14,* 271–276.

Rada, R. T., Meyer, G. G., & Kellner, R. (1978). Visual conversion reaction in children and adults. *Journal of Nervous and Mental Disease, 166,* 580–587.

Rada, R. T., Meyer, G. G., & Krill, A. E. (1969). Visual conversion reaction in children: I. Diagnosis. *Psychosomatics, 10,* 23–28.

Radbill, S. X. (1980). Children in a world of violence: A history of child abuse. In C. H. Kempe & R. E. Helfer (Eds.), *The battered child* (pp. 3–20). Chicago: University of Chicago Press.

Rado, S. (1956). On the psychoanalytic exploration of fear and other emotions. In S. Rado (Ed.), *Collected papers: Vol. 1. Psychoanalysis of behavior* (pp. 243–247). New York: Grune & Stratton.

Rado, S. (1959). Obsessive behavior: So-called obsessive-compulsive neurosis. In S. Arieti (Ed.), *American handbook of psychiatry* (Vol. 1, pp. 324–344). New York: Basic Books.

Ragan, P. V., & McGlashan, T. H. (1986). Childhood parental death and adult psychopathology. *American Journal of Psychiatry, 143,* 153–157.

Rahe, R. H. (1975). Epidemiological studies of life change and illness. *International Journal of Psychiatry in Medicine, 6,* 133–146.

Raiten, D. J., & Massaro, T. F. (1987). Nutrition and developmental disabilities: An examination of the orthomolecular hypothesis. In D. J. Cohen & A. M. Donnellan (Eds.), *Handbook of autism and pervasive developmental disorders* (pp. 566–583). New York: Wiley.

Rako, S., & Mazer, H. (Eds.) (1980). *Semrad: The heart of a therapist.* New York: Jason Aronson.

Rank, B. (1949). Adaptation of the psychoanalytic technique for the treatment of young children with atypical development. *American Journal of Orthopsychiatry, 19,* 130–139.

Rank, B. (1955). Intensive study and treatment of preschool children who show marked personality deviations or "atypical development" and their parents. In G. Caplan (Ed.), *Emotional problems of early childhood.* New York: Basic Books.

Rapoport, J. L. (1977). Pediatric psychopharmacology and childhood depression. In J. G. Schulterbrandt & A. Raskin (Eds.), *Depression in childhood: Diagnosis, treatment, and conceptual models* (pp. 87–100). New York: Raven Press.

Rapoport, J. L. (1983). The use of drugs: Trends in research. In M. Rutter (Ed.), *Developmental neuropsychiatry* (pp. 385–403). New York: Guilford.

Rapoport, J. L. (1985). Childhood obsessive-compulsive disorder. In D. Shaffer, A. A. Ehrhardt, & L. L. Greenhill (Eds.), *The clinical guide to child psychiatry* (pp. 208–217). New York: Free Press.

Rapoport, J. L. (1986). Childhood obsessive-compulsive disorder. *Journal of Child Psychology and Psychiatry, 27,* 289–295.

Rapoport, J. L. (Ed.) (1989). *Obsessive-compulsive disorder in children and adolescents.* Washington, DC: American Psychiatric Press.

Rapoport, J. L., Berg, C. J., Ismond, D. R., Zahn, T. P., & Neims, A. (1984). Behavioral effects of caffeine in children. *Archives of General Psychiatry, 41,* 1073–1079.

Rapoport, J. L., Buchsbaum, M. S., Weingartner, H., Zahn, T. P., Ludlow, C., & Mikkelsen, E. J. (1980a). Dextroamphetamine: Its cognitive and behavioral effects in normal and hyperactive boys and normal men. *Archives of General Psychiatry, 37,* 933–943.

Rapoport, J. L., Buchsbaum, M. S., Zahn, T. P., Weingartner, H., Ludlow, C., & Mikkelsen, E. J. (1978). Dextroamphetamine: Cognitive and behavioral effects in normal prepubertal boys. *Science, 199,* 560–563.

Rapoport, J. L., Donnelly, M., Zametkin, A., & Carrougher, J. (1986a). 'Situational hyperactivity' in a U.S. clinical setting. *Journal of Child Psychology and Psychiatry, 27,* 639–646.

Rapoport, J. L., Elkins, R., Langer, D. H., Sceery, W., Buchsbaum, M. S., Gillin, J. C., Murphy, D. L., Zahn, T. P., Lake, R., Ludlow, C., & Mendelson, W. (1981). Childhood obsessive-compulsive disorder. *American Journal of Psychiatry, 138,* 1545–1554.

Rapoport, J. L., Mikkelsen, E. J., Zavadil, A., Nee, L., Gruenau, C., Mendelson, W., & Gillin, J. C. (1980b). Childhood enuresis: II. Psychopathology, tricyclic concentration in plasma, and antienuretic effect. *Archives of General Psychiatry, 37,* 1146–1152.

Rapoport, J. L., & Quinn, P. O. (1975). Minor physical anomalies (stigmata) and early developmental deviation: A major biological subgroup of "hyperactive children." In R. Gittelman-Klein (Ed.), *Recent advances in child psychopharmacology* (pp. 31–46). New York: Human Sciences Press.

Rapoport, J. L., Quinn, P. O., Bradbard, G., Riddle, K. D., & Brooks, E. (1974a). Imipramine and methylphenidate treatments of hyperactive boys. *Archives of General Psychiatry, 30,* 789–793.

Rapoport, J. L., Quinn, P. O., Burg, C., & Bartley, L. (1979). Can hyperactives be identified in infancy? In R. L. Trites (Ed.), *Hyperactivity in children* (pp. 103–115). Baltimore: University Park Press.

Rapoport, J. L., Quinn, P. O., & Lamprecht, F. (1974b). Minor physical anomalies and plasma dopamine-beta-hydroxylase activity in hyperactive boys. *American Journal of Psychiatry, 131,* 386–390.

Rappaport, L., Landman, G., Fenton, T., & Levine, M. D. (1986b). Locus of control as predictor of compliance and outcome in treatment of encopresis. *Journal of Pediatrics, 109,* 1061–1064.

Raskin, M., Talbott, J. A., & Meyerson, A. T. (1966). Diagnosis of conversion reactions: Predictive value of psychiatric criteria. *Journal of the American Medical Association, 197,* 102–106.

Rauste-von Wright, M., & von Wright, J. (1981). A longitudinal study of psychosomatic symptoms in healthy 11–18 year old girls and boys. *Journal of Psychosomatic Research, 25,* 525–534.

Ravenscroft, K., Jr. (1980, October). Acute phobic hallucinosis of childhood. Paper presented at the American Academy of Child Psychiatry Convention, Chicago.

Ravenscroft, K., Jr. (1988). Psychoanalytic family therapy approaches to the adolescent bulimic. In H. J. Schwartz (Ed.), *Bulimia: Psychoanalytic treatment and theory* (pp. 443–488). Madison, CT: International Universities Press.

Raymer, D., Weininger, O., & Hamilton, J. R. (1984). Psychological problems in children with abdominal pain. *Lancet, 1,* 439–440.

Realmuto, G. M., Jensen, J. B., Wescoe, S. (1990). Specificity and sensitivity of sexually anatomically correct dolls in substantiating abuse: A pilot study. *Journal of the American Academy of Child and Adolescent Psychiatry, 29,* 743–746.

Reckless, W. C. (1943). The etiology of delinquent and criminal behavior: A planning report for research. *Social Science Research Council Bulletin, 50,* 1–169.

Redl, F., & Wineman, D. (1957). *The aggressive child.* New York: Free Press.

Redmond, D. E., Jr. (1979). New and old evidence for the involvement of a brain norepinephrine system in anxiety. In W. E. Fann, I. Karacan, A. D. Porkorny, & R. L. Williams (Eds.), *Phenomenology and treatment of anxiety* (pp. 153–203). New York: Spectrum.

Redmond, D. E., Jr. (1982). Does clonidine alter anxiety in humans? *Trends in pharmacological sciences, 3,* 477–480.

Redmond, D. E., Jr., & Huang, Y. H. (1979). New evidence for a locus coeruleus-norepinephrine connection with anxiety. *Life Sciences, 25,* 2149–2162.

Reeves, J. C., Werry, J. S., Elkind, G. S., & Zametkin, A. (1987). Attention deficit, conduct, oppositional, and anxiety disorders in children: II. Clinical characteristics. *Journal of the American Academy of Child and Adolescent Psychiatry, 26,* 144–155.

Reich, T., James, J. W., & Morris, C. A. (1972). The use of multiple threshold in determining the mode of transmission of semi-continuous traits. *Annals of Human Genetics, 36,* 163–184.

Reid, A. H. (1980). Psychiatric disorders in mentally handicapped children: A clinical and follow-up study. *Journal of Mental Deficiency Research, 24,* 287–298.

Reiman, E. M., Raichle, M. E., Robins, E., Butler, F. K., Herscovitch, P., Fox, P., & Perlmutter, J. (1986). The application of positron emission tomography to the study of panic disorder. *American Journal of Psychiatry, 143,* 469–477.

Reiser, M. F. (1984). *Mind, brain, body: Toward a convergence of psychoanalysis and neurobiology.* New York: Basic Books.

Reiss, D. (1976). The family and schizophrenia. *American Journal of Psychiatry, 133,* 181–185.

Reiss, D. (1981). *The family's construction of reality.* Cambridge: Harvard University Press.

Reite, M., & Caine, N. G. (Eds.). (1983). *Child abuse: The nonhuman primate data.* New York: Alan R. Liss.

Rekers, G., & Lovaas, O. I. (1974). Behavioral treatment of deviant sex-role behaviors in a male child. *Journal of Applied Behavioral Analysis, 7,* 173–190.

Renne, C. M., & Creer, T. L. (1976). Training children with asthma to use inhalation therapy equipment. *Journal of Applied Behavioral Analysis, 9,* 1–11.

Renne, C. M., & Creer, T. L. (1985). Asthmatic children and their families. *Advances in Developmental and Behavioral Pediatrics, 6,* 41–81.

Renshaw, D. C. (1987). Evaluating suspected cases of child sexual abuse. *Psychiatric Annals, 17,* 262–270.

Reznick, J. S., Kagan, J., Snidman, N., Gersten, M., Baak, K., & Rosenberg, A. (1986). Inhibited and uninhibited children: A follow-up study. *Child Development, 57,* 660–680.

Richards, W., Church, J. A., Roberts, M. J., Newman, L. J., & Garon, M. R. (1981). A self-help program for childhood asthma in a residential treatment center. *Clinical Pediatrics, 20,* 453–457.

Richman, N., Stevenson, J., & Graham, P. J. (1982). *Pre-school to school: A behavioral study.* London: Academic Press.

Richmond, J. B., Eddy, E. J., & Garrard, S. D. (1954). The syndrome of fecal soiling and megacolon. *American Journal of Orthopsychiatry, 24,* 391–401.

Richmond, J. B., Eddy, E. J., & Green, M. (1958). Rumination: A psychosomatic syndrome of infancy. *Pediatrics, 22,* 49–55.

Riddle, K. D., & Rapoport, J. L. (1976). A 2-year follow-up of 72 hyperactive boys. *Journal of Nervous and Mental Disease, 162,* 126–134.

Riddle, M. A. (1987). Individual and parental psychotherapy in autism. In D. J. Cohen & A. M. Donnellan (Eds.), *Handbook of autism and pervasive developmental disorders* (pp. 528–540). New York: Wiley.

Riddle, M. A., Hardin, M. T., Cho, S. C., Woolston, J. L., & Leckman, J. F. (1988a). Desipramine treatment of boys with attention-deficit hyperactivity disorder and tics: Preliminary clinical experience. *Journal of the American Academy of Child and Adolescent Psychiatry, 27,* 811–814.

Riddle, M. A., Hardin, M. T., King, R. A., Scahill, L., & Woolston, J. L. (1990a). Fluoxetine treatment of children and adolescents with Tourette's and obsessive-compulsive disorders: Preliminary clinical experience. *Journal of the American Academy of Child and Adolescent Psychiatry, 29,* 45–48.

Riddle, M. A., King, R., Hardin, M., Scahill, L., Ort, S., & Leckman, J. (1990b, October). *Behavioral side effects of fluoxetine.* New research poster presented at the 37th annual meeting of the American Academy of Child and Adolescent Psychiatry, Chicago, IL.

Riddle, M. A., Leckman, J. F., Hardin, M. T., Anderson, G. M., & Cohen, D. J. (1988b). Fluoxetine treatment of obsessions and compulsions in patients with Tourette's syndrome [Letter]. *American Journal of Psychiatry, 145,* 1173–1174.

Riddle, M. A., Nelson, J. C., Kleinman, C. S., Rasmusson, A., Leckman, J. F., King, R. A., & Cohen, D. J. (1991). Sudden death in children receiving norpramin: Review of three reported cases and commentary. *Journal of the American Academy of Child and Adolescent Psychiatry, 30*.

Riddle, M. A., Scahill, L., King, R., Hardin, M. T., Towbin, K. E., Ort, S. I., Leckman, J. F., & Cohen, D. (1990c). Obsessive-compulsive disorder in children and adolescents: Phenomenology and family history. *Journal of the American Academy of Child and Adolescent Psychiatry, 29,* 766–772.

Rimland, B. (1978). Savant capabilities of autistic children and their cognitive implications. In G. Serban (Ed.), *Cognitive defects in the development of mental illness* (pp. 43–65). New York: Brunner/Mazel.

Rimland, B., Callaway, E., & Dreyfus, P. (1978). The effect of high doses of vitamin B6 on autistic children: A double-blind crossover study. *American Journal of Psychiatry, 135,* 472–475.

Rimland, B., & Musinger, H. (1977). Burt's IQ data. *Science, 195,* 248.

Rinsley, D. B. (1980). Diagnosis and tretment of borderline and narcissistic children and adolescents. *Bulletin of the Menninger Clinic, 44,* 147–170.

Rinsley, D. B. (1982). *Borderline and other self disorders: A developmental and object-relations perspective.* New York: Jason Aronson.

Ritvo, E. R., & Freeman, B. J. (1978). The National Society for Autistic Children's definition of the syndrome of autism. *Journal of the American Academy of Child Psychiatry, 17,* 565–575.

Ritvo, E. R., Freeman, B. J., Geller, E., & Yuwiler, A. (1983). Effects of fenfluramine on 14 outpatients with the syndrome of autism. *Journal of the American Academy of Child Psychiatry, 22,* 549–558.

Ritvo, E. R., Freeman, B. J., Mason-Brothers, A., Mo, A., & Ritvo, A. M. (1985a). Concordance for the syndrome of autism in 40 pairs of afflicted twins. *American Journal of Psychiatry, 142,* 74–77.

Ritvo, E. R., Freeman, B. J., Scheibel, A. B., Duong, T., Robinson, H., Guthrie, D., & Ritvo, A. (1986). Lower Purkinje cell counts in the cerebella of four autistic subjects: Initial findings of the UCLA-NSAC Autopsy Research Report. *American Journal of Psychiatry, 143,* 862–866.

Ritvo, E. R., Spence, M. A., Freeman, B. J., Mason-Brothers, A., Mo, A., & Marazita, M. L. (1985b). Evidence for autosomal recessive inheritance in 46 families with multiple incidences of autism. *American Journal of Psychiatry, 142,* 187–192.

Ritvo, S. (1984). The image and uses of the body in psychic conflict. *Psychoanalytic Study of the Child, 39,* 449–469.

Rivinus, T. M., Jamison, D. L., & Graham, P. J. (1975). Childhood organic neurological disease presenting as psychiatric disorder. *Archives of Disease in Childhood, 50,* 115–119.

Robbins, D. R., & Alessi, N. E. (1985). Depressive symptoms and suicidal behavior in adolescents. *American Journal of Psychiatry, 142,* 588–592.

Robertson, H. A., Martin, I. L., & Candy, J. M. (1978). Differences in benzodiazepine receptor binding in Maudsley reactive and Maudsley non-reactive rats. *European Journal of Pharmacology, 50,* 455–457.

Robertson, James, & Robertson, Joyce (1971). Young children in brief separation: A fresh look. *Psychoanalytic Study of the Child, 26,* 264–315.

Robertson, M. (1987). Molecular genetics of the mind. *Nature, 325,* 755.

Robin, M. (1982). Sheltering arms: The roots of child protection. In E. H. Newberger (Ed.), *Child abuse* (pp. 1–21). Boston: Little, Brown.

Robins, L. N. (1966). *Deviant children grown up: A sociologic and psychologic study of sociopathic personality.* Baltimore, MD: Williams & Wilkens.

Robins, L. N. (1974). *Deviant children grown up* (2nd ed.). Huntington, NY: Krieger.

Robins, L. N., Helzer, J. E., Weissman, M. M., Orvaschel, H., Gruenberg, E., Burke, J. D., Jr., & Regier, D. A. (1984). Lifetime prevalence of specific psychiatric disorders in three sites. *Archives of General Psychiatry, 41,* 949–958.

Robins, L. N., & Wish, E. (1977). Childhood deviance as a developmental process. *Social Forces, 56,* 448–471.

Robson, K. S. (1983). *The borderline child: Approaches to etiology, diagnosis, and treatment.* New York: McGraw-Hill.

Rochlin, G. (1959). The loss complex: A contribution to the etiology of depression. *Journal of the American Psychoanalytic Association, 7,* 299–316.

Rodriguez, A., Rodriguez, M., & Eisenberg, L. (1959). The outcome of school phobia: A follow-up study based on 41 cases. *American Journal of Psychiatry, 116,* 540–544.

Rogeness, G. A., Amrung, S. A., Macedo, C. A., Harris, W. R., & Fisher, C. (1986). Psychopathology in abused or neglected children. *Journal of the American Academy of Child Psychiatry, 25,* 659–665.

Rogers, M. P., Dubey, D., & Reich, P. (1979). The influence of the psyche and the brain on immunity and disease suspectibility: A critical review. *Psychosomatic Medicine, 41,* 147–164.

Roiphe, H., & Galenson, E. (1973). The infantile fetish. *Psychoanalytic Study of the Child, 28,* 147–166.

Rose, R. M. (1980). Endocrine responses to stressful psychological events. *Psychiatric Clinics of North America, 3,* 251–276.

Rosen, A. C., Rekers, G. A., & Friar, L. R. (1977). Theoretical and diagnostic issues in child gender disturbances. *Journal of Sexual Research, 13,* 89–103.

Rosenbaum, J. F., Biederman, J., Gersten, M., Hirshfeld, D. R., Meminger, S. R., Herman, J. B., Kagar, J., Resnick, S., & Snidman, N. (1988). Behavioral inhibition in children of parents with panic disorder and agoraphobia: A controlled study. *Archives of General Psychiatry, 45,* 463–470.

Rosenberg, B., & Silverstein, H. (1969). *The varieties of delinquent experience.* Waltham, MA: Blaisdell.

Rosenberger, P. B., & Hier, D. B. (1980). Cerebral asymmetry and verbal intellectual deficits. *Annals of Neurology, 8,* 300–304.

Rosenblum, L. A. (1984). Monkeys' responses to separation and loss. In M. Osterweis, F. Solomon, & M. Green (Eds.), *Bereavement: Reactions, consequences, and care* (pp. 179–196). Washington, DC: National Academy Press.

Rosenfeld, A. A. (1979a). The clinical management of incest and sexual abuse of children. *Journal of the American Medical Association, 242,* 1761–1764.

Rosenfeld, A. A. (1979b). Endogamic incest and the victim–perpetrator model. *American Journal of Diseases of Children, 133,* 406–410.

Rosenfeld, A. A., Nadelson, C. C., & Krieger, M. (1979). Fantasy and reality in patients' reports of incest. *Journal of Clinical Psychiatry, 40,* 159–164.

Rosenfeld, A. A., & Newberger, E. H. (1977). Compassion vs. control: Conceptual and practical pitfalls in the broadened definition of child abuse. *Journal of the American Medical Association, 237,* 2086–2088.

Rosenfeld, S. K., & Sprince, M. P. (1963). An attempt to formulate the meaning of the concept "borderline." *Psychoanalytic Study of the Child, 18,* 603–635.

Rosenfeld, S. K., & Sprince, M. P. (1965). Some thoughts on the technical handling of borderline children. *Psychoanalytic Study of the Child, 20,* 495–517.

Rosenn, D. W., Loeb, L. S., & Jura, M. B. (1980). Differentiation of organic from nonorganic failure to thrive syndrome in infancy. *Pediatrics, 66,* 698–704.

Rosenthal, D. (1970). *Genetic theory and abnormal behavior.* New York: McGraw-Hill.

Rosenthal, D. (1971). A program of research on heredity in schizophrenia. *Behavioral Science, 16,* 191–201.

Rosenthal, D., Wender, P. H., Kety, S. S., Schulsinger, F., Welner, J., & Rieder, R. O. (1975). Parent–child relationship and psychopathological disorder in the child. *Archives of General Psychiatry, 32,* 466–476.

Rosenthal, D., Wender, P. H., Kety, S. S., Welner, J., & Schulsinger, F. (1971). The adopted-away offspring of schizophrenics. *American Journal of Psychiatry, 128,* 307–311.

Rosenthal, N. E., Carpenter, C. J., James, S. P., Parry, B. L., Rogers, S. L. B., & Wehr, T. A. (1986). Seasonal affective disorder in children and adolescents. *American Journal of Psychiatry, 143,* 356–358.

Rosenthal, P. A., & Doherty, M. B. (1984). Serious sibling abuse by preschool children. *Journal of the American Academy of Child Psychiatry, 23,* 186–190.

Ross, A. O. (1972). Behavior therapy. In B. B. Wolman (Ed.), *Manual of child psychopathology.* New York: McGraw-Hill.

Ross, D. M., & Ross, S. A. (1982). *Hyperactivity: Current issues, research, and theory* (2nd ed.). New York: Wiley.

Ross, M. W., Walinder, J., Lundstrom, R., & Thuwe, I. (1981). Cross cultural approaches to transsexualism: A comparison between Sweden and Australia, *Acta Psychiatrica Scandanavica, 63,* 75–82.

Rothstein, A. (1981). Hallucinatory phenomena in childhood: A critique of the literature. *Journal of the American Academy of Child Psychiatry, 20,* 623–635.

Rothstein, A. (1982). An integrative perspective on the diagnosis of learning disorders. *Journal of the American Academy of Child Psychiatry, 21,* 420–426.

Rourke, B. P., & Strang, J. D. (1983). Subtypes of reading and arithmetical disabilities: A neuropsychological analysis. In M. Rutter (Ed.), *Developmental neuropsychiatry* (pp. 473–488). New York: Guilford.

Routh, D. K., & Ernst, A. R. (1984). Somatization disorder in relatives of children and adolescents with functional abdominal pain. *Journal of Pediatric Psychology, 9,* 427–437.

Rowe, D. C., & Plomin, R. (1978). The Burt controversy: A comparison of Burt's data on IQ with data from other studies. *Behavior Genetics, 8,* 81–83.

Roy-Byrne, P. P., Geraci, M., & Uhde, T. W. (1986). Life events and the onset of panic disorder. *American Journal of Psychiatry, 143,* 1424–1427.

Rubinstein, R. A., & Brown, R. T. (1984). An evaluation of the validity of the diagnostic category of attention-deficit disorder. *American Journal of Ortho-psychiatry, 54,* 398–414.

Rumsey, J. M., Berman, K. F., Denckla, M. B., Hamburger, S. D., Kruesi, M. J., & Weinberger, D. R. (1987). Regional cerebral blood flow in severe developmental dyslexia. *Archives of Neurology, 44,* 1144–1150.

Rumsey, J. M., Dorwart, R., Vermess, M., Denckla, M. B., Kruesi, M. J., & Rapoport, J. L. (1986). Magnetic resonance imaging of brain anatomy in severe develop-mental dyslexia. *Archives of Neurology, 43,* 1045–1046.

Rumsey, J. M., Rapoport, J. L., & Sceery, W. R. (1985). Autistic children as adults: Psychiatric, social, and behavioral outcomes. *Journal of the American Academy of Child Psychiatry, 24,* 465–473.

Rush, F. (1980). *The best kept secret.* Englewood Cliffs, NJ: Prentice-Hall.

Russell, A. T., Bott, L., & Sammons, C. (1987, October). *The phenomenology of schizotypal disorder of childhood: A schizophrenia spectrum disorder?* Paper presented at the annual meeting of the American Academy of Child and Adolescent Psychiatry, Washington, D. C.

Russell, A. T., Bott, L., & Sammons, C. (1989). The phenomenology of schizo-phrenia occurring in childhood. *Journal of the American Academy of Child and Adolescent Psychiatry, 28,* 399–407.

Russell, D. E. H. (1983). The incidence and prevalence of intrafamilial and extrafamilial sexual abuse of female children. *Child Abuse and Neglect, 7,* 133–146.

Russell, D. E. H. (1986). *The secret trauma: Incest in the lives of girls and women.* New York: Basic Books.

Russell, G. (1979). Bulimia nervosa: An ominous variant of anorexia nervosa. *Psychological Medicine, 9,* 429–448.

Russell, G. F. M., Szmukler, G. I., Dare, C., & Eisler, I. (1987). An evaluation of family therapy in anorexia nervosa and bulimia nervosa. *Archives of General Psychiatry, 44,* 1047–1056.

Rutter, M. (1971). Parent–child separation. *Journal of Child Psychology and Psychiatry, 12,* 233–260.

Rutter, M. (1972). Childhood schizophrenia reconsidered. *Journal of Autism and Childhood Schizophrenia, 2,* 315–337.

Rutter, M. (1975). *Helping troubled children.* New York: Plenum.

Rutter, M. (1978a). Developmental issues and prognosis. In M. Rutter & E. Schopler (Eds.), *Autism: A reappraisal of concepts and treatment* (pp. 497–506). New York: Plenum.

Rutter, M. (1978b). Prevalence and types of dyslexia. In A. L. Benton & D. Pearl (Eds.), *Dyslexia: An appraisal of current knowledge* (pp. 3–28). New York: Oxford University Press.

Rutter, M. (1979). Protective factors in children's responses to stress and disadvantage. In M. Kent & J. E. Rolf (Eds.), *Primary prevention of psychopathology: Vol. 3. Social competence in children* (p. 64). Hanover, NH: University Press of New England.

Rutter, M. (1981a). *Maternal deprivation reassessed* (2nd ed.). Harmondsworth, England: Penguin.

Rutter, M. (1981b). Psychological sequelae of brain damage in childhood. *American Journal of Psychiatry, 138,* 1533–1544.

Rutter, M. (1982). Syndromes attributed to "minimal brain dysfunction" in childhood. *American Journal of Psychiatry, 139,* 21–33.

Rutter, M. (1983a). Behavioral studies: Questions and findings on the concept of a distinctive syndrome. In M. Rutter (Ed.), *Developmental neuropsychiatry* (pp. 259–279). New York: Guilford.

Rutter, M. (1983b). Cognitive deficits in the pathogenesis of autism. *Journal of Child Psychology and Psychiatry, 24,* 513–531.

Rutter, M. (1983c). Introduction: Concepts of brain dysfunction syndromes. In M. Rutter (Ed.), *Developmental neuropsychiatry* (pp. 1–11). New York: Guilford.

Rutter, M. (1983d). Stress, coping, and development: Some issues and some questions. In N. Garmezy & M. Rutter (Eds.), *Stress, coping, and development in children* (pp. 1–41). New York: McGraw-Hill.

Rutter, M. (1985a). Infantile autism and other pervasive developmental disorders. In M. Rutter & L. Hersov (Eds.), *Child and adolescent psychiatry: Modern approaches* (pp. 545–566). Oxford: Blackwell.

Rutter, M. (1985b). Infantile autism. In D. Shaffer, A. A. Ehrhardt, & L. L. Greenhill (Eds.), *The clinical guide to child psychiatry* (pp. 48–78). New York: Free Press.

Rutter, M. (1985c). The treatment of autistic children. *Journal of Child Psychology and Psychiatry, 26,* 193–214.

Rutter, M. (1986a). The developmental psychopathology of depression: Issues and perspectives. In M. Rutter, C. E. Izard, & P. B. Read (Eds.), *Depression in young people: Developmental and clinical perspectives* (pp. 3–30). New York: Guilford.

Rutter, M. (1986b). Depressive feelings, cognitions, and disorders: A research postscript. In M. Rutter, C. E. Izard, & P. B. Read (Eds.), *Depression in young people: Developmental and clinical perspectives* (pp. 491–519). New York: Guilford.

Rutter, M. (1987a). Psychosocial resilience and protective mechanisms. *American Journal of Orthopsychiatry, 57,* 316–331.

Rutter, M. (1987b). Temperament, personality and personality disorder. *British Journal of Psychiatry, 150,* 443–458.

Rutter, M. (1988). Depressive disorders. In M. Rutter, A. H. Tuma, & I. S. Lann (Eds.), *Assessment and diagnosis in child psychopathology* (pp. 347–376). New York: Guilford.

Rutter, M., Chadwick, O., & Shaffer, D. (1983). Head injury. In M. Rutter (Ed.), *Developmental neuropsychiatry* (pp. 83–111). New York: Guilford.

Rutter, M., Cox, A., Tupling, C., Burger, M., & Yule, W. (1975). Attainment and adjustment in two geographical areas: I. Prevalence of psychiatric disorder. *British Journal of Psychiatry, 126,* 493–509.

Rutter, M., & Giller, H. (1984). *Juvenile delinquency: Trends and perspectives.* New York: Guilford.

Rutter, M., & Lockyer, L. (1967). A five to fifteen year follow-up study of infantile psychosis: I. Description of sample. *British Journal of Psychiatry, 113,* 1169–1182.

Rutter, M., & Schopler, E. (1987). Autism and pervasive developmental disorders: Concepts and diagnostic issues. *Journal of Autism and Developmental Disorders, 17,* 159–186.

Rutter, M., Tizard, J., & Whitmore, K. (1981). *Education, health and behaviour.* Huntington, NY: Krieger. (Original work published 1970)

Rutter, M., & Yule, W. (1975). The concept of specific reading retardation. *Journal of Child Psychology and Psychiatry, 16,* 181–197.

Rutter, M., Yule, W., & Graham, P. (1973). Enuresis and behavioural deviance: Some epidemiological considerations. In I. Kolvin, R. C. MacKeith, & S. R. Meadow (Eds.), *Bladder control and enuresis* (pp. 137–147) (Clinics in Developmental Medicine, Nos. 48/49). London: Heinemann.

Ryan, N. D., Puig-Antich, J., Ambrosini, P., Rabinovich, H., Robinson, D., Nelson, B., Iyengar, S., & Twomey, J. (1987a). The clinical picture of major depression in children and adolescents. *Archives of General Psychiatry, 44,* 854–861.

Ryan, N. D., Puig-Antich, J., Cooper, T., Rabinovich, H., Ambrosini, P., Davies, M., King, J., Torres, D., & Fried, J. (1986). Imipramine in adolescent major depression: Plasma level and clinical response. *Acta Psychiatrica Scandinavica, 73,* 275–288.

Ryan, N. D., Puig-Antich, J., Cooper, T. B., Rabinovich, H., Ambrosini, P., Fried, J., Davies, M., Torres, D., & Suckow, R. F. (1987b). Relative safety of single versus divided dose imipramine in adolescent major depression. *Journal of the American Academy of Child and Adolescent Psychiatry, 26,* 400–406.

Sack, W. H., Mason, R., & Higgins, J. E. (1985). The single-parent family and abusive child punishment. *American Journal of Orthopsychiatry, 55,* 252–259.

Sacks, O. (1985, February 28). The twins. *New York Review of Books, 32*(3), 16–20.

Safer, D. J., Allen, R. P., & Barr, E. (1975). Growth rebound after termination of stimulant drugs. *Journal of Pediatrics, 86,* 113–116.

Saghir, M. T., & Robins, E. (1973). *Male and female homosexuality: A comprehensive investigation.* Baltimore: Williams & Wilkins.

Sahley, T. L., & Panksepp, J. (1987). Brain opioids and autism: An updated analysis of possible linkages. *Journal of Autism and Developmental Disorders, 17,* 201–216.

Salzman, L. (1968). *The obsessive personality: Origins, dynamics and therapy.* New York: Science House.

Salzman, L. (1983). The value of psychotherapy over antidepressants in treating phobias and obsessive-compulsive disorders. *Integrative Psychiatry, 1,* 28–29.

Salzman, L. E., Levenson, A., & Smith, J. C. (1988). Suicides among persons 15–24 years of age, 1970–1984. *Morbidity and Mortality Weekly Report, CDC Surveillance Summaries, 37*(55-1), 61–68.

Salzinger, S., Samit, C., Krieger, R., Kaplan, S., & Kaplan, T. (1986). A controlled study of the life events of the mothers of maltreated children in suburban families. *Journal of the American Academy of Child Psychiatry, 25,* 419–426.

Samenow, S. E. (1984). *Inside the criminal mind.* New York: Times Books.

Sameroff, A. J. (1975). Early influences on development: Fact or fancy? *Merrill-Palmer Quarterly, 21,* 267–294.

Sameroff, A. J. (1986). Environmental context of child development. *Journal of Pediatrics, 109,* 192–200.

Sameroff, A. J., & Chandler, M. J. (1975). Reproductive risk and the continuum of caretaking casualty. In F. D. Horowitz, E. M. Hetherington, S. Scarr-Salapatek, & G. M. Siegel, *Review of child development research* (Vol. 4, pp. 187–244). Chicago: University of Chicago Press.

Sameroff, A. J., & Seifer, R. (1983). Familial risk and child competence. *Child Development, 54,* 1254–1268.

Sameroff, A., Seifer, R., Zax, M., & Barocas, R. (1987). Early indicators of developmental risk: Rochester longitudinal study. *Schizophrenia Bulletin, 13,* 383–394.

Sandberg, S. T., Rutter, M., & Taylor, E. (1978). Hyperkinetic disorder in psychiatric clinic attenders. *Developmental Medicine and Child Neurology, 20,* 279–299.

Sandberg, S. T., Wieselberg, M., & Shaffer, D. (1980). Hyperkinetic and conduct problem children in a primary school population: Some epidemiological considerations. *Journal of Child Psychology and Psychiatry, 21,* 293–311.

Sanders, L. W., Stechler, G., Julia, H., & Burns, P. (1976). Primary prevention and some aspects of temporal organization in early infant–caretaker interaction. In E. N. Rexford, L. W. Sander, & T. Shapiro (Eds.), *Infant psychiatry* (pp. 187–204). New Haven: Yale University Press.

Sanders, M. R., Rebgetz, M., Morrison, M., Por, W., Gordon, A., Dadds, M., & Shepherd, R. (1989). Cognitive-behavioral treatment of recurrent nonspecific abdominal pain in children: An analysis of generalization, maintenance, and side effects. *Journal of Consulting and Clinical Psychology, 57,* 294–300.

Sandler, J., & Joffe, W. G. (1965a). Notes on childhood depression. *International Journal of Psychoanalysis, 46,* 88–96.

Sandler, J., & Joffe, W. G. (1965b). Notes on obsessional manifestations in children. *Psychoanalytic Study of the Child, 20,* 425–438.

Sandoval, J., & Lambert, S. E. (1984). Hyperactive and learning disabled children: Who gets help? *Journal of Special Education, 18,* 495–503.

Sargent, J., Liebman, R., & Silver, M. (1985). Family therapy for anorexia nervosa. In D. M. Garner & P. E. Garfinkel (Eds.), *Handbook of psychotherapy for anorexia nervosa and bulimia* (pp. 257–279). New York: Guilford.

Sarnoff, C. (1976). *Latency.* New York: Jason Aronson.

Satterfield, J. H., Cantwell, D. P., & Satterfield, B. T. (1974). Pathophysiology of the hyperactive child syndrome. *Archives of General Psychiatry, 31,* 839–844.

Satterfield, J. H., Hoppe, C. M., & Schell, A. M. (1982). A prospective study of delinquency in 110 adolescent boys with attention-deficit disorder and 88 normal adolescent boys. *American Journal of Psychiatry, 139,* 795–798.

Satterfield, J. H., Satterfield, B. T., & Cantwell, D. P. (1981). Three-year multi-modality treatment study of 100 hyperactive boys. *Journal of Pediatrics, 98,* 650–655.

Satterfield, J. H., Satterfield, B. T., & Schell, A. M. (1987). Therapeutic interventions to prevent delinquency in hyperactive boys. *Journal of the American Academy of Child and Adolescent Psychiatry, 26,* 56–64.

Satterfield, J. H., Schell, A. M., Backs, R. W., & Hidaka, K. C. (1984). A cross-sectional and longitudinal study of age effects of electrophysiological measures in hyperactive and normal children. *Biological Psychiatry, 19,* 973–990.

Sauzier, M., & Mitkus, C. (1986). Sexual abuse and rape in childhood. In K. S. Robson (Ed.), *Manual of clinical child psychiatry* (pp. 213–240). Washington, DC: American Psychiatric Press.

Scarr, S., & Kidd, K. K. (1983). Developmental behavior genetics. In P. H. Mussen (Ed.), *Handbook of child psychology* (Vol. 2, pp. 345–433). New York: Wiley.

Schachar, R., Rutter, M., & Smith, A. (1981). The characteristics of situationally and pervasively hyperactive children: Implications for syndrome definition. *Journal of Child Psychology and Psychiatry, 22,* 375–392.

Schachar, R., Taylor, E., Wieselberg, M., Thorley, G., & Rutter, M. (1987). Changes in family function and relationships in children who respond to methylphenidate. *Journal of the American Academy of Child and Adolescent Psychiatry, 26,* 728–732.

Schaefer, C. E., Millman, H. L., & Levine, G. F. (1979). *Therapies for psychosomatic disorders in children.* San Francisco: Jossey-Bass.

Schaffer, H. R. (1958). Objective observations of personality development in early infancy. *British Journal of Medical Psychology, 31,* 174–183.

Schaffer, H. R. (1971). Cognitive structure and early social behaviour. In H. R. Schaffer (Ed.), *The origins of human social relations.* New York: Academic.

Schaffer, H. R., & Callender, W. M. (1959). Psychological effects of hospitalization in infancy. *Paediatrics, 24,* 528–539.

Schalock, R. L., Harper, R. S., & Genung, T. (1981). Community integration of mentally retarded adults: Community placement and program success. *American Journal of Mental Deficiency, 85,* 478–488.

Schanberg, S. M., Evoniuk, G., & Kuhn, C. M. (1984). Tactile and nutritional aspects of maternal care: Specific regulators of neuroendocrine function and cellular development. *Proceedings of the Society for Experimental Biology and Medicine, 175,* 135–146.

Schandry, R. (1981). Heart beat perception and emotional experience. *Psychophysiology, 8,* 483–488.

Scharff, D. E., & Scharff, J. S. (1987). *Object relations family therapy.* New York: Jason Aronson.

Schechter, M. D., & Roberge, L. (1976). Sexual exploitation. In R. E. Helfer & C. H. Kempe (Eds.), *Child abuse and neglect: The family and the community* (pp. 127–142). Cambridge, MA: Ballinger.

Scheerenberger, R. C. (1983). *Public residential services for the mentally retarded: 1982.* Washington, DC: National Association of Superintendents of Public Residential Facilities for the Mentally Retarded.

Schetky, D. H. (1986). Emerging issues in child sexual abuse. *Journal of the American Academy of Child Psychiatry, 25,* 490–492.

Schiff, M., & Lewontin, R. (1986). *Education and class: The irrelevance of IQ genetic studies.* Oxford: Oxford University Press.

Schilder, P. (1938). The organic background of obsessions and compulsions. *American Journal of Psychiatry, 94,* 1397–1416.

Schleifer, M., Weiss, G., Cohen, N., Elman, M., Cvejic, H., & Kruger, E. (1975). Hyperactivity in preschoolers and the effect of methylphenidate. *American Journal of Orthopsychiatry, 45,* 38–50.

Schmale, A. H., & Engel, G. L. (1975). The role of conservation-withdrawal in depressive reactions. In E. J. Anthony & T. Benedek (Eds.), *Depression and human existence* (pp. 183–198). Boston: Little, Brown.

Schmauk, F. J. (1970). Punishment, arousal and avoidance learning in sociopaths. *Journal of Abnormal Psychology, 76,* 325–335.

Schmideberg, M. (1959). The borderline patient. In S. Arieti (Ed.), *American handbook of psychiatry* (Vol. 1, pp. 398–418). New York: Basic Books.

Schmitt, B. D. (1981). Child neglect. In N. S. Ellerstein (Ed.), *Child abuse and neglect: A medical reference* (pp. 297–306). New York: Wiley.

Schmitt, B. D. (1982). Nocturnal enuresis: An update on treatment. *Pediatric Clinics of North America, 29,* 21–30.

Schopler, E., Chess, S., & Eisenberg, L. (1981). Our memorial to Leo Kanner. *Journal of Autism and Developmental Disorders, 11,* 257–269.

Schotte, D. E., & Stunkard, A. J. (1987). Bulimia vs. bulimic behaviors on a college campus. *Journal of the American Medical Association, 258,* 1213–1215.

Schuler, A. L., & Prizant, B. M. (1987). Facilitating communication: Pre-language approaches. In D. J. Cohen & A. M. Donnellan (Eds.), *Handbook of autism and pervasive developmental disorders* (pp. 301–315). New York: Wiley.

Schumaker, J. B., Deshler, D. D., & Ellis, E. S. (1986). Intervention issues related to the education of LD adolescents. In J. K. Torgesen & B. Y. L. Wong (Eds.), *Psychological and educational perspectives on learning disabilities* (pp. 329–365). New York: Academic.

Schuman, D. C. (1987). Psychodynamics of exaggerated accusations: Positive feedback in family systems. *Psychiatric Annals, 17,* 242–247.

Schwab, E. K., & Conners, C. K. (1986). Nutrient–behavior research with children: Methods, considerations, and evaluation. *Journal of American Dietetic Association, 86,* 319–324.

Schwartz, D. M., Thompson, M. G., & Johnson, C. L. (1982). Anorexia nervosa and bulimia: The socio-cultural context. *International Journal of Eating Disorders, 1,* 20–36.

Schwartz, G. E., Weinberger, D. A., & Singer, J. A. (1981). Cardiovascular differentiation of happiness, sadness, anger, and fear following imagery and exercise. *Psychosomatic Medicine, 43,* 343–364.

Schwartz, H. J. (Ed.) (1988). *Bulimia: Psychoanalytic treatment and theory.* Madison, CT: International Universities Press.

Schwartz, R. C., Barrett, M. J., & Saba, G. (1985). Family therapy for bulimia. In D. M. Garner & P. E. Garfinkel (Eds.), *Handbook of psychotherapy for anorexia nervosa and bulimia* (pp. 280–307). New York: Guilford.

Scott, D. W. (1986). Anorexia nervosa in the male: A review of clinical, epidemiological and biological findings. *International Journal of Eating Disorders, 5,* 799–819.

Sears, R. R. (1965). Development of gender role. In F. A. Beach (Ed.), *Sex and behavior* (p. 133). New York: Wiley.

Sears, R. R., Maccoby, E. E., & Levin, H. (1957). *Patterns of child rearing.* Evanston, IL: Row, Peterson.

Sechahaye, M. A. (1951). *Symbolic realization.* New York: International Universities Press.

Sechahaye, M. A. (1956). The transference in symbolic realization. *International Journal of Psychoanalysis, 37,* 270–277.

Segal, H. (1980). *Introduction to the work of Melanie Klein.* (2nd ed.). New York: Basic Books.

Seidl, T., & Paradise, J. E. (1984). Child sexual abuse: Effective case management by a multidisciplinary team. *Resident and Staff Physician, 30,* 48–51.

Selfe, L. (1977). *Nadia: A case of extraordinary drawing ability in an autistic child.* London: Academic.

Seligman, M. E. P., Maier, S. P., & Solomon, R. L. (1971). Unpredictable and uncontrollable aversive events. In F. R. Brush (Ed.), *Aversive conditioning and learning.* New York: Academic.

Seligman, M. E. P., & Peterson, C. (1986). A learned helplessness perspective on childhood depression: Theory and research. In M. Rutter, C. E. Izard, & P. B. Read (Eds.), *Depression in young people: Developmental and clinical perspectives* (pp. 223–249). New York: Guilford.

Seligman, S. P., & Pawl, J. H. (1984). Impediments to the formation of the working alliance in infant–parent psychotherapy. In J. D. Call, E. Galenson, & R. L. Tyson (Eds.), *Frontiers of infant psychiatry* (Vol. 2, pp. 232–237). New York: Basic Books.

Sellin, T. (1938). *Culture conflict and crime.* New York: Social Science Research Council.

Selner, J. C., & Staudenmayer, H. (1979). Parents' subjective evaluation of a self-help education–exercise program for asthmatic children and their parents. *Journal of Asthma Research, 17,* 13–21.

Selvini-Palazzoli, M. (1965). Interpretation of mental anorexia. In J. E. Meyer & H. Feldman (Eds.), *Anorexia nervosa* (pp. 96–103). Stuttgart: Georg Thieme Verlag.

Selvini-Palazzoli, M. (1978). *Self starvation: From individual to family therapy in the treatment of anorexia nervosa.* New York: Jason Aronson.

Senf, G. M. (1986). LD research in sociological and scientific perspective. In J. K. Torgeson & B. Y. L. Wong (Eds.), *Psychological and educational perspectives on learning disabilities* (pp. 27–53). New York: Academic.

Sgroi, S. M. (1975). Sexual molestation of children: The last frontier in child abuse. *Children Today, 4,* 18–21.

Sgroi, S. M. (1982). *Handbook of clinical intervention in child sexual abuse.* Lexington, MA: Lexington Books.

Sgroi, S. M., Porter, F. S., & Blick, L. C. (1982). Validation of child sexual abuse. In S. M. Sgroi (Ed.), *Handbook of clinical intervention in child sexual abuse* (pp. 39–79). Lexington, MA: Lexington Books.

Shaffer, D. (1973). The association between enuresis and emotional disorder: A review of the literature. In I. Kolvin, R. C. MacKeith, & S. R. Meadow (Eds.), *Bladder control and enuresis* (pp. 118–136). (Clinics in Developmental Medicine, Nos. 48/49). London: Heinemann.

Shaffer, D. (1974). Suicide in childhood and early adolescence. *Journal of Child Psychology and Psychiatry, 15,* 275–291.

Shaffer, D. (1982). Diagnostic considerations in suicidal behavior in children and adolescents. *Journal of the American Academy of Child Psychiatry, 21,* 414–415.

Shaffer, D. (1985a). Depression, mania and suicidal acts. In M. Rutter & L. Hersov (Eds.), *Child and adolescent psychiatry: Modern approaches* (2nd ed.). Oxford: Blackwell.

Shaffer, D. (1985b). Enuresis. In M. Rutter & L. Hersov (Eds.), *Child and adolescent psychiatry* (pp. 465–481). Boston: Blackwell.

Shaffer, D. (1985c). Nocturnal enuresis: Its investigation and treatment. In D. Shaffer, A. A. Ehrhardt, & L. L. Greenhill (Eds.), *The clinical guide to child psychiatry* (pp. 29–47). New York: Free Press.

Shaffer, D. (1986a). Developmental factors in child and adolescent suicide. In M. Rutter, C. E. Izard, & P. B. Read (Eds.), *Depression in young people: Developmental and clinical perspectives* (pp. 383–396). New York: Guilford.

Shaffer, D. (1986b). Learning theories of anxiety. In R. Gittelman (Ed.), *Anxiety disorders of childhood* (pp. 157–167). New York: Guilford.

Shaffer, D., & Ambrosini, P. J. (1985). Enuresis and sleep disorders. In J. M. Weiner (Ed.), *Diagnosis and psychopharmacology of childhood and adolescent disorders* (pp. 305–331). New York: Wiley.

Shaffer, D., Costello, A. J., & Hill, I. D. (1968). Control of enuresis with imipramine. *Archives of Disease in Childhood, 43,* 665–671.

Shaffer, D., Gardner, A., & Hedge, B. (1984). Classification of enuretic children. *Developmental Medicine and Child Neurology, 26,* 781–792.

Shaffer, D., Garland, A., Gould, M., Fisher, P., & Trautman, P. (1988). Preventing teenage suicide: A critical review. *Journal of the American Academy of Child and Adolescent Psychiatry, 27,* 675–687.

Shaffer, D., & Greenhill, L. (1979). A critical note on the predictive validity of "the hyperkinetic syndrome." *Journal of Child Psychology and Psychiatry, 20,* 61–72.

Shaffer, D., & Schonfeld, I. (1984). A critical note on the value of attention deficit as a basis for a clinical syndrome. In L. M. Bloomingdale (Ed.), *Attention deficit disorder: Diagnostic, cognitive, and therapeutic understanding* (pp. 119–131). New York: SP Medical and Scientific Books.

Shaffer, D., Schonfeld, I., O'Connor, P. A., Stokman, C., Trautman, P., Shafer, S., & Ng, S. (1985). Neurological soft signs. *Archives of General Psychiatry, 42,* 342–351.

Shafii, M., Carrigan, S., Whittinghill, J. R., & Derrick, A. (1985). Psychological autopsy of completed suicide in children and adolescents. *American Journal of Psychiatry, 142,* 1061–1064.

Shapiro, D. (1965). *Neurotic styles.* New York: Basic Books.

Shapiro, E. G., & Rosenfeld, A. A. (1987). *The somatizing child: Diagnosis and treatment of conversion and somatization disorders.* New York: Springer-Verlag.

Shapiro, E. R. (1978a). The psychodynamics and developmental psychology of the borderline patient: A review of the literature. *American Journal of Psychiatry, 135,* 1305–1315.

Shapiro, E. R. (1978b). Research on family dynamics: Clinical implications for the family of the borderline adolescent. *Adolescent Psychiatry, 6,* 360–376.

Shapiro, E. R., & Freedman, J. (1987). Family dynamics of adolescent suicide. *Adolescent Psychiatry, 14,* 191–207.

Shapiro, E. R., Shapiro, R. L., Zinner, J., & Berkowitz, D. A. (1977). The borderline ego and the working alliance: Indications for family and individual treatment in adolescence. *International Journal of Psycho-Analysis, 58,* 77–93.

Shapiro, E. R., Zinner, J., Shapiro, R. L., & Berkowitz, D. A. (1975). The influence of family experience on borderline personality development. *International Review of Psychoanalysis, 2,* 399–411.

Shapiro, E. S., Shapiro, A. K., Fulop, G., Hubbard, M., Mandeli, J., Nordlie, J., Phillips, R. A. (1989). Controlled study of haloperidol, pimozide, and placebo for the treatment of Gilles de la Tourette's syndrome. *Archives of General Psychiatry, 46,* 722–730.

Shapiro, R. L. (1979). Family dynamics and object-relations theory: An analytic group-interpretive approach to family therapy. *Adolescent Psychiatry, 7,* 118–135.

Shapiro, S. K., & Garfinkel, B. D. (1986). The occurrence of behavior disorders in children: The interdependence of attention deficit disorder and conduct disorder. *Journal of the American Academy of Child Psychiatry, 25,* 809–819.

Shapiro, T. (1977). The quest for a linguistic model to study the speech of autistic children: Studies on echoing. *Journal of the American Academy of Child Psychiatry, 16,* 608–619.

Shapiro, T. (1983). The borderline syndrome in childhood: A critique. In K. S. Robson (Ed.), *The borderline child* (pp. 11–29). New York: McGraw-Hill.

Shapiro, T. (1990). Resolved: Borderline personality exists in children under twelve. *Journal of the American Academy of Child and Adolescent Psychiatry, 29,* 480–483.

Shapiro, T., Frosch, E., & Arnold, S. (1987). Communicative interaction between mothers and their autistic children: Application of a new instrument and changes after treatment. *Journal of the American Academy of Child and Adolescent Psychiatry, 26,* 485–490.

Shapiro, T., & Perry, R. (1976). Latency revisited. The age of 7 plus or minus 1. *Psychoanalytic Study of the Child, 31,* 79–105.

Shapiro, T., Sherman, M., Calamari, G., & Koch, D. (1987). Attachment in autism and other developmental disorders. *Journal of the American Academy of Child and Adolescent Psychiatry, 26,* 480–484.

Shaver, B. A. (1974). Maternal personality and early adaptation as related to infantile colic. In P. M. Shereshefsky & L. J. Yarrow (Eds.), *Psychological aspects of a first pregnancy and early postnatal adaptation* (pp. 209–215). New York: Raven Press.

Shaywitz, B. A., Cohen, D. J., & Bowers, M. B. (1977). CSF monoamine metabolites in children with minimal brain dysfunction: Evidence for alteration of brain dopamine. *Journal of Pediatrics, 90,* 67–71.

Shaywitz, B. A., Shaywitz, S. E., Byrne, T., Cohen, D. J., & Rothman, S. (1983). Attention deficit disorder: Quantitative analysis of CT. *Neurology, 33,* 1500–1503.

Shaywitz, S. E., Cohen, D. J., & Shaywitz, B. A. (1978). The biochemical basis of minimal brain dysfunction. *Journal of Pediatrics, 92,* 179–187.

Shaywitz, S. E., Cohen, D. J., & Shaywitz, B. A. (1980). Behavior and learning difficulties in children of normal intelligence born to alcoholic mothers. *Journal of Pediatrics, 96*, 978–982.

Shaywitz, S. E., Hunt, R. D., Jatlow, P., Cohen, D. J., Young, J. G., Pierce, R. N., Anderson, G. M., & Shaywitz, B. A. (1982). Psychopharmacology of attention deficit disorder: Pharmacokinetic, neuroendocrine, and behavioral measures following acute and chronic treatment with methylphenidate. *Pediatrics, 69*, 688–694.

Shaywitz, S. E., Schnell, C., Shaywitz, B. A., & Towle, V. R. (1986). Yale Children's Inventory (YCI): An instrument to assess children with attentional deficits and learning disabilities: I. Scale development and psychometric properties. *Journal of Abnormal Child Psychology, 14*, 347–364.

Shaywitz, S. E., & Shaywitz, B. A. (1984). Diagnosis and management of attention deficit disorder: A pediatric perspective. *Pediatric Clinics of North America, 31*, 429–457.

Shaywitz, S. E., Shaywitz, B. A., Cohen, D. J., & Young, J. G. (1983). Monoaminergic mechanisms in hyperactivity. In M. Rutter (Ed.), *Developmental neuropsychiatry* (pp. 330–347). New York: Guilford.

Shaywitz, S. E., Shaywitz, B. A., Fletcher, J. M., & Escobar, M. D. (1990). Prevalence of reading disability in boys and girls. *JAMA, 264*, 998–1002.

Shaywitz, S. E., Shaywitz, B. A., McGraw, K., & Groll, S. (1984). Current status of the neuromaturational examination as an index of learning disability. *Journal of Pediatrics, 104*, 819–825.

Shaywitz, S. E., Shaywitz, B. A., Schnell, C., & Towle, V. R. (1988). Concurrent and predictive validity of the Yale Children's Inventory: An instrument to assess children with attentional deficits and learning disabilities. *Pediatrics, 81*, 562–571.

Shear, M. K. (1986). Pathophysiology of panic: A review of pharmacologic provocative tests and naturalistic monitoring data [Supplement]. *Journal of Clinical Psychiatry, 47*(6), 18–26.

Shekim, W. O., Javaid, J., Davis, J. M., & Bylund, D. B. (1983). Urinary MHPG and HVA excretion in boys with attention deficit disorder and hyperactivity treated with *d*-amphetamine. *Biological Psychiatry, 18*, 707–714.

Sheldon, W. H. (1942). *Varieties of temperament.* New York: Harper.

Shelton, R. C., & Weinberger, D. R. (1986). X-ray computerized tomography studies in schizophrenia: A review and synthesis. In H. A. Nasrallah & D. R. Weinberger (Eds.), *The neurology of schizophrenia* (Vol. 1, pp. 207–250). Amsterdam: Elsevier.

Sherif, M., & Sherif, C. W. (1964). *Reference groups: Explorations into conformity and deviation of adolescents.* New York: Harper & Row.

Sherrington, R., Brynjolfsson, J., Petursson, H., Potter, M., Dudleston, K., Barraclough, B., Wasmuth, J., Dobbs, M., & Gurling, H. (1988). Localization of a susceptibility locus for schizophrenia on chromosome 5. *Nature, 336*, 164–167.

Short, J. F., Tennyson, R. A., & Howard, K. I. (1963). Behavior dimensions of gang delinquency. *American Sociological Review, 28*, 411–428.

Showers, J., & Pickrell, E. (1987). Child firesetters: A study of three populations. *Hospital and Community Psychiatry, 38*, 495–501.

Siegel, B., Anders, T. F., Ciaranello, R. D., Bienenstock, B., & Kraemer, H. C. (1986). Empirically derived subclassification of the autistic syndrome. *Journal of Autism and Developmental Disorder, 16,* 275–293.

Siegelman, E. (1969). *Children who set fires: An exploratory study.* Resources Agency of California, Department of Conservation, Division of Forestry.

Siever, L. J., & Davis, K. L. (1985). Overview: Toward a dysregulation hypothesis of depression. *American Journal of Psychiatry, 142,* 1017–1031.

Sifneos, P. E. (1973). The prevalence of "alexithymic" characteristics in psycho-somatic patients. *Psychotherapy and Psychosomatics, 22,* 255–262.

Sigman, M., Ungerer, J. A., Mundy, P., & Sherman, T. (1987). Cognition in autistic children. In D. J. Cohen & A. M. Donnellan (Eds.), *Handbook of autism and pervasive developmental disorders* (pp. 103–120). New York: Wiley.

Silbergeld, E. K., & Goldberg, A. M. (1974). Lead-induced behavioral dysfunction: An animal model of hyperactivity. *Experimental Neurology, 42,* 146–157.

Silbert, A., Wolff, P. H., & Lilienthal, J. (1977). Spatial and temporal processing in patients with Turner's syndrome. *Behavior Genetics, 7,* 11–21.

Sills, R. H. (1978). Failure to thrive: The role of clinical and laboratory evaluation. *American Journal of Diseases of Children, 132,* 967–969.

Silver, L. B. (1984). *The misunderstood child: A guide for parents of learning disabled children.* New York: McGraw-Hill.

Silver, L. B. (1989). Psychological and family problems associated with learning disabilities: Assessment and intervention. *Journal of the American Academy of Child and Adolescent Psychiatry, 28,* 319–325.

Simcha-Fagan, O., Langner, T. S., Gersten, J. C., & Eisenberg, J. G. (1975). *Violent and antisocial behavior: A longitudinal study of urban youth.* Unpublished report of the Office of Child Development (OCD-CB-480, p. 7).

Simpson, E. (1979). *Reversals: A personal account of victory over dyslexia.* New York: Washington Square Press.

Singer, M. T., Wynne, L. C., & Toohey, M. L. (1978). Communication disorders and the families of schizophrenics. In L. C. Wynne, R. L. Cromwell, & S. Matthysse (Eds.), *The nature of schizophrenia: New approaches to research and treatment* (pp. 499–511). New York: Wiley.

Skeels, H. M. (1966). Adult status of children with contrasting early life experiences: A follow-up study. *Monographs of the Society for Research in Child Development, 105*(31), 1–65.

Skinner, B. F. (1953). *Science and human behavior.* New York: Macmillan.

Skodak, M., & Skeels, H. M. (1949). A final follow-up study of one-hundred adopted children. *Journal of Genetic Psychology, 75,* 85–125.

Skynner, A. C. R. (1974). School phobia: A reappraisal. *British Journal of Medical Psychology, 47,* 1–16.

Slater, E. O., Beckwith, R., & Behnke, L. (1939). Types, levels, and irregularities of response to a nursery school situation of 40 children observed with special reference to the home environment. *Monographs of the Society for Research in Child Development, 21*(2), i–148.

Slater, E. O., & Glithero, E. (1965). A follow-up of patients diagnosed as suffering from "hysteria." *Journal of Psychosomatic Research, 9,* 9–13.

Smith, C. R. (1986). The future of the LD field: Intervention approaches. *Journal of Learning Disabilities, 19,* 461–472.

Smith, M. (1985). Recent work on low level lead exposure and its impact on behavior, intelligence and learning: A review. *Journal of the American Academy of Child Psychiatry, 24,* 24–32.

Smith, R. C., Baumgartner, R., & Calderon, M. (1987). Magnetic resonance imaging studies of the brains of schizophrenic patients. *Psychiatry Research, 20,* 33–46.

Smith, S. (1981). *No easy answers.* New York: Bantam Books.

Smith, S. D., Kimberling, W. J., Pennington, B. F., & Lubs, H. A. (1983). Specific reading disability: Identification of an inherited form through linkage analysis. *Science, 219,* 1345–1347.

Smith, S. D., Pennington, B. F., Kimberling, W. J., & Ing, P. S. (1990). Familial dyslexia: Use of genetic linkage data to define subtypes. *Journal of the American Academy of Child and Adolescent Psychiatry, 29,* 204–213.

Snyder, J. C., Hampton, R., & Newberger, E. H. (1983). Family dysfunction: Violence, neglect, and sexual misuse. In M. D. Levine, W. B. Carey, A. C. Crocker, & R. T. Gross (Eds.), *Developmental–behavioral pediatrics* (pp. 259–275). Philadelphia: Saunders.

Snyder, S. H. (1980). *Biological aspects of mental disorder.* New York: Oxford University Press.

Solanto, M. V., & Wender, E. H. (1989). Does methylphenidate constrict cognitive functioning? *Journal of the American Academy of Child and Adolescent Psychiatry, 28,* 897–902.

Soloff, P. H. (1987). Neuroleptic treatment in the borderline patient: Advantages and techniques. *Journal of Clinical Psychiatry, 48*(Suppl. 8), 26–30.

Soloff, P. H., & Millward, J. W. (1983). Psychiatric disorders in the families of borderline patients. *Archives of General Psychiatry, 40,* 37–44.

Solomon, R. L., Kamin, L. J., & Wynne, L. C. (1953). Traumatic avoidance learning: The outcomes of several extinction procedures with dogs. *Journal of Abnormal Social Psychology, 48,* 291–302.

Sorce, J. F., & Emde, R. N. (1981). Mother's presence is not enough: Effect of emotional availability on infant exploration. *Developmental Psychology, 17,* 737–745.

Sorce, J. F., Emde, R. N., Campos, J., & Klinnert, M. D. (1985). Maternal emotional signaling: Its effect on the visual cliff behavior of 1-year-olds. *Developmental Psychology, 21,* 195–200.

Sours, J. A. (1979). The primary anorexia nervosa syndrome. In J. D. Noshpitz (Ed.), *Basic handbook of child psychiatry* (Vol. 2, pp. 568–580). New York: Basic Books.

Sours, J. A. (1980). *Starving to death in a sea of objects: The anorexia nervosa syndrome.* New York: Jason Aronson.

Sparrow, S., Balla, D., & Cicchetti, D. (1984). *Vineland Adaptive Behavior Scales (survey form).* Circle Pines, MN: American Guidance Service.

Special Report: Schizophrenia 1987, *Schizophrenia Bulletin, 13*(1), 1–214.

Sperling, M. (1964). The analysis of a boy with transvestite tendencies: A contribution to the genesis and dynamics of transvestism. *Psychoanalytic Study of the Child, 19,* 470–493.

Sperling, M. (1968). Asthma in children: An evaluation of concepts and therapies. *Journal of the American Academy of Child Psychiatry, 7,* 44–58.

Sperling, M. (1978). *Psychosomatic disorders in childhood.* New York: Jason Aronson.

Spitz, R. A. (1945). Hospitalism: An inquiry into the genesis of psychiatric conditions in early childhood. *Psychoanalytic Study of the Child, 1,* 53–74.

Spitz, R. A. (1946). Anaclitic depression. *Psychoanalytic Study of the Child, 2,* 313–342.

Spitz, R. A. (1965). *The first year of life.* New York: International Universities Press.

Spitz, R. A., & Wolf, K. M. (1946). Anaclitic depression. An inquiry into the genesis of psychiatric conditions in early childhood: II. *Psychoanalytic Study of the Child, 2,* 313–342.

Spitzer, R. L., Endicott, J., & Gibbon, M. (1979). Crossing the border into borderline personality and borderline schizophrenia. *Archives of General Psychiatry, 36,* 17–24.

Spitzer, R. L., Endicott, J., & Robins, E. (1978). Research diagnostic criteria: Rationale and reliability. *Archives of General Psychiatry, 35,* 773–782.

Sprague, R. L. (1983). Behavior modification and educational techniques. In M. Rutter (Ed.), *Developmental neuropsychiatry* (pp. 404–421). New York: Guilford.

Sprague, R. L., & Sleator, E. K. (1975). What is the proper dose of stimulant drugs in children? In R. Gittelman-Klein (Ed.), *Recent advances in child psychopharmacology* (pp. 79–108). New York: Human Sciences Press.

Sprague, R. L., & Sleator, E. K. (1977). Methylphenidate in hyperkinetic children: Differences in dose effects on learning and social behavior. *Science, 198,* 1274–1276.

Spreen, O., & Haaf, R. G. (1986). Empirically derived learning disability subtypes: A replication attempt and longitudinal patterns over fifteen years. *Journal of Learning Disabilities, 19,* 170–180.

Sreenivasan, U. (1985). Effeminate boys in a child psychiatric clinic: Prevalence and associated factors. *Journal of the American Academy of Child Psychiatry, 24,* 689–694.

Sroufe, L. A., Fox, N. E., & Pancake, V. R. (1983). Attachment and dependency in developmental perspective. *Child Development, 54,* 1615–1627.

Stanley, E. J., & Barter, J. T. (1970). Adolescent suicidal behavior. *American Journal of Orthopsychiatry, 40,* 87–96.

Stanley, M., & Mann, J. J. (1988). Biological factors associated with suicide. In A. J. Frances & R. E. Hales (Eds.), *Review of psychiatry* (pp. 334–352). Washington, DC: American Psychiatric Press.

Stanovich, K. E. (1986). Cognitive processes and the reading problems of learning-disabled children: Evaluating the assumption of specificity. In J. K. Torgesen & B. Y. L. Wong (Eds.), *Psychological and educational perspective on learning disabilities* (pp. 85–131). New York: Academic.

Steele, B. F. (1976). Violence within the family. In R. E. Helfer, & C. H. Kempe, (Eds.), *Child abuse and neglect: The family and the community.* Cambridge, MA: Ballinger.

Steele, B. F., & Pollock, C. B. (1968). A psychiatric study of parents who abuse infants and small children. In R. E. Helfer & C. H. Kempe (Eds.), *The battered child* (pp. 103–147). Chicago: University of Chicago Press.

Stein, M. (1986). A reconsideration of specificity in psychosomatic medicine: From olfaction to the lymphocyte. *Psychosomatic Medicine, 48,* 3–21.

Stein, S. P., & Charles, E. (1971). Emotional factors in juvenile diabetes mellitus: A study of early life experience of adolescent diabetics. *American Journal of Psychiatry, 128,* 700–704.

Stein, Z. A., & Susser, M. W. (1963). The social distribution of mental retardation. *American Journal of Mental Deficiency, 67,* 811–821.

Stein, Z. A., & Susser, M. W. (1965). Socio-medical study of enuresis among delinquent boys. *British Journal of Preventive and Social Medicine, 19,* 174–181.

Stein, Z. A., & Susser, M. W. (1966). Nocturnal enuresis as a phenomenon of institutions. *Developmental Medicine and Child Neurology, 8,* 677–685.

Stein, Z. A., & Susser, M. W. (1967). Social factors in the development of sphincter control. *Developmental Medicine and Child Neurology, 9,* 692–706.

Stein, Z. A., & Susser, M. W. (1971). Mutability of intelligence and epidemiology of mild mental retardation. In S. Chess & A. Thomas (Eds.), *Annual Progress in Child Psychiatry and Child Development* (pp. 367–407). New York: Brunner/Mazel.

Steinberg, D. (1985). Psychotic and other severe disorders in adolescence. In M. Rutter & L. Hersov (Eds.), *Child and adolescent psychiatry: Modern approaches* (pp. 567–583). Oxford: Blackwell.

Steinhausen, H-C., Schindler, H-P., & Stephan, H. (1983). Correlates of psychopathology in sick children: An empirical model. *Journal of the American Academy of Child Psychiatry, 22,* 559–564.

Stern, D. N. (1977). *The first relationship: Infant and mother.* Cambridge: Harvard University Press.

Stern, D. N. (1985). *The interpersonal world of the infant: A view from psychoanalysis and developmental psychology.* New York: Basic Books.

Stevens, H. (1969). Conversion hysteria-revisited by the pediatric neurologist. *Clinical Procedures of Children's Hospital (D.C.), 25,* 27–39.

Stevens, J. (1987). Brief psychoses: Do they contribute to the good prognosis and equal prevalence of schizophrenia in developing countries? *British Journal of Psychiatry, 151,* 393–396.

Stewart, M. A., Cummings, C., Singer, S., & DeBlois, C. S. (1981). The overlap between hyperactive and unsocialized aggressive children. *Journal of Child Psychology and Psychiatry, 22,* 35–45.

Stewart, M. A., & Olds, S. W. (1973). *Raising a hyperactive child.* New York: Harper & Row.

Stewart, M. A., Pitts, F. N., Craig, A. G., & Dieruf, W. (1966). The hyperactive child syndrome. *American Journal of Orthopsychiatry, 36,* 861–867.

Stickler, G. B., & Murphy, D. B. (1979). Recurrent abdominal pain. *American Journal of Diseases of Children, 133,* 486–489.

Still, G. F. (1902). Some abnormal psychical conditions in children. *Lancet, I,* 1008–1012, 1077–1082, 1163–1168.

Stokes, A., Bawden, H., Camfield, P., Backman, J., & Dooley, J. (1988, October). *Factors associated with the adjustment of children with Tourette's syndrome.* Paper presented at the Annual Meeting of the American Academy of Child and Adolescent Psychiatry, Seattle.

Stoller, R. J. (1964). A contribution to the study of gender identity. *International Journal of Psychoanalysis, 45,* 220–226.

Stoller, R. J. (1968). Male childhood transsexualism. *Journal of the American Academy of Child Psychiatry, 7,* 193–209.

Stoller, R. J. (1974). Symbiosis anxiety & the development of masculinity. *Archives of General Psychiatry, 30:* 164–172.

Stoller, R. J. (1978). Boyhood gender aberrations: Treatment issues. *Journal of the American Psychoanalytic Association, 26,* 541–558.

Stone, A. (1984). Violence and temporal lobe epilepsy [Letter to the editor]. *American Journal of Psychiatry, 141,* 1641.

Stone, C., & Bernstein, L. (1980). Case management with borderline children: Theory and practice. *Clinical Social Work Journal, 8,* 147–160.

Stone, M. H. (1980). *The borderline syndromes: Constitution, adaptation and personality.* New York: McGraw-Hill.

Stone, M. H. (1984). Critical and unresolved issues of borderline personality. *Integrative Psychiatry, 2,* 177–181.

Stone, M. H. (1985). Schizotypal personality: Psychotherapeutic aspects. *Schizophrenia Bulletin, 11,* 576–589.

Strachey, J. (1934). The nature of the therapeutic action of psychoanalysis. *International Journal of Psycho-Analysis, 15,* 127–159.

Straus, M. A., Gelles, R. J., & Steinmetz, S. K. (1980). *Behind closed doors: Violence in the American family.* New York: Anchor Press.

Strauss, A. A., & Kephart, N. C. (1955). *Psychopathology and education of the brain-injured child: Vol. 2. Progress in theory and clinic.* New York: Grune & Stratton.

Strauss, A. A., & Lehtinen, L. E. (1947). *Psychopathology and education of the brain-injured child: Vol. 1.* New York: Grune & Stratton.

Strauss, J. S., & Carpenter, Jr., W. T. (1981). *Schizophrenia.* New York: Plenum Medical.

Strober, M. (1985). Depressive illness in adolescence. *Psychiatric Annals, 15,* 375–378.

Strober, M., & Carlson, G. A. (1982). Bipolar illness in adolescents with major depression. Clinical, genetic and psychopharmacologic predictors in a 3–4 year prospective follow-up investigation. *Archives of General Psychiatry, 39,* 549–555.

Strober, M., Salkin, B., Burroughs, J., & Morrell, W. (1982). Validity of the bulimia-restricter distinction in anorexia nervosa. *Journal of Nervous and Mental Disease, 170,* 345–351.

Strunk, R. C., Mrazek, D. A., Fuhrmann, G. S., & LaBrecque, J. F. (1985). Physiologic and psychological characteristics associated with deaths due to asthma in childhood. A case-controlled study. *Journal of the American Medical Association, 254,* 1193–1198.

Sullivan, H. S. (1953). *The interpersonal theory of psychiatry.* New York: Norton.

Summers, F., & Walsh, F. (1977). The nature of the symbiotic bond between mother and schizophrenic. *American Journal of Orthopsychiatry, 47,* 484–494.

Summit, R. (1982). Beyond belief—the reluctant discovery of incest. In M. Kirkpatrick (Ed.), *Women's sexual experience: Explorations of the dark continent* (pp. 127–150). New York: Plenum.

Suomi, S. J. (1986). Anxiety-like disorders in young nonhuman primates. In R. Gittelman (Ed.), *Anxiety disorders of childhood* (pp. 1–23). New York: Guilford.

Suomi, S. J., Kraemer, G. W., Baysinger, C. M., & DeLizio, R. D. (1981). Inherited and experiential factors associated with individual differences in anxious behavior displayed by rhesus monkeys. In D. F. Klein & J. Rabkin (Eds.), *Anxiety: New research and changing concepts* (pp. 179–200). New York: Raven Press.

Suomi, S. J., Seaman, S. F., Lewis, J. K., DeLizio, R. D., & McKinney, W. T., Jr. (1978). Effects of imipramine treatment on separation-induced social disorders in rhesus monkeys. *Archives of General Psychiatry, 35,* 321–325.

Susman, E. J., Trickett, P. K., Iannotti, R. J., Hollenbeck, B. E., & Zahn-Waxler, C. (1985). Child-rearing patterns in depressed, abusive, and normal mothers. *American Journal of Orthopsychiatry, 55,* 237–251.

Sutherland, E. H., & Cressey, D. (1974). *Criminology* (9th ed.). Philadelphia: Lippincott.

Swanson, H. L. (1988). Toward a metatheory of learning disabilities. *Journal of Learning Disabilities, 21,* 196–209.

Swanson, J. M., & Kinsbourne, M. (1980). Food dyes impair performance of hyperactive children on a laboratory learning test. *Science, 207,* 1485–1487.

Swanson, L., & Biaggio, M. K. (1985). Therapeutic perspectives on father-daughter incest. *American Journal of Psychiatry, 142,* 667–674.

Swedo, S. E. (1989). Rituals and releasers: An ethological model of obsessive-compulsive disorder. In J. L. Rapoport (Ed.), *Obsessive-compulsive disorder in children and adolescents* (pp. 269–288). Washington, DC: American Psychiatric Press.

Swedo, S. E., & Rapoport, J. L. (1990). Neurobiology of obsessive-compulsive disorder in childhood. In S. I. Deutsch (Ed.), *Application of basic neuroscience to child psychiatry.* New York: Plenum.

Swedo, S. E., Rapoport, J. L., Cheslow, D. L., Leonard, H. L., Ayoub, E. M., Hosier, D. M., & Wald, E. R. (1989b). High prevalence of obsessive-compulsive symptoms in patients with Sydenham's chorea. *American Journal of Psychiatry, 146,* 246–249.

Swedo, S. E., Rapoport, J. L., Leonard, H., Lenane, M., & Cheslow, D. (1989a). Obsessive-compulsive disorder in children and adolescents. Clinical phenomenology of 70 consecutive cases. *Archives of General Psychiatry, 46,* 335–341.

Swedo, S. E., Schapiro, M. B., Grady, C. L., Cheslow, D. L., Leonard, H. L., Kumar, A., Friedland, R., Rapoport, S. I., & Rapoport, J. (1989c). Cerebral glucose metabolism in childhood-onset obsessive-compulsive disorder. *Archives of General Psychiatry, 46,* 518–523.

Swift, W. J. (1982). The long-term outcome of early onset anorexia nervosa: A critical review. *Journal of the American Academy of Child Psychiatry, 21,* 38–46.

Swift, W. J. (1985). Assessment of the bulimic patient. *American Journal of Orthopsychiatry, 55,* 384–396.

Swift, W. J., Andrews, D., & Barklage, N. E. (1986). The relationship between affective disorder and eating disorders: A review of the literature. *American Journal of Psychiatry, 143*, 290–299.

Szatmari, P., Boyle, M., & Offord, D. R. (1989). ADDH and conduct disorder: Degree of diagnostic overlap and differences among correlates. *Journal of the American Academy of Child and Adolescent Psychiatry, 28*, 865–872.

Szatmari, P., Tuff, L., Finlayson, A. J., & Bartolucci, G. (1990). Asperger's syndrome and autism: Neurocognitive aspects. *Journal of the American Academy of Child and Adolescent Psychiatry, 29*, 130–136.

Szurek, S. A., & Berlin, I. N. (Eds.) (1973). *Clinical studies in childhood psychoses.* New York: Brunner/Mazel.

Szymanski, L. S. (1977). Psychiatric diagnostic evaluation of mentally retarded individuals. *Journal of the American Academy of Child Psychiatry, 16*, 67–87.

Tal, A., & Miklich, D. (1976). Emotionally induced decreases in pulmonary flow rates in asthmatic children. *Psychosomatic Medicine, 38*, 190–200.

Talbot, M. (1957). Panic in school phobia. *American Journal of Orthopsychiatry, 27*, 286–295.

Tanguay, P. E. (1982). In S. Cantor (Ed.), *The schizophrenic child* (pp. iii–vii). Montreal: Eden.

Tanguay, P. E., & Asarnow, R. (1986). Schizophrenia in children. In R. Michels & J. O. Cavenar (Eds.), *Psychiatry* (Vol. 2, pp. 1–9). Philadelphia: Lippincott.

Tanguay, P. E., & Cantor, S. L. (1986). Schizophrenia in children. *Journal of the American Academy of Child Psychiatry, 25*, 591–594.

Tarjan, G., Wright, S. W., Eyman, R. K., & Keeran, C. V. (1973). Natural history of mental retardation: Some aspects of epidemiology. *American Journal of Mental Deficiency, 77*, 369–379.

Tardieu, A. (1868). *Etude medico-legale sur l'infanticide.* Paris: J-B Bailliére et Fils.

Tarter, R. E., Hegedus, A. M., Winsten, N. E., & Alterman, A. I. (1984). Neuropsychological, personality, and familial characteristics of physically abused delinquents. *Journal of the American Academy of Child Psychiatry, 23*, 668–674.

Taylor, E. A. (1983). Drug response and diagnostic validation. In M. Rutter (Ed.), *Developmental neuropsychiatry* (pp. 348–368). New York: Guilford.

Taylor, E. A. (1985). Syndromes of overactivity and attention deficit. In M. Rutter & L. Hersov (Eds.), *Child and adolescent psychiatry: Modern approaches* (pp. 424–443). Oxford: Blackwell.

Taylor, E. A. (1986). Overactivity, hyperactivity and hyperkinesis: Problems and prevalence. In E. Taylor (Ed.), *The overactive child.* Philadelphia: Lippincott.

Taylor E. A., & Sandberg, S. (1984). Hyperactive behavior in English schoolchildren: A questionnaire survey. *Journal of Abnormal Child Psychology, 12*, 143–156.

Taylor, R. L., & Warren, S. A. (1984). Educational and psychological assessment of children with learning disorders. *The Pediatric Clinics of North America, 31*, 281–296.

Tennant, C. (1988). Parental loss in childhood: Its effect in adult life. *Archives of General Psychiatry, 45*, 1045–1050.

Tennes, K., Downey, K., & Vernadakis, A. (1977). Urinary cortisol excretion rates and anxiety in normal one-year-old infants. *Psychosomatic Medicine, 39,* 178–187.

Terman, L. M. & Merrill, M. A. (1973). *Stanford-Binet Intelligence Scale: Manual for the Third Revision, Form L-M.* Boston: Houghton Mifflin.

Terr, L. C. (1986). The child psychiatrist and the child witness: Traveling companions by necessity, if not by design. *Journal of the American Academy of Child Psychiatry, 25,* 462–472.

Terr, L. C. (1987). Childhood psychic trauma. In J. D. Noshpitz (Ed.), *Basic handbook of child psychiatry* (Vol. 5, pp. 262–272). New York: Basic Books.

Terr, L. C. (1988a). Debate Forum. Anatomically correct dolls: Should they be used as the basis for experts testimony? *Journal of the American Academy of Child and Adolescent Psychiatry, 27,* 255–257.

Terr, L. C. (1988b). Debate Forum. Anatomically correct dolls: Should they be used as the basis for experts testimony? *Journal of the American Academy of Child and Adolescent Psychiatry, 27,* 387–388.

Theander, S. (1970). Anorexia nervosa: A psychiatric investigation of 94 female patients. *Acta Psychiatrica Scandinavica Supplementum, 214,* 5–194.

Thomas, A., & Chess, S. (1977). *Temperament and development.* New York: Brunner/ Mazel.

Thomas, A., & Chess, S. (1984). Genesis and evolution of behavioral disorders: From infancy to early adult life. *American Journal of Psychiatry, 141,* 1–9.

Thomas, A., Chess, S., & Birch, H. G. (1968). *Temperament and behavior disorders in children.* New York: New York University Press.

Thompson, J. K., & Thompson, C. M. (1986). Body size distortion and self-esteem in asymptomatic, normal weight males and females. *International Journal of Eating Disorders, 5,* 1061–1068.

Thompson, R. J. (1986). *Behavior problems in children with developmental and learning disabilities.* Ann Arbor: University of Michigan Press.

Thoren, P., Asberg, M., Cronholm, B., Jornestedt, L., & Traskman, L. (1980). Clomipramine treatment of obsessive-compulsive disorder: I. A controlled clinical trial. *Archives of General Psychiatry, 37,* 1281–1285.

Tienari, P., Sorri, A., Lahti, I., Naarala, M., Wahlberg, K-E., Moring, J., Pohjola, J., & Wynne, L. C. (1987). Genetic and psychosocial factors in schizophrenia: The Finnish Adoptive Family Study. *Schizophrenia Bulletin, 13,* 477–484.

Tienari, P., Sorri, A., Lahti, I., Naarala, M., Wahlberg, K-E., Ronkko, T., Pohjola, J., & Moring, J. (1985). The Finnish Adoptive Family Study of schizophrenia. *The Yale Journal of Biology and Medicine, 58,* 227–237.

Tinbergen, N. (1966). *Social behavior in animals* (2nd ed.). London: Methuen.

Tishler, C. L., & McKenry, P. C. (1982). Parental negative self and adolescent suicide attempts. *Journal of the American Academy of Child Psychiatry, 21,* 404–408.

Tizard, B., & Hodges, J. (1978). The effect of early institutional rearing on the development of eight-year-old children. *Journal of Child Psychology and Psychiatry, 19,* 99–118.

Tomasson, K. & Kuperman, S. (1990). Bipolar disorder in a prepubescent child. *Journal of the American Academy of Child and Adolescent Psychiatry, 29,* 308–310.

Torgersen, S. (1983). Genetic factors in anxiety disorders. *Archives of General Psychiatry, 40,* 1085–1089.

Torgersen, S. (1984). Genetic and nosological aspects of schizotypal and borderline personality disorders. *Archives of General Psychiatry, 41,* 546–554.

Torgersen, S. (1985). Relationship of schizotypal personality disorder to schizophrenia: Genetics. *Schizophrenia Bulletin, 11,* 554–563.

Torgergen, S. (1986a). Childhood and family characteristics in panic and generalized anxiety disorders. *American Journal of Psychiatry, 143,* 630–632.

Torgersen, S. (1986b). Genetic factors in moderately severe and mild affective disorders. *Archives of General Psychiatry, 43,* 222–226.

Torgersen, S. (1986c). Genetics of somatoform disorders. *Archives of General Psychiatry, 43,* 502–505.

Torrey, E. F. (1986). Functional psychoses and viral encephalitis. *Integrative Psychiatry, 4,* 224–236.

Touwen, B. C. L., & Prechtl, H. F. R. (1970). *The neurological examination of the child with minor nervous dysfunction.* London: Spastics International Medical Publications.

Towbin, K. E., Leckman, J. F., & Cohen, D. J. (1987). Drug treatment of obsessive-compulsive disorder: A review of findings in the light of diagnostic and metric limitations. *Psychiatric Development, 5,* 25–50.

Towbin, K. E., Riddle, M. A., Leckman, J. F., Brunn, R. D., & Cohen D. J. (1988). The clinical care of individuals with Tourette's syndrome. In D. J. Cohen, R. D. Brunn, & J. F. Leckman (Eds.), *Tourette's syndrome and tic disorders: Clinical understanding and treatment* (pp. 329–352). New York: Wiley.

Treffert, D. A. (1989). *Extraordinary people: Understanding "idiot savants."* New York: Harper & Row.

Trites, R. L. (1979). *Hyperactivity in children: Etiology, measurement, and treatment implications.* Baltimore: University Park Press.

Trites, R. L., & Laprade, K. (1983). Evidence for an independent syndrome of hyperactivity. *Journal of Child Psychology and Psychiatry, 24,* 573–586.

Troisi, A., & D'Amato, F. R. (1984). Ambivalence in monkey mothering: Infant abuse combined with maternal possessiveness. *Journal of Nervous and Mental Disease, 172,* 105–108.

Tronick, E. Z., & Gianino, A. R. (1986). The transmission of maternal disturbance to the infant. In E. Z. Tronick & T. Fields (Eds.), *Maternal depression and infant disturbance* (pp. 5–11). New York: Wiley.

Tsai, L., Stewart, M. A., & August, G. (1981). Implication of sex differences in the familial transmission of infantile autism. *Journal of Autism and Developmental Disorders, 11,* 165–173.

Tsuang, M. T. (1978). Genetic counseling for psychiatric patients and their families. *American Journal of Psychiatry, 135,* 1465–1475.

Turner, R. K. (1973). Conditioning treatment of nocturnal enuresis: Present status. In I. Kolvin, R. C., MacKeith, & S. R. Meadow (Eds.), *Bladder control and enuresis* (pp. 195–210). (Clinics in Developmental Medicine, Nos. 48/49). London: Heinemann.

Turner, S. M., Jacob, R. G., Beidel, D. C., & Himmelhoch, J. (1985). Fluoxetine treatment of obsessive-compulsive disorder. *Journal of Clinical Psychopharmacology*, *5*, 207–212.

Tyrer, P. (1985). Neurosis divisible? *Lancet*, *1*, 685–688.

U.S. Department of Education. (1987). *Ninth annual report to Congress on the implementation of the Education of the Handicapped Act* (pp. 3–5). Washington, DC: U.S. Department of Education.

U.S. Department of Health and Human Services. (1982). *Television and behavior: Ten years of scientific progress and implications for the eighties*. Washington, DC: U.S. Department of Health and Human Services.

Ushakov, G. K., & Girich, Y. P. (1971). Special features of psychogenic depressions in children and adolescents. In A. L. Annell (Ed.), *Depressive states in childhood and adolescence* (pp. 510–516). Stockholm: Almqvist & Wiksell.

Valente, M. (1971). Autism: symptomatic and idiopathic—and mental retardation. *Pediatrics*, *48*, 495–496.

Van Winter, J. T., & Stickler, G. B. (1984). Panic attack syndrome. *Journal of Pediatrics*, *105*, 661–665.

Vandenberg, S. G., Singer, S. M., & Pauls, D. L. (1986). *The heredity of behavior disorders in adults and children*. New York: Plenum Medical.

Vandereycken, W., & Pierloot, R. (1983). The significance of subclassification in anorexia nervosa: A comparative study of clinical features in 141 patients. *Psychological Medicine*, *13*, 543–549.

Vandersall, T., & Wiener, J. (1971). Children who set fires. *Archives of General Psychiatry*, *22*, 53–71.

Varley, C. K. (1983). Effects of methylphenidate in adolescents with attention deficit disorder. *Journal of the American Academy of Child Psychiatry*, *22*, 351–354.

Vela, R., Gottlieb, H., & Gottlieb, E. (1983). Borderline syndromes in childhood: A critical review. In K. S. Robson (Ed.), *The borderline child: Approaches to etiology, diagnosis, and treatment* (pp. 31–48). New York: McGraw-Hill.

Vellutino, F. R. (1987). Dyslexia. *Scientific American*, *256*, 34–41.

Venault, P., Chapouthier, G., de Carvalho, L. P., Simiand, J., Morre, M., Dodd, R. H., & Rossier, J. (1986). Benzodiazepine impairs and beta-carboline enhances performance in learning and memory tasks. *Nature*, *321*, 864–866.

Verhulst, F. C., Van der Lee, J. H., Akkerhuis, G. W., Sanders-Woudstra, J. A. R., Timmer, F. C., & Donkhorst, I. D. (1985). The prevalence of nocturnal enuresis: Do DSM-III criteria need to be changed? A brief research report. *Journal of Child Psychology and Psychiatry*, *26*, 989–993.

Vietze, P., Falsey, S., O'Connor, S., Sandler, H., Sherrod, K., & Altemeier, W. (1980). Newborn behavioral and interactional characteristics of nonorganic failure-to-thrive infants. In T. Field, S. Goldberg, D. Stern, & A. Sostek (Eds.), *High-risk infants and children* (pp. 5–23). New York: Academic.

Vinogradov, S., Dishotsky, N. I., Doty, B. A., & Tinklenberg, J. R. (1988). Patterns of behavior in adolescent rape. *American Journal of Orthopsychiatry*, *58*, 179–187.

Viorst, J. (1986). *Necessary losses*. New York: Simon & Schuster.

Volkan, V. D. (1981). *Linking objects and linking phenomena*. New York: International Universities Press.

Volkmar, F. R. (1987). Social development. In D. J. Cohen & A. M. Donnellan (Eds.), *Handbook of autism and pervasive developmental disorders* (pp. 41–60). New York: Wiley.

Volkmar, F. R., & Cohen, D. J. (1985). The experience of infantile autism: A first-person account by Tony W. *Journal of Autism and Developmental Disorders, 15*, 47–54.

Volkmar, F. R., & Cohen, D. J. (1988). Classification and diagnosis of childhood autism. In E. Schopler, & G. B. Mesibov, (Eds.), *Diagnosis and assessment in autism* (pp. 71–89). New York: Plenum.

Volkmar, F. R., & Cohen, D. J. (1989). Disintegrative disorder or "late onset" autism. *Journal of Child Psychology and Psychiatry, 30*, 717–724.

Volkmar, F. R., Cohen, D. J., Bregman, J. D., Hooks, M. Y., & Stevenson, J. M. (1989). An examination of social typologies in autism. *Journal of the American Academy of Child and Adolescent Psychiatry, 28*, 82–86.

Volkmar, F. R., Cohen, D. J., Hoshino, Y., Rende, R., Paul, R. (1988). Phenomenology and classification of the childhood psychoses. *Psychological Medicine, 18*, 191–201.

Volkmar, F. R., Cohen, D. J., & Paul, R. (1986). An evaluation of DSM-III criteria for infantile autism. *Journal of the American Academy of Child Psychiatry, 25*, 190–197.

Volkmar, F. R., & Nelson, D. S. (1990). Seizure disorders in autism. *Journal of the American Academy of Child and Adolescent Psychiatry, 29*, 127–129.

Volkmar, F. R., Paul, R., & Cohen, D. J. (1985a). The use of "Asperger's syndrome." *Journal of Autism and Developmental Disorders, 15*, 437–439.

Volkmar, F. R., Poll, J., & Lewis, M. (1984). Conversion reactions in childhood and adolescence. *Journal of the American Academy of Child Psychiatry, 23*, 424–430.

Volkmar, F. R., Stier, D. M., & Cohen, D. J. (1985b). Age of onset of pervasive developmental disorder. *American Journal of Psychiatry, 142*, 1450–1452.

Vrough, K., & Handrich, M. (1966). *Sex-typing in the preschool years: An overview* (Report No. 13). Chicago, IL: Institute of Juvenile Research, Department of Mental Health.

Waldfogel, S., Coolidge, J. C., & Hahn, P. B. (1957). The development, meaning and management of school phobia. *American Journal of Orthopsychiatry, 27*, 754–780.

Waldron, S., Shrier, D. K., Stone, B., & Tobin, F. (1975). School phobia and other childhood neuroses: A systematic study of the children and their families. *American Journal of Psychiatry, 132*, 802–808.

Waldrop, M. F., Bell, R. Q., McLaughlin, B., & Halverson, C. F. (1978). Newborn minor physical anomalies predict short attention span, peer aggression, and impulsivity at age 3. *Science, 199*, 563–565.

Walinder, J. (1967). *Transsexualism: A study of 43 cases.* Goteborg: Scandinavian University Books.

Wallerstein, J. S., & Kelly, J. B. (1980). *Surviving the breakup: How children and parents cope with divorce.* New York: Basic Books.

Walsh, B. T., Gladis, M., Roose, S. P., Stewart, J. W., Stetner, F., & Glassman, A. H. (1988). Phenelzine vs. placebo in 50 patients with bulimia. *Archives of General Psychiatry, 45,* 471–475.

Walters, A. S., Barrett, R. P., Feinstein, C., Mercurio, A., & Hole, W. T. (1990). A case report of naltrexone treatment of self-injury and social withdrawal in autism. *Journal of Autism and Developmental Disorders, 20,* 169–176.

Ward, C. D. (1988). Transient feelings of compulsion caused by hemispheric lesions: Three cases. *Journal of Neurology, Neurosurgery and Psychiatry, 51,* 266–268.

Ward, I. L. (1977). Exogenous androgen activates female behavior in non-copulating, prenatally stressed male rats. *Journal of Comparative and Physiologic Psychology, 91,* 465–471.

Warren, W. (1960). Some relationships between the psychiatry of children and of adults. *Journal of Mental Science, 106,* 815–826.

Warren, W. (1965). A study of adolescent psychiatric inpatients and the outcome six or more years later: II. The follow-up study. *Journal of Child Psychology and Psychiatry, 6,* 141–160.

Wasman, M., & Flynn, J. (1962). Directed attack elicited from hypothalamus. *Archives of Neurology, 6,* 220–227.

Wasserman, A. L., Whitington, P. F., & Rivara, F. P. (1988). Psychogenic basis for abdominal pain in children and adolescents. *Journal of the American Academy of Child and Adolescent Psychiatry, 27,* 179–184.

Wasserman, G. A., Gardier, K., Allen, R., & Shilansky, M. (1987). Interactions between abused infants and strangers. *Journal of the American Academy of Child and Adolescent Psychiatry, 26,* 504–509.

Wasserman, G. A., Green, A., & Allen, R. (1983). Going beyond abuse: Maladaptive patterns of interaction in abusing mother–infant pairs. *Journal of American Academy of Child Psychiatry, 22,* 245–252.

Wasserman, S., & Rosenfeld, A. (1985). Decision-making in child abuse and neglect. *Bulletin of the American Academy of Psychiatry and the Law, 13,* 259–271.

Waterhouse, L., Fein, D., Nath, J., & Snyder, D. (1983). Critique of DSM-III diagnosis of pervasive developmental disorders. In G. Tischler (Ed.), *DSM-III: An interim appraisal.* Washington, DC: American Psychiatric Association.

Watkins, J. M., Asarnow, R. F., Tanguay, P. E. (1988). Symptom development in childhood onset schizophrenia. *Journal of Child Psychology and Psychiatry, 29,* 865–878.

Watson, J. B., & Rayner, R. (1920). Conditioned emotional reactions. *Journal of Experimental Psychology, 3,* 1–14.

Watt, N. F. (1978). Patterns of childhood social development in adult schizophrenics. *Archives of General Psychiatry, 35,* 160–165.

Watt, N. F., Anthony, E. J., Wynne, L. C., & Rolf, J. E. (Eds.) (1984). *Children at risk for schizophrenia: A longitudinal perspective.* New York: Cambridge University Press.

Weil, A. P. (1953). Certain severe disturbances of ego development in childhood. *Psychoanalytic Study of the Child, 8,* 271–287.

Weinberg, W. A., & Brumback, R. A. (1976). Mania in childhood—Case studies and literature review. *American Journal of Diseases of Children, 130,* 380–385.

Weinberg, W. A., Rutman, J., Sullivan, L., Penick, E. C., & Deitz, S. G. (1973). Depression in children referred to an educational diagnostic center: Diagnosis and treatment. *Journal of Pediatrics, 83,* 1065–1072.

Weinberg, S. K. (1955). *Incest behavior.* New York: Citadel.

Weinberger, D. R. (1987). Implications of normal brain development for the pathogenesis of schizophrenia. *Archives of General Psychiatry, 44,* 660–669.

Weinberger, D. R., & Kleinman, J. E. (1986). Observations on the brain in schizophrenia. In R. E. Hales & A. J. Frances (Eds.), *Psychiatry update: American Psychiatric Association annual review* (Vol. 5, pp. 42–67). Washington, DC: American Psychiatric Association Press.

Weiner, H. (1977). *Psychobiology and Human Disease.* New York: Elsevier.

Weiner, I. B. (1967). Behavior therapy in obsessive-compulsive neurosis: Treatment of an adolescent boy. *Psychotherapy: Theory, Research and Practice, 4,* 27–29.

Weintraub, M. I. (1983). *Hysterical conversion reactions.* New York: Spectrum.

Weintraub, S., Winters, K. C., & Neale, J. M. (1986). Competence and vulnerability in children with an affectively disordered parent. In M. Rutter, C. E. Izard, & P. B. Read (Eds.), *Depression in young people: Developmental and clinical perspectives* (pp. 205–220). New York: Guilford.

Weiss, B., Williams, J. H., Margen, S., Abrams, B., Caan, B., Citron, L. J., Cox, C., McKibben, J., Ogar, D., & Schultz, S. (1980). Behavioral responses to artificial food colors. *Science, 207,* 1487–1489.

Weiss, E. (1947). Psychogenic rheumatism. *Annals of Internal Medicine, 26,* 890–900.

Weiss, G. (1983). Long-term outcome: Findings, concepts and practical implications. In M. Rutter (Ed.), *Developmental neuropsychiatry* (pp. 422–436). New York: Guilford.

Weiss, G. (1984). Biopsychosocial aspects of the hyperactive child syndrome. In L. L. Greenhill & B. Shopsin (Eds.), *The psychobiology of childhood* (pp. 1–17). New York: Spectrum.

Weiss, G. (1985). Follow-up studies on outcome of hyperactive children. *Psychopharmacology Bulletin, 21,* 169–177.

Weiss, G., & Hechtman, L. T. (1979). The hyperactive child syndrome. *Science, 205,* 1348–1354.

Weiss, G., & Hechtman, L. T. (1986). *Hyperactive children grown up: Empirical findings and theoretical considerations.* New York: Guilford.

Weiss, G., Hechtman, L., Milroy, T., & Perlman, T. (1985). Psychiatric status of hyperactives as adults: A controlled prospective 15-year follow-up of 63 hyperactive children. *Journal of the American Academy of Child Psychiatry, 24,* 211–220.

Weiss, G., Hechtman, L., Perlman, T., Hopkins, J., & Wener, A. (1979). Hyperactives as young adults: A controlled prospective ten-year follow-up of 75 children. *Archives of General Psychiatry, 36,* 675–681.

Weiss, J. M., Bailey, W. H., Goodman, P. A., Hoffman, L. J., Ambrose, M. J., Salman, S., & Charry, J. M. (1982). A model for neurochemical study of depression. In M. V. Spigelstein & A. Levy (Eds.), *Behavioral models and the analysis of drug action.* Amsterdam: Elsevier.

Weiss, M., & Burke, A. (1970). A 5- to 10-year follow-up of hospitalized school phobic children and adolescents. *American Journal of Orthopsychiatry, 40,* 672–676.

Weiss, M., & Cain, B. (1964). The residential treatment of children and adolescents with school phobia. *American Journal of Orthopsychiatry, 34,* 103–112.

Weiss, S. R. B., & Uhde, T. W. (1990). Animal models of anxiety. In J. Ballenger (Ed.), *Neurobiology of panic disorder.* New York: Wiley-Liss.

Weiss, S. W., and Ebert, M. H. (1983). Psychological and behavioral characteristics of normal-weight bulimics and normal-weight controls. *Psychosomatic Medicine, 45,* 293–303.

Weissman, M. M., Gammon, G. D., John, K., Merikangas, K. R., Warner, V., Prusoff, B. A., & Sholomskas, D. (1987). Children of depressed parents. Increased psychopathology and early onset of major depression. *Archives of General Psychiatry, 44,* 847–853.

Weissman, M. M., Gershon, E. S., Kidd, K. K., Prusoff, B. A., Leckman, J. F., Dibble, E., Hamovit, J., Thompson, W. D., Pauls, D. L., & Guroff, J. J. (1984a). Psychiatric disorders in the relatives of probands with affective disorders. *Archives of General Psychiatry, 41,* 13–21.

Weissman, M. M., Leckman, J. F., Merikangas, K. R., Gammon, G. D., & Prusoff, B. A. (1984b). Depression and anxiety disorders in parents and children. *Archives of General Psychiatry, 41,* 845–852.

Weissman, M. M., Prusoff, B. A., Gammon, G. D., Merikangas, K. R., Leckman, J. F., & Kidd, K. K. (1984c). Psychopathology in the children (ages 6–18) of depressed and normal parents. *Journal of the American Academy of Child Psychiatry, 23,* 78–84.

Weller, E. B. (1988, September). *Childhood Bereavement.* Paper presented at annual meeting of Consortium on Childhood Depression, New Haven, CT.

Weller, E. B., & Weller, R. A. (Eds.). (1984). *Major depressive disorders in children.* Washington, DC: American Psychiatric Press.

Wells, K. C., & Vitulano, L. A. (1984). Anxiety disorders in childhood. In S. M. Turner (Ed.), *Behavioral theories and treatment of anxiety* (pp. 413–434). New York: Plenum.

Welner, A., Reich, T., Robins, E., Fishman, R., & Van Doren, J. (1976). Obsessive-compulsive neurosis: Record, follow-up and family studies: I. Inpatient record study. *Comprehensive Psychiatry, 17,* 527–539.

Welner, Z., Welner, A., Stewart, M., Palkes, H., & Wish, E. (1977). A controlled study of siblings of hyperactive children. *Journal of Nervous and Mental Disease, 165,* 110–117.

Wender, P. H. (1971). *Minimal brain dysfunction in children.* New York: Wiley.

Wender, P. H. (1973). Some speculations concerning a possible biochemical basis of minimal brain dysfunction. *Annals of the New York Academy of Sciences, 205,* 18–28.

Wender, P. H., Kety, S. S., Rosenthal, D., Schulsinger, F., Ortmann, J., & Lunde, I. (1986). Psychiatric disorders in the biological and adoptive families of adopted individuals with affective disorders. *Archives of General Psychiatry, 43,* 923–929.

Wender, P. H., Reimherr, F. W., & Wood, D. R. (1981). Attention deficit disorder ('minimal brain dysfunction') in adults: A replication study of diagnosis and drug treatment. *Archives of General Psychiatry, 38,* 449–456.

Wender, P. H., Reimherr, F. W., Wood, D., & Ward, M. (1985). A controlled study of methylphenidate in the treatment of attention deficit disorder, residual type, in adults. *American Journal of Psychiatry, 142,* 547–552.

Wender, P. H., Rosenthal, D., Kety, S. S., Schulsinger, F., & Welner, J. (1974). Crossfostering: A research strategy for clarifying the role of genetic and experimental factors in the etiology of schizophrenia. *Archives of General Psychiatry, 30,* 121–128.

Wender, P. H., & Wender, E. H. (1978). *The hyperactive child and the learning disabled child: A handbook for parents.* New York: Crown.

Werner, E. E., Bierman, J. M., & French, F. E. (1971). *The children of Kauai.* Honolulu: University of Hawaii Press.

Werner, E. E., Honzik, M. P., & Smith, R. S. (1968). Prediction of intelligence and achievement at ten years from twenty months pediatric and psychologic examinations. *Child Development, 39,* 1063–1075.

Werner, E. E., & Smith, R. S. (1977). *Kauai's children come of age.* Honolulu: University of Hawaii Press.

Werry, J. S. (1986). Diagnosis and assessment. In R. Gittelman (Ed.), *Anxiety disorders of childhood* (pp. 73–100). New York: Guilford.

Werry, J. S., & Cohrssen, J. (1965). Enuresis: An etiologic and therapeutic study. *Journal of Pediatrics, 67,* 423–431.

Werry, J. S., & Quay, H. C. (1971). The prevalence of behavior symptoms in younger elementary school children. *American Journal of Orthopsychiatry, 41,* 136–143.

Werry, J. S., Reeves, J. C., & Elkind, G. S. (1987). Attention deficit, conduct, oppositional, and anxiety disorders in children: I. A review of research on differentiating characteristics. *Journal of the American Academy of Child and Adolescent Psychiatry, 26,* 133–143.

Werry, J. S., Sprague, R. L., & Cohen, M. N. (1975). Conners' teacher rating scale for use in drug studies with children: An empirical study. *Journal of Abnormal Child Psychology, 3,* 217–229.

Whalen, C. K., Collins, B. E., Henker, B., Alkus, S. R., Adams, D., & Stapp, J. (1978). Behavior observations of hyperactive children and methylphenidate (Ritalin) effects in systematically structured classroom environments: Now you see them, now you don't. *Journal of Pediatric Psychology, 3,* 177–187.

Whalen, C. K., & Henker, B. (Eds.). (1980). *Hyperactive children: The social ecology of identification and treatment.* New York: Academic.

Whalen, C. K., & Henker, B. (1984). Hyperactivity and the attention deficit disorders: Expanding frontiers. *The Pediatric Clinics of North America, 31,* 397–427.

Whalen, C. K., Henker, B., Castro, J., & Granger, D. (1987a). Peer perceptions of hyperactivity and medication effects. *Child Development, 58,* 816–828.

Whalen, C. K., Henker, B., Collins, B. E., Finck, D., & Dotemoto, S. (1979a). A social ecology of hyperactive boys: Medication effects in structured classroom environments. *Journal of Applied Behavioral Analysis, 12,* 65–81.

Whalen, C. K., Henker, B., Collins, B. E., McAulliffe, S., & Vaux, A. (1979b). Peer interaction in a structured communication task: Comparisons of normal and hyperactive boys and of methylphenidate (Ritalin) and placebo effects. *Child Development, 50,* 388–401.

Whalen, C. K., Henker, B., & Hinshaw, S. P. (1985). Cognitive-behavioral therapies for hyperactive children: Premises, problems and prospects. *Journal of Abnormal Child Psychology, 13,* 391–410.

Whalen, C. K., Henker, B., Swanson, J. M., Granger, D., Kliewer, W., & Spencer, J. (1987b). Natural social behaviors in hyperactive children: Dose effects of methylphenidate. *Journal of Consulting Clinical Psychologists, 55,* 187–193.

Wheeler, M. J., Crisp, A. H., Hsu, L. K. G., & Chen, C. N. (1983). Reproductive hormone changes during weight gain in male anorectics. *Clinical Endocrinology, 18,* 423–429.

White, R., Benedict, M. I., Wulff, L., & Kelley, M. (1986). Physical disabilities as risk factors for child maltreatment: A selected review. *American Journal of Orthopsychiatry, 57,* 93–101.

Whiting, J. W. M., & Child, I. L. (1953). *Child training and personality.* New Haven: Yale University Press.

Whitten, C. F. (1981). Growth failure. In N. S. Ellerstein (Ed.), *Child abuse and neglect: A medical reference* (pp. 197–219). New York: Wiley.

Whybrow, P. C., Akiskal, H. S., & McKinney, Jr., W. T. (1984). *Mood disorders: Toward a new psychobiology.* New York: Plenum.

Widiger, T. A., Frances, A., & Trull, T. J. (1987a). A psychometric analysis of the social-interpersonal and cognitive-perceptual items for the schizotypal personality disorder. *Archives of General Psychiatry, 44,* 741–745.

Widiger, T. A., Trull, T. J., Hurt, S. W., Clarkin, J., & Frances, A. (1987b). A multidimensional scaling of the DSM-III personality disorders. *Archives of General Psychiatry, 44,* 557–563.

Wiener, J. M. (1976). Identical male twins discordant for anorexia nervosa. *Journal of the American Academy of Child Psychiatry, 15,* 523–534.

Wierzbicki, M. (1987). Similarity of monozygotic and dizygotic child twins in level and lability of subclinically depressed mood. *American Journal of Orthopsychiatry, 57,* 33–40.

Willerman, L. (1973). Activity level and hyperactivity in twins. *Child Development, 44,* 288–293.

Willerman, L. (1979). Effects of families on intellectual development. *American Psychologist, 34,* 923–929.

Williams, D. T., Gold, A. P., Shrout, P., Shaffer, D., & Adams, D. (1979). The impact of psychiatric intervention on patients with uncontrolled seizures. *Journal of Nervous and Mental Disease, 167,* 626–631.

Williams, D. T., & Singh, M. (1976). Hypnosis as a facilitating therapeutic adjunct in child psychiatry. *Journal of the American Academy of Child Psychiatry, 15,* 326–342.

Williams, D. T., Spiegel, H., & Mostofsky, D. I. (1978). Neurogenic and hysterical seizures in children and adolescents: Differential diagnosis and therapeutic considerations. *American Journal of Psychiatry, 135,* 82–86.

Williams, K., Goodman, M., & Green, R. (1985). Parent-child factors in gender role socialization in girls. *Journal of the American Academy of Child Psychiatry, 24,* 720–731.

Williams, P., & King, M. (1987). The "epidemic" of anorexia nervosa: another medical myth? *Lancet, 24,* 205–207.

Wilson, G. T., & Lindholm, L. (1987). Bulimia nervosa and depression. *International Journal of Eating Disorders, 6,* 725–732.

Windheuser, H. J. (1977). Anxious mothers as models for coping with anxiety. *Behavioral Analysis and Modification, 2,* 62–63.

Wing, L. (1981a). Asperger's syndrome: A clinical account. *Psychological Medicine, 11,* 115–129.

Wing, L. (1981b). Sex ratios in early childhood autism and related conditions. *Psychiatry Research, 5,* 129–137.

Wing, L. (1985). *Autistic children: A guide for parents and professionals* (2nd ed.). New York: Brunner/Mazel.

Wing, L., & Attwood, A. (1987). Syndromes of autism and atypical development. In D. J. Cohen & A. M. Donnellan (Eds.), *Handbook of autism and pervasive developmental disorders* (pp. 3–19). New York: Wiley.

Wing, L., & Gould, J. (1979). Severe impairments of social interaction and associated abnormalities in children: Epidemiology and classification. *Journal of Autism and Developmental Disorders, 9,* 11–29.

Winnicott, D. W. (1964). *The child, the family, and the outside world.* Harmondsworth: Penguin.

Winnicott, D. W. (1965). *The maturational processes and the facilitating environment.* London: Hogarth Press.

Winnicott, D. W. (1975). *Through paediatrics to psycho-analysis.* New York: Basic Books.

Winokur, A., March, V. & Mendels, J. (1980). Primary affective disorder in relatives of patients with anorexia nervosa. *American Journal of Psychiatry, 137,* 695–698.

Wise, S. P., & Rapoport, J. L. (1989). Obsessive-compulsive disorders: Is it basal ganglia dysfunction? In J. L. Rapoport (Ed.), *Obsessive-compulsive disorder in children and adolescents* (pp. 327–344). Washington, DC: American Psychiatric Press.

Wittig, M. A., & Petersen, A. C. (Eds.). (1979). *Sex-related differences in cognitive function.* New York: Academic.

Wolfenstein, M. (1966). How is mourning possible? *Psychoanalytic Study of the Child, 21,* 93–123.

Wolff, H. G. (1950). Life stress and bodily disease—A formulation. In H. G. Wolff, S. Wolf, Jr., & C. E. Hare (Eds.), *Life stress and bodily disease.* Baltimore: Williams & Wilkins.

Wolff, S., & Barlow, A. (1979). Schizoid personality in childhood: A comparative study of schizoid, autistic, and normal children. *Journal of Child Psychology and Psychiatry, 20,* 29–46.

Wolfgang, M. E. (1978). Real and perceived changes of crime and punishment. *Deadalus, 108,* 143–157.

Wong, B. Y. L. (1986). Problems and issues in the definition of learning disabilities. In J. K. Torgesen & B. Y. L. Wong (Eds.), *Psychological and educational perspectives on learning disabilities* (pp. 1–26). New York: Academic.

Wong, D. F., Wagner, H. N., Jr., Tune, L. E., Dannals, R. F., Pearlson, G. D., Links, J. M., Tamminga, C. A., Broussolle, E. P. , Ravart, H. T., Wilson, A. A., Toung, J. K. T., Malat, J., Williams, J. A., O'Tuama, L. A., Synder, S. H., Kuhar, M. J., & Gjedde, A. (1986). Positron emission tomography reveals elevated D2 dopamine receptors in drug naive schizophrenics. *Science, 234,* 1558–1563.

Wood, D. R., Reimherr, F. W., Wender, P. H., & Johnson, G. E. (1976). Diagnosis and treatment of minimal brain dysfunction in adults. *Archives of General Psychiatry, 33,* 1453–1460.

Wooden, W., & Berkey, M. (1984). *Children and arson: America's middle class nightmare.* New York: Plenum.

Woolston, J. L., Rosenthal, S. L., Riddle, M. A., Sparrow, S. S., Cicchetti, D., & Zimmerman, L. D. (1989). Childhood comorbidity of anxiety/affective disorders and behavior disorders. *Journal of the American Academy of Child and Adolescent Psychiatry, 28,* 707–713.

Work, H. H. (1979). Mental retardation. In J. D. Noshpitz (Ed.), *Basic handbook of child psychiatry* (Vol. 2, pp. 402–415). New York: Basic Books.

Wright, L., & Walker, C. E. (1978). A simple behavioral treatment program for psychogenic encopresis. *Behaviour Research and Therapy, 16,* 209–212.

Wurtman, R. J. (1987). Nutrients affecting brain composition and behavior. *Integrative Psychiatry, 5,* 226–257.

Wynne, L. C., Cole, R. E., & Perkins, P. (1987). University of Rochester Child and Family Study: Risk research in progress. *Schizophrenia Bulletin, 13,* 463–476.

Wynne, L. C., Singer, M. T., Bartko, J. J., & Toohey, M. L. (1977). Schizophrenics and their families: Research on parental communication. In J. M. Tanner (Ed.), *Developments in psychiatric research* (pp. 254–286). London: Hodder & Stoughton.

Yablonsky, L. (1962). *The violent gang.* New York: Macmillan.

Yager, J., & Edelstein, C. K. (1985). The outpatient management of bulimia. In W. H. Kaye & H. E. Gwirtsman (Eds.), *The treatment of normal weight bulimia* (pp. 47–100). Washington, DC: American Psychiatric Press.

Yager, J., & Strober, M. (1985). Family aspects of eating disorders. *Annual Review, 4,* 481–502.

Yalom, I. Green, R., & Fisk, N. (1973). Prenatal exposure to female hormones: Effect on psychosexual development in boys. *Archives of General Psychiatry, 28,* 554–561.

Yando, R., & Kagan, J. (1968). The effect of teacher tempo on the child. *Child Development, 39,* 27–34.

Yarrow, L. J. (1963). Research in dimensions of early maternal care. *Merrill-Palmer Quarterly, 9,* 101–114.

Yates, A. (1987a). Eating disorders and long-distance running: The ascetic condition. *Integrative Psychiatry, 5,* 201–211.

Yates, A. (1987b). Psychological damage associated with extreme eroticism in young children. *Psychiatric Annals, 17,* 257–261.

Yates, A. (1988a). Debate Forum. Anatomically correct dolls: Should they be used as the basis for expert testimony? *Journal of the American Academy of Child and Adolescent Psychiatry, 27,* 254–255.

Yates, A. (1988b). Debate Forum. Anatomically correct dolls: Should they be used as the basis for expert testimony? *Journal of the American Academy of Child and Adolescent Psychiatry, 27,* 387.

Yates, A. (1989). Current perspectives on the eating disorders: I. History, psychological and biological aspects. *Journal of the American Academy of Child and Adolescent Psychiatry, 28,* 81 828.

Yates, A. (1990). Current perspectives on the eating disorders: II. Treatment, outcome, and research directions. *Journal of the American Academy of Child and Adolescent Psychiatry, 29,* 1–9.

Yeates, W. K. (1973). Bladder function in normal micturition. In I. Kolvin, R. C. MacKeith, & S. R. Meadow (Eds.), *Bladder control and enuresis* (pp. 28–36). (Clinics in Developmental Medicine, Nos. 48/49). London: Heinemann.

Yesavage, J. A., & Widrow, L. (1985). Early parental discipline and adult self-destructive acts. *The Journal of Nervous and Mental Disease, 173,* 74–77.

Yochelson, S., & Samenow, S. E. (1976). *The criminal personality: Vol. 1. A profile for change.* New York: Jason Aronson.

Yochelson, S., & Samenow, S. E. (1977). *The criminal personality: Vol. 2. The change process.* New York: Jason Aronson.

Yochelson, S., & Samenow, S. E. (1986). *The criminal personality: Vol. 3. The drug user.* New York: Jason Aronson.

Young, J. G., Brasic, J. R., & Leven, L. (1990). Genetic causes of autism and the pervasive developmental disorders. In S.I. Deutsch, A. Weizman, & R. Weizman (Eds.), *Application of basic neuroscience to child psychiatry* (pp. 183–216). New York: Plenum Medical.

Young, J. G., & Cohen, D. J. (1979). The molecular biology of development. In J. D. Noshpitz (Ed.), *Basic handbook of child psychiatry* (Vol. 1, pp. 22–62). New York: Basic Books.

Young, J. G., Cohen, D. J., Anderson, G. M., & Shaywitz, B. A. (1984). Neurotransmitter ontogeny as a perspective for studies of child development and pathology. In L. L. Greenhill & B. Shopsin (Eds.), *The psychobiology of childhood* (pp. 51–84). New York: Spectrum.

Young, I. L., & Goldsmith, A. O. (1972). Treatment of encopresis in a day treatment program. *Psychotherapy: Theory, Research and Practice, 9,* 231–235.

Young, S., Goy, R., & Phoenix, C. (1964). Hormones and behavior. *Science, 143,* 212–218.

Young, J. G., Kavanagh, M. E., Anderson, G. M., Shaywitz, B. A., & Cohen, D. J. (1982). Clinical neurochemistry of autism and associated disorders. *Journal of Autism and Developmental Disorders, 12,* 147–165.

Yule, W., & Rutter, M. (1985). Reading and other learning difficulties. In M. Rutter & L. Hersov (Eds.), *Child and adolescent psychiatry: Modern approaches* (pp. 444–464). Boston: Blackwell.

Yuwiler, A., Geller, E., & Ritvo, E. (1985). Biochemical studies on autism. In A. Lajtha (Ed.), *Handbook of neurochemistry* (pp. 671–691). New York: Plenum.

Zahn-Waxler, C., Cummings, E. M., McKnew, D. H., & Radke-Yarrow, M. (1984a). Altruism, aggression, and social interaction in young children with a manic-depressive parent. *Child Development, 55,* 112–122.

Zahn-Waxler, C., McKnew, D. H., Cummings, E. M., Davenport, Y. B., & Radke-Yarrow, M. (1984b). Problem behaviors and peer interactions of young children with a manic-depressive parent. *American Journal of Psychiatry, 141,* 236–240.

Zahn-Waxler, C., Radke-Yarrow, M., & King, R. A. (1979). Child rearing and children's prosocial initiations toward victims of distress. *Child Development, 50,* 319–330.

Zahner, G. E. P., Clubb, M. M., Leckman, J. F., & Pauls, D. L. (1988). The epidemiology of Tourette's syndrome. In D. J. Cohen, R. D. Brunn, & J. F. Leckman (Eds.), *Tourette's syndrome and tic disorders: Clinical understanding and treatment* (pp. 79–89). New York: Wiley.

Zahner, G. E. P., & Pauls, D. L. (1987). Epidemiological surveys of infantile autism. In D. J. Cohen & A. M. Donnellan (Eds.), *Handbook of autism and pervasive developmental disorders* (pp. 199–207). New York: Wiley.

Zametkin, A. J., & Rapoport, J. L. (1987). Neurobiology of attention deficit disorder with hyperactivity: Where have we come in 50 years? *Journal of the American Academy of Child and Adolescent Psychiatry, 26,* 676–686.

Zametkin, A. J., Rapoport, J. L., Murphy, D. L., Linnoila, M., & Ismond, D. (1985). Treatment of hyperactive children with monoamine oxidase inhibitors: 1. Clinical efficacy. *Archives of General Psychiatry, 42,* 962–966.

Zeitlin, H. (1986). *The natural history of psychiatric disorder in children.* New York: Oxford University Press.

Zetzel, E. R. (1970a). Anxiety and the capacity to bear it. In E. R. Zetzel, *The capacity for emotional growth* (pp. 33–52). New York: International Universities Press. (Original work published 1949 in *International Journal of Psychoanalysis, 30,* 1–12)

Zetzel, E. R. (1970b). *The capacity for emotional growth.* New York: International Universities Press.

Ziegler, R., & Holden, L. (1988). Family therapy for learning disabled and attention deficit disordered children. *American Journal of Orthopsychiatry, 58,* 196–210.

Zigler, E. (1979). Controlling child abuse in America: An effort doomed to failure. In R. Bourne & E. H. Newberger (Eds.), *Critical perspectives on child abuse* (pp. 171–213). Lexington, MA: Lexington Books.

Zigler, E., & Balla, D. A. (1977a). Impact of institutional experience on the behavior and development of retarded persons. *American Journal of Mental Deficiency, 82,* 1–11.

Zigler, E., & Balla, D. (1977b). Personality factors in the performance of the retarded: Implications for clinical assessment. *Journal of the American Academy of Child Psychiatry, 16,* 19–37.

Zigler, E., & Balla, D. (1982). *Mental retardation: The developmental-difference controversy.* Hillsdale, NJ: Erlbaum.

Zigler, E., Balla, D., & Hodapp, R. (1984). On the definition and classification of mental retardation. *American Journal of Mental Deficiency, 89,* 215–230.

Zigler, E., & Hodapp, R. M. (1986). *Understanding mental retardation.* London: Cambridge University Press.

Zilboorg, G. (1957). Further observations on ambulatory schizophrenias. *American Journal of Orthopsychiatry, 27,* 677–682.

Zinner, J., & Shapiro, E. R. (1975). Splitting in families of borderline adolescents. In J. Mack (Ed.), *Borderline states in psychiatry* (pp. 103–122). New York: Grune & Stratton.

Zohar, J., & Insel, T. R. (1987). Psychobiology of obsessive-compulsive disorder. *Biological Psychiatry, 22,* 667–687.

Zohar, J., Insel, T. R., Zohar-Kadouch, R. C., Hill, J. L., & Murphy, D. L. (1988). Serotonergic responsivity in obsessive-compulsive disorder. *Archives of General Psychiatry, 45,* 167–172.

Zubin, J., & Spring, B. (1977). Vulnerability—a new view of schizophrenia. *Journal of Abnormal Psychology, 86,* 103–126.

Zucker, K. J. (1982). Childhood gender disturbance: Diagnostic issues. *Journal of the American Academy of Child Psychiatry, 21,* 274–280.

Zucker, K. J. (1985). Cross-gender identified children. In B. W. Steiner (Ed.), *Gender dysphoria: Development, research and management* (pp. 75–174). New York: Plenum.

Zucker, K. J., Bradley, S. J., Doering, R. W., & Lozinski, J. A. (1985). Sextyped behavior in cross-gender-identified children: Stability and change at a one-year follow-up. *Journal of the American Academy of Child Psychiatry, 24,* 710–719.

Zucker, K. J., Finegan, J. K., Doering, R. W., & Bradley, S. J. (1983). Human figure drawings of gender problem children: A comparison to sibling, psychiatric and normal controls. *Journal of Abnormal Child Psychology, 11,* 287–298.

Zuger, B. (1966). Effeminate behavior present in boys from early childhood: I. The clinical syndrome and follow-up studies. *The Journal of Pediatrics, 69,* 1098–1107.

Zuger, B. (1970). The role of familial factors in persistent effeminate behavior in boys. *American Journal of Psychiatry, 126,* 1167–1170.

Zuger, B. (1974). Effeminate behavior in boys. *Archives of General Psychiatry, 30,* 173–177.

Zuger, B. (1978). Effeminate behavior present in boys from childhood: Ten additional years of follow-up. *Comprehensive Psychiatry, 19,* 363–369.

Zuger, B., & Taylor, P. (1969). Effeminate behavior present in boys from early childhood: II. Comparison with similar symptoms in non-effeminate boys. *Pediatrics, 44,* 375–380.

Author Index

Subject Index